World Health Organization Classification of Tumours

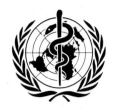

WHO   OMS

International Agency for Research on Cancer (IARC)

Pathology and Genetics of Tumours of the Breast and Female Genital Organs

Edited by

Fattaneh A. Tavassoli

Peter Devilee

IARC*Press*

Lyon, 2003

World Health Organization Classification of Tumours

Series Editors   Paul Kleihues, M.D.
Leslie H. Sobin, M.D.

Pathology and Genetics of Tumours of the Breast and Female Genital Organs

Editors   Fattaneh A. Tavassoli, M.D.
Peter Devilee, Ph.D.

Coordinating Editors   Lawrence M. Roth, M.D.
Rosemary Millis, M.D.

Editorial Assistants   Isabelle Forcier
Christine Zorian

Layout   Lauren A. Hunter
Sibylle Söring
Pascale Dia

Illustrations   Georges Mollon
Lauren A. Hunter

Printed by   Druckhaus Tecklenborg
48565 Steinfurt, Germany

Publisher   IARC*Press*
International Agency for
Research on Cancer (IARC)
69008 Lyon, France

This volume was produced in collaboration with the

International Academy of Pathology (IAP)

The WHO Classification of Tumours of the Breast and Female Genital Organs
presented in this book reflects the views of Working Groups that convened for
Editorial and Consensus Conferences in Lyon, France,
January 12-16 and March 16-20, 2002.

Members of the Working Groups are indicated
in the List of Contributors on page 365

*The Working Group on Gynaecological Tumours greatly
appreciates the participation of, and guidance by
Dr. Robert E. Scully, Harvard Medical School*

Published by IARC Press, International Agency for Research on Cancer,
150 cours Albert Thomas, F-69008 Lyon, France

Format for bibliographic citations:
Tavassoli F.A., Devilee P. (Eds.): World Health Organization Classification of
Tumours. Pathology and Genetics of Tumours of the Breast
and Female Genital Organs. IARC Press: Lyon 2003

IARC Library Cataloguing in Publication Data

Pathology and genetics of tumours of the breast and female genital organs /
        editors, Fattaneh A. Tavassoli, Peter Devilee.

    (World Health Organization classification of tumours ; 5)

    1. Breast Neoplasms—genetics. 2. Breast Neoplasms—pathology
    3. Genital Neoplasms, Female—genetics 4. Genital Neoplasms, Female—pathology
    I. Tavassoli, Fattaneh A. II. Devilee, Peter III. Series

    ISBN 92 832 2412 4   (NLM Classification W 1)

Contents

CHAPTER 1

Tumours of the Breast

Cancer of the breast is one of the most common human neoplasms, accounting for approximately one quarter of all cancers in females. It is associated with the Western lifestyle, and incidence rates are, therefore, highest in countries with advanced economies. Additional risk factors include early menarche and late childbirth. Breast cancer is further characterized by a marked genetic susceptibility. Early detection and advances in treatment have begun to reduce mortality rates in several countries. Through the use of cDNA expression profiles, it may become possible to predict clinical outcome in individual patients.

The typing of invasive breast cancer and its histological variants is well established. More difficult is the classification of pre-invasive breast lesions which are now increasingly detected by mammography. The WHO Working Group agreed that more clinical follow-up and genetic data are needed for a better understanding of the natural history of these lesions.

WHO histological classification of tumours of the breast

Epithelial tumours
Invasive ductal carcinoma, not otherwise specified   8500/3
    Mixed type carcinoma
    Pleomorphic carcinoma   8022/3
    Carcinoma with osteoclastic giant cells   8035/3
    Carcinoma with choriocarcinomatous features
    Carcinoma with melanotic features
Invasive lobular carcinoma   8520/3
Tubular carcinoma   8211/3
Invasive cribriform carcinoma   8201/3
Medullary carcinoma   8510/3
Mucinous carcinoma and other tumours with abundant mucin
    Mucinous carcinoma   8480/3
    Cystadenocarcinoma and columnar cell mucinous carcinoma   8480/3
    Signet ring cell carcinoma   8490/3
Neuroendocrine tumours
    Solid neuroendocrine carcinoma
    Atypical carcinoid tumour   8249/3
    Small cell / oat cell carcinoma   8041/3
    Large cell neuroendocrine carcinoma   8013/3
Invasive papillary carcinoma   8503/3
Invasive micropapillary carcinoma   8507/3
Apocrine carcinoma   8401/3
Metaplastic carcinomas   8575/3
    Pure epithelial metaplastic carcinomas   8575/3
      Squamous cell carcinoma   8070/3
      Adenocarcinoma with spindle cell metaplasia   8572/3
      Adenosquamous carcinoma   8560/3
      Mucoepidermoid carcinoma   8430/3
    Mixed epithelial/mesenchymal metaplastic carcinomas   8575/3
Lipid-rich carcinoma   8314/3
Secretory carcinoma   8502/3
Oncocytic carcinoma   8290/3
Adenoid cystic carcinoma   8200/3
Acinic cell carcinoma   8550/3
Glycogen-rich clear cell carcinoma   8315/3
Sebaceous carcinoma   8410/3
Inflammatory carcinoma   8530/3
Lobular neoplasia
    Lobular carcinoma in situ   8520/2
Intraductal proliferative lesions
    Usual ductal hyperplasia
    Flat epithelial atypia
    Atypical ductal hyperplasia
    Ductal carcinoma in situ   8500/2
Microinvasive carcinoma
Intraductal papillary neoplasms
    Central papilloma   8503/0
    Peripheral papilloma   8503/0
    Atypical papilloma
    Intraductal papillary carcinoma   8503/2
    Intracystic papillary carcinoma   8504/2
Benign epithelial proliferations
    Adenosis including variants
      Sclerosing adenosis
      Apocrine adenosis
      Blunt duct adenosis
      Microglandular adenosis
      Adenomyoepithelial adenosis
    Radial scar / complex sclerosing lesion

Adenomas
    Tubular adenoma   8211/0
    Lactating adenoma   8204/0
    Apocrine adenoma   8401/0
    Pleomorphic adenoma   8940/0
    Ductal adenoma   8503/0

Myoepithelial lesions
Myoepitheliosis
Adenomyoepithelial adenosis
Adenomyoepithelioma   8983/0
Malignant myoepithelioma   8982/3

Mesenchymal tumours
Haemangioma   9120/0
Angiomatosis
Haemangiopericytoma   9150/1
Pseudoangiomatous stromal hyperplasia
Myofibroblastoma   8825/0
Fibromatosis (aggressive)   8821/1
Inflammatory myofibroblastic tumour   8825/1
Lipoma   8850/0
  Angiolipoma   8861/0
Granular cell tumour   9580/0
Neurofibroma   9540/0
Schwannoma   9560/0
Angiosarcoma   9120/3
Liposarcoma   8850/3
Rhabdomyosarcoma   8900/3
Osteosarcoma   9180/3
Leiomyoma   8890/0
Leiomyosarcoma   8890/3

Fibroepithelial tumours
Fibroadenoma   9010/0
Phyllodes tumour   9020/1
    Benign   9020/0
    Borderline   9020/1
    Malignant   9020/3
Periductal stromal sarcoma, low grade   9020/3
Mammary hamartoma

Tumours of the nipple
Nipple adenoma   8506/0
Syringomatous adenoma   8407/0
Paget disease of the nipple   8540/3

Malignant lymphoma
Diffuse large B-cell lymphoma   9680/3
Burkitt lymphoma   9687/3
Extranodal marginal-zone B-cell lymphoma of MALT type   9699/3
Follicular lymphoma   9690/3

Metastatic tumours

Tumours of the male breast
Gynaecomastia
Carcinoma
    Invasive   8500/3
    In situ   8500/2

---

[1] Morphology code of the International Classification of Diseases for Oncology (ICD-O) {921} and the Systematized Nomenclature of Medicine (http://snomed.org).
Behaviour is coded /0 for benign tumours, /2 for in situ carcinomas and grade 3 intraepithelial neoplasia, /3 for malignant tumours, and /1 for borderline or uncertain behaviour.

TNM classification of carcinomas of the breast

TNM Clinical Classification[1,2]

T – Primary Tumour

TX	Primary tumour cannot be assessed
T0	No evidence of primary tumour
Tis	Carcinoma in situ
Tis (DCIS)	Ductal carcinoma in situ
Tis (LCIS)	Lobular carcinoma in situ
Tis (Paget)	Paget disease of the nipple with no tumour

Note: Paget disease associated with a tumour is classified according to the size of the tumour.

T1	Tumour 2 cm or less in greatest dimension
T1mic	Microinvasion 0.1 cm or less in greatest dimension[a]
T1a	More than 0.1 cm but not more than 0.5 cm in greatest dimension
T1b	More than 0.5 cm but not more than 1 cm in greatest dimension
T1c	More than 1 cm but not more than 2 cm in greatest dimension
T2	Tumour more than 2 cm but not more than 5 cm in greatest dimension
T3	Tumour more than 5 cm in greatest dimension
T4	Tumour of any size with direct extension to chest wall or skin only as described in T4a to T4d

Note: Chest wall includes ribs, intercostal muscles, and serratus anterior muscle but not pectoral muscle.

T4a	Extension to chest wall
T4b	Oedema (including peau d'orange), or ulceration of the skin of the breast, or satellite skin nodules confined to the same breast
T4c	Both 4a and 4b, above
T4d	Inflammatory carcinoma[b]

Notes: [a] Microinvasion is the extension of cancer cells beyond the basement membrane into the adjacent tissues with no focus more than 0.1cm in greatest dimension. When there are multiple foci of microinvasion, the size of only the largest focus is used to classify the microinvasion (Do not use the sum of all individual foci). The presence of multiple foci of microinvasion should be noted, as it is with multiple larger invasive carcinomas.
[b] Inflammatory carcinoma of the breast is characterized by diffuse, brawny induration of the skin with an erysipeloid edge, usually with no underlying mass. If the skin biopsy is negative and there is no localized measurable primary cancer, the T category is pTX when pathologically staging a clinical inflammatory carcinoma (T4d). Dimpling of the skin, nipple retraction, or other skin changes, except those in T4b and T4d, may occur in T1, T2, or T3 without affecting the classification.

N – Regional Lymph Nodes[3]

NX	Regional lymph nodes cannot be assessed (e.g. previously removed)
N0	No regional lymph node metastasis
N1	Metastasis in movable ipsilateral axillary lymph node(s)
N2	Metastasis in fixed ipsilateral axillary lymph node(s) or in clinically apparent* ipsilateral internal mammary lymph node(s) in the absence of clinically evident axillary lymph node metastasis
N2a	Metastasis in axillary lymph node(s) fixed to one another or to other structures
N2b	Metastasis only in clinically apparent* internal mammary lymph node(s) and in the absence of clinically evident axillary lymph node metastasis
N3	Metastasis in ipsilateral infraclavicular lymph node(s) with or without axillary lymph node involvement; or in clinically apparent* ipsilateral internal mammary lymph node(s) in the presence of clinically evident axillary lymph node metastasis; or metastasis in ipsilateral supraclavicular lymph node(s) with or without axillary or internal mammary lymph node involvement
N3a	Metastasis in infraclavicular lymph node(s)
N3b	Metastasis in internal mammary and axillary lymph nodes
N3c	Metastasis in supraclavicular lymph node(s)

Note: * clinically apparent = detected by clinical examination or by imaging studies (excluding lymphoscintigraphy)

M – Distant Metastasis

MX	Distant metastasis cannot be assessed
M0	No distant metastasis
M1	Distant metastasis

pTNM Pathological Classification

pT – Primary Tumour

The pathological classification requires the examination of the primary carcinoma with no gross tumour at the margins of resection. A case can be classified pT if there is only microscopic tumour in a margin.
The pT categories correspond to the T categories.

Note: When classifying pT the tumour size is a measurement of the invasive component. If there is a large in situ component (e.g. 4 cm) and a small invasive component (e.g. 0.5 cm), the tumour is coded pT1a.

pN – Regional Lymph Nodes[4]

pNX	Regional lymph nodes cannot be assessed (not removed for study or previously removed)
pN0	No regional lymph node metastasis*
pN1mi	Micrometastasis (larger than 0.2 mm, but none larger than 2 mm in greatest dimension)
pN1	Metastasis in 1 - 3 ipsilateral axillary lymph node(s), and/or in internal mammary nodes with microscopic metastasis detected by sentinel lymph node dissection but not clinically apparent**
pN1a	Metastasis in 1-3 axillary lymph node(s), including at least one larger than 2 mm in greatest dimension
pN1b	Internal mammary lymph nodes with microscopic metastasis detected by sentinel lymph node dissection but not clinically apparent
pN1c	Metastasis in 1 - 3 axillary lymph nodes and internal mammary lymph nodes with microscopic metastasis detected by sentinel lymph node dissection but not clinically apparent
pN2	Metastasis in 4 - 9 ipsilateral axillary lymph nodes, or in clinically apparent*** ipsilateral internal mammary lymph node(s) in the absence of axillary lymph node metastasis
pN2a	Metastasis in 4-9 axillary lymph nodes, including at least one that is larger than 2 mm
pN2b	Metastasis in clinically apparent internal mammary lymph node(s), in the absence of axillary lymph node metastasis
pN3	Metastasis in 10 or more ipsilateral axillary lymph nodes; or in infraclavicular lymph nodes; or in clinically apparent ipsilateral internal mammary lymph nodes in the presence of one or more positive axillary lymph nodes; or in more than 3 axillary lymph nodes with clinically negative, microscopic metastasis in internal mammary lymph nodes; or in ipsilateral supraclavicular lymph nodes
pN3a	Metastasis in 10 or more axillary lymph nodes (at least one larger than 2 mm) or metastasis in infraclavicular lymph nodes
pN3b	Metastasis in clinically apparent internal mammary lymph node(s) in the presence of one or more positive axillary lymph node(s); or metastasis in more than 3 axillary lymph nodes and in internal mammary lymph nodes with microscopic metastasis detected by sentinel lymph node dissection but not clinically apparent
pN3c	Metastasis in supraclavicular lymph node(s)

Note: * Cases with only isolated tumour cells (ITC) in regional lymph nodes are classified as pN0. ITC are single tumour cells or small clusters of cells, not more than 0.2 mm in greatest dimension, that are usually detected by immunohistochemistry or molecular methods but which may be verified on H&E stains. ITCs do not typically show evidence of metastatic activity (e.g., proliferation or stromal reaction).
** not clinically apparent = not detected by clinical examination or by imaging studies (excluding lymphoscintigraphy).
*** clinically apparent = detected by clinical examination or by imaging studies (excluding lymphoscintigraphy) or grossly visible pathologically.

pM – Distant Metastasis
The pM categories correspond to the M categories.

Stage Grouping

Stage 0	Tis	N0	M0
Stage I	T1	N0	M0
Stage IIA	T0	N1	M0
	T1	N1	M0
	T2	N0	M0
Stage IIB	T2	N1	M0
	T3	N0	M0
Stage IIIA	T0	N2	M0
	T1	N2	M0
	T2	N2	M0
	T3	N1, N2	M0
Stage IIIB	T4	N0,N1,N2	M0
Stage IIIC	Any T	N3	M0
Stage IV	Any T	Any N	M1

---

[1] {51,2976}.

[2] A help desk for specific questions about the TNM classification is available at http://tnm.uicc.org.

[3] The regional lymph nodes are:

1. Axillary (ipsilateral): interpectoral (Rotter) nodes and lymph nodes along the axillary vein and its tributaries, which may be divided into the following levels:
   (i)   Level I (low-axilla): lymph nodes lateral to the lateral border of pectoralis minor muscle.
   (ii) Level II (mid-axilla): lymph nodes between the medial and lateral borders of the pectoralis minor muscle and the interpectoral (Rotter) lymph nodes.
   (iii) Level III (apical axilla): apical lymph nodes and those medial to the medial margin of the pectoralis minor muscle, excluding those designated as subclavicular or infraclavicular.

   Note: Intramammary lymph nodes are coded as axillary lymph nodes, level I.

2. Infraclavicular (subclavicular) (ipsilateral).
3. Internal mammary (ipsilateral): lymph nodes in the intercostal spaces along the edge of the sternum in the endothoracic fascia.
4. Supraclavicular (ipsilateral).

[4] The pathological N classification requires the resection and examination of at least the low axillary lymph nodes (level I). Examination of one or more sentinel lymph nodes may be used for pathological classification. If classification is based solely on sentinel node biopsy without subsequent axillary lymph node dissection it should be designated (sn) for sentinel node, e.g. pN1(sn).

Invasive breast carcinoma

I.O. Ellis
S.J. Schnitt
X. Sastre-Garau
G. Bussolati
F.A. Tavassoli
V. Eusebi
J.L. Peterse
K. Mukai
L. Tabár
J. Jacquemier

C.J. Cornelisse
A.J. Sasco
R. Kaaks
P. Pisani
D.E. Goldgar
P. Devilee
M.J. Cleton-Jansen
A.L. Børresen-Dale
L. van't Veer
A. Sapino

Definition

Invasive breast carcinoma is a group of malignant epithelial tumours characterized by invasion of adjacent tissues and a marked tendency to metastasize to distant sites. The vast majority of these tumours are adenocarcinomas and are believed to be derived from the mammary parenchymal epithelium, particularly cells of the terminal duct lobular unit (TDLU). Breast carcinomas exhibit a wide range of morphological phenotypes and specific histopathological types have particular prognostic or clinical characteristics.

Epidemiology

Invasive breast cancer is the most common carcinoma in women. It accounts for 22% of all female cancers, 26% in affluent countries, which is more than twice the occurrence of cancer in women at any other site {2188}. The areas of high risk are the affluent populations of North America, Europe and Australia where 6% of women develop invasive breast cancer before age 75. The risk of breast cancer is low in the less developed regions of sub-Saharan Africa and Southern and Eastern Asia, including Japan, where the probability of developing breast cancer by age 75 is one third that of rich countries. Rates are intermediate elsewhere. Japan is the only rich country that in year 2000 still showed low incidence rates.
The prognosis of the disease is very good if detected at an early stage. Significant improvements in survival have been recorded in western countries since the late 1970s {37,485}, but advancements have been dramatic in the 1990s due to the combined effect of population screening and adjuvant hormonal treatment. As a result, the increasing mortality trend observed until the 1980s leveled off or declined in several high risk countries e.g. the United States of America (USA), the United Kingdom and the Netherlands {3155}.

The risk of the disease had been increasing until the early 1980s in both developed and developing countries and continues to increase in particular in the developing countries {3068}. Thereafter, in developed countries, the advent of mammography and the previously mentioned improvements in survival altered both incidence and mortality; the latter no longer appropriately reflect trends in the underlying risk of the disease.
Breast cancer incidence, as with most epithelial tumours, increases rapidly with age. Figure 1.02 shows age-specific incidence rates for three selected populations representing countries with low (Japan), intermediate (Slovenia) and high incidence rates (USA), just before screening was implemented. The curves show a characteristic shape, rising steeply up to menopausal age and less rapidly or not at all afterwards. The different behaviour at older ages is due to a cohort effect in the populations of Japan

and Slovenia experiencing an increase in risk that affects mainly younger generations. If current trends persist, these generations will maintain their higher risk and the age-specific curve will approach that of Americans.
Around 1990, breast cancer incidence varied 10-fold world wide, indicating important differences in the distribution of the underlying causes {2189}. Geographical variations, time trends, and studies of populations migrating from low to high risk areas which show that migrant populations approach the risk of the host country in one or two generations {174,1478,3266}, clearly suggest an important role of environmental factors in the aetiology of the disease.

Aetiology

The aetiology of breast cancer is multifactorial and involves diet, reproductive factors, and related hormonal imbalances. From descriptive epidemiological

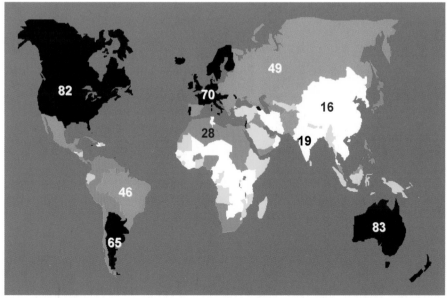

Fig. 1.01 Global incidence rates of breast cancer. Age-standardized rates (ASR) per 100,000 population and year. From Globocan 2000 {846}.

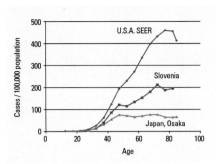

Fig. 1.02 Incidence of female breast cancer by age in selected populations 1988-1993. From M. Parkin et al. {2189}.

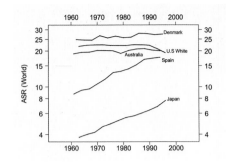

Fig. 1.04 Female breast cancer mortality trends. Source: WHO/NCHS.

data it has clearly emerged that breast cancer is a disease of affluent societies which have acquired the Western lifestyle, characterized by a high-caloric diet rich in animal fat and proteins, combined with a lack of physical exercise. Regions which have featured this lifestyle for a long period of time (North America, Northern Europe, Australia) have reached a plateau of an incidence rate of 70 to 90 new cases per 100,000 population/year while countries that have more recently become industrialized and affluent show a marked increase in incidence and mortality. In addition to breast cancer, the Western lifestyle carries a high risk of cancer of the prostate, colon/rectum, and endometrium. Specific environmental exposures operative in the development of breast cancer (e.g. radiation, alcohol, exogenous hormones) have been identified but carry a lower risk.

More than most other human neoplasms, breast cancer often shows familial clustering. Two high penetrance genes have been identified (*BRCA1/2*) which greatly increase the breast cancer risk (see Chapter 8). However, it is anticipated that multigenic traits also play a significant role in the inherited susceptibility to breast cancer.

Reproductive lifestyle

For almost half a century, the events of reproductive life have been considered to be risk factors for breast cancer in women. Breast cancer occurs more frequently among women who have an early menarche, remain nulliparous or, if parous, have few children with a late age at first delivery. Infertility per se appears to be a risk factor as may be lack of breast-feeding. Finally, late age at menopause also increases the risk {1430}.

Most of these factors have also been found relevant in populations at low risk of breast cancer such as the Japanese and Chinese. Although the data is limited in Africa, at least one study confirmed the negative impact of late age at first delivery, reduced number of pregnancies and shorter breast feeding time {2770}. Recent data indicates that the age at any delivery, not just the first is associated with breast cancer risk, with deliveries occurring before the age of 30 having a protective effect {3137}.

Controversies still surround the issue of abortion, some studies, but not others,

finding an increased risk for induced abortion. Similarly, the protective effect of lactation, once considered quite a strong factor, was later given less importance; its impact appears limited to long-term cumulative breast feeding, preferably exceeding two years {435}.

Exogenous hormones

Two major types of hormonal compounds have been evaluated in relation to breast cancer: oral contraceptives and menopausal replacement therapy.

The evidence suggests a small increase in the relative risk associated with the use of combined oral contraceptives, especially among current and recent users, which is not related to duration of use and type or dose of preparation, and may be partly linked to detection bias {1296}. Data on injectable pure progestogen contraceptives shows relative risks from 1.0 to 1.3, which are not statistically significant {1294}.

Epidemiological studies on postmenopausal estrogen therapy show a small increase in risk with longer duration of use in current and recent users {1298}. Information on the effect of postmenopausal estrogen-progestogen therapy was provided in only a minority of studies, but indicates that the increased relative risk in long-term users is not significantly different from that for long-term use of estrogens alone {1297}. Yet it should be noted that, among hormone replacement therapy users, there is an over representation of tumours that, with regard to tumour stage, type and grade are associated with a more favourable prognosis {1760}.

Nutrition

High intakes of fruit and vegetables are probably associated with a slightly reduced risk of breast cancer {3153}.

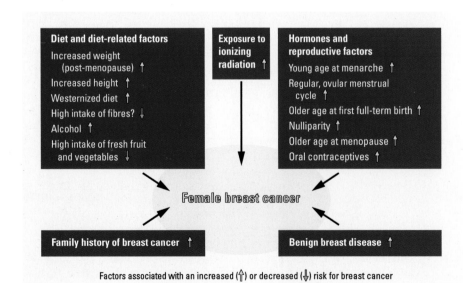

Fig. 1.03 Aetiological factors involved in the development of breast cancer.

Rapid growth and greater adult height, reflecting in part, the total food intake in early years, are associated with an increased risk {674}. Similarly a high body mass, also linked to a high total caloric intake, or intake not counterbalanced by caloric expenditure, is a risk factor for postmenopausal breast cancer. Total fat, as well as saturated animal fat, also possibly increases the risk {674, 3153}.

Meat consumption is possibly associated with an increased risk. Red meat was more frequently cited as a risk factor and diets rich in poultry possibly have no links {3153}. In countries with different meat consumption levels within the population, higher risks were associated with higher total meat, red meat or processed meat intake in most studies, although this was not always statistically significant. In conclusion there is considerable consistent evidence that higher meat consumption, particularly red or fried/browned meat is associated with a higher risk of breast cancer {674}.

Recent studies, however, tend to suggest that several associations, either preventive for vegetables and fruit, or risk for fat may have been overstated {804,815,817}.

Other questions remaining unsolved include the long term cumulative effects of exposure to contaminants, either formed during cooking, such as heterocyclic amines in well-done meat or pesticide residues.

Alcohol

The consumption of alcohol has been relatively consistently found to be associated with a mild increase in risk of breast cancer {2729,3153}. A dose-response

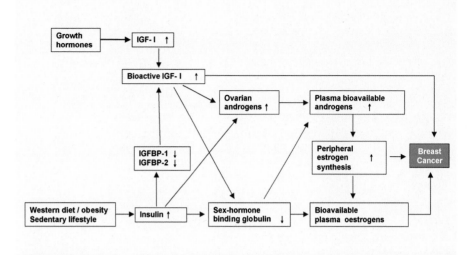

Fig. 1.06 Insulin, IGF-I, bioavailable sex steroids, and breast cancer.

was found with number of drinks per day, including a low level of consumption {1691}. Hormone use or other factors potentially including genetic polymorphism {2182} may modify the risk.

Smoking

The evidence on smoking and breast cancer remains inconclusive {787,816, 784,402}. Tobacco has been viewed as an anti-estrogen and a potential protective factor {182}.

Body weight

It has long been known that the influence of weight on breast cancer risk depends on the menopausal status {1292}. More than 100 studies over nearly 30 years in many countries have established that higher body weight increases breast cancer risk among postmenopausal women. This is largely independent of reproductive and lifestyle risk factors and of the effect of physical activity. The association appears to increase in a stepwise fashion with advancing age after menopause.

The increase in risk with body-mass index (BMI) has been somewhat modest in the majority of studies {1292}. Above a BMI of 24 kg/m^2, the incidence rate increases among postmenopausal women. The greatest slope of increases in risk across higher BMI levels is in low and moderate risk countries suggesting that increases in BMI now being observed in those countries may become a major factor contributing to future increases in breast cancer rates.

While risk ratios have levelled off at BMI levels near 25 kg/m^2 in high risk countries, this is not the case in low to moderate risk countries, where risk has continued to increase across a wider range of body weight. The association between BMI and breast cancer is stronger among women who have never used postmenopausal hormone replacement therapy, suggesting that the risk from being overweight may be mediated by the elevations in endogenous estrogen production among heavier women. Adult weight gain is a strong and consistent predictor of postmenopausal breast cancer risk particularly among women who have never used hormone replacement therapy {1292}.

In populations with a high incidence of breast cancer, the overall association between BMI and breast cancer risk among premenopausal women is the inverse. The reduction in risk with excessive weight is modest and not observed until a BMI of 28 kg/m^2. Despite this, however, the breast cancer mortality rate is not lower among heavier premenopausal women {1292}.

Physical activity

The association between physical activity and breast cancer risk is independent of menopausal status {1292}. The decrease in risk among the most physically active women was about 20-40%. Activity that is sustained throughout lifetime, or at a minimum performed after menopause, may be particularly beneficial. It appears that physical activity has

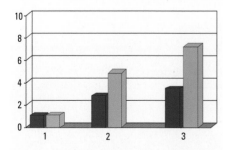

Fig. 1.05 Breast cancer risk by increasing levels of circulating insulin-like growth factor (IGF-1) in women <50 years. Blue columns, IGF-1, orange columns, IGF-1 binding protein (IGFBP-3). From S.E. Hankinson et al. {1127}.

similar effects within different populations. Although lifetime physical activity is desirable, beginning recreational physical activity after the menopause can probably be beneficial for both weight control and breast cancer risk reduction {1292}.

Endogenous hormones
There is overwhelming evidence from epidemiological studies that sex steroids (androgens, estrogens, progestogens) have an important role in the development of breast tumours. Breast cancer incidence rates rise more steeply with age before menopause than after, when ovarian synthesis of estrogens and progesterone ceases and ovarian androgen production gradually diminishes {1447}. The estrogen excess hypothesis is central, stipulating that breast cancer risk depends directly on breast tissue exposure to estrogens. In vitro studies show increased breast cell proliferation and inhibition of apoptosis. Animal studies show increased rates of tumour development when estrogens are administered. The risk is higher among postmenopausal women who have elevated plasma levels of testosterone and androstenedione, reduced levels of sex hormone-binding globulin (SHBG), and increased levels of oestrone, oestradiol, and bioavailable oestradiol not bound to SHBG.
A second major theory, the estrogen plus progestogen hypothesis {255, 1446}, postulates that, compared to exposure to estrogens alone (as in postmenopausal women not using exogenous hormones), risk of breast cancer is further increased in women who have elevated plasma and tissue levels of estrogens in combination with progestogens. This theory is supported by observations that proliferation of mammary epithelial cells is increased during the luteal phase of the menstrual cycle, compared to the follicular phase.
Among premenopausal women, several studies have not shown any clear association between breast cancer risk and circulating levels of androgens, estrogens, or progesterone {255,1183,2448, 2613,2909}.
A metabolic consequence of excess body weight and lack of physical activity is development of insulin resistance. Elevated insulin levels, may lead to increased ovarian and/or adrenal synthesis of sex steroids, particularly of andro-

gens, and decrease the hepatic synthesis of and circulating levels of SHBG {1376}. Especially in postmenopausal women, elevated plasma androgens lead to increased estrogen formation in adipose tissue, and hence to increased levels of oestrone and oestradiol. The hypothesis that chronic hyperinsulinemia might explain the observed associations of breast cancer risk with low plasma SHBG and elevated androgens and estrogens, among postmenopausal women {1376} has, however, received only limited support {661,1377}. Insulin-growth factor-I (IGF-I) and IGF-binding proteins (IGFBP) appear to be significant risk predictors {1127,1377}.
Future adult cancer risk is in part set by conditions of exposure in utero. The preventive effect of gravidic toxaemia is recognized {1288} and since the 1950s studies have incriminated high birth weight as a risk factor for cancer, in particular of the breast {1857}. Similarly, among twins, the risk of breast cancer may be affected by the type of twinning (dizygotic versus monozygotic) and sex of the dizygotic twin {429}. A study of maternal pregnancy hormone levels in China and the United States of America (USA) did not find, however, the expected higher levels in the USA but rather the reverse {1676}. Another important period is adolescence, where diet may play a role either directly or possibly indirectly through a modification of growth velocity {242}.

Some specific exposures
Only limited data is available on specific exposures in relation to breast cancer. Long-term follow-up of women exposed to the Hiroshima or Nagasaki nuclear explosions indicates an increased risk of breast cancer, in particular for women exposed around puberty {2938}. Similarly, exposure as a result of treatment and surveillance of tuberculosis is associated with risk {304}. Yet there is little evidence for a different pattern of risk as a function of fractionated versus one time only irradiation {1678}. Systematic reviews on occupation and breast cancer are few, indicating an increased risk for selected occupations and specific chemical and physical exposures. This data contrasts with the long-held view that risk of breast cancer is related to social class, with higher risk for execu-

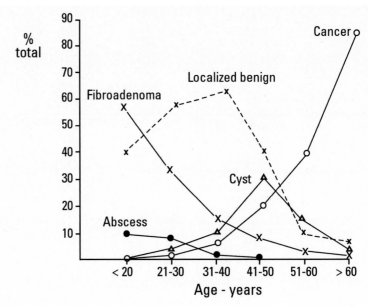

Fig. 1.07 Age distribution of benign and malignant breast lesions in patients presenting with a discrete breast lump. From Dixon and Sainsbury {707}.

Table 1.01
Frequency of symptoms of women presenting in a breast clinic {288,698}.

Lump	60-70%
Pain	14-18%
Nipple problems	7-9%
Deformity	1%
Inflammation	1%
Family history	3-14%

tives, administrative and clerical jobs {387}. A recent hypothesis deals with circadian disruption through night work, with an increased risk in women working predominantly at night {632,2556}.

Over the last ten years concerns have arisen as to the potential risks of exposure to, not only hormones, but to artificial products mimicking hormonal activities. This led to the concept of xeno-hormones, mostly represented so far by xeno-estrogens. The exact role they play is unknown. Most epidemiological studies deal with various pesticides, essentially organochlorines which remain in the environment for a very long time and the residues of which may be found in adipose tissue of various species, including humans {628}. Studies have produced conflicting results with some suggesting a possibly increased risk, some no risk and others showing a negative effect. For the time being, many consider these links as speculative and unfounded {1951,2503} or as markers of susceptibility {1951}.

Finally, based on animal experience, a viral hypothesis has been put forward. In mice, a retrovirus, the murine mammary

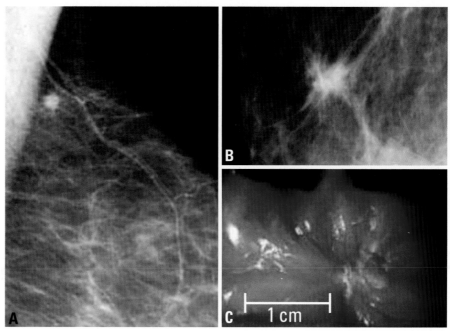

Fig. 1.08 A Mammogram of infiltrating carcinoma, clinically occult, less than 1 cm. **B** Mammographic detail of small, non-palpable, infiltrating carcinoma (<1 cm). **C** Macroscopic picture.

tumour virus, is a recognized cause of mammary tumours, transmitted with milk from mothers to daughters. Another candidate is the Epstein-Barr virus, although data from the USA are not particularly supportive {1015}. Other potential viral candidates remain to be searched for.

Localization

Breast carcinoma arises from the mammary epithelium and most frequently the epithelial cells of the TDLU. There is a slightly higher frequency of invasive breast cancer in the left breast with a reported left to right ratio of approximately 1.07 to 1 {1096}. Between 40 and 50% of tumours occur in the upper outer quadrant of the breast and there is a decreasing order of frequency in the other quadrants from the central, upper inner, lower outer to the lower inner quadrant {1096}.

Clinical features
Symptoms and signs

The majority of women with breast cancer present symptomatically, although the introduction of breast screening has led to an increasing proportion of asymtomatic cases being detected mammographically. Breast cancer does not have specific signs and symptoms, which allow reliable distinction from various forms of benign breast disease. However, the frequency distribution of

benign and malignant disease does differ between age cohorts, benign conditions being more common in younger women and breast cancer the commonest cause of symptoms in older women. The most common findings in symptomatic women are breast lumps, which may or may not be associated with pain. Nipple abnormalities (discharge, retraction, distortion or eczema) are less common and other forms of presentation are rare.

Some symptoms have a higher risk of underlying malignancy for which hospital referral is recommended.

Breast abnormalities should be evaluated by triple assessment including clinical examination, imaging (mammography and ultrasound) and tissue sampling by either fine needle aspiration cytology or needle core biopsy.

Clinical examination should be systematic and take account of the nature of the lump and, if present, any skin dimpling or change in contour of the breast and also assessment of the axilla.

Imaging

Imaging should include mammography except in women under age 35, where it is rarely of value, unless there is strong clinical suspicion or tissue/needle biopsy evidence of malignancy.

The mammographic appearances of breast carcinoma are varied and include well defined, ill defined and spiculate

Table 1.02
Conditions requiring referral to a specialist clinic.

Lump
Any new discreet mass
A new lump in pre-existing nodularity
Asymmetrical nodularity that persits at review after menstruation
Abscess on breast inflammation which does not settle after one course of antibiotics
Cyst persistently refilling or recurrent cyst (if the patient has recurrent multiple cysts and the GP has the necessary skills, then aspiration is acceptable)
Pain
If associated with a lump
Intractable pain that interferes with a patient's lifestyle or sleep and which has failed to respond to reassurance, simple measures such as wearing a well supporting brassiere and common drugs
Unilateral persistent pain in postmenopausal women
Nipple discharge
All women > 50
Women < 50 with:
bilateral discharge sufficient to stain clothes
bloodstained discharge
persistent single duct discharge
Nipple retraction, distortion, eczema
Change in skin contour
Family history of breast cancer

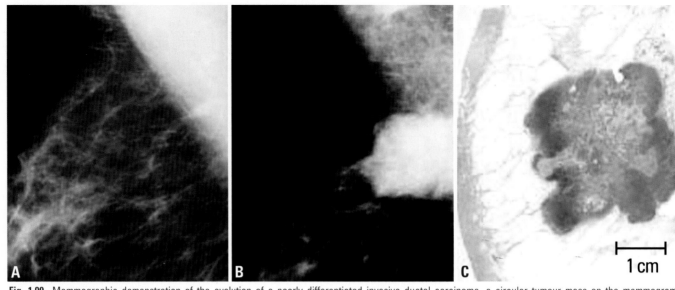

Fig. 1.09 Mammographic demonstration of the evolution of a poorly differentiated invasive ductal carcinoma, a circular tumour mass on the mammogram. **A** Non-specific density in the axillary tail of the right breast, undetected at screening. **B** 18 Months later: >30 mm ill defined, high density lobulated tumour, mammographically malignant. Metastatic lymph nodes are seen in the axilla. **C** Large section histology of the tumour.

masses, parenchymal deformity and calcification with or without a mass lesion. By far the most common manifestation of breast cancer on the mammogram is tumour mass without calcifications. The mammographic histological correlation of 1,168 open surgical biopsies at Falun Central Hospital, Sweden, included 866

Table 1.03
Mammographic appearance of histologically malignant breast lesions.

Stellate and circular without calcifications	64%
Stellate and circular with calcifications	17%
Calcifications only	19%

Table 1.04
Spectrum of histological diagnosis corresponding to mammographic circular/oval lesions.

Invasive ductal carcinoma, NOS	59%
Medullary carcinoma	8%
Mucinous carcinoma	7%
Intracystic carcinoma	5%
Tubular carcinoma	4%
Invasive lobular carcinoma	4%
Other diagnoses	13%

histologically proven malignancies. As seen in Table 1.03, the mammograms of these breasts cancer showed:
1) Stellate or circular tumour mass with no associated calcifications in 64% of the cases.
2) An additional 17% had both calcifications and tumour mass.
3) Only calcifications without associated tumour mass accounted for less than 20% of all malignancies detectable on the mammogram.

Grading of invasive carcinoma
Invasive ductal carcinomas and all other invasive tumours are routinely graded based on an assessment of tubule/gland formation, nuclear pleomorphism and mitotic counts.
Many studies have demonstrated a significant association between histological grade and survival in invasive breast carcinoma. It is now recognized as a powerful prognostic factor and should be included as a component of the minimum data set for histological reporting of breast cancer {779,1190}. Assessment of histological grade has become more objective with modifications of the Patley & Scarff {2195} method first by Bloom and Richardson {293} and more recently by Elston and Ellis {777,2385}.

Method of grading
Three tumour characteristics are evaluated; tubule formation as an expression of glandular differentiation, nuclear pleomor-

phism and mitotic counts. A numerical scoring system of 1-3 is used to ensure that each factor is assessed individually. When evaluating tubules and glandular acini only structures exhibiting clear central lumina are counted; cut off points of 75% and 10% of glandular/tumour area are used to allocate the score.
Nuclear pleomorphism is assessed by reference to the regularity of nuclear size and shape of normal epithelial cells in adjacent breast tissue. Increasing irregularity of nuclear outlines and the number and size of nucleoli are useful additional features in allocating scores for pleomorphism.
Evaluation of mitotic figures requires care and observers must count only defined mitotic figures; hyperchromatic and pyknotic nuclei are ignored since they are more likely to represent apoptosis than proliferation. Mitotic counts require standardization to a fixed field area or by using a grid system {1984}. The total number of mitoses per 10 high power fields. Field selection for mitotic scoring should be from the peripheral leading edge of the tumour. If there is heterogeneity, regions exhibiting a higher frequency of mitoses should be chosen. Field selection is by random meander through the chosen area. Only fields with a representative tumour cell burden should be assessed.
The three values are added together to produce scores of 3 to 9, to which the grade is assigned as follows:

Grade 1 - well differentiated: 3-5 points
Grade 2 - moderately differentiated:
6-7 points
Grade 3 - poorly differentiated: 8-9 points

Invasive ductal carcinoma, not otherwise specified (NOS)

Definition
Invasive ductal carcinoma, not otherwise specified (ductal NOS) comprises the largest group of invasive breast cancers. It is a heterogeneous group of tumours that fail to exhibit sufficient characteristics to achieve classification as a specific histological type, such as lobular or tubular carcinoma.

ICD-O code   8500/3

Synonyms and historical annotation
Invasive ductal carcinoma, no specific type (ductal NST); infiltrating ductal carcinoma.
Many names have been used for this form of breast carcinoma including scirrhous carcinoma, carcinoma simplex and spheroidal cell carcinoma. Infiltrating ductal carcinoma is used by the Armed Forces Institute of Pathology {1832,2442} and was the nomenclature adopted in the previous WHO classifica-

Table 1.05
Semi-quantitative method for assessing histological grade in breast. From Elston and Ellis {777}.

Feature			Score
Tubule and gland formation			
Majority of tumour (>75%)			1
Moderate degree (10-75%)			2
Little or none (<10%)			3
Nuclear pleomorphism			
Small, regular uniform cells			1
Moderate increase in size and variability			2
Marked variation			3
Mitotic counts			
Dependent on microscope field area			1-3
Examples of assignment of points for mitotic counts for three different field areas:			
Field diameter (mm)	0.44	0.59	0.63
Field area (mm²)	0.152	0.274	0.312
Mitotic count*			
1 point	0-5	0-9	0-11
2 points	6-10	10-19	12-22
3 points	>11	>20	>23

tion {2548,3154}. This perpetuates the traditional concept that these tumours are derived exclusively from mammary ductal epithelium in distinction from lobular carcinomas, which were deemed to have arisen from within lobules for which there is no evidence. In addition it has been shown that the terminal duct-lobular unit (TDLU) should be regarded as a single entity from the point of view of the site of origin of most breast carcinomas {147,3091}. Some groups {874,2325} have retained the term ductal but added the phrase 'not otherwise specified (NOS)', whilst others {2147} prefer to use 'no specific type (NST)' to emphasize their distinction from specific type tumours. This latter view is increasingly

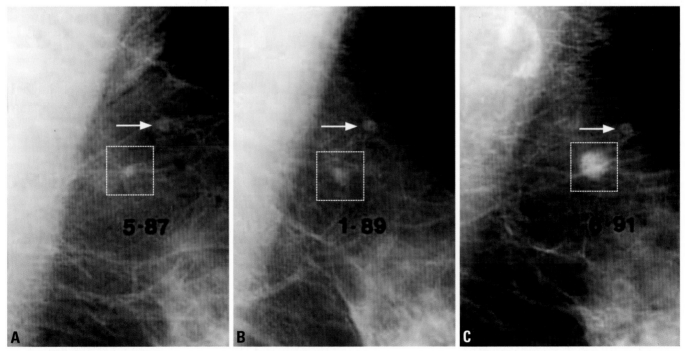

Fig. 1.10 Well differentiated infiltrating ductal carcinoma, Grade 1. **A** First screen. Intramammary lymph node and small (<5 mm), nonspecific density. **B** Second screen: 20 months later. The density has grown a little. **C** Third screen: after another 29 months. The 10 mm tumour is more obvious but still not palpable.

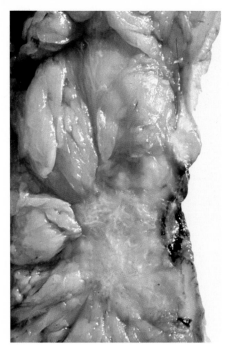

Fig. 1.11 Invasive ductal carcinoma, not otherwise specified. 84 year old patient, mastectomy specimen.

accepted internationally, but since 'ductal' is still widely used the terms invasive ductal carcinoma, ductal NOS or NST are preferred terminology options.

Epidemiology

Ductal NOS carcinoma forms a large proportion of mammary carcinomas and its epidemiological characteristics are similar to those of the group as a whole (see epidemiology). It is the most common 'type' of invasive carcinoma of the breast comprising between 40% and 75% in published series {774}. This wide range is possibly due to the lack of application of strict criteria for inclusion in the special types and also the fact that some groups do not recognize tumours with a combination of ductal NOS and special type patterns as a separate

mixed category, preferring to include them in the no special type (ductal NOS) group.

Ductal NOS tumours, like all forms of breast cancer, are rare below the age of 40 but the proportion of tumours classified as such in young breast cancer cases is in general similar to older cases {1493}. There are no well recognized differences in the frequency of breast cancer type and proportion of ductal NOS cancers related to many of the known risk factors including geographical, cultural/lifestyle, reproductive variables (see aetiology). However, carcinomas developing following diagnosis of conditions such as atypical ductal hyperplasia and lobular neoplasia, recognized to be associated with increased risk include a higher proportion of tumours of specific type specifically tubular and classical lobular carcinoma {2150}. Familial breast cancer cases associated with *BRCA1* mutations are commonly of ductal NOS type but have medullary carcinoma like features, exhibiting higher mitotic counts, a greater proportion of the tumour with a continuous pushing margin, and more lymphocytic infiltration than sporadic cancers {1572}. Cancers associated with *BRCA2* mutations are also often of ductal NOS type but exhibit a high score for tubule formation (fewer tubules), a higher proportion of the tumour perimeter with a continuous pushing margin and a lower mitotic count than sporadic cancers {1572}.

Macroscopy

These tumours have no specific macroscopical features. There is a marked variation in size from under 10 mm to over 100 mm. They can have an irregular, stellate outline or nodular configuration. The tumour edge is usually moderately or ill defined and lacks sharp circumscription.

Classically, ductal NOS carcinomas are firm or even hard on palpation, and may have a curious 'gritty' feel when cut with a knife. The cut surface is usually greywhite with yellow streaks.

Histopathology

The morphological features vary considerably from case to case and there is frequently a lack of the regularity of structure associated with the tumours of specific type. Architecturally the tumour cells may be arranged in cords, clusters and trabeculae whilst some tumours are characterized by a predominantly solid or syncytial infiltrative pattern with little associated stroma. In a proportion of cases glandular differentiation may be apparent as tubular structures with central lumina in tumour cell groups. Occasionally, areas with single file infiltration or targetoid features are seen but these lack the cytomorphological characteristics of invasive lobular carcinoma. The carcinoma cells also have a variable appearance. The cytoplasm is often abundant and eosinophilic. Nuclei may be regular, uniform or highly pleomorphic with prominent, often multiple, nucleoli, mitotic activity may be virtually absent or extensive. In up to 80% of cases foci of associated ductal carcinoma in situ (DCIS) will be present {147,2874}. Associated DCIS is often of high grade comedo type, but all other patterns may be seen.

Some recognize a subtype of ductal NOS carcinoma, infiltrating ductal carcinoma with extensive in situ component.

The stromal component is extremely variable. There may be a highly cellular fibroblastic proliferation, a scanty connective tissue element or marked hyalinisation. Foci of elastosis may also be present, in a periductal or perivenous distribution. Focal necrosis may be pres-

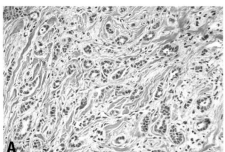
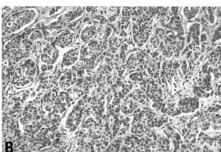
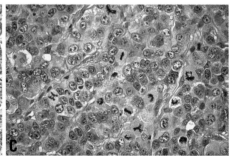

Fig. 1.12 A Infiltrating ductal carcinoma, grade I. **B** Infiltrating ductal carcinoma, grade II. **C** Invasive ductal NOS carcinoma, grade III with no evidence of glandular differentiation. Note the presence of numerous cells in mitosis, with some abnormal mitotic figures present.

ent and this is occasionally extensive. In a minority of cases a distinct lympho-plasmacytoid infiltrate can be identified.

Mixed type carcinoma

For a tumour to be typed as ductal NOS it must have a non-specialized pattern in over 50% of its mass as judged by thorough examination of representative sections. If the ductal NOS pattern comprises between 10 and 49% of the tumour, the rest being of a recognized special type, then it will fall into one of the mixed groups: mixed ductal and special type or mixed ductal and lobular carcinoma. Apart from these considerations there are very few lesions that should be confused with ductal NOS carcinomas.

Pleomorphic carcinoma

ICD-O code   8022/3

Pleomorphic carcinoma is a rare variant of high grade ductal NOS carcinoma characterized by proliferation of pleomorphic and bizarre tumour giant cells comprising >50% of the tumour cells in a background of adenocarcinoma or adenocarcinoma with spindle and squamous differentiation {2683}. The patients range in age from 28 to 96 years with a median of 51. Most patients present with a palpable mass; in 12% of cases, metastatic tumour is the first manifestation of disease. The mean size of the tumours is 5.4 cm. Cavitation and necrosis occur in larger tumours.

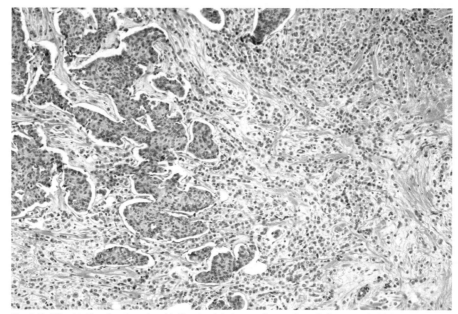
Fig. 1.13 Mixed infiltrating ductal and infiltrating lobular carcinoma. Two distinct morphologic patterns are seen in this tumour, ductal on the left and lobular on the right.

The tumour giant cells account for more than 75% of tumour cells in most cases. Mitotic figures exceed 20 per 10 high power fields. All these tumours qualify as grade 3 carcinomas. The intraepithelial component displays a ductal arrangement and is often high grade with necrosis. Lymphovascular invasion is present in 19% of cases.

Generally BCL2, ER and PR negative, two thirds of these pleomorphic carcinomas are TP53 positive, and one third are S-100 protein positive. All are positive for CAM5.2, EMA and pan-cytokeratin (AE1/AE3, CK1). A majority (68%) is aneuploid with 47% of them being triploid. A high S-phase (>10%) is found in 63%. Axillary node metastases are present in 50% of the patients with involvement of 3 or more nodes in most. Many patients present with advanced disease.

Carcinoma with osteoclastic giant cells

ICD-O code   8035/3

The common denominator of all these carcinomas is the presence of osteoclastic giant cells in the stroma {1089}. The giant cells are generally associated with an inflammatory, fibroblastic, hyper-

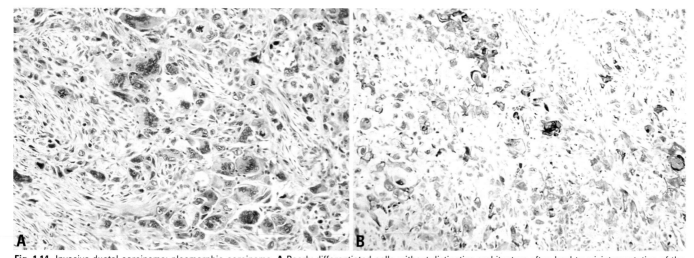
Fig. 1.14 Invasive ductal carcinoma: pleomorphic carcinoma. **A** Poorly differentiated cells without distinctive architecture often lead to misinterpretation of the lesion as a sarcoma. **B** Immunostain for keratin (AE1/AE3 and LP34) confirms the epithelial nature of the process.

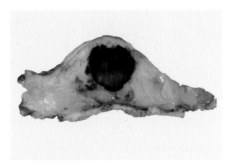

Fig. 1.15 Invasive carcinomas with stromal osteoclastic giant cells often have vascular stromal tissue with haemosiderin pigment accumulation giving them a brown macroscopic appearance.

vascular stroma, with extravasated red blood cells, lymphocytes, monocytes along with mononucleated and binucleated histiocytes some containing haemosiderin. The giant cells are variable in size and appear to embrace the epithelial component or are found within lumena formed by the cancer cells. The giant cells contain a variable number of nuclei. The giant cells and hypervascular reactive stroma can be observed in lymph node metastases and in recurrences {2952}.

The carcinomatous part of the lesion is most frequently a well to moderately differentiated infiltrating ductal carcinoma but all the other histological types have been observed particularly invasive cribriform carcinoma {2003,2241}, and also tubular, mucinous, papillary {3062}, lobular {1274,2837}, squamous and other metaplastic patterns {1200,2044, 3062}.

About one-third of the reported cases had lymph nodes metastasis. The five year survival rate is around 70%, similar to, or better than, patients with ordinary infiltrating carcinomas {3062}. Prognosis is related to the characteristics of the associated carcinoma and does not appear to be influenced by the presence of stromal giant cells.

The giant cells show uniform expression of CD68 (as demonsrated by KP1 antibody on paraffin sections) {1200} and are negative for S100 protein, actin, and negative for cytokeratin, EMA, estrogen and progesterone receptors {2869}.

The giant cells are strongly positive for acid phosphatase, non-specific esterase and lysosyme, but negative for alkaline phosphatase indicative of morphological similarity to histiocytic cells and osteoclasts {2423,2869,2952, 3025}.

A number of ultrastructural and immunohistochemical studies have confirmed the histiocytic nature of the osteoclastic cells present in these unusual carcinomas {2632,2869,2952,3025}. In vitro studies have recently shown that osteoclasts may form directly from a precursor cell population of monocytes and macrophages. Tumour associated macrophages (TAMs) are capable of differentiating into multinucleated cells, which can affect bone resorption in metastases {2313}. Osteoclastic giant cells in carcinoma are probably also related to TAMs. Angiogenesis and chemotactic agents produced by the carcinoma may be responsible for the migration of histiocytes to the area involved by cancer and their ultimate transformation to osteoclastic giant cells {2638,2869}.

Carcinoma with choriocarcinomatous features

Patients with ductal NOS carcinoma may have elevated levels of serum human β–chorionic gonadotrophin (β-HCG) {2649} and as many as 60% of ductal NOS carcinoma have been found to contain β-HCG positive cells {1243}. Histological evidence of choriocarcinomatous differentiation, however, is exceptionally rare with only a few cases reported {993,1061,2508}. All were in women between 50 and 70 years old.

Carcinoma with melanotic features

A few case reports have described exceptional tumours of the mammary parenchyma that appear to represent combinations of ductal carcinoma and malignant melanoma {2031,2146,2485} and in some of these cases, there appeared to be a transition from one cell type to the other. A recent genetic analysis of one such case showed loss of heterozygosity at the same chromosomal loci in all the components of the tumour, suggesting an origin from the same neoplastic clone {2031}.

The mere presence of melanin in breast cancer cells should not be construed as evidence of melanocytic differentiation, since melanin pigmentation of carcinoma cells can occur when breast cancers invade the skin and involve the dermo-epidermal junction {150}. In addition, care must be taken to distinguish tumours showing melanocytic differentiation from breast carcinomas with prominent cytoplasmic lipofuscin deposition {2663}.

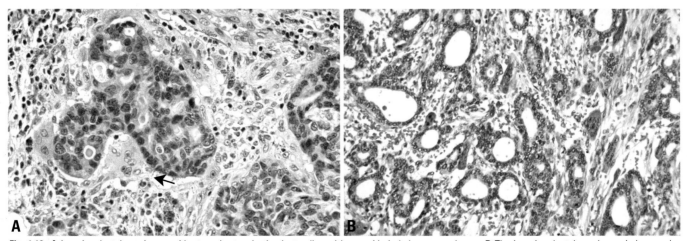

Fig. 1.16 **A** Invasive ductal carcinoma with stromal osteoclastic giant cells and haemosiderin-laden macrophages. **B** The invasive ductal carcinoma is low grade. Multinucleated giant cells are evident in the stroma.

Most melanotic tumours of the breast represent metastases from malignant melanomas originating in extra-mammary sites {2694}. Primary melanomas may arise anywhere in the skin of the breast, but an origin in the nipple-areola complex is extremely rare {2168}. The differential diagnosis of malignant melanoma arising in the nipple areolar region must include Paget disease, the cells of which may on occasion contain melanin pigment {2544}. This is discussed in the section on Paget disease.

Genetics
The genetic variation seen in breast cancer as a whole is similarly reflected in ductal NOS tumours and has until recently proved difficult to analyse or explain. The increasing accumulation of genetic alterations seen with increasing grade (decreasing degree of differentiation) has been used to support the hypothesis of a linear progression model in this type and in invasive breast cancer as a whole. The recent observation by a number of groups that specific genetic lesion or regions of alteration are associated with histological type of cancer or related to grade in the large ductal NOS group does not support this view. It implies that breast cancer of ductal NOS type includes a number of tumours of unrelated genetic evolutionary pathways {365} and that these tumours show fundamental differences when compared to some special type tumours including lobular {1085} and tubular carcinoma {2476}. Furthermore, recent cDNA microarray analysis has demonstrated that ductal NOS tumours can be classified in to subtypes on the basis of expression patterns {2218,2756}.

Prognosis and predictive factors
Ductal NOS carcinoma forms the bulk (50-80%) of breast cancer cases and its prognostic characteristics and management are similar or slightly worse with a 35-50% 10 year survival {771} compared to breast cancer as a whole with around a 55% 10 year survival. Prognosis is influenced profoundly by the classical prognostic variables of histological grade, tumour size, lymph node status and vascular invasion (see general discussion of prognosis and predictive factors at the end of this chapter) and by predictors of therapeutic response such as estrogen receptor and ERBB2 status.

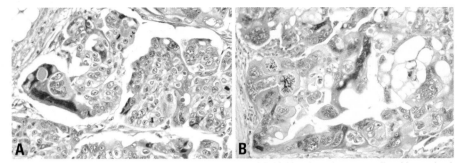

Fig. 1.17 Carcinoma with choriocarcinomatous features. **A,B** Multinucleated tumour cells with smudged nuclei extend their irregular, elongated cytoplasmic processes around clusters of monocytic tumour cells, mimicking the biphasic growth pattern of choriocarcinoma. **B** Note the abnormal mitotic figures in this high grade carcinoma.

Approximately 70-80% of ductal NOS breast cancers are estrogen receptor positive and between 15 and 30% of cases ERBB2 positive. The management of ductal NOS carcinomas is also influenced by these prognostic and predictive characteristics of the tumour as well as focality and position in the breast.

Invasive lobular carcinoma

Definition
An invasive carcinoma usually associated with lobular carcinoma in situ is composed of non-cohesive cells individually dispersed or arranged in single-file linear pattern in a fibrous stroma.

ICD-O code   8520/3

Epidemiology
Invasive lobular carcinoma (ILC) represents 5-15% of invasive breast tumours {725,771,1780,2541,2935,3133}. During the last 20 years, a steady increase in its incidence has been reported in women over 50 {1647}, which might be attributable to the increased use of hormone replacement therapy {312,1648,2073}. The mean age of patients with ILC is 1-3 years older than that of patients with infiltrating ductal carcinoma (IDC) {2541}.

Clinical features
The majority of women present with a palpable mass that may involve any part of the breast although centrally located tumours were found to be slightly more common in patients with ILC than with IDC {3133}. A high rate of multicentric tumours has been reported by some {699,1632} but this has not been found in other series based on clinical {2541} or

radiological {1599} analysis (see bilateral breast carcinoma section). An 8-19% incidence of contralateral tumours has also been reported {699,725,834}, representing an overall rate of 13.3 %. This may be higher than that for IDC {1241,2696}. However, no significant difference in the rate of bilaterality was observed in other series of cases {648, 1168,2186}. At mammography, architectural distortion is more commonly observed in ILC than in IDC whereas microcalcifications are less common in ILC {895,1780,3066}.

Macroscopy
ILC frequently present as irregular and poorly delimited tumours which can be difficult to define macroscopically because of the diffuse growth pattern of the cell infiltrate {2696}. The mean diameter has been reported to be slightly larger than that of IDC in some series {2541,2696,3133}.

Histopathology
The classical pattern of ILC {895, 1780,3066} is characterized by a proliferation of small cells, which lack cohesion

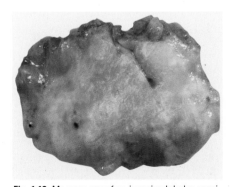

Fig. 1.18 Macroscopy of an invasive lobular carcinoma displays an ill defined lesion.

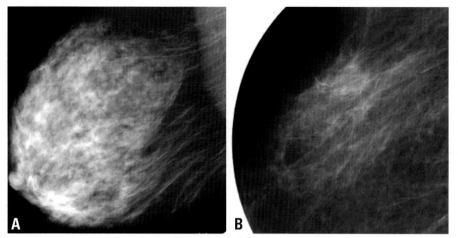
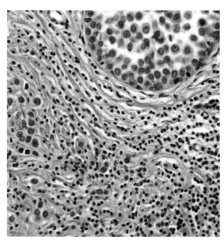

Fig. 1.19 Mammography of invasive lobular carcinoma. **A** Architectural distortion in the axillary tail, corresponding to a palpable area of thickening. **B** Magnification view of the architectural axillary distortion.

Fig. 1.20 In situ and invasive lobular carcinoma. The larger cells on the left and lower part of the field are invasive tumour cells.

and appear individually dispersed through a fibrous connective tissue or arranged in single file linear cords that invade the stroma. These infiltrating cords frequently present a concentric pattern around normal ducts. There is often little host reaction or disturbance of the background architecture. The neoplastic cells have round or notched ovoid nuclei and a thin rim of cytoplasm with an occasional intracytoplasmic lumen {2312} often harbouring a central mucoid inclusion. Mitoses are typically infrequent. This classical form of ILC is associated with features of lobular carcinoma in situ in at least 90% of the cases {705,2001}.

In addition to this common form, variant patterns of ILC have been described. The *solid pattern* is characterized by sheets of uniform small cells of lobular morphology {835}. The cells lack cell to cell cohesion and are often more pleomorphic and have a higher frequency of mitoses than the classical type. In the *alveolar variant*, tumour cells are mainly arranged in globular aggregates of at least 20 cells {2668}, the cell morphology and growth pattern being otherwise typical of lobular carcinoma. *Pleomorphic lobular carcinoma* retains the distinctive growth pattern of lobular carcinoma but exhibits a greater degree of cellular atypia and pleomorphism than the classical form {808,1858,3082}. Intra-lobular lesions composed of signet ring cells or pleomorphic cells are features frequently associated with it. Pleomorphic lobular carcinoma may show apocrine {808} or histiocytoid {3047} differentiation. A mixed group is composed of cases showing an admixture of the classical type with one or more of these patterns {705}. In about 5% of invasive breast cancers, both ductal and lobular features of differentiation are present {1780} (see Mixed type carcinoma, page 21). Analysis of E-cadherin expression may help to divide these cases between ductal and lobular tumours but the immunophenotype remains ambiguous in a minority of cases {34}.

The admixture of tubular growth pattern and small uniform cells arranged in a linear pattern defines tubulo-lobular carcinoma (TLC) (ICD-O 8524/3) {875}. LCIS is observed in about one third of TLC. Comparison of the clinico-pathological features of TLC and pure tubular carcinoma (TC) has shown that axillary metastases were more common in TLC (43%) than in TC (12%) {1062}. A high rate of estrogen receptor (ER) positivity has also been reported in TLC {3141}. Further analysis of TLC, especially regarding E-cadherin status, should help to determine whether TLC should be categorized as a variant of tubular or of lobular tumours. Without this data these tumours are best classified as a variant of lobular carcinoma.

Immunoprofile
About 70-95% of lobular carcinomas are ER positive, a rate higher than the 70-80% observed in IDC {2541,3235}. Progesterone receptor (PR) positivity is 60-70% in either tumour type {2541,

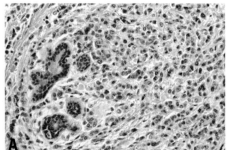
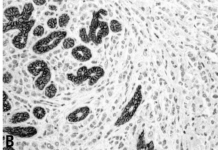
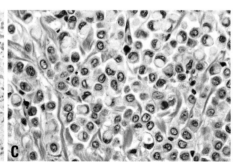

Fig. 1.21 A Invasive lobular carcinoma. **B** Loss of E-cadherin expression is typical of lobular carcinoma cells. Note immunoreactivity of entrapped normal lobules. **C** Large number of signet ring cells and intracytoplasmic lumina (targetoid secretion).

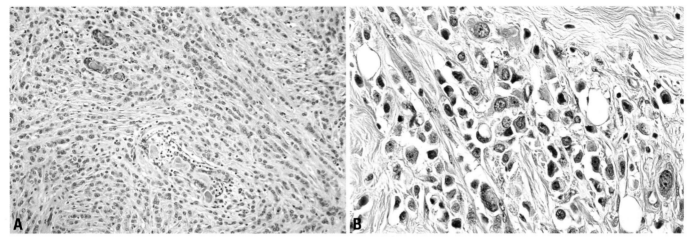

Fig. 1.22 A Classic invasive lobular carcinoma with uniform, single cell files compared to (B). **B** Invasive pleomorphic lobular carcinoma with characteristic pleomorphic, atypical nuclei.

3235}. ER was found to be expressed in the classical form and in variants {1994}, but the rate of positivity was higher (100%) in alveolar {2668} and lower (10%) in pleomorphic ILC {2318} than in the classical type. The proliferation rate in ILC is generally low {2027}. With the exception of pleomorphic lobular carcinoma ERBB2 overexpression in ILC {2274,2477,2750}, is lower than reported in IDC {2358}.

Genetics

Using flow cytometry, ILCs were found near diploid in about 50% of the cases {887}. This fits with the finding that chromosomal abnormalities, assessed by cytogenetical {887} or comparative genomic hybridization (CGH) analysis {2027}, are less numerous in ILC than in IDC. In ILC, the most common genetic alteration, found in 63-87% of the cases {887,2027}, is a loss of the long arm of chromosome 16.

The E (epithelial)-cadherin gene, which maps in 16q22, is implicated in maintaining coherence of adult epithelial tissues {1217}, and acts as a cell differentiation and invasion suppressor factor {922,3030}. A correlation has been found between deletion of 16q and the loss of E-cadherin expression {2027}. Immunohistochemical analysis has shown complete loss of E-cadherin expression in 80-100% of ILC {956,1892,2094, 2152,2336}. This contrasts with the mere decrease in staining intensity observed in 30-60% of IDC.

Molecular analysis has shown that, in most cases, the lack of E-cadherin immunostaining can be related to the presence of protein truncation mutations {260,1394,2380}, together with the inactivation of the wild type allele. Alternative mechanisms may also be involved in the alteration of E-cadherin {723,3190} and/or E-cadherin-associated proteins {723,1892,2337,2374}.

Analysis of neoplastic lesions corresponding to early steps of tumour development has shown that both loss of heterozygosity of the 16q chromosomal region {800} and of E-cadherin expression {649,3034} were also observed in LCIS and in mixed ductal-lobular carcinoma {34}. Inactivation of the E-cadherin gene may thus represent an early event in oncogenesis and this biological trait indicates that LCIS is a potential precursor of ILC. However, other molecular events must be involved in the transition from in situ to invasive lobular tumours. Furthermore, genetic losses concerning other parts of the long arm of chromosome 16 than the locus of E-cadherin have been found in IDC and in ILC {2960}, as well as in DCIS {460}. This strongly suggests that several genes localized in this chromosomal region, and presenting tumour suppressive properties, may be involved in breast oncogenesis.

A combination of mutation analysis and E-cadherin protein expression may offer a method for identification of lobular carcinoma.

Prognosis and predictive factors

A lower frequency of axillary nodal metastasis in ILC than in IDC has been reported in several series, the difference ranging from 3-10% {1327,1578,2541, 2696,2935}. Metastatic involvement by scattered isolated cells may simulate sinusoidal histiocytes and require immunohistochemical detection.

The metastatic pattern of ILC differs from that of IDC. A higher frequency of tumour extension to bone, gastro-intestinal tract, uterus, meninges, ovary and diffuse serosal involvement is observed in ILC while extension to lung is more frequent in IDC {319,1142,1327,2541,2696,2935}. IHC using antibodies raised against GCDFP-15, cytokeratin 7, ER, and E-cadherin may help establish a female genital tract tumour as a metastatic ILC. Several studies have reported a more favourable disease outcome for ILC than for IDC {705,725,771,2696,2935} whereas others found no significant differences {2205,2541,2696,2731} or a worse prognosis for ILC {126}.

When the histological subtypes of ILC were analysed separately, a more favourable outcome was reported for the classical type than for variants {699, 705,725}. However, alveolar ILC has been considered as a low grade tumour {2668}, whereas a poor prognosis of pleomorphic ILC has been reported in some series {808,3082}. No difference in the outcome of different subtypes has been observed in other series {2935}.

Furthermore, a large extent of lymph node involvement has not been found to increase significantly the risk of local relapse {2570}. A link between lack of E-cadherin expression and adverse outcome of the disease has also been reported {125,1176}.

Treatment of ILC should depend on the stage of the tumour and parallel that of IDC. Conservative treatment has been shown to be appropriate for ILC {327, 2205,2269,2541,2570,2696}.

Tubular carcinoma

Definition
A special type of breast carcinoma with a particularly favourable prognosis composed of distinct well differentiated tubular structures with open lumina lined by a single layer of epithelial cells.

ICD-O code   8211/3

Epidemiology
Pure tubular carcinoma accounts for under 2% of invasive breast cancer in most series. Higher frequencies of up to 7% are found in series of small T1 breast cancers. Tubular cancers are often readily detectable mammographically because of their spiculate nature and associated cellular stroma and are seen at higher frequencies of 9-19%, in mammographic screening series {1853, 2192,2322}.

When compared with invasive carcinomas of no special type (ductal NOS), tubular carcinoma is more likely to occur in older patients, be smaller in size and have substantially less nodal involvement {691,1379,2166}.

These tumours are recognized to occur in association with some epithelial proliferative lesions including well differentiated/low grade types of ductal carcinoma in situ (DCIS), lobular neoplasia and flat epithelial atypia {915,1034}. In addition, an association with radial scar has been proposed {1668,2725}.

Macroscopy
There is no specific macroscopical feature which distinguishes tubular carcinoma from the more common ductal no special type (NOS) or mixed types, other than small tumour size. Tubular carcinomas usually measure between 0.2 cm and 2 cm in diameter; the majority are 1 cm or less {772,1829,2081}.

Two morphological subtypes have been described, the 'pure' type which has a pronounced stellate configuration with radiating arms and central yellow flecks due to stromal elastosis and the sclerosing type characterized by a more diffuse, ill defined structure {410,2190}.

Histopathology
The characteristic feature of tubular carcinoma is the presence of open tubules composed of a single layer of epithelial cells enclosing a clear lumen. These tubules are generally oval or rounded and, typically, a proportion appears angulated. The epithelial cells are small and regular with little nuclear pleomorphism and only scanty mitotic figures. Multilayering of nuclei and marked nuclear pleomorphism are contraindications for diagnosis of pure tubular carcinoma, even when there is a dominant tubular architecture. Apical snouts are seen in as many as a third of the cases {2874}, but are not pathognomonic. Myoepithelial cells are absent but some tubules may have an incomplete surrounding layer of basement membrane components.

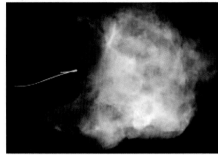

Fig. 1.23 Tubular carcinoma. Specimen X-ray.

A secondary, but important feature is the cellular desmoplastic stroma, which accompanies the tubular structures. Calcification may be present in the invasive tubular, associated in situ or the stromal components.

DCIS is found in association with tubular carcinoma in the majority of cases; this is usually of low grade type with a cribriform or micropapillary pattern. Occasionally, the in situ component is lobular in type. More recently an association has been described with flat epithelial atypia and associated micropapillary DCIS {915,1034}.

There is a lack of consensus concerning the proportion of tubular structures required to establish the diagnosis of tubular carcinoma. In the previous WHO Classification {1,3154} and a number of published studies {410,1350, 1832} no specific cut-off point is indicated although there is an assumption that all the tumour is of a tubular configuration. Some authors have applied a strict 100% rule for tubular structures {409,552, 2190}, some set the proportion of tubular structures at 75% {1668,1829, 2224,2442}, and

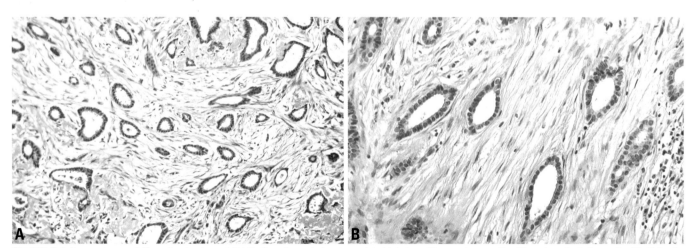

Fig. 1.24 Tubular carcinoma. **A** There is a haphazard distribution of rounded and angulated tubules with open lumens, lined by only a single layer of epithelial cells separated by abundant reactive, fibroblastic stroma. **B** The neoplastic cells lining the tear-drop shaped tubules lack significant atypia.

yet others at 90% {97,2147}. For pragmatic reasons, a 90% purity requirement offers a practical solution.

Tumours exhibiting between 50 and 90% tubular growth pattern with other types should be regarded as mixed type of carcinoma (see Mixed type carcinomas).

Differential diagnosis

Sclerosing adenosis (SA) can be distinguished from tubular carcinoma by its overall lobular architecture and the marked compression and distortion of the glandular structures. Myoepithelial cells are always present in sclerosing adenosis and can be highlighted by immunostaining for actin. Similarly, a fully retained basement membrane can be shown by immunohistological staining for collagen IV and laminin in tubules of SA. Microglandular adenosis (MA) can be more difficult to differentiate because of the rather haphazard arrangement of the tubules, and lack of myoepithelial cells in the tubules. However, the tubules of MA are more rounded and regular and often contain colloid-like secretory material, at least focally, compared to the often angulated tubules of tubular carcinoma. Furthermore a ring of basement membrane is present around tubules of MA. Complex sclerosing lesions/radial scars have a typical architecture with central fibrosis and elastosis containing a few small, often distorted, tubular structures in which myoepithelial cells can be demonstrated. The surrounding glandular structures show varying degrees of dilatation and ductal epithelial hyperplasia.

Immunophenotype

Tubular carcinoma is nearly always estrogen and progesterone receptor positive, has a low growth fraction, and is ERBB2 and EGFR negative {691, 1379,2166}.

Genetics

Tubular carcinomas of the breast have a low frequency of genetic alterations when compared to other types of breast carcinoma. Using LOH and CGH techniques, alterations have been found most frequently at chromosomes 16q (loss), 1q (gain), 8p (loss), 3p FHIT gene locus, and 11q ATM gene locus {1754,1779,2476, 3046}. Of particular interest is the observation that other sites of chromosomal alteration previously found at high levels in other types

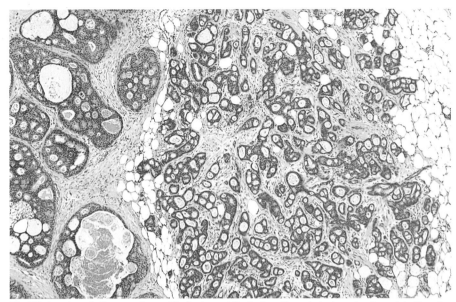

Fig. 1.25 Invasive cribriform carcinoma. The haphazard distribution of irregularly shaped and angulated invasive areas is in contrast with the rounded configuration of the ducts with cribriform DCIS on the left side of the field.

of breast cancer are not seen, which implies that tubular carcinoma of the breast is genetically distinct.

Prognosis and predictive factors

Pure tubular carcinoma has an excellent long term prognosis {409,410,552,771, 1829,2081,2224} which in some series is similar to age matched women without breast cancer {691}. Recurrence following mastectomy or breast conservation treatment is rare and localized tubular carcinomas are considered to be ideal candidates for breast conservation techniques. Following breast conservation, the risk of local recurrence is so low that some centres consider adjuvant radiotherapy unnecessary. Axillary node metastases occur infrequently, and when observed rarely involve more than one low axillary lymph node. There is little adverse effect of node positivity in tubular carcinoma {691,1471} and the use of systemic adjuvant therapy and axillary node dissection are considered unnecessary by some groups {691,2166}.

Invasive cribriform carcinoma

Definition

An invasive carcinoma with an excellent prognosis that grows in a cribriform pattern similar to that seen in intraductal cribriform carcinoma; a minor (<50%) component of tubular carcinoma may be admixed.

ICD-O code 8201/3

Epidemiology

Invasive cribriform carcinoma (ICC) accounts for 0.8-3.5% of breast carcinomas. The mean age of patients is 53-58 years {2148,2670,3017}.

Clinical features

The tumour may present as a mass but is frequently clinically occult. At mammography, tumours typically form a spiculated mass frequently containing microcalcifications {2670,2806}. Multifocality is observed in 20% of the cases {2148}.

Histopathology

The pure ICC consists almost entirely (>90%) of an invasive cribriform pattern. The tumour is arranged as invasive islands, often angulated, in which well defined spaces are formed by arches of cells (a sieve-like or cribriform pattern). Apical snouts are a regular feature. The tumour cells are small and show a low or moderate degree of nuclear pleomorphism. Mitoses are rare. A prominent, reactive appearing, fibroblastic stroma is present in many ICC. Intraductal carcinoma, generally of the cribriform type, is observed in as many as 80% of cases {2148}. Axillary lymph node metastases occur in 14.3% {2148}, the cribriform pattern being retained at these sites. Lesions showing a predominantly cribriform arrangement associated with a minor (<50%) component of tubular carcinoma are also included in the group of classic ICC {2148}. Cases with a component (10-40%) of another carcinoma type, other than tubular carcinoma, should be called mixed type of carcinoma {2148,3017}.

Immunoprofile
ICC is estrogen receptor positive in 100% and progesterone receptor in 69% of cases {3017}.

Differential diagnosis
ICC should be differentiated from carcinoid tumour and adenoid cystic carcinoma; the former has intracytoplasmic argyrophilic granules, while the latter has a second cell population in addition to a variety of intracystic secretory and basement membrane-like material. The lack of laminin around the cribriform structures also differentiates ICC from adenoid cystic carcinoma {3092}. ICC is distinguished from extensive cribriform DCIS by the lack of a myoepithelial cell layer around its invasive tumour cell clusters, its haphazard distribution and irregular configuration.

Prognosis and predictive factors
ICC has a remarkably favourable outcome {771,2148,3017}. The ten-year overall survival was 90% {771} to 100% {2148}. The outcome of mixed invasive cribriform carcinoma has been reported to be less favourable than that of the classic form, but better than that of common ductal carcinoma {2148}. The biological behaviour of ICC is very similar to that of tubular carcinoma {771}. It has been suggested that cribriform elements might correspond to tubules {2148}. However, many ICC have no definite tubular structures and separation of this tumour as a distinct clinicopathological entity is justified.

Medullary carcinoma

Definition
A well circumscribed carcinoma composed of poorly differentiated cells arranged in large sheets, with no glandular structures, scant stroma and a prominent lymphoplasmacytic infiltrate.

ICD-O code   8510/3

Epidemiology
Medullary carcinoma (MC) represents between 1 and 7% {294,2334} of all breast carcinomas, depending on the stringency of diagnostic criteria used. The mean age of women with MC ranges from 45 to 52 years {623,2204,2334, 3064}.

Clinical features
The tumour is well delineated and soft on palpation. Mammographically MC is typically well circumscribed and may be confused with a benign lesion.

Macroscopy
MC has distinctive rounded, well defined margins and a soft consistency. Fleshy tan to grey in appearance, foci of necrosis and haemorrhage are frequent. The median diameter varies from 2.0-2.9 cm {2334,2370,3064}.

Histopathology
Since the early descriptions of MC {895,1908,2367}, the histological features of this tumour have been further specified {2334,2370,3064}.
Classically, five morphological traits characterize MC.
1. A syncytial architecture should be observed in over 75% of the tumour mass. Tumour cells are arranged in sheets, usually more than four or five cells thick, separated by small amounts of loose connective tissue. Foci of necrosis and of squamous differentiation may be seen.
2. Glandular or tubular structures are not present, even as a minor component.
3. Diffuse lymphoplasmacytic stromal infiltrate is a conspicuous feature. The density of this infiltrate varies among cases, mononuclear cells may be scarce or so numerous that they largely obliterate the carcinoma cells. Lymphoid follicles and/or epithelioid granuloma may be present.
4. Carcinoma cells are usually round with abundant cytoplasm and vesicular nuclei containing one or several nucleoli. The nuclear pleomorphism is moderate or marked, consistent with grade 2 or 3. Mitoses are numerous. Atypical giant cells may be observed.
5. Complete histological circumscription of the tumour is best seen under low magnification. Pushing margins may delimit a compressed fibrous zone at the periphery of the lesion.

Besides these typical histologic traits, the presence of an intraductal component is considered as a criterion for exclusion by some authors {2370,3064}, but acceptable by others {2334}, especially when it is located in the surrounding tissue or reduced to small areas within the tumour mass.
These diagnostic criteria, particularly the status of the margin, may be difficult to assess in practice, and may explain the low reproducibility in the diagnosis of MC observed in certain series {950,2203, 2372}. To overcome this difficulty, a simplified scheme has been proposed {2202}. Syncytial growth pattern, lack of tubule formation and lymphoplasmacytic infiltrate, together with sparse tumour necrosis (<25%) were found to be the most reproducible and characteristic features of MC. However, the prognostic significance of this simplistic scheme needs to be assessed {1339}.
Tumours showing the association of a predominantly syncytial architecture with only two or three of the other criteria are usually designated as atypical medullary carcinoma (AMC) {2334,2370}. However, strictly defined morphological criteria are necessary to preserve the entity of MC characterized by its relatively favourable prognosis {2334,2478} which is not shared by AMC. Several works {2334, 3064} have advocated the elimination of the AMC category in order to avoid confusion with MC and the term infiltrating ductal carcinoma with medullary features seems to be more appropriate for these tumours.

Immunoprofile and ploidy
Flow cytometry and immunohistochemical analysis has shown that most MC are aneuploid and highly proliferative tumours {551,1244,1345,1766,2108, 2201}. A high apoptosis rate has also

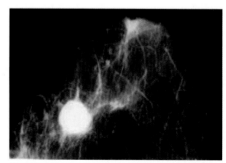
Fig. 1.26 Medullary carcinoma. Mammogram showing a typical rounded, dense tumour without calcifications.

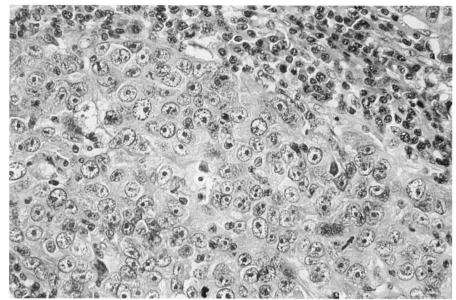

Fig. 1.27 Medullary carcinoma. The tumour is composed of a syncytial sheet of large pleomorphic cells. There is no glandular differentiation. The adjacent stroma contains numerous plasma cells and mature lymphocytes.

been reported {1386,3170}. MC typically lack estrogen receptors (ER) expression {1244,1340,2204,2272}, and have a low incidence of ERBB2 overexpression {2439,2746,2750}.

The cytokeratin profile is similar in typical and atypical MC, and does not differ significantly from that of common ductal tumours {610,1340,2943}. The cell cohesiveness of MC, contrasting with the poorly differentiated pattern and high mitotic index, has been characterized by the expression of the intercellular adhesion molecule-1 {156} and of E-cadherin {444}. This feature might account for the good limitation of the tumour and the late axillary lymph node extension.

Immunophenotyping of the lymphoid infiltrate of MC has shown that most cells correspond to mature T lymphocytes, a profile similar to that observed in common ductal carcinomas {214}. Evidence of polyclonality of the B-cell infiltrate has been obtained {1510}. Plasma cells were found to express IgG {1310} or IgA {1254}. The recent finding of an increased number of activated cytotoxic lymphocytes in MC may correspond to an active host versus tumour response {3169}. Expression of HLA class I and class II molecules by carcinoma cells, as a cause or a consequence of the immune response, was reported to characterize MC {840}. Although EBV-associated lymphoepithelioma shares some morphological features with MC, only a few cases were found associated with EBV, in contrast with the 31-51% rate of EBV-positive common ductal carcinomas {310,857}.

Genetics

A high frequency of MC has been reported in patients with *BRCA1* germ line mutation, whereas this observation was less common among patients with *BRCA2* mutation or with no known germ line mutation. Typical MC were observed in 7.8% {1767} to 13% {8} of BRCA1-associated carcinomas, versus 2% in control populations. However, the presence of medullary features was found in 35% {1767} to 60% {121} of tumours arising in BRCA1 carriers. Reciprocally, in a population of MC, germ line mutations of *BRCA1* was observed in 11% of the cases {764}. There is thus a large overlap between medullary features and the phe-

notype of *BRCA1* germline associated tumours, but not all *BRCA1* mutations lead to medullary phenotype.

MC are also characterized by a high rate of *TP53* alterations. Somatic mutations were found in 39% {1766} to 100% {643} of MC, together with protein accumulation in 61-87% of the cases {643, 711,1345}. This contrasts with the 25-30% rate of *TP53* alterations found in common ductal carcinomas {643,711, 1345}. No specific *TP53* mutation was found to characterize MC {643} but TP53 overstaining may be considered as a biological marker of MC. Both *TP53* and *BRCA1* are involved in the process of DNA repair and the alteration of these genes, together with a high proliferation rate, may account for the high sensitivity of MC to radio- and/or chemotherapy.

Prognosis and predictive factors

MC has been reported to have a better prognosis than the common IDC {1339, 1740,1908,2204,2334,2352,2367,2370, 3064} but this has been questioned by others {285,771,876}. The overall 10-year-survival reported for MC varies between about 50% {285,771,1740} to more than 90% {1339,2334,3064}. Differences in diagnostic criteria may account for this disparity and several reports underline that stringency in diagnostic criteria is required to preserve the anatomo-clinical identity of MC {876,2334,2370,3064} which is justified by the characteristic prognosis of this tumour. The outcome of MC associated with more than three metastatic axillary lymph nodes has been reported to be poor {285,1740,2202} or no different from that of common ductal tumours {876,2352}. However, less than 10% of MC {876,1339,2334,2352,2370} present with node metastases, and this might account in part for the relatively favourable overall prognosis of MC.

Table 1.06
Histological criteria required for a diagnosis of MC.

> Syncytial growth pattern (> 75%)

> Absence of glandular structures

> Diffuse lymphoplasmacytic infiltrate, moderate to marked

> Nuclear pleomorphism, moderate to marked

> Complete histological circumscription

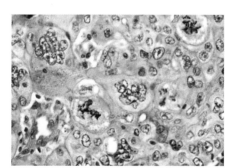

Fig. 1.28 Medullary carcinoma. Note multinucleated malignant cells with atypical mitoses.

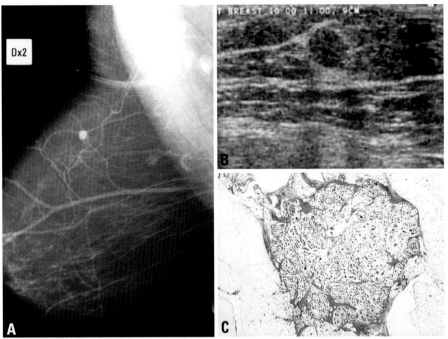

Fig. 1.29 Mucinous carcinoma. **A** Mammogram showing small rounded density of less than 10 mm diameter in the upper-outer quadrant. **B** Ultrasound suggests mucinous carcinoma. **C** Low power view of the mucinous carcinoma.

Mucin producing carcinomas

Definition
A variety of carcinomas in the breast are characterized by production of abundant extracellular and/or intracellular mucin. Among these are mucinous (colloid) carcinoma, mucinous cystadenocarcinoma, columnar cell mucinous carcinoma and signet ring cell carcinoma.

Mucinous carcinoma

Mucinous carcinoma is characterized by a proliferation of clusters of generally small and uniform cells floating in large amounts of extracellular mucus often visible to the naked eye.

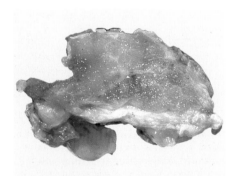

Fig. 1.30 Mucinous carcinoma. 38 year old patient, tumour excision.

ICD-O code   8480/3

Synonyms
Colloid carcinoma, mucoid carcinoma, gelatinous carcinoma.

Epidemiology
Pure mucinous carcinoma accounts for about 2% of all breast carcinomas {2338,2590,2934}. It occurs in a wide age range, but the mean and median age of patients with mucinous carcinoma in some studies is somewhat higher than that of regular infiltrating carcinomas, being often over 60 years {2447,2590}.

Clinical features
The tumours usually present as a palpable lump. The location is similar to that of breast carcinomas in general. Mammographically, mucinous carcinoma appears as a well defined, lobulated lesion. On magnification or compression views {547}, a less defined margin may become more evident. The mammographic resemblance to a benign process (circumscription and lobulation) increases with increasing mucin content.

Macroscopy
The typical glistening gelatinous appearance with bosselated, pushing margins and a soft consistency make the lesion

readily recognizable. The tumours range in size from less than 1 cm to over 20 cm, with an average of 2.8 cm {1498,2338, 2447,2934}.

Histopathology
Mucinous carcinoma is characterized by proliferation of clusters of generally uniform, round cells with minimal amounts of eosinophilic cytoplasm, floating in lakes of mucus. Delicate fibrous septae divide the mucous lake into compartments. The cell clusters are variable in size and shape; sometimes with a tubular arrangement; rarely, they assume a papillary configuration. Atypia, mitotic figures and microcalcifications are not common, but occur occasonaly. An intraepithelial component characterized by a micropapillary to solid pattern is present in 30-75% of the tumours. The lakes of mucin are mucicarmine positive, but intracytoplasmic mucin is rarely present. A notable proportion of the lesions have neuroendocrine differentiation {150,855} easily demonstrable by Grimelius stain or immunoreaction for chromogranin and synaptophysin (see also neuroendocrine carcinoma of breast).

The descriptive term cellular mucinous carcinoma has been used by some {1751} to differentiate the endocrine variant of mucinous carcinoma from the non-endocrine one; presence of intracytoplasmic neuroendocrine granules does not always correlate with the degree of cellularity, however.

Traditionally, pure and mixed variants of mucinous carcinoma have been described {1498,2934}. A pure tumour must be composed entirely of mucinous carcinoma. The pure mucinous carcinomas are further subdivided into cellular and hypocellular variants. The former is more likely to have intracytoplasmic mucin and argyrophilic granules. As soon as another pattern becomes evident as a component of the tumour mass, the lesions qualifies as a mixed tumour (the proportion of the different components should be noted). The most common admixture is with regular invasive duct carcinoma.

Differential diagnosis
The two lesions most likely to be confused with mucinous carcinoma are myxoid fibroadenoma and mucocoele like lesion {2417}. The presence of compressed spaces lined by epithelial and

myoepithelial cells in fibroadenomas, along with mast cells within the myxoid stroma, helps in its recognition.

In mucocoele-like lesions, the presence of myoepithelial cells adhering to the strips of cells floating in the lakes of mucus serves as an important clue to their benign nature; the cell clusters in mucinous carcinoma are purely epithelial. The presence of ducts variably distended by mucinous material adjacent to a mucocoele is another helpful clue in distinguishing mucocoele-like lesions from mucinous carcinomas.

Immunoprofile and ploidy
Typically mucinous carcinoma is estrogen receptor positive {2669}, while less than 70% {691} are progesterone receptor positive. Nearly all pure mucinous carcinomas are diploid, while over 50% of the mixed variety are aneuploid {2933}.

Prognosis and predictive factors
Prognostic factors relevant to breast carcinomas in general are also applicable to pure mucinous carcinomas. Tumour cellularity has also been implicated in that cellular tumours are associated with a worse prognosis {502}. The presence or absence of argyrophilic granules had no prognostic significance in two studies

{2590,2934}. In general, pure mucinous carcinomas have a favourable prognosis {844,2590,2934}. The ten-year survival ranges from 80% {1498} to 100% {844,2053}. Pure mucinous carcinomas have a far better prognosis than the mixed variety with at least a 18% difference in survival rates noted in several studies {1498,2053,2934}. About 10% of women with the pure form die of their cancer compared to 29% of those with the mixed type {1498,2053}. A similar difference also exists in the incidence of axillary node metastases for pure and mixed types; only 3-15% of the pure variety show axillary node metastases compared to 33-46% of the mixed type {82,1498,2338}. Late distant metastases may occur {502,2447,2934}.

A rare cause of death among women with mucinous carcinoma is cerebral infarction due to mucin embolism to the cerebral arteries {2944}.

Mucinous cystadenocarcinoma and columnar cell mucinous carcinoma

Definition
A carcinoma composed of generally tall, columnar cells with basally located bland nuclei and abundant intracytoplasmic

mucin that appears either cystic (mucinous cystadenocarcinoma) or solid (columnar cell mucinous carcinoma) to the naked eye.

ICD-O code
Mucinous cystadenocarcinoma   8470/3

Epidemiology
Only four examples of mucinous cystadenocarcinoma and two of the solid columnar cell type have been reported {1486}. They occurred in women 49 to 67 years of age.

Clinical features
The clinical features of mucinous cystadenocarcinomas are similar to common infiltrating ductal carcinomas.

Macroscopy
The tumours vary in size from 0.8 to 19 cm, are cystic and display a gelatinous appearance with abundant mucoid material simulating an ovarian mucinous tumour.

Histopathology
Microscopically, both of these variants, are composed of tall columnar mucinous cells with abundant intracytoplasmic mucin and basal nuclei. In the

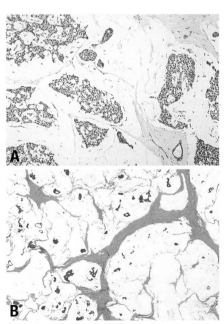

Fig. 1.31 Mucinous carcinoma. **A** Hypercellular variant with large clusters of densely packed malignant cells. **B** Hypocellular variant. Lakes of mucus are separated by fibrous septae. A few isolated or clusters of carcinoma cells are floating in the mucus lakes.

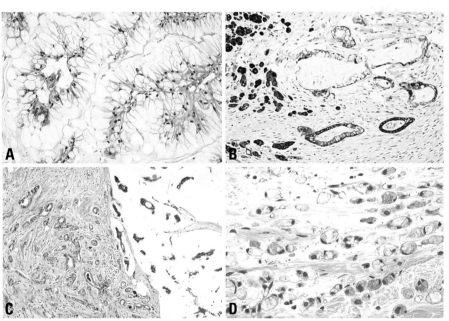

Fig. 1.32 A Mucinous cystadenocarcinoma. Papillary processes lined by mucinous columnar cells protude into cystic spaces. **B** Mucinous cystadenocarcinoma. Many of the invasive cells are immunoreactive to CK34βE12. **C** Combined mucinous and infiltrating ductal carcinoma. A favourable prognosis associated with pure mucinous carcinoma is no longer expected when it is admixed with regular infiltrating duct carcinoma. **D** Signet ring cell carcinoma. The invasive cells assume a lobular growth pattern and contain abundant intracytoplasmic mucin conferring a signet-ring cell appearance to the cells.

Table 1.07
Criteria for the differential diagnosis of mucin producing carcinomas.

Histological type	Location of mucin	Growth pattern	In situ component
Mucinous (colloid) carcinoma	Extracellular	Clusters of cells in mucus lakes	Ductal
Mucinous cystadenocarcinoma	Intracellular and extracellular	Large cysts, columnar cells, epithelial stratification, papillae, solid areas	Ductal
Columnar mucinous carcinoma	Intracellular	Round and convoluted glands lined by a single layer of columnar cells	Ductal
Signet ring cell carcinoma	Intracellular	Isolated cells, cords, clusters	Mainly lobular

cystic variant numerous cysts of variable size are formed, some with papillary fronds lined by a single layer of predominantly bland appearing, columnar mucinous cells. Focal atypia characterized by nuclear pleomorphism (but sparse mitotic activity), loss of polarity and eosinophilic cellular transformation is invariably present, as is invasion of surrounding stroma by most often the eosinophilic cells. Axillary node metastases occur in a quarter of mucinous cystadenocarcinomas.

The columnar cell variant is composed of a compact to loose aggregation of round and convoluted glands lined by a single layer of generaly tall, columnar mucimous epithelium with bland, basal nuclei and rare mitotic figures.

Prognosis and predictive factors
After a maximum follow-up of only 2 years, none of the patients has developed a recurrence or metastasis.

Signet ring cell carcinoma

ICD-O code   8490/3

Signet ring cell carcinomas are of two types. One type is related to lobular carcinoma and is characterized by large intracytoplasmic lumina which compress the nuclei towards one pole of the cell {1849}. Their invasive component has the targetoid pattern of classical lobular carcinoma. The other type is similar to diffuse gastric carcinoma, and is characterized by acidic mucosubstances that diffusely fill the cytoplasm and dislodge the nucleus to one pole of

the cell. This type of signet ring cell carcinoma can be seen in association with the signet ring cell variant of DCIS {1143}.

Neuroendocrine tumours

Definition
Primary neuroendocrine (NE) carcinomas of the breast are a group, which exhibits morphological features similar to those of NE tumours of both gastrointestinal tract and lung. They express neuroendocrine markers in more than 50% of the cell population. Breast carcinoma, not otherwise specified, with focal endocrine differentiation, revealed by immunocytochemical expression of neuroendocrine markers in scattered cells, is not included this group.

Synonym
Endocrine carcinoma.

Epidemiology
NE breast carcinomas represent about 2-5% of breast carcinomas. Most patients are in the 6th or 7th decades of life {2535}. Neuroendocrine differentiation also occurs in male breast carcinoma {2591}.

Clinical features
There are no notable or specific differences in presentation from other tumour types. Patients often present with a palpable nodule, which usually appears as a circumscribed mass on mammographic and ultrasound examination. Patients with small cell carcinoma often present at an advanced stage.

Endocrine hormone related syndromes are exceptionally rare. Of interest is the increase in the blood of neuroendocrine markers such as chromogranin A.

Macroscopy
NE breast carcinomas can grow as infiltrating or expansile tumours. The consistency of tumours with mucin production is soft and gelatinous.

Histopathology
Most NE breast carcinomas form alveolar structures or solid sheets of cells with a tendency to produce peripheral palisading. However, they may present as different subtypes, depending on the cell type, grade, degree of differentiation and presence of mucin production. The latter is observed in 26% of cases {2535}.

Solid neuroendocrine carcinoma

These tumours consist of densely cellular, solid nests and trabeculae of cells that vary from spindle to plasmacytoid and large clear cells {2536} separated by delicate fibrovascular stroma. In some tumours, the nests are packed into a solitary, well defined to lobulated mass; the tumour cells rarely form rosette-like structures and display peripheral palisading reminiscent of *carcinoid* tumour.

Some of these appear to originate from solitary, solid papillary intraductal carcinomas. Others form multiple, often rounded solid nests separated by a dense, collagenous stroma resembling the alveolar pattern of invasive lobular carcinoma. Mitotic activity ranges from 4 in the carcinoid-like tumour to 12 in the alveolar variant; focal necrosis may be seen. The tumour cells contain NE granules.

Small cell / oat cell carcinoma

ICD-O codes
Small cell carcinoma   8041/3
Oat cell carcinoma   8042/3

This is morphologically indistinguishable from its counterpart in the lung on the basis of histological and immunohistochemical features {2662}. The tumours are composed of densely packed hyperchromatic cells with scant cytoplasm and display an infiltrative growth pattern. An in situ component with the same cytological features may

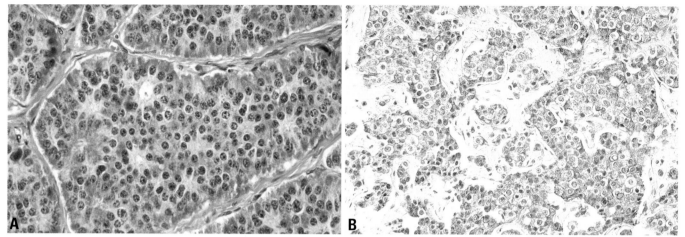

Fig. 1.33 Neuroendocrine carcinoma. **A** Tumour cells are polarized around lumina; some cells show eosinophilic granules – carcinoid-like pattern. **B** IHC staining is positive for chromogranin.

be present. Areas of tumour necrosis containing pyknotic hyperchromatic nuclei are rarely detectable. Crush artefact and nuclear streaming occur, but are more typical of aspiration cytology samples. Lymphatic tumour emboli are frequently encountered.

Large cell neuroendocrine carcinoma

ICD-O code   8013/3

These poorly differentiated tumours are composed of crowded large clusters of cells, with moderate to abundant cytoplasm, nuclei with vesicular to finely granular chromatin and a high number of mitotic figures ranging from 18 to 65 per 10 hpf. Focal areas of necrosis are present {2535}. These tumours exhibit neuroendocrine differentiation similar to those encountered in the lung (see also below).

Differential diagnosis

A nodule of NE carcinoma in the breast may reflect metastatic carcinoid or small cell carcinoma from another site {2022}. Immunohistochemistry may help to distinguish between metastatic and primary small cell carcinomas. Mammary small cell carcinomas are cytokeratin 7-positive and cytokeratin 20-negative, whereas, for example, pulmonary small cell carcinomas are negative for both {2662}. The presence of DCIS with similar cytological features is supportive of breast origin. In addition, the expression of estrogen (ER) and progesterone receptors (PR) and of the

apocrine marker GCDFP-15, which is frequently expressed by well and moderately differentiated endocrine breast carcinomas {2535}, are supportive of a primary breast carcinoma.

Mammary small cell carcinoma can be confused histologically with lobular carcinoma. The negative immunoreaction for E-cadherin in lobular carcinomas, in contrast to a positive reaction in 100% of small cell carcinomas, is useful in the differential diagnosis {2661}.

It is also important to differentiate neuroendocrine breast carcinomas from carcinomas with neuroendocrine differentiation. The latter have immunoex-

pression for neuroendocrine markers in scattered cells; this feature is noted in 10-18% of breast carcinomas of the usual type. Such focal neuroendocrine differentiation does not seem to carry a special prognostic or therapeutic significance {1876}.

Immunoprofile

Argyrophilia demonstrated by Grimelius silver precipitation is a feature of neuroendocrine breast carcinomas. Only darkly granulated cells should be considered as argyrophilic {2536}.

Expression of chromogranin proteins and/or synaptophysin also confirmed

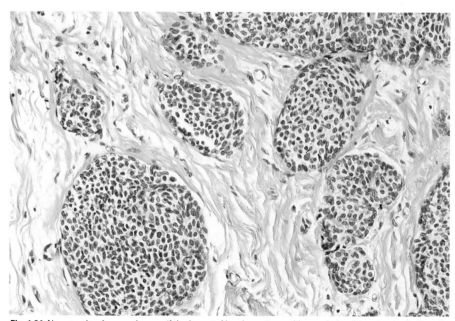

Fig. 1.34 Neuroendocrine carcinoma of the breast. Alveolar pattern with rounded solid nests of spindle cells invading a dense collagenous stroma.

evidence of neuroendocrine differentiation {2533}. These proteins are identifiable by immunohistochemical and immunoblot analysis. Poorly and moderately differentiated endocrine breast carcinomas of the alveolar subtype, in general, express chromogranin A. The mRNA specific for chromogranin A is detectable by in situ hybridization technique {2535}. About 50% of well or moderately differentiated tumours express chromogranin B and A and only 16% express synaptophysin {2535}. A monoclonal antibody against neurone-specific enolase (NSE) has also been used and is expressed in 100% of small cell carcinomas of the breast {2662}, whereas chromogranin A and synaptophysin are expressed in about 50% of such cases. In addition, 20% of small cell mammary carcinomas express thyroid transcription factor-1 (TTF-1) {2661}.

Immunodetection of pan-endocrine markers may fail to recognize endocrine tumours, which produce but do not retain the specific antigen in the cells. Estrogen (ER) and progesterone receptors (PR) are expressed in the majority of tumour cells in well differentiated tumours {2535}, and in more than 50% of small cell carcinomas {2662}.

Expression of somatostatin receptors (SSR), a known feature of tumours showing neuroendocrine differentiation, has been demonstrated in endocrine breast carcinomas as well {2169}.

Ultrastructure

Different types of dense core granules, whose neurosecretory nature is confirmed by ultrastructural immunolocalization of chromogranin A have been identified by electron microscopy in endocrine breast carcinomas {397}.

The presence of clear vesicles of pre-synaptic type is correlated with the expression of synaptophysin.
Both dense core granules and mucin vacuoles are present in neuroendocrine mucinous carcinomas {1265}.

Genetics

Neuroendocrine breast carcinomas have not been correlated to specific gene mutations.

Postulated normal counterpart

Argyrophilic and chromogranin A-reactive cells, located between the basal myoepithelial and the luminal epithelial cells, have been demonstrated in histologically normal breast tissue surrounding infiltrating and in situ neuroendocrine breast carcinomas {382,1995, 2542,2956}.

Prognosis and predictive factors

Histological grading is one of the most important prognostic parameters.
NE breast carcinomas may be graded using classical criteria described elsewhere.
Excluding the rare small cell variety, 45% of NE breast carcinomas are well differentiated, 40% are moderately differentiated, and only 15% are poorly differentiated. Small cell NE carcinomas should be considered as undifferentiated carcinomas {2535}.
Mucinous differentiation is a favourable prognostic factor {2535}.
The prognosis of primary small cell carcinomas of the breast depends on the stage of disease at the time of diagnosis. It has been demonstrated that low stage small cell carcinomas respond to conventional treatment without progression of the disease at a follow up of 33 to 48 months {2662}.

Invasive papillary carcinoma

Definition

When papillary intraductal carcinomas invade, they generally assume the pattern of infiltrating duct carcinoma and lack a papillary architecture. Most of the published literature concerning papillary carcinomas of the breast probably include both invasive and in situ papillary lesions as they do not generally specify features of an invasive process {413, 603,969,1269,1604,1618,1834}. In this section, however, only data concerning invasive papillary carcinomas will be reviewed. Invasive papillary carcinomas comprise less than 1-2% of invasive breast cancers, and are characterized by a relatively good prognosis {879,2567}.

ICD-O code   8503/3

Clinical features

Invasive papillary carcinomas are diagnosed predominantly in postmenopausal patients. Fisher et al. {879} noted a disproportionate number of cases in non-Caucasian women. Similar to medullary carcinomas, Fisher et al. noted that a significant proportion of patients with invasive papillary carcinoma exhibit axillary lymphadenopathy suggestive of metastatic disease, but which on pathological examination is due to benign reactive changes {879}.
Mammographically, invasive papillary carcinoma is usually characterized by nodular densities which may be multiple, and are frequently lobulated {1880, 2567}. These lesions are often hypoechoic on ultrasound {1827}. One study noted the difficulty in distinguishing between intracystic papillary carcinoma, intracystic papillary carcinoma with invasion, and invasive papillary carcinoma {1827}.

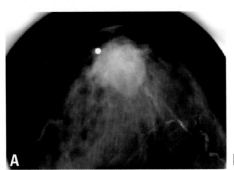 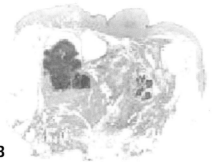 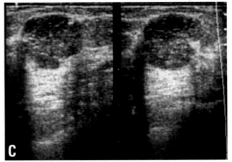

Fig. 1.35 Invasive papillary carcinoma. **A** Microfocus magnification image of a papillary carcinoma shows a low density rounded tumour. **B** Large section histology. **C** Ultrasonography shows a lobulated, well delineated lesion.

Macroscopy

Fisher et al. reported that invasive papillary carcinoma is grossly circumscribed in two-thirds of cases {879}. Other invasive papillary carcinomas are grossly indistinguishable from invasive breast cancers of no special type.

Histopathology

Of the 1,603 breast cancers reviewed in the NSABP-B04 study, 38 had papillary features, and all but 3 of these were "pure," without an admixture of other histologic types {879}. Microscopically, expansile invasive papillary carcinomas are characteristically circumscribed, show delicate or blunt papillae, and show focal solid areas of tumour growth. The cells typically show amphophillic cytoplasm, but may have apocrine features, and also may exhibit apical "snouting" of cytoplasm similar to tubular carcinoma. The nuclei of tumour cells are typically intermediate grade, and most tumours are histologic grade 2 {879}. Tumour stroma is not abundant in most cases, and occasional cases show prominent extracellular mucin production. Calcifications, although not usually evident mammographically, are commonly seen histologically, but usually are present in associated DCIS. DCIS is present in more than 75% of cases, and usually, but not exclusively, has a papillary pattern. In rare lesions in which both the invasive and in situ components have papillary features, it may be difficult to determine the relative proportion of each. Lymphatic vessel invasion has been noted in one third of cases. Microscopic involvement of skin or nipple was present in 8 of 35 cases (23%), but Paget disease of the nipple was not observed {879}.

Estrogen receptor positivity was observed in all 5 cases of invasive papillary carcinoma examined in one study, and progesterone receptor positivity in 4 of 5 (80%) {2351}. In a review of cytogenetic findings in 5 examples of invasive papillary carcinoma, 60% exhibited relatively simple cytogenetic abnormalities {40}. In addition, none of the 4 examples of papillary carcinomas examined in two recent reports were associated with either TP53 protein accumulation or ERBB2 oncoprotein overexpression {2440,2750}.

Clinical course and prognosis

There are only limited data on the prognostic significance of invasive papillary

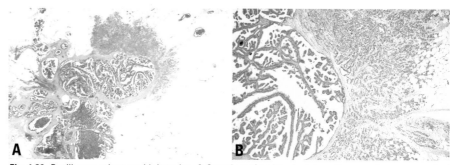

Fig. 1.36 Papillary carcinoma with invasion. **A** Overview of an intraductal papillary carcinoma, present at the centre, with invasive carcinoma apparent in the upper right side of the lesion. **B** Higher magnification shows an infiltrating duct carcinoma pattern by the invasive component of the lesion while the in situ region is clearly papillary.

carcinoma {868,871,879}. Among 35 patients with this tumour in the NSABP-B04 trial, after 5 years median follow-up, there were only 3 treatment failures, including 1 patient who died from metastatic papillary carcinoma. These survival data were similar to those reported in patients with pure tubular and mucinous carcinomas in this study {879}. A later publication updating the NSABP-B04 results at 15 years revealed that patients with "favourable" histology tumours (including invasive papillary carcinomas) still had significantly better survival in univariate analysis, but tumour histology was not an independent predictor of survival in multivariate analysis {871}. However, node-negative patients with invasive papillary carcinomas enrolled in the NSABP-B06 trial experienced improved survival after 10 years follow-up compared to patients with carcinomas of no special type, and tumour histology was an independent predictor of survival in multivariate analysis {868}.

Invasive micropapillary carcinoma

Definition

A carcinoma composed of small clusters of tumour cells lying within clear stromal spaces resembling dilated vascular channels.

ICD-O code   8507/3

Epidemiology

Carcinomas with a dominant micropapillary growth pattern account for less than 2% of all invasive breast cancers {707, 1715,1982,2194,2229}. The term invasive micropapillary carcinoma was coined by Siriaunkgul and Tavassoli who first described nine examples of this lesion {707}. While quite rare in its pure form, focal micropapillary growth has been reported in 3-6% of more common types of invasive carcinomas {1982,2194}. It occurs in the same age range as invasive ductal carcinoma of no special type.

Clinical features

Invasive micropapillary carcinoma usually presents as a solid mass. Axillary lymph node metastases are present at first presentation in 72-77% {707,1715, 1982,2194,2229,3049} .

Macroscopy

Pure micropapillary carcinoma has a lobulated outline due to the expansive mode of growth.

Histopathology

Micropapillary carcinoma consists of hollow aggregates of malignant cells, which on cross section have the appearance of tubules with diminished or obliterated lumens rarely containing pyknotic nuclei. These tumour cell cluster lie within artifactual stromal spaces caused by shrinkage of the surrounding tissue. The stromal spaces lack an endothelial lining and may be part of a speculated "missing lymphatic labyrinth" in mammary stroma {1152}. Nuclear pleomorphism is moderate, mitotic activity low, and there is neither necrosis nor lymphocytic reaction. In non-pure tumours, gradual or abrupt transitions from typical invasive ductal carcinoma to the micropapillary components are found. Peritumoural angioinvasion may be present in up to 60% of cases. Intravascular tumour emboli,

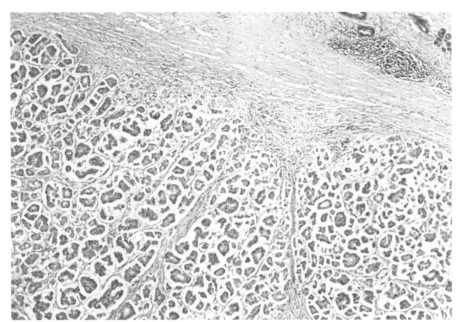

Fig. 1.37 Invasive micropapillary carcinoma. Tumour cell clusters with irregular central spaces proliferate within empty stromal spaces. Some clusters have reversed polarity with an "inside out" morphology.

lymph node metastases and malignant cells in pleural fluids all show the same arrangement found in the primary tumour.

Prognostic and predictive features

This unusual growth pattern is correlated with the presence of vascular invasion and axillary lymph node metastases. In multivariate analyses, however, a micropapillary growth pattern has no independent significance for survival {1982,2194}.

Apocrine carcinoma

Definition

A carcinoma showing cytological and immunohistochemical features of apocrine cells in >90% of the tumour cells.

ICD-O code   8401/3

Epidemiology

The reported incidence of apocrine carcinoma depends on the method of detection. Based on light microscopy alone it is only 0.3-4% {149,910}. An ultrastructural study found a frequency of 0.4% for apocrine carcinomas in a prospective series {1926}.
Immunohistochemical studies using anti GCDFP-15, a putative marker of apocrine differentiation {1800} gave conflicting data with an incidence ranging from 12% {809} to 72% {3113}. Twenty seven per cent of cases were positive with an in situ hybridization method using a mRNA probe against the sequence of the GCDFP-15 {1700}. In conclusion, carcinomas composed predominantly of apocrine cells constitute at the most 4% of all invasive carcinomas; focal apocrine cells diagnosed either by histology, immunohistochemistry or genetic techniques are frequent and occur in at least 30% of "ordinary" invasive carcinomas {1700}.

Clinical features

There is no difference between the clinical or mammographic features, size and site of carcinomas among apocrine and non-apocrine lesions. Bilaterality is rare in apocrine carcinomas.

Histopathology

Any type and grade of breast carcinoma can display apocrine differentiation including ordinary invasive duct carcinomas, tubular, medullary, papillary, micropapillary and neuroendocrine types {17,569,809,1700}, as well as classical and pleomorphic invasive lobular carcinomas {802,808}. However, recognition of apocrine carcinoma at present has no practical importance and is only of academic value.
Apocrine lobular in situ neoplasias {802,2534}, and apocrine ductal in situ carcinomas (ADCIS) are also well recognized {17,1605,2887}. Apocrine carcinomas, whatever their origin, are usually composed by two types of cells variously intermingled {804}. Type A cell recognized first by most authors has abundant granular intensely eosinophilic cytoplasm. The granules are periodic acid-Schiff positive after diastase digestion. Their nuclei vary from globoid with prominent nucleoli to hyperchromatic. Some tumours, when constituted by a pure proliferation of type A cells, superficially mimic granular cell tumours. This type of apocrine carcinoma has sometimes been referred

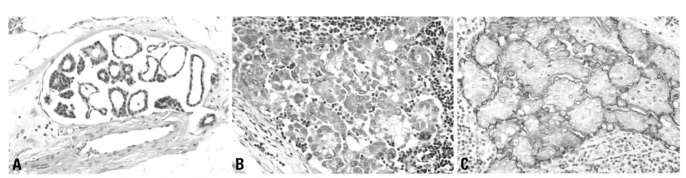

Fig. 1.38 Invasive micropapillary carcinoma. A Note the prominent vascular invasion and occasional pyknotic nuclei within the central spaces. B Lymph node metastasis. C EMA staining of of the peripheral cell membranes suggestive of an 'inside out' morphology.

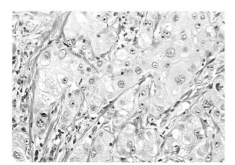
Fig. 1.39 Apocrine carcinoma. Note abundant eosinophilic cytoplasm and vesicular nuclei.

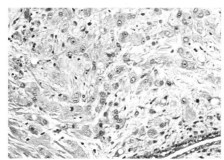
Fig. 1.40 Apocrine carcinoma, surperficially resembling a granular cell tumour.

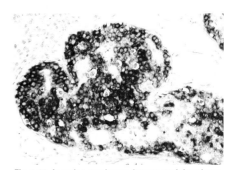
Fig. 1.41 Apocrine carcinoma. Immunostaining shows intense positivity for GCDFP-15.

to as myoblastomatoid {806}. Type B cell shows abundant cytoplasm in which fine empty vacuoles are seen. These latter result in foamy appearance so that the cells may resemble histiocytes and sebaceous cells. Nuclei are similar to those in type A cells. These same cells have been designated as sebocrine {2876}. (See also Sebaceous carcinoma, page 46). Carcinomas composed purely of foamy apocrine cells may surperfically resemble a histiocytic proliferation or even an inflammatory reaction {806}. In difficult cases, both granular cell tumours and histiocytic proliferations can be easily distinguished by staining the tumours with keratin antibodies that are positive only in apocrine carcinomas.

Immunoprofile
Apocrine carcinomas are typically GCDFP-15 positive and BCL2 protein negative. Expression of GCDFP-15 is a feature common to many variants of breast carcinoma, however, and has been used to support breast origin in metastatic carcinomas of unknown primary site. Estrogen and progesterone receptors are usually negative in apocrine carcinoma by immonuhistochemical assessment. Interestingly, many ER-, PR- apocrine carcinomas do have the ERmRNA, but fail to produce the protein {336}. The expression of other biological markers is in general similar to that of other carcinomas {177,1605,2425}. Androgen receptors have been reported as positive in 97% of ADCIS in one series {1605} and 81% in another {2624}. Sixty-two percent of invasive duct carcinomas were positive in the latter series {2624} and in 22% of cases in another study {1874}. The significance of AR in apocrine carcinomas is uncertain.

Genetics
Molecular studies in benign, hyperplastic and neoplastic apocrine lesions parallel those seen in non apocrine tumours {1357,1673}.

Prognosis and predictive factors
Survival analysis of 72 cases of invasive apocrine duct carcinoma compared with non apocrine duct carcinoma revealed no statistical difference {17,809}.

Metaplastic carcinomas

Definition
Metaplastic carcinoma is a general term referring to a heterogeneous group of neoplasms generally characterized by an intimate admixture of adenocarcinoma with dominant areas of spindle cell, squamous, and/or mesenchymal differentiation; the metaplastic spindle cell and squamous cell carcinomas may present in a pure form without any admixture with a recognizable adenocarcinoma. Metaplastic carcinomas can be classified into broad subtypes according to the phenotypic appearance of the tumour.

ICD-O code   8575/3

Synonyms
Matrix producing carcinoma, carcinosarcoma, spindle cell carcinoma.

Epidemiology
Metaplastic carcinomas account for less than 1% of all invasive mammary carcinomas {1273}. The average age at presentation is 55.

Clinical features
Clinical presentation is not different from that of infiltrating duct NOS carcinoma.

Most patients present with a well circumscribed palpable mass, with a median size of 3-4 cm, in some reports more than half of these tumours measure over 5 cm, with some massive lesions (>20 cm) which may displace the nipple and ulcerate through the skin.
On mammography, most metaplastic carcinomas appear as well delineated mass densities. Microcalcifications are not a common feature, but may be present in the adenocarcinomatous areas; ossification, when present, is, of course, apparent on mammography.

Macroscopy
The tumours are firm, well delineated and often solid on cut surface. Squamous or chondroid differentiation is reflected as pearly white to firm glistening areas on the cut surface. One large and/or multiple small cysts may be apparent on the cut surface of larger squamous tumours.

Table 1.08
Classification of metaplastic carcinomas.

Purely epithelial
Squamous
Large cell keratinizing
Spindle cell
Acantholytic
Adenocarcinoma with spindle cell differentiation
Adenosquamous, including mucoepidermoid
Mixed epithelial and Mesenchymal
(specify components)
Carcinoma with chondroid metaplasia
Carcinoma with osseous metaplasia
Carcinosarcoma (specify components)

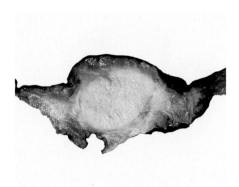

Fig. 1.42 Squamous cell carcinoma. A well circumscribed mass shows numerous irregularly shaped depressions on cut surface.

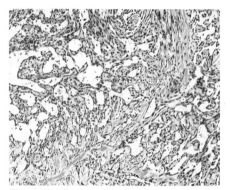

Fig. 1.43 Squamous cell carcinoma, acantholytic variant, which is often mistaken for angiosarcoma.

Squamous cell carcinoma

A breast carcinoma entirely composed of metaplastic squamous cells that may be keratinizing, non-keratinizing or spindled; they are neither derived from the overlying skin nor represent metastases from other sites.

ICD-O codes
Squamous cell carcinoma	8070/3
Large cell keratinizing variant	8071/3
Spindle cell variant	8074/3
Acantholytic variant	8075/3

Histopathology
Squamous cell carcinomas assume several phenotypes including large cell keratinizing, non-keratinizing, and less frequently spindle cell and acantholytic types; some show a combination of these patterns {752,987,1022, 1928,2520,2932,3061}. The most bland appearing and well differentiated cells often line cystic spaces; as the tumour cells emanate out to infiltrate the surrounding stroma, they become spindle shaped and lose their squamous features. A pronounced stromal reaction is often admixed with the spindled squamous carcinoma. The squamous differentiation is retained in metastatic foci. Squamous cell carcinoma can be graded based mainly on nuclear features and, to a lesser degree, cytoplasmic differentiation.

Immunoprofile
The spindle cell and acantholytic variants require immunohistochemical confirmation of their epithelial nature. The epithelial tumour cell components are positive for broad spectrum and high molecular weight cytokeratins (CK5 and CK34betaE12), but negative for vascular endothelial markers. Nearly all squamous cell carcinomas are negative for both estrogen (ER) and progesterone receptors (PR) {3059,3061}.

Adenocarcinoma with spindle cell metaplasia

Definition
An invasive adenocarcinoma with abundant spindle cell transformation. The spindle cells are neither squamous, nor mesenchymal, but rather glandular in nature.

ICD-O code   8572/3

Clinical features
This tumour occurs mainly in postmenopausal women and presents as a discrete mass.

Pathologic features
Macroscopically, a well circumscribed, solid mass, the tumour is composed of tubules of adenocarcinoma admixed with neoplastic spindle cells. The spindle cells immunoreact with epithelial markers including CK7, but not with CK5,6 or other markers of squamous/myoepithelial differentiation. At the ultrastructural level, the spindle

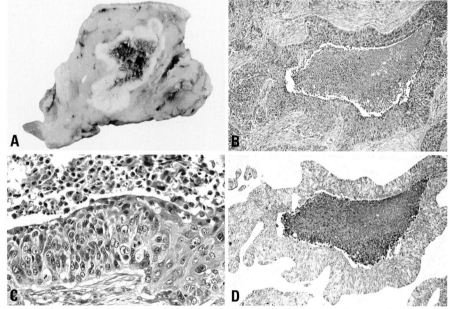

Fig. 1.44 Squamous cell carcinoma of the breast. A Macroscopically, there are often central cystic areas. B Variously shaped spaces lined by squamous epithelium are characteristic of the more common mammary squamous cell carcinoma. C Higher magnification showing a range of squamous cell differentiation with the most differentiated at the right. D Immunostain for cytokeratins 5, 6 is positive as expected for squamous epithelium.

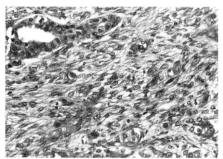

Fig. 1.45 Adenocarcinoma with spindle cell metaplasia. The spindle cells are neither squamous nor mesenchymal, but rather glandular, intermixed with glands.

cells contain intracytoplasmic lumens confirming a glandular cell population.

Adenosquamous carcinoma

Definition
An invasive carcinoma with areas of well developed tubule/gland formation intimately admixed with often widely dispersed solid nests of squamous differentiation.

ICD-O code   8560/3

Histopathology
While focal squamous differentiation has been observed in 3.7% of infiltrating duct carcinomas {878}, a prominent admixture of invasive ductal and squamous cell carcinoma is rarely observed. The squamous component is often keratinizing, but ranges from very well differentiated keratinizing areas to poorly differentiated non-keratinizing foci.

Eight tumours described as examples of low grade *mucoepidermoid carcinoma*, comparable to those occuring in the salivary glands, have been reported in the breast; these behave as low grade carcinomas {1130,1156,1515, 1629,1709,2191,2234}.

Immunoprofile
The squamous component is negative for both ER and PR, while the positivity of the ductal carcinoma component for ER and PR depends on its degree of differentiation.

Low grade adenosquamous carcinoma
Low grade adenosquamous carcinoma {2431} is a variant of metaplastic carcinoma which is morphologically similar to adenosquamous carcinoma of the skin and has been classified by some as syringomatous squamous tumour {2816}. The same lesion has been interpreted as an infiltrating syringomatous adenoma by others who prefer to avoid designation of carcinoma for a group of lesions which mainly recur after local excision.

ICD-O code   8560/1

Synonym
Infiltrating syringomatous adenoma. This entity is also discussed in Tumours of the Nipple.

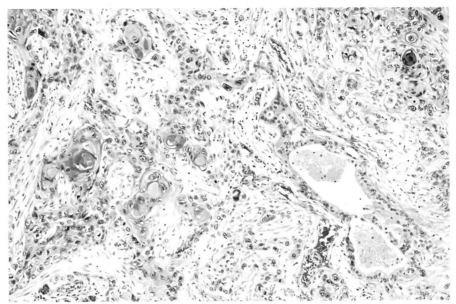

Fig. 1.46 Adenosquamous carcinoma. Both glandular and squamous differentiation coexist in this carcinoma.

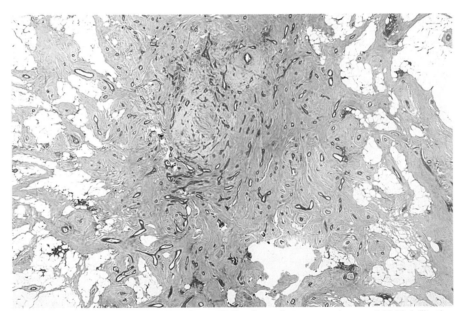

Fig. 1.47 Low grade adenosquamous carcinoma / infiltrating syringomatous adenoma. A highly infiltrative growth pattern is responsible for the high frequency of local recurrence associated with many lesions.

Clinical features
The age range at presentation is wide. These lesions usually present as a small palpable mass between 5 and 80 mm in size.

Histology
These tumours are composed of small glandular structure and solid cords of epithelial cells haphazardly arranged in an infiltrative spindle celled stromal component {2421,2995}. The proportions of these three components is variable between cases. The solid nests of cells may contain squamous cells, squamous pearls or squamous cyst formation. The stroma is typically "fibromatosis-like" being cellular and composed of bland spindle cells. The stromal component can, however, be collagenous, hyalinized or variably cellular, and osteocartilagenous foci can occur rarely. It has been recognized that some low grade adenosquamous carcinomas may be found in association with a central sclerosing proliferation such as a radial scar, sclerosing papillary lesion or sclerosing adenosis {672,2421,2995}. The frequen-

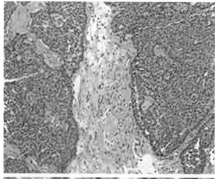

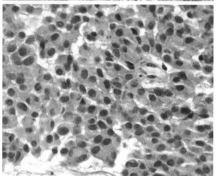

Fig. 1.48 Mucoepidermoid carcinoma.This low grade invasive carcinoma is morphologically similar to its counterpart in the salivary glands.

cy of ductal carcinoma in situ in association with adenosquamous carcinomas is variable. These tumours lack estrogen receptor expression {672,3142}.

Prognosis and predictive factors
The majority of case have an excellent prognosis, but a proportion of cases can behave in a locally aggressive manner {2995}, recurrence appears to be related to adequacy of local excision. Lymph node metastatic spread is extremely rare and noted in a single case that was 3.5 cm {2995}.

Mixed epithelial / mesenchymal metaplastic carcinomas

ICD-O code   8575/3

Synonyms
Carcinoma with osseous metaplasia (8571/3), carcinoma with chondroid metaplasia (8571/3), matrix producing carcinoma, carcinosarcoma (8980/3).

Histopathology
This wide variety of tumours, some of which are also regarded as "matrix producing carcinomas" {1414,2953}, show infiltrating carcinoma mixed with often heterologous mesenchymal elements ranging from areas of bland chondroid and osseous differentiation to frank sarcoma (chondrosarcoma, osteosarcoma, rhabdomyosarcoma, liposarcoma, fibrosarcoma). When the mesenchymal component is malignant, the designation of carcinosarcoma is used. Undifferentiated spindle cell elements may form part of the tumour. Grading is based mainly on nuclear features and, to a lesser degree, cytoplasmic differentiation.

Immunoprofile
The spindle cell elements may show positive reactivity for cytokeratins, albeit focally. Chondroid elements are frequently S-100 positive and may coexpress cytokeratins, but are negative for actin. Many of these tumours are negative for ER and PR both in the adenocarcinoma and the mesenchymal areas, but the adenocarcinoma component may be ER and PR positive if well to moderately differentiated. In carcinosarcomas, the mesenchymal component fails to immunoreact with any epithelial marker.

Differential diagnosis
The differential diagnosis varies for the different subtypes of metaplastic carcinoma.
Angiosarcoma may be confused with the acantholytic variant of squamous cell carcinoma, but focal areas of squamous differentiation can be found when sampled thoroughly. A negative immunoreaction with vascular endothelial markers and a positive reaction with cytokeratins will support the diagnosis of an epithelial neoplasm.
Fibromatosis and a variety of spindled mesenchymal tumours may be confused with spindle cell squamous carcinoma; these are all generally negative for epithelial markers.
Myoepithelial carcinoma is the most difficult lesion to distinguish from spindle cell squamous carcinoma. The former often has ducts with prominent to hyperplastic myoepithelial cells at its periphery, while the latter may have clear cut focal squamous differentiation. Reactions to a variety of immunostains may be similar, with the possible exception of those myoepithelial carcinomas that are diffusely S-100 positive. Electron microscopy may be needed to distinguish some of these lesions. Squamous carcinoma cells have abundant tonofilaments and well developed desmosomes whether spindled or polygonal. Intercellular bridges are abundant in the well differentiated areas In contrast, the spindle cell myoepithelial carcinomas often have pinocytotic vesicles, myofibrils and basal lamina in addition to tonofilaments and desmosomes.

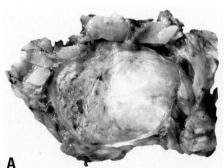
A

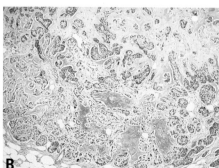
B

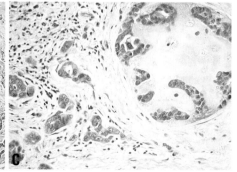
C

Fig. 1.49 A Metaplastic carcinoma with chondroid differentiation, 77 year old patient, mastectomy. **B** Carcinoma with mesenchymal (benign osseous and chondroid) differentiation. Typically, these carcinomas have a well delineated pushing margin. Areas of osseous and/or chondroid differentiation are variably scattered in an otherwise typical infiltrating ductal carcinoma. **C** Carcinoma with mesenchymal (benign osseous and chondroid) differentiation. The adenocarcinoma is admixed, in part, with chondroid matrix containing lacunar spaces and rare chondrocytes.

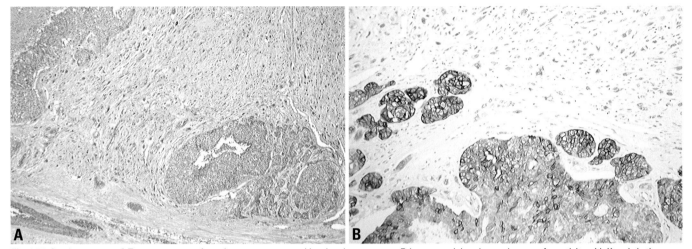

Fig. 1.50 Carcinosarcoma. **A** Two aggregates of carcinoma are separated by abundant sarcoma. **B** Immunostaining shows absence of reactivity with Kermix in the mesenchymal component, while the epithelial cells are positive.

The squamous and adenosquamous carcinoma should be distinguished from pleomorphic carcinomas that may have either pattern admixed with a large number of bizarre tumour giant cells; this distinction is important as pleomorphic carcinomas are far more aggressive than either squamous or adenosquamous carcinoma.

Adenocarcinomas with chondroid differentiation should be distinguished from pleomorphic adenomas. Pleomorphic adenomas invariably have a myoepithelial cell component (that may be dominant in some tumours) growing around spaces lined by benign epithelial cells. Myoepithelial cells are not evident in adenocarcinomas with chondroid differentiation.

Prognosis and predictive factors of metaplastic carcinomas

Given the tumour size of >3-4 cm in many cases, metastases to axillary nodes are relatively uncommon; approximately 10-15% of pure squamous cell carcinomas have axillary node metastases {503,1928}. About 19-25% of those with chondro-osseous elements have axillary node metastases {752,1273, 2259}, and 21% have distant metastases {752}. Axillary node metastases were more common (56%) among tumours with spindle and squamous metaplasia in Huvos's study {239}, however. When metaplastic carcinomas metastasize to the axillary nodes or beyond, they retain and often manifest their metaplastic potential. In studies combining carcinomas with chondroid and osseous meta-

plasia, the five year survival has ranged from 28-68% {474,1273,3060}; those with spindle or squamous differentiation have a 63% 5-year survival {1273}. Advanced stage and lymph node involvement is associated with a more aggressive course as anticipated. Among squamous cell carcinomas, the acantholytic variant may exhibit a more aggressive behaviour {807}.

The carcinosarcomas are very aggressive tumours. Some metastasize as mixed epithelial and mesenchymal tumours, while only the epithelial or the sarcomatous component may metastasize in others.

There is not much information available on the efficacy of current therapies in the management of metaplastic carcinomas.

Lipid-rich carcinoma

Definition
A breast carcinoma in which approximately 90% of neoplastic cells contain abundant cytoplasmic neutral lipids.

ICD-O code   8314/3

Synonym
Lipid secreting carcinoma.

Epidemiology
Using conventional morphological features only (i.e. foamy to vacuolated clear cells), incidences of <1-6%, have been reported {28,2330,2988}. Four cases only were seen within a 12-year period at

the AFIP {2876}. A frequency of 0.8% was found in a study using Sudan III on frozen sections {3158}.

The age of patients with putative lipid rich carcinoma ranges from 33 to 81 years. All except one were female, the exception being a 55-year-old man {1803}.

Clinical features
Most patients have palpable nodules. One case presented as Paget disease of the nipple {28}.

Macroscopy
The tumour size in the cases reported varies from 1.2 to 15 cm {3158}.

Histopathology
Lipid-rich carcinoma should be distinguished from other carcinomas with vacuolated, clear cytoplasm {702}. If histochemical methods are employed on frozen breast carcinomas, up to 75% contain cytoplasmic lipid droplets, but only 6% in large quantities {873}; only these cases should be designated lipid-rich carcinoma.

Histology shows a grade III invasive carcinoma in most cases. There may be associated in situ lobular or ductal carcinoma {28,2330}. The neoplastic cells have large, clear, foamy to vacuolated cytoplasm in which neutral lipids should be demonstrable {2876}. The tumour cells are devoid of mucins. Alpha lactalbumin and lactoferrin were found in five cases while fat globule membrane antigen was evident in occasional cells only {3158}.

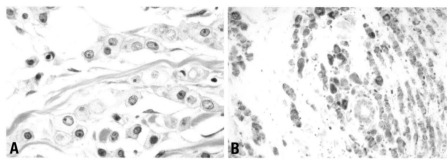

Fig. 1.51 Lipid rich carcinoma. **A** The cells have abundant eosinopohilic or microvacuolated cytoplasm with round nuclei displaying prominent nucleoli. **B** Oil red O stain shows abundant intracytoplasmic lipids within every cell.

Immunoprofile

There is limited data in hormone receptor expression but all tumours from one series were negative {3158}.

Ultrastructure

Well developed Golgi apparatus and lipid droplets of different sizes are recognized in the cytoplasm {1546}.

Prognosis and predictive factors

Despite the positive correlation of lipid content with high histological grade {873} and extensive lymph node metastases in 11 of 12 patients {2330}, at the present it is not possible to establish with certainty that lipid rich carcinomas are aggressive tumours. The reported series include very heterogeneous lesions and have very short follow up.

Secretory carcinoma

Definition

A rare, low grade carcinoma with a solid, microcystic (honeycomb) and tubular architecture, composed of cells that produce abundant intracellular and extracellular secretory (milk-like) material.

ICD-O code   8502/3

Synonym

Juvenile carcinoma.

Epidemiology

This is a rare tumour, with a frequency below 0.15% of all breast cancers {323,1579}. The tumour usually occurs in females, but has also been seen in males including a 3-year-old boy {1401}.
It occurs in children {1831} as well as adults {1519,2080}. A recent report {2430} disclosed 67 patients. Twenty-five

(37%) were aged less than 20 years, 21 (31%) older than 30 years and the remaining 21 in between. Therefore, the term secretory carcinoma is preferred {2080}. Mucoid carcinoma, invasive lobular carcinoma and signet ring cell carcinoma are "secretory" carcinomas "in sensu strictu", but are all well defined distinct entities and therefore it is preferred to restrict the use of the term secretory carcinoma to this rare tumour type {2080}.

Clinical features

The tumours manifest as indolent, mobile lumps, located near the areola in about half of the cases, this being especially so in men and children.

Macroscopy

SC usually presents as circumscribed nodules, greyish-white or yellow to tan in colour measuring from 0.5 to 12 cm. Larger tumours occur in older patients.

Histopathology

Microscopically SC is generally circumscribed, but areas of invasion of the adipose tissue are frequent. Sclerotic tissue in the centre of the lesion may be observed. The lesions are structurally composed of 3 patterns present in varying combinations:
1. A microcystic (honeycombed) pattern composed of small cysts often merge into larger spaces closely simulate thyroid follicles {2722},
2. A compact more solid, and
3. A tubular pattern consisting of numerous tubular spaces containing secretions {1519}.
The neoplastic cells have been subdivided into two types {2881} with all possible combinations. One has a large amount of pale staining granular cytoplasm, which on occasions can appear foamy. The nuclei are ovoid and have a small nucleolus. Intracytoplasmic lumina (ICL) are numerous and vary from small to "enormous" {1579}. Fusion of ICL generates the microcystic structures. The secretion located within the ICL or in the extracytoplasmic compartment is intensely eosinophilic and PAS positive after diastase digestion in most of the cases; Alcian blue positive material is also seen. The two types of mucosubstances are usually independently produced and a combination of the two

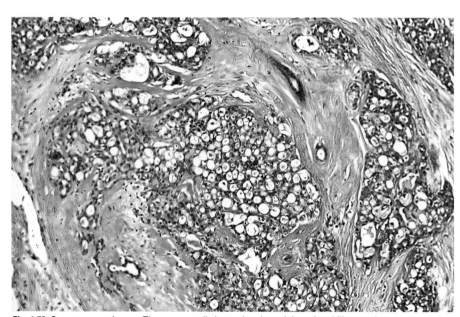

Fig. 1.52 Secretory carcinoma. The tumour cells have abundant pink eosinophilic cytoplasm.

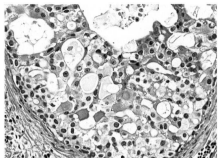

Fig. 1.53 Secretory carcinoma. The tumour cells have abundant pink eosinophilic cytoplasm.

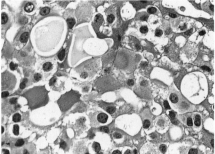

Fig. 1.54 Secretory carcinoma. Abundant secretory material is evident.

as seen in the "tagetoid pattern" of ICL described by Gad and Azzopardi {943} is rarely evident.

Mitoses and necrotic areas are rare. Ductal in situ carcinoma of either the secretory or low grade type may be present, either at the margins or within the tumour {2430}.

Immunoprofile

EMA, alpha lactalbumin and S-100 protein are frequently expressed in SC {323,1579,2430}. Estrogen receptors are mostly undetectable.

Prognosis and predictive factors

SC has an extremely favourable prognosis in children and adolescents but seems slightly more aggressive in older patients {2881}. Isolated recurrences in children are exceptional {52}, but the risk of nodal involvement is similar in young and older patients {2430}. Axillary lymph node metastases are found in approximately 15% of patients {2814} but metastases are confined to 4 lymph nodes at the most {52}.

Tumours less than 2 cm in size are unlikely to progress {2881}. Simple mastectomy, as opposed to excision of the tumour, has led to a cure, with the exception of the case reported by Meis {1860}. Recurrence of the tumour may appear after 20 years {1519}, and prolonged follow up is advocated. Fatal cases are the exception {1519,2881} and have never been reported in children.

Oncocytic carcinoma

Definition

A breast carcinoma composed of more than 70% oncocytic cells.

ICD-O code   8290/3

Historical annotation

Oncocyte (a Greek derived word) means "swollen cell", in this case due to an accumulation of mitochondria. The term oncocyte is used when mitochondria occupy 60% of the cytoplasm {990}. Oncocytic tumours can be seen in various organs and tissues {2271, 2405}.

In oncocytes, mitochondria are diffusely dispersed throughout the cytoplasm while in mitochondrion-rich cells they are grouped to one cell pole {2948}.

The proportion of oncocytes present within a tumour required to call it oncocytic has been arbitrarily proposed by various authors and varies from organ to organ. In a small series of breast oncocytic carcinomas, Damiani et al. {616}, using immunohistochemistry with an anti

mitochondrial antibody, found 70-90% of the neoplastic cells packed massively with immunoreactive granules.

Epidemiology

Only occasional cases have been described {566,616}. However, the incidence in the breast is probably underestimated as oncocytes are easily overlooked or misdiagnosed as apocrine elements {615}. All described patients have been over 60 years old. There is no predilection for site. One case occurred in a man {566}.

Macroscopy

The largest tumour measured 2.8 cm {616}.

Histopathology

The tumours are all similar with defined, circumscribed borders and vary from glandular to solid. The cells have abundant cytoplasm filled with small eosinophilic granules. Nuclei are monotonous and round to ovoid with a conspicuous nucleolus. Mitoses are not frequent. In situ carcinomas with a papillary appearance have been described {616}.

Differential diagnosis

Oncocytic carcinomas can be distinguished from apocrine, neuroendocrine carcinomas and oncocytic myoepithelial lesions {615,945,2013} by their immunophenotype.

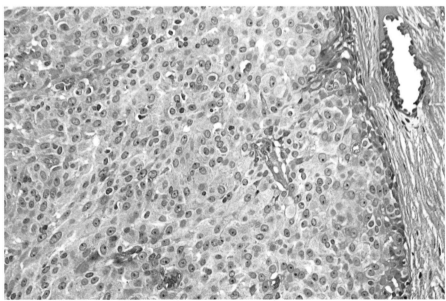

Fig. 1.55 Oncocytic carcinoma. Note well circumscribed nodule and cells with abundant eosinophilic cytoplasm.

Immunoprofile

Immunoprofile
The cases studied by Damiani et al. {616} showed diffuse and strong immunoreactivity with an anti mitochondrial antibody. Epithelial membrane antigen outlined the luminal borders of neoplastic glands when these were present. GCDFP-15 was absent in 3 cases and ER was observed in 90% of the cells in one {616}.

Prognosis and predictive factors

The follow up and number of reported cases is too small to allow meaningful discussion of prognosis.

Adenoid cystic carcinoma

Definition

A carcinoma of low aggressive potential, histologically similar to the salivary gland counterpart.

ICD-O code   8200/3

Synonyms

Carcinoma adenoides cysticum, adenocystic basal cell carcinoma, cylindromatous carcinoma.

Epidemiology

Adenoid cystic carcinoma (ACC) represent about 0.1% of breast carcinomas {149,1581}. It is important that stringent criteria are adopted to avoid misclassified lesions as found in about 50% of the cases recorded by the Connecticut Tumor Registry {2815}. The age distribution, is similar to that seen in infiltrating duct carcinomas in general {2419}.

Clinical features

The lesions are equally distributed between the two breasts and about 50% are found in the sub-periareolar region {149}. They may be painful or tender and unexpectedly cystic. A discrete nodule is the most common presentation.

Macroscopy

The size varies from 0.7 to 12 cm, with an average amongst most reported cases of 3 cm. Tumours are usually circumscribed, and microcysts are evident. They are pink, tan or grey in appearance {2309, 2419}.

Histopathology

ACC of the breast is very similar to that of the salivary gland, lung and cervix {1838}.

Three basic patterns are seen: trabecular-tubular, cribriform and solid. The 3 patterns have been used by Ro et al. {2381} to develop their grading system. The cribriform pattern is the most characteristic as the neoplastic areas are perforated by small apertures like a sieve. The "apertures" are of two types: The first, also referred to as pseudolumens {1406}, results from intratumoral invaginations of the stroma (stromal space). Accordingly, this type of space is of varying shape, mostly round, and contains myxoid acidic stromal mucosubstances which stain with Alcian blue {152} or straps of collagen with small capillaries. Sometimes the stromal spaces are filled by hyaline collagen and the smallest are constituted by small spherules or cylinders of hyaline material which has been shown ultrastructurally and immunohistochemically to be basal lamina {463}. With immunohistochemistry a rim of laminin and collagen IV positive material outlines the stromal spaces. The second type of space is more difficult to see as it is less numerous and usually composed of small lumina. These are genuine secre-

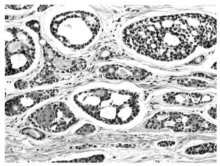

Fig. 1.56 Adenoid cystic carcinoma. The typical fenestrated nests composed of two cell types (dominant basaloid and few eosinophilic) are shown.

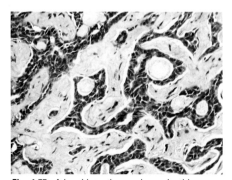

Fig. 1.57 Adenoid cystic carcioma. In this case, there is a predominant tubular architecture.

tory glandular structures (glandular space) which contain eosinophilic granular secretion of neutral mucosubstances, and are periodic acid-Schiff positive after diastase digestion {152}. The dual structural pattern reflects a dual cell component. The basaloid cell has scanty cytoplasm, a round to ovoid nucleus and one to two nucleoli {1581}. It constitutes the bulk of the lesion and also lines the cribriform stromal spaces. The second type of cell lines the true glandular lumina, and has eosinophilic cytoplasm and round nuclei similar to those of the basaloid cells. A third type of cell seen in 14% of cases by Tavassoli and Norris {2885} consists of sebaceous elements that can occasionally be numerous.

ACC contains a central core of neoplastic cells, surrounded by areas of invasion; ductal carcinoma in situ is absent at the periphery. The stroma varies from tissue very similar to that seen in the normal breast to desmoplastic, myxoid or even extensively adipose.

ACC has been seen in association with adenomyoepithelioma {2994} and low grade syringomatous (adenosquamous) carcinoma {2419} which suggests a close relationship among these combined epithelial and myoepithelial tumours.

Differential diagnosis
ACC must be distinguished from benign collagenous spherulosis {519} and from cribriform carcinoma, which more closely simulates ACC. Cribriform carcinoma is characterized by proliferation of one type of neoplastic cell only, and one type of mucosubstance. In addition, estrogen and progesterone receptors are abundant in cribriform carcinomas and absent from virtually all cases of ACC {2381}.

Immunoprofile and ultrastructure
The two main cell types are different at both ultrastructural and immunohistochemical levels.
Ultrastructurally, the basaloid cells have myoepithelial features particularly when located at the interstitial surface that lines the pseudoglandular spaces {3244}. They show thin cytoplasmic filaments with points of focal condensation {3094}. These cells have been shown to be positive for actomyosin {105} and similar to myoepithelial cells are posi-

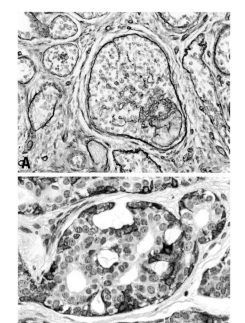

Fig. 1.58 Adenoid cystic carcinoma. Immunostain for laminin **(A)** decorates the basement membranes, while cytoplasmic immunoreaction with actin **(B)** unmasks the neoplastic myoepithelial cell component of the tumour.

tive for smooth muscle actin and calponin {902} as well as keratin 14. Nevertheless, most basaloid cells are nondescript elements showing at electron microscopy level few filaments and organelles without specific features {1507,2885}.

The cells that line the glandular lumina are cuboidal to spindle-shaped. When cuboidal, they have blunt microvilli along the luminal margins (secretory type). When spindle-shaped, they show abundant tonofilaments along with microvillous cytoplasmic processes such as to merit the design {2885}. Accordingly, the secretory type of cell

is keratin 7 positive, while the adenosquamous cell is both keratin 7 and 14 positive {902}. These cells can undergo squamous metaplasia as seen in two of the cases reported by Lamovec et al. {1581}. Squamous metaplasia is more common in breast ACC, but is virtually never seen in salivary gland ACC.

Prognosis and predictive factors
ACC is a low grade malignant tumour generally cured by simple mastectomy. Like its analogue in the salivary gland, it rarely spreads via the lymphatic stream. Local recurrence is related to incomplete excision, but patients have been reported to survive 16 years after the excision of the recurrence {2223}. Only two cases of axillary node metastases have been reported {2381,3094}. Distant metastases occur in about 10% of cases {544} and the lungs are frequently involved.

Acinic cell carcinoma

Definition
Acinic cell carcinoma (ACCA) is the breast counterpart of similar tumours that occur in the parotid gland and show acinic cell (serous) differentiation.

ICD-O code   8550/3

Epidemiology
ACCA is a rare tumour. Seven cases have been recorded {619,2561}. Other carcinomas showing serous secretion, probably related to ACCA, have also been reported {1287,1483}. It affects women between 35 and 80 years (mean 56 years) {619}.

Clinical features
ACCA presents as a palpable nodule ranging from 2 to 5 cm size. One case was discovered at mammography {619}.

Histopathology
The tumours show a combination of solid, microcystic and microglandular areas. One case {619} was mostly solid, and another {2404} had comedo-like areas with a peripheral rim of microglandular structures.

Cytologically, the cells have abundant, usually granular, amphophilic to eosinophilic cytoplasm. The granules may be coarse and, bright red, reminiscent of those in Paneth cells or amphophilic. However, clear "hypernephroid" cytoplasm is not unusual. The nuclei are irregular, round to ovoid, with a single nucleolus. The mitotic count varies and can be as high as 15 mitoses/10 high power fields {619}.

Immunoprofile
Most of the cells stain intensely with anti-amylase, lysozyme chymotrypsin, EMA and S-100 protein antisera {619}. GCDFP-15, the mucoapocrine marker, may also be focally positive.

Ultrastructure
Three cases published were composed of cells with cytoplasm filled by zymogen-like granules measuring from 0.08 to 0.9 μm {619,2404,2561}.

Prognosis and predictive factors
None of the 7 reported cases has died of the tumour, although follow up was limited (maximum 5 years). In two cases axillary lymph nodes contained metastases. Treatments varied from neoadjuvant chemotherapy with radical mastectomy to lumpectomy alone.

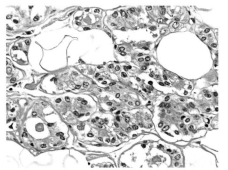

Fig. 1.59 Acinic cell carcinoma showing aggregates of cells with granular cytoplasm.

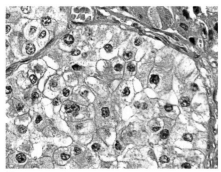

Fig. 1.60 Acinic cell carcinoma. Note the absence of nuclear atypia.

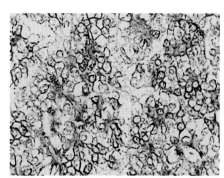

Fig. 1.61 Acinic cell carcinoma, immunostain is positive for lysozyme.

Glycogen–rich, clear cell carcinoma (GRCC)

Definition
A carcinoma in which more than 90% of the neoplastic cells have abundant clear cytoplasm containing glycogen.

ICD-O code   8315/3

Synonyms
Clear cell carcinoma   8310/3
Glycogen-rich carcinoma   8315/3

Epidemiology
The frequency is from 1-3% of breast carcinomas {880,1264}, with an age range of 41-78 years, median 57 years {2870}.

Clinical features
These tumours show similar presentation features to ductal NOS carcinoma.

Macroscopy
The clear cell glycogen-rich carcinoma does not differ grossly from that of usual invasive or intraductal carcinoma {1165}. The neoplasm ranges from 1 to 8 cm in size {2422,2754,2870}.

Histopathology
A strict definition for clear cell glycogen-rich is necessary for two reasons. Carcinomas in the breast with a clear cell appearance are uncommon and are due to an artefact produced by extraction of intracytoplasmic substances during tissue processing. However, as the substances that are extracted differ, they may be of different biological significance. In addition, intracytoplasmic glycogen has

been observed without significant clear cell in 58% of breast carcinoma {880}.
The lesions usually have the structural features of intraductal and infiltrating ductal neoplasms but rarely those of lobular, medullary or tubular types have been noted. GRCCs has either circumscribed or infiltrative borders {880,165, 2754,2870}.
The in situ component, either in the pure form or in association with most invasive cases has a compact solid, comedo or papillary growth pattern. The invasive tumour is generally composed of solid nests, rarely of tubular or papillary structures.
The tumour cells tend to have sharply defined borders and polygonal contours. The clear or finely granular cytoplasm contains PAS positive diastase labile glycogen. The nuclei are hyperchromatic, with clumped chromatin and prominent nucleoli.

Differential diagnosis
To differentiate this tumour from other clear cell tumours, including lipid rich carcinoma, histiocytoid carcinoma, adenomyoepithelioma, clear cell hidradenoma and metastatic clear cell carcinoma (particularly of renal origin), enzyme cytochemistry and immunohistochemistry are useful {702,1165,1549,2754}.

Immunoprofile
Hormone receptor status is similar to ductal NOS {880}.

Prognosis and predictive factors
Most reports suggest that GRCC is more aggressive than typical ductal carcinoma

{2313,2754}. The incidence of axillary lymph node invasion is significantly higher than in the other non-GRCC forms {1264}. The histologic grade is intermediate to high with a paucity of grade I tumours {1165}.
Although follow up studies confirm that disease free and overall survival is significantly worse in GRCC, due to the low incidence, there are no multiparametric analyses to compare GRCC stage by stage with the other histological types of breast carcinoma.

Sebaceous carcinoma

Definition
A primary breast carcinoma of the skin adnexal type with sebaceous differentiation. There should be no evidence of derivation from cuteneous adnexal sebaceous glands.

ICD-O code   8410/3

Epidemiology
Only 4 examples of this rare mammary tumour have been observed {2876}. The women, three of whom were white, were aged 45-62 years {2876,3006}.

Clinical features
All the patients presented with a palpable mass.

Macroscopy
The tumours range in size from 7.5-20 cm. The margins are sharply delineated, and the cut surface is solid and bright yellow.

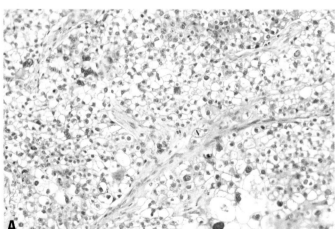
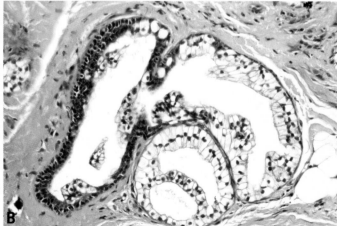

Fig. 1.62 Glycogen-rich carcinoma. **A** Cells with abundant clear cytoplasm and relatively uniform round nuclei grow in a solid pattern supported by branching vessels. **B** Note transition from typical ductal epithelial cells to clear cells in a duct adjacent to the invasive carcinoma.

Table 1.09
Glycogen-rich (GRCC) and non glycogen-rich clear cell tumours of the breast.

	GRCC	Lipid rich carcinoma	Histiocytoid lobular carcinoma	Apocrine carcinoma	Hidradenoma	Secretory carcinoma	Adenomyo-epithelioma	Metastatic clear cell carcinoma from the kidney
Cell type	One	One	One	One	Two	One	Two	One
Cytoplasm	Empty	Foamy	Foamy	Foamy	Empty	Foamy/empty/granular		Empty
Nuclei	High grade	High grade	Low grade	Low grade	Low grade	Low grade	Low grade	Low grade
PAS	+	-	-	+	+	+	+	+
PAS diastase	-	-	-	+	+	-	+/-	-
Mucicarmine	-	-	+	+	-	+	-	-
Oil red-O	-	+	-	-	-	-	-	-
Smooth actin	-	-	-	-	-	-	+	- Vimentin +
S100	-	-	-	-	+	+	+	-
GCDFP-15	+/-	-	+	+	-	-	+ (apocrine)	-

Histopathology

The tumour is characterized by a lobulated or nested proliferation of a varying admixture of sebaceous cells with abundant finely vacuolated cytoplasm surrounded by smaller ovoid to spindle cells with a small amount of eosinophilic cytoplasm and without any vacuolization. The nuclei in both cell types are irregularly shaped to rounded, vesicular with 0 to 2 nucleoli. Mitotic figures are sparse, but may be focally abundant. Focal squamous morules may be present focally. Sebocrine cells with features of both apocrine and sebaceous cells and noted in a variety of apocrine lesions have not been a notable feature of sebaceous carcinomas.

Immunoprofile

The tumour cells stain positively with pancytokeratin (AE1/AE3/LP34). In the three cases assessed, immunostains for progesterone receptor (PR) were positive in all, two were estrogen receptor (ER) positive, and one was ER negative.

Differential diagnosis

Apocrine carcinoma with a large population of sebocrine cells and lipid rich carcinomas enter the differential diagnosis. The former invariably has typical apocrine cells admixed and the latter forms cords and irregular cell clusters with a more subtle vacuolization of the cells.

Neither has the smaller second cell population or the squamous metaplasia that may be present in sebaceous carcinoma.

Prognosis and predictive factors

Not much is known about the behaviour of these tumours. The 7.5 cm tumour was treated by radical mastectomy, but none of the 20 axillary nodes was positive {2876}. Another recently reported case was associated with extensive metastases with sebaceous differentiation evident at the distant sites {3006}.

Inflammatory carcinoma

Definition

A particular form of mammary carcinoma with a distinct clinical presentation {1607} believed to be due to lymphatic obstruction from an underlying invasive adenocarcinoma; the vast majority of cases have a prominent dermal lymphatic infiltration by tumour. Inflammatory carcinoma is a form of advanced breast carcinoma classified as T4d {51, 2976}. Dermal lymphatic invasion without the character-

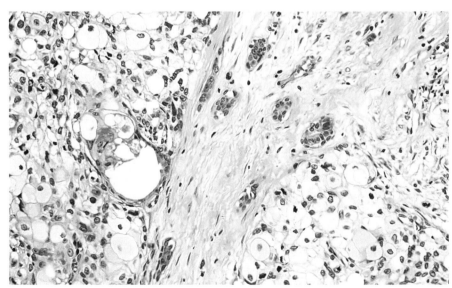

Fig. 1.63 Sebaceous carcinoma. The cells have abundant finely vacuolated cytoplasm and form rounded aggregates with a few amphophilic cells present in the periphery.

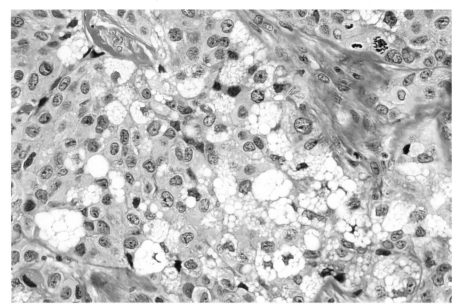

Fig. 1.64 Sebaceous carcinoma. Cells with moderate amounts of eosinophilic or abundant microvacuolated cytoplasm and variably compressed nuclei resembling lipoblasts are admixed.

istic clinical picture is insufficient to qualify as inflammatory carcinoma.

ICD-O code   8530/3

Epidemiology
The age distribution is similar to ductal NOS carcinoma and breast carcinoma in general {1095,2384}. There is no recognized specific association with younger age and pregnancy but the phenomenon of peritumoural lymphatic vascular invasion is found more frequently in younger women {1095,2795}. The reported frequency of an inflammatory presentation of primary breast carcinoma varies between 1 and 10%, being influenced by the diagnostic criteria (clinical or pathological) and the nature of the reporting centre (local population clinical centre versus tertiary referral centre) {769,1641,2517}.

Clinical features
The clinical findings include diffuse erythema, oedema, peau d'orange, tenderness, induration, warmth, enlargement and in some cases a palpable ill defined mass. The diagnosis is based on clinical features and should be confirmed by biopsy. Dermal lymphatic tumour emboli are not always found in small diagnostic skin biopsy samples {724,2384}.

Histopathology
Despite the name, inflammatory carcinoma is not associated with any significant degree of inflammatory cell infiltration and is not an inflammatory condition. The cutaneous signs are produced as a consequence of lymphatic obstruction and consequent oedema, which produce signs mimicking an inflammatory process. Inflammatory signs can be the primary clinical presenting abnormality (primary inflammatory carcinoma) or develop as a consequence of tumour recurrence (secondary inflammatory carcinoma).

Histologically the underlying invasive carcinoma is not regarded as having specific histological features, the majority of tumours have ductal NOS and are of grade 3 morphology {1708,1851}. These tumours often have an associated lymphoid infiltrate usually of mature lymphocytes and plasma cells, a low frequency of estrogen receptor positivity {445,1490} and ERBB2 overexpression {1074}. The skin often shows co-existing features associated with lymphatic obstruction including separation of collagen fibres with broadening of the reticular dermal layer due to oedema. Involved dermal lymphatics may have an associated lymphoplasmacytic infiltrate {2427}. Secondary or recurrent inflammatory carcinoma has been shown to be associated more with ductal NOS and apocrine histological types of breast carcinoma and is rare following presentation with other types, papillary, medullary and mucinous {2384}. The skin may also show stromal metastatic deposits of tumour particularly in secondary or recurrent inflammatory carcinoma.

Differential diagnosis
There may be a discrepancy between clinical presentation with inflammatory features and presence of dermal lymphatic emboli. Dermal vascular emboli may not be present in a biopsy taken from erythematous or oedematous area, or may be present in skin beyond the clinical skin changes. The skin biopsy will usually also show dermal lymphatic dilatation. The clinical features of inflammatory carcinoma are generally regarded as specific but underlyng true inflammatory conditions should be excluded if histological confirmation is not achieved.

Prognosis and predictive factors
Prior to the introduction of systemic therapy the prognosis of inflammatory carcinoma even when treated by mastectomy, was very poor with 5 year survival under 5% {1052,2384}. Use of systemic chemotherapy has produced an improvement in survival figures reported as 25 to 50% at 5 years {406,828,1805, 1907,2154}. In cases treated with neoadjuvant chemotherapy or radiotherapy, residual tumour, including intravascular emboli, are usually present in the mastectomy specimen even when a clinical response has been observed {2427}. Mastectomy and radiotherapy are considered beneficial for initial local control and palliation of symptoms {406,582, 2243}. There are no consistent findings with respect to influence of additional clinical features such as presence of a clinical mass or findings in skin biopsy on survival. However, response to chemotherapy and radiotherapy, and pathological response have been shown to be associated with improved disease free survival {473,828,841,1826}.

Bilateral breast carcinoma

Definition
A synchronous breast cancer is one detected within two months of the initial primary tumour.

Approximately 5-10% of women treated for breast cancer will have either synchronous bilateral cancers or will develop a subsequent contralateral breast cancer (CBC) {448,872,1219,1491, 2383}. The prevalence of synchronous bilateral breast cancer is approximately 1% of all breast cancers {448,648,872, 1491,1936}. An increase in the detection of synchronous cancers has been reported following the introduction of bilateral mammography for the investigation of symptomatic breast disease and for population based breast screening {751,872,1491,1492}.

It is well recognized that a previous history of breast cancer increases the risk of subsequent breast cancer in the contralateral breast. The reported annual hazard rates of between 0.5-1% per year {448,872,1491,2383,2798} appear relatively constant up to 15 years {1491} giving a cumulative incidence rate for survivors of around 5% at 10 years and 10% at 15 years.

Family history {253,448,1219} and early age of onset {35,1168,2798} have been reported to increase the risk of CBC development in some studies but others have found no such associations with either early age of onset {252,253,872} or family history {35,872}. One study has reported that family history, early age of onset and lobular histology are independent predictors of metachronous contralateral breast cancer development {1492}.

These characteristics suggest a possible genetic predisposition. Women with a strong family history who develop breast cancer at an early age are at considerable risk of contralateral breast cancer as a first event of recurrence particularly if the first primary is of lobular histology or is of favourable prognostic type {1491, 1492}.

Patients with metachronous CBC are younger at the age of onset of the original primary. Many, but not all, series report that a higher percentage of the tumours are of lobular type {35,252,872, 1219,1241,1492,2383}. This observation does not imply that tumours of lobular type, in isolation from other risk factors such as young age and family history, should be considered to have a higher risk of bilateral breast involvement {1491}. A greater frequency of multicentricity in one or both breast tumours has also been reported {355}. There does not appear to be any association with histological grade, other tumour types or the stage of the disease {355,1491,1492}.

Prognosis and predictive features

Theoretically women with synchronous CBC have a higher tumour burden than women with unilateral disease which may jeopardize their survival prospects {1035}. Indeed, synchronous CBC

appears to have a worse prognosis than unilateral cohorts or women with metachronous CBC {164,1092,1233}. Others have failed to demonstrate any survival difference between women with unilateral and those with synchronous CBC {911,1053,2555}.

Tumour spread and staging

Tumour spread

Breast cancer may spread via lymphatic and haematogenous routes and by direct extension to adjacent structures. Spread via the lymphatic route is most frequently to the ipsilateral axillary lymph nodes, but spread to internal mammary nodes and to other regional nodal groups may also occur. Although breast cancer may metastasize to any site, the most common are bone, lung, and liver. Unusual sites of metastasis (e.g. peritoneal surfaces, retroperitoneum, gastrointestinal tract, and reproductive organs) and unusual presentations of metastatic disease are more often seen with invasive lobular carcinomas than with other histological types {319,704,1142,1578}.

Several models have been proposed to explain the spread of breast cancer. The Halsted model, assumes a spread from the breast to regional lymph nodes and from there to distant sites. This hypothesis provided the rationale for radical en bloc resection of the breast and regional lymph nodes. Others suggest a systemic disease from inception, which implies that survival is unaffected by local treatment. However, clinical behaviour suggests that metastases occur as a function of tumour growth and progression {1181}. This concept is supported by the results of axillary sentinel lymph nodes, which show that metastatic axillary lymph node involvement is a progressive process.

Tumour staging

Both clinical and pathological staging is used in breast carcinoma. Clinical staging is based on information gathered prior to first definitive treatment, including data derived from physical examination, imaging studies, biopsy, surgical exploration, and other relevant findings. Pathological staging is based on data used for clinical staging supplemented or modified by evidence obtained during surgery, particularly from the pathologi-

cal examination of the resected primary tumour, regional lymph nodes, and/or more distant metastases, when relevant. The staging system currently in most widespread use is the TNM Classification {51,2976}. The most recent edition is provided at the beginning of this chapter. The pathological tumour status ("pT") is a measurement only of the invasive component. The extent of the associated intraductal component should not be taken into consideration. In cases of microinvasive carcinoma (T1mic) in which multiple foci of microinvasion are present, multiplicity should be noted but the size of only the largest focus is used, i.e. the size of the individual foci should not be added together. The pathological node status ("pN") is based on information derived from histological examination of routine haematoxylin and eosin-stained sections. Cases with only isolated tumour cells are classified as pN0 (see relevant footnote in the TNM Table which also indicates how to designate sentinel lymph node findings). A sub-classification of isolated tumour cells is provided in TNM publications {51,1195, 2976}.

Measurement of tumour size

The microscopic invasive tumour size (I) is used for TNM Classification (pT). The dominant (largest) invasive tumour focus is measured, except in multifocal tumours where no such large single focus is apparent. In these cases the whole tumour size (w) is used.

Somatic genetics of invasive breast cancer

As in other organ sites, it has become evident that breast cancers develop through a sequential accumulation of genetic alterations, including activation of oncogenes (e.g. by gene amplification), and inactivation of tumour suppressor genes, e.g. by gene mutations and deletions.

Cytogenetics

As yet no karyotypic hallmarks of breast cancer have been identified, such as the t(8;14) in chronic myelogenous leukaemia (CML), or the i(12p) in testicular cancer. There is not even a cytogenetic marker for any of the histological subtypes of breast cancer. One reason for this is certainly the technical difficulty of obtaining sufficient numbers of good quality metaphase spreads from an individual tumour. However, it may also relate to the genetic complexity of this tumour. Nonetheless, several hundred primary tumours have been karyotyped to date, allowing some general patterns to be discerned {1879}. An increased modal chromosome number is the most conspicuous characteristic in many tumours, in keeping with the finding that approximately two-thirds of all breast cancers have a hyperploid DNA-content in flow-cytometric analysis. Unbalanced translocations are most often seen as recurrent changes, with the i(1)(q10) and the der(1;16)(q10;p10) the most prominent. For the latter, it is not clear whether loss of 16q or gain of 1q is the selective change, or whether both are. Other conspicuous changes are i(8)(q10), and subchromosomal deletions on chromosomes 1 (bands p13, p22, q12, q42), 3 (p12-p14), and 6 (q21). No specific genes have been associated with any of these changes.

DNA amplification

Classic cytogenetic analysis had already indicated that double minute chromosomes and homogeneously staining regions, are a frequent occurrence in breast cancer. These regions were later shown to contain amplified oncogenes (see below). Comparative genomic hybridization (CGH) has identified over 20 chromosomal subregions with increased DNA-sequence copy-number, including 1q31-q32, 8q24, 11q13, 16p13, 17q12, 17q22-q24 and 20q13. For many of these regions, the critically amplified genes are not precisely known. Chromosomal regions with increased copy-number often span tens of megabases, suggesting the involvement of more than one gene. Loss of chromosomal material is also detected by CGH, and this pattern is largely, though not completely, in agreement with loss of heterozygosity data (see below).

Oncogenes

A number of known oncogenes were initially found to be amplified in subsets of breast cancer by Southern blot analyses and fluorescent in situ hybridization. Subsequently, a number of genes have been identified as critical targets for DNA amplifications by a combination of CGH and gene expression analysis. Oncogenic activation by point-mutation seems to be rare in breast tumours. Listed by chromosome region, the following (onco)gene amplifications seem to be involved in the progression of breast cancer.

1p13-21: *DAM1* has been found amplified in two breast cancer cell lines, but it is not certain whether this gene is driving the amplification {1962}.

7p13: The epidermal growth factor receptor gene (*EGFR*), encoding a cell membrane localized growth factor receptor, is amplified in less than 3% of breast carcinomas.

8p12: The fibroblast growth factor receptor 1 gene (*FGFR1*; formerly called *FLG*) encoding a cell membrane located receptor for fibroblast growth factor, is amplified in approximately 10% of breast carcinomas {41}.

8q24: *MYC* encodes a nuclear protein involved in regulation of growth and apoptosis. *MYC* amplification is found in approximately 20% of breast {250,596}. The MYC protein has a very short half-life, precluding the assessment of protein

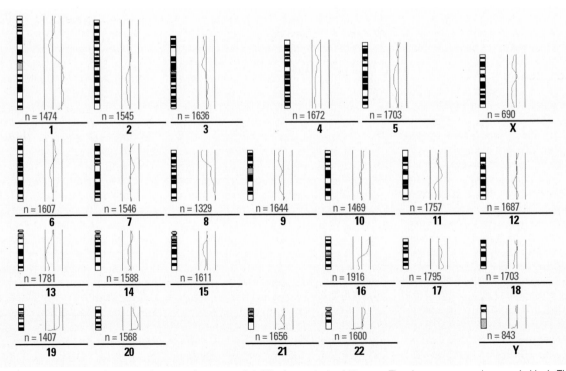

Fig. 1.65 Invasive ductal carcinoma. Summary of comparative genome hybridization analysis of 80 cases. The chromosome numbers are in black. The red curves depict the average ratio profiles between tumour-derived and normal-derived fluorescence signals. Of the three lines to the right of each chromosome, the middle represents a ratio of 1.0; deviations of the curve to the left or right indicate loss or gain of chromosomal material, respectively. Average ratios were computed from "n" single chromosomes from different metaphases. Data were retrieved from the Online CGH Tumour Database (http://amba.charite.de/~ksch/cghdatabase/index.htm). For details on methodology see F. Richard et al. {2366}.

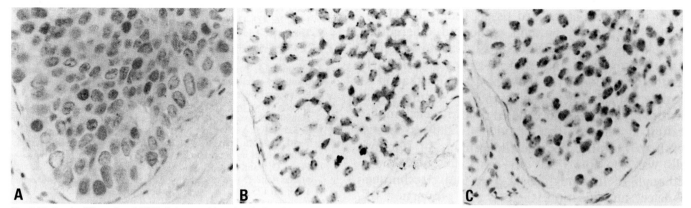

Fig. 1.66 Poorly differentiated DCIS. **A** Immunohistochemical staining and bright field in situ hybridization (BRISH) of cyclin D1 in the same case of DCIS. Strong staining of poorly differentiated DCIS. **B** Immunohistochemical staining and BRISH of cyclin D1 in the same case of DCIS. BRISH with a chromosome 11-specific (peri)centromeric probe. **C** BRISH with the cyclin D1 specific cosmid. Immunohistochemical staining and BRISH of cyclin D1 in the same case of DCIS. BRISH with the cyclin D1 specific cosmid. Reprinted with permission from C.B. Vos et al. {3035}.

overexpression as a substitute for the analysis of gene amplification. Amplification of subregions of 8q can be complex. There appears to be at least one additional oncogene mapping to chromosome 8q12-22, which has not been identified yet.

10q26: The fibroblast growth factor receptor 2 (*FGFR2*; formerly: *BEK*) gene encodes a cell membrane located receptor for fibroblast growth factor. This gene is amplified in approximately 12% of breast carcinomas {41}.

11q13: Amplification of the cyclin D1 gene (*CCND1*), encoding a nuclear protein involved in cell cycle regulation, has been found in 15-20% of breast tumours, in association with estrogen receptor positivity. Cyclin D1 can also bind to the estrogen receptor, resulting in ligand-independent activation of the receptor {3273}. Immunohistochemically, cyclin D1 appears to be overexpressed in 80% of invasive lobular carcinomas, but is not always accompanied by *CCND1* gene amplification {2133}.

17q12: The human epidermal growth factor receptor-2 (*ERBB2*) proto-oncogene (also known as *HER2*, and equivalent to the rodent neu gene) encodes a 185-kD transmembrane glycoprotein with intrinsic tyrosine kinase activity. A ligand for ERBB2 has not been identified but it is hypothesized that ERBB2 amplifies the signal provided by other receptors of this family by heterodimerizing with them. Ligand-dependent activation of ERBB1, ERBB3, and ERBB4 by EGF or heregulin results in heterodimerization and, thereby, ERBB2 activation. *ERBB2* amplification results in overexpression of

ERBB2 protein, but not all tumours with overexpression have amplified 17q12. Overexpression is found in approximately 20-30% of human breast carcinomas {2962}. In breast cancers with normal *ERBB2* copy number, expression of ERBB2 may be variable but is very rarely as high as that in tumours with *ERBB2* amplification (usually 10-fold to 100-fold higher and equivalent to millions of monomers). Numerous studies have investigated the relationship between *ERBB2* status and clinicopathological characteristics in breast cancer {2962}.

17q22-q24: At least three genes (*RPS6KB1*, *PAT1*, and *TBX2*) have been found to be co-amplified and overexpressed in ~10% of breast cancers {181}. Further analysis identified *RPS6KB1*, *MUL*, *APPBP2*, *TRAP240* and one unknown gene to be consistently overexpressed in two commonly amplified subregions {1896}. The ribosomal protein S6 kinase (RPS6KB1) is a serine-threonine kinase whose activation is thought to regulate a wide array of cellular processes involved in the mitogenic response including protein synthesis, translation of specific mRNA species, and cell cycle progression from G1 to S phase.

20q13: It is presently unknown whether the *CSE1L/CAS* gene, the *NCOA3* gene or any other gene in this region serves as the target for the amplification, which is found in approximately 15% of breast carcinomas. Three independent regions of amplification have been identified and their co-amplification is common. Cellular apoptosis susceptibility (CAS) encodes a protein, which may have a function in the control of apoptosis and

cell proliferation {346}. *NCOA3* gene encodes a co-activator of the estrogen receptor {109}, and its amplification has been found to be associated with estrogen receptor positivity. High resolution mapping of the amplified domains has suggested that a putative oncogene, *ZNF217*, and *CYP24* (encoding vitamin D 24 hydroxylase), whose overexpression is likely to lead to abrogation of growth control mediated by vitamin D, may be targets for the amplification {60}.

The *STK15* gene (also known as BTAK and Aurora-A) is amplified in approximately 12% of primary breast tumours, as well as in breast, ovarian, colon, prostate, neuroblastoma, and cervical cancer cell lines {3259}. *STK15* encodes a centrosome-associated serine-threonine kinase, and may also be overexpressed in tumours without amplification of 20q13 {1885}. Centrosomes appear to maintain genomic stability through the establishment of bipolar spindles during cell division, ensuring equal segregation of replicated chromosomes to daughter cells. Deregulated duplication and distribution of centrosomes are implicated in chromosome segregation abnormalities, leading to aneuploidy seen in many cancer cell types. Elevated *STK15* expression induces centrosome amplification and overrides the checkpoint mechanism that monitors mitotic spindle assembly, leading to chromosomal instability {83,1885,3259}.

Loss of heterozygosity (LOH)

Loss of heterozygosity (LOH) has been found to affect all chromosome arms

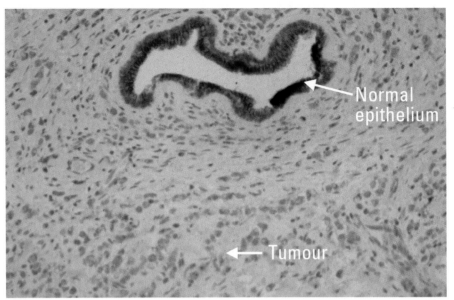

Fig. 1.67 Lobular carcinoma of breast. Immunohistochemical staining of a lobular breast carcinoma with a mutated *CDH1* gene. Normal duct epithelium shows positive staining for membrane associated E-cadherin, which is lacking in tumour cells.

in breast cancer to varying degrees {265,680}. Unfortunately, collation of LOH data into a coherent map has been complicated enormously by the use of different terminology and technology in this area {679}. A tumour specific loss of an allele, but also an imbalance in allele intensities (allelic imbalance) are both called LOH. LOH is often equated with 'deletion' although it may also be caused by somatic recombination. Complete loss of an allele can only be reliably and unequivocally measured in tumour DNA samples with very low levels of contamination from non-malignant cells (i.e. <25%). Without microdissection or flow sorting of tumour cells, this cannot be obtained from many primary breast cancer tissues. In addition, allelic imbalance can also be caused by chromosomal aneuploidy (trisomies etc), or low-copy amplification of certain chromosome regions, which is fundamentally different from 'classical' LOH. These factors impede meta-analysis of published allelic imbalance/LOH data in breast cancer, although it is clear that there are chromosome arms where LOH occurs at very high rates.

LOH is interpreted in the light of Knudson's two-hit model for the inactivation of a tumour suppressor gene {679}. Numerous studies have attempted to map common regions of LOH on chromosome arms with frequent LOH. Such a region could flag the position of

a tumour suppressor gene more accurately, aiding its identification.

Tumour suppressor genes

Several chromosome regions showing frequent LOH have been extensively investigated because of the presence of appealing candidate tumour suppressor genes. Many of these regions are supported by CGH and cytogenetic analyses. They include 1p32-36, 3p14-21, 6q25, 7q31, 8p12-21, 9p21, 13q12-q14, 16q22, 16q24, 17p13, 18q21. Several interesting candidate tumour suppressor genes lie in these regions (for example, *FANCA* in 16q24, *HIC1* in 17p13, *PDGFRL* in 8p21, *FHIT* in 3p14, *CDKN2A* in 9p21, *TP73* in 1p36), but their role in breast cancer remains to be established.

By definition, a tumour suppressor gene is a gene whose normal function inhibits the initiation or progression of tumour growth. This can be demonstrated by cell biological, biochemical or genetic evidence, which are not always in full agreement. For example, transfection of the retinoblastoma gene *RB1* into some breast cancer cell lines reverts their tumourigenic phenotype in vitro, yet no inactivating *RB1* mutations have been reported in primary breast tumours. *RASSF1A* is located in the region 3p21, which is frequently deleted in breast cancer. It might serve as a Ras effector, mediating the apoptotic effects of onco-

genic RAS {621}. In breast tumour cell lines, the promoter of *RASSF1A* is highly methylated and its expression is down-regulated {622}. In primary tumours, the proportion with promotor-hypermethylation is lower, and so is the effect on expression down-regulation {42}. No inactivating mutations in the coding regions have been detected, and the relationship between LOH and promotor-methylation status is presently unclear {1368}. To avoid these difficulties in interpreting the available data, we shall restrict ourselves here to those genes for which acquired inactivating mutations in the coding region have been demonstrated in a proportion of primary breast cancers or breast cancer cell lines. Using these criteria, very few tumour suppressor genes have been identified in breast cancer. Listed by chromosomal site, they are:

6q26: *IGF2R*. The *M6P/IGF2R* gene, encoding the insulin-like growth factor II (IGF-II)/mannose 6-phosphate receptor, is frequently inactivated during carcinogenesis. IGF2R is postulated to be a tumour suppressor due to its ability to bind and degrade the mitogen IGF-II, promote activation of the growth inhibitor TGFβ, and regulate the targeting of lysosomal enzymes. Several missense mutations in *M6P/IGF2R* disrupt the ligand binding functions of the intact IGF2R. Missense mutations have been found in about 6% of primary breast tumours {1125}.

7q31: *ST7* (for suppression of tumourigenicity 7) is a gene with unknown cellular function. Transfection of *ST7* into the prostate-cancer-derived cell line PC3, abrogated its tumourigenicity in vivo. Three breast tumour cell lines harboured frame shifting mutations in *ST7*, which was accompanied by LOH in at least one of them. A role of *ST7* in primary breast cancer has been questioned {358,2912}.

8q11: *RB1CC1*. The RB1CC1 protein is a key regulator of the tumour suppressor gene *RB1*. It is localized in the nucleus and has been proposed to be a transcription factor because of its leucine zipper motif and coiled-coil structure. Seven of 35 (20%) primary breast cancers examined contained mutations in *RB1CC1*, including 9 large interstitial deletions predicted to yield markedly truncated RB1CC1 proteins {440}. In all 7 cases, both *RB1CC1* alleles were inactivated, and in each case both mutations were acquired somatically.

16q22: *CDH1.* The cell-cell adhesion molecule E-cadherin acts as a strong invasion suppressor in experimental tumour cell systems. Frequent inactivating mutations have been identified in *CDH1* in over 60% of infiltrating lobular breast cancers, but not in ductal carcinomas {261}. Most mutations cause translational frame shifting, and are predicted to yield secreted truncated E-cadherin fragments. Most mutations occur in combination with LOH, so that no E-cadherin expression is detectable immunohistochemically. This offers a molecular explanation for the typical scattered tumour cell growth in infiltrative lobular breast cancer. Lobular carcinoma in situ (LCIS) has also been found to contain *CDH1* mutations {3034}.

17p13: *TP53* encodes a nuclear protein of 53 kD, which binds to DNA as a tetramer and is involved in the regulation of transcription and DNA replication. Normal p53 may induce cell cycle arrest or apoptosis, depending on the cellular environment {3147}. Mutations, which inactivate or alter either one of these functions, are found in approximately 20% of breast carcinomas {2237}. Most of these are missense changes in the DNA-binding domain of the protein; a small proportion (~20%) are frame shifting. The large majority of these mutations are accompanied by loss of the wildtype allele (LOH). Missense mutations in *TP53* can be detected immunohistochemically because mutated p53 fails to activate expression of MDM2. The MDM2 protein normally targets p53 for ubiquitin-mediated degradation, constituting a feedback loop to maintain low levels of p53 protein in the cell.

Microsatellite instability

Microsatellite instability (MSI) is a genetic defect caused by mutations in mismatch repair genes (*MLH1*, *MSH2*, *MSH6*, *PMS1*, and *PMS2*), reflected by the presence of multiple alleles at loci consisting of small tandem repeats or mononucleotide runs. MSI in breast cancer is negligible, with the possible exception of breast cancer arising in the context of the HNPCC inherited colon cancer syndrome. The most convincing study is probably that of Anbazhagan et al., who have analysed 267 breast carcinomas at 104 microsatellite loci {85}; not one single case of MSI was detected. Somatic mutations in the mismatch repair

genes have not yet been detected in breast cancer.

Gene expression patterns

Expression profiling is expression-analysis of thousands of genes simultaneously using microarrays {69,1072,1171, 2218,2756,3104}. Tumours show great multidimensional variation in gene expression, with many different sets of genes showing independent patterns of variation. These sets of genes relate to biological processes such as proliferation or cell signalling. Despite this variation, there are also striking similarities between tumours, providing new opportunities for tumour classification. ER-positive and ER-negative cancers show distinct expression profiles {1072,2986, 3104}. Breast cancers arising in women carrying a *BRCA1* mutation could be distinguished from sporadic cases, and from those that developed in *BRCA2* carriers {1171,2986}. Although this field is still in its infancy, 5 distinct gene expression patterns were discerned among 115 tumours {2218,2756,2757}, one basal-like, one ERBB2-overexpressing, two luminal-like, and one normal breast tissue-like subgroup. Approximately 25% of the tumours did not fit any of these classifications. The luminal-like tumours express keratins 8 and 18, and show

strong expression of the estrogen receptor cluster of genes. The tumours of the other groups were mainly ER-negative. The basal-like group is characterized by high expression of keratins 5/6 and 17 and laminin. The ERBB2-group also expresses several other genes in the ERBB2 amplicon, such as GRB7. The normal breast-like group shows a high expression of genes characteristic of adipose tissue and other non-epithelial cell types. Cluster analyses of 2 published, independent data sets representing different patient cohorts from different laboratories, uncovered the same breast cancer subtypes {2757}.

Somatic genetics of breast cancer metastases

According to the present view, metastasis marks the end in a sequence of genomic changes underlying the progression of an epithelial cell to a lethal cancer. Not surprisingly, therefore, lymph node metastases and distant metastases in general contain more genomic aberrations than their cognate primary tumours {1117,2028}. Flow cytometric DNA content measurements have demonstrated extensive DNA ploidy heterogeneity in primary breast carcinomas, with the concurrent presence of diploid and multiple aneuploid DNA stemlines. Identical het-

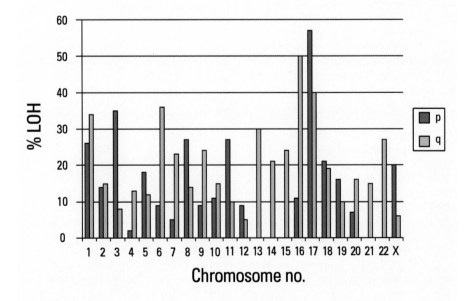

Fig. 1.68 Allelotyping of breast cancer. The percentage LOH is calculated as the ratio between the number of tumours with loss of an allele at a given chromosome arm and the total number of cases informative (i.e. heterozygous) for the analysis. Red bars: p-arm; green bars: q-arm.

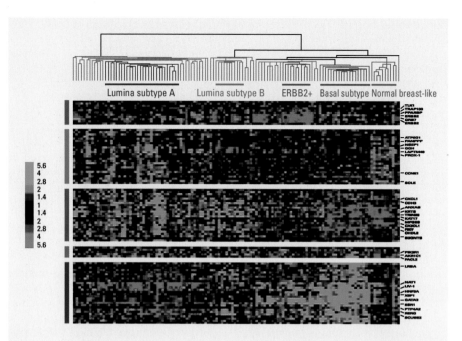

Fig. 1.69 Hierarchical clustering of 115 tumour tissues and 7 nonmalignant tissues using gene expression profiling. Experimental dendrogram showing the clustering of the tumours into five subgroups (top panel). Gene clusters associated with the ERBB2 oncogene, luminal subtype B, basal subtype, normal breast-like group, luminal subtype A with high estrogen receptor expression. Scale bar represents fold change for any given gene relative to the median level of expression across all samples. From T. Sorlie et al. {2757}.

erogeneity is often present in their cognate lymph node metastases, suggesting that the generation of DNA ploidy diversity has taken place prior to metastasis {197}. LOH analysis of these DNA ploidy stemlines showed that all allelic imbalances observed in the diploid clones recurred in the cognate aneuploid clones, but were, in the latter, accompanied by additional allelic imbalances at other loci and/or chromosome arms {313}. This indicates that the majority of allelic imbalances in breast carcinomas are established during generation of DNA ploidy diversity. Identical allelic imbalances in both the diploid and aneuploid clones of a tumour suggests linear tumour progression. But the simultaneous presence of early diploid and advanced aneuploid clones in both primary and metastatic tumour sites suggested that acquisition of metastatic propensity can be an early event in the genetic progression of breast cancer. Intriguingly, single disseminated cancer cells have been detected in the bone marrow of 36% of breast cancer patients {339}. Using single-cell CGH, it was demonstrated that disseminated cells from patients without a clinically detectable distant metastasis displayed significantly fewer chromosomal aberrations than primary tumours or cells from patients with manifest metastasis, and their aberrations appeared to be randomly generated {2560}. In contrast, primary tumours and disseminated cancer cells from patients with manifest metastasis harboured different and characteristic chromosomal imbalances. Thus, contrary to the widely held view that the precursors of metastasis are derived from the most advanced clone within the primary tumour, these data suggest that breast tumour cells may disseminate in a far less progressed genomic state than previously thought, and that they acquire genomic aberrations typical of metastatic cells thereafter. These findings have two major clinical implications. First, all adjuvant therapies that do not target genetic or epigenetic events occurring early during tumourigenesis are unlikely to eradicate minimal residual disease, because disseminated cancer cells may not uniformly share mutations that are acquired later on. Second, because disseminated cells progress independently from the primary tumour, a simple extrapolation from primary tumour data to disseminated cancer cells is impossible.

Genetic susceptibility: familial risk of breast cancer

Introduction

Breast cancer has been recognized for over 100 years as having a familial component {349}. Epidemiological investigations have attempted to quantify the risks associated with a positive family history and to examine whether the pattern of related individuals is consistent with the effects of a single gene of large effect, shared environmental effects, many genes acting in an additive manner, or most likely, a combination of two or more of these. In addition a number of specific genes have been identified as playing a role. The most important ones are *BRCA1* and *BRCA2* which are discussed in Chapter 8. However, these two genes account for only about a fifth of overall familial breast cancer {107,592,2230} and explain less than half of all high risk, site-specific breast cancer families {898, 2631}.

Familial risk of breast cancer

Virtually every study has found significantly elevated relative risks of breast cancer for female relatives of breast cancer patients. However, the magnitude has varied according to the number and type of affected relatives, age at diagnosis of the proband(s), laterality, and the overall study design. Most studies have found relative risks between 2 and 3 for first-degree relatives selected without regard to age at diagnosis or laterality. A comprehensive study, using the Utah Population Database, of

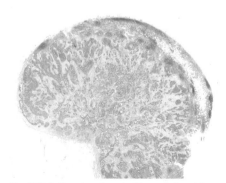

Fig. 1.70 Axillary lymph node. The nodal architecture is destroyed by massive metastatic ductal carcinoma.

first-degree relatives of breast cancer probands diagnosed before age 80 estimated a relative risk of 1.8 in the relatives {1029}. When the breast cancer was of early onset (diagnosed before age 50), the relative risk among first-degree relatives increased to 2.6 and the risk for early-onset breast cancer among these relatives was 3.7 (95% CI. 2.8—4.6). The risk to subsequent relatives in families with two affected sisters was increased to 2.7 with a particularly high risk of 4.9 of early onset breast cancer. A second registry-based study in Sweden found essentially identical results to the Utah study {715}.

Perhaps the largest population-based study (the Cancer and Steroid Hormone (CASH) case-control study) of probands with breast cancer diagnosed between the ages of 20 and 54 estimated the risk of breast cancer in first-degree relatives compared with controls was 2.1 {501}.

A study of cancer at a number of sites in a large set of twins in Scandinavia {1658}, estimated the proportion of variance due to genetic (heritability), shared environment, and random (individual-specific) environmental effects for each cancer site. Based on this data, the authors calculated a co-twin relative risk of 2.8 in DZ and 5.2 in MZ twins, and estimated that 27% of breast cancer is due to inherited cause while only 6% could be attributed to shared environment.

The role of other factors with respect to family history has been examined. Larger familial effects among relatives of young bilateral probands compared with young probands with unilateral breast cancer have been found {93,1246,2129}. The relationship of histology to familial breast cancer is less clear {500,2989}.

Another feature, which conveys strong familial risk of breast cancer, is the occurrence of breast cancer in a male. It has been estimated that female relatives of probands with male breast cancer have a two-fold to three-fold increased risk of breast cancer {94,2449}.

Familial associations of breast and other cancers

A number of studies have found increased risks for other cancers among relatives of breast cancer probands. The most commonly reported are ovarian, uterine, prostate and colon cancers. In

Table 1.10
Estimates of relative risks for breast cancer.

Relative affected, status of proband	Estimate of relative risk	{Reference} (Study Type)
Mother	3.0	{1321a} (a)
Sister	3.0	{1321a} (a)
Mother	2.0	{2214} (a)
Sister	3.0	{2214} (a)
Sister, premenopausal proband	5.0	{92a} (b)
Sister, postmenopausal proband	2.0	{92a} (b)
First-degree relative (FDR)	2.0	{346a} (c)
Sister, bilateral proband	6.0	{2129} (c)
Sister	2.0	{412a} (d)
Mother	2.0	{412a} (d)
First-degree relative (FDR)	2.0	{2556a} (a)
FDR<45, proband<45	3.0	{2556a} (a)
FDR>45, proband>45	1.5	{2556a} (a)
First degree relative	2.1	{501} (c)
First degree relative, proband <55	2.3	{1246} (a)
First degree relative, proband >55	1.6	{1246} (a)
FDR, bilateral proband	6.4	{1246} (a)
First degree relative	2.3	{2720a} (c)
Second degree relative	1.8	{2720a} (c)
First degree relative	1.8	{896} (a)
FDR<50, proband<50	3.7	{896} (a)
FDR, 2 affected probands	2.7	{896} (a)
Mother	1.9	{715} (a)
Sister	2.0	{715} (a)

(a) Ratio of observed frequencies in cancer families to expected frequencies in the general population;
(b) Ratio of observed rate of cancer in relatives of cases to observed rate of cancer in relatives of cases to observed rate of cancer in relatives of selected controls;
(c) Odds ratio from case-control study with non-cancer controls
(d) Relative risk from prospective study.

the Utah Population Database, when risks to all other sites among such probands were examined statistically significant familial associations were found between breast cancer and cancers of the prostate (relative risk = 1.2, P<0.0001), colon (1.35, P<0.0001), thyroid (1.7, P<0.001) and non-Hodgkin lymphoma (1.4, P<0.001) {1029}. The Swedish registry study also found a significant familial relationship between breast and prostate cancer of similar magnitude.

Other studies have also shown relationships between breast cancer and ovarian, colon and uterine cancers, although the results have not been consistent across studies {95,1992,2172,2918}.

Undoubtedly, the majority of the associa-

tions detected in these population studies is due to the BRCA1 gene, known to be involved in a large proportion of extended kindreds with clearly inherited susceptibility to breast and ovarian cancer. It is likely that some of the discrepancies in results are linked to the frequency of BRCA1 deleterious alleles in the respective datasets.

Possible models to explain the familial risk of breast cancer

BRCA1 and BRCA2 explain only a minority (about 20%) of the overall familial risk of breast cancer although they may contribute much more substantially to the four-fold increased risk at younger ages. Assuming an overall two-fold increased risk among first-degree female relatives

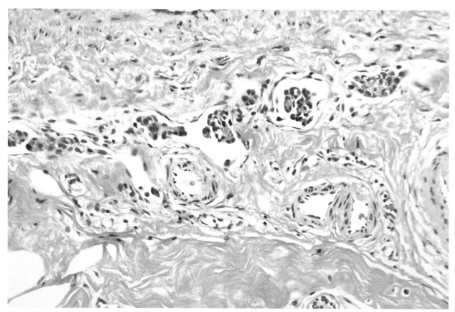

Fig. 1.71 Lymphatic vessel invasion. Several tumour cell nests are present in endothelial lined spaces.

of breast cancer cases and that, as is likely, these genes act in an additive manner with the other loci involved in familial aggregation, then we are left with a residual familial risk of 1.8 to be explained by other genes and/or correlated family environment. There could be several genes similar in action to *BRCA1* and *BRCA2*, with lower breast cancer risks, or a set of more common polymorphisms in biologically relevant genes, each associated with only a small increased risk, or something in-between. Genes are not the only factor which could cause the observed familial correlation. Shared lifestyle or environmental risk factors would also cause some degree of familial clustering, however it can be demonstrated that the known environmental risk factors for breast cancer are unlkely to contribute significantly to the overall familial risk {1238}.

Based on a model of the contribution of genetic variation to the overall familial risk, it can be estimated that variation in as few as 70 of the 30,000 genes in the human genome may contribute to breast cancer susceptibility. Of course, this model is based on a number of unverifiable assumptions and does not include potential gene-gene and gene-environment interactions, so should be interpreted cautiously. However, it seems clear that there are not going to be hundreds of loci involved (or if there are, they will be impossible to find given

the weakness of the effects). Only until more of these loci are identified, and their interaction with known epidemiological risk factors assessed, will we be able to untangle the underlying causes of the observed familial risk.

Prognosis and predictive factors

Clinical features
Age
The prognostic significance of age and menopausal status in patients with breast carcinoma is controversial. Younger patients have been found to have a poor prognosis {59,2029}, a favourable outcome {2500} or no correlation has been found with age at all {1207}. These discrepancies may be due to differences in patient selection, age grouping, and other factors, including high grade, vascular invasion, extensive in situ component, steroid receptor negativity, high proliferation, *TP53* abnormalities. An increased incidence of node positivity was found in two large studies of patients under 35 years.

Pregnancy
Breast cancer developing during pregnancy is generally considered to have an unfavourable prognosis. There is, however, conflicting data as to whether this is an independent factor. It may be partly, or entirely, due to the poor prognosis associated with young age and also the fact that the cancer is often

detected at a late stage as small tumours are not felt in the pregnant or lactating breast {91,311,1079}. Pregnancy in women who have been treated for breast cancer does not appear to affect prognosis {119}.

Morphological factors
The traditional pathological factors of lymph node status, tumour size, histological type, and histological grade are the most useful prognostic factors in breast cancer patients {886,1763}, although this is now challenged by gene expression profiling.

Lymph node status
The status of the axillary lymph nodes is the most important single prognostic factor for patients with breast cancer. Numerous studies have shown that disease-free and overall survival rates decrease as the number of positive nodes increases {886}. The clinical significance of micrometastases and isolated tumour cells in the nodes, particularly those identified exclusively by immunohistochemistry, remains a matter of debate {71,1655} although virtually all studies with more than 100 patients have shown that micrometastases are associated with a small but significant decrease in disease-free and/or overall survival {1655}.

Approximately 10-20% of patients considered to be node-negative by routine pathological examination have identifiable tumour cells as determined by serial sectioning, immunohistochemical staining for epithelial markers, or both. However, at present, it appears premature to recommend the routine use of step sections and/or immunohistochemistry to evaluate sentinel or non-sentinel lymph nodes {71}.

Tumour size
Tumour size is an important prognostic factor. Even among patients with breast cancers 1 cm and smaller (T1a and T1b), size is an important prognostic factor for axillary lymph node involvement and outcome {461}. However, the manner in which the pathological tumour size is reported varies. Some pathologists report the macroscopic size, some a microscopic size that includes both the invasive and in situ components, and others report the microscopic size of the invasive compo-

nent only. There is often poor correlation between the tumour size determined by gross pathological examination and the size of the invasive component as determined by histological measurement {27}. The size of the invasive component is clinically significant, and so the pathological tumour size for classification (pT) is a measurement of only the invasive component {51}. Therefore, when there is a discrepancy between the gross and the microscopic size of the invasive component, the microscopic size takes precedence, and should be indicated in the pathology report and used for pathological staging.

Histological type
Some special histological types of breast cancer are associated with a particularly favourable clinical outcome {771,2433}. These include tubular, invasive cribriform, mucinous, and adenoid cystic carcinomas. Some authors also include tubulolobular and papillary carcinomas. The 20-year recurrence-free survival of special type tumours 1.1 to 3.0 cm in size is similar to that of invasive ductal carcinomas of no special type 1 cm and smaller (87% and 86%, respectively) {2433}. The prognostic significance of medullary carcinoma remains controvertial and is discussed elsewhere (see medullary carcinoma).

Histological grade
Grading is recommended for all invasive carcinomas of the breast, regardless of morphological type {1984, 2216,2905}. This practice has been criticized by some pathologists who feel that grading is not appropriate for the special histological types such as pure tubular, invasive cribriform, mucinous, medullary and infiltrating lobular carcinomas. For example, most infiltrating lobular carcinomas, especially those of classical subtype, are assessed as grade 2 and the overall survival curve of lobular carcinoma overlies that of all other types of grade 2 carcinoma. In mucinous carcinoma and in carcinoma of mixed morphological type, grading provides a more appropriate estimate of prognosis than type alone {2216}. In medullary carcinoma no additional prognostic value has been found.
Higher rates of distant metastasis and poorer survival are seen in patients with higher grade (poorly differentiated) tu-

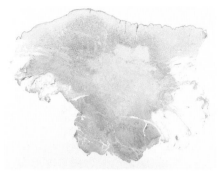

Fig. 1.72 Carcinoma with central fibrosis. There is extensive central fibrosis with only a rim of invasive carcinoma left around the fibrotic area.

mours, independent of lymph node status and tumour size {550,777,836, 868,886,1031,1763,2030,2434}. Tumour grading has prognostic value even in breast cancers 1 cm and smaller {461}. The optimal grading method {777} has been detailed earlier in this chapter. The combination of histological type and grade provides a more accurate assessment of prognosis than does histological type alone {2216}.
Histological grade may also provide useful information with regard to response to chemotherapy and, therefore, be a predictive factor as well as a prognostic indicator. Several studies have suggested that high histological grade is associated with a better response to certain chemotherapy regimens than low histological grade {2254}. However, additional studies are required to define this relationship more clearly {612}.

Tumour cell proliferation
Markers of proliferation have been extensively investigated to evaluate prognosis {886,1304}. Mitotic count is part of histological grading. Other methods include DNA flow cytometry measurement of S-phase fraction (SPF). Many studies indicate that high SPF is associated with inferior outcome.
Ki-67/MIB-1 is a labile, non-histone nuclear protein detected in the G1 through M phases of the cell cycle, but not in resting cells and is therefore a direct indicator of the growth fraction. The percentage of Ki-67 positive cells can be used to stratify patients into good and poor survivors. Quantitative RT-PCR in detecting the mRNA level has also been introduced as well as array based quantification of proliferation (see below).

Lymphatic and blood vessel invasion
Lymphatic vessel invasion has been shown to be an important and independent prognostic factor, particularly in patients with T1, node-negative breast cancers {461,1606,1623, 2433,2445,2452}. Its major value is in identifying patients at increased risk of axillary lymph node involvement {627,839,1592,2253,2415} and adverse outcome {186a,627,1623, 2415,2434}. As with histological grade, the ability of pathologists to reproducibly identify lymphatic vessel invasion has been challenged {998} but can be improved if stringent criteria are employed {627,2109,2253,2415, 2452}. Lymphatic vessel invasion must be distinguished from tumour cell nests within artifactual tissue spaces created by shrinkage or retraction of the stroma during tissue processing.
Blood vessel invasion has been reported to have an adverse effect on clinical outcome. However, there is a broad range in the reported incidence, from under 5% to almost 50% {1470,1592, 2444,2445,2452, 3083}. This is due to a variety of factors including the patient population, the criteria and methodology used, and difficulty in identifying blood vessels.

Perineural invasion
Perineural invasion is sometimes observed in invasive breast cancers, but it has not been shown to be an independent prognostic factor {2426}.

Tumour necrosis
In most studies {2452}, the presence of necrosis has been associated with an adverse effect on clinical outcome {414, 877,999,2175}, although in one, necrosis was associated with a worse prognosis only within the first two years after diagnosis {999}.

Inflammatory cell infiltrates
The presence of a prominent mononuclear cell infiltrate has been correlated in some studies with high histological grade {2030}. However, the prognostic significance of this finding is controversial, with some studies noting an adverse effect on clinical outcome {67,286,2785} and others observing either no significant effect or a beneficial effect {635,1601,2445,2785}.

Extent of ductal carcinoma in situ

The presence of an extensive intraductal component is a prognostic factor for local recurrence in patients treated with conservative surgery and radiation therapy, when the status of the excision margins is unknown. However, this is not an independent predictor when the microscopic margin status is taken into consideration {2569}. Its relationship with metastatic spread and patient survival remains unclear {2176,2437,2689}.

Tumour stroma

Prominent stromal elastosis has variously been reported to be associated with a favourable prognosis {2664,2858}, an unfavourable prognosis {84,1016}, and to have no prognostic significance {626, 1266,2393}. The presence of a fibrotic focus in the centre of an invasive carcinoma has also been reported to be an independent adverse prognostic indicator {545,1153}

Combined morphologic prognostic factors

The best way to integrate histological prognostic factors is an unresolved issue {1833}. The Nottingham Prognostic Index takes into consideration tumour size, lymph node status and histological grade, and stratifies patients into good, moderate and poor prognostic groups with annual mortality rates of 3%, 7%, and 30%, respectively {954}. Another proposal for a prognostic index includes tumour size, lymph node status and mitotic index (morphometric prognostic index) {2993}.

Molecular markers and gene expression

A large number of genetic alterations have been identified in invasive breast carcinomas, many of which are of potential prognostic or predictive value. Some provide treatment-independent information on patient survival, others predict the likelihood that a patient will benefit from a certain therapy. Some alterations may have both prognostic and predictive value.

Steroid hormone receptors (Estrogen receptor (ER) and Progesterone receptor PR)

Estrogen is an important mitogen exerting its activity by binding to its receptor (ER). Approximately 60% of breast carcinomas express the ER protein. Initially,

ER-positive tumours were associated with an improved prognosis, but studies with long-term follow-up have suggested that ER-positive tumours, despite having a slower growth rate, do not have a lower metastatic potential. Nonetheless, ER status remains very useful in predicting the response to adjuvant tamoxifen {4, 368,1304,1833,2120}. Measurement of both ER and PR has been clinical practice for more than 20 years. PR is a surrogate marker of a functional ER. In estrogen target tissues, estrogen treatment induces PR. Both can be detected by ligand binding assay, or more commonly nowadays, by immunohistochemical (IHC) analysis using monoclonal antibodies. ER/PR-positive tumours have a 60-70% response rate compared to less than 10% for ER/PR-negative tumours. ER-positive/PR-negative tumours have an intermediate response of approximately 40%. Hormone receptor status is the only recommended molecular marker to be used in treatment decision {9,886, 1030}. The impact of hormone receptor status on prognosis and treatment outcome prediction is complex. The finding, in cell lines, that tamoxifen can interact with the recently identifed ERβ receptor (ERB) may provide new clues towards improvement of predicting tamoxifen responsiveness {1526,1925,3269}.

Epidermal growth factor receptor (EGFR) and transforming growth factor alpha (TGFα), antiapoptotic protein bcl-2, cyclin dependent kinase inhibitor p27 are other potential prognostic markers that look promising. Elevated expression of EGFR, in the absence of gene amplification, has been associated with estrogen receptor negativity {2509}.

The ERBB2 / HER2 oncogene

The prognostic value of ERBB2 overexpression, first reported in 1987 {2719}, has been extensively studied {2962,3173}. ERBB2 over-expression is a weak to moderately independent predictor of survival, at least for node-positive patients. Gene amplification or over-expression of the ERBB2 protein can be measured by Southern blot analysis, FISH, differential PCR, IHC and ELISA {2958}. Studies of the predictive value of ERBB2-status have not been consistent. A recent review {3173} concluded that ERBB2 seems to be a weak to moderately strong negative

predictor for response to alkylating agents and a moderately positive predictive factor for response to anthracyclines. There was insufficient data to draw conclusions on the response to taxanes or radiotherapy. In an adjuvant setting, ERBB2 status should not be used to select adjuvant systemic chemotherapy or endocrine therapy. Conversely, when adjuvant chemotherapy is recommended, anthracycline-based therapy should be preferred for ERBB2 positive patients. A humanized anti-ERBB2 monoclonal antibody, trastuzumab (Herceptin), has been developed as a novel anti-cancer drug targeting overexpressed ERBB2 {529}. This has been shown to be effective in 20% of patients with ERBB2 amplified tumours.

TP53 mutations

Approximately 25% of breast cancers have mutations in the tumour suppressor gene TP53, most of which are missense mutations leading to the accumulation of a stable, but inactive protein in the tumour cells {1196,2759,2761}. Both DNA sequencing and IHC have been used to assess TP53-status in the tumour. However, some 20% of the mutations do not yield a stable protein and are thus not detected by IHC, while normal (wildtype) protein may accumulate in response to DNA damage or cellular stress signals. Studies using DNA sequencing all showed a strong association with survival whereas those using only IHC did not, or did so only weakly {5,886,1304,2237,2760}. Given the diverse cellular functions of the p53 protein and the location and type of alteration within the gene, specific mutations might conceivably be associated with a particularly poor prognosis. Patients with mutations in their tumours affecting the L2/L3 domain of the p53 protein, which is important for DNA binding, have a particularly poor survival {251,317,976,1523}.

The role of p53 in the control of the cell cycle, DNA damage repair, and apoptosis, provides a strong biological rationale for investigating whether mutations are predictors of response to DNA damaging agents. Several studies using DNA sequencing of the entire gene have addressed this in relation to different chemotherapy and radiotherapy regimes {16,241,249,976}. A strong

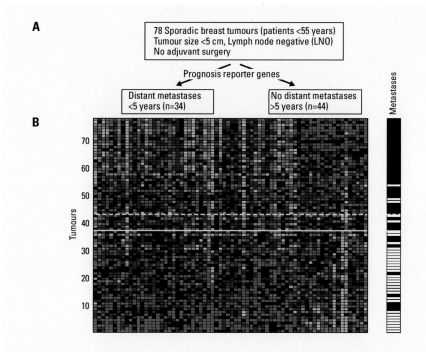

Fig. 1.73 A Supervised classification on prognosis signatures, using a set of prognostic reporter genes to identify optimally two types of disease outcome from 78 sporadic breast tumours into a poor prognosis and good prognosis group. **B** Each row represents a tumour and each column a gene. Genes are ordered according to their correlation coefficient with the two prognostic groups. Tumours are ordered by the correlation to the average profile of the good prognosis group. Solid line, prognostic classifier with optimal accuracy; dashed line, with optimized sensitivity. Above the dashed line patients have a good prognosis signature, below the dashed line the prognosis signature is poor. The metastasis status for each patient is shown in the right panel: white indicates patients who developed distant metastases within 5 years after the primary diagnosis; black indicates patients who continued to be disease-free for at least 5 years. From L.J. van't Veer et al. {2986}.

association between specific mutations and short survival and poor response to treatment was seen, emphasizing the importance of DNA sequence analysis of the entire coding region of *TP53* when evaluating its prognostic and predictive value.

Loss of heterozygosity (LOH)
LOH at the *TP53* gene has been shown to be a marker for prognosis and predictor of response to certain therapies (see above). Other regions with LOH that appear to correlate to short survival include 11q23 and several regions on 3p {1216,1552}. Deletion of 9q13 is also associated with shorter survival. The target gene(s) in these areas have still to be identified {1326}.

DNA amplification
Conventional as well as array-based CGH have identified a number of amplified regions containing putative oncogenes with prognostic potential. Ampli-

fication of the *FGFR1* gene on 8p12 has been correlated with reduced disease-free survival, especially if the gene is amplified together with the cyclin D1 gene {596}. The *MYC* gene on 8q24 is amplified in approximately 20% of breast carcinomas, which is associated with estrogen receptor negativity {596}, locally advanced disease and poor prognosis {250}. On 11q13, cyclin D1 (*CCND1*) is amplified in 15-20% of breast tumours. In ER-positive tumours, *CCND1* amplification is associated with a relatively poor prognosis {596,2582}, and is more frequent in lobular carcinomas compared to ductal carcinomas.

Expression profiling
Much recent work has been focused on the potential of gene expression profiles to predict the clinical outcome of breast cancer {257,1257,2328,2757, 2986,2990}. These studies, although heterogeneous in patient selection and numbers of tumours analysed, have indi-

cated that gene expression patterns can be identified that associate with lymph node or distant metastasis, and that are capable of predicting disease course in individual patients with high accuracies (circa 90%). In the largest study to date {2990}, analysing 295 tumours, the expression profile was a strong independent factor and outcompeted lymph node status as a predictor of outcome. These findings suggest that some primary tumours express a "metastasis signature", which is difficult to reconcile with the classic tumour progression model in which a rare subpopulation of tumour cells have accumulated the numerous alterations required for metastasis to occur. Interestingly, some of the genes in the signature seem to be derived from non-epithelial components of the tumour {2328}, suggesting that stromal elements represent an important contributing factor to the metastatic phenotype. Survival differences were also noted between the different subtypes of breast tumours as defined by expression patterns {2756, 2757}. The patients with basal-like and ERBB2+ subtypes were associated with the shortest survival, while a difference in the outcome for tumours classified as luminal A versus luminal B was also evident. The luminal subtype B may represent a class of ER-positive tumours with poor outcome, possibly not responding to tamoxifen. This strongly supports the idea that many of these breast tumour subtypes represent biologically distinct disease entities with different clinical outcome.

A remarkable feature of the expression signatures identified in these studies is that they usually involve fewer than 100 genes {257,2986}, in one instance even only 17 genes {2328}. However, somewhat confusing is that the overlap between the different sets of genes thus defined is incomplete {1257,2757}. Further comparative studies are required to elucidate the critical components of the poor prognosis signature, while the clinical utility of this new diagnostic tool must now be demonstrated in a prospective trial setting. At a more fundamental level, it will be interesting to establish whether the observed association between expression signatures and survival reflects an intrinsic biological behaviour of breast tumour cells or a differential response to therapy.

Lobular neoplasia

F.A. Tavassoli
R.R. Millis
W. Boecker
S.R. Lakhani

Definition

Characterized by a proliferation of generally small and often loosely cohesive cells, the term lobular neoplasia (LN) refers to the entire spectrum of atypical epithelial proliferations originating in the terminal duct-lobular unit (TDLU), with or without pagetoid involvement of terminal ducts. In a minority of women after long-term follow-up, LN constitutes a risk factor and a nonobligatory precursor for the subsequent development of invasive carcinoma in either breast, of either ductal or lobular type.

ICD-O code

Lobular carcinoma in situ (LCIS) 8520/2

Synonyms and historical annotation

The designations atypical lobular hyperplasia (ALH) and lobular carcinoma in situ (LCIS) have been widely used for variable degrees of the lesion.

Two series published in 1978 {1100, 2438} concluded that the features generally used to subdivide the lobular changes into LCIS and ALH were not of prognostic significance. To avoid overtreatment, Haagensen suggested the designation lobular neoplasia (LN) for these lesions {1100}. To emphasize their non-invasive nature, the term lobular intraepithelial neoplasia (LIN) has been proposed. Based on morphological criteria and clinical outcome, LIN has been categorized into three grades {338}.

Epidemiology

The frequency of LN ranges from less than 1% {3106,3107} to 3.8 % {1099} of all breast carcinomas. It is found in 0.5-4% of otherwise benign breast biopsies {2150}. Women with LN range in age from 15 {32} to over 90 years old {2876}, but most are premenopausal.

Clinical features

The lesion is multicentric in as many as 85% of patients {2446,2876} and bilateral in 30% {1096} to 67% {2001} of women who had been treated by bilateral mastectomy. No mammographic abnormalities are recognized {2128,2273}, except in the occasional variant of LN characterized by calcification developing within central necrosis {2534}.

Macroscopy

LN is not associated with any grossly recognizable features.

Histopathology

The lesion is located within the terminal duct-lobular unit {3091} with pagetoid involvement of the terminal ducts evident in as many as 75% of cases {86,1096}. On low power examination, while lobular architecture is maintained, the acini of one or more lobules are expanded to varying degrees by a monomorphic proliferation of loosely cohesive, usually small cells, with uniform round nuclei, indistinct nucleoli, uniform chromatin and rather indistinct cell margins with sparse cytoplasm. Necrosis and calcification are uncommon and mitoses are infrequent. Intracytoplasmic lumens are often present but are not specific to LN {89}. In some lesions, however, the proliferating cells are larger and more pleomorphic or of signet ring type. Apocrine metaplasia occurs but the existence of endocrine variant of LN {801} is disputed.

Two types of LN have been recognized {1100}: Type A with the more usual morphology described above and Type B composed of larger, more atypical cells with less uniform chromatin and conspicuous nucleoli. The two cell types may be mixed. When composed of pleomorphic cells, the term pleomorphic LN has been used. The neoplastic cells either replace or displace the native epithelial cells in the TDLU. The myoepithelial cells may remain in their original basal location or they may be dislodged and admixed with the neoplastic cells. The basement membrane is generally intact although this is not always visible in all sections. Pagetoid involvement of adjacent ducts between intact overlying flattened epithelium and underlying basement membrane is frequent and can result in several different patterns including a 'clover leaf' or 'necklace' appearance {1099}. Solid obliteration of acini may occur, sometimes with massive distension and central necrosis. LN may involve a variety of lesions including sclerosing adenosis, radial scars, papillary lesions, fibroadenomas and collagenous spherulosis.

Immunoprofile

LN is positive for estrogen receptor (ER) in 60-90% of cases and in a slightly lower percentage for progesterone receptor (PR) {62,369,1010,2159,2483}. The classical variety of LN is more likely to be positive than the pleomorphic variant {223,2683}. Unlike high grade DCIS, however, classic LN rarely expresses ERBB2 or TP53 protein {62,2327a,2483, 2746}. Positivity is more likely with the pleomorphic variant {1859,2683}. Intra-

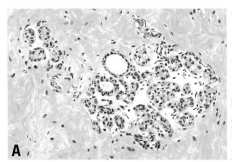
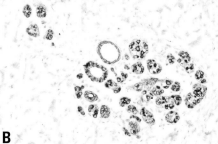

Fig. 1.74 Early lobular neoplasia. **A** The few neoplastic lobular cells are hardly apparent on a quick examination of the TDLU. **B** Double immunostaining with E-cadherin (brown) and CK34BE12 (purple) unmasks the few neoplastic cells (purple) proliferating in this lobule. These early lesions are often missed on H&E stained sections.

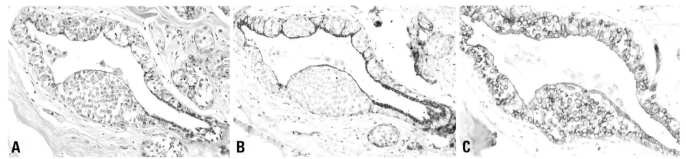

Fig. 1.75 Lobular neoplasia. **A** Aggregates of loosely cohesive neoplastic cells proliferate beneath the native epithelial cell lining (pagetoid growth pattern). **B** Typically, the neoplastic cells are E-cadherin negative. **C** Immunostain for CK34BE12 shows a polarized positive reaction in the cytoplasm.

cytoplasmic immunoreactivity for casein has also been reported {1994,2149}. E-cadherin, commonly identified in ductal lesions, is generally absent from both LN and invasive lobular carcinoma {1892,2336}.

Grading
A three tiered grading system has been suggested, based on the extent and degree of proliferation and/or cytological features. Those lesions with markedly distended acini, often with central necrosis, and those composed of either severely pleomorphic cells or pure signet ring cells with or without acinar distension, were designated LIN 3; they have been reported to be often associated with invasive carcinoma {2876}. This grading system requires validation by other centres and is not endorsed at this time.

Differential diagnosis
Poor tissue preservation may give a false impression of loosely cohesive cells leading to over-diagnosis of LN.
Distinction from a solid DCIS can be difficult on morphological grounds alone, particularly when DCIS remains confined

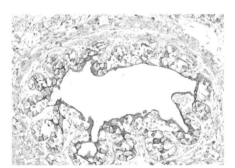

Fig. 1.76 Lobular neoplasia. CK5/6 immunohisto-chemistry demonstrating the pagetoid spread of tumour cells infiltrating the positively stained original epithelium, leading to a reticulated staining pattern.

to the lobule without unfolding it (so called lobular cancerization). The presence of secondary lumina or a rosette-like arrangement of cells indicates a ductal lesion. In problematic cases, the immunoprofile may be helpful. LN is typically E-cadherin and CK 5,6 negative, but HMW CK34BE12 positive {337}. DCIS, on the other hand, is typically E-cadherin positive, but CK34BE12 negative. Occasional lesions are negative or positive for both HMWCK34BE12 and E-cadherin markers. Since, at present, it is uncertain how these morphologically and immuno-histochemically hybrid lesions with ductal and lobular features would behave, it is important that they are recognized so that more can be learned about their nature in the future {337}.
When LN involves sclerosing adenosis or other sclerosing lesions, it can be confused with an invasive carcinoma. The presence of a myoepithelial cell layer around the neoplastic cell clusters excludes the possibility of an invasive carcinoma; immunostaining for actin can unmask the myoepithelial cells, thus facilitating the distinction.
Presence of isolated cells invading the stroma around a focus of LN can cause diagnostic problems. Absence of myoepithelial cells around the individual cells and their haphazard distribution accentuated by any of the epithelial markers (optimally with double immunos-taining techniques) can help establish the presence of stromal invasion by individual or small clusters of neoplastic cells.

Molecular genetics
Loss of heterozygosity (LOH) at loci frequently observed in invasive carcinoma has also been reported in LN, ranging from 8% on chromosome 17p to 50% on 17q {1569}. LOH on chromosome 16q,

the site of the E-cadherin gene, was found in approximately 30%. LOH was identified in LN associated with invasive carcinoma and in pure LN, suggesting that it may be a direct precursor of invasive lobular cancer. Further support for this hypothesis has come from a report that showed LOH in 50% of LN associated with invasive carcinoma at markers on chromosome 11q13 {1988}. LOH was seen in 10% of ALH and 41% of invasive lobular carcinomas. Using comparative genomic hybridization (CGH), loss of chromosomal material from 16p, 16q, 17p and 22q and gain of material to 6q was identified in equal frequency in 14 ALH and 31 LCIS

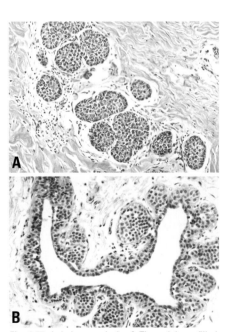

Fig. 1.77 Lobular neoplasia. **A** The acini are filled and moderately distended by neoplastic cells; the acinar outlines are retained. **B** Clover-leaf pattern. This is one of the classic patterns of LN, with the acini distended by neoplastic cells pulling away from the intralobular segment of the terminal duct, creating a clover-leaf or necklace appearance.

lesions {1707}, suggesting that both are 'neoplastic' and at a similar stage of genetic evolution.

The most direct evidence for a precursor role of LN comes from mutational analysis of the E-cadherin gene {259,260}. In one study {261}, 27 of 48 (56%) invasive lobular carcinomas had mutation in the E-cadherin gene, while none of 50 breast cancers of other types showed any alteration. It was subsequently demonstrated that truncating mutations identified in invasive lobular carcinoma were also present in the adjacent LN, providing direct proof that LN was a precursor lesion {3034}.

Prognosis and predictive factors

The relative risk (RR) for subsequent development of invasive carcinoma among patients with LN ranges from 6.9 to about 12 times that expected in women without LN {87,88,1100}.

Amongst 1174 women in 18 separate retrospective studies, diagnosed as having LN and treated by biopsy alone, 181 (15.4%) eventually developed invasive carcinoma {88,1096,1100,2150,2428, 2438}. Of these, 102 (8.7%) developed in the ipsilateral breast, and 79 (6.7%) in the contralateral breast, demonstrating an almost equal risk for either breast. However, in a prospective study of 100 cases of LN with 10 years of follow-up, 11 of 13 invasive recurrences were ipsilateral {2127}.

With extended follow-up, the risk of development of invasive cancer continues to increase to 35% for those women who survive 35 years after their initial diagnosis of LN. Furthermore, the RR increases substantially from 4.9 (95% CI: 3.7–6.4) after one biopsy with LN to 16.1 (95% CI:6.9–31.8) after a second biopsy with LN {298}.

Early studies suggested that among LN lesions, there are no clinical or pathological features associated with increased risk of subsequent invasive carcinoma {2150,2438}. However, a more recent study using the three tiered grading system, but with a comparatively short follow-up of 5 years, found that LIN 3 and, to a lesser extent LIN 2, were associated with an increased risk {869}, but LIN 1 was not. In another study, 86% of invasive carcinomas associated with LIN 3 were lobular in type, in contrast to 47% of those associated with LIN 2 and only 11% of those associated with LIN 1 {338}.

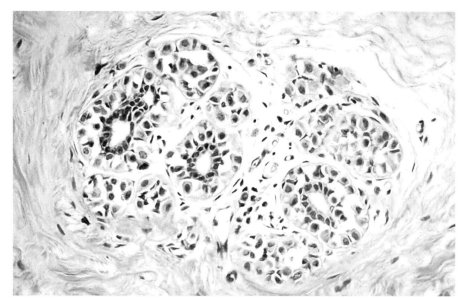

Fig. 1.78 Lobular neoplasia. Loosely cohesive neoplastic cells are proliferating in this lobule, but they have not distended the acini.

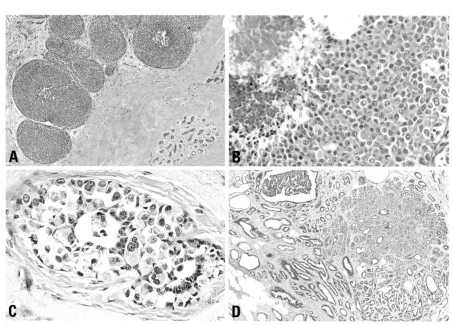

Fig. 1.79 Lobular neoplasia. **A** Necrotic type with massive distention of the acini. **B** Note the loosely cohesive cells and the necrosis. **C** Lobular neoplasia, pleomorphic type. Even though there is not a significant distention of the involved TDLU, the neoplastic cells are highly pleomorphic and loosely cohesive. This is the intraepithelial counterpart of pleomorphic invasive lobular carcinoma. **D** LN involving sclerosing adenosis. The lobulated configuration of the sclerosing adenosis is apparent at low magnification. The ductules in part of the lesion are filled and expanded by proliferation of a monotonous neoplastic cell population. This setting may be confused with invasive carcinoma, particularly when the sections are suboptimal.

Management of LN has evolved with increased understanding of the disease {1082}. The current consensus is that LN constitutes a risk factor and a non obligate precursor for subsequent development of invasive carcinoma in either breast, of either ductal or lobular type, but only in a minority of women after long-term follow-up. The current recommended management for LN is, therefore, life long follow-up with or without tamoxifen treatment. Re-excision should be considered in cases of massive acinar distension, and when pleomorphic, signet ring or necrotic variants are identified at or close to the margin.

Intraductal proliferative lesions

F.A. Tavassoli   S.J. Schnitt
H. Hoefler   W. Boecker
J. Rosai   S.H. Heywang-Köbrunner
R. Holland   F. Moinfar
I.O. Ellis   S.R. Lakhani

Definition

Intraductal proliferative lesions are a group of cytologically and architecturally diverse proliferations, typically originating from the terminal duct-lobular unit and confined to the mammary duct lobular system. They are associated with an increased risk, albeit of greatly different magnitudes, for the subsequent development of invasive carcinoma.

ICD-O codes

In the ICD-O classification, /2 is used for in situ carcinomas. The code 8500/2 covers all grades of ductal carcinoma in situ and ductal intraepithelial neoplasia, grade 3.

Site of origin and route of lesion progression

A vast majority of intraductal proliferative lesions originate in the terminal duct-lobular unit (TDLU) {3091}. A substantially smaller proportion originates in larger and lactiferous ducts.

Segmentally distributed, ductal carcinoma in situ (DCIS) progression within the duct system is from its origin in a TDLU toward the nipple and into adjacent branches of a given segment of the duct system. The rare lesions that develop within the lactiferous ducts may progress toward the nipple resulting in Paget disease or to the adjacent branches of a reference duct {2089,2090,2093}.

Terminology

Intraductal proliferative lesions of the breast have traditionally been divided into three categories: usual ductal hyperplasia (UDH), atypical ductal hyperplasia (ADH) and ductal carcinoma in situ (DCIS). It should be noted, however, that the term "DCIS" encompasses a highly heterogeneous group of lesions that differ with regard to their mode of presentation, histopathological features, biological markers, and risk for progression to invasive cancer. In most cases, the histopathological distinction between different types of intraductal proliferation can be made on morphological grounds alone, particularly with standardization of histopathological criteria. However, even then, the distinction between some of the lesions (particularly between ADH and some low grade forms of DCIS) remains problematic. In addition, population-based mammography screening has resulted in increased detection of lesions that show cytological atypia with or without intraluminal proliferation but do not fulfil the diagnostic criteria for any of the existing categories. Those lesions lacking intraluminal projection have been described in the past as clinging carcinoma and more recently referred to under a variety of names including flat epithelial atypia, atypical cystic lobules, atypical columnar alteration with prominent apical snouts and secretions.

Progression to invasive breast cancer

Clinical follow-up studies have indicated that these intraductal proliferative lesions are associated with different levels of risk for subsequent development of invasive breast cancer, that ranges from approximately 1.5 times that of the reference population for UDH, to 4-5-fold (range, 2.4-13.0-fold) for ADH, and 8-10-fold for DCIS {886}. Recent immunophenotypic and molecular genetic studies have provided new insights into these lesions indicating that the long-held notion of a linear progression from normal epithelium through hyperplasia, atypical hyperplasia and carcinoma in situ to invasive cancer is overly simplistic; the inter-relationship between these various intraductal proliferative lesions and invasive breast cancer is far more complex. In brief, these data have suggested that: (1) UDH shares few similarities with most ADH, DCIS or invasive cancer; (2) ADH shares many similarities with low grade DCIS; (3) low grade DCIS and high grade DCIS appear to represent genetically distinct disorders leading to distinct forms of invasive breast carcinoma, further emphasizing their heterogeneity; and (4) at least some lesions with flat epithelial atypia are neoplastic. These data support the notion that ADH and all forms of DCIS represent intraepithelial neoplasias which in the WHO classification of tumours of the digestive system have been defined as 'lesions characterized by morphological changes that include altered architecture and abnormalities in cytology and differentiation; they result from clonal alterations in genes and carry a predisposition, albeit of variable magnitude, for invasion and metastasis' {1114}. The WHO Working Group felt that UDH is not a significant risk factor and that at the time of the meeting, there was insufficient genetic evidence to classify it as a precursor lesion. However, a recent CGH study suggests that a subset of UDH can be a precursor of ADH {1037}.

Classification and grading

These emerging genetic data and the increasingly frequent detection of ADH and low grade DCIS by mammography have raised important questions about the manner in which intraductal proliferative lesions are currently classified.

Although used by pathology laboratories worldwide, the traditional classification system suffers from high interobserver variability, in particular, in distinguishing between atypical ductal hyperplasia (ADH) and some types of low grade ductal carcinoma in situ (DCIS). Some members of the Working Group proposed that the traditional terminology be replaced by ductal intraepithelial neoplasia (DIN), reserving the term carcinoma for invasive tumours. This would help to avoid the possibility of overtreatment, particularly in the framework of population-based mammography screening programmes. In several other organ sites, the shift in terminology has already occurred e.g. cervix (CIN), prostate (PIN) and in the recent WHO classification of tumours of the digestive system {1114}.

The majority of participants in the WHO Working Group was in favour of maintaining the traditional terminology which in Table 1.11 is shown next to the corresponding terms of the DIN classification. For purposes of clinical management and tumour registry coding, when the

DIN terminology is used, the traditional terminology should be mentioned as well. The classification of intraductal proliferative lesions should be viewed as an evolving concept that may be modified as additional molecular genetic data become available.

Diagnostic reproducibility
Multiple studies have assessed reproducibility in diagnosing the range of intraductal proliferative lesions, some with emphasis on the borderline lesions {299, 503,2155,2157,2411,2571,2723,2724}. These studies have clearly indicated that interobserver agreement is poor when no standardized criteria are used {2411}. Although diagnostic reproducibility is improved with the use of standardized criteria {2571} discrepancies in diagnosis persist in some cases, particularly in the distinction between ADH and limited forms of low grade DCIS. In one study, consistency in diagnosis and classification did not change significantly when interpretation was confined to specific images as compared with assessment of the entire tissue section on a slide, reflecting inconsistencies secondary to differences in morphological interpretation {780}. While clinical follow-up studies have generally demonstrated increasing levels of breast cancer risk associated with UDH, ADH and DCIS respectively, concerns about diagnostic reproducibility have led some to question the practice of utilizing these risk estimates at the individual level {299}.

Aetiology
In general, the factors that are associated with the development of invasive breast carcinoma are also associated with increased risk for the development of intraductal proliferative lesions {1439a, 1551a,2536a}. (See section on epidemiology of breast carcinoma).

Genetics of precursor lesions
To date, several genetic analyses have been performed on potential precursor lesions of carcinoma of the breast. The sometimes contradictory results (see below) may be due to: (i) small number of cases analysed, (ii) the use of different histological classification criteria, (iii) histomorphological heterogeneity of both the normal and neoplastic breast tissue and (iv) genetic heterogeneity, as identified by either conventional cytogenetics {1175} or by fluorescence in situ hybridization

Table 1.11
Classification of intraductal proliferative lesions.

Traditional terminology	Ductal intraepithelial neoplasia (DIN) terminology
Usual ductal hyperplasia (UDH)	Usual ductal hyperplasia (UDH)
Flat epithelial atypia	Ductal intraepithelial neoplasia, grade 1A (DIN 1A)
Atypical ductal hyperplasia (ADH)	Ductal intraepithelial neoplasia, grade 1B (DIN 1B)
Ductal carcinoma in situ, low grade (DCIS grade 1)	Ductal intraepithelial neoplasia, grade1C (DIN 1C)
Ductal carcinoma in situ, intermediate grade (DCIS grade 2)	Ductal intraepithelial neoplasia, grade 2 (DIN 2)
Ductal carcinoma in situ, high grade (DCIS grade 3)	Ductal intraepithelial neoplasia, grade 3 (DIN 3)

(FISH) analysis {1949}. Further evidence for genetic heterogeneity comes from comparative genomic hybridization (CGH) data of microdissected tissue in usual ductal hyperplasia (UDH), atypical ductal hyperplasia (ADH) {135} and DCIS {134,366}.
There has been a tendency to interpret loss of heterozygosity as evidence for clonal evolution and neoplastic transformation. However, histologically normal ductal epithelium closely adjacent to invasive ductal carcinoma may share an LOH pattern with the carcinoma, while normal ducts further away in the breast do not {671}. LOH has been reported in normal epithelial tissues of the breast, in association with carcinoma and in reduction mammoplasties, however, the significance of these finding remains to be evaluated {671,1586,1945}. LOH has also been identified in the stromal component of in situ {1889} and invasive breast carcinoma {1545,1889}, in non-neoplastic tissue from reduction mammoplasty specimens {1568}, and in normal-appearing breast ducts {1586}. The biological significance of these alterations are still poorly understood, but the available data suggest that genetic alterations may occur very early in breast tumorigenesis prior to detectable morphological changes and that epithelial/stromal interactions play a role in progression of mammary carcinoma.

Clinical features
The age range of women with intraductal proliferative lesions is wide, spanning 7 to 8 decades post adolescence. All these lesions are extremely rare prior to puberty; when they do occur among infants and children, they are generally a reflection of exogenous or abnormal endogenous hormonal stimulation. The mean age for DCIS is between 50-59 years. Though most often unilateral, about 22% of women with DCIS in one breast develop either in situ or invasive carcinoma in the contralateral breast {3055}.

Macroscopy
A vast majority of intraductal proliferative lesions, particularly those detected mammographically, are not evident on macroscopic inspection of the specimen. A small proportion of high grade DCIS may be extensive enough and with such an abundance of intraluminal necrosis or associated stromal reaction that it would present as multiple areas of round, pale comedo necrosis or a firm, gritty mass.

Usual ductal hyperplasia (UDH)

Definition
A benign ductal proliferative lesion typically characterized by secondary lumens, and streaming of the central proliferating cells. Although not considered a precursor lesion, long-term follow-up of patients with UDH suggests a slightly elevated risk for the subsequent development of invasive carcinoma.

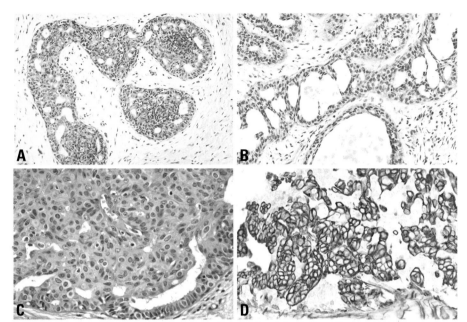

Fig. 1.80 Usual ductal hyperplasia. **A** Florid type. The peripheral distribution of irregularly sized spaces is a characteristic of UDH readily apparent at low magnification. **B** The proliferating cells may form epithelial bridges, but the bridges are delicate and formed by spindled stretched cells. **C** Intensive, predominantly solid intraductal proliferation of a heterogeneous cell population. Note spindling of the cells. Several irregular peripheral luminal spaces. **D** Intraluminal proliferation with many CK5-positive and occasional CK5-negative cells.

Synonyms
Intraductal hyperplasia, hyperplasia of the usual type, epitheliosis, ordinary intraductal hyperplasia.

Mammography
UDH does not have a mammographic presentation, except in rare cases with microcalcification.

Risk of progression
Long-term follow up of patients with UDH in one study showed that 2.6% develop subsequent invasive carcinoma after an average interval of over 14 years, compared to 8.3 years for those with ADH {2886}. In another study, the absolute risk of a woman with UDH developing breast cancer within 15 years was 4% {732}. The Cancer Committee of the College of American Pathologists has assigned UDH a slightly increased risk (RR of 1.5-2.0) for subsequent development of invasive carcinoma {885}.

Histopathology
UDH is characterized by irregularly shaped and sized secondary lumens, often peripherally distributed, and streaming of the central bolus of proliferating cells. Epithelial bridges are thin and stretched; nuclei are unevenly distributed.

In some cases, the proliferation has a solid pattern and no secondary lumens are evident. Cytologically, the lesion is composed of cells with indistinct cell margins, variation in the tinctorial features of the cytoplasm and variation in shape and size of nuclei. Admixture of epithelial, myoepithelial or metaplastic apocrine cells is not uncommon. The presence or

Table 1.12
Usual ductal hyperplasia.

Architectural features
1. Irregular fenestrations
2. Peripheral fenestrations
3. Stretched or twisted epithelial bridges
4. Streaming
5. Uneven distribution of nuclei and overlapped nuclei

Cellular features
1. Multiple cell types
2. Variation in appearance of epithelial cells
3. Indistinct cell margins and deviation from a round contour
4. Variation in the appearance of nuclei

One of the most important indicators of UDH is the presence of an admixture of two or more cell types (epithelial, myoepithelial and/or metaplastic apocrine cells).

absence of either microcalcifications or necrosis does not impact the diagnosis. UDH with necrosis, a rare event, may be mistaken for DCIS; the diagnosis should be based on the cytological features and not the presence of necrotic debris. UDH generally displays either diffuse or a mosaic pattern of positivity with high molecular weight cytokeratins {1963, 2126} such as CK5, CK1/5/10/14 (clone CK34betaE12 or clone D5/16 B4); it is also positive for E-cadherin. In UDH, the percentage of ER-positive cells was found slightly increased compared to the normal breast {2667}. Increased levels of cyclin D1 expression were recently described in 11-19% of UDH cases {1172,3264}.

Genetic alterations
Approximately 7% of UDH show some degree of aneuploidy. Loss of heterozygosity (LOH) for at least one locus, has been noted in one-third of UDH {2071}. On chromosome 11p, LOH was present in 10-20% of UDH cases {72,2071}. Losses on 16q and 17p were identified in UDH lesions without evidence of adjacent carcinoma {1037} whereas no alterations were reported by others {301}. In UDH adjacent to carcinoma, polysomy of chromosome 1 as well as increased signal frequencies for the 20q13 region (typically present in DCIS) were identified by FISH {593,3100}. By CGH, UDH lesions adjacent to carcinoma showed gain on chromosome 20q and loss on 13q in 4 of 5 cases {136}, although no alteration was reported in another study {301}. Some recent CGH studies suggest that a proportion of UDH lesions is monoclonal {1037,1358}, and that a subset shows alterations similar to those observed in ADH {1037}; however, the frequency of genetic alterations seen in UDH using LOH and CGH is much lower than in ADH. TP53 protein expression has not been demonstrated in UDH or in any other benign proliferative lesions {1567}. Mutations of the *TP53* gene are also absent, except as inherited mutations in Li-Fraumeni patients {72}.

Flat epithelial atypia

Definition
A presumably neoplastic intraductal alteration characterized by replacement of the native epithelial cells by a single or 3-5 layers of mildly atypical cells.

Synonyms

Ductal intraepithelial neoplasia 1A (DIN 1A); clinging carcinoma, monomorphous type; atypical cystic lobules; atypical lobules, type A; atypical columnar change.

Risk of progression

Some cases of flat epithelial atypia may progress to invasive breast cancer but no quantitative epidemiological data are currently available for risk estimation.

Histopathology

A flat type of epithelial atypia, this change is characterized by replacement of the native epithelial cells by a single layer of mildly atypical cells often with apical snouts, or proliferation of a monotonous atypical cell population in the form of stratification of uniform, cuboidal to columnar cells generally up to 3-5 cell layers with occasional mounding. Arcades and micropapillary formations are absent or very rare. The TDLUs involved are variably distended and may contain secretory or floccular material that often contains microcalcifications.

Genetic alterations

Data on genetic alterations in flat epithelial atypia are limited. LOH has been found in at least one locus in 70% of cases in a study evaluating eight loci in thirteen lesions {1889}. LOH on 11q (D11S1311) was the most commonly noted in 50% of the pure flat atypia,

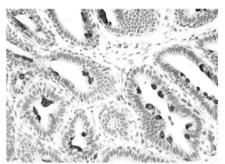

Fig. 1.82 Flat epithelial atypia. Immunostain for CK34βE12 shows no staining in the neoplastic cells lining the ductules, but the residual luminal epithelial cells adherent along the luminal surface show intense staining.

while among seven flat atypias associated with infiltrating carcinomas, the frequency of LOH on 11q (D11S1311) was 57% {1889}.

Atypical ductal hyperplasia (ADH)

Definition

A neoplastic intraductal lesion characterized by proliferation of evenly distributed, monomorphic cells and associated with a moderately elevated risk for progression to invasive breast cancer.

Synonyms

Ductal intraepithelial neoplasia 1B (DIN 1B), atypical intraductal hyperplasia.

Risk of progression

The Cancer Committee of the College of American Pathologists has assigned ADH a moderately increased risk (RR of 4.0-5.0) for subsequent development of invasive breast cancer {885}. Following a breast biopsy diagnosis of ADH, 3.7-22% of the women develop invasive carcinomas {299,733,1520,2886}. On the other hand, ADH has also been present in 2.2% {2158} to 10.5% {1688} of controls who did not develop subsequent carcinoma. The average interval to the subsequent development of invasive carcinoma is 8.3 years compared to 14.3 years for women with UDH {2886}.

However, drastically different relative risk (RR) estimations have been reported for ADH, ranging from a low of 2.4 to a high of 13 {412,732,1688,1775,1830,2155, 2158}. The upper values are even higher than the RR of 8-11 suggested for DCIS {732,885}. On the other hand, the RR of 2.4 for ADH reported in one study {1775} is much closer to the RR of 1.9 associated with UDH.

Histopathology

The most distinctive feature of this lesion is the proliferation of evenly distributed, monomorphic cells with generally ovoid to rounded nuclei. The cells may grow in micropapillae, tufts, fronds, arcades, rigid bridges, solid and cribriform patterns. Cytologically, ADH corresponds to low grade DCIS.

ADH is diagnosed when characteristic cells coexist with patterns of UDH, and/or there is partial involvement of TDLU by classic morphology. There is currently no general agreement on whether quantitative criteria should be applied to separate ADH from low grade DCIS. Some define the upper limit of ADH as one or more completely involved duct/ductular cross sections measuring ≤2 mm in aggregate, while others require that the characteristic cytology and architecture be present completely in two spaces. Microcalcifications may be absent, focal or extensive within the lumen of involved ducts; its presence does not impact diagnosis.

Immunoprofile
ERBB2 protein overexpression is rare in ADH {72,1172}, in contrast to high amplification rates in high grade DCIS, suggesting that ERBB2 alterations are either

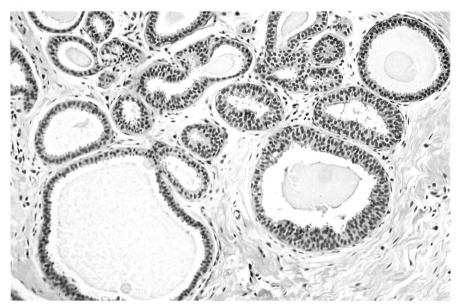

Fig. 1.81 Flat epithelial atypia. A terminal duct-lobular unit with distended acini and a floccular secretory luminal content. The spaces are lined by one to three layers of monotonous atypical cells.

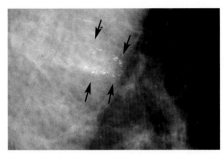

Fig. 1.83 Atypical ductal hyperplasia. Several rounded calcifications, possibly including 1-2 "tea cup" shaped calcifications are seen. Usually such calcifications indicate benign changes. However, the calcifications appear to follow two ducts. Furthermore, a faint group of very fine microcalcifications can barely be perceived.

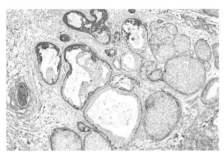

Fig. 1.84 Atypical ductal hyperplasia. A terminal duct-lobular unit with dilated ductules that are partly filled with a CK5/6 negative ductal proliferation which on H&E had the characteristics of a low grade DCIS. Note on the left side some cytokeratin positive ductules.

not an early event in malignant transformation or that they are largely restricted to high grade DCIS. Increased levels of cyclin D1 expression were recently described in 27-57% of ADH {1172, 3264}. Nuclear accumulation of the TP53 protein is absent in ADH and low grade DCIS {1567}. Nearly 90% of ADH are negative for high molecular weight cytokeratins 1/5/10/14 (clones CK34BetaE12 and D5/16 B4), an important feature in separating ADH from UDH {1963,2126}.

Genetic alterations
Fifty percent of ADH cases share their LOH patterns with invasive carcinomas from the same breast, strongly supporting a precursor relationship between these lesions {1567}. LOH has been identified frequently on chromosomes 16q, 17p, and 11q13 {1567,1570}. *TP53* mutations are restricted to affected members of Li-Fraumeni families.

Ductal carcinoma in situ (DCIS)

Definition
A neoplastic intraductal lesion characterized by increased epithelial proliferation, subtle to marked cellular atypia and an inherent but not necessarily obligate tendency for progression to invasive breast cancer.

ICD-O code   8500/2

Synonyms
Intraductal carcinoma, ductal intraepithelial neoplasia (DIN 1C to DIN 3).

Risk of progression
DCIS is considered a precursor lesion (obligate or non-obligate), with a relative risk (RR) of 8-11 for the development of invasive breast cancer {732,885}. However, there is evidence that conser-

vative treatment (complete local eradication) is usually curative (see below).

Epidemiology
A striking increase in the detection of DCIS has been noted with the introduction of widespread screening mammography and increasing awareness of breast cancer in the general population since 1983. The average annual increase in the incidence rate of DCIS in the decade of 1973 to 1983 was 3.9% compared to 17.5% annually in the decade between 1983 to 1992, increasing from 2.4 per 100,000 women in 1973 to 15.8 per 100,000 in 1992 for women of all races, an overall increase of 557% {794}. In the US, data from the National Cancer Institute's Surveillance, Epidemiology and End Results (SEER) program noted that the proportion of breast carcinomas diagnosed as DCIS increased from 2.8% in 1973 to 14.4% in 1995 {794}. While close to 90% of pre-mammography DCIS were of the high grade comedo type, nearly 60% of mammographically detected lesions are non-comedo and this percentage is increasing.

Interestingly, despite the more limited surgical excisions, mortality from "DCIS" has declined. Of women with DCIS diagnosed between 1978 and 1983 (pre-mammographic era), 3.4% died of breast cancer at 10 years, despite having been treated by mastectomy in the vast majority of cases. On the other hand, only 1.9% of women diagnosed with DCIS between 1984 and 1989 died of breast cancer at 10 years, despite the increasing trend toward lumpectomy {794}. Judging from the 10-year follow-

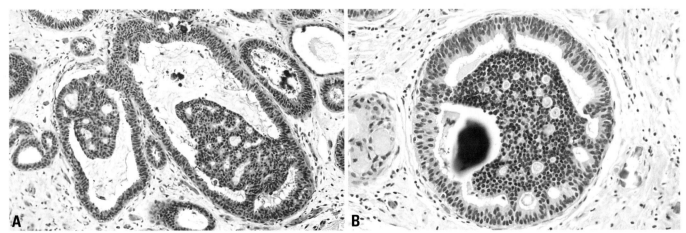

Fig. 1.85 Atypical ductal hyperplasia. **A** Two adjacent ducts showing partial cribriform involvement in a background of flat epithelial atypia. **B** Partial involvement of a duct by a cribriform proliferation of uniform, rounded cells in the setting of a flat epithelial atypia. Microcalcification is also present.

up period currently available for these women, it appears as if "DCIS per se is not a life threatening disease" {794}. The deaths that do occur are related to an undetected invasive carcinoma present at the time of the initial diagnosis of DCIS, progression of residual incompletely excised DCIS to invasive carcinoma, or development of a de novo invasive carcinoma elsewhere in the breast {794}.

Clinical features

In countries where population screening is performed, the vast majority of DCIS (>85%) are detected by imaging alone. Only approximately 10% of DCIS are associated with some clinical findings and up to 5% is detected incidentally in surgical specimens, obtained for other reasons. Clinical findings, which may be associated with DCIS include (i) palpable abnormality, (ii) pathological nipple discharge and (iii) nipple alterations associated with Paget disease.

Imaging

Mammography constitutes by far the most important method for the detection of DCIS. In current screening programs, 10-30% of all detected 'malignancies' are DCIS {810,1280}. In the majority of cases, mammographic detection is based on the presence of significant microcalcifications that are associated with most of these lesions {1206, 1231,2796}.

Calcifications associated with well differentiated DCIS are usually of the laminated, crystalline type resembling psammoma bodies. They often develop as pearl-like particles in the luminal spaces within the secretion of the tumour and appear on the mammogram as multiple clusters of granular microcalcifications that are usually fine. These multiple clusters reflect the frequent lobular arrangement of this type of DCIS.

Calcifications associated with poorly differentiated DCIS, are, histologically, almost exclusively of the amorphous type developing in the necrotic areas of the tumour. They appear on the mammogram as either linear, often branching, or as coarse, granular microcalcifications.

Calcifications associated with the intermediately differentiated DCIS may be of either the amorphous or the laminated type.

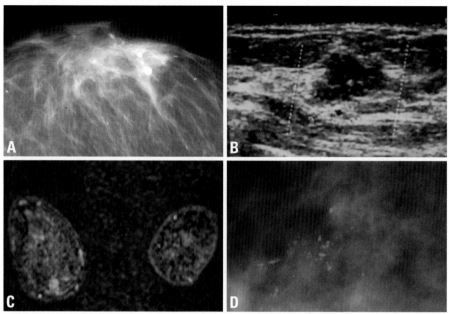

Fig. 1.86 Ductal carcinoma in situ images. **A** This galactogram was performed because of pathologic discharge from a single duct. On the galactogram multiple filling defects and truncation of the duct (approx. 4 cm behind the nipple) are demonstrated. **B** Low grade cribriform DCIS. In this patient, an ill circumscribed nodular nonpalpable (8 mm) low grade cribriform DCIS was detected by ultrasound. **C** MRI of an intermediate grade papillary DCIS. A strongly enhancing somewhat ill circumscribed lesion is visualized at 6 o'clock in the patient's right breast (coronal plane). **D** High grade comedo-type DCIS. Highly suspicious coarse granular and pleomorphic microcalcifications are shown, which follow the ductal course indicating presence of a DCIS.

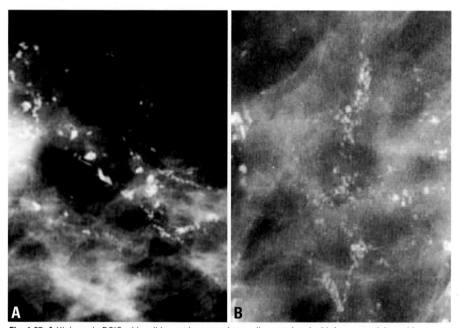

Fig. 1.87 A High grade DCIS with solid growth pattern is usually associated with fragmented, branching, casting type calcifications. Microfocus magnification, detail image. The rod-like, "casting-type" calcifications are characterisitc for Grade 3 DCIS. **B** High grade DCIS with micropapillary growth pattern is usually associated with dotted casting type calcifications.

About 17% of the lesions lack histologic evidence of microcalcifications; they are either mammographically occult or manifest as an architectural distortion, a nodular mass or nonspecific density {1206}.

Size, extent and distribution

Size/extent is an important factor in the management of DCIS. The assessment of extent of DCIS is complex and needs in optimal conditions the correlation of the

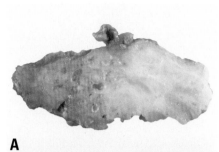

A

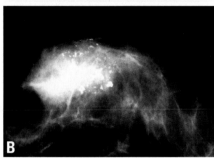

B

Fig. 1.88 Large excision biopsy of a high grade ductal carcinoma in situ. **A** Note the sharp demarcation between DCIS, comedo type (left), and adjacent fibrous stroma. **B** Mammography showing a large area with highly polymorphic microcalcifications.

mammogram, the specimen X-ray and the histologic slides. Since the majority of DCIS is non palpable, the mammographic estimate is the sole guide for resection. Therefore, data on the mammographic pathological correlation of the tumour size are essential for guiding the extent of surgery. The mammographic extent of a DCIS is defined as the greatest distance between the most peripherally located clusters of suspicious microcalcifications, and the histologic extent as the greatest distance between the most peripherally located, histologically verified, DCIS foci. Histologic evaluation supported by correlation with the X-ray of the sliced specimen allows a precise and reproducible assessment of the extent of any DCIS present. Whole organ studies have shown that mammography, on the basis of significant microcalcifications, generally underestimates the histologic or "real" size of DCIS by an average of 1-2 cm. In a series of DCIS cases with mammographic sizes up to 3 cm, the size difference was less than 2 cm in more than 80% of the cases {1231}.

DCIS may appear as a multifocal process due to the presence of multiple tumour foci on two-dimensional plane sections. However, these tumour spots may not necessarily represent separate foci. Intraductal tumour growth on three-

dimensional studies appears to be continuous rather than discontinuous {831}. More specifically, whereas poorly differentiated DCIS shows a predominantly continuous growth, the well differentiated DCIS, in contrast, may present a more discontinuous (multifocal) distribution.

These results have a direct implication on the reliability of the margin assessment of surgical specimens. In cases of poorly differentiated DCIS, margin assessment should, theoretically, be more reliable than well differentiated DCIS. In a multifocal process with discontinuous growth, the surgical margin may lie between the tumour foci, giving the false impression of a free margin.

The distribution of DCIS in the breast is typically not multicentric, defined as tumour involvement in two or more remote areas separated by uninvolved glandular tissue of 5 cm. On the contrary, DCIS is typically 'segmental' in distribution {1230}. In practical terms, this implies that two apparently separate areas of "malignant" mammographic microcalcifications usually do not represent separate fields of DCIS but rather a larger tumour in which the two mammographically identified fields are connected by DCIS, which is mammographically invisible due to the lack of detectable size of microcalcifications. One should be aware that single microscopic calcium particles smaller than about 80μ cannot be seen on conventional mammograms.

Grading

Although there is currently no universal agreement on classification of DCIS, there has been a move away from traditional architectural classification. Most modern systems use cytonuclear grade alone or in combination with necrosis and or cell polarization. Recent international consensus conferences held on this subject endorsed this change and recommended that, until more data emerges on clinical outcome related to pathology variables, grading of DCIS should form the basis of classification and that grading should be based primarily on cytonuclear features {6,7,1565,2346}.

Pathologists are encouraged to include additional information on necrosis, architecture, polarization, margin status, size and calcification in their reports.

Depending primarily on the degree of nuclear atypia, intraluminal necrosis and, to a lesser extent, on mitotic activity and

Table 1.13
Features of DCIS to be documented for the surgical pathology report.

Major lesion characteristics
1. Nuclear grade
2. Necrosis
3. Architectural patterns
Associated features
1. Margins If positive, note focal or diffuse involvement. Distance from any margin to the nearest focus of DCIS.
2. Size (either extent or distribution)
3. Microcalcifications (specify within DCIS or elsewhere)
4. Correlate morphological findings with specimen imaging and mammographic findings

calcification, DCIS is generally divided into three grades; the first two features constitute the major criteria in the majority of grading systems. It is not uncommon to find admixture of various grades of DCIS as well as various cytological variants of DCIS within the same biopsy or even within the same ductal space. When more than one grade of DCIS is present, the proportion (percentage) of various grades should be noted in the diagnosis {2876}. It is important to note that a three tiered grading system does not necessarily imply progression from grade 1 or well differentiated to grade 3 or poorly differentiated DCIS.

Histopathology
Low grade DCIS
Low grade DCIS is composed of small, monomorphic cells, growing in arcades, micropapillae, cribriform or solid patterns. The nuclei are of uniform size and have a regular chromatin pattern with inconspicuous nucleoli; mitotic figures

Table 1.14
Minimal criteria for low grade DCIS.

Cytological features
1. Monotonous, uniform rounded cell population
2. Subtle increase in nuclear-cytoplasmic ratio
3. Equidistant or highly organized nuclear distribution
4. Round nuclei
5. Hyperchromasia may or may not be present
Architectural features
Arcades, cribriform, solid and/or micropapillary pattern

are rare. Some require complete involvement of a single duct cross section by characteristic cells and architecture, while others require either involvement of two spaces or one or more duct cross sections exceeding 2 mm in diameter. Microcalcifications are generally of the psammomatous type. There may be occasional desquamated cells within the ductal lumen but the presence of necrosis and comedo histology are unacceptable within low grade DCIS.

DCIS with micropapillary pattern may be associated with a more extensive distribution in multiple quadrants of the breast compared to other variants {2584}. The working group's minimal criteria for diagnosis of low grade DCIS are shown in Table 1.14.

Intermediate grade DCIS

Intermediate grade DCIS lesions are often composed of cells cytologically similar to those of low grade DCIS, forming solid, cribriform or micropapillary patterns, but with some ducts containing intraluminal necrosis. Others display nuclei of intermediate grade with occasional nucleoli and coarse chromatin; necrosis may or may not be present. The distribution of amorphous or laminated microcalcifications is generally similar to that of low grade DCIS or it may display characteristics of both low grade and high grade patterns of microcalcification.

High grade DCIS

High grade DCIS is usually larger than 5 mm but even a single <1 mm ductule with the typical morphological features is sufficient for diagnosis. It is composed of highly atypical cells proliferating as one layer, forming micropapillae, cribriform or solid patterns. Nuclei are high grade, markedly pleomorphic, poorly polarized, with irregular contour and distribution, coarse, clumped chromatin and prominent nucleoli. Mitotic figures are usually common but their presence is not required. Characteristic is the comedo necrosis with abundant necrotic debris in duct lumens surrounded by a generally solid proliferation of large pleomorphic tumour cells. However, intraluminal necrosis is not obligatory. Even a single layer of highly anaplastic cells lining the duct in a flat fashion is sufficient. Amorphous microcalcifications are common.

Unusual variants

A minority of the DCIS lesions is composed of spindled {827}, apocrine {2887}, signet ring, neuroendocrine, squamous or clear cells. There is no consensus or uniform approach to grading of these unusual variants. Some believe assessment of nuclear features and necrosis can be applied to grading of the

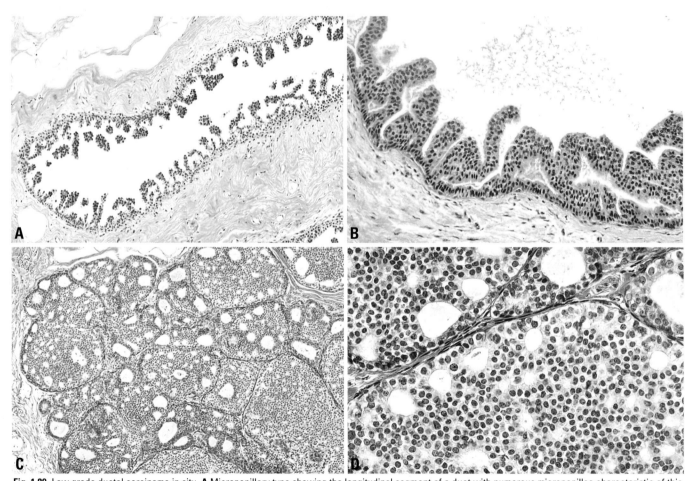

Fig. 1.89 Low grade ductal carcinoma in situ. **A** Micropapillary type showing the longitudinal segment of a duct with numerous micropapillae characteristic of this variant. **B** Micropapillary type. The micropapillae lack a fibrovascular core and are composed of a piling of uniform cells with rounded nuclei. **C** Cribriform type. Multiple adjacent ducts are distended by a sieve-like proliferation of monotonous uniform cells. The multiple spaces are rounded and distributed in an organized fashion. **D** Cribriform type. A highly uniform population of cells with round nuclei distributed equidistant from one another grow in a cribriform pattern.

unusual variants as well. Using this approach many apocrine DCIS lesions qualify as high grade, while a minority would qualify as intermediate or, rarely, high grade DCIS. The clear and spindle cell DCIS are sometimes found coexistent and continuous with typical low grade DCIS, but often the nuclei are moderately atypical qualifying the lesions as intermediate grade DCIS. High nuclear grade spindle or clear cell DCIS is extremely rare. A vast majority of apocrine carcinomas are ER, PR and BCL2 negative, but androgen receptor positive {2888}.

Proliferation

In vivo labelling with bromodeoxyuridine (BrdU) has found no significant differences between proliferating cell fraction among UDH and ADH, but the proliferating cell fraction is significantly increased in DCIS {412}. With the Ki67 antibody, the highest proliferating index (PI) of 13% has been noted among the comedo DCIS, while the PI for low grade DCIS, cribriform type is 4.5% and for micropapillary type, it is 0% {61}.

DNA Ploidy: Aneuploidy has been found in 7% of UDH, 13-36% of ADH, and 30-72% of low to high grade DCIS respectively {408,579,792}.

Hormone receptor expression

Estrogen plays a central role in regulating the growth and differentiation of breast epithelium as well as in the expression of other genes including the progesterone receptor (PR) {72}. The presence and concentration of the two receptors are used, not only as a clinical index of potential therapeutic response, but also as markers of prognosis for invasive breast carcinomas {196}. Only a few

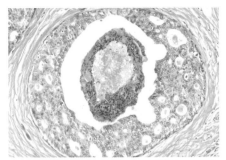

Fig. 1.91 DCIS, intermediate grade (DCIS grade 2). This typical and most common intermediate grade DCIS is characterized by a cribriform growth pattern and intraluminal necrosis.

studies have evaluated estrogen receptor (ER) in intraductal proliferative breast lesions. Among DCIS, about 75% of the cases show ER expression {72,1399}, and an association between ER positivity and the degree of differentiation has been described {1399}. There is agreement that nearly all examples of ADH express high levels of ER in nearly all the cells {72,1301,2667}. The relationship between ER positive cell numbers and patient age, as found in normal breast epithelium, is lost in these ADH lesions, indicating autonomy of ER expression or of the cells expressing the receptor {2667}.

Differential diagnosis

The solid variant of low grade DCIS may be misinterpreted as lobular neoplasia (LN). Immunohistochemistry for E-cadherin and CK1/5/10/14 (clone CK34BetaE12) are helpful in separating the two. Low grade DCIS is E-cadherin positive in 100% of cases {337, 1090,3034} and CK34BetaE12 negative in 92% of cases {337,1890}, whereas lobular neoplasia (LN) is E-cadherin negative {337,1033} and CK34BetaE12 positive in nearly all cases {337}. The presence of individual or clusters of cells invading the stroma (microinvasion) around a duct with DCIS is a frequent source of diagnostic problems. The difficulty is compounded by the frequent presence of dense lymphoplasmacytic infiltrate around the involved ducts. Immunostains for an epithelial and myoepithelial marker are helpful optimally in the form of double immunostaining; the epithelial cell marker can unmask the haphazard distribution of the cells, while the absence of a myoepithelial cell layer would generally ascertain the invasive nature of the cells in question. Despite all

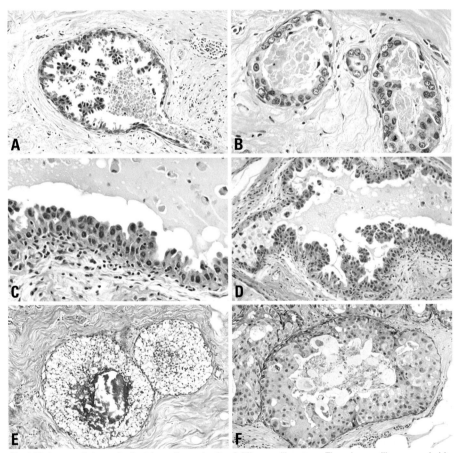

Fig. 1.90 Intermediate grade ductal carcinoma in situ. **A** Micropapillary type. The micropapillae are varied in shape and composed of cells with moderately atypical, pleomorphic nuclei. A few apoptotic cells are present in the lumen. **B** Flat type, approaching high grade DCIS. Two adjacent ductal spaces are lined by atypical cells, rare mitotic figures and a few apoptotic nuclei. **C, D** Duct/part of a duct with micropapillary atypical epithelial proliferation. Note secretory material in the lumen that should not be mixed up with comedo-type necrosis. **E** Clear cell type. The neoplastic cells have clear cytoplasm with moderate nuclear pleomorphism. **F** Apocrine type with moderate nuclear size variation. The abundant pink, granular cytoplasm suggests an apocrine cell type.

these added studies, the distinction can remain impossible in some cases.

An unknown, but relatively small, proportion of intraepithelial neoplasias cannot be easily separated into ductal or lobular subtypes on the basis of pure H&E morphology. Using immunostains for E-cadherin and CK34βE12, some of these will qualify as ductal (E-cadherin+, CK34BetaE12-), some as lobular (E-cadherin-, CK34βE12+), while others are either negative for both markers (negative hybrid) or positive for both (positive hybrid) {337}. This important group requires further evaluation as it may reflect a neoplasm of mammary stem cells or the immediate post-stem cells with plasticity and potential to evolve into either ductal or lobular lesions {338}.

Expression profiling

Gene expression profiling has become a powerful tool in the molecular classification of cancer. Recently, the feasibility and reproducibility of array technology in DCIS was demonstrated {1721}. More than 100 changes in gene expression in DCIS were identified in comparison with control transcripts. Several genes, previously implicated in human breast cancer progression, demonstrated differential expression in DCIS versus non-malignant breast epithelium, e.g. up-regulation of lactoferrin (a marker of estrogen stimulation), PS2 (an estrogen-responsive marker), and SIX1 (a homeobox protein frequently up-regulated in metastatic breast cancer), and down-regulation of oxytocin receptor {3148}.

Genetic alterations

Most studies on somatic gene alterations in premalignant breast lesions are based on small sample numbers and have not been validated by larger series {72}, with the exceptions of the *TP53* tumour suppressor gene and the oncogenes *ERBB2* and *CCND1* {72,196}. Other genes, not discussed here (e.g. oncogenes *c-myc*, *fes*, *c-met*, and tumour suppresser gene *RB1*) may also play an important role in breast carcinogenesis (for review see {3048}).

Cytogenetics

Conventional cytogenetic analysis of premalignant lesions of the breast has been carried out in only a small number of cases, and, as with invasive ductal

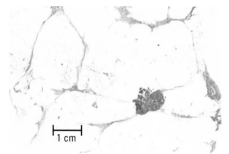

Fig. 1.92 High grade ductal carcinoma in situ forming a tumour mass. Large section, H&E.

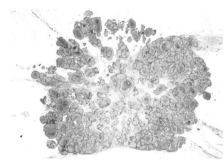

Fig. 1.93 High grade ductal carcinoma in situ. Low power view shows extensive DCIS with calcification.

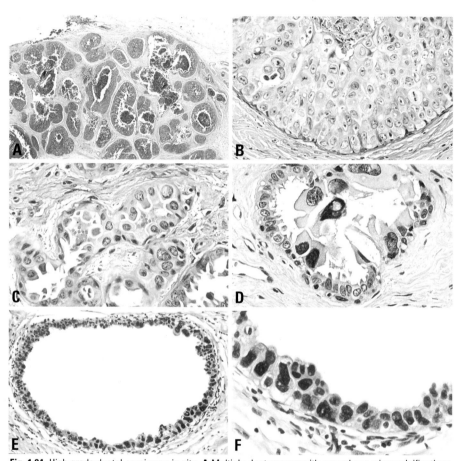

Fig. 1.94 High grade ductal carcinoma in situ. **A** Multiple duct spaces with amorphous microcalcifications and peripheral epithelial proliferations. **B** Comedo type. The proliferating cells show significant nuclear atypia, mitotic figures and there is intraluminal necrosis. **C** Flat type. Significantly atypical cells have replaced the native, normal mammary epithelium. **D** Flat type. A highly anaplastic cell population has replaced the native epithelial cell layer. **E** Flat type with significant nuclear pleomorphism. **F** Flat type. A highly anaplastic cell population has replaced the native epithelial layer, but there is no significant intraluminal proliferation.

carcinoma, abnormalities of chromosomes 1 and 16 have been identified in DCIS {1146,1567}. FISH-analyses using DNA probes to centromeric sequences of almost all chromosomes frequently identified polysomy of chromosome 3, 10, and 17 and loss of chromosome 1, 16, and 18 in DCIS {1949}.

Chromosomal imbalance

CGH studies of DCIS have demonstrated a large number of chromosomal alterations including frequent gains on 1q, 6q, 8q, 17q, 19q, 20q, and Xq, and losses on 8p, 13q, 16q, 17p, and 22q {134,301,365,366,1333,1548,3045}. Most of these chromosomal imbalances resemble those identified in invasive ductal carcinoma, adding weight to the theory that DCIS is a direct precursor.

LOH

In DCIS, loss of heterozygosity (LOH) was frequently identified at several loci on chromosomes 1 {1942}, 3p21 {1743}, and chromosomes 8p, 13q, 16q, 17p, 17q, and 18q {924,2317,3036}. The highest reported rates of LOH in DCIS are between 50% and 80% and involve loci on chromosomes 16q, 17p, and 17q, suggesting that altered genes in these regions may be important in the development of DCIS {72,924,3036}. Among more than 100 genetic loci studied so far on chromosome 17, nearly all DCIS lesions showed at least one LOH {72,301,924,1942,2071,2317,2475}. By CGH and FISH, low and some intermediate grade DCIS and invasive tubular carcinoma (G1) show loss of 16q, harbouring one of the cadherin gene clusters, whereas some intermediate grade and high grade DCIS and nearly all G2 and G3 invasive ductal carcinomas show no loss of genetic material on this locus but have alterations of other chromosomes (-13q, +17p, +20q). Based upon this data, a genetic progression model was proposed {301}.

ERBB2

The ERBB2 (Her2/neu) oncogene has received attention because of its association with lymph node metastases, short relapse free time, poor survival, and decreased response to endocrine and chemotherapy in breast cancer patients {72,1567}. Studies of ERB B2 have used mainly FISH technique to identify amplification and immunohistochemistry (IHC) to detect over expression of the oncogene, which are highly correlated {72}. Amplification and/or over expression was observed on average in 30% of DCIS, correlating directly with differentiation {72}; it was detected in a high proportion of DCIS of high nuclear grade (60-80%) but was not common in low nuclear grade DCIS {196}. Patients with ERBB2 positive tumours may benefit from adjuvant treatment with monoclonal antibody (Herceptin).

Cyclin D1

This protein plays an important part in regulating the progress of the cell during the G1 phase of the cell cycle. The gene

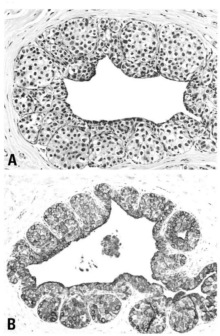

Fig. 1.95 Unusual intraductal proliferation. **A** The lesion shows a uniform cell population proliferating in a solid pagetoid pattern similar to lobular neoplasia, but the cells appear more adherent than in typical lobular neoplasia (LN). **B** Double immunostain is positive for both CK34βE12 (purple) and E-cadherin (brown), qualifying the lesion as a hybrid positive type that may suggest the diagnosis of DCIS.

(CCND1) is considered a potential oncogene, but in clinical studies of invasive breast cancer, overexpression of cyclin D1 was found to be associated with estrogen receptor expression and low histological grade, both markers of good prognosis {1007}. Amplification of CCND1 occurs in about 20% of DCIS and is more commonly found in high grade than in low grade DCIS (32% versus 8%) {2700}. The cyclin D1 protein was detected in 50% of cases, and high levels were more likely in low grade than in the intermediate and high grade DCIS {2700}. Although so far no oncogene has been identified on chromosome 20q13, amplification of this region was frequently found in DCIS {134,856}.

TP53 mutations

The TP53 protein is a transcription factor involved in the control of cell proliferation, response to DNA damage, apoptosis and several other signaling pathways. It is the most commonly mutated tumour suppressor gene in sporadic breast cancer {196} and this is generally associated with aggressive biological features and poor clinical outcome. Most TP53 mutations are missense point mutations resulting in an inactivated protein that accumulates in the cell nucleus {72,712}. In DCIS, TP53 mutations were found with different frequency among the three histological grades, ranging from rare in low grade DCIS, 5% in intermediate-grade, and common (40%) in high grade DCIS {712,3048}.

Prognosis and predictive factors

The most important factor influencing the possibility of recurrence is persistence of neoplastic cells post-excision; primary and recurrent DCIS generally have the same LOH pattern, with acquisition of additional alterations in the latter {1670} The significance of margins is mainly to ascertain complete excision. In randomized clinical trials, comedo necrosis was found to be an important predictor of local recurrence in the NSABP-B17 trial {2843}, while solid and cribriform growth patterns along with involved margin of excision were found to be predictive of local recurrence in EORTC-10853 trial {270,271}. In retrospective trials, on the other hand, high nuclear grade, larger lesion size, comedo necrosis and involved margins of excision were all found to be predictive of local recurrence following breast conservative treatment for DCIS.

Although mastectomy has long been the traditional treatment for this disease, it likely represents over-treatment for many patients, particularly those with small, mammographically detected lesions. Careful mammographic and pathologic evaluation are essential to help assess patient suitability for breast conserving treatment.

While excision and radiation therapy of DCIS (with or without Tamoxifen) have significantly reduced the chances of recurrence {866,870}, some patients with small, low grade lesions appear to be adequately treated with excision alone, whereas those with extensive lesions may be better served by mastectomy. Better prognostic markers are needed to help determine which DCIS lesions are likely to recur or to progress to invasive cancer following breast conserving treatment. The optimal management is evolving as data accumulates from a variety of prospective studies.

Microinvasive carcinoma

I.O. Ellis
F.A. Tavassoli

Definition

A tumour in which the dominant lesion is non-invasive, but in which there are one or more clearly separate small, microscopic foci of infiltration into non-specialized interlobular stroma. If there is doubt about the presence of invasion, the case should be classified as an in situ carcinoma.

ICD-O code

Microinvasive carcinoma is not generally accepted as a tumour entity and does not have an ICD-O code.

Epidemiology

Microinvasive carcinomas are rare and occur mostly in association with an in situ carcinoma. They account for far less than 1% of breast carcinomas even in pure consultation practices where the largest number of microinvasive carcinoma is reviewed {2680}.

Clinical features

There are no specific clinical features associated with microinvasive carcinoma. These lesions are typically associated with ductal carcinoma in situ which is often extensive. The features associated with the associated in situ component are responsible for detection as a mass lesion, mammographic calcification or a nipple discharge. (See clinical features of ductal and lobular carcinoma in situ).

Histopathology

There is no generally accepted agreement on the definition of microinvasive carcinoma. This is particularly true for the maximum diameter compatible with the diagnosis of microinvasive carcinoma.

Size limits

Microinvasive carcinoma has been defined as having a size limit of 1 mm {1984,2425,2739,2905}. Consequently, diagnosis of microinvasive carcinoma is rare in routine practice, in contrast to larger (>1 mm) foci of invasion. Alternatively, it has also been defined as a single focus no larger than 2 mm in maximum dimension or 2-3 foci, none exceeding 1 mm in maximum dimension. Some studies have provided no maximum size {2579,3140} or criteria {1467, 2703}. Others have defined the microinvasive component as a percentage of the surface of the histologic sections {2583}. Some have described subtypes separating those purely composed of single cells and those also containing cell clusters and/or tubules of non-gradable tumour without providing information about maximum size, extent, or number of microinvasive foci {656}. More precise definitions accept an unlimited number of clearly separate foci of infiltration into the stroma with none exceeding 1 mm in diameter {80}, 1 or 2 foci of microinvasion with none exceeding 1 mm {2695}, a single focus not exceeding 2 mm or three foci, none exceeding 2 mm in maximum diameter {2680}.

Some authors propose that the definition of microinvasive carcinoma requires extension of the invasive tumour cells beyond the specialized lobular stroma {774,2905} despite the definitive presence of vascular channels both within

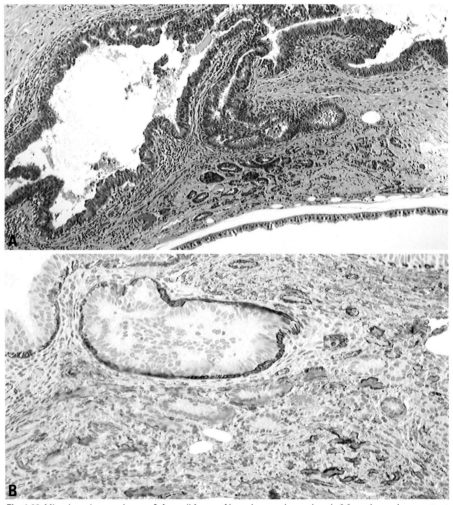

Fig. 1.96 Microinvasive carcinoma. **A** A small focus of invasive carcinoma barely 0.8 mm in maximum extent is present adjacent to an aggregate of ducts displaying mainly flat epithelial atypia. **B** Immunostain for actin shows no evidence of a myoepithelial (ME) cell layer around the invasive tubules, in contrast to persistence of a distinct ME cell layer around the adjacent tubules with flat epithelial atypia.

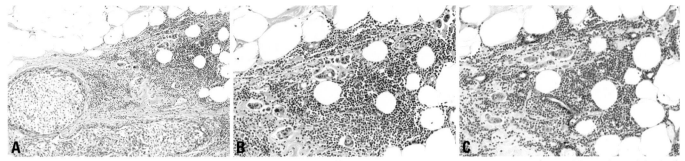

Fig. 1.97 Microinvasive carcinoma. **A** Two ducts are filled by DCIS, while small clusters of carcinoma cells invade the stroma (upper right quadrant of the field) admixed with a dense lymphocytic infiltrate. **B** Higher magnification shows small invasive cell clusters within stromal spaces distributed over a 0.7 mm area and surrounded by a dense lymphocytic infiltrate. **C** Immunostain for actin decorates the vessel walls, while absence of myoepithelial cells around the tumour cell clusters confirms their invasive nature.

the specialized lobular stroma and immediately surrounding the basement membrane that invests the ducts.

Associated lesions
Typically, microinvasive carcinoma occur in larger areas of high grade DCIS in which the tumour cell population extends to involve lobular units or areas of benign disease.
Microinvasion occurs in association not only with all grades of DCIS, including papillary DCIS, but also with other precursor lesions of invasive breast cancer, e.g. lobular neoplasia (LN) {1226,1249, 1993}, indicating that at least some forms of lobular neoplasia behave as true precursors of invasive lesions.

Stromal reaction
Microinvasion is most often present in a background of significant periductal / perilobular lymphocytic infiltrate or an altered desmoplastic stroma, features often present in cases of comedo DCIS. Angulation of mesenchymal structures may be emphasized by the plane of sectioning and can produce features reminiscent of invasive carcinoma. Basement membrane structures in such foci may be discontinuous but it is unusual to lose the entire basement membrane around such a lesion. Similarly myoepithelial cells may be scarce but are rarely totally absent in such areas.

Change in morphology
When true invasion extends into non-specialized stroma, the islands of tumour cells frequently adopt a different morphological character which is more typical of well established invasive mammary carcinoma of ductal NOS

type and is distinct from the patterns seen with cancerization of lobules.

Differential diagnosis
When there is doubt about the presence of invasion and particularly, if uncertainty persists even after recuts and immunostains for detection of myoepithelial cells, the case should be diagnosed as an in situ carcinoma. Similarly, suspicious lesions which disappear on deeper levels should be regarded as unproven, with no definite evidence of established invasion.
Invasion is associated with a loss of immunoreactivity to myoepithelial cells. A variety of markers is available for the identification of myoepithelial cells {3181}. The most helpful include smooth muscle actin, calponin, and smooth muscle myosin (heavy chain); the latter in particular shows the least cross-reactivity with myofibroblasts that may mimic a myoepithelial cell layer when apposed to the invasive cells.

Prognosis and predictive factors
In true microinvasive carcinomas of the breast, the incidence of metastatic disease in axillary lymph nodes is very low and the condition is generally managed clinically as a form of DCIS.
However, given the lack of a generally accepted standardized definition of microinvasive carcinoma, there is little evidence on the behaviour of microinvasive carcinoma. A recent detailed review of the literature {2425} concluded that a variety of different diagnostic criteria and definitions have been used and as a consequence it is difficult to draw any definitive conclusions.
There are studies that have found no evidence of axillary node metastases asso-

ciated with a finite number of invasive foci <1 mm in maximum dimension or a single invasive focus <2 mm {2680, 2695}. Others have shown a small percentage (up to 5%) with axillary node metastases {2453,2744} or have described up to 20% axillary node metastases {656,1472,2282,2579,2583}. Of 38 women who had undergone mastectomy for their minimally invasive carcinomas (a single focus <2 mm or up to 3 invasive foci, none exceeding 1 mm, with no axillary node metastases), developed recurrences or metastases {2680}. The few other studies with comparable, but not exactly the same definition, and follow-up data support the excellent prognosis for these tumours within the short periods of available follow-up {2453, 2695,3140}.
In practice, it may be impossible for pathologists to routinely examine an entire sample exhaustively. Therefore, it is quite possible that small foci of invasive carcinoma may be missed, particularly in the setting of extensive in situ carcinoma. For this reason, it may be appropriate to sample the lowest axillary lymph nodes, or sentinel node as a matter of routine, when treating patients by mastectomy for extensive DCIS with or without accompanying microinvasive carcinoma {1472}. The pathology report should provide the size of the largest focus along with the number of foci of invasion, noting any special studies utilized to arrive at the diagnosis, ie. 1.3 mm, 2 foci, immunocytochemistry.
Until there is a generally accepted definition with reliable follow-up data, microinvasive carcinoma of the breast remains an evolving concept that has not reached the status of a WHO-endorsed disease entity.

Intraductal papillary neoplasms

G. MacGrogan
F. Moinfar
U. Raju

Definition

Papillary neoplasms are characterized by epithelial proliferations supported by fibrovascular stalks with or without an intervening myoepithelial cell layer. They may occur anywhere within the ductal system from the nipple to the terminal ductal lobular unit (TDLU) and may be benign (intraductal papilloma), atypical, or malignant (intraductal papillary carcinoma).

Intraductal papilloma

A proliferation of epithelial and myoepithelial cells overlying fibrovascular stalks creating an arborescent structure within the lumen of a duct.

Intraductal papilloma of the breast is broadly divided into central (large duct) papilloma, usually located in the subareolar region, and peripheral papilloma arising in the TDLU {2092}. The confusing term "papillomatosis" should be avoided as it has been used for usual ductal hyperplasia as well as for multiple papillomas.

ICD-O code   8503/0

Central papilloma

Synonyms

Large duct papilloma, major duct papilloma.

Epidemiology

The incidence of the various forms of intraductal papillary lesions is uncertain due to the lack of consistent terminology. Overall, less than 10% of benign breast neoplasms correspond to papillomas {413,1098}. Central papillomas can occur at any age, but the majority present during the fourth and fifth decades {1098,1945}.

Clinical features

Unilateral sanguineous, or sero-sanguineous, nipple discharge is the most frequent clinical sign, and is observed in 64-88% of patients {3148}. A palpable mass is less frequent. Mammographic abnormalities include a circumscribed retro-areolar mass of benign appearance, a solitary retro-areolar dilated duct and, rarely, microcalcifications {401,3148}. Small papillomas may be mammographically occult because of their location in the central dense breast and usually lack of calcification. Typical sonographic features include a well defined smooth-walled, solid, hypoechoic nodule or a lobulated, smooth-walled, cystic lesion with solid components. Duct dilatation with visible solid intraluminal echoes is common {3176}.

Galactography shows an intraluminal smooth or irregular filling defect associated with obstructed or dilated ducts, or a complete duct obstruction with ret-

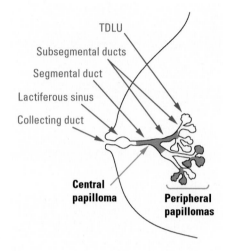

Fig. 1.98 Distribution of papillomas in breast.

rograde flow of contrast material. Galactography may be useful to the breast surgeon in identifying and localizing the discharging duct, prior to duct excision {3148}.

Macroscopy

Palpable lesions may form well circumscribed round tumours with a cauliflower-like mass attached by one or more pedicles to the wall of a dilated duct containing serous and/or sanguineous fluid. The size of central papillomas varies considerably from a few millimetres to 3-4 cm or larger and they can extend along the duct for several centimetres.

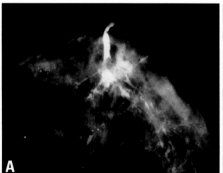
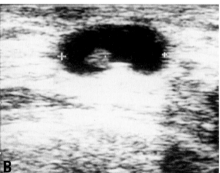

Fig. 1.99 Central papilloma. **A** Smooth intraluminal filling defect associated with duct dilatation. **B** Well defined smooth wall cystic lesion with a solid component.

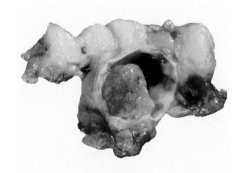

Fig. 1.100 Papilloma, gross. Nodular mass in a cystic duct.

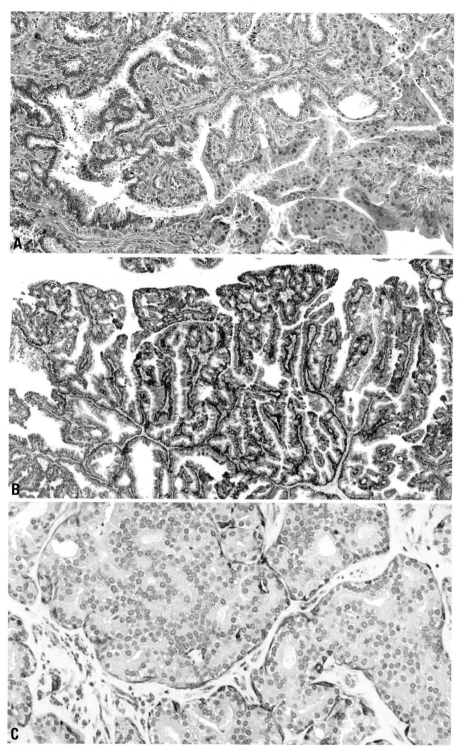

Fig. 1.101 A Typical morphology of a papilloma of the breast. **B** Cytokeratin (34βE12) staining decorates myoepithelial and some epithelial cells. **C** Papilloma with atypical ductal hyperplasia (ADH). Note HHF-35 immunoreactive myoepithelial cells at the periphery of ADH.

Histopathology

Papillomas are characterized by an arborescent structure composed of fibrovascular stalks covered by a layer of myoepithelial cells with overlying epithelial cells. In some lesions papillary and ductal patterns coexist. When the ductal pattern predominates and is associated with marked sclerosis, the term sclerosing papilloma may be used. Ductal adenoma is considered by some as a variant of generally sclerosing papilloma.

Papilloma may be subject to morphological changes such as inflammation, necrosis, myoepithelial hyperplasia, apocrine, squamous, sebaceous, mucinous, osseous and chondroid metaplasia as well as usual intraductal hyperplasia {148,893,1350,1945,2327,2420,2873}.

A pseudo-infiltrative pattern may be observed at the periphery of these lesions particularly in the sclerosing variant.

The myoepithelial cell layer may have an uneven distribution both in areas of UDH, ADH, and DCIS {2325}.

The entire range of ductal intraepithelial proliferations may arise within, or secondarily involve, a central papilloma. The clinical implications of such lesions have not at this time been fully established and should be considered in the context of the surrounding breast tissue.

Peripheral papilloma

Synonym
Microscopic papilloma.

Epidemiology
The average age at presentation of peripheral papillomas is similar to that of central papillomas or slightly younger {401,1097,1945}.

Clinical features
Peripheral papillomas are often clinically occult. They rarely present as a mass and nipple discharge is far less frequent in this group {401}. They are also usually mammographically occult, but they may manifest as peripherally situated microcalcifications, nodular prominent ducts or multiple small peripheral well circumscribed masses {401}. Microcalcifications may be located in the peripheral papillomas or in adjacent non-papillary intraductal proliferative lesions, e.g. ADH.

Macroscopy
Unless they are associated with other changes, peripheral papillomas are usually a microscopic finding.

Histopathology
Peripheral papillomas are usually multiple. They originate within the TDLUs from where they may extend into the larger ducts {2092}. The histological features are basically the same as for central papillomas. Compared to central papillomas, however, peripheral papillomas are more frequently observed in association

Table 1.15
Differential diagnosis of benign papilloma and intraductal papillary carcinoma.

Feature	Papilloma	Papillary intraductal carcinoma
Cell types covering fibrovascular stalks	Epithelial and myoepithelial	Epithelial (myoepithelial cells may be seen at periphery of duct wall)*
Nuclei	Normochromatic vesicular chromatin; variable in size and shape	May be hyperchromatic, with diffuse chromatin: relatively uniform in size and shape
Apocrine metaplasia	Frequent	Absent
Fibrovascular stalks	Usually broad and present throughout lesion; may show sclerosis	Often fine and may be absent in some areas; sclerosis uncommon
Immunohistochemical markers for myoepithelial cells (e.g. smooth muscle actin, HMW-CK [such as CK 5/6])	Positive	Negative*

* Myoepithelial cells may be present in some papillary carcinomas–see text for explanation.

with concomitant usual ductal hyperplasia, atypical intraductal hyperplasia, ductal carcinoma in situ or invasive carcinoma as well as with sclerosing adenosis or radial scar {1097,1945,2091,2092}. The term micropapilloma has been applied to the smallest type of peripheral papillomas corresponding to multiple microscopic papillomas that grow in foci of adenosis. Collagenous spherulosis, consisting of round eosinophilic spherules of basement membrane (type IV collagen), edged by myoepithelial cells may be seen in some peripheral papillomas.

Atypical papilloma

Atypical intraductal papillomas are characterized by the presence of a focal atypical epithelial proliferation with low grade nuclei. Such intraepithelial proliferations may occasionally resemble atypical ductal hyperplasia (ADH) or small foci of low grade DCIS.

Prognosis and predictive features of benign and atypical papillomas

The risk of subsequent invasive carcinoma associated with papillomas or atypical papillomas should be appreciated in the context of the surrounding breast tissue. A benign papilloma without surrounding changes is associated with a slightly increased relative risk of subsequent invasive breast carcinoma, similar to that of moderate or florid usual ductal hyperplasia in the breast proper {885,2151}. The relative risk associated

with peripheral papilloma may be higher compared to central papilloma. However, this risk also depends on the concurrent presence of other forms of proliferative disease and as yet no study has been designed to specifically answer this question {2151}. There is disagreement as to whether the risk of subsequent invasive breast carcinoma applies only to the same site in the ipsilateral breast or applies to both breasts {2151,2326}. The significance of atypia within a papilloma is still not clear and is obscured by the frequent concurrent presence of atypia within the surrounding breast parenchyma. It appears that if epithelial atypia is confined to the papilloma without surrounding proliferation or atypia the risk of subsequent invasive breast carcinoma is similar to that of non-atypical papilloma. As expected, epithelial atypia when present simultaneously both within and outside a papilloma is associated with a moderate to highly increased relative risk {2151}; this is not a reflection of the risk associated with pure atypical papilloma, however.

The standard treatment for papillomas has been complete excision with microscopic assessment of surrounding breast tissue. Because of potential variability within a papillary lesion, complete excision is prudent, regardless of the findings in a previous core biopsy.

The differential diagnosis of benign and malignant papillary lesions on frozen section can be extremely difficult and a definitive diagnosis should always be made only after examination of paraffin embedded material.

Intraductal papillary carcinoma

ICD-O code   8503/2

Synonym
Papillary carcinoma, non-invasive.

Definition
This lesion is located within a variably distended duct and may extend into its branches. It is characterized by proliferation of fibrovascular stalks and its diagnosis requires that 90% or more of

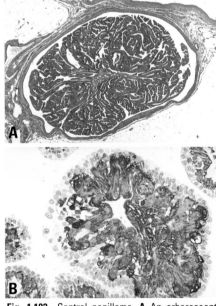

Fig. 1.102 Central papilloma. **A** An arborescent structure composed of papillary fronds within a dilated duct. **B** Myoepithelial hyperplasia with SMA positive "myoid" transformation.

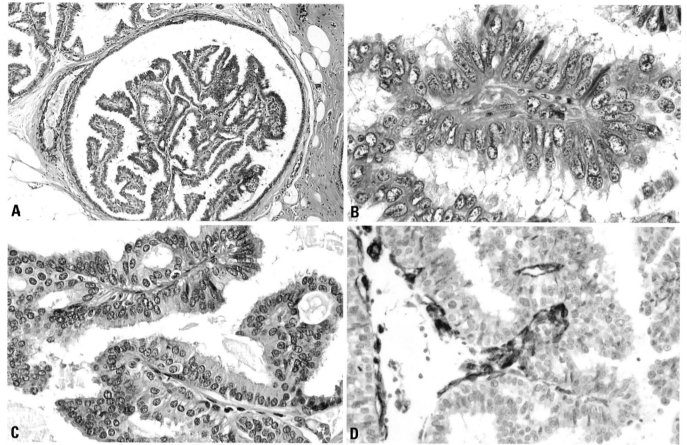

Fig. 1.103 Papillary intraductal carcinoma. **A** Cystically dilated duct with arborescent papillary tumour. **B** Papillary structure lined by epithelial columnar cells. **C** Two papillary structures lined by atypical cylindrical cells with formation of arcades. **D** Papillary structures are devoid of myoepithelial cells. Smooth muscle actin (SMA) immunostaining highlights vascular structures in papillary fronds. Epithelial cells lining the papillary fronds are CK 5/6 negative (not shown).

the papillary processes are totally devoid of a myoepithelial cell layer regardless of presence or absence of notable epithelial proliferation, and/or that any of the recognized patterns of low grade DCIS occupies 90% or more of the lesion.

These neoplasms can be either solitary and central in location corresponding to intracystic papillary carcinoma, or multifocal within the TDLU and correspond to the papillary type of DCIS.

Intracystic papillary carcinoma

Definition
This lesion is a variant of intraductal papillary carcinoma, located within a large cystic duct and characterized by thin fibrovascular stalks devoid of a myoepithelial cell layer and of a neoplastic epithelial cell population with histopathological features characteristic of low grade DCIS.

ICD-O code   8504/2

Synonyms
Intracystic papillary carcinoma, non-invasive; papillary intraductal carcinoma; papillary ductal carcinoma in situ; encysted papillary carcinoma.

Epidemiology
Less than 2% of breast carcinomas correspond to intraductal papillary carcinomas {413,1945}. The average age of occurrence is around 65 (range, 34-92 years) {413,1618}.

Clinical and macroscopic features
On the basis of clinical presentation and macroscopy, there are no distinctive features that can separate papilloma from papillary carcinoma, nonetheless, intracystic papillary carcinomas tend to be larger.

Histopathology
Intraductal papillary carcinoma is a papillary lesion usually of large size

(mean 2 cm, range 0.4-10 cm) located within a large cystic duct characterized by thin fibrovascular stalks devoid of a myoepithelial cell layer and a neoplastic epithelial cell population usually presenting characteristics of low grade DCIS. These cells are arranged in either solid, cribriform, micropapillary or stratified spindle cell patterns {413,1618, 1945}. Some may show a dimorphic cell

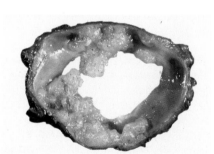

Fig. 1.104 Gross appearance of an intracystic papillary breast carcinoma. Macroscopically, the distinction between papilloma and papillary carcinoma may be difficult.

population (featuring epithelial and myo-epithelial differentiation) which may be mistaken for two cell types {1618}. Less frequently, the epithelial cell component presents the characteristics of intermediate or high grade DCIS. Concomitant DCIS may be present in the surrounding breast tissue. A complete absence of the myoepithelial cell layer in the papillary processes indicates a carcinoma; the presence of myoepithelial cells does not invariably exclude the diagnosis of intraductal papillary carcinoma, however. A myoepithelial cell layer is usually present in the lining of the duct wall into which the papillary carcinoma proliferates.

Solid and transitional cell variants have been described {1752,1905}. The distinctive features of the former are production of extracellular and intracellular mucin, association with mucinous carcinoma and often a spindle cell population. Argyrophilia and neuroendocrine features have been noted in a large number of the solid cases {694,1752,2955}. The transitional cell variant is characterized by proliferation of sheets of transitional type cells overlying the fibrovascular cores.

As with benign papillomas entrapment of epithelial structures within the wall can result in a pseudoinvasive pattern. A definitive diagnosis of invasive carcinoma associated with intracystic papillary carcinoma should only be considered when neoplastic epithelial structures infiltrate the breast tissue beyond the fibrous wall and have one of the recognized patterns of invasive carcinoma. Following a needle biopsy (fine needle aspiration or core biopsy), epithelial displacement into the needle tract, scar tissue or lymphatic spaces can mimic invasion {3231}.

Genetic alterations

Genetic alterations in the form of interstitial deletions {701}, LOH {1671}, numerical and structural alterations at chromosomes 16q and 1q with fusion of chromosomes 16 and 1 [der(1;16)] {2961} have been described, but the significance of these alterations are as yet, unclear.

Prognosis and predictive factors

Intraductal papillary carcinoma in the absence of concomitant DCIS or invasive carcinoma in the surrounding breast tissue has a very favourable prognosis with no reported lymph node metastases or disease-related deaths. The presence of

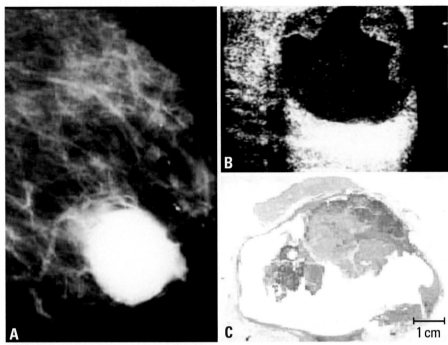

Fig. 1.105 Intracystic papillary carcinoma. **A** Left breast, medio-lateral oblique projection showing a 3x3 cm, solitary, high density circular mass in the lower half of the breast. **B** Breast ultrasound demonstrates intracystic growth. **C** Intracystic papillary carcinoma in situ. Large section histology.

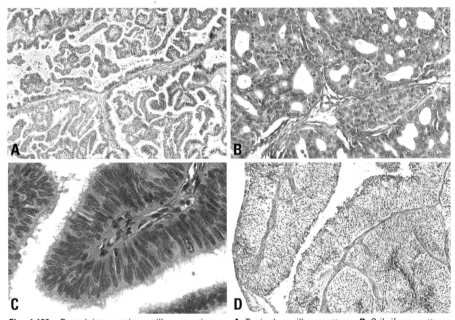

Fig. 1.106 Ductal intracystic papillary carcinoma. **A** Typical papillary pattern. **B** Cribriform pattern. **C** Stratified columnar cells, in the absence of myoepithelial cells. **D** Transitional cell-type pattern.

DCIS or invasive carcinoma in the surrounding breast tissue are associated with an increase in frequency of local recurrence (in situ or invasive) in the former, and an increase in local and metastatic rates in the latter {413}.

Complete excision of intraductal papillary carcinoma with adequate sampling

of the lesion and surrounding breast tissue is mandatory for treatment and appreciation of subsequent breast cancer risk.

Prognosis and management of papillary type of DCIS is similar to that of common DCIS and is dealt with in the corresponding chapter.

Benign epithelial proliferations

G. Bussolati
F.A. Tavassoli
B.B. Nielsen
I.O. Ellis
G. MacGrogan

Localization

There is little data on location or laterality of most benign breast lesions. As with carcinoma, the majority arise within the terminal duct lobular unit (TDLU). A major exception is the benign solitary intraductal papilloma, approximately 90% of which occurs in the large ducts in the central region of the breast {1098}. Other benign lesions specific to the nipple areolar complex include nipple adenoma and syringoma and are discussed in the chapter on nipple.

Clinical features

The predominant presenting symptoms in women attending a breast clinic are described in the section on Invasive Carcinoma, where signs and symptoms most likely to be associated with a low risk of malignancy are described. The frequency of benign conditions varies considerably with the age of the patient. Fibroadenoma is most frequent in younger patients, other localized benign lesions and cysts occur most frequently in women between the ages of 30 and 50. This contrasts with carcinoma, which is rare below the age of 40. The mammographic appearances of benign epithelial lesions are varied but common lesions such as cysts are typically seen as well defined or lobulated mass lesions. Calcification is also a common feature of fibrocystic change and sclerosing adenosis. Other benign lesions such as radial scar, complex sclerosing lesion and fat necrosis can produce ill defined or spiculate mass lesions, which are indistinguishable from some forms of breast carcinoma.

Adenosis

Definition

A frequent, benign, proliferative process that affects mainly the lobular (acinar) component of the breast parenchyma. It can be accompanied by fibrosis causing considerable distortion of the glands simulating an invasive process.

Frequently it is a small and microscopic change, but it may be widespread. In some instances, it may form a palpable mass and has been called nodular adenosis or adenosis tumour. Several histological types have been described, but there is not complete agreement on their designation. Only the most frequent variants are discussed.
Radial scar/complex sclerosing lesion which incorporates a combination of benign changes including adenosis is also included in this section.

Epidemiology

This lesion occurs most frequently in women in their third and fourth decade.

Macroscopy

Adenosis may be non-distinctive, showing unremarkable fibrous or cystic breast tissue. A few cases assume the appearance of a firm rubbery grey mass.

Histopathology

Adenosis in its simplest form is characterized by a usually loosely structured proliferation of acinar or tubular structures, composed of an epithelial and myoepithelial cell layer and surrounded by a basement membrane.

Sclerosing adenosis

Sclerosing adenosis (SA) is characterized by a compact proliferation of acini with preservation of the luminal epithelial and the peripheral myoepithelial (ME) cell layers along with a surrounding basement membrane. These elements can easily be demonstrated by immunohistochemical staining for keratin, smooth-muscle actin and laminin, respectively. Although compression or attenuation of the acini by surrounding fibrosis may be marked, sclerosing adenosis nearly always retains an organic or lobulated configuration often best observed at low power view. Microcalcifications are common within

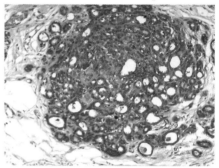

Fig. 1.107 Sclerosing adenosis. Typical organic configuration of the lesion.

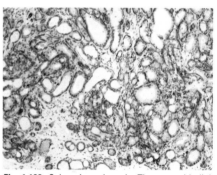

Fig. 1.108 Sclerosing adenosis. The myoepithelial cells are prominent with immunostain for smooth muscle actin.

the glands. Areas of apocrine metaplasia are also common. Rarely neural invasion is encountered and vascular invasion has been reported {149}. Lesions which form a mass show adenosis with a mixture of growth patterns {2015}, the most frequent of which is sclerosing adenosis.
In rare cases sclerosing adenosis may be involved by DCIS or LIN {1046, 1275a,1846a,2015,2336a,3104a}.

Differential diagnosis

Sclerosing adenosis can mimic invasive carcinoma. The overall lobulated architecture, persistence of ME cells, and lack of epithelial atypia help to exclude carcinoma {321,1046}. In cases involved by in situ carcinoma, the immunohistochemical demonstration of persistent myoepithelial cells is crucial in excluding invasion.

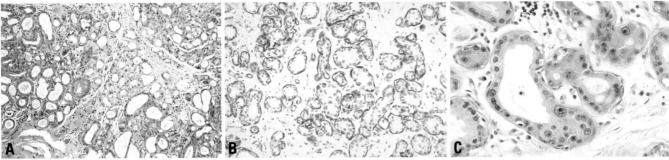

Fig. 1.109 A Apocrine adenosis/sclerosing adenosis with apocrine metaplasia and focal atypia. **B** Immunostain for actin demonstrating myoepithelial cells around the tubules. **C** Typical apocrine metaplasia in sclerosing adenosis, characterized by a three-fold nuclear size variation.

Apocrine adenosis

Synonym
Adenosis with apocrine metaplasia.

Apocrine adenosis (AA) is an ambiguous term, as it has been used for several different lesions {805,2698,2699}. In this context, it is used for adenosis, particularly sclerosing adenosis, with widespread apocrine metaplasia constituting at least 50% of the adenotic area {3093}. The apocrine epithelium may exhibit cytological atypia, so that the histological appearance mimics invasive carcinoma {2621,2698,2699}.

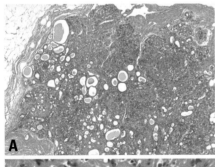

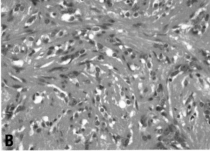

Fig. 1.110 A Nodular sclerosing adenosis. Note the well delineated margins. **B** High power view of the lesion in A, showing distorted and compressed tubular structures and intervening hyaline stroma. Such lesions may pose difficulties in the differential diagnosis to invasive lobular carcinoma.

Blunt duct adenosis

The term blunt duct adenosis (BDA) has been used for an organoid microscopic form of adenosis with variable distension of lumens showing columnar cell metaplasia {2015}.

Microglandular adenosis

Microglandular adenosis (MGA) is a rare lesion, characterized by a diffuse haphazard proliferation of small round glands {507,692,2413,2884}. These may be clustered, but without sclerosis or compression {507,3081}. The surrounding collagenous stroma may be hypocellular or hyalinized. There is no elastosis. The glands have a round lumen, which frequently contains periodic acid-Schiff (PAS) positive, eosinophilic secretory material. The epithelium is cuboid and without snouts. The cytoplasm may be clear or eosinophilic and granular. There is no nuclear atypia. There are no myoepithelial cells {184,321,797,2884}, but a surrounding basement membrane, not always recognizable without immunohistochemical staining for laminin or collagen IV {692,2884, 3081}, is present. Electron microscopy shows a multilayered basement membrane surrounding the tubules of MGA {2884}.

The epithelium of MGA is positive for S-100 in addition to cytokeratin {1372}. When carcinoma arises in association with MGA it may retain an alveolar pattern {1331} or be of ductal or one of the special types {2016}; the vast majority of these invasive carcinomas retain S-100 immunoreactivity regardless of their subtype {1484}.

Adenomyoepithelial adenosis

Adenomyoepithelial adenosis (AMEA) is an extremely rare type of adenosis, which seems to be associated with adenomyoepithelioma {803,805,1454} (see section on adenomyoepithelial lesions).

Prognosis and predictive factors of adenosis
Most types of adenosis are not associated with increased risk of subsequent carcinoma. However, there are exceptions, as nearly one third of cases of MGA harbour an invasive carcinoma {803,1454}, and apocrine adenosis has been found to be monoclonal and perhaps a putative precancerous lesion {3093}.

Radial scar / Complex sclerosing lesion

Definition
A benign lesion that on imaging, grossly and at low power microscopy resembles invasive carcinoma because the lobular architecture is distorted by the sclerosing process. The term radial scar (RS) has been applied to small lesions and com-

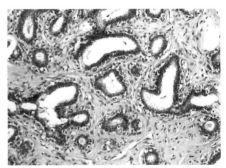

Fig. 1.111 Blunt duct adenosis, typical morphology.

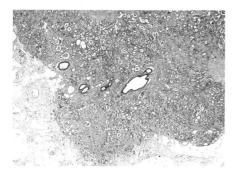

Fig. 1.112 Microglandular adenosis. An extensive lesion that presented as a palpable mass; the characteristic open lumens of the tubules and the colloid-like secretory material are apparent, providing clues to the nature of the process.

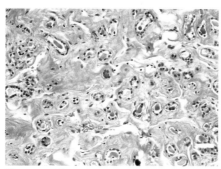

Fig. 1.113 Microglandular adenosis with diffusely arranged small uniform glands, separated by a densely collagenous background.

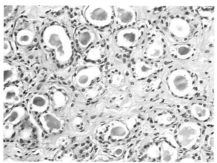

Fig. 1.114 Microglandular adenosis. The tubules are lined by a single layer of attenuated to cuboidal epithelial cells with vacuolated cytoplasm; colloid-like secretory material is present within the lumen.

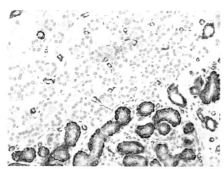

Fig. 1.115 Microglandular adenosis. Immunostain for smooth muscle actin confirms absence of a myoepithelial cell layer in MGA; the adjacent TDLUs show actin-positive myoepithelial cells.

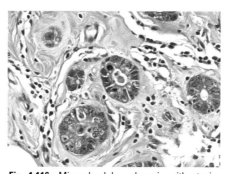

Fig. 1.116 Microglandular adenosis with atypia. There is diminished intraluminal colloid-like secretion, enlarged cells displaying mild to moderate nuclear pleomorphism and mitotic figures.

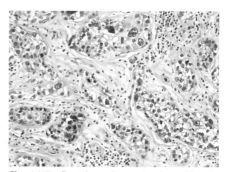

Fig. 1.117 Ductal carcinoma in situ arising in microglandular adenosis. Note the significant atypia of the cells proliferating within the obliterated tubules.

plex sclerosing lesion (CSL) to larger ones that contain a variety of ductal epithelial hyperplasia along with sclerosis.

Synonyms
Radial scar, sclerosing papillary lesion, radial sclerosing lesion, scleroelastotic scar, stellate scar, benign sclerosing ductal proliferation, non-encapsulated sclerosing lesion, infiltrating epitheliosis.

Epidemiology
The reported incidence varies depending on the mode of detection and how detected by mammography when the appearance mimics that of an infiltrating carcinoma producing an irregular stellate density. Very occasionally they are of sufficient size to produce a palpable mass {2725}. They are often multiple and frequently bilateral.

Macroscopy
These lesions may be undetected on gross examination or may be of sufficient size to produce an irregular area of firmness which can exhibit yellow streaks

reflecting the elastotic stroma. The appearance may be indistinguishable from that of a carcinoma.

Histopathology
RSs are composed of a mixture of benign changes of which adenosis forms a major part. They have a stellate outline with central dense hyalinized collagen and sometimes marked elastosis. Entrapped in the scar are small irregular tubules. The two cell layer is usually retained although this may not always be visible on haematoxylin and eosin staining and the myoepithelial layer is occasionally inapparent. The tubules sometimes contain eosinophilic secretions. Around the periphery of the lesion there are various degrees of ductal dilatation, ductal epithelial hyperplasia, apocrine metaplasia and hyperplasia. In the more complex larger CSLs, several of these lesions appear to combine and then converge with prominent areas of sclerosing adenosis, and small, frequently sclerosing, peripheral papillomas and various patterns of intraepithelial proliferation.

Differential diagnosis
Distinction from carcinoma depends on the characteristic architecture of a CSL, the lack of cytological atypia, the presence of a myoepithelial layer (in most cases) and basement membrane around the tubular structures (demonstration by immunohistochemistry may be necessary), the presence of a dense hyalinized stroma and lack of a reactive fibroblastic stroma.

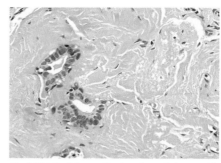

Fig. 1.118 Radial scar. Centre of a radial scar with two tubular structures, surrounded by hyalinized and elastotic tissue. Note the atrophic myoepithelial layer.

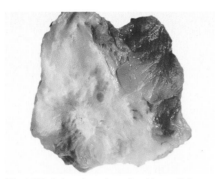

Fig. 1.119 Sclerosing adenosis with a radial scar.

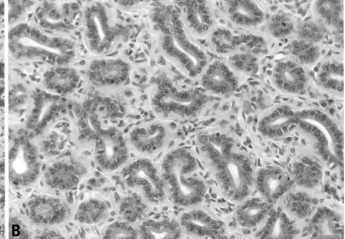

Fig. 1.120 Radial scar. A central fibrous scar is surrounded by epithelial proliferation.

Prognosis and predictive factors

It has been suggested that these lesions are pre-neoplastic or even represent early invasive carcinomas {1668} and also that they may represent a marker of risk for the subsequent development of carcinoma. Follow up studies, however, have been few and contradictory {843,1320} suggesting that an apparent risk is related to the various patterns of associated intraductal hyperplasia. It is doubtful that, without epithelial proliferation, there is a risk of the subsequent development of invasive carcinoma. In larger lesions the risk may be slightly higher as the increase in size is usually due to various forms of epithelial hyperplasia. A high incidence of atypical hyperplasia and carcinoma (both in situ and invasive) has been reported in CSLs detected by mammography, particularly in lesions measuring over 0.6 cm, and in women over 50 years old {719,2725}.

Tubular adenoma

Definition

Benign, usually round, nodules formed by a compact proliferation of tubular structures composed of the typical epithelial and myoepithelial cell layers. The epithelial cells are similar to those of the normal resting breast, but adenoma variants have been described where these show apocrine or lactating features.

ICD-O code   8211/0

Epidemiology

Tubular adenomas occur mainly in young females {1202,1211,1919,2074}. They rarely occur before menarche or after menopause {1600,2025}. They reportedly account for 0.13 to 1.7% of benign breast lesions {1202,1211,2874}. Patients with lactating adenomas are nursing mothers who have noted an area of increased firmness, either during lactation or, earlier, during pregnancy.

Clinical features

The clinical and imaging features are usually those of fibroadenoma.

Macroscopy

The tumours are firm, well circumscribed and homogeneous with a uniform, yellowish, cut surface.

Histopathology

The lesion is composed entirely of small, round tubules with little intervening stroma. The latter may contain a few lymphocytes. The epithelial cells are uniform, Mitotic activity is usually low. The tubular lumen is small and often empty, but eosinophilic proteinaceous material can be present. Occasional larger tubules give rise to thin branches. Combined tubular adenoma and fibroadenoma has been described {1202,2874}. Rare cases have been described of in situ and/or invasive carcinoma involving adenomas (tubular or lactating) {561,1202,1211, 2442}, a phenomenon also known to occur in fibroadenomas.

Lactating adenoma

ICD-O code   8204/0

During pregnancy and lactation, the epithelial cells of a tubular type adenoma may show extensive secretory changes warranting a designation of lactating adenoma {1332,2074}. It has been suggested that such lesions represent focal accumulation of hyperplastic lobules.

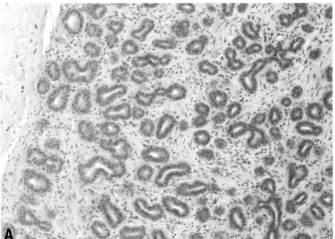

Fig. 1.121 Tubular adenoma. **A** The fibrous capsule is present in the left upper corner. **B** Higher magnification displays epithelial and myoepithelial cell lining of the tubules.

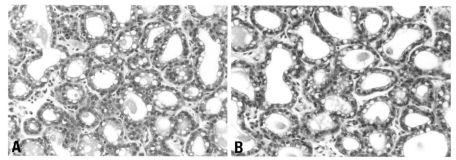

Fig. 1.122 Lactating adenoma. Epithelial cells show extensive secretory changes (**A, B**).

Apocrine adenoma

ICD-O code   8401/0

Synonym
Nodular adenosis with apocrine metaplasia.

Sometimes the epithelial cells of nodular adenosis show extensive apocrine metaplasia; these lesions may be termed apocrine adenoma {561,1713,2442}.

Immunoprofile
The immunophenotype of adenomas is similar to normal breast and reflects the various metaplastic and or secretory changes affecting them.

Differential diagnosis
Differentiation of adenomas from fibroadenomas is based on the prominent proliferating stromal component and the often elongated and compressed epithelial elements in the intracanalicular variant of the latter.

Pleomorphic adenoma

Definition
A rare lesion morphologically similar to pleomorphic adenoma (benign mixed tumour) of the salivary glands.

ICD-O code   8940/0

Epidemiology
These lesions have been reported in patients (mainly females) over a wide range of age {172,454}. Multiple tumours have been described {454,2874}. Calcification is common and gives a diagnostically important sign on mammography.

Histopathology
The histological picture is the same as that seen in pleomorphic adenomas of

salivary glands Some authors {2442, 2730,2753} consider pleomorphic adenoma to be a form of intraductal papilloma with extensive cartilaginous metaplasia. Because of the presence of a chondroid stromal component, pleomorphic adenomas pose a difficult differential diagnosis from metaplastic carcinomas with a mesenchymal component and primary sarcomas of the breast. The presence of foci of intraductal or invasive carcinoma points to the diagnosis of metaplastic carcinoma, while extensive cellular anaplasia characterizes sarcomas.

Ductal adenoma

Definition
A well circumscribed benign glandular proliferation located, at least in part, within a duct lumen {151}.

ICD-O code   8503/0

Synonym
Sclerosing papilloma.

Epidemiology
These lesions occur over a wide age range but are most frequent in women over 40 years {151,1577}. It is debatable whether these lesions represent the sclerotic evolution of an intraductal papilloma or are a distinct entity.

Clinical features
They may present as a mass or rarely as a nipple discharge. Imaging shows a density which can mimic a carcinoma.

Histopathology
Arranged mainly at the periphery are glandular structures with typical dual cell layer while in the centre there is dense scar-like fibrosis. The compact

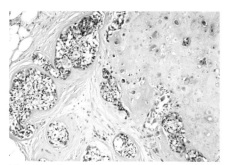

Fig. 1.123 Pleomorphic adenoma. Nests of clear myoepithelial cells proliferate around few, barely apparent darker epithelial cells; abundant cartilage is present on the right.

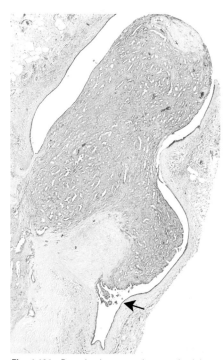

Fig. 1.124 Ductal adenoma, characterized by a "polypoid" protrusion into a distended duct; a few papillary projections are evident (arrow).

proliferating tubules, compressed or slightly dilated, and surrounded by fibrosis may impart a pseudoinfiltrative appearance. Epithelial and stromal changes similar to those observed in intraductal papillomas can occur; apocrine metaplasia is frequent. {1577}. Papillary fronds are not always detectable in a given plane of section.

Prognosis and predictive factors of mammary adenomas
All adenomas of the breast are benign lesions that do not recur if adequately excised and do not predispose to carcinoma.

Myoepithelial lesions

F.A. Tavassoli
J. Soares

Definition

Lesions either derived from, or composed of, a dominant to pure population of myoepithelial (ME) cells. They include adenoid cystic carcinoma, pleomorphic adenoma, myoepitheliosis, adenomyoepithelial adenosis, adenomyoepithelioma (benign or malignant) and malignant myoepithelioma (myoepithelial carcinoma). The first two lesions are discussed elsewhere. In this section, the focus will be on the others.

Immunohistochemical profile of myoepithelial cells

Myoepithelial cells show positive immunoreaction with alpha smooth muscle actin, calponin, caldesmon, smooth muscle myosin heavy chain (SMM-HC) maspin S-100 protein and high MW cytokeratins 34betaE12, CK5 and CK14. Nuclear immunoreactivity with p63 is also a feature of ME cells. Rarely there is staining with glial fibrillary acidic protein (GFAP). Myoepithelial cells are negative for low MW cytokeratins (CK 8/18), estrogen receptor (ER), progesterone receptor (PR), and desmin {191,1516,1573, 1741,2418,2702,2738,2953,3099}.

Epidemiology

Patients range in age from 22 to 87 years {2418,2868,2875,3192}.

Clinical features

Apart from myoepitheliosis, which is rarely palpable, these lesions usually present as a palpable tumour and/or mammographic density without distinctive features.

Myoepitheliosis

Definition

A multifocal, often microscopic, proliferation of spindle to cuboidal myoepithelial cells growing into and/or around small ducts and ductules.

Macroscopy

Myoepitheliosis generally appears as a firm irregular area.

Histopathology

The intraductal proliferating spindle cells may develop a prominent palisading pattern. The cuboidal cells may have longitudinal nuclear grooves resembling transitional cells. Rarely atypia and mitotic activity appear, warranting a designation of atypical myoepitheliosis.

The periductal variant of myoepitheliosis is often associated with sclerosis and is considered by some to be a variant of sclerosing adenosis; the cells have varied phenotypes.

When completely excised, recurrences do not develop.

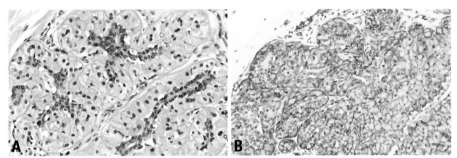

Fig. 1.125 Myoepitheliosis, periductal type. **A** The myoepithelial cells with abundant eosinophilic cytoplasm proliferate around the epithelial cells compressing the ductular lumens. This change is often multifocal. **B** Immunostain for actin is positive in the myoepithelial cells, but negative in the epithelial-lined compressed ductular spaces.

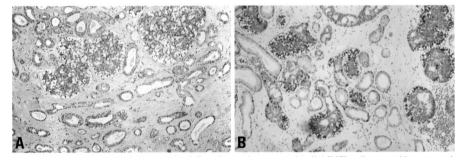

Fig. 1.126 Adenomyoepithelial adenosis. **A** Prominent clear myoepithelial (ME) cells are evident around several ductules. **B** Both the clear and normal ME cells are intensely imunoreactive for S-100 protein.

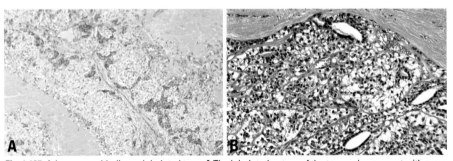

Fig. 1.127 Adenomyoepithelioma, lobulated type. **A** The lobulated nature of the tumour is apparent with massive central infarction in the two adjacent nodules. The lighter cells reflect the proliferating ME cells, while the darker cells represent the epithelial cells. **B** Adenomyoepithelioma. In this case, the proliferating ME cells have a clear cell phenotype and surround a few spaces lined by darker epithelial cells.

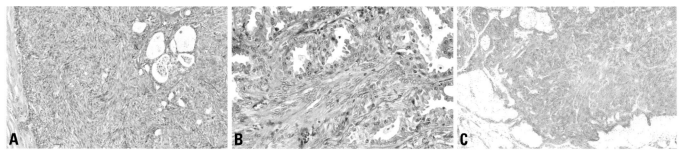

Fig. 1.128 Adenomyoepithelioma, spindle cell type. **A** There is a solid proliferation of spindled myoepithelial cells surrounding irregular epithelial lined spaces. **B** The epithelial spaces may show apocrine metaplasia. **C** Immunostain for S-100 protein shows positivity in the proliferating myoepithelial cells, while the epithelial cells fail to react.

Adenomyoepithelial adenosis

Definition
An extremely rare type of adenosis associated with adenomyoepithelioma {803, 805,1454}.

Histopathology
Adenomyoepithelial adenosis (AMEA) consists of a diffuse proliferation of round or irregular tubular structures lined by a cuboidal to columnar epithelium, which may show apocrine metaplasia. There is a prominent, focally hyperplastic myoepithelial cell layer with strikingly clear cytoplasm. There is no significant nuclear atypia or mitotic activity, but most described cases blend with or surround an adenomyoepithelioma {803,805,1454}.

Adenomyoepithelioma

Definition
Composed of a predominantly and usually solid proliferation of phenotypically variable myoepithelial cells around small epithelial lined spaces, in rare instances, the epithelial, the myoepithelial or both components of an adenomyoepithelioma (AME) may become malignant (malignant AME).

ICD-O codes
Benign   8983/0
Malignant   8983/3

Macroscopy
Well delineated, benign adenomyoepitheliomas are rounded nodules with a median size of 2.5 cm.

Histopathology
Histologically, AMEs they are characterized by a proliferation of layers or sheaths of ME cells around epithelial lined spaces. The tumour may display a spindle cell, a tubular, or, most often, a lobulated growth pattern. Fibrous septae with central hyalinization or infarction are common in the lobulated lesions. The ME cell phenotype is most variable in the lobulated pattern ranging from clear to eosinophilic and hyaline (plasmacytoid) types. Satellite nodules, seen adjacent to the lobulated variant in some cases reflect an intraductal extension of the lesion. The tubular variant has an ill defined margin. Mitotic activity of the proliferating myoepithelial cells in benign lesions is generally in the range of 1-2/10, always ≤2/10 high power field (hpf). Either the epithelial, the myoepithelial or both components of an adenomyoepithelioma may become malignant and

give rise to a carcinoma while the background lesion retains its adenomyoepitheliomatous appearance {793,900,903, 1695,2868,2953}. The aggressive myoepithelial component may assume a spindle configuration and develop into nodules resembling myofibroblastic lesions. A variety of epithelial derived carcinomas, sarcomas and carcinosarcomas occur in this setting (Table 1.16) {2868}. Rarely, both components develop into either separate malignancies or a single malignant infiltrative process composed of angulated tubules lined by both epithelial and myoepithelial cells.

Differential diagnosis
The tubular variant of AME should be distinguished from a tubular adenoma; the latter may have prominent ME cells, but lacks the myoepithelial proliferation typical of an AME. Furthermore, tubular adenoma is sharply circumscribed unlike the ill defined tubular AME.
The lobulated and spindle cell variants of AME should be distinguished from

Table 1.16
Classification of myoepithelial lesions.

1. Myoepitheliosis
  a. Intraductal
  b. Periductal
2. Adenomyoepithelial adenosis
3. Adenomyoepithelioma
  a. Benign
  b. With malignant change (specify the subtype)
  – Myoepithelial carcinoma arising in an adenomyoepithelioma
  – Epithelial carcinoma arising in an adenomyoepithelioma
  – Malignant epithelial and myoepithelial components
  – Sarcoma arising in adenomyoepithelioma
  – Carcinosarcoma arising in adenomyoepithelioma
4. Malignant myoepithelioma (ME carcinoma)

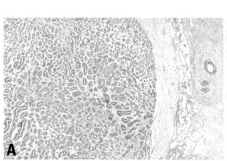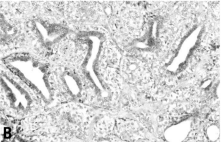

Fig. 1.129 Adenomyoepithelioma, adenosis type. **A** At least focally well delineated, these tumours superficially resemble a tubular adenoma. **B** Higher magnification shows proliferation of ME cells in the tubules beyond the normal single layer.

Table 1.17
Immunoprofile of various spindle cell tumours of the breast.

Tumour	Smooth muscle actin	Calponin	S-100	Kermix*	CAM5.2**	ER	Desmin	CD34	HMB45
Myoepithelioma	+	+	+	+	–	–	–	–	–
Spindle cell carcinoma	–	–	–	++	+	+/–	–	–	–
Smooth muscle cell tumours	+	+/–	–	+/–	+/–	+/–	+	–	–
Myofibroblastic lesions	+	+/–	+/–	–	–	–	–*	+	–
Melanoma	–	–	+	–	–	–	–	–	–

* Kermix a cocktail of AE1/AE3 (cytokeratin 1-19), and LP34 (CK5,6 & 18)
**Cam 5.2 (CK8 & 18)

pleomorphic adenoma; the latter generally has prominent areas of chondroid and/or osseous differentiation.

Prognosis and predictive factors
The majority of AME are benign {1573, 1695,2418,2581,2868}. Lesions that contain malignant areas, those with high mitotic rate, or infiltrating margins have a potential for recurrence and metastases. Local recurrence {1440, 2868,3192} as well as distant metastasis {2875} have been described, mainly among those with agressive features.

Malignant myoepithelioma

Definition
An infiltrating tumour composed purely of myoepithelial cells (predominantly spindled) with identifiable mitotic activity.

Synonyms
Infiltrating myoepithelioma, myoepithelial carcinoma.

ICD-O code   8982/3

Macroscopy
Ranging from 1.0 to 21 cm in size, these tumours are generally well defined with focal marginal irregularity, although some are stellate. There may be foci of necrosis and haemorrhage on the firm rubbery cut surface in larger tumours and sometimes nodular areas of hyalinization even in smaller tumours.

Histopathology
Histologically, there is an infiltrating proliferation of spindle cells often lacking

significant atypia. Mitotic activity may not exceed 3-4 mf/10hpf. The spindled tumour cells appear to emanate from the myoepithelial cells of ductules entrapped in the periphery of the lesion. Aggregates of collagen and prominent central hyalinization may be evident.

Differential diagnosis
The differential diagnosis includes spindle cell carcinomas, fibromatosis and a variety of myofibroblastic lesions. The presence of a dominant nodule with

irregular and shallow infiltration at the margins is helpful in distinguishing this lesion from fibromatosis and myofibroblastic tumours. Immunohistochemistry is, and, rarely, electron microscopy may be, required to confirm the myoepithelial nature of the neoplastic cells.

Prognosis and predictive factors
Local recurrence or distant metastases have rarely been documented {1573, 2581,2875}. Complete excision with uninvolved margins is recommended.

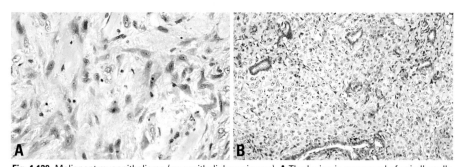

Fig. 1.130 Malignant myoepithelioma (myoepithelial carcinoma). **A** The lesion is composed of spindle cells lacking significant atypia or mitotic activity. **B** At the periphery of the same lesion, often a more epithelioid or plump cell population is evident emanating from the myoepithelial cell layer of the entrapped ductules.

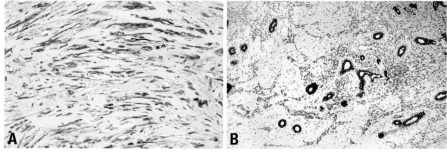

Fig. 1.131 Malignant myoepithelioma. **A** Immunostain for smooth muscle actin is positive in the neoplastic spindle cells. **B** Immunostain for kermix (AE1/AE3/LP34) shows intense staining of the entrapped normal ductules; a less intense immunoreaction is evident in the neoplastic spindle cells.

Mesenchymal tumours

M. Drijkoningen
F.A. Tavassoli
G. Magro
V. Eusebi
M. Devouassoux-Shisheboran

J.P. Bellocq
S. Lanzafame
G. MacGrogan
J.L. Peterse

Definition
Benign and malignant mesenchymal tumours morphologically similar to those occurring in the soft tissues as well as those occurring predominantly in the breast.

Benign vascular tumours

Haemangioma

Definition
A benign tumour or malformation of mature vessels.

ICD-O code   9120/0

Epidemiology
Haemangiomas of the breast have been described in both male and female patients from 18 months to 82 years old {1373,2874}. They rarely present as palpable lesions but an increasing number of non-palpable mammary haemangiomas are nowadays detected by breast imaging {3077}. Incidental "perilobular" haemangiomas are found in 1.2% of mastectomies and 4.5% of benign breast biopsies {2443} and 11% in a series of post mortem cases (age range 29–82 years) {1633}.

Macroscopy
Rarely palpable, the lesions are well circumscribed and vary from 0.5-2 cm with a reddish-brown spongy appearance.

Histopathology
Symptomatic haemangiomas may be of cavernous, capillary or venous subtypes {2435,2611}. Cavernous haemangioma is the most common type; it consists of dilated thin walled vessels lined by flattened endothelium and congested with blood. Thrombosis may be present with papillary endothelial hyperplasia (Masson's phenomenon) {1946}. Dystrophic calcification may be found in organizing thrombi as well as in the stroma between the vascular channels. Capillary haemangiomas are composed of nodules of small vessels with a lobular arrangement around a larger feeding vessel. The intervening stroma is fibrous. The endothelial lining cells may have prominent hyperchromatic nuclei but without tufting or a solid spindle cell growth pattern. Venous haemangiomas consist of thick walled vascular channels with smooth muscle walls of varying thickness {2435}.

In perilobular haemangiomas, the lobulated collections of thin-walled, wide vascular channels are seen within the intralobular stroma. Expansion into the extralobular stroma and adjacent adipose tissue is often present. The vascular channels are lined by flattened endothelium without a surrounding muscle layer {1373}. Occasional cases with prominent hyperchromatic endothelial nuclei have been described and designated atypical haemangiomas {1225}. An anastomosing growth pattern, papillary endothelial proliferations and mitoses are absent and their presence should arouse suspicion and careful exclusion of an angiosarcoma.

Prognosis and predictive factors
Recurrence, even after incomplete excision, has not been reported. Careful evaluation of the whole lesion to exclude a well differentiated angiosarcoma is indicated in all symptomatic vascular breast lesions.

Angiomatosis

Definition
A diffuse excessive proliferation of well formed vascular channels affecting a large area in a contiguous fashion.

Synonym
Diffuse angioma.

Epidemiology
This very rare benign vascular lesion may be congenital. Most cases have been described in women between 19 and 61 years old {1921,2416}. One case was in a male.

Clinical features
Angiomatosis presents as a breast mass. Rapid increase in size has been described in a woman during pregnancy {76}.

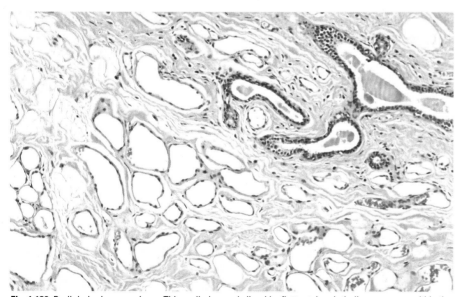

Fig. 1.132 Perilobular haemangioma. Thin walled vessels lined by flattened endothelium are seen within the intralobular stroma.

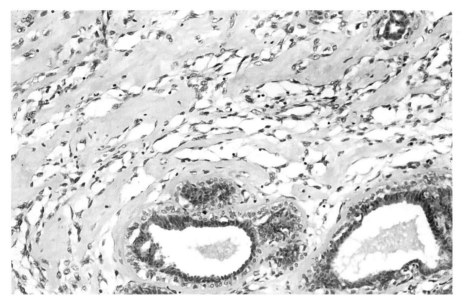

Fig. 1.133 Pseudoangiomatous stromal hyperplasia (PASH). Interanastomosing, empty, slit-like spaces within breast stroma are typical.

Pathology
Macroscopic and histopathological appearances are similar to angiomatosis at other sites. The haemorrhagic spongy lesions are composed of usually thin walled large blood or lymphatic vessels diffusely extending throughout the parenchyma of the breast.

Prognosis and predictive factors
Recurrence after incomplete excision has been reported, and may occur after a long disease-free interval {2416}. In many cases, complete excision requires a mastectomy.

Haemangiopericytoma

Definition
A circumscribed area of bland ovoid to spindled cells proliferating around branching and "stag-horn" vessels.

ICD-O codes
Benign	9150/0
NOS	9150/1
Malignant	9150/3

Epidemiology
This is a rare mesenchymal tumour. Around 20 primary haemangiopericytomas have been reported in the breast. The patients are mostly women aged 22–67, but a few cases have been reported in children (5 and 7 years old) and in men {118,2889}.

Clinical features
Patients usually present with a mass that appears as a well circumscribed area of density on mammography.

Macroscopy
The tumours are round to oval, well circumscribed and range in size from 1 to 19 cm {118,1415,2855,2889}. They are firm with a solid, yellow-tan to grey-white cut surface. Myxoid areas alternate with small cysts filled with watery fluid. Haemorrhage and necrosis are evident in some larger tumours.

Histopathology
The histological and immunophenotype appearances are similar to haemangiopericytomas described elsewhere {2889}. They are composed of a compact proliferation of plump ovoid to spindle cells with indistinct cell margins arranged around an abundance of usually thin-walled, irregularly branching vascular channels. Some of the branching vessels assume a "stag-horn" configuration. Mammary ducts and ductules are often trapped focally in the periphery of the lesion.

Prognosis and predictive factors
Most cases of mammary haemangiopericytoma have been benign. There is no well documented example of metastatic disease or even recurrence {118, 1415,2855,2889}. Wide local excision rather than mastectomy is often sufficient for complete tumour excision.

Pseudoangiomatous stromal hyperplasia

Definition
A benign lesion consisting of complex anastomosing slit-like pseudovascular spaces, that are either acellular or lined by slender spindle-shaped stromal cells.

Epidemiology
The clinicopathological spectrum of mammary pseudoangiomatous stromal hyperplasia (PASH) extends from insignificant microscopic changes, often associated with either benign or malignant breast disease, to diffuse involvement of the breast or cases where a localized palpable or non-palpable breast mass is produced (nodular PASH) {1275,2270,3037}. The latter is uncommon and reported to occur in 0.4% of breast biopsies {2270}. Focal or multifocal PASH without mass formation has been reported in 23% of breast biopsies, usually as an incidental finding. PASH has been reported in at least 25% of cases of gynaecomastia {157,1865}.

Aetiology
The immunophenotype of the proliferating cells confirms that PASH is of myofibroblastic origin {1113,2279,2510,3249}. The pseudoangiomatous spaces are also discernible in frozen sections, indicating that they are not a fixation artefact {157,3037}.

Clinical features
Nodular PASH usually present as a painless, well circumscribed, mobile palpable mass, clinically indistinguishable from fibroadenoma {532,1275, 2270,2279,3037,3249}. Smaller lesions may be detected by mammography {532, 2270}. On imaging, nodular PASH is indistinguishable from fibroadenoma {2270}. Diffuse lesions are an incidental finding {1275}. Bilateral lesions may occur {157}. Rapid growth has been reported {532,2270,2765,3026}.

Macroscopy
Macroscopically, nodular PASH is usually indistinguishable from fibroadenoma ranging in size from 1 to 17 cm. The cut surface is pale tan-pink to yellow {92, 1275,2279,2622,3037}.

Histopathology
PASH may be present in normal breast tissue or in various benign lesions {867,

1113,1275}. There is a complex pattern of interanastomosing empty slit-like spaces, present within and between breast lobules with a perilobular concentric arrangement {1275,2279}. In gynaecomastia, a periductal pattern is found {157}. The spaces are formed by separation of collagen fibres and are either acellular or lined by spindle cells, simulating endothelial cells. Mitoses, tufting, atypia and pleomorphism are absent {92,1275,2279, 3037,3249}. There is no destruction of normal breast tissue, no necrosis, nor invasion of fat {1275} and collagen IV cannot identify a basement membrane around the spaces {867}. The intervening stroma often consists of dense, hyalinized collagen and spindle cells with nuclei displaying pointed ends {1275, 2510}. In rare more proliferative lesions, a fascicular pattern is found: the stroma is composed of bundles of plump spindle cells that may obscure the underlying pseudoangiomatous architecture {2279}. At low power, PASH may resemble low-grade angiosarcoma but can be distinguished by its growth pattern and cytological features. The immunohistochemical characteristics are also different.

Immunoprofile
The spindle cells adjacent to the clefts are positive for CD34, vimentin, actin, calponin, but negative for the endothelial cell markers Factor VIII protein, Ulex europaeus agglutinin-1 and CD31. They are also negative for S100, low and high MW cytokeratins, EMA and CD68. Desmin is usually negative, but may be positive in fascicular lesions {157,928,1865,2279,3037}.

Prognosis and predictive factors
PASH is not malignant but local recurrence has been rarely reported possibly attributable to growth after incomplete excision, or the presence of multiple lesions that were not all excised {2270,2279,3037}.

Myofibroblastoma

Definition
A benign spindle cell tumour of the mammary stroma composed of myofibroblasts.

ICD-O code   8825/0

Epidemiology
Myofibroblastoma (MFB) occurs in the breast of both women and men aged

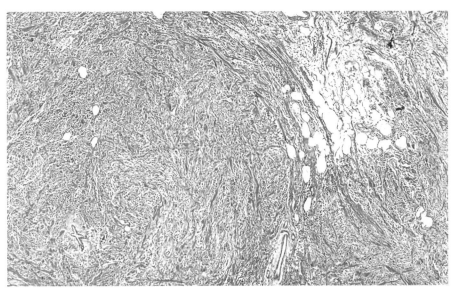
Fig. 1.134 Myofibroblastoma. An expansile tumour composed of spindle to oval cells arranged in intersecting fascicles interrupted by thick bands of collagen. Some adipose tissue is present in the right upper corner.

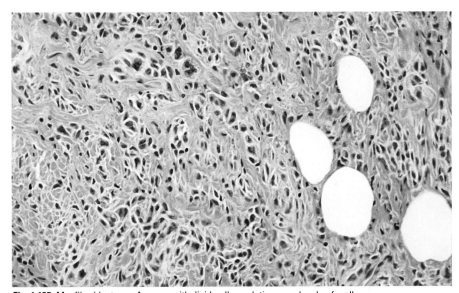
Fig. 1.135 Myofibroblastoma. A more epithelioid cell population may develop focally.

between 40 and 87 years {1023,1735}. In a few cases, an association with gynaecomastia has been documented.

Clinical features
MFB presents as a solitary slowly growing nodule. Synchronous bilaterality and unilateral multicentricity is rarely observed {1113}. Imaging shows a well circumscribed, homogeneously solid and hypoechoic mass devoid of microcalcifications {1113,1374,2252}.

Macroscopy
MFB is usually a well circumscribed encapsulated tumour raging in size from 0.9 to 10 cm.

Histopathology
An expansile tumour with pushing borders, myofibroblastroma is composed of spindle to oval cells arranged in short, haphazardly intersecting fascicles interrupted by thick bands of brightly eosinophilic collagen. The cells have relatively abundant, ill defined, pale to deeply eosinophilic cytoplasm with a round to oval nucleus containing 1 or 2 small nucleoli. Necrosis is usually absent and mitoses are only rarely observed (up to 2 mitoses x 10 high power fields). There is no entrapment of mammary ducts or lobules within the tumour. Variable numbers of scattered mast cells may be seen in the stroma but otherwise inflammatory

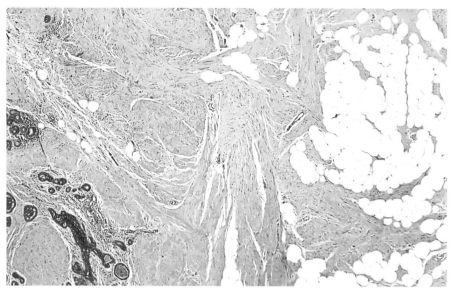

Fig. 1.136 Fibromatosis. Fascicles of spindle myofibroblast invade the adipose tissue and extend between lobules (on the left).

cells are absent. Variations include the occurrence of infiltrating margins, a prominent epithelioid cell component, mono- or multinucleated giant cells with a mild to severe degree of nuclear pleomorphism and extensive myxoid or hyaline change in the stroma. Occasionally, lipomatous, smooth muscle, cartilaginous or osseous components form additional integral parts of the tumour {934, 1734-1736}. MFB should be distinguished from nodular fasciitis, inflammatory myofibroblastic tumour, fibromatosis, benign peripheral nerve sheath tumours, haemangiopericytomas and leiomyomas {1736}. The differential diagnosis is based on immunophenotype but even so may be difficult in some cases.

Immunoprofile
The neoplastic cells react positively for vimentin, desmin, α-smooth muscle actin and variably for CD34, bcl-2 protein, CD99 and sex steroid hormone receptors (estrogen, progesterone and androgen receptors) {1023,1733,1913}.

Fibromatosis

Definition
This uncommon, locally aggressive, lesion without metastatic potential originates from fibroblasts and myofibroblasts within the breast parenchyma, excluding mammary involvement by extension of a fibromatosis arising from the pectoral fascia.

ICD-O code   8821/1

Synonym
Desmoid tumour.

Epidemiology
Fibromatosis accounts for less than 0.2% of all breast lesions {390,681,1083, 2432,3063}. It is seen in women from 13 to 80 years (average 46 and median 40) and is more common in the childbearing age than in perimenopausal or postmenopausal patients {681}. A few cases have been reported in men {378,2482}.

Clinical features
The lesion presents as a solitary, painless, firm or hard palpable mass. Bilateral tumours are rare {681,2432,3063}. Skin or nipple retraction may be observed {294} and rarely nipple discharge {3063}. Mammographically, fibromatosis is indistinguishable from a carcinoma {681}.

Macroscopy
The poorly demarcated tumour measures from 0.5 to 10 cm (average 2.5 cm) {681,2432,3063} with a firm, white-grey cut surface.

Histopathology
Mammary fibromatoses are histologically similar to those arising from the fascia or aponeuroses of muscles elsewhere in the body with the same immunophenotype. Proliferating spindled fibroblasts and myofibroblasts form sweeping and interlacing fascicles; the periphery of the lesion reveals characteristic infiltrating finger-like projections entrapping mammary ducts and lobules {3063}.

Fibromatosis must be distinguished from several entities in the breast.

Fibrosarcomas are richly cellular, with nuclear atypia and a much higher mitotic rate than fibromatosis. Spindle cell carcinomas disclose more typical areas of carcinoma and, in contrast to fibromatosis, the cells are immunoreactive for both epithelial markers and vimentin {1022}. Myoepithelial carcinomas are actin and/or S-100 protein positive. While CAM 5.2 positivity may be weak, pancytokeratin (Kermix) is strongly expressed in at least some tumour cells, and there is diffuse staining with CK34Beta E12 and CK 5,6.

Lipomatous myofibroblastomas show a finger-like infiltrating growth pattern, reminiscent of fibromatosis {1736}. However, the cells are estrogen (ER), progesterone (PR) and androgen receptor (AR) positive in 70% of cases, while fibromatosis does not stain with these antibodies.

Nodular fasciitis is also composed of immature appearing fibroblasts but tends to be more circumscribed, and has a higher mitotic rate. The prominent inflammatory infiltrate is scattered throughout the lesion and is not limited to the periphery as in fibromatosis.

Reactive spindle cell nodules and scars at the site of a prior trauma or surgery demonstrate areas of fat necrosis, calcifications and foreign body granulomas, features that are not common in fibromatosis.

Immunoprofile
The spindle cells are vimentin positive and a small proportion of them are also actin positive, while they are invariably negative for cytokeratin and S-100 protein. In contrast to one-third of extramammary desmoid tumours {1662,1888, 2353}, fibromatoses in the breast are ER, PR, AR, and pS2 (assessed as a measure of functional ER) negative {681,2335}.

Prognosis and predictive factors
Mammary fibromatoses display a low propensity for local recurrence, with a reported frequency of 21% {1083}, 23% {3063}, and 27% {2432} of cases compared with that of 57% {790} for extramammary lesions. When it does occur, one or more generally develop within two to three years of initial surgery {1083, 3063}, but local recurrence may develop after a 6-year interval {3063}.

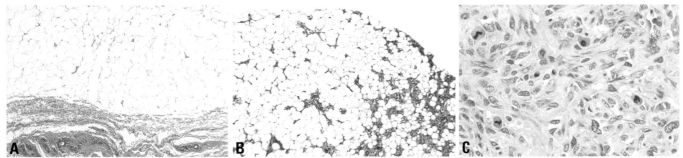

Fig. 1.137 A Lipoma. Intraparenchymal well circumscribed mature fat tissue. **B** Angiolipoma. Well circumscribed mature fat tissue separated by a network of small vessels. **C** Cellular angiolipoma. Patches of solid, spindle cell proliferation are typically present.

Inflammatory myofibroblastic tumour

Definition
A tumour composed of differentiated myofibroblastic spindle cells accompanied by numerous inflammatory cells.

ICD-O code   8825/1

Synonyms
Inflammatory pseudotumour, plasma cell granuloma.

Epidemiology
Inflammatory myofibroblastic tumour (IMT) is a heterogeneous clinicopathological entity {1845} that may occur at any anatomical location. There is uncertainty as to whether IMT is reactive or neoplastic in nature. Some authors regard IMT as a low grade sarcoma {1845}. Only rare cases of IMT have been reported in the breast {276,467,2235,3183}.

Clinical features
IMT usually presents as a palpable circumscribed firm mass.

Macroscopy
Gross examination usually shows a well circumscribed firm white to grey mass.

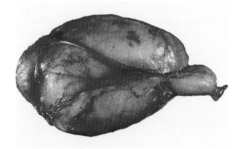

Fig. 1.138 Lipoma. Well circumscribed, lobulated mass of 11 cm.

Histopathology
The lesion consists of a proliferation of spindle cells with the morphological and immunohistochemical features of myofibroblasts, arranged in interlacing fascicles or in a haphazard fashion, and variably admixed with an inflammatory component of lymphocytes, plasma cells and histiocytes.
IMT should be distinguished from other benign and malignant spindle cell lesions occurring in the breast. The hallmark of IMT is the significant inflammatory cell component.

Prognosis and predictive factors
Although the clinical behaviour of IMT cannot be predicted on the basis of histological features, in the breast most reported cases have followed a benign clinical course after complete surgical excision {276,467,2235}, with the exception of a bilateral case with local recurrence in both breasts after 5 months {3183}. Additional cases with longer follow-up are needed to define the exact clinical behaviour.

Lipoma

Definition
A tumour composed of mature fat cells without atypia.

ICD-O code   8850/0

Epidemiology
Although adipose tissue is quantitatively an important component of the normal breast tissue, pathologists rarely encounter intramammary lipomas. Subcutaneous lipomas are more often resected. Most common lipomas become apparent in patients 40-60 years of age.

Clinical features
Lipomas usually present as a slow growing solitary mass with a soft doughy consistency.

Macroscopy
Lipomas are well circumscribed, thinly encapsulated round or discoid masses; usually less than 5 cm in diameter.

Histopathology
Lipomas differ little from the surrounding fat. They may be altered by fibrous tissue, often hyalinized or show myxoid changes. Secondary alterations like lipogranulomas, lipid cysts, calcifications, may occur as a result of impaired blood supply or trauma.

Variants of lipoma
These include angiolipoma {1268,2876, 3232} which, unlike angiolipomas at other sites, in the breast are notoriously painless. Microscopy reveals mature fat cells separated by a branching network of small vessels that is more pronounced in the sub capsular areas.
Characteristically, thrombi are found in some vascular channels. Some lesions rich in vessels are called cellular angiolipomas.
Other variants which have been described in the breast include spindle cell

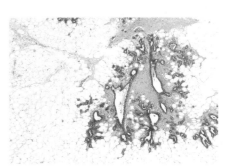

Fig. 1.139 Adenolipoma. Well circumscribed mature fat containing organoid glandular tissue.

lipoma {1645}, hibernoma {2425} and chondrolipoma {1774a}. Adenomas containing glandular breast tissue such as adenolipoma are considered as hamartomas by some and variants of lipoma by others.

Granular cell tumour

Definition
A tumour of putative schwannian origin consisting of cells with eosinophlic granular cytoplasm.

ICD-O code   9580/0

Epidemiology
Granular cell tumour (GCT) can occur in any site of the body. It is relatively uncommon in the breast {2114}. It occurs more often in females than in males {430} with a wide age range from 17-75 years {325, 617,668,3090} GCT is a potential mimicker of breast cancer, clinically, radiologically and grossly {608,617,995,2549}.

Clinical features
GCT generally presents as a single, firm, painless mass in the breast parenchyma but may be superficial causing skin retraction and even nipple inversion, whereas location deep in the breast parenchyma may lead to secondary involvement of the pectoralis fascia. Rarely, patients have simultaneous GCTs occurring at multiple sites in the body, including the breast {1920,1922}. Imaging typically shows a dense mass with stellate margin.

Macroscopy
GCT appears as a well circumscribed or infiltrative firm mass of 2–3 cm or less with a white to yellow or tan cut surface.

Histopathology
The histology is identical to that seen in GCT at other sites of the body. There is an infiltrating growth pattern, even in lesions, which appear circumscribed on gross examination. The cellular component is composed of solid nests, clusters or cords of round to polygonal cells with coarsely granular, eosinophilic periodic acid-Schiff (PAS) positive (diastase resistant) cytoplasm. due to the presence of abundant intracytoplasmic lysosomes. Awareness that GCT can occur in the breast is essential. Immunoreactivity with S-100 is important in confirming the diagnosis of GCT; lack of positivity for cytokeratins excludes breast carcinoma.

Prognosis and predictive factors
The clinical behaviour of GCT is usually benign following complete surgical excision. Rarely, lymph node metastases have been reported {668}. In contrast, a malignant course should be expected in the extremely rare malignant mammary GCTs which show nuclear pleomorphism, mitoses and necrosis {468}.

Benign peripheral nerve sheath tumours

Definition
Benign peripheral nerve sheath tumours (BPNST) include three distinct lesions usually occurring in the peripheral nerves or soft tissues: schwannomas composed of differentiated Schwann cells; neurofibromas consisting of a mixture of Schwann cells, perineurial like cells and fibroblasts and perineuromas composed of perineural cells.

ICD-O codes
Schwannoma   9560/0
Neurofibroma   9540/0

Epidemiology
The breast is only rarely the primary site of BPNST. There are only a few case reports of schwannomas {881,953,1081} and neurofibromas {1223,1675,2645}, but to our knowledge primary perineuroma of the breast has not been recorded. Since neurofibromas may be part of neurofibromatosis type I (NF1), follow-up is needed because of the potential for malignant degeneration. The occurrence of breast cancer in the context of breast neurofibromas has been reported {1948}. The age of patients at diagnosis is wide, ranging from 15 to 80 years with a prevalence of females.

Clinical features
The lesions present as a painless nodule and the pathology and immunophenotype is identical to their counterparts at other sites of the body.

Angiosarcoma

Definition
A malignant tumour composed of neoplastic elements with the morphological properties of endothelial cells.

ICD-O code   9120/3

Synonyms
These tumours include lesions which were formerly termed haemangiosarcoma, haemangioblastoma, lymphangiosarcoma and metastasizing haemangioma. Lymphangiosarcomas probably exist as a specific sarcoma of lymphatic endothelium but, at present, there is no

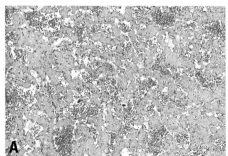
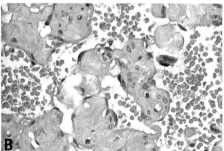
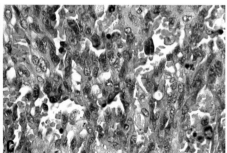

Fig. 1.140 Primary mammary angiosarcoma. **A, B** Grade I (well differentiated) angiosarcoma showing interanastomosing channels containing red blood cells. The endothelial nuclei are prominent and hyperchromatic, but mitotic figures are absent. **C** High grade (poorly differentiated) angiosarcoma. Solid aggregates of pleomorphic endothelial cells surround vascular channels.

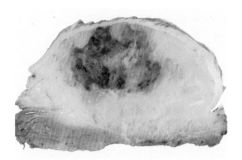

Fig. 1.141 Angiosarcoma after breast conserving treatment. The spongy, haemorrhagic mass contains occasional solid areas. In this case, the neoplasm involves the breast parenchyma as well as the skin.

reliable criterion upon which to make a histological distinction between tumours derived from endothelia of blood and lymphatic vessels.

Epidemiology

Mammary angiosarcoma can be subdivided into 1) Primary (de novo) forms in the breast parenchyma; 2) Secondary in the skin and soft tissues of the arm following ipsilateral radical mastectomy and subsequent lymphoedema - the Stewart Treves (S-T) syndrome; 3) Secondary in the skin and chest wall following radical mastectomy and local radiotherapy; 4) Secondary in the skin or breast parenchyma or both following conservation treatment and radiotherapy. Angiosarcomas, as with other sarcomas of the breast, are rare and their incidence is about 0.05% of all primary malignancies of the organ {2876}. While the incidence of primary breast angiosarcomas has remained constant, the incidence of secondary forms has changed. S-T syndrome has dramatically declined in recent years in institutions in which more conservation surgical treatments have been adopted, while angiosarcomas of the breast developing after conserving surgery with supplementary radiation therapy have been diagnosed since the late 1980s {570}.

Primary (de novo) angiosarcoma of breast parenchyma

In patients with primary angiosarcoma, the age ranges from 17 to 70 years (median 38 years) with no prevalence of laterality {2436}. The tumours are deeply located in the breast tissue {2784}. Approximately 12% of patients present with diffuse breast enlargement {2876}. When the tumour involves the overlying skin a bluish-red discoloration may ensue. Imaging is of little help {1656, 2564,3118}.

Macroscopy

Angiosarcomas vary in size from 1 to 20 cm, averaging 5 cm {2425}, have a spongy appearance and a rim of vascular engorgement which corresponds to a zone of well differentiated tumour. Poorly differentiated tumours appear as an ill defined indurated fibrous lesion similar to that of any other poorly differentiated sarcoma. Angiosarcomas must be sampled extensively to look for poorly differentiated areas that on occasion constitute the minority of a tumour.

Histopathology

Two systems have been used to grade angiosarcomas of the breast {717,1847}. Although very similar, the one proposed by Donnell et al. {717} has gained wide impact as it was tested in a large number of patients with adequate follow up {2436}.

Grade I (well differentiated) angiosarcomas consist of interanastomosing vascular channels that dissect the interlobular stroma. The neoplastic vessels have very wide lumina filled with red blood cells. The nuclei of the endothelium lining the neoplastic vessels are prominent and hyperchromatic. Care must be taken to differentiate grade I angiosarcoma from benign vascular tumours.

Grade III (poorly differentiated) angiosarcomas are easy to diagnose as interanastomosing vascular channels are intermingled with solid endothelial or spindle cell areas that show necrotic foci and numerous mitoses. In a grade III angiosarcoma, more than 50% of the total neoplastic area is composed of solid and spindle cell components without evident vascular channels {2425}.

A tumour qualifies as grade II (intermediately differentiated) angiosarcoma when at least 75% of the bulk of the tumour is formed by the well differentiated pattern seen in grade I, but in addition there are solid cellular foci scattered throughout the tumour.

Clinical feature

The average age of patients with grade I angiosarcomas is 43 years while 34 and 29 years are the respective figures for grade II and III angiosarcomas {717}.

Immunoprofile

Factor VIII, CD34 and CD31 are the most widely used antibodies that characterize endothelial differentiation. While present

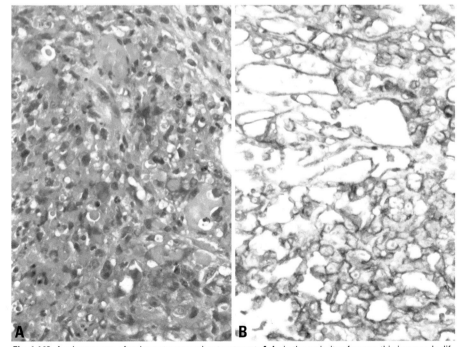

Fig. 1.142 Angiosarcoma after breast conserving treatment. **A** As in the majority of cases, this is a poorly differentiated angiosarcoma in which vascular channels are hard to see. **B** Immunostaining for the endothelial marker CD31 clearly demonstrates the solid areas of endothelial cells with occasional vascular channels.

in all grade I and most grade II angiosarcomas these markers may be lost in more poorly differentiated tumours or areas of tumour.

Prognosis and predictive factors

If well differentiated angiosarcomas (Grade I) were excluded, this breast tumour is usually lethal {457}.

Grading systems highlight the relative benignity of well differentiated angiosarcomas. The survival probability for grade I tumours was estimated as 91% at 5 years and 81% at 10 years. For grade III tumours the survival probability was 31% at 2 years and 14% at 5 and 10 years. Grade II lesions had a survival of 68% at 5 and 10 years. Recurrence free survival at 5 years was 76% for grade I, 70% for grade II and 15% for grade III angiosarcomas {2436}. Metastases are mainly to lungs, skin bone and liver. Very rarely axillary lymph nodes show metastases at presentation {457}. The grade can vary between the primary tumour and its metastases {2876}. Radio and chemotherapy are ineffective.

Angiosarcoma of the skin of the arm after radical mastectomy followed by lymphoedema

Stewart and Treves in 1949 gave a lucid description of a condition subsequently named S-T syndrome {2793}. They reported six patients who had: 1) undergone mastectomy for breast cancer including axillary dissection; 2) developed an "immediate postmastectomy oedema" in the ipsilateral arm; 3) received irradiation to the breast area together with the axilla; 4) developed oedema which started in the arm and extended to the forearm and finally the dorsum of the hands and digits.

The patients ranged in age from 37-60 years, with a mean age of 64 years {3149}. The angiosarcomatous nature of S-T syndrome has been conclusively proved by ultrastructure and immunohistochemistry in most of the cases studied {1049, 1462,1862,2690}.

The oedema is preceded by radical mastectomy for breast carcinoma including axillary dissection {275} and develops within 12 months. Nearly 65% of patients also had irradiation of the chest wall and axilla {2425}. The interval to tumour appearance varies from 1-49 years {2425}, but most become evident about 10 years

following mastectomy {2752,3149}.
S-T syndrome is a lethal disease with a median survival of 19 months {3149}. Lungs are the most frequent site of metastasis.

Post-radiotherapy angiosarcoma

Angiosarcoma can manifest itself after radiotherapy in two separate settings.
1) In the chest wall when radiotherapy has been administered after mastectomy for invasive breast carcinoma with a latency time ranging from 30 to 156 months (mean 70 months). The age is more advanced than that of de novo angiosarcoma ranging from 61 to 78 years {2223}. In these cases the neoplastic endothelial proliferation is necessarily confined to the skin {392}.
2) In the breast after conservation treatment for breast carcinoma. Fifty two cases had been reported as of December 1997. The first case was described in 1987 {1764}. This type of angiosarcoma involves only the skin in more than half the cases, while exclusive involvement of breast parenchyma is very rare. Most tumours (81%) are multifocal and a large majority of patients harbour grade II to III angiosarcomas. Radiotherapy and chemotherapy are ineffective {2876}.

Liposarcoma

Definition

A variably cellular or myxoid tumour containing at least a few lipoblasts.

ICD-O code   8850/3

Epidemiology

Primary liposarcoma should be distinguished from liposarcomatous differentiation in a phyllodes tumour. It occurs predominantly in women ranging in age from 19-76 years (median, 47 years) {116, 138}. The tumour only rarely occurs in the male breast {3027}. Liposarcoma following radiation therapy for breast carcinoma has been reported.

Clinical features

Patients present most often with a slowly enlarging, painful mass. In general, skin changes and axillary node enlargement are absent. Rarely the tumour is bilateral {3027}.

Macroscopy

Liposarcomas are often well circumscribed or encapsulated, about one-third have infiltrative margin. With a median size of 8 cm, liposarcomas may become enormous exceeding 15 cm {116,138}. Necrosis and haemorrhage may be present on the cut surface of larger tumours.

Histopathology

The histopathology and immunophenotype is identical to that of liposarcoma at other sites. The presence of lipoblasts establishes the diagnosis. Practically every variant of soft tissue liposarcoma has been reported in the breast, including the pleomorphic, dedifferentiated and myxoid variants. Despite the well delineated gross appearance, many mammary liposarcomas have at least partial infiltrative margins on histological examination. Atypia is often present at least focally. The well differentiated and myxoid variants have a delicate arborizing vascular network and few lipoblasts. These may assume a signet-ring appearance in the myxoid variant. The pleomorphic variant is composed of highly pleomorphic cells and bears significant resemblance to malignant fibrous histiocytoma; the presence of lipoblasts identifies the lesion as a liposarcoma. Mitotic figures are readily identifiable in this variant.

Differential diagnosis
Vacuolated cells in a variety of lesions may be confused with lipoblasts. Typical lipoblasts have scalloped irregular nuclei with sharply defined vacuoles that contain lipid rather than glycogen or mucin. Clear nuclear pseudo-inclusions are a characteristic of the bizarre large cells in atypical lipomatous tumours and help distinguish these atypical cells from true lipoblasts that are diagnostic of a liposarcoma.

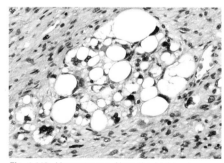
Fig. 1.143 Liposarcoma. Note the highly pleomorphic nuclei and multiple lipoblasts.

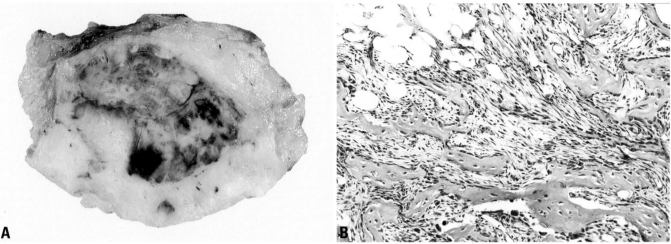

Fig. 1.144 Mammary osteosarcoma. **A** The sectioned surface shows a well delineated, solid mass with focal haemorrhage. **B** The spindle cell component of the tumour invades the adipose tissue and is admixed with abundant bony frabeculae.

Prognosis and predictive factors
Both the myxoid and pleomorphic variants of liposarcoma can recur and metastasize. Axillary node metastases are exceptionally rare. Recurrences generally develop within the first year and patients who die from their disease usually do so within a year of the diagnosis. Because of the high frequency of marginal irregularity, complete excision with tumour free margins is necessary. Liposarcomas behave particularly aggressively when associated with pregnancy.

Rhabdomyosarcoma

Definition
A tumour composed of cells showing varying degrees of skeletal muscle differentiation.

ICD-O codes
Rhabdomyosarcoma   8900/3
Alveolar type   8920/3
Pleomorphic type   8901/3

Epidemiology
Pure primary rhabdomyosarcoma of the breast is very uncommon, and, although primary mammary rhabdomyosarcoma has been described, it usually represents a metastasis from a soft tissue rhabdomyosarcoma occuring in children, young females or males {2402}. More frequently, rhabdomyosarcomatous differentiation may be observed in older women as an heterologous component of a malig-

nant phyllodes tumour or a metaplastic carcinoma.

Pathology
Primary rhabdomyosarcoma has been reported in adolescents {773,1166,1198, 2402}, when it is predominantly of the alveolar subtype; the pleomorphic subtype has been reported in older women over forty {2871}.
Metastatic rhabdomyosarcoma to the breast is again predominantly of the alveolar subtype {1166,1248}. The primary lesion is usually located on the extremities, in the nasopharynx/paranasal sinuses or on the trunk {1166}. A metastasis from an embryonal rhabdomyosarcoma to the breast is less frequent {1166, 2531}.
Metastatic breast tumours may occur as part of disseminated disease or as an isolated lesion.

Mammary osteosarcoma

Definition
A malignant tumour composed of spindle cells that produce osteoid and/or bone together with cartilage in some cases.

ICD-O code   9180/3

Synonym
Mammary osteogenic sarcoma.

Epidemiology
Accounting for about 12% of all mammary sarcomas, pure osteosarcomas must be distinguished from those origi-

nating in phyllodes tumours or carcinosarcomas. Absence of connection to the skeleton, which should be confirmed by imaging studies, is required for a diagnosis of a primary mammary osteosarcomas.
Osteosarcomas occur mainly in older women with a median age of 64.5 years; the age range is 27–89 years {2681}. The vast majority of patients are women who are predominantly Caucasian. A prior history of radiation therapy or trauma has been noted in some women {331}.

Clinical features
The tumour presents as an enlarging mass which is associated with pain in one-fifth of cases. Bloody nipple discharge or nipple retraction occurs in 12% of the women. Mammographically, osteosarcomas present as a well circumscribed mass with focal to extensive coarse calcification. Because of their predominantly circumscribed nature, they may be misinterpreted as a benign lesion {3072}.

Macroscopy
Osteosarcomas vary in size from 1.4 to 13 cm; most are about 5 cm in size and are sharply delineated. The consistency varies from firm to stony hard depending on the proportion of osseous differentiation. Cavitation and necrosis are seen in larger tumours.

Histopathology
The histopathological appearance and immunophenotype are similar to that of

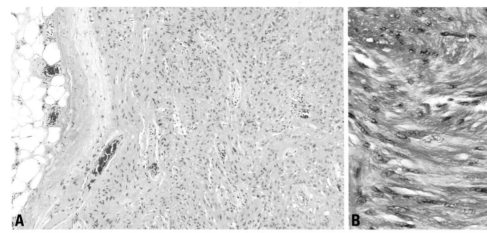

Fig. 1.145 Leiomyoma. **A** The well circumscribed margin (left) is apparent. **B** The bland smooth muscle cells proliferate in whorls and fascicles.

extraosseous osteosarcoma at other sites of the body. Despite the predominantly circumscribed margins, characteristically, at least focal infiltration is present. The tumour is composed of a spindle to oval cell population with variable amounts of osteoid or osseous tissue; cartilage is present in over a third of the cases {2681} but no other differentiated tissues.

The appearance of the tumours varies depending on the cellular composition (fibroblastic, osteoblastic, osteoclastic) as well as the type and amount of matrix (osteoid, osseous, chondroid).

The osteoclastic giant cells are immunoreactive with the macrophage marker CD68 (clone KP1) while the spindle cells fail to immunoreact with either estrogen receptor (ER) or progesterone receptor (PR) or epithelial markers.

Prognosis and predictive factors

Mammary osteosarcomas are highly aggressive lesions with an overall five-year survival of 38% {2681}. Recurrences develop in over two-thirds of the patients treated by local excision and 11% of those treated by mastectomy. Metastases to the lungs and absence of axillary node involvement are typical of osteosarcomas. Many of the patients who develop metastases die of the disease within 2 years of initial diagnosis {2681}.

Fibroblastic osteosarcomas are associated with a better survival compared to the osteoblastic or osteoclastic variants. Large tumour size at presentation, prominent infiltrating margins and necrosis are associated with more aggressive behaviour.

Leiomyoma and leiomyosarcoma

Definition

Benign and malignant tumours composed of intersecting bundles of smooth muscle which is mature in benign lesions. Malignant lesions are larger in size and show more mitotic activity in the neoplastic cells.

ICD-O codes

Leiomyoma	8890/0
Leiomyosarcoma	8890/3

Epidemiology

Benign and malignant smooth muscle tumours of the breast are uncommon and represent less than 1% of breast neoplasms. The majority of leiomyomas originate from the areolar-nipple complex and a minority occur within the breast proper {1981}. Leiomyosarcomas arise mainly within the breast {821}.

The age at presentation of leiomyomas and leiomyosarcomas overlaps, extending from the fourth to the seventh decades. However, cases of both have been reported in adolescents {2000} and patients over eighty years old {821}.

Clinical features

Both leiomyomas and leiomyosarcomas usually present as a slowly growing palpable mobile mass that may be painful. Incidental asymptomatic leiomyomas discovered in mastectomy specimens have been reported {1981}.

Macroscopy

These lesions appear as well circumscribed firm nodules with a whorled or lobulated cut surface. Their size ranges from 0.5 to 15 cm {770,2000}.

Histopathology

The histopathology and immunophenotype are identical to that seen in smooth muscle tumours elsewhere in the body. These neoplasms may be well circumscribed {1981} or show irregular infiltrative borders {2000}. Both are composed of spindle cells arranged in interlacing fascicles.

In leiomyomas, these cells have elongated cigar-shaped nuclei and eosinophilic cytoplasm without evidence of atypia. Mitoses are sparse and typically fewer than 3 per 10 high power fields {458}. In leiomyosarcomas, nuclear atypia and mitotic activity are more prominent {821}. Tumour necrosis may also be observed. Infiltrating margins may not be evident in some leiomyosarcomas.

Differential diagnosis

A diagnosis of a smooth muscle tumour of the breast should be considered only after excluding other breast lesions that may show benign or malignant smooth muscle differentiation i.e. fibroadenoma, muscular hamartoma and sclerosing adenosis should be distinguished from leiomyoma; spindle cell myoepithelioma and sarcomatoid carcinoma from leiomyosarcoma.

Prognosis and predictive factors

Leiomyomas are best treated by complete excision whereas, wide excision with tumour-free margins is recommended for leiomyosarcomas. Late local recurrence and metastatasis have been reported in cases of mammary leiomyosarcoma {458,2014}.

Fibroepithelial tumours

J.P. Bellocq
G. Magro

Definition

A heterogeneous group of genuine biphasic lesions combining an epithelial component and a quantitatively predominant mesenchymal component (also called stromal component) which is responsible for the gross appearance. Depending on the benign or malignant nature of each component, various combinations may occur. They are classified into two major categories: fibroadenomas and phyllodes tumours.

Hamartomas are not fibroepithelial tumours, but represent pseudotumoral changes. As they contain glandular and stromal tissue, and sometimes may resemble fibroadenomas, they have been included in this chapter.

Fibroadenoma

Definition

A benign biphasic tumour, fibroadenoma (FA) occurs most frequently in women of childbearing age, especially those under 30.

ICD-O code

9010/0

Aetiology

Usually considered a neoplasm, some believe FA results from hyperplasia of normal lobular components rather than being a true neoplasm.

Clinical features

FA presents as a painless, solitary, firm, slowly growing (up to 3 cm), mobile, well defined nodule. Less frequently it may occur as multiple nodules arising synchronously or asynchronously in the same or in both breasts and may grow very large (up to 20 cm) mainly when it occurs in adolescents. Such lesions, may be called "giant" fibroadenomas. With the increasing use of screening mammography, small, non-palpable FAs are being discovered.

Macroscopy

The cut surface is solid, firm, bulging, greyish in colour, with a slightly lobulated

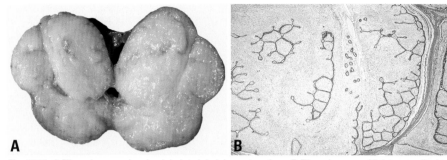

Fig. 1.146 A Fibroadenoma showing lobulated, bulging cut surface. **B** Fibroadenoma with intracanalicular growth pattern.

pattern and slit like spaces. Variations depend on the amount of hyalinization and myxoid change in the stromal component. Calcification of sclerotic lesions is common.

Histopathology

The admixture of stromal and epithelial proliferation gives rise to two distinct growth patterns of no clinical significance. The pericanalicular pattern is the result of proliferation of stromal cells around ducts in a circumferential fashion; this pattern is observed most frequently during the second and third decades of life. The intracanalicular pattern is due to compression of the ducts into clefts by the proliferating stromal cells. The stromal component may sometimes exhibit focal or diffuse hypercellularity (especially in women less than 20 years of age), atypical bizarre multinucleated giant cells {233,2278}, extensive myxoid changes or hyalinization with dystrophic calcification and, rarely, ossification (especially in postmenopausal women). Foci of lipomatous, smooth muscle {1040}, and osteochondroid {1852,2762} metaplasia may rarely occur. Mitotic figures are uncommon. Total infarction has been reported, but rarely.

The epithelial component can show a wide spectrum of typical hyperplasia, mainly in adolescents {411,1525,1861, 2250}, and metaplastic changes such as apocrine or squamous metaplasia may be seen. Foci of fibrocystic change, sclerosing adenosis and even extensive myoepithelial proliferation can also occur in FA. In situ lobular, and ductal carcinoma occasionally develop within FAs {693,1525}.

Juvenile (or cellular) fibroadenomas are characterized by increased stromal cellularity and epithelial hyperplasia {1861, 2250}. The term giant FA has been used as a synonym for juvenile fibroadenoma by some, but is restricted to massive fibroadenomas with usual histology by others.

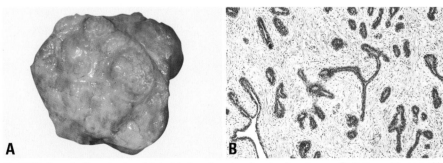

Fig. 1.147 Juvenile fibroadenoma. **A** Lobulated sectioned surface in a 8 cm tumour. Patient was 16 years old. **B** Periductal growth pattern with moderate stromal hypercellularity.

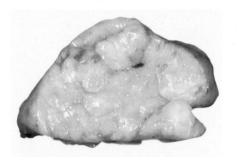

Fig. 1.148 Phyllodes tumour. A well circumscribed 6.5 cm mass with a few clefts was histologically benign.

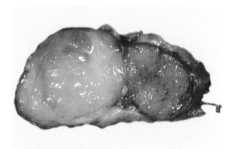

Fig. 1.149 Phyllodes tumour. A circumscribed 9 cm tumour contained a large yellow nodule of liposarcoma (yellow) adjacent to a nodule of malignant phyllodes tumour (pink).

Differential diagnosis

Most FAs, especially those of large size, cellular stroma and epithelial clefts need to be distinguished from phyllodes tumours (see below). Another breast lesion, which can simulate FA, is hamartoma.

Prognosis and predictive features

Most FAs do not recur after complete surgical excision. In adolescents, there is a tendency for one or more new lesions to develop at another site or even close to the site of the previous surgical treatment.

The risk of developing cancer within a FA or in breasts of patients previously treated for FA is low, although a slightly increased risk has been reported {734, 1640}.

Phyllodes tumours

Definition

A group of circumscribed biphasic tumours, basically analogous to fibroadenomas, characterized by a double layered epithelial component arranged in clefts surrounded by an overgrowing hypercellular mesenchymal component typically organized in leaf-like structures.

Phyllodes tumours (PTs) are usually benign, but recurrences are not uncommon and a relatively small number of patients will develop haematogenous metastases. Depending on the bland or overtly sarcomatous characteristics of their mesenchymal component (also called stromal component), PTs display a morphological spectrum lying between fibroadenomas (FAs) and pure stromal sarcomas.

Still widespread in the literature, the generic term "cystosarcoma phyllodes", is currently considered inappropriate and potentially dangerous since the majority of these tumours follow a benign course. It is highly preferable to use the neutral term "phyllodes tumour", according to the view already expressed in the WHO classification of 1981 {3154}, with the adjunction of an adjective determining the putative behaviour based on histological characteristics.

ICD-O codes

Phyllodes tumour, NOS	9020/1
Phyllodes tumour, benign	9020/0
Phyllodes tumour, borderline	9020/1
Phyllodes tumour, malignant	9020/3
Periductal stromal sarcoma, low grade	9020/3

Epidemiology

In western countries, PTs account for 0,3-1% of all primary tumours and for 2,5% of all fibroepithelial tumours of the breast. They occur predominantly in middle-

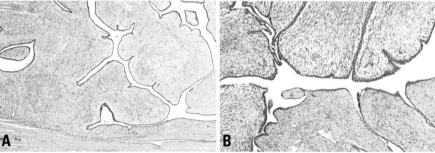

Fig. 1.150 Benign phyllodes tumour. **A** Leaf-like pattern and well defined interface with the surrounding normal tissue. **B** Higher magnification shows stromal cellularity.

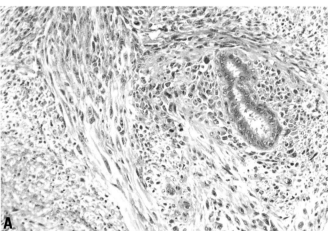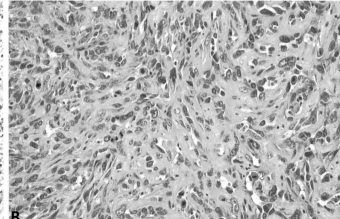

Fig. 1.151 Malignant phyllodes tumour. **A** Periductal stromal growth with malignant features. **B** Note severe stromal atypia and multiple mitoses.

aged women (average age of presentation is 40-50 years) around 15-20 years older than for FAs.

In Asian countries, PTs occur at a younger age (average 25-30 years) {487}.

Malignant PTs develop on average 2-5 years later than benign PTs. Among Latino whites, especially those born in Central and South America, malignant phyllodes is more frequent {254}.

Isolated examples of PTs in men have been recorded {1424a,2023}.

Aetiology

PTs are thought to be derived from intralobular or periductal stroma. They may develop de novo or from FAs. It is possible, in rare cases, to demonstrate the presence of a pre-existing FA adjacent to a PT.

Clinical features

Usually, patients present with a unilateral, firm, painless breast mass, not attached to the skin. Very large tumours (>10 cm) may stretch the skin with striking distension of superficial veins, but ulceration is very rare. Due to mammographic screening, 2-3 cm tumours are becoming more common, but the average size remains around 4-5 cm {775,2425}. Bloody nipple discharge caused by spontaneous infarction of the tumour has been described in adolescent girls {1781, 2833}. Multifocal or bilateral lesions are rare {1932}.

Imaging reveals a rounded, usually sharply defined, mass containing clefts or cysts and sometimes coarse calcifications.

Macroscopy

PTs form a well circumscribed firm, bulging mass. Because of their often clearly defined margins, they are often shelled out surgically.

The cut surface is tan or pink to grey and may be mucoid. The characteristic whorled pattern with curved clefts resembling leaf buds is best seen in large lesions, but smaller lesions may have an homogeneous appearance. Haemorrhage or necrosis may be present in large lesions.

Histopathology

PTs typically exhibit an enhanced intracanalicular growth pattern with leaf-like projections into dilated lumens. The epithelial component consists of luminal

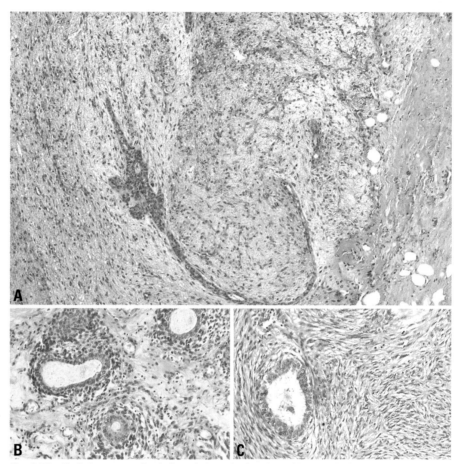

Fig. 1.152 Phyllodes tumour, borderline. **A** A predominantly pushing margin in a borderline tumour. **B** Periductal stromal condensation. **C** Dense spindle-cell stroma with a few mitotic figures.

epithelial and myoepithelial cells. Apocrine or squamous metaplasia is occasionally present and hyperplasia is not unusual. In benign phyllodes tumours, the stroma is more cellular than in FAs, the spindle cell nuclei are monomorphic and mitoses are rare. The stromal cellularity may be higher in zones in close contact with the epithelial component. Areas of sparse stromal cellularity, hyalinisation or myxoid changes are not uncommon. Necrotic areas may be seen in very large tumours. The presence of occasional bizarre giant cells should not be taken as a mark of malignancy. Lipomatous, cartilagenous and osseous metaplasia have been reported {2057,2730}. The margins are usually well delimited, although very small tumour buds may protrude into the surrounding tissue. Such expansions may be left behind after surgical removal and are a source of local recurrence.

Malignant PTs have infiltrative rather than pushing margins. The stroma shows frankly sarcomatous, usually fibrosarco-

matous changes. Heterologous differentiation such as liposarcoma, osteosarcoma, chondrosarcoma or rhabdomyosarcoma may occur {536,1161,2057,2249, 2308}. Such changes should be indicated in the diagnostic report. Due to overgrowth of the sarcomatous components, the epithelial component may only be identified after examining multiple sections.

Borderline PTs (or low grade malignant PTs) display intermediate features and the stroma often resembles low-grade fibrosarcoma.

Malignant epithelial transformation (DCIS or LIN and their invasive counterparts) is uncommon {2136}.

Differential diagnosis

Benign PTs may be difficult to distinguish from fibroadenomas. The main features are the more cellular stroma and the formation of leaf-like processes. However, the degree of hypercellularity that is required to qualify a PT at its lower limit is difficult to define. Leaf-like

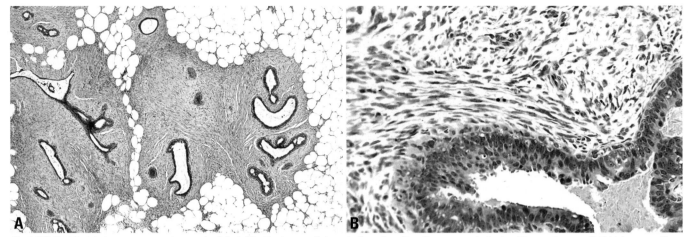

Fig. 1.153 Periductal stroma sarcoma, low grade. **A** An infiltrative hypercellular spindle cell proliferation surrounds ducts with open lumens. **B** At higher magnification, the neoplastic spindle cells contain at least three mitotic figures per 10 high power fields.

processes may be found in intracanalicular FAs with hypocellular and oedematous stroma, but the leaf-like processes are few in number and often poorly formed.

The term giant FA as well as juvenile (or cellular) FA have often been used inappropriately as a synonym for benign PT. Although the term periductal stromal sarcoma has been used as a synonym for PTs {2079}, it is better restricted to a very rare non circumscribed biphasic lesion characterized by a spindle cell proliferation localized around tubules that retain an open lumen and absence of leaf-like processes {2876}. These often low grade lesions may recur and rarely progress to a classic PT.

Malignant PTs may be confused with pure sarcomas of the breast. In such case, diagnosis depends on finding residual epithelial structures. However, the clinical impact of these two entities appears to be similar {1887}.

Grading
Several grading systems have been proposed with either two subgroups {1596,2876}, or three subgroups {1473, 1887}. None is universally applied since prediction of the behaviour remains difficult in an individual case.

Grading is based on semi-quantitative assessment of stromal cellularity, cellular pleomorphism, mitotic activity, margin appearance and stromal distribution.

Because of the structural variability of PTs, the selection of one block for every 1 cm of maximal tumour dimension is appropriate {2876}. PTs should be subclassified according to the areas of highest cellular activity and most florid architectural pattern. The different thresholds of mitotic indices vary substantially from author to author. Since the size of high power fields is variable among different microscope brands, it has been suggested that the mitotic count be related to the size of the field diameter {1887}. Stromal overgrowth has been defined as stromal proliferation to the point where the epithelial elements are absent in at least one low power field (40x) {3058}. So defined, stromal overgrowth is not uncommon.

Prognosis and predictive factors
Local recurrence occurs in both benign and malignant tumours. Recurrence may mirror the microscopic pattern of the original tumour or show dedifferentiation (in 75% of cases) {1067}. Metastases to nearly all internal organs have been reported, but the lung and skeleton are the most common sites of spread. Axillary lymph node metastases are rare, but have been recorded in 10-15% in cases of systemic disease {1887,2876}. Recurrences generally develop within 2 years, while most deaths from tumour occur within 5 years of diagnosis, sometimes after mediastinal compression through direct chest wall invasion.
The frequency of local recurrence and metastases correlate with the grade of PTs but vary considerably from one series to another. The average in pub-

Table 1.18
Main histologic features of the 3 tiered grading subgroups for phyllodes tumours.

	Benign	Borderline	Malignant
Stromal hypercellularity	modest	modest	marked
Cellular pleomorphism	little	moderate	marked
Mitosis	few if any	intermediate	numerous (more than 10 per 10 HPF)
Margins	well circumscribed, pushing	intermediate	invasive
Stromal pattern	uniform stromal distribution	heterogeneous stromal expansion	marked stromal overgrowth
Heterologeous stromal differentiation	rare	rare	not uncommon
Overall average distribution {1887}	60%	20%	20%

lished data suggests a 21% rate of local recurrence overall, with a 17%, 25% and 27% rate in benign, borderline and malignant PTs, respectively, and a 10% rate of metastases overall, with a 0%, 4% and 22% rate in benign, borderline and malignant PTs, respectively {1887}. Local recurrence after surgery is strongly dependent on the width of the excision margins {186}.

Mammary hamartomas

Definition
A well demarcated, generally encapsulated mass, composed of all components of breast tissue.

Epidemiology
Hamartomas occur predominantly in the peri-menopausal age group, but may be found at any age, including teenagers and post-menopausal women.

Clinical features
Hamartomas are frequently asymptomatic and only revealed by mammography {3042}. They are detected in 0.16% of mammograms {1204}. Very large lesions can deform the breast. Due to their well defined borders they are easily enucleated.

Macroscopy
Hamartomas are round, oval, or discoid, ranging in size from 1 cm to more than 20 cm. Depending on the composition of the lesion the cut surface may resemble nor-

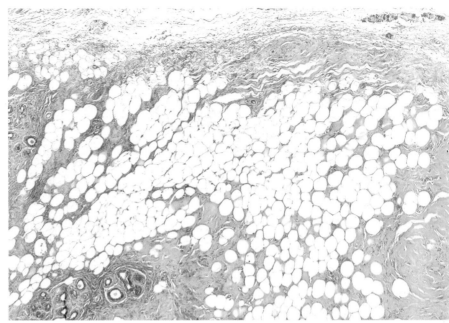

Fig. 1.154 Hamartoma. Intraparenchymal mass of common breast tissue with well defined margin.

mal breast tissue, a lipoma or may be rubbery and reminiscent of a FA.

Histopathology
Generally encapsulated, this circumscribed mass of breast tissue may show fibrocystic or atrophic changes; pseudoangiomatous hyperplasia (PASH) is frequent {446}. The lesion gives the impression of "breast within breast". In adolescents, differentiation between the appearance of the normal adolescent breast and FAs or asymmetric virginal hypertrophy can be difficult. Rare examples resembling phyllodes tumours, have been observed {2876}.

Variants of hamartoma

Adenolipoma {867}, adenohibernoma {618}, and myoid hamartoma {624} could all be considered variants of mammary hamartoma.

Prognosis
The lesion is benign with no tendency to recur.

Tumours of the nipple

V. Eusebi
K.T. Mai
A. Taranger-Charpin

Nipple adenoma

Definition
A compact proliferation of small tubules lined by epithelial and myoepithelial cells, with or without proliferation of the epithelial component, around the collecting ducts of the nipple.

ICD-O code   8506/0

Synonyms
Nipple duct adenoma; papillary adenoma; erosive adenomatosis; florid papillomatosis; papillomatosis of the nipple, subareolar duct papillomatosis.

Historical annotation
Under the designation of nipple adenoma (NA), several morphological lesions (some of which overlap) have been included {1356,2222,2429,2894}.
1. The largest group consists of cases showing an adenosis pattern in its classical form, with sclerosis and/or pseudoinvasive features, sclerosing papillomatosis {2429}, and infiltrative epitheliosis {149}).
2. Epithelial hyperplasia (papillomatosis {2429}; epitheliosis {149}) of the collecting ducts.
3. Lesions composed of a combination of epithelial hyperplasia and sclerosing adenosis.

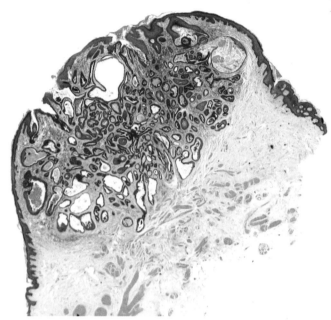

Fig. 1.155 Adenoma of the nipple. A compact aggregate of tubules replaces the nipple stroma.

Epidemiology
NA is rare with a wide age range from 20 to 87 years) {2894} and may occur in males {2429}.

Clinical features
Presenting symptoms are most frequently a sanguineous or serous discharge and occasionally erosion of the nipple or underlying nodule {2222}.

Histopathology
In the adenosis type, proliferating two cell layered glands sprout from and compress the collecting ducts {2222} resulting in cystic dilatation of the latter and formation of a discrete nodule. The epidermis may undergo hyperkeratosis. Rarely the adenosis expands to cause erosion of the epidermis {2429}.
When the sclerosis and pseudoinfiltrative patterns are prominent, an invasive carcinoma is closely simulated. The background stroma shows loose myxoid features, large collagenous bands or elastosis {149}.

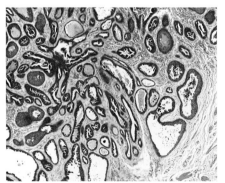

Fig. 1.156 Adenoma of the nipple. There is no significant epithelial proliferation in the tubules in this case.

Epithelial hyperplasia may be florid within the tubules of adenosis or mainly within the collecting ducts. Enlargement of the galactophore ostia and exposure of the epithelial proliferation to the exterior in a fashion reminiscent of "ectropion" of the uterine cervix may occur.

Prognosis and predictive factors
Occasional recurrences have been described after incomplete excision {2425}. Association with carcinoma has been reported but is rare {1367, 2429}.

Syringomatous adenoma

Definition
A non metastasizing, locally recurrent, and locally invasive tumour of the nipple/areolar region showing sweat duct differentiation.

ICD-O code   8407/0

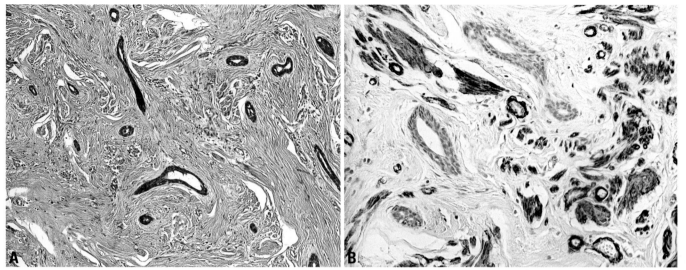

Fig. 1.157 Syringomatous adenoma of the nipple. **A** Irregular shaped glandular structures are present between smooth muscle bundles. **B** Actin stains the fascicles of smooth muscle but the syringoma is unstained.

Synonym
Infiltrating syringomatous adenoma.

Epidemiology
Syringomatous adenoma (SyT) is a rare lesion {1365,2414,2816}. While only 24 cases have been reported under this designation {98}, other cases have been reported as examples of low grade adenosquamous carcinoma {2431,2816, 2995}. The age range is from 11 to 67 years with an average age of 40 years.

Clinical features
SyA presents as a firm discrete mass (1–3 cm) situated in the nipple and sub-areolar region {269,1365}.

Macroscopy
The lesion appears as a firm, ill defined nodule.

Histopathology
SyA consists of nests and branching cords of cells, glandular structures and small keratinous cysts permeating the nipple stroma in between bundles of muscle as well as in perineural spaces {1365,3056}. Extensions of the tumour may be present at a great distance from the main mass with intervening normal tissue. Cytologically, most of the proliferating elements appear bland with scant eosinophilic cytoplasm and regular round nuclei. The cells lining the gland lumina are cuboidal or flat. Frequently the glandular structures display two layers of cells: i.e. inner luminal and outer cuboidal basal cells occasionally containing smooth muscle actin. Mitoses are rare and necrotic areas are absent. The stroma is usually sclerotic, but myxoid areas containing spindle cells are frequent.

Differential diagnosis
This includes tubular carcinoma (TC) which rarely involves the nipple and low grade adenosquamous carcinoma which occurs in the breast parenchyma {2431}.

Prognosis and predictive factors
Recurrence has been reported {269}. Optimal treatment is excision with generous margins.

Paget disease of the nipple

Definition
The presence of malignant glandular epithelial cells within the squamous epithelium of the nipple, is almost always associated with underlying intraductal carcinoma, usually involving more than one lactiferous duct and more distant ducts, with or without infiltration, deep in the underlying breast. Paget disease (PD) of the nipple without an underlying carcinoma is rare.

ICD-O code   8540/3

Epidemiology
PD may be bilateral and may occur in either gender but at a relatively higher rate in men. The incidence is estimated at 1-4.3% of all breast carcinomas.

Aetiology
The glandular nature of the neoplastic cells in PD is confirmed by electron microscopic studies that show intra-cytoplasmic lumen with microvilli {2505}. Immunohistochemical studies confirm that Paget cells have the same phenotype as the underlying intra-ductal carcinoma cells {530,1423}. Suggested mechanisms of development are: a) intraepithelial epider-motropic migration of malignant cells of intraductal carcinoma to the epidermis; b) direct extension of underlying intra-ductal carcinoma to the nipple and overlying skin; and c) in situ neoplastic transformation of multi-potential cells located in the basal layer of the lactiferous duct and epidermis.

Clinical features
Depending on the extent of epidermal involvement, the skin may appear unremarkable or show changes ranging from focal reddening to a classical eczematous appearance, which may extend to the areola and adjacent epidermis. There is sometimes retraction of the nipple.

Histopathology
In the epidermis, there is proliferation of atypical cells with large nuclei and abundant clear or focally dense cytoplasm. They are disposed in small clus-

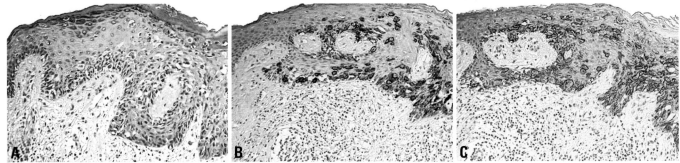

Fig. 1.158 Paget disease of the nipple. **A** Atypical cells with clear cytoplasm admixed with those with dense cytoplasm. **B, C** Immunostaining for cytokeratin 7 **(B)** and ERBB2 **(C)** decorate the neoplastic cells predominantly located in the lower portion of the epidermis.

ters which are often closely packed in the centre of the lesion and lower portion of the epidermis but tend to be dispersed in single cells at the periphery and upper portion of the epidermis. The underlying lactiferous ducts contain a usually high grade DCIS that merges with the PD. Rarely, lobular intraepithelial neoplasia is encountered. Even when the in situ carcinoma is in the deep breast tissue, an involved lactiferous duct with or without skip areas can almost always be identified by serial sectioning.

An associated infiltrating carcinoma occurs in one-third of patients who present without a palpable mass and in more than 90% of those with a palpable mass. Special stains reveal the presence of mucin in the Paget cells in a large number of cases. Paget cells occasionally contain melanin pigment granules as a result of phagocytosis.

Immunoprofile
Immunohistochemically, Paget cells demonstrate similar properties to the underlying intraductal carcinoma cells with positive immunoreactivity for carcinoembryonic antigen, low molecular weight cytokeratin and ERBB2. On occasion, one of these antisera may be negative. Squamous carcinoma is commonly non-reactive for these antisera, but rarely may be immunoreactive for cytokeratin 7 {3128}. Contrary to malignant melanoma, PD is usually S-100 protein and HMB45 negative. In PD, TP53 and estrogen receptor may be negative or positive, depending on the immunoprofile of the corresponding underlying carcinoma.

Differential diagnosis
PD occasionally poses differential diagnostic problems with malignant melanoma due to the pagetoid pattern of spread and the presence of pigment granules and also with squamous cell carcinoma in situ, due to the proliferation of atypical dark cells. The application of histochemical techniques and the use of immunostains will solve the question in most cases.

Prognosis and predictive factors
The prognosis is dependent on the presence or absence of underlying intraductal carcinoma and associated invasive carcinoma in the deep breast tissue.

Malignant lymphoma and metastatic tumours

J. Lamovec
A. Wotherspoon
J. Jacquemier

Malignant lymphoma

Definition

Malignant lymphoma of the breast may present as a primary or secondary tumour; both are rare. There is no morphological criterion to differentiate between the two {117,1792}.

The criteria for defining and documentation of primary breast lymphoma, first proposed by Wiseman and Liao {3136} and, with minor modifications, accepted by others, are as follows:

1. Availability of adequate histological material.
2. Presence of breast tissue in, or adjacent to, the lymphoma infiltrate.
3. No concurrent nodal disease except for the involvement of ipsilateral axillary lymph nodes.
4. No previous history of lymphoma involving other organs or tissues.

As such criteria seem too restrictive and leave no room for primary breast lymphomas of higher stages, some authors include cases in which the breast is the first or major site of presentation, even if, on subsequent staging procedures, involvement of distant nodal sites or bone marrow is discovered {359,1261,1753}.

Epidemiology

Primary breast lymphoma may appear at any age, but the majority of patients are postmenopausal women. A subset of patients is represented by pregnant or lactating women with massive bilateral breast swelling; most of these cases were reported from Africa {2643} although non-African cases are also on record {1753}. The disease is exceedingly rare in men {2540}.

Clinical features

Clinical presentation of primary breast lymphoma usually does not differ from that of breast carcinoma. It usually presents with a painless lump sometimes multinodular, which is bilateral in approximately 10% of cases. Imaging usually reveals no feature which helps to distinguish primary from secondary lymphoma {1657,2199}. The value of MR imaging in breast lymphomas has not been clearly determined {1952,1961}.

Macroscopy

Primary and secondary breast lymphomas most commonly appear as a well circumscribed tumour of varying size, up to 20 cm in largest diameter. On cut surface, the neoplastic tissue is white to white-grey, soft or firm, with occasional haemorrhagic or necrotic foci {994, 1580,1753,3136}.

Histopathology

Microscopically, the majority of primary breast lymphomas are diffuse large B cell lymphomas, according to the most recent WHO classification {352,1144}. In older literature, cases designated as reticulum cell sarcoma, histiocytic lymphoma and at least some lymphosarcoma cases would nowadays most probably be included in the above category. More recently, such lymphomas were diagnosed as centroblastic or immunoblastic by the Kiel classification or diffuse large cell cleaved or noncleaved and immunoblastic lymphomas by the Lukes-Collins classification and Working Formulation {18,296,534,706,994,1261, 1346,1580,1665}.

A minor proportion of primary lymphomas of the breast reflect Burkitt lymphoma, extranodular marginal-zone B-cell lymphoma of mucosa associated lymphoid tissue (MALT) type, follicular lymphoma, lymphoblastic lymphoma of either B or T type, and, extremely rarely, T-cell lymphomas of variable subtypes by the current WHO classification.

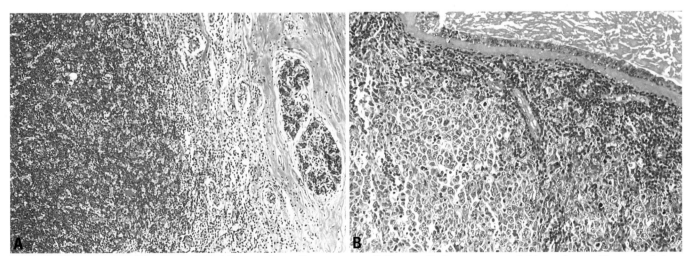

Fig. 1.159 Diffuse large B-cell lymphoma. **A** Medullary carcinoma-like appearance. **B** Circumscribed mass, composed of large pleomorphic neoplastic lymphoid cells.

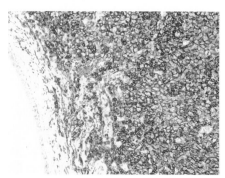

Fig. 1.160 CD20 immunoexpression in diffuse large B-cell lymphoma.

The relationship of the surrounding mammary tissue to the lymphomatous infiltration differs from case to case. In some, the bulk of the lesion is located in the subcutaneous tissue, and breast parenchyma is found only peripherally. In others, numerous ducts and lobules are embedded in the infiltrate but clearly separated from it. Sometimes lymphoma cells infiltrate the ducts to different degrees and, in rare cases, the latter are overgrown by lymphoma cells and barely visible, sometimes revealed only by using keratin immunostaining. The stroma may be scant or abundant and the infiltrates may have a "medullary" appearance. In some cases, lymphoma cells form cords and ribbons simulating an infiltrating lobular carcinoma.

Diffuse large B-cell lymphoma

ICD-O code   9680/3

Lymphoma of this type is characterized by a diffuse pattern of infiltration of breast tissue by large lymphoma cells varying in appearance from quite uniform to pleomorphic. Generally, the lymphoma cells resemble centroblasts or immunoblasts. The nuclei are oval, indented or even lobated, usually with distinct, single or multiple nucleoli, and the amount of cytoplasm is variable. Mitoses are usually numerous, various numbers of cells are apoptotic and necrotic foci may be found. Lymphoma cells are often admixed with smaller reactive lymphocytes of B or T type; macrophages may be prominent, imparting a "starry sky" appearance to the tumour. In some cases, pseudofollicular structures are seen due to selective infiltration of ductal-lobular units {18}. Adjacent mammary tissue may exhibit lobular atrophy or lymphocytic lobulitis

{18,113}; the latter may be prominent and widespread, featuring lymphocytic mastopathy {113}.

Lymphoma cells are immunoreactive for CD20, CD79a, and CD45RB and negative for CD3 and CD45RO. Cases with immunoblastic features may demonstrate light chain restriction. Exceptionally, lymphoma cells express CD30 antigen {18}.

Burkitt lymphoma

ICD-O code   9687/3

The morphological features of Burkitt lymphoma of the breast are identical with those seen in such a lymphoma in other organs and tissues: the infiltrate is composed of sheets of uniform, primitive looking, cells of medium size, with round nuclei, multiple nucleoli, coarse chromatin and a rather thick nuclear membrane. The cells are cohesive and the cytoplasm is moderate in amount with fine vacuoles containing lipids; it squares off with the cytoplasm of adjacent cells. Mitoses are very numerous. Numerous tingible-body macrophages are evenly dispersed among the neoplastic cells producing the characteristic, but by no means pathognomonic, "starry sky" appearance of the lymphoma. The breast tissue is usually hyperplastic and secretory.

Patients are usually pregnant or lactating women, particularly from tropical Africa where Burkitt lymphoma is endemic {2643}. Less frequently, non-endemic, sporadic cases, primarily presenting in the breasts, have been observed {1378}. Tumours typically present with massive bilateral breast swelling {2643}.

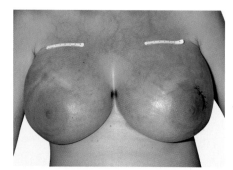

Fig. 1.161 Burkitt lymphoma. Bilateral breast involvement may be the presenting manifestation during pregnancy and puberty. BL cells have prolactin receptors.

Immunohistochemically, pan-B markers are positive, surface Ig, usually of IgM type, is also positive. In addition, CD10 and bcl-6 are commonly positive, while CD5, bcl-2 and TdT are negative. EBV is frequently demonstrated in endemic but not in sporadic cases. IgH and IgL genes are rearranged.

Extranodal marginal-zone B-cell lymphoma of MALT type

ICD-O code   9699/3

At least some breast lymphomas appear to belong to the category of MALT lymphomas although the data on their frequency vary substantially. The breast was suggested to be one component of a common mucosal immune system {268} and may acquire lymphoid tissue as a part of an autoimmune process {2585} within which the lymphoma may develop. A number of recent series on breast lymphoma include examples of MALT lymphoma {534,994,1261,1580,1792}; they were not encountered in other series {117, 296,1346,1665}.

Classically, MALT lymphomas are composed of small lymphocytes, marginal zone (centrocyte-like) and/or monocytoid B-cells, often interspersed with larger blastic cells. Monotypic plasma cells may be numerous and sometimes predominant. The infiltrate is diffuse and neoplastic colonization of pre-existent reactive follicles may be seen. A lymphoepithelial lesion, defined originally as an infiltration of glandular epithelium by clusters of neoplastic centrocyte-like cells {1305}, is rarely seen. Neoplastic infiltration and destruction of mammary ducts by lymphoma cells, most commonly encountered in large B-cell lymphomas or infiltration of ductal epithelium by non-neoplastic T cells should not be confused with a true lymphoepithelial lesion. However, the presence of such a lesion is not a prerequisite for a diagnosis of MALT lymphoma.

Inflammatory reactive conditions may mimic MALT lymphomas; perhaps many cases previously described as pseudolymphoma were in reality MALT lymphomas given enough time to follow their evolution.

Immunohistochemically, MALT lymphoma expresses pan-B cell markers

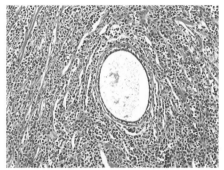

Fig. 1.162 Lymphoblastic T-cell lymphoma, secondary with lobular carcinoma-like appearance.

such as CD20 and CD79a; it is usually bcl-2 positive but negative for CD10, CD5 and CD23.

The translocation t(11;18)(q21;q21) has been identified in many MALT lymphomas although not in the few analysed breast cases {2125}. Furthermore, trisomy 3 has been identified in a number of MALT lymphomas at different sites but breast cases were not included in the study {3157}.

Follicular lymphoma

ICD-O code   9690/3

Follicular lymphoma is another type of lymphoma, which is included in recent primary breast lymphoma series {113, 296,534,994,1261,1346,1580,1665, 1792}. It features neoplastic follicles composed of centrocytes and centroblasts in different proportions and may be either grade 2 or 3, depending on the number of centroblasts inside the neoplastic follicles.

Immunohistochemically, the lymphoma cells show positivity for pan B antigens, CD10 and bcl-2 but are negative for CD5 and CD23. Follicular dendritic cells in tight clusters positive for CD21 delineate neoplastic follicles

Differential diagnosis

Malignant lymphoma of the breast may, on routine haematoxilin and eosin stained slides without using immunohistochemical methods, be misdiagnosed as carcinoma, particularly infiltrating lobular or medullary carcinoma {18}. In addition, some cases of granulocytic sarcoma (myeloid cell tumour) may be confused with T cell lymphomas if only a limited number of immunoreactions are

used. Inflammatory conditions in the breast may mimic MALT lymphoma.

Prognosis and predictive factors

Primary breast lymphomas behave in a way similar to lymphomas of corresponding type and stage in other sites.

Metastasis to the breast from extramammary malignancies

Epidemiology

Metastatic involvement of the breast is uncommon as an initial symptom of a non-mammary malignant neoplasm {2424} accounting for 0.5-6% of all breast malignancies {982,3029}. Women are affected five to six times more frequently than men are {982, 3029}.

The clinically reported incidence is lower than that found at autopsy. It is also higher when lymphoma and leukaemia are included {2940,3029}. Metastases within the breast are more frequent in patients with known disseminated malignancy (25-40%) {2424}.

After lymphoma and leukaemia, malignant melanoma {2135,2424,2872, 3020,3163} is the most common source from an extramammary site followed by rhabdomyosarcoma in children or adolescents {393,1129}, and tumours of lung, ovary, kidney, thyroid, cervix, stomach and prostate {344,393, 982,1111,1129,1530,1758,2134,2481, 3020,3029,3038}.

Clinical features

The patient usually presents with a palpable lesion, generally well circumscribed and rapidly growing to a size of 1-3 cm. Tumours are solitary in 85% of cases {2424}, usually situated in the upper outer quadrant {778} and located superficially. The lesions may be bilateral (8-25%) {982} or multinodular. They can rarely simulate an inflammatory breast carcinoma {3020}. Axillary lymph node involvement is frequent {3029}. Mammographically, metastatic lesions are well circumscribed and without calcification excluding those from ovarian lesions, making mammographic differentiation from medullary or intracystic carcinoma difficult {1758, 2134,3038}.

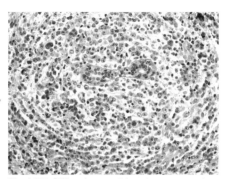

Fig. 1.163 Diffuse large cell lymphoma, secondary to the breast.

Macroscopy

Typically the tumour is nodular, solitary and well circumscribed.

Multinodularity, when is present, would be an important feature favouring a metastatic carcinoma.

Histopathology

It is important to recognize that the morphology is not that of a primary mammary carcinoma and to consider the possibility of a metastasis from an extramammary primary. This is particularly crucial with the increasing use of fine needle and tissue core biopsies {982}.

However, some metastatic tumours may have some similarities to primary breast neoplasms such as squamous, mucinous, mucoepidermoid, clear cell or spindle cell neoplasms, but they lack an intraductal component and are generally well circumscribed {2424}.

Differential diagnosis

Immunohistochemistry is useful in separating metastatic from primary carcinoma. The expression of hormonal receptor and GCFDP-15 is in favour of a breast primary carcinoma. A panel of antibodies such as those to cytokeratin 7, 20, CA19-9, CA125, S100, vimentin and HMB45 can be helpful depending on the morphological appearance of the lesion {778,2424}.

Prognosis and predictive factors

Metastatic involvement of the breast is a manifestation of generalized metastases in virtually all cases {2424,3020}. The prognosis of patients with metastatic disease in the breast is dependent on the site of the primary and the histological type {3029}.

Tumours of the male breast

K. Prechtel   P. Pisani
F. Levi   H. Hoefler
C. La Vecchia   D. Prechtel
A. Sasco   P. Devilee
B. Cutuli

Definition

Breast tumours occur much less frequently in men than in women. The most common male breast lesions are gynaecomastia, carcinoma, and metastatic cancers. Other benign or malignant lesions also occur, but much more rarely.

Gynaecomastia

Definition

Gynaecomastia is a non-neoplastic, often reversible, enlargement of the rudimentary duct system in male breast tissue with proliferation of epithelial and mesenchymal components resembling fibroadenomatous hyperplasia of the female breast.

Synonym

Fibrosis mammae virilis (no longer used).

Epidemiology

There are three typical, steroid dependent, age peaks; neonatal, adolescent (2nd/3rd decade) and the so-called male climacteric phase (6th/7th decade). There is always relative or absolute endogeneous or exogeneous estrogenism. Gynaecomastia is frequent in Klinefelter syndrome and also occurs in association with liver cirrhosis, endocrine tumours and certain medications {1263, 2572}.

Clinical features

Gynaecomastia generally involves both breasts but is often clinically more distinct in one. Nipple secretion is rare. There is a palpable retroareolar nodule or plaque like induration. Occasionally there is aching pain.

Macroscopy

There is generally circumscribed enlargement of breast tissue which is firm and grey white on the cut surface.

Histopathology

There is an increased number of ducts lined by epithelial and myoepithelial cells. The surrounding cellular, myxoid stroma contains fibroblasts and myofibroblasts, intermingled with lymphocytes and plasma cells. Lobular structures, with or without secretory changes, are rare and mostly occur in response to exogenous hormonal stimulation such as transsexual estrogen therapy. This florid phase is followed by an inactive fibrous phase with flat epithelial cells and hyalinized periductal stroma. An intermediate phase with a combination of features also occurs. Occasionally, duct ectasia, apocrine or squamous metaplasia develop. An increase in the amount of adipose breast tissue alone may be called lipomatous pseudogynaecomastia.

Immunoprofile

Patients with Klinefelter syndrome exhibit elevated amounts of estrogen (ER) and progesterone (PR) receptors but other examples of gynaecomastia do not demonstrate significant elevation {2215, 2666}.

In gynaecomastia induced by antiandrogen therapy, but not in carcinoma of the breast, there may be strong focal prostate specific antigen (PSA) immunoreactivity in normal or hyperplastic duct epithelium, while PSAP activity is negative. These findings should not be misinterpreted as indicating a metastasis from a prostatic carcinoma {968}.

Prognosis and predictive factors

Recurrence of gynaecomastia is possible. Atypical ductal epithelial hyperplasia and carcinoma in situ are rarely seen in cases of gynaecomastia but there is no convincing evidence that gynaecomastia, per se, is precancerous.

Carcinoma

Definition

Carcinoma of the male breast is a rare malignant epithelial tumour histologically identical to that seen in the female breast. Both in situ and invasive carcinoma occur, at a ratio of about 1:25 {713}.

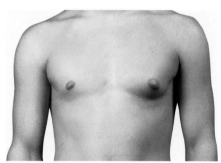

Fig. 1.164 Gynaecomastia of the male breast (left > right).

ICD-O code   8500/3

Epidemiology

Male breast cancer is extremely rare, representing less than 1% of all breast cancers, and less than 1% of all cancer deaths in men. Not surprisingly, therefore, little is known about its epidemiology. The incidence of and mortality from male breast cancer have been reported to be rising. Reviews of incidence trends in Scandinavia {814} and mortality trends in Europe {1551} give no support to the existence of such upward trends. Mortality rates, for most countries, in the late 1980s and 1990s tended to be lower than those registered three decades earlier, suggesting that advances in diagnosis and treatment may have improved the prognosis {1551}.

In the 1990s, mortality rates from male breast cancer were around 2 per million

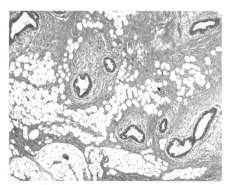

Fig. 1.165 Gynaecomastia of the male breast, with proliferating ducts and periductal stroma.

male population both in the USA and the European Union (EU). A higher incidence with a lower average age and more cases in an advanced stage is reported in native Africans and Indians {39,1281,1329,1330,2539,2985}. This is reinforced by the consistently higher incidence rates for the black compared to the white male population in the US cancer registries {2189}.

Aetiology

Some aspects of the aetiology of male breast cancer are similar to those of the much more common female counterpart. Thus, a direct association has been suggested with socio-economic class (i.e. increased risk in higher socio-economic classes) {607,1551,2539}, although this remains controversial {1627,2906}. Likewise, it has been reported that both never married men and Jewish men are at higher risk {1726,2539,2906}.

Family history of breast cancer in female and male first degree relatives has repeatedly been associated with male breast cancer risk, although quantification of relative and attributable risks on a population level remains undefined {418, 607,1185,1551,2449, 2539,2799}. It has been estimated that there is a family history in about 5% of male breast cancer patients, but these patients do not present at a younger age {1210,2297}. Hereditary factors are discussed elsewhere (see genetic chapter).

Again, as for female breast cancer, anthropometric characteristics have been investigated, and body mass index (BMI) was directly associated with male breast cancer risk {418,607, 1551,2539}. In a large case-control study {1253}, the relative risk was 2.3 for the highest quartile of BMI. This study also suggested an association with height but the relative risk was only 1.5 and of borderline significance {1253}.

Previous breast or testicular disease and gynaecomastia have been related to male breast cancer, and associations have been reported with an undescended testis {2231,2577,2906}, orchiectomy, orchitis, testicular injury, late puberty and infertility {2539}.

Male breast cancer is more common among those with Klinefelter syndrome {418,2539} and infertility or low fertility,

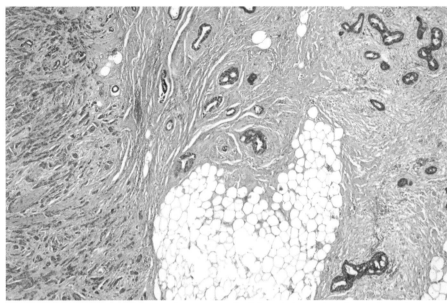

Fig. 1.166 Invasive ductal carcinoma and gynaecomastia of the male breast. Invasive carcinoma is present in the left third of the field.

possibly as a consequence of Klinefelter syndrome or other hormonal abnormalities {607,1551,2539,2906}. Similar to the role of estrogen in female breast cancer {36,225,540,1128}, high estrogen and prolactin levels have been reported as risk factors for male breast cancer {2539}, and several small studies have found higher serum or urinary estrogen levels in cases than in controls {386,2024,2107,2363}. This is supported by retrospective cohort studies in Denmark, indicating an excess occurrence of breast cancer among men with cirrhosis and relative hyperestrogenism {2755}. However, not all the results were consistent with this pattern of hormonal influence {173,3110}.

Other endocrine factors may play an important role in the aetiology {815, 1253,2539}. It has been suggested that diabetes mellitus may increase risk, possibly through hormonal mechanisms {815,1253,2539}.

Reports on lifestyle factors have shown in general no material association with smoking, alcohol or coffee consumption {1253,2231,2449}, although one study found a significant protective effect of smoking {2231}. A higher risk was associated with limited physical exercise and frequent consumption of red meat, while consumption of fruit and vegetables was related to a decreased risk, although the trends were not significant

{1253}. In another large study from ten population-based cancer registries {2449}, no trends in risk were observed with increased dietary intakes of several foods and nutrients, and no association was found with the use of any dietary supplement. Dietary factors are unlikely to be strong determinants of breast cancer in men {2449}, though moderate associations, as described for female breast cancer {1636,1639}, remain possible.

Although an association with electromagnetic field exposure has been suggested in the past {669,1784,2791}, the Report of an Advisory Group on Non-Ionising Radiation to the National Radiological Protection Board (2001) concluded that there is no evidence that electromagnetic fields are related to adult male breast cancer {2355}.

Invasive carcinoma

Clinical features

The most frequent sign is a palpable subareolar mass. Nipple ulceration or sanguineous secretion is seen in 15–30%. In 25–50% of patients, there is fixation to or ulceration of the overlying skin. A quarter of patients complain of pain.

Male breast cancer is usually unilateral and occurs more frequently in the left breast. Synchronous bilateral tumours are found in less than 5% of cases.

Macroscopy

The majority of male breast cancers measure between 2 and 2.5 cm. Multiple separate nodules are rare as is involvement of the entire breast.

Histopathology

The histological classification and grading of male and female invasive breast carcinoma are identical, but lobular carcinoma does not usually occur in men even in those exposed to endogenous or exogenous hormonal stimulation {1855,2521,2552} and should only be diagnosed if E-cadherin expression is absent {34}.

Immunoprofile

Compared to breast carcinoma in women, male breast carcinomas have a somewhat higher frequency of ER positivity in the 60-95% range, while PR positivity occurs in 45-85% of cases {315, 578,1836,1917}. The concentrations are independent of patient age and similar to those found in postmenopausal women {2297}. Androgen receptors are expressed in up to 95% of cases.

Prognosis and predictive factors

The prognosis and predictive factors are the same as for female breast cancer at comparative stages.

Metastasis to the breast

The ratio of primary breast cancer and a metastasis from another primary site to the breast is about 25:1. The most fre-

quent primaries are prostatic carcinoma, adenocarcinoma of the colon, carcinoma of the urinary bladder, malignant melanoma and malignant lymphoma.

Carcinoma and sarcoma secondary to previous treatment

As in women, carcinoma following previous chemotherapy and/or irradiation has been reported {326,601}, as has post irradiation sarcoma {2644}.

Carcinoma in situ

ICD-O code   8500/2

Clinical features

In the absence of mammographic screening in men, the two most frequent symptoms are sero-sanguineous nipple discharge and/or subareolar tumour.

Histopathology

The histological features are in general similar to those in the female breast but two major studies have found that the most frequent architectural pattern is papillary, while comedo DCIS occurs rarely {602,1221}. Lobular intraepithelial neoplasia is also extremely rare. Paget disease may be relatively more common among men compared to women due to the shorter length of the duct system in male breast.

Other tumours

Almost all breast tumours which occur in women have also, been reported in men, albeit rarely.

Genetics in male breast cancer

Very little is currently known about the molecular events leading to the development and progression of sporadic breast cancer in males. Loss of heterozygosity (LOH) and comparative genomic hybridisation (CGH) studies and cytogenetic analysis have shown that somatic genetic changes in sporadic male breast carcinomas are quantitatively and qualitatively similar to those associated with sporadic female breast cancer {2532,2927,3134,3265}. Tumour phenotypic markers, such as ERBB2 and TP53 expression, are also

quite similar between the sexes {3129}. Ki-ras mutations are not significantly increased in male breast cancer {636}. LOH on chromosome 8p22 and 11q13 are frequently identified in male breast cancer {490,1073} suggesting that the presence of one or more tumour suppressor genes in these regions may play a role in the development or progression of the disease. LOH at 11q13 is found more often in carcinomas with positive nodal status than in carcinomas without lymph node metastasis {1073}. Frequent allelic losses on chromosome 13q are reported in familial, as well as in sporadic, male breast cancer {2296, 3134}. Chromosome 13q is the region containing the BRCA2, BRUSH-1, and retinoblastoma gene. Depending on the population, studies demonstrated that 4-38% of all male breast cancers are associated with BRCA2 alterations {918,1550, 2921}. Other putative target genes are also situated here, including protocadherin 9 and EMK (serine/threonine protein kinase). Possibly, multiple tumour suppressor genes may influence the observed pattern of loss of heterozygosity {1383}.

The role of aberrant hormone secretion or hormone receptor function in the development or progression of the disease remains controversial. Hormonal imbalances, such as those in Klinefelter syndrome or Reifenstein syndrome (mutation of the androgen receptor gene: Xq11-12) are known risk factors for breast cancer in males {427, 1213,2484}. In three men, germline mutations in the androgen receptor gene was reported including two brothers with Reifenstein syndrome {1686,3152}. However it has been shown that mutations of the androgen receptor are not obligatory for the development of male breast cancer {1213}.

Cytogenetic studies reveal clonal chromosomal anomalies: Loss of the Y chromosome and gain of an X chromosome, as well as the gain of chromosome 5, are all frequently observed {1213,2484}. Taken together with previous data, the present findings suggest close similarities between the molecular pathogenesis of male and female breast cancers.

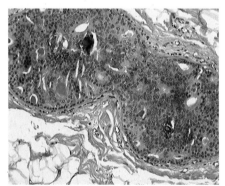

Fig. 1.167 Male breast carcinoma, DCIS. The in situ carcinomas are generally of the non-necrotic cribriform or papillary types. Though necrosis develops in some cases composed of either micropapillary or the cribriform types, true comedo DCIS is rare.

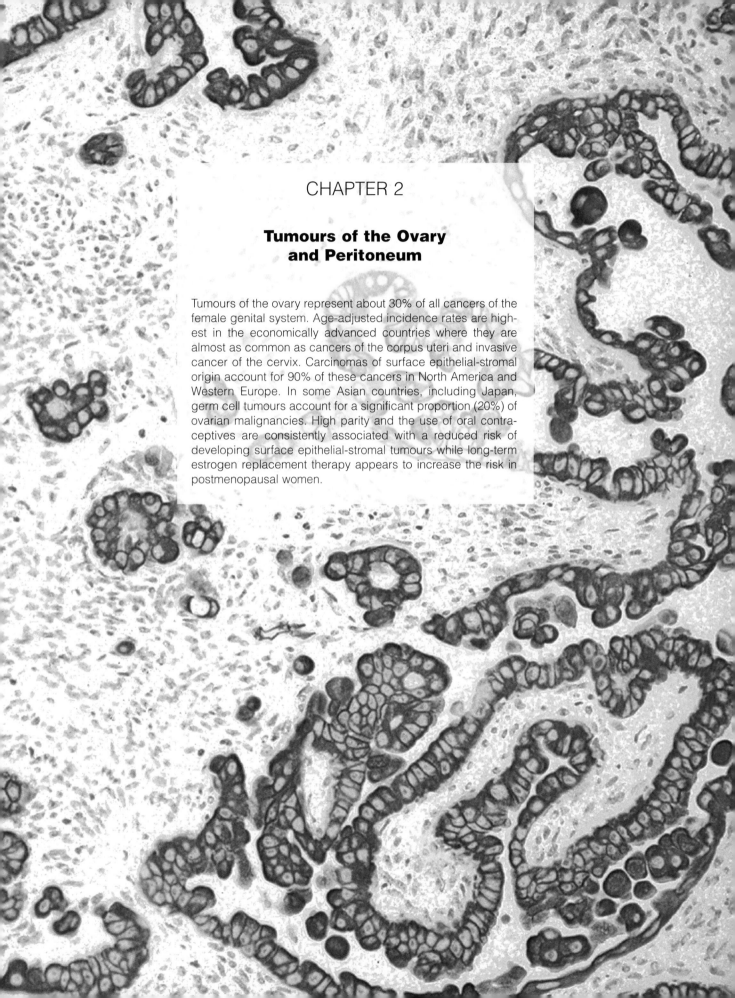

CHAPTER 2

Tumours of the Ovary and Peritoneum

Tumours of the ovary represent about 30% of all cancers of the female genital system. Age-adjusted incidence rates are highest in the economically advanced countries where they are almost as common as cancers of the corpus uteri and invasive cancer of the cervix. Carcinomas of surface epithelial-stromal origin account for 90% of these cancers in North America and Western Europe. In some Asian countries, including Japan, germ cell tumours account for a significant proportion (20%) of ovarian malignancies. High parity and the use of oral contraceptives are consistently associated with a reduced risk of developing surface epithelial-stromal tumours while long-term estrogen replacement therapy appears to increase the risk in postmenopausal women.

WHO histological classification of tumours of the ovary

Surface epithelial-stromal tumours
Serous tumours
  Malignant
    Adenocarcinoma — 8441/3'
    Surface papillary adenocarcinoma — 8461/3
    Adenocarcinofibroma (malignant adenofibroma) — 9014/3
  Borderline tumour — 8442/1
    Papillary cystic tumour — 8462/1
    Surface papillary tumour — 8463/1
    Adenofibroma, cystadenofibroma — 9014/1
  Benign
    Cystadenoma — 8441/0
    Papillary cystadenoma — 8460/0
    Surface papilloma — 8461/0
    Adenofibroma and cystadenofibroma — 9014/0
Mucinous tumours
  Malignant
    Adenocarcinoma — 8480/3
    Adenocarcinofibroma (malignant adenofibroma) — 9015/3
  Borderline tumour — 8472/1
    Intestinal type
    Endocervical-like
  Benign
    Cystadenoma — 8470/0
    Adenofibroma and cystadenofibroma — 9015/0
  Mucinous cystic tumour with mural nodules
  Mucinous cystic tumour with pseudomyxoma peritonei — 8480/3
Endometrioid tumours including variants with squamous differentiation
  Malignant
    Adenocarcinoma, not otherwise specified — 8380/3
    Adenocarcinofibroma (malignant adenofibroma) — 8381/3
    Malignant müllerian mixed tumour — 8950/3
    (carcinosarcoma)
    Adenosarcoma — 8933/3
    Endometrioid stromal sarcoma (low grade) — 8931/3
    Undifferentiated ovarian sarcoma — 8805/3
  Borderline tumour
    Cystic tumour — 8380/1
    Adenofibroma and cystadenofibroma — 8381/1
  Benign
    Cystadenoma — 8380/0
    Adenofibroma and cystadenofibroma — 8381/0
Clear cell tumours
  Malignant
    Adenocarcinoma — 8310/3
    Adenocarcinofibroma (malignant adenofibroma) — 8313/3
  Borderline tumour
    Cystic tumour — 8310/1
    Adenofibroma and cystadenofibroma — 8313/1
  Benign
    Cystadenoma — 8310/0
    Adenofibroma and cystadenofibroma — 8313/0
Transitional cell tumours
  Malignant
    Transitional cell carcinoma (non-Brenner type) — 8120/3
    Malignant Brenner tumour — 9000/3
  Borderline
    Borderline Brenner tumour — 9000/1
      Proliferating variant — 9000/1
  Benign
    Brenner tumour — 9000/0

      Metaplastic variant — 9000/0
Squamous cell tumours
    Squamous cell carcinoma — 8070/3
    Epidermoid cyst
Mixed epithelial tumours (specify components)
    Malignant — 8323/3
    Borderline — 8323/1
    Benign — 8323/0
Undifferentiated and unclassified tumours
    Undifferentiated carcinoma — 8020/3
    Adenocarcinoma, not otherwise specified — 8140/3

Sex cord-stromal tumours
Granulosa-stromal cell tumours
  Granulosa cell tumour group
    Adult granulosa cell tumour — 8620/1
    Juvenile granulosa cell tumour — 8622/1
  Thecoma-fibroma group
    Thecoma, not otherwise specified — 8600/0
      Typical — 8600/0
      Luteinized — 8601/0
    Fibroma — 8810/0
    Cellular fibroma — 8810/1
    Fibrosarcoma — 8810/3
    Stromal tumour with minor sex cord elements — 8593/1
    Sclerosing stromal tumour — 8602/0
    Signet-ring stromal tumour
    Unclassified (fibrothecoma)
Sertoli-stromal cell tumours
  Sertoli-Leydig cell tumour group (androblastomas)
    Well differentiated — 8631/0
    Of intermediate differentiation — 8631/1
      Variant with heterologous elements (specify type) — 8634/1
    Poorly differentiated (sarcomatoid) — 8631/3
      Variant with heterologous elements (specify type) — 8634/3
    Retiform — 8633/1
      Variant with heterologous elements (specify type) — 8634/1
  Sertoli cell tumour — 8640/1
  Stromal-Leydig cell tumour
Sex cord-stromal tumours of mixed or unclassified cell types
  Sex cord tumour with annular tubules — 8623/1
  Gynandroblastoma (specify components) — 8632/1
  Sex cord-stromal tumour, unclassified — 8590/1
Steroid cell tumours
  Stromal luteoma — 8610/0
  Leydig cell tumour group
    Hilus cell tumour — 8660/0
    Leydig cell tumour, non-hilar type — 8650/1
    Leydig cell tumour, not otherwise specified — 8650/1
  Steroid cell tumour, not otherwise specified — 8670/0
    Well differentiated — 8670/0
    Malignant — 8670/3

Germ cell tumours
Primitive germ cell tumours
  Dysgerminoma — 9060/3
  Yolk sac tumour — 9071/3
    Polyvesicular vitelline tumour
    Glandular variant
    Hepatoid variant
  Embryonal carcinoma — 9070/3

Polyembryoma	9072/3
Non-gestational choriocarcinoma	9100/3
Mixed germ cell tumour (specify components)	9085/3
Biphasic or triphasic teratoma	
Immature teratoma	9080/3
Mature teratoma	9080/0
Solid	
Cystic	
Dermoid cyst	9084/0
Fetiform teratoma (homunculus)	

Monodermal teratoma and somatic-type tumours associated
with dermoid cysts

Thyroid tumour group	
Struma ovarii	
Benign	9090/0
Malignant (specify type)	9090/3
Carcinoid group	
Insular	8240/3
Trabecular	8240/3
Mucinous	8243/3
Strumal carcinoid	9091/1
Mixed	
Neuroectodermal tumour group	
Ependymoma	9391/3
Primitive neuroectodermal tumour	9473/3
Medulloepithelioma	9501/3
Glioblastoma multiforme	9440/3
Others	
Carcinoma group	
Squamous cell carcinoma	8070/3
Adenocarcinoma	8140/3
Others	
Melanocytic group	
Malignant melanoma	8720/3
Melanocytic naevus	8720/0
Sarcoma group (specify type)	
Sebaceous tumour group	
Sebaceous adenoma	8410/0
Sebaceous carcinoma	8410/3
Pituitary-type tumour group	
Retinal anlage tumour group	9363/0
Others	

Germ cell sex cord-stromal tumours	
Gonadoblastoma	9073/1
Variant with malignant germ cell tumour	
Mixed germ cell-sex cord-stromal tumour	
Variant with malignant germ cell tumour	
Tumours of the rete ovarii	
Adenocarcinoma	9110/3
Adenoma	9110/0
Cystadenoma	
Cystadenofibroma	
Miscellaneous tumours	
Small cell carcinoma, hypercalcaemic type	8041/3
Small cell carcinoma, pulmonary type	8041/3
Large cell neuroendocrine carcinoma	8013/3
Hepatoid carcinoma	8576/3
Primary ovarian mesothelioma	9050/3
Wilms tumour	8960/3
Gestational choriocarcinoma	9100/3
Hydatidiform mole	9100/0
Adenoid cystic carcinoma	8200/3
Basal cell tumour	8090/1
Ovarian wolffian tumour	9110/1
Paraganglioma	8693/1
Myxoma	8840/0
Soft tissue tumours not specific to the ovary	
Others	
Tumour-like conditions	
Luteoma of pregnancy	
Stromal hyperthecosis	
Stromal hyperplasia	
Fibromatosis	
Massive ovarian oedema	
Others	
Lymphoid and haematopoetic tumours	
Malignant lymphoma (specify type)	
Leukaemia (specify type)	
Plasmacytoma	9734/3

Secondary tumours

---

[1] Morphology code of the International Classification of Diseases for Oncology (ICD-O) {921} and the Systematized Nomenclature of Medicine (http://snomed.org). Behaviour is coded /0 for benign tumours, /3 for malignant tumours, and /1 for borderline or uncertain behaviour.

WHO histological classification of tumours of the peritoneum

Peritoneal tumours	
Mesothelial tumours	
Diffuse malignant mesothelioma	9050/3
Well differentiated papillary mesothelioma	9052/0
Multicystic mesothelioma	9055/1
Adenomatoid tumour	9054/0
Smooth muscle tumour	
Leiomyomatosis peritonealis disseminata	

Tumour of uncertain origin	
Desmoplastic small round cell tumour	8806/3
Epithelial tumours	
Primary peritoneal serous adenocarcinoma	8461/3
Primary peritoneal borderline tumour (specify type)	
Others	

---

[1] Morphology code of the International Classification of Diseases for Oncology (ICD-O) {921} and the Systematized Nomenclature of Medicine (http://snomed.org). Behaviour is coded /0 for benign tumours, /3 for malignant tumours, and /1 for borderline or uncertain behaviour.

TNM and FIGO classification of tumours of the ovary

TNM and FIGO classification[1,2,3]

T – Primary Tumour

TNM Categories	FIGO Stages	
TX		Primary tumour cannot be assessed
T0		No evidence of primary tumour
T1	I	Tumour limited to the ovaries
T1a	IA	Tumour limited to one ovary; capsule intact, no tumour on ovarian surface; no malignant cells in ascites or peritoneal washings
T1b	IB	Tumour limited to both ovaries; capsule intact, no tumour on ovarian surface; no malignant cells in ascites or peritoneal washings
T1c	IC	Tumour limited to one or both ovaries with any of the following: capsule ruptured, tumour on ovarian surface, malignant cells in ascites or peritoneal washings
T2	II	Tumour involves one or both ovaries with pelvic extension
T2a	IIA	Extension and/or implants on uterus and/or tube(s); no malignant cells in ascites or peritoneal washings
T2b	IIB	Extension to other pelvic tissues; no malignant cells in ascites or peritoneal washings
T2c	IIC	Pelvic extension (2a or 2b) with malignant cells in ascites or peritoneal washings
T3 and/or N1	III	Tumour involves one or both ovaries with microscopically confirmed peritoneal metastasis outside the pelvis and/or regional lymph node metastasis
T3a	IIIA	Microscopic peritoneal metastasis beyond pelvis
T3b	IIIB	Macroscopic peritoneal metastasis beyond pelvis 2 cm or less in greatest dimension
T3c and/or N1	IIIC	Peritoneal metastasis beyond pelvis more than 2 cm in greatest dimension and/or regional lymph node metastasis
M1	IV	Distant metastasis (excludes peritoneal metastasis)

Note: Liver capsule metastasis is T3/stage III, liver parenchymal metastasis M1/stage IV. Pleural effusion must have positive cytology for M1/stage IV.

N – Regional Lymph Nodes[4]

NX	Regional lymph nodes cannot be assessed
N0	No regional lymph node metastasis
N1	Regional lymph node metastasis

M – Distant Metastasis

MX	Distant metastasis cannot be assessed
M0	No distant metastasis
M1	Distant metastasis

Stage Grouping

Stage IA	T1a	N0	M0
Stage IB	T1b	N0	M0
Stage IC	T1c	N0	M0
Stage IIA	T2a	N0	M0
Stage IIB	T2b	N0	M0
Stage IIC	T2c	N0	M0
Stage IIIA	T3a	N0	M0
Stage IIIB	T3b	N0	M0
Stage IIIC	T3c	N0	M0
	Any T	N1	M0
Stage IV	Any T	Any N	M1

---

[1] {51,2976}.
[2] A help desk for specific questions about the TNM classification is available at http://tnm.uicc.org.
[3] The classification applies to malignant surface epithelial-stromal tumours including those of borderline malignancy. Non-epithelial ovarian cancers may also be classified using this scheme.
[4] The regional lymph nodes are the hypogastric (obturator), common iliac, external iliac, lateral sacral, para-aortic, and inguinal nodes.

Surface epithelial-stromal tumours

K.R. Lee
F.A. Tavassoli
J. Prat
M. Dietel
D.J. Gersell
A.I. Karseladze
S. Hauptmann
J. Rutgers

P. Russell
C.H. Buckley
P. Pisani
P. Schwartz
D.E. Goldgar
E. Silva
R. Caduff
R.A. Kubik-Huch

Definition

Surface epithelial-stromal tumours are the most common neoplasms of the ovary. They originate from the ovarian surface epithelium or its derivatives and occur in women of reproductive age and beyond. They are histologically composed of one or more distinctive types of epithelium, admixed with a variable amount of stroma.Their biological behaviour varies with histological type.

Epidemiology

Cancer of the ovary represents about 30% of all cancers of the female genital organs. In developed countries it is about as common as cancers of the corpus uteri (35%) and invasive cancer of the cervix (27%). The age-adjusted incidence rates vary from less than 2 new cases per 100,000 women in most of Southeast Asia and Africa to over 15 cases in Northern and Eastern Europe. The economically advanced countries of North America, Europe, Australia, New Zealand and temperate South America show the highest rates. In the United States more women die from ovarian cancer today than from all other pelvic gynaecological cancer sites combined {1066}. Incidence rates have been either stable or have shown slow increases in most western countries, whereas they have risen steadily in parts of Eastern Asia.

Aetiology

Two factors consistently associated with a reduced risk of the disease are high parity and the use of oral contraceptives {1295,2474}. Three recent studies have shown an increased risk of ovarian cancer in postmenopausal women treated with high-dose estrogen replacement therapy for 10 years or greater {963, 2373,2399}. Very little is known of the aetiology of non-familial cases. The protective effects of pregnancies and of oral contraception suggest a direct role for ovulation in causing the disease, but no convincing mechanism linking the risk factors with malignant transformation has been proposed.

Several dietary factors have been related to ovarian cancer {819}. There is emerging evidence that the Western lifestyle, in particular, obesity, is associated with an increased risk {388}.

Clinical features

Signs and symptoms

Women with ovarian cancer have a poor prognosis. The mean 5-year survival rate in Europe is 32% {256}. This unfavourable outcome is largely ascribed to a lack of early warning symptoms and a lack of diagnostic tests that allow early detection. As a result, approximately 70% of patients present when this cancer is in an advanced stage, i.e. it has metastasized to the upper abdomen or beyond the abdominal cavity {394}. It is now recognized that the overwhelming majority of women diagnosed with ovarian cancer actually have symptoms, but they are subtle and easily confused with those of various benign entities, particularly those related to the gastrointestinal tract {1024,2106}.

Physical signs associated with early stage ovarian cancer may be limited to palpation by pelvic examination of a mobile, but somewhat irregular, pelvic mass (stage I). As the disease spreads into the pelvic cavity, nodules may be found in the cul-de-sac, particularly on bimanual rectovaginal examination (stage II). Ascites may occur even when the malignancy is limited to one or both ovaries (stage IC). As the disease involves the upper abdomen, ascites may be evident. A physical examination of the abdomen may demonstrate flank bulging and fluid waves associated with the ascites. Metastatic disease is commonly found in the omentum, such that the latter may be readily identified in the presence of advanced stage (stage III) ovarian cancer as a ballottable or palpable mass in the mid-abdomen, usually superior to the umbilicus and above the palpable pelvic mass. Finally, the

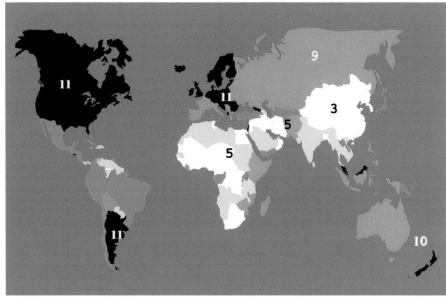

Fig. 2.01 Global incidence rates of ovarian cancer. Age-standardized rates (ASR) per 100,000 population and year. From Globocan 2000 {846}.

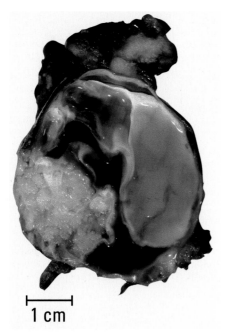

Fig. 2.02 Serous adenocarcinoma. The sectioned surface of the tumour shows two solid nodules within a multiloculated cyst.

disease may spread through lymphatics to either the inguinal or left supraclavicular lymph nodes, which may be readily palpable. It may advance into the pleural cavity as a malignant effusion, usually on the right side or bilateral, in which case the lung bases exhibit dullness to percussion and decreased breath sounds and egophony to auscultation (stage IV). Advanced intra-abdominal ovarian carcinomatosis may also present with signs of intestinal obstruction including nausea, vomiting and abdominal pain.

Imaging
Due to its wide availability, ultrasound (US) is the imaging method of choice to assess an ovarian lesion and to determine the presence of solid and cystic elements. The distinction between benign, borderline and malignant tumours is generally not possible by US, either alone or in combination with magnetic resonance imaging (MRI) or computed tomography (CT). None of these methods has a clearly established role in preoperative tumour staging. Surgical exploration remains the standard approach for staging {1116,1417,1522,1795,2898}.

Tumour spread and staging
About 70-75% of patients with ovarian cancer have tumour spread beyond the pelvis at the time of diagnosis {1770}. Ovarian cancers spread mainly by local extension, by intra-abdominal dissemination and by lymphatic dissemination, but rarely also through the blood stream. The International Federation of Gynecology and Obstetrics (FIGO) Committee on Gynecologic Oncology is responsible for the staging system that is used internationally today {217}. The pTNM-system is based on the postoperative pathological staging for histological control and confirmation of the disease. {51,2976}.

Histogenesis
The likely origin of ovarian surface epithelial-stromal tumours is the mesothelial surface lining of the ovaries and/or invaginations of this lining into the superficial ovarian cortex that form inclusion cysts {838}.

Genetic susceptibility
Familial clustering
Numerous epidemiological investigations of ovarian cancer have attempted to quantify the risks associated with a positive family history. Whereas ovarian cancer has not been as extensively studied as breast cancer, several studies point to familial clustering. The relative risk of ovarian cancer for first degree relatives varies from 1.94 to 25.5, the latter if both a mother and sister are affected {1029,2557,2801}.

BRCA1/2
A number of specific genes have been identified as playing a role. The most important of these, BRCA1 and BRCA2, are discussed in chapter 8. In contrast to breast cancer in which only a minority of the familial clustering could be explained by known major susceptibility loci such as BRCA1 and BRCA2, it is likely that the majority of the familial risk of ovarian cancer is explained by BRCA1 and to a lesser extent BRCA2, MLH1 and MSH2. Using statistical modelling and the results from BRCA1 and BRCA2 mutation testing in 112 families with at least two cases of ovarian cancer (allowing for insensitivity of the mutation detection assay), BRCA1 and BRCA2 accounted for nearly all of the non-chance familial aggregation {973}.

HNPCC
Ovarian cancer is a minor feature of the hereditary nonpolyposis colon cancer syndrome caused by mutations in genes associated with DNA base mismatch repair, the most frequent of which are *MLH1* and *MSH2*.

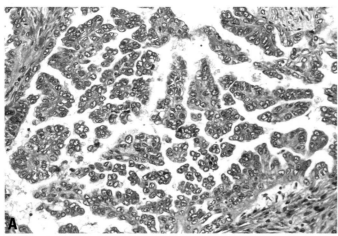
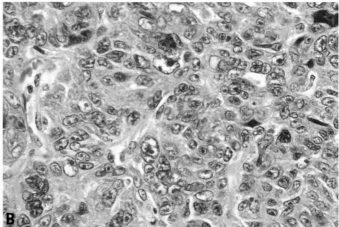

Fig. 2.03 Serous adenocarcinoma. **A** The tumour is composed of closely packed papillae most of which lack fibrous cores lined by cells with atypical nuclei and high nuclear to cytoplasmic ratios. **B** This poorly differentiated tumour shows relatively solid papillary aggregates without fibrovascular cores and scattered bizarre, pleomorphic nuclei. Cherry red nucleoli are apparent in some nuclei.

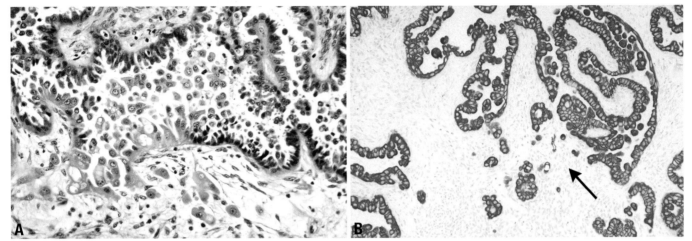

Fig. 2.04 A Serous borderline tumour with microinvasion. There is a transition from the typical small serous cells to cells with more abundant eosinophilic cytoplasm associated with disruption of the epithelial/stromal interface; the latter cell population invades the underlying stroma as isolated cells and small cell clusters in the lower part of the field. **B** Small clusters of cells and single cells within the stroma indicating microinvasion (arrow) in the lower central part of the field are demonstrated by cytokeratin immunohistochemistry.

Association with endometrial cancer
Several studies provide evidence of associations between ovarian and other cancers, particularly endometrial {715, 1029}. The relative risk of developing endometrial cancer is about 1.5 among mothers and sisters of ovarian cancer cases, although in both studies the risk fell just short of statistical significance.

Serous tumours

Definition
Ovarian tumours characterized in their better-differentiated forms by cell types resembling those of the fallopian tube.

ICD-O codes
Serous adenocarcinoma	8441/3
Serous borderline tumour	8442/1
Benign serous tumours	
Serous papillary cystadenoma	8460/0
Serous cystadenoma	8441/0
Serous surface papilloma	8461/0
Serous adenofibroma,	
cystadenofibroma	9014/0

Serous adenocarcinoma

Definition
An invasive ovarian epithelial neoplasm composed of cells ranging in appearance from those resembling fallopian tube epithelium in well differentiated tumours to anaplastic epithelial cells with severe nuclear atypia in poorly differentiated tumours.

Macroscopy
The tumours range from not being macroscopically detectable to over 20-cm in diameter and are bilateral in two-thirds of all cases, but only in one-third of stage I cases. Well differentiated tumours are solid and cystic with soft papillae within the cystic spaces or on the surface. The papillae tend to be softer and more confluent than in cases of borderline tumours. Rare tumours are confined to the ovarian surface. Poorly differentiated tumours are solid, friable, multinodular masses with necrosis and haemorrhage.

Histopathology
The architecture of the tumour varies from glandular to papillary to solid. The glands are typically slit-like or irregular. The papillae are usually irregularly branching and highly cellular. In poorly differentiated tumours solid areas are usually extensive and composed of poorly differentiated cells in sheets with small papillary clusters separated by myxoid or hyaline stroma. Psammoma bodies may be present in varying numbers. The stroma may be scanty or desmoplastic. Serous carcinomas may contain a variety of other cell types as a minor component (less than 10%) that may cause diagnostic problems but do not influence the outcome. Serous psammocarcinoma is a rare variant of serous carcinoma characterized by massive psammoma body formation and low grade cytological features. The epithelium is arranged in small nests with no areas of solid epithelial proliferation, and at least 75% of the epithelial nests are associated with psammoma body formation {1001}.

Immunoprofile
Serous carcinomas are always cytokeratin 7 positive and cytokeratin 20 negative. They are also positive for epithelial membrane antigen, CAM5.2, AE1/AE3, B72.3 and Leu M1 and for CA125 in 85% of the cases, but negative for calretinin and other mesothelial markers.

Grading
Various grading systems have been proposed for serous carcinomas. The utilization of a three-tiered grading system is recommended since the tumour grade has important prognostic and therapeutic implications {2687}.

Somatic genetics
The prevailing view of the pathogenesis of serous adenocarcinoma is that it arises directly from the ovarian surface epithelium, invaginations or epithelial inclusions and progresses rapidly {205}. At present, serous carcinoma is regarded as a relatively homogeneous group of tumours from the standpoint of pathogenesis. Thus, although these neoplasms are graded as well, moderately and poorly differentiated, they are thought to represent a spectrum of differentiation reflecting progression from a low grade to a high grade malignancy. Whereas in colorectal carcinoma a

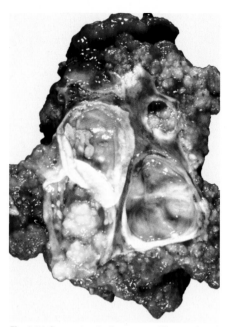

Fig. 2.05 Serous borderline tumour. The sectioned surface shows a solid and cystic neoplasm with numerous papillary excrescences.

tumour progression model in which sequential accumulation of molecular genetic alterations leading to morphologically recognizable stages is well established {1468}, a similar model for ovarian serous carcinoma has not been proposed because well defined precursor lesions have not been identified.

It has been reported that even the earliest histological serous carcinomas are already high grade and morphologically resemble their advanced stage counterparts {205}. The histological similarities are paralleled by recent molecular genetic findings demonstrating *TP53* mutations in very small stage I serous carcinomas and in the adjacent "dysplastic" surface epithelium {2275}. Most studies have shown that approximately 60% of advanced stage ovarian serous carcinomas have mutant *TP53* {230,3095}. Thus, although the molecular genetic findings in these early carcinomas are preliminary, they suggest that serous carcinoma in its very earliest stage of development resembles advanced stage serous carcinoma at the molecular level. This would support the view that there are no morphologically recognized intermediate steps in the progression of the conventional type of ovarian serous carcinoma. Serous borderline tumours (SBTs), non-invasive and invasive micropapillary types, frequently display *KRAS* mutations but rarely mutant *TP53*. Increased allelic

imbalance of chromosome 5q is associated with the progression from typical SBT to micropapillary SBT and increased allelic imbalance of chromosome 1p with the progression from micropapillary SBT to invasive serous carcinoma {2706}. In contrast, *KRAS* mutations are very rare in conventional serous carcinoma, but *TP53* mutations occur in approximately 60%. Recently, mutations were also identified in the *BRAF* gene, a downstream mediator of *KRAS*. *BRAF* and *KRAS* mutations appear to be mutually exclusive. These mutations were only detected in low grade ovarian serous carcinomas {2707}. Thus, there appears to be more than one pathway of tumorigenesis for serous carcinoma. In one pathway, conventional serous carcinoma, a high grade neoplasm, develops "de novo" from the surface epithelium of the ovary, grows rapidly and is highly aggressive {205}. These tumours, even at their earliest stage, display *TP53* mutations but not *KRAS* mutations. In the other pathway a SBT progresses in a "stepwise" fashion through a non-invasive micropapillary stage before becoming invasive {2706} or through microinvasion in a background of typical SBT. The indolent micropapillary tumours frequently display *KRAS* mutations, but *TP53* mutations are only rarely detected.

Genetic susceptibility
The neoplasms that develop in women with germline *BRCA1* mutations are mostly serous carcinomas of the ovary, fallopian tube and peritoneum.

Prognosis and predictive factors
The overall 5-year survival is approximately 40%; however, many of those alive at 5 years are alive with disease. Up to 85% of cases present with widespread metastatic disease. Survival at 5 years in this group is 10-20%. Patients with disease confined

Table 2.01
Histological criteria for the diagnosis of serous borderline tumours.

- Epithelial hyperplasia in the form of stratification, tufting, cribriform and micropapillary arrangements
- Atypia (usually mild to moderate)
- Detached cell clusters
- Variable and usually minimal mitotic activity
- Absence of destructive stromal invasion

to the ovary or pelvis have a 5-year survival of 80%. Patients with serous psammocarcinoma have a protracted clinical course and a relatively favourable prognosis; their clinical behaviour more closely resembles that of SBT than serous carcinoma of the usual type.

Serous borderline tumour with microinvasion

Definition
An ovarian serous tumour of low malignant potential exhibiting early stromal invasion characterized by the presence in the stroma of individual or clusters of neoplastic cells cytologically similar to those of the associated non-invasive tumour. One or more foci may be present; none should exceed 10 mm^2.

Synonyms
Serous tumour of low malignant potential with microinvasion, serous tumour of borderline malignancy with microinvasion.

Epidemiology
Present in about 10-15% of SBTs, microinvasion occurs in women ranging in age from 17-83 years with a median age of 34.5 years {203,2867}.

Clinical features
Most symptomatic women present with a pelvic mass or pain. About 28% of the 39 women in the 2 major series were pregnant at the time of presentation {203,2867}.

Macroscopy
The macroscopic features are similar to those of SBT without microinvasion.

Tumour spread and staging
At presentation about 60% of the neoplasms are stage IA, 13% stage 1B, 5% stage IC, 8% stage IIC, 10% stage III (mostly IIIC) and 2.5% stage IV (liver metastases).

Histopathology
The hallmark of serous borderline tumours with microinvasion is the presence within the tumour stroma of single cells and cell clusters with generally abundant eosinophilic cytoplasm morphologically identical to those of the adjacent non-invasive tumour. The microinvasive foci form micropapillary, solid or rarely cribriform arrangements without or with only minimal stromal or cellular reaction. These cells are often

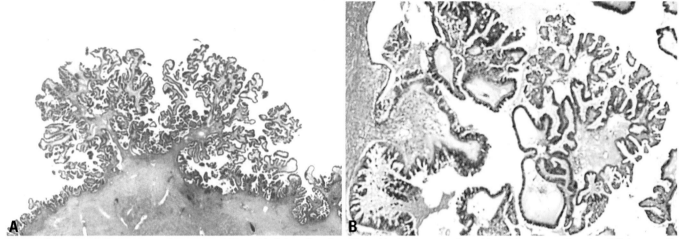

Fig. 2.06 Serous borderline tumour, typical pattern. **A** The epithelial papillae show hierarchical and complex branching without stromal invasion. **B** Higher magnification shows stratification and tufting of the epithelium with moderate atypia.

located within empty stromal spaces, but vascular space invasion occurs in 10% of cases. In 87% of the 39 reported cases the invasive cells were of the eosinophilic cell type {203,2867}. The lymph nodes were rarely assessed as part of staging for these tumours. Tumour cells, mainly of the eosinophilic cell type, were found in three nodes (obturator, external iliac, and para-aortic) from two women {203,2867}.

Prognosis and predictive factors
The behaviour of SBTs with microinvasion is similar to that of SBTs without microinvasion. In one series long-term follow-up was available in 11 cases with a 5-year survival of 100% and a 10-year survival of 86% {2285}. Unilateral salpingo-oophorectomy is currently acceptable therapy for young women who wish to preserve fertility.

Serous borderline tumour

Definition
An ovarian tumour of low malignant potential exhibiting an atypical epithelial proliferation of serous type cells greater than that seen in their benign counterparts but without destructive stromal invasion.

Synonyms
Serous tumour of low malignant potential, serous tumour of borderline malignancy. The designation "atypical proliferative serous tumour" is not recommended because it discourages complete surgical staging {2285} and because long term follow up indicates that some patients with typical SBT do not follow a benign course {3946}.

Epidemiology
Patients with SBT are approximately 10-15 years younger than those with serous carcinoma (i.e. 45 years vs. 60 years). About 30-50% of SBTs are bilateral.

Clinical features
Signs and symptoms
The tumour is often asymptomatic but may rarely present with abdominal enlargement or pain due to rupture of a cystic tumour or torsion. In younger women SBT has been associated with a high rate of infertility {2894a}.

Macroscopy
The tumour may be cystic with a variable number of excrescences, form a solid purely surface papillary growth or have a combination of these appearances. In

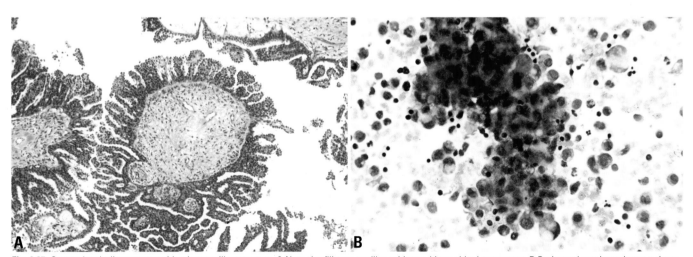

Fig. 2.07 Serous borderline tumour with micropapillary pattern. **A** Note the filigree papillae with non-hierarchical processes. **B** Peritoneal cytology shows a three-dimensional papillary-like tumour cell formation with low grade nuclear atypia mixed with mesothelial and inflammatory cells.

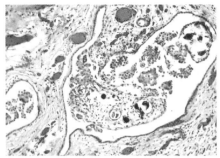

Fig. 2.08 Non-invasive peritoneal implant, epithelial type. The implant consists of hierarchical branching papillae within cystic spaces.

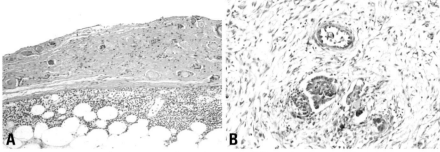

Fig. 2.09 Non-invasive peritoneal implant, desmoplastic type. **A** The implant is plastered on the peritoneal surface without destructive invasion of the underlying tissue. **B** The epithelial aggregates show moderate cellular atypia, and only a small portion of the implant is made up of epithelial cells.

contrast to carcinomas, SBTs generally lack areas of necrosis and haemorrhage. The cysts usually contain serous fluid, but occasionally it is mucinous.

Tumour spread and staging

Stage I SBTs are confined to the inner surface of the cyst with no spread beyond the ovary. The staging of SBT follows the TNM/FIGO system for carcinomas {51, 2976}.

Histopathology

The hallmarks of SBT that distinguish it from a cystadenoma are the presence of epithelial hyperplasia forming papillae (with fibroedematous stalks), micropapillae associated with "detached" or "floating" cell clusters and mild to moderate nuclear atypia. It is distinguished from serous carcinoma by the lack of destructive stromal invasion. The proliferating cells vary from uniform, small cells with hyperchromatic nuclei to larger cells displaying eosinophilic cytoplasm with variable and generally low mitotic activity. Psammoma bodies may be present but are less abundant than in serous carcinomas.

SBTs are divided into typical and micropapillary types. The typical type makes up the vast majority (90%) of SBTs and has a classic branching papillary architecture and epithelial tufts overlying the papillae. The micropapillary type accounts for a small proportion (5-10%) of tumours. This type shows focal or diffuse proliferation of the tumour cells in elongated, thin micropapillae with little or no stromal support emerging directly from the lining of a cyst, from large papillae in a non-hierarchical pattern or from the surface of the ovary. The micropapillae are at least five times as long as they are wide, arising directly from papillae with a thick fibrous stalk (non-hierarchical branching creating a "Medusa head-like appearance"). Less common patterns are cribriform and almost solid proliferations of non-invasive cells overlying papillary stalks. A continuous 5-mm growth of any of these three patterns is required for the diagnosis of micropapillary SBT.

Up to 30% of SBTs are associated with tumour on the outer surface of the ovary, and about two-thirds are associated with peritoneal implants {376,2615}.

Serous surface borderline tumour
In this variant, polypoid excrescences formed by fine papillae with features of SBT occupy the outer surface of the ovary.

Serous borderline adenofibroma and cystadenofibroma
In this variant, the epithelial lining of the glands and/or cysts of the adenofibroma or cystadenofibroma has the features of SBT instead of benign epithelium.

Peritoneal implants

Two prognostically different types of peritoneal implants have been identified, non-invasive and invasive. The former is further subdivided into desmoplastic and epithelial types. Whereas the non-invasive implants (regardless of their type) have almost no negative influence on the

Table 2.02
Serous borderline tumours. Histology of non-invasive vs. invasive peritoneal implants.

Non-invasive implants
Extension into interlobular fibrous septa of the omentum
Lacks disorderly infiltration of underlying tissue
Desmoplastic type
Proliferation appears plastered on peritoneal surface
Nests of cells, glands and or papillae proliferate in a prominent (>50%) background of dense fibroblastic or granulation tissue with well defined margins
Epithelial type
Fills submesothelial spaces
Exophytic proliferations with hierarchical branching papillae
Composed predominantly of epithelial cells
No stromal reaction
Frequent psammoma bodies
Invasive implants (Sampling of underlying tissues is crucial for assessment of invasion)
Haphazardly distributed glands invading normal tissues such as omentum
Loose or dense fibrous reaction without significant inflammation
Generally dominant epithelial proliferation
Nuclear features resembling a low grade serous adenocarcinoma
Irregular borders
Aneuploidy

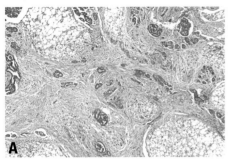 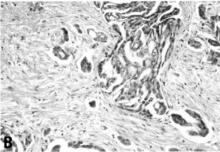

Fig. 2.10 Invasive peritoneal implant of the omentum. **A** Adipose tissue is invaded by haphazardly distributed glands and small cell clusters accompanied by a dense fibrous stromal reaction. **B** Haphazardly distributed glands and small cell clusters exhibit marked nuclear atypia and are accompanied by a dense fibrous stromal reaction.

Fig. 2.11 Serous borderline tumour. A lymph node contains epithelial inclusions of serous borderline tumour showing the typical papillary growth pattern.

10 year survival rates, the invasive form is associated with a poor prognosis, i.e. more than 50% have recurrences, and the 10 year survival rate is only about 35%. Therefore, the morphology of the peritoneal implants is the main prognostic factor for patients with stage II-III SBT. When underlying tissue is absent in a biopsy specimen, the lesion is classified as non-invasive on the assumption that it has been stripped away with ease {2605}. It is important to note that implants are heterogeneous, and various types may coexist in different areas; therefore, sampling of as many implants as feasible is recommended. The omentum is the most likely site for invasive implants. Therefore, surgeons must take a sufficient amount of omental tissue to enable the pathologist to distinguish non-invasive from invasive implants. In turn, the pathologist must assess multiple samples of macroscopically "normal" appearing omentum to ascertain adequate sampling.

Invasive implants should be distinguished from benign epithelial inclusions and foci of endosalpingiosis. The latter are uncommon, occurring between a fifth and a tenth as often as implants {207}. Benign epithelial inclusions are characterized by small, generally round glands lined by a single layer of flat to low columnar cells without atypia or mitotic activity, often associated with a fibrous stroma. Small rounded glands also characterize endosalpingiosis, but the latter may be papillary and the lining cells show the typical appearance of tubal epithelium (ciliated, secretory and intercalated cells).

Lymph node involvement
Pelvic and para-aortic lymph nodes are involved by SBT in about 20% of cases;

this finding appears to be without clinical significance. These lesions may be true metastases in peripheral sinuses, mesothelial cells in sinuses misinterpreted as tumour cells or independent primary SBTs arising in müllerian inclusion glands that are present in 25-30% of pelvic and para-aortic lymph nodes.

Somatic genetics
The pattern of genetic alterations described in SBTs (for review see {1159}) differs from that of invasive carcinomas, e.g. *TP53* mutations are most often absent in typical {838,1408} and micropapillary SBTs {1408}, but are present in up to 88% of cases of invasive serous carcinoma. Loss of heterozygosity on the long arm of the inactivated X chromosome {464} is characteristic for SBT and rare in carcinomas (for review see {838}). Chromosomal imbalances have been identified in 3 of 9 SBTs, 4 of 10 micropapillary SBTs and 9 of 11 serous carcinomas by comparative genomic hybridization; some changes in micropapillary SBT are shared with SBT and others with serous carcinomas only suggesting a relationship among them {2771}. The genetic profile indicates that SBTs are a separate category with little capacity to transform into a malignant phenotype. The situation concerning micropapillary SBTs has to be clarified.

Prognosis and predictive factors
Clinical criteria
Stage 1 SBTs do not progress and have an indolent clinical course with a 5-year survival rate of up to 99% {1542} and a 10-year survival which is not much worse. In stage III SBTs, i.e. distributed throughout the abdominal cavity with peritoneal implants (for details see below), the 5-year survival rate ranges between

55-75%, and the probability of a 10-year survival is not significantly worse.

Histopathological criteria
Compared to typical SBTs, it has been suggested that micropapillary SBTs have a higher frequency of bilaterality (59-71% vs. 25-30%) {754,2727}, an increased risk of recurrence among higher stage lesions {2727}, more frequent ovarian surface involvement (50-65% vs. 36%) and probably a higher frequency of advanced stage at presentation (48-66% vs. 32-35%) at least among referral cases {376,754}.
Several reports based on large series of cases, however, have demonstrated no difference in survival among patients with typical SBT and those with a micropapillary pattern among specific stages {658, 754,1000,1412,2285,2727}, indicating a need for further investigation of the significance of the micropapillary pattern. In addition to its indolent course, micropapillary SBT differs from conventional serous carcinoma by its lack of responsiveness to platinum-based chemotherapy {210}.

Cytophotometric predictive factors
The most reliable approach is the application of DNA-cytophotometry (preferably the static variant) according to the guidelines of the 1997 ESACP consensus report {1011,1141}. About 95% of SBTs display a diploid DNA-histogram with only a few cells in the 4c region indicating their low proliferative activity and only minor genetic alterations associated with an excellent clinical outcome {1380}. On the other hand, aneuploid SBTs characterized by a stemline deviation have a high recurrence rate, and the patients die frequently of their disease.
For peritoneal implants DNA-cytophotometry is also of prognostic importance because aneuploid implants were found

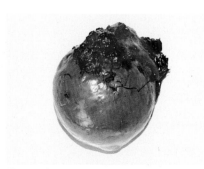

Fig. 2.12 Serous surface papilloma. A portion of the external surface of the ovary is covered by papillary excrescences.

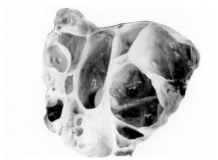

Fig. 2.13 Serous cystadenoma. Sectioned surface shows a multiloculated cystic tumour with smooth cyst walls.

to be associated with a poor prognosis {652,2145}. Although rare, transformation of a SBT into a bona fide frankly invasive carcinoma may occur.

Benign serous tumours

Definition
Benign tumours composed of epithelium resembling that of the fallopian tube or in some cases the surface epithelium of the ovary.

Epidemiology
Benign serous tumours of the ovary account for approximately 16% of all ovarian epithelial neoplasms. The majority of benign serous tumours arise in adults in the fourth to sixth decades, although they may occur in patients younger than twenty or older than eighty years.

Localization
Benign serous tumours arise preferentially in the cortex of the ovary or on its surface (8%). They are usually bilateral, especially in older women. Often the tumours are metachronous with intervals that range from three to fourteen years.

Similar tumours in extraovarian sites occasionally accompany benign serous tumours.

Clinical features
Signs and symptoms
The most common symptoms are pain, vaginal bleeding and abdominal enlargement, but usually the tumour is asymptomatic and discovered incidentally during ultrasound investigation of another gynaecological disorder.

Macroscopy
Benign serous tumours are usually 1-10 cm in diameter but occasionally reach up to 30 cm or more. They are typically unilocular or multilocular cystic lesions, the external surface is smooth, and the inner surface may contain small papillary projections. The cyst contents are watery and very rarely opaque or bloody. Adenofibromas are solid and have a spongy sectioned surface with minute, colourless fluid-containing cysts. Cystadenofibromas contain both solid areas and cysts. Surface papillomas appear as warty excrescences of different sizes on the surface of the ovary.

Histopathology
Benign serous tumours typically are lined by an epithelium similar to that of the fallopian tube with ciliated and less frequently nonciliated secretory cells. Of special diagnostic interest are the cysts with flattened lining, some of which may represent benign serous neoplasms with a desquamated lining. The only effective method to establish their nature is the application of scanning electron microscopy, which easily detects the ciliated cells, allowing a definitive diagnosis to be made.

Histogenesis
Benign serous tumours result from the proliferation of the surface epithelium of the ovary, {272,1403,2605} producing surface papillary excrescences or invaginating into the cortex of the ovary, forming so called inclusion cysts. Some morphological data support the possibility that a number of benign serous tumours arise from remnants in the hilar region of the ovary, possibly from rete cysts {726,1403,1823}.

Prognosis and predictive factors
Serous cystadenomas are benign.

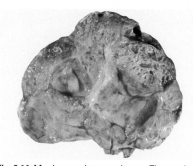

Fig. 2.14 Mucinous adenocarcinoma. The sectioned surface shows a multiloculated cystic tumour with more solid areas containing small cysts.

Mucinous tumours

Definition
Ovarian tumours some or all of whose epithelial cells contain intracytoplasmic mucin. They may resemble those of the endocervix, gastric pylorus or intestine. In some tumours only scattered goblet cells are present in an epithelium that is otherwise non-mucinous.

ICD–O codes
Mucinous adenocarcinoma	8480/3
Mucinous cystadenocarcinofibroma	9015/3
Mucinous borderline tumour	8472/1
Mucinous cystadenoma	8470/0
Mucinous adenofibroma	9015/0

Mucinous adenocarcinoma and related tumours

Definition
A malignant epithelial tumour of the ovary that in its better differentiated areas resembles intestinal or endocervical epithelium. Ovarian mucinous adenocarcinomas differ from borderline tumours by having evidence of ovarian stromal invasion.

Macroscopy
Mucinous carcinomas are usually large, unilateral, smooth surfaced, multilocular or unilocular cystic masses containing watery or viscous mucoid material. They are bilateral in approximately 5% of cases. Haemorrhagic, necrotic, solid or papillary areas are relatively frequent, and some tumours may be predominantly solid {1613,2605}. Because areas of malignancy may be limited, generous sampling of all mucinous cystic tumours to include up to one histological section per 1-2 cm of tumour diameter with sam-

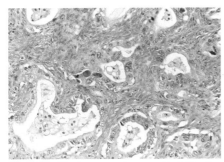

Fig. 2.15 Mucinous carcinoma with infiltrative invasive pattern. Irregular glands lined by cells with malignant features infiltrate the stroma.

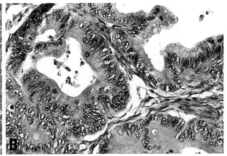

Fig. 2.16 Mucinous adenocarcinoma with expansile invasive pattern. **A** Note the complex glandular proliferation. **B** The glands are lined by cells that have highly atypical nuclei and some intracytoplasmic mucin.

pling of all macroscopically suspicious areas has been recommended.

Histopathology

In the absence of obvious infiltration of the stroma, invasion is assumed if there are complex papillary areas or back-to-back glands lined by malignant-appearing cells with little or no discernible intervening stroma. To qualify as frankly invasive, such areas should be at least 10 mm^2 and at least 3 mm in each of 2 linear dimensions {1613}. Alternatively, invasion may be in the form of infiltrative glands, tubules, cords or cell nests. The stroma may resemble ovarian stroma or be desmoplastic. In most cases there are also areas that are benign or borderline in appearance {1147,1150,1228,2047,2401}. Rarely, mucinous tumours contain areas of mucinous adenofibroma with malignant epithelial cells and foci of stromal invasion.

Differential diagnosis
The most important differential diagnosis of mucinous ovarian carcinoma is with metastatic mucinous carcinoma that may present clinically as a primary ovarian tumour. Most of these originate in the large intestine, appendix, pancreas, biliary tract, stomach or cervix {237,639, 1587,1703,2377,2406,3200,3221}. Since this problem has been emphasized relatively recently, it is likely that early reports of the histological appearance and behaviour of ovarian mucinous carcinomas have been contaminated by metastatic carcinomas masquerading as primary ovarian neoplasms (see Table 2.03). Common features that favour a primary mucinous carcinoma are an expansile pattern of invasion and a complex papillary pattern {1614}. Common features favouring a metastatic mucinous carcinoma are bilaterality, a multinodular

growth pattern microscopically, histological surface involvement by epithelial cells (surface implants) and vascular space invasion {1614}.

Somatic genetics

Tumour heterogeneity is common and probably is a reflection of the progression from benign to malignant neoplasia that occurs in the development of mucinous carcinomas. Recent studies strongly suggest that in the sequence of malignant transformation from benign and borderline mucinous tumours to infiltrative carcinoma intraepithelial (non-invasive) carcinomas and carcinomas with purely expansile (not obvious) invasion represent transitional stages of mucinous carcinogenesis {1613}. This hypothesis is also supported by recent molecular studies of genetic alterations in mucinous tumours {591,964,1755,1891}. An increasing frequency of codon 12/13 *KRAS* mutations in benign, borderline and carcinomatous mucinous ovarian tumours has been reported supporting the viewpoint that *KRAS* mutational activation is an early event in mucinous ovarian tumorigenesis. Mucinous borderline tumours have a higher frequency of *KRAS* mutations than that of mucinous cystadenomas but a lower rate than that of mucinous carcinomas {591,1755,1891}. Using microdissection, the same *KRAS* mutation has been detected in separate areas exhibiting different histological grades within the same neoplasm {591}.

Prognosis and predictive factors
Clinical criteria
Stage I mucinous carcinomas have an excellent prognosis. However, the prognosis in cases with extraovarian spread is very poor {1076,1228,1458,1613,2377, 2401,3069}.

Histopathological criteria
With the exception of one recent series {3769}, grading of mucinous carcinomas has not been shown to be predictive of behaviour or response to therapy independent of the surgical stage {1076, 1228,1458,1613,2377,3069}. Infiltrative stromal invasion proved to be biologically more aggressive than expansile invasion. If individual invasive foci are all less than 10 mm^2, they have been termed "microinvasive," and cases with this finding have had a favourable outcome {1453,1613, 1987,2047,2401,2713}.

Mucinous borderline tumour, intestinal type

Definition
Ovarian tumours of low malignant potential exhibiting an epithelial proliferation of mucinous type cells greater than that seen in their benign counterparts but without evidence of stromal invasion. The epithelial component resembles intestinal epithelium, almost always contains goblet cells, usually contains neuroendocrine cells and rarely contains Paneth cells.

Synonyms
Mucinous tumour of low malignant potential, intestinal type; mucinous tumour of borderline malignancy, intestinal type.

Epidemiology
These account for 85-90% of mucinous borderline tumours.

Macroscopy
Mucinous borderline tumours of intestinal type are bilateral in approximately 5% of cases and usually are large, multilocular or unilocular cystic masses containing watery or viscous mucoid material.

Table 2.03
Primary vs. metastatic mucinous ovarian carcinomas.

Features favouring primary carcinoma
Unilaterality
Large size, smooth surface
Expansile pattern of growth
Features favouring metastatic carcinoma
Bilaterality
Known primary mucinous carcinoma at another site
Macroscopically friable and necrotic
Variable or nodular pattern of growth
Ovarian surface involvement
Ovarian vascular invasion
Cytokeratin 7-negative
Non-contributory
Benign or borderline-appearing areas
Infiltrative pattern of growth
Luminal necrotic debris
Tumour grade

Velvety excrescences may line the cysts. Haemorrhagic, necrotic, solid or papillary areas are occasionally present {1613,2605}.

Histopathology

Areas resembling mucinous cystadenoma are common. In the borderline areas the cells lining the cysts are stratified (usually to no more than 3 layers) and may form filiform intracystic papillae with at least minimal stromal support. Nuclei are slightly larger with more mitotic figures than in cystadenomas. Goblet cells and sometimes Paneth cells are present. The overall appearance resembles a hyperplastic or adenomatous colonic polyp {322,653,1076,1147,1150,1613,2377, 2491,2605,2713}. Some or most of the epithelial cells lining the cysts of intestinal type borderline tumours may appear

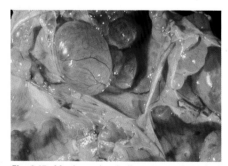

Fig. 2.17 Mucinous borderline tumour, intestinal type. The sectioned surface shows a multiloculated tumour with large cysts.

cytologically malignant and may be stratified to four or more layers in a solid, papillary or cribriform pattern. Whether tumours with such foci should be classified as non-invasive carcinomas or as borderline tumours has been a subject of controversy for many years. To provide for uniformity in reporting, it has been recommended that they be classified as borderline with intraepithelial carcinoma {2605}.

Prognosis and predictive factors

When the tumour is confined to the ovaries at initial staging, the prognosis is excellent with only rarely reported recurrences {1150}. It is likely that most tumours diagnosed as intestinal-type mucinous borderline tumour that are associated with pseudomyxoma peritonei are actually metastatic from a similar-appearing tumour in the appendix (see section on pseudomyxoma peritonei). In the remaining cases with advanced disease, the metastases are usually in the form of invasive pelvic or abdominal implants rather than pseudomyxoma peritonei. In these cases the prognosis is similar to that of ovarian mucinous carcinomas with metastases, and it is likely that areas of invasion within the ovarian tumour were not sampled {1076,1147,1150,1613,2401}. Table 2.04 summarizes the differences in appearance and outcome among neoplasms having the appearance of mucinous borderline tumours.

Mucinous borderline tumour, endocervical-like

Definition

Ovarian tumours of low malignant potential exhibiting an epithelial proliferation of mucinous type cells greater than seen in their benign counterparts but without destructive stromal invasion. The mucinous epithelial cells resemble endocervical epithelium.

Synonyms

Mucinous tumour of low malignant potential, endocervical-like; mucinous tumour of borderline malignancy, endocervical-like; müllerian mucinous borderline tumour.

Epidemiology

These tumours make up 10-15% of mucinous borderline tumours {1613,2497,2713}.

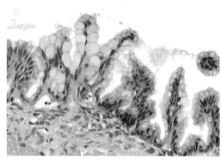

Fig. 2.18 Mucinous borderline tumour, intestinal type. Goblet cells and nuclear stratification are evident.

Macroscopy

Mucinous endocervical-like borderline tumours usually are multilocular or unilocular cystic masses containing watery or viscous mucoid material. Haemorrhagic, necrotic, solid or papillary areas may be present {1613,2605}. They are smaller than the intestinal type and have fewer cysts. They are bilateral in approximately 40% of cases and sometimes arise within an endometriotic cyst {2497}.

Tumour spread and staging

Endocervical-like borderline tumours may be associated with abdominal or pelvic implants, some of which may appear invasive {2497,2713}.

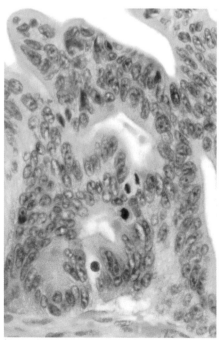

Fig. 2.19 Mucinous borderline tumour, intestinal type, with intraepithelial carcinoma. Malignant mucinous epithelium with a cribriform pattern and mitotic figures lines a cyst.

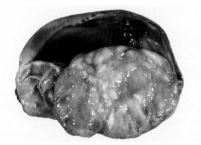

Fig. 2.20 Mucinous endocervical-like borderline tumour. The sectioned surface shows a solid and cystic mucin-containing tumour arising in an endometriotic cyst.

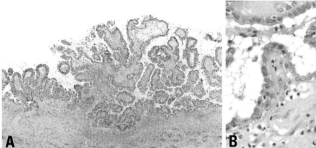

Fig. 2.21 Mucinous endocervical-like borderline tumour. **A** Note the papillae lined by atypical cells with stratification and budding. **B** Some cells contain intracytoplasmic mucin, and the stroma of the papillae is infiltrated by neutrophils.

Histopathology

They differ from intestinal-type borderline tumours in that the intracystic growth is composed of broad bulbous papillae similar to those of serous borderline tumours. The epithelial cells lining the papillae are columnar mucinous cells and rounded cells with eosinophilic cytoplasm; the latter are often markedly stratified with detached cell clusters. The nuclei are only slightly atypical. Characteristically, there are many acute inflammatory cells within the papillae or free-floating in extracellular spaces.

Precursor lesions

Endocervical-like borderline tumours likely arise from endometriosis {2497}. At least in some cases the peritoneal implants may arise from independent foci of endometriosis with in situ transformation.

Prognosis and predictive features

Endocervical-like borderline tumours may be associated with abdominal or pelvic implants, some of which may appear invasive, but the clinical behaviour has been indolent in the relatively few cases that have been reported {2497,2713}. However, more cases in this category need to be studied.

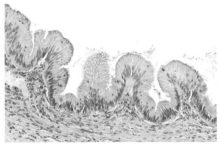

Fig. 2.22 Mucinous cystadenoma. The presence of pseudostratified epithelium with low cellular proliferation in the absence of nuclear atypia does not justify the borderline category.

Benign mucinous tumours

Definition

Benign mucinous tumours composed of epithelium resembling endocervical or gastrointestinal epithelium. The latter almost always contains goblet cells, usually contains neuoendocrine cells and rarely contains Paneth cells.

Macroscopy

Mucinous cystadenomas are usually large, unilateral, multilocular or unilocular cystic masses containing watery or viscous mucoid material. Cystadenofibromas and adenofibromas are partially to almost completely solid with only small cysts {200}.

Histopathology

Benign mucinous tumours consist of cystadenomas, cystadenofibromas and adenofibromas These contain glands and cysts lined by mucinous columnar epithelium {2605}. Cellular stratification is minimal, and nuclei are basally located with only slight, if any, atypia. Cystadenomas may have mucin extravasation with or without a stromal reaction. An ipsilateral dermoid cyst is present in 3-5% of cases. The uncommon mucinous adenofibroma is composed predominantly of fibromatous stroma {200}.

Mucinous cystic tumours with mural nodules

Rare mucinous cystic tumours contain one or more solid mural nodules in which the histological features differ markedly from the background of either an intestinal-type borderline tumour or carcinoma {2007,2288,2290,2605}. The nodules are yellow, pink or red with areas of haemorrhage or necrosis and range up to 12 cm in size. They may be malignant (anaplastic carcinoma, sarcoma or carcinosarcoma) or benign (sarcoma-like). Mucinous cystic tumours containing more than 1 type of mural nodule as well as mixed nodules have been described. Anaplastic carcinomatous nodules usually contain a predominant population of cytokeratin-positive, large, rounded or spindle-shaped cells with abundant eosinophilic cytoplasm and high grade malignant nuclei. The few sarcomas that have been reported have been fibrosarcomas or rhabdomyosarcomas or have not been otherwise classified. Sarcoma-like nodules are sharply circumscribed and without vascular invasion but otherwise may appear alarming, containing pleomorphic cells with bizarre nuclei and many mitotic figures, often accompanied by spindle-shaped cells, epulis-type giant cells, acute and chronic inflammatory cells and foci of haemorrhage and necrosis. The sarcoma-like cells may be weakly or focally cytokeratin-positive, but this finding, in itself, does not indicate a carcinomatous component {2605}. The distinction is important because patients with anaplastic carcinoma in a mural nodule may follow a malignant course {2290}, whereas the outcome of

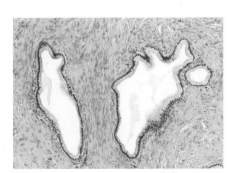

Fig. 2.23 Mucinous adenofibroma. Uniform mucinous glands are associated with a prominent fibrous stroma.

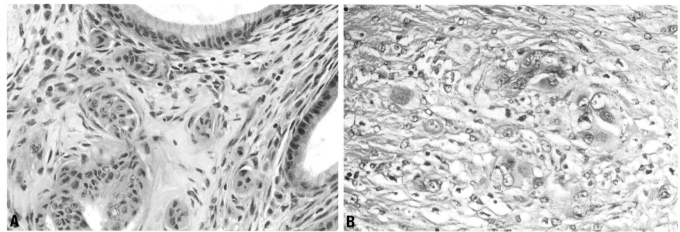

Fig. 2.24 Mucinous borderline tumour (MBT). **A** Note the microinvasive focus in a MBT. **B** Mural nodule from another MBT. The mural nodule is composed of epithelial cells with anaplastic nuclei, abundant cytoplasm and some intracytoplasmic mucin in a fibrous stroma.

those with only sarcoma-like nodules is the same as the corresponding category of mucinous tumour without the nodules {163}. Although the foci of anaplastic carcinoma are found more often in advanced stage tumours, it is now apparent that when they are confined to intact stage IA tumours, they are not necessarily associated with an adverse outcome {2401}.

Mucinous cystic tumours associated with pseudomyxoma peritonei

Since there is strong evidence that ovarian mucinous tumours associated with pseudomyxoma peritonei (PP) are almost all metastatic rather than primary, it is important that such tumours are not diagnosed as stage II or III mucinous borderline tumours or carcinomas without first excluding an appendiceal or other gastrointestinal primary. Present evidence suggests that almost all genuine ovarian mucinous borderline tumours are stage

1. The number of stage 2 and 3 tumours in this category has been greatly exaggerated by including cases in which PP is associated with an undetected primary tumour in the appendix. Also, there is probably an unwarranted apparent increase in the number of high stage ovarian mucinous carcinomas because of undetected primary intestinal mucinous carcinomas associated with the clinical syndrome of PP.

Pseudomyxoma peritonei is a clinical term used to describe the finding of abundant mucoid or gelatinous material in the pelvis and abdominal cavity surrounded by fibrous tissue. The mucus may be acellular or may contain mucinous epithelial cells. Mucinous ascites, the presence of free-floating mucinous fluid, in the peritoneal cavity, almost never leads to pseudomyxoma peritonei. Areas of pseudomyxoma peritonei should be thoroughly sampled and examined histologically. The degree of atypia (benign, borderline or malignant)

of any epithelial cells that are present should be reported, as well as whether the mucin dissects into tissues with a fibrous response or is merely on the surface. Pseudomyxoma peritonei with epithelial cells that are benign or borderline-appearing has been termed "disseminated peritoneal adenomucinosis" by some authors {2409}, and patients with this finding have had a benign or protracted clinical course. In cases where the epithelial cells of the pseudomyxoma peritonei appear malignant, termed "peritoneal mucinous carcinomatosis" {2409}, the source has usually been the appendix or colon, and the clinical course has usually been fatal.

Pseudomyxoma peritonei may be present in women without a cystic ovarian tumour or in men. In such cases the source is almost always a gastrointestinal mucinous neoplasm, most commonly from the appendix {2409}. In cases where there is an appendiceal tumour and a mucinous cystic ovarian tumour,

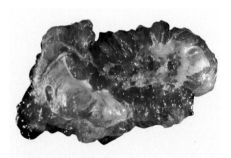

Fig. 2.25 Mucinous cystic tumour associated with pseudomyxoma peritonei. The sectioned surface shows a multiloculated cystic tumour associated with areas of haemorrhage.

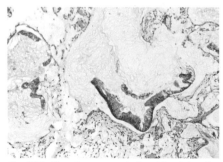

Fig. 2.26 Pseudomyxoma peritonei involving the omentum. Strips of low grade neoplastic mucinous epithelium are associated with abundant extracellular mucin.

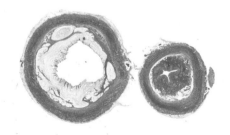

Fig. 2.27 Mucinous appendiceal tumour associated with pseudomyxoma peritonei. Note on the left, the dilatation of the wall and distention of the mucosa by mucin-producing tumour cells.

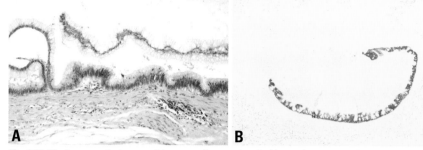

Fig. 2.28 Mucinous cystic tumour of the appendix associated with synchronous mucinous ovarian tumours. **A** The appendiceal lesion shows pseudostratified mucinous epithelium (colonic type) with mild nuclear atypia. **B** The mucinous epithelium of the ovarian lesion shows strong immunoreactivity for cytokeratin 20 and was negative for cytokeratin 7, strongly supporting the appendiceal origin of the tumour.

the origin of the pseudomyxoma peritonei has been disputed. A majority of investigators believe that the ovarian tumour(s) are secondary in almost all such cases {2294,2407,3199}. However, a synchronous origin in both organs has also been proposed {2623}.

Clonality studies have demonstrated identical *KRAS* mutations or the lack of them in both the appendiceal and the simultaneous ovarian tumours {590, 2830}. LOH analysis has shown similar findings in three cases and divergent findings in three; this latter observation appears to indicate that some simultaneous tumours are independent primaries

{590}, though genetic progression of the metastatic tumours could also account for the disparity of these results.

The ovarian tumours are usually classified as either mucinous cystadenomas or intestinal-type borderline tumours. The epithelial cells within them are often found floating in mucin that dissects into the ovarian stroma (pseudomyxoma ovarii). They are well differentiated and often have a tall columnar appearance with abundant mucinous cytoplasm that is positive for cytokeratin 7 in approximately one-half of the cases {1075, 2408}. The latter finding differs from that of primary ovarian mucinous cystadeno-

ma or intestinal-type borderline tumours most of which are cytokeratin 7-positive. The appendiceal tumour may be quite small relative to the ovarian tumour(s) and may not be appreciated macroscopically. Thus, removal and thorough histological examination of the appendix is indicated in cases of pseudomyxoma peritonei with a mucinous cystic ovarian tumour. In cases where an appendiceal mucinous neoplasm is found, it should be considered as the primary site and the ovaries as secondary. If the appendix has not been examined histologically and the ovarian tumours are bilateral, or unilateral in the absence of an ipsilateral dermoid cyst, the appendix should also be considered primary. If an appendiceal mucinous neoplasm is not found after thorough histological examination, if the appendix had been removed previously in the absence of pseudomyxoma peritonei or if the ovarian tumour is accompanied by a dermoid cyst in the absence of either a macroscopic or histological appendiceal lesion, the ovarian tumour may be considered to be the source of the pseudomyxoma peritonei {1613}. In equivocal cases cytokeratin 7 negativity in the ovarian tumour strongly suggests that it is metastatic.

Table 2.04
Behaviour of problematic mucinous ovarian neoplasms with invasive implants or pseudomyxoma peritonei.

Tumour type	Macroscopy	Histopathology	Appearance of extraovarian disease	Usual behaviour in cases with extraovarian disease
Intestinal type MBT	Large, smooth surfaced multilocular cyst, bilateral in 5%	Cysts are lined with slightly stratified intestinal type cells with mild nuclear atypia and no detached cell clusters Usually CK7 positive	Invasive peritoneal implants without PP This is a rare finding	Prognosis is poor. Cases with invasive implants are likely due to unsampled invasive areas in the ovarian tumour.
Intestinal type MBT with intraepithelial carcinoma	Same	Same, with foci of malignant-appearing nuclei and often highly stratified, solid or cribriform areas	Invasive peritoneal implants without PP	Same as above
Endocervical-like MBT	Smaller with fewer cysts and may be associated with endometriosis, bilateral in 40%	Cysts composed of complex, bulbous papillae with highly stratified, benign-appearing mucinous and eosinophilic cells, detached cell clusters and numerous neutrophils	Invasive or noninvasive peritoneal implants	Benign
Mucinous ovarian tumours associated with PP	Bilateral in a high percentage of cases	Usually resembles intestinal type of MBT often with pseudomyxoma ovarii	PP Often primary appendiceal tumour	Variable, depending on the degree of atypia of the tumour cells in PP
PP = Pseudomyxoma peritonei; MBT = mucinous borderline tumour				

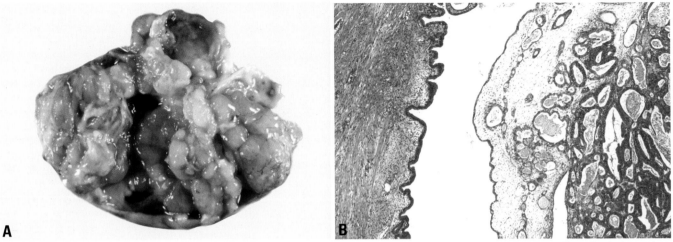

Fig. 2.29 Ovarian endometrioid adenocarcinoma arising from an endometriotic cyst. **A** This solid and cystic tumour forms polypoid structures. The patient had a synchronous endometrioid adenocarcinoma of the uterine corpus. **B** Well differentiated endometrioid adenocarcinoma is seen to the right and an endometriotic cyst on the left.

Endometrioid tumours

Definition
Tumours of the ovary, benign, low malignant potential or malignant, that closely resemble the various types of endometrioid tumours (epithelial and/or stromal) of the uterine corpus. Although an origin from endometriosis can be demonstrated in some cases, it is not required for the diagnosis.

ICD-O codes

Endometrioid adenocarcinoma, not otherwise specified	8380/3
Variant with squamous differentiation	8570/3
Ciliated variant	8383/3
Oxyphilic variant	8290/3
Secretory variant	8382/3
Adenocarcinofibroma	8381/3
Malignant müllerian mixed tumour	8950/3
Adenosarcoma	8933/3
Endometrioid stromal sarcoma	8930/3
Endometrioid borderline tumour	8380/1
Cystadenoma	8380/0
Adenofibroma; cystadenofibroma	8381/0

Endometrioid adenocarcinoma

Definition
A malignant epithelial tumour of the ovary that closely resembles the common variant of endometrioid carcinoma of the uterine corpus. Although an origin from endometriosis can be demonstrated in some cases, it is not required for the diagnosis.

Epidemiology
Endometrioid carcinomas account for 10-20% of ovarian carcinomas {1409, 2489} and occur most commonly in women in the fifth and sixth decades of life {2773}.

Aetiology
Up to 42% of the tumours are associated with endometriosis in the same ovary or elsewhere in the pelvis {676,932,1927, 2489,2287a} and 15-20% are associated with endometrial carcinoma {1477,1479, 1683,3239}. These associations suggest that some endometrioid ovarian carcinomas may have the same risk factors for their development as endometrial carcinomas {613}. Patients whose tumours occur in association with endometriosis are 5-10 years younger on average than patients without associated ovarian endometriosis {2600}.

Clinical features
Like most ovarian carcinomas, many endometrioid carcinomas are asymptomatic. Some present as a pelvic mass, with or without pain and may be associated with endocrine symptoms secondary to steroid hormone secretion by the specialized ovarian stroma {1790}. Serum CA125 is elevated in over 80% of the cases {946,1603}.

Macroscopy
The tumours, typically measuring 10-20 cm in diameter, are solid, soft, friable or cystic with a fungating mass protruding into the lumen. They are bilateral in 28% of the cases.

Tumour spread and staging
Stage I carcinomas are bilateral in 17% of the cases {2233}. The stage distribution of endometrioid carcinomas differs from that of serous carcinomas. According to the FIGO annual report, 31% of the tumours are stage I; 20%, stage II; 38%, stage III; and 11%, stage IV {2233}.

Histopathology
Ovarian endometrioid carcinomas closely resemble endometrioid carcinomas of the uterine corpus. The well differentiated form shows round, oval or tubular glands lined by stratified nonmucin-containing epithelium. Cribriform or villoglandular patterns may be present. Squamous differentiation occurs in 30-50% of the cases, often in the form of morules (cytologically benign-appearing squamous cells) {341,2605}. The designation "endometrioid carcinoma with squamous differentiation" (rather than adenoacanthoma and adenosquamous carcinoma) is favoured {2604,2605}. Aggregates of spindle-shaped epithelial cells are an occasional finding in endometrioid carcinoma {2942}. Occasionally, the spindle cell nests undergo a transition to clearly recognizable squamous cells suggesting that the former may represent abortive squamous differentiation {2605}.
Rare examples of mucin-rich, secretory, ciliated cell and oxyphilic types have been described {759,1187,2258}. In the mucin-rich variant glandular lumens and the apex of cells are occupied by mucin {2605}. The secretory type contains vacuolated cells resembling those of an

early secretory endometrium {2605}. The oxyphilic variant has a prominent component of large polygonal tumour cells with abundant eosinophilic cytoplasm and round central nuclei with prominent nucleoli {2258}.

Occasional tumours contain solid areas punctuated by tubular or round glands or small rosette-like glands (microglandular pattern) simulating an adult granulosa cell tumour {3206}. In contrast to Call-Exner bodies, however, the microglands contain intraluminal mucin. The nuclei of endometrioid carcinomas are usually round and hyperchromatic, whereas those of granulosa cell tumours are round, oval, or angular, pale and grooved. Rare cases of endometrioid carcinomas of the ovary show focal to extensive areas resembling Sertoli and Sertoli-Leydig cell tumours {2111,2466,3206}. They contain small, well differentiated hollow tubules, solid tubules or, rarely, thin cords resembling sex cords. When the stroma is luteinized, this variant may be mistaken for a Sertoli-Leydig cell tumour, particularly in cases in which the patient is virilized. Nevertheless, typical glands of endometrioid carcinoma and squamous differentiation are each present in 75% of the tumours, facilitating their recognition as an endometrioid carcinoma {3206}. Furthermore, immunostains for alpha-inhibin are positive in Sertoli cells but negative in the cells of endometrioid carcinoma {1789}.

Immunoprofile
Endometrioid carcinomas are vimentin, cytokeratin, epithelial membrane antigen, estrogen and progesterone recep-

tor and B72.3 positive but alpha-inhibin negative {1789}.

Grading
Grading of endometrioid carcinoma uses the same criteria as endometrial adenocarcinoma {3238} (see chapter 4).

Histogenesis
Most endometrioid carcinomas are thought to arise from surface epithelial inclusions, and up to 42% are accompanied by ipsilateral ovarian or pelvic endometriosis {676,932,1927,2489} that may display the entire spectrum of endometrial hyperplasia (simple, complex, typical and atypical). Atypical ipsilateral endometriosis occurs in up to 23% of endometrioid carcinomas {932} and may have a role in the evolution of some endometrioid carcinomas {2618}.

Somatic genetics
Somatic mutations of beta-catenin (*CTNNB1*) and *PTEN* are the most common genetic abnormalities identified in sporadic endometrioid carcinomas. The incidence of *CTNNB1* mutations ranges from 38-50% {1909,2153}. Mutations have been described in exon 3 (codons 32, 33, 37, and 41) and involve the phosphorylation sequence for glycogen synthase kinase 3β. These mutations probably render a fraction of cellular beta-catenin insensitive to APC-mediated down-regulation and are responsible for its accumulation in the nuclei of the tumour cells. Beta-catenin is immunohistochemically detectable in carcinoma cells in more than 80% of the cases. Endometrioid carcinomas with beta-

catenin mutations are characteristically early stage tumours associated with a good prognosis {955}.

PTEN is mutated in approximately 20% of endometrioid ovarian tumours and in 46% of those with 10q23 loss of heterozygosity (LOH) {2075}. *PTEN* mutations occur between exons 3 to 8. The majority of endometrioid carcinomas with *PTEN* mutations are well differentiated and stage I tumours, suggesting that in this subset of ovarian tumours *PTEN* inactivation is an early event {2075}. The finding of 10q23 LOH and *PTEN* mutations in endometriotic cysts that are adjacent to endometrioid carcinomas with similar genetic alterations provides additional evidence for the precursor role of endometriosis in ovarian carcinogenesis {2543}.

Microsatellite instability (MI) also occurs in sporadic endometrioid carcinomas of the ovary although less frequently than in uterine endometrioid carcinomas. The reported frequency of MI in the former tumours ranges from 12.5-19% {1055,1909}. Like endometrial carcinomas, many ovarian carcinomas with MI follow the same process of MLH1 promoter methylation and frameshift mutations at coding mononucleotide repeat microsatellites {1055}.

Simultaneous endometrioid carcinomas of the ovary and endometrium
Endometrioid carcinoma of the ovary is associated in 15-20% of the cases with carcinoma of the endometrium {767,822,1479,2651,3239}. The very good prognosis in those cases in which the tumour is

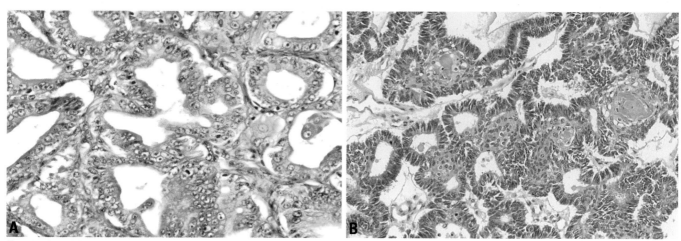

Fig. 2.30 Well differentiated endometrioid adenocarcinoma of the ovary. **A** Confluent growth of glands is evident with replacement of stroma. **B** Note the squamous differentiation in the form of squamous morules and keratin pearls.

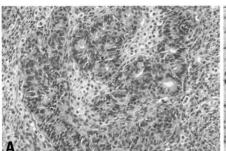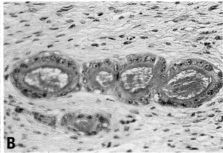

Fig. 2.31 Sertoliform endometroid carcinoma. **A** The tubular glands contain high grade nuclei. The luteinized ovarian stromal cells resemble Leydig cells. **B** Small endometrioid glands contain luminal mucin. (Mucicarmine stain).

limited to both organs provides strong evidence that these neoplasms are mostly independent primaries arising as a result of a müllerian field effect {822}. Less frequently, one of the carcinomas represents a metastasis from the other tumour.

The criteria for distinguishing metastatic from independent primary carcinomas rely mainly upon conventional clinico-pathologic findings, namely stage, size, histological type and grade of the tumours, the presence and extent of blood vessel, tubal and myometrial invasion, bilaterality and pattern of ovarian involvement, coexistence with endometrial hyperplasia or ovarian endometriosis and, ultimately, patient follow-up {762, 2286,2978}. By paying attention to these findings, the precise diagnosis can be established in most cases. Occasionally, however, the differential diagnosis may be difficult or impossible as the tumours may show overlapping features.

In difficult cases comparative analysis of the immunohistochemical and DNA flow cytometric features of the two neoplasms may be of some help {822,2286}. The presence of identical aneuploid DNA indexes in two separate carcinomas suggests

that one of them is a metastasis from the other {2286}. In contrast, when the two neoplasm have different DNA indexes, the possibility of two independent primaries has to be considered {2286}. The latter results, however, do not completely exclude the metastatic nature of 1 of the tumours, since metastatic tumours or even different parts of the same tumour may occasionally have different DNA indexes reflecting tumour progression {2728}.

Molecular pathology techniques can also be helpful {1788}. These include LOH, {783,923,1664,2641}, gene mutation {923,1664,1909} and clonal X-inactivation analyses {926}. Although LOH pattern concordance in two separate carcinomas is highly suggestive of a common clonal origin (i.e. one tumour is a metastasis from the other), the finding of different LOH patterns does not necessarily indicate that they represent independent tumours. Some studies have shown varying LOH patterns in different areas of the same tumour as a consequence of tumour heterogeneity {287}. Discordant *PTEN* mutations and different microsatellite instability (MI) patterns in the two neoplasms are suggestive of independent primary carcinomas; nevertheless,

metastatic carcinomas may also exhibit gene mutations that differ from those of their corresponding primary tumours as a result of tumour progression {923}. Alternatively, two independent primary carcinomas may present identical gene mutations reflecting induction of the same genetic abnormalities by a common carcinogenic agent acting in two separate sites of a single anatomic region {1786,1788}. In other words, the genetic profile can be identical in independent tumours and different in metastatic carcinomas {1788}. Therefore, clonality analysis is useful in the distinction of independent primary carcinomas from metastatic carcinomas provided the diagnosis does not rely exclusively on a single molecular result and the molecular data are interpreted in the light of appropriate clinical and pathologic findings {1786,1788,2283}.

According to FIGO when the site of origin remains in doubt after pathological examination, the primary site of the tumour should be determined by its initial clinical manifestations.

Genetic susceptibility

Most endometrioid carcinomas occur sporadically, but occasional cases develop in families with germline mutations in DNA mismatch repair genes, mainly *MSH2* and *MLH1* (Muir-Torre syndrome) {535}. This syndrome, thought to be a variant of the hereditary nonpolyposis colon cancer syndrome, is characterized by an inherited autosomal dominant susceptibility to develop cutaneous and visceral neoplasms {796}.

Prognosis and predictive factors

The 5-year survival rate (FIGO) of patients with stage I carcinoma is 78%; stage II, 63%; stage III, 24%; and stage

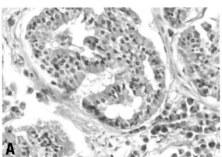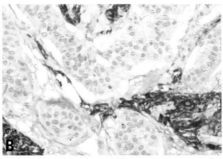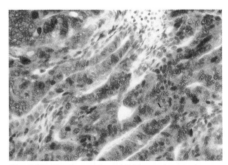

Fig. 2.32 Endometrioid adenocarcinoma resembling a granulosa cell tumour. **A** Note the microglandular pattern. **B** Immunostains for alpha-inhibin are positive in the luteinized stromal cells and negative in the epithelial cells.

Fig. 2.33 Ovarian endometrioid carcinoma. Immunostain for beta-catenin shows intense and diffuse positivity.

IV, 6% {2233}. Patients with grade 1 and 2 tumours have a higher survival rate than those with grade 3 tumours {1479}. Peritoneal foreign body granulomas to keratin found in cases of endometrioid carcinoma with squamous differentiation do not seem to affect the prognosis adversely in the absence of viable-appearing tumour cells on the basis of a small series of cases {1459}. Endometrioid carcinomas with a mixed clear cell, serous or undifferentiated carcinoma component are reported to have a worse prognosis {2941}.

Malignant müllerian mixed tumour

Definition
A highly aggressive neoplasm containing malignant epithelial and mesenchymal elements.

Synonyms
Carcinosarcoma, malignant mesodermal mixed tumour, metaplastic carcinoma.

Epidemiology
Malignant müllerian mixed tumours (MMMTs) are rare, representing less than 1% of ovarian malignancies. They occur most commonly in postmenopausal women of low parity, the median age being around 60.

Clinical features
The clinical presentation is similar to that of carcinoma of the ovary.

Aetiology
An increased incidence has been reported in women who have had pelvic irradiation {3080}.

Macroscopy
The neoplasms form large (10-20 cm diameter), partly solid and partly cystic, or, less commonly, solid, grey-brown, unilateral or bilateral, bosselated masses with foci of haemorrhage and necrosis {479}. The sectioned surface is fleshy and friable, and cartilage and bone may be apparent. The tumours are bilateral in 90% of cases.

Tumour spread and staging
There is extraovarian spread to the pelvic peritoneum, omentum, pelvic organs and regional lymph nodes in more than 75% of cases at the time of diagnosis.

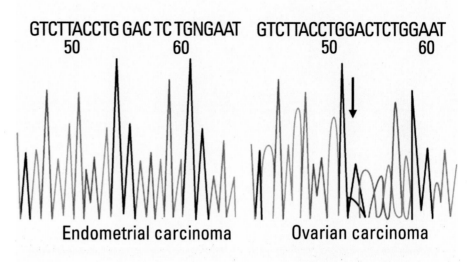

Fig. 2.34 Genetic differences in concurrent endometrial and ovarian adenocarcinoma. DNA sequencing of exon 3 of the beta-catenin (CTNNB1) gene showing a GGA to GCA change at codon 32 (Asp>His) in the ovarian endometrioid adenocarcinoma (right, arrow). The mutation was not identified in the uterine endometrial carcinoma (left).

Histopathology
The histological and immunoprofile are similar to those of its uterine counterpart and those occurring elsewhere in the female genital system (see chapter 4).

Histogenesis
MMMT is believed to develop from the ovarian surface epithelium or from foci of endometriosis and, therefore, may be regarded as a high grade carcinoma with metaplastic sarcomatous elements. The positive tumour response to chemotherapy directed at ovarian carcinoma also supports this viewpoint.

Somatic genetics
There is evidence that MMMTs are monoclonal {26,2748} as the phenotypically different elements share similar allelic losses and retentions {925} and a cell line developed from an MMMT expresses both mesenchymal and epithelial antigens {195}. Furthermore, a heterogeneous pattern of allelic loss at a limited number of chromosomal loci in either the carcinomatous or sarcomatous component of the neoplasm is consistent with either genetic progression or genetic diversion occurring during the clonal evolution of the tumour.

Genetic susceptibility
There is anecdotal evidence of BRCA2 mutation {2748}.

Prognosis and predictive factors
Improved cytoreductive surgery and platinum based chemotherapy has resulted in a median survival of 19 months {2715} and an overall 5-year survival of 18-27% {120,1182}. The survivors almost invariably have early stage disease at the time of diagnosis, and low stage is a statistically significant indicator of outcome {120,436,1182,2749}. No other histopathological factors are significant indicators of outcome.

Adenosarcoma

Definition
A biphasic tumour characterized by a proliferation of müllerian-type epithelium with a benign or occasionally markedly atypical appearance embedded in or

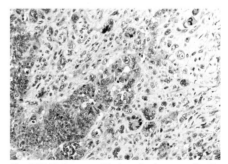

Fig. 2.35 Malignant müllerian mixed tumour. Poorly differentiated glands are surrounded by spindle-shaped, rounded and multinucleated cells.

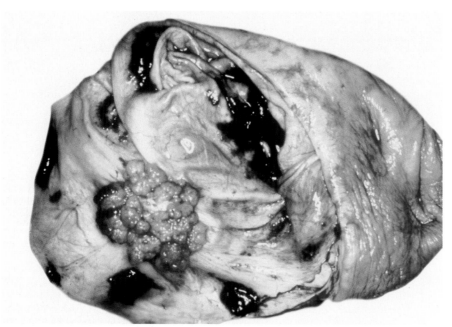

Fig. 2.36 Endometrioid borderline tumour. Whereas most endometrioid borderline tumours have an adenofibromatous appearance, the adenofibromatous lesion is rarely evident within a large cystic mass.

overlying a dominant sarcomatous mesenchyme.

Clinical features

Most of the tumours reported so far have been unilateral, occurring in the 4th and 5th decades. Abdominal discomfort and distension are the usual complaints.

Macroscopy and histopathology

The tumour is frequently adherent to the surrounding tissue {512,604,929}. The macroscopic and histological features are described in detail in the uterine counterpart (see chapter 4).

Prognosis and predictive factors

Occasional reports have linked the spread of adenosarcomas into the abdominal cavity with a poor clinical outcome {510}. The stroma is often predominantly fibrotic, oedematous or hyalized with characteristic foci of perivascular cuffing seen only focally (sometimes, the foci are very small) and still the tumours recur and kill the patient {760}. Unfortunately, there exist no established morphological criteria to predict such biological behaviour. However, if during the course of the disease sarcomatous overgrowth develops, signifying invasive potential, the patient requires careful monitoring. In a series of 40 cases, the 5-year survival was 64%, the 10-year survival 46% and the 15-year survival 30% {760}. Age greater than 53 years, tumour rupture, high grade and the presence of high grade sarcomatous overgrowth appear to be associated with recurrence or extraovarian spread. Ovarian adenosarcoma has a worse prognosis than its uterine counterpart, presumably because of the greater ease of peritoneal spread {760}. Therapeutically, an aggressive surgical approach with wide excision is most often recommended {510}. Chemotherapy and radiation may be applied in individual cases; however, no established protocols exist.

Endometrioid stromal and undifferentiated ovarian sarcoma

Definition

Endometrioid stromal sarcoma (ESS) is a monophasic sarcomatous tumour characterized by a diffuse proliferation of neoplastic cells similar to stromal cells of proliferative endometrium. At its periphery the tumour exhibits a typical infiltrative growth pattern. Those neoplasms that have moderate to marked pleomorphism, significant nuclear anaplasia and more cytoplasm than is found in endometrial stromal cells should be classified as undifferentiated ovarian sarcoma.

Clinical features

More than 70% of the tumours are unilateral. The age range is 11-76 years with the majority of tumours occurring around the 5th and 6th decade. The clinical symptoms do not differ from those recognized for other ovarian tumours.

Macroscopy

Most tumours are solid and firm, but some may show variably sized cysts, sometimes filled with mucoid or haemorrhagic fluid or debris. The sectioned surface appears yellow-white or tan, sometimes interspersed with grey fibrous bundles or septa.

Histopathology

Roughly half of the cases of ESS are associated with either endometriosis or a similar sarcomatous lesion of the endometrial stroma or both {2605}. The dominant cell type of ESS consists of small, round to oval, or occasionally spindle shaped cells with round nuclei and scanty, sometimes barely visible pale cytoplasm. The cells may be arranged haphazardly in a diffuse pattern or may form parallel cell sheets mimicking fibroma. Hypocellular areas with a distinct oedematous appearance can be present. Lipid droplets may be present within tumour cells, which are often associated with foam cells. A hallmark of ESS is the presence of abundant small thick-walled vessels resembling spiral arteries of the late secretory endometrium. The vessels often are surrounded by whorls of neoplastic cells. Reticulin stain discloses delicate fibrils characteristically enveloping individual tumour cells. The cellularity can vary markedly within the same specimen. The tumour can be partly intersected by fibrous bands forming more or less distinct nodules. Sometimes, hyaline plaques are present. Rarely, cord-like or plexiform arrangements of tumour cells similar to the growth patterns seen in ovarian sex cord tumours such as granulosa cell tumours or thecomas are observed. In these areas reticulin fibrils are more or less absent. Rarely, glandular elements are interspersed, but they never represent a dominant feature. At its periphery the tumour exhibits a typical infiltrative growth pattern. In cases where the tumour has spread into extraovarian sites, a tongue-like pattern of invasion

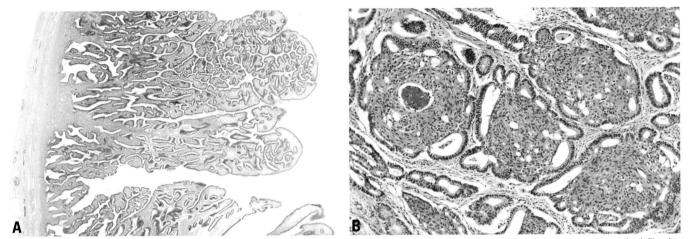

Fig. 2.37 A This polypoid intracystic tumour consists of complex villoglandular structures with abundant stroma. Neither confluence of glands nor destructive infiltrative growth is present. **B** Endometrioid borderline tumour of the ovary. Squamous morules appear to form bridges within dilated endometrial glands.

into the adjacent tissue and intravascular growth appears.

Most neoplasms are low grade, whereas approximately 10% of cases are high grade and are classified as undifferentiated ovarian sarcoma. In the past, tumours with less than 10 mitoses per 10 high power fields were classified as low grade ESS, whereas tumours with more than 10 mitoses per 10 high power fields were traditionally designated high grade {3208}. However, there is no evidence that mitotic rate alone alters the outcome, and all tumours with an appearance resembling that of endometrial stroma should be designated endometrioid stromal sarcoma {438}, whereas those that lack endometrial stromal differentiation should be diagnosed as undifferentiated ovarian sarcoma. The latter is a high grade neoplasm that is composed of pleomorphic mesenchymal cells with distinct variablility in size and shape. The nuclei are highly atypical with prominent nucleoli and occasionally resemble rhabdomyosarcoma or fibrosarcoma.

Immunoprofile
Immunostaining demonstrates the expression of vimentin and CD10 in ESS. Muscle-associated proteins are only focally expressed. Alpha-inhibin was negative in all cases examined {1681}.

Differential diagnosis
ESS must be differentiated from other ovarian lesions, including some small cell tumours. The major problem is to distinguish ESS from adult granulosa cell-tumour, foci of stromal hyperplasia, ovarian fibroma or ovarian thecoma.

On morphological grounds alone, it is not always possible to decide whether the ovarian lesion is a primary ESS of the ovary or a metastatic lesion from a uterine ESS. Thus, an ovarian ESS should never be diagnosed unless the uterus is carefully examined to exclude a uterine primary. Should ESS be found in both organs, it is more or less impossible to decide which tumour is the primary and which is metastatic. One criterion that establishes a primary site in the ovary is its continuity with endometriotic foci in the ovary.

Somatic genetics
Mutation of the *TP53* tumour suppressor gene associated with overexpression of TP53 protein has been frequently observed in ovarian sarcomas. These mutations may occur on the basis of an impaired DNA repair system in these tumours {1681}.

Prognosis and predictive factors
Since over one-half of the ESSs have already spread to pelvic or upper abdominal sites at the time of diagnosis, the tumour stage remains the major prognostic criterion {438}. Whether the neoplasm is an ESS or undifferentiated ovarian sarcoma also influences the clinical course {3208}. ESS often has a favourable outcome with survival in excess of 5 years even in the context of extraovarian spread. After 10 years, however, the tumour-related mortality increases, particularly if extraovarian manifestations were noted at the time of diagnosis. Tumour relapse represents an ominous prognostic sign. Undifferentiated ovarian sarcomas have a rapid course and a

poor prognosis {3208}.
Radical panhysterectomy is the recommended therapy. Successful treatment with progesterone, non-hormonal cytostatic drugs or radiation has been reported occasionally in ESS.

Endometrioid borderline tumour

Definition
An ovarian tumour of low malignant potential composed of atypical or histologically malignant endometrioid type glands or cysts often set in a dense fibrous stroma with an absence of stromal invasion.

Synonyms
Endometrioid tumour of low malignant potential, endometrioid tumour of borderline malignancy.

Epidemiology
Endometrioid tumours with atypical epithelial proliferations and lacking stromal invasion are rare. Their precise prevalence is not known because of variation in diagnostic criteria, but reportedly they account for 3-18% of malignant ovarian neoplasms {137,2490,2528}.

Aetiology
These tumours appear to be predominantly derived from the surface epithelium of the ovary or endometriosis.

Clinical features
Patients range in age from 22-77 years {201,2737}. A pelvic mass is palpable in a majority of patients, and others present with uterine bleeding. The tumours are

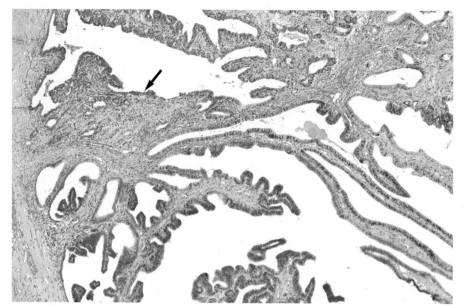

Fig. 2.38 Endometrioid borderline tumour of the ovary with microinvasion. Cystic tumour contains complex papillae. A small area has densely packed glands indicative of microinvasion (arrow).

predominantly unilateral, but rare bilateral lesions occur.

Macroscopy
Tumours range in size from 2-40 cm, have a tan to grey-white sectioned surface that varies from solid to predominantly solid with cysts ranging from a few mm to 8 cm in diameter {201,2737}. Haemorrhage and necrosis are present mainly in larger tumours.

Histopathology
Three patterns have been described {201,2737}. The most common is adenofibromatous. Islands of crowded endometrioid glands or cysts lined by cells displaying grade 1 to, rarely, grade 3 cytological atypia proliferate in an adenofibromatous stroma. Stromal invasion is absent. Mitotic activity is usually low.

Squamous metaplasia is common, and necrosis may develop in the metaplastic epithelium. The second pattern is villoglandular or papillary with an atypical cell lining similar to atypical hyperplasia of the endometrium again in a fibromatous background. The third form shows a combination of villoglandular and adenofibromatous patterns. Anywhere from 15% to over half of the patients have endometriosis in the same ovary as well as at extraovarian sites {201,2737}.

Prognosis and predictive factors
The prognosis is excellent. Recurrences and metastases are rare. Even in the rare case of an extraovarian tumour nodule involving the colonic serosa {2737}, no subsequent problems developed 9 years after surgery, radiation and chemotherapy. Since a few patients treated by unilat-

eral salpingo-oophorectomy developed endometrioid carcinoma in the contralateral ovary, and 1 died from it, bilateral salpingo-oophorectomy would be prudent when retention of fertility is no longer an issue. Unilateral salpingo-oophorectomy along with follow-up for early detection of any subsequent ovarian or endometrial adenocarcinoma is acceptable for women of childbearing age.

Benign endometrioid tumours

Definition
Ovarian tumours with histological features of benign glands or cysts lined by well differentiated cells of endometrial type.

Epidemiology
Because of the rarity of these neoplasms no convincing epidemiological data can be quoted. The reported patients are mainly of the reproductive age.

Localization
Benign endometrioid tumours are usually unilateral, though in rare cases involvement of both ovaries is encountered.

Clinical features
Signs and symptoms
There are no specific clinical symptoms of benign endometrioid tumours. Small neoplasms are incidental findings, sometimes in the wall of an ovarian endometriotic cyst. Large tumours are manifested by pain and abdominal swelling.

Imaging
Imaging techniques, including US, CT and MRI, cannot effectively establish the specific nosological character of the process. They can visualize endometriotic foci and thus indirectly indicate the presumptive endometrioid nature of the neoplasm; otherwise the results of imaging technique show the formal characteristics, i.e. cystic or cystic-fibrous architecture of the lesion {234}.

Histopathology
The histological diagnosis of endometrioid adenomas and cystadenomas is based on the presence of well differentiated, benign appearing glands or cysts lined by endometrial type cells with or without squamous differentiation. In the adenofibromatous variant fibrous stroma predominates. Though adenofibromas

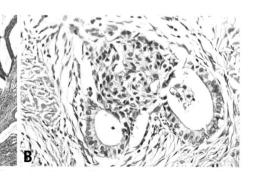

Fig. 2.39 **A** Endometrioid cystadenoma. The cystic neoplasm forms villiform structures lined by well differentiated endometrioid type epithelium. **B** Endometrioid adenofibroma. A squamous morule bridges two endometrioid type glands lined by uniform cells set in a fibrous stroma.

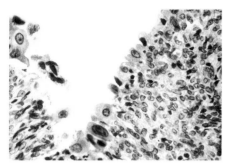

Fig. 2.40 Endometrioid cyst with atypia. The cyst wall is lined by markedly atypical cells surrounded by endometrial stroma.

can have minimal periglandular endometrial stroma, cases in which endometrial stroma is present throughout the lesion are classified as endometriosis. The latter can have all forms of endometrial hyperplasia including those with atypia.

Clear cell tumours

Definition
Ovarian tumours, benign, borderline or malignant, with an epithelial component consisting most commonly of clear and hobnail cells, but often containing other cell types, which rarely predominate.

Histopathology
Clear cell tumours may by predominantly epithelial or may also contain a prominent fibromatous component. The epithelium may consist of one or more cell types. The most common cells are clear cells and hobnail cells. Other cells that may be present include cuboidal, flat, oxyphilic and rarely, signet-ring cells. Most clear cell tumours are carcinomas, and many have an adenofibromatous background. Benign and borderline clear cell tumours are rare and almost always adenofibromatous.

ICD-O codes
Clear cell adenocarcinoma	8310/3
Clear cell adenocarcinofibroma	8313/3
Clear cell tumour of borderline malignancy	8310/1
Clear cell adenofibroma of borderline malignancy	8313/1
Clear cell cystadenoma	8310/0
Clear cell cystadenofibroma	8313/0

Clear cell adenocarcinoma

Definition
A malignant ovarian tumour composed of glycogen-containing clear cells and hobnail cells and occasionally other cell types.

Epidemiology
The mean age of patients is 57 years.

Aetiology
Tumours may arise directly from the ovarian surface epithelium, from inclusion cysts or from an endometriotic cyst.

Clinical features
Clear cell tumours among all surface epithelial cancers have the highest association of ovarian and pelvic endometriosis and paraendocrine hypercalcaemia {3204}.

Macroscopy
The mean diameter of clear cell adenocarcinomas is 15 cm. The tumours may be solid, but more commonly the sectioned surface reveals a thick-walled unilocular cyst with multiple yellow fleshy nodules protruding into the lumen or multiloculated cysts containing watery or mucinous fluid. Tumours associated with endometriosis typically contain chocolate-brown fluid.

Tumour spread and staging
Patients with clear cell adenocarcinomas present as stage I disease in 33% of cases, as stage II in 19%, as stage III in 29% and as stage IV in 9% {2233}.

Histopathology
Clear cell adenocarcinomas display tubulocystic, papillary and solid patterns that may be pure or mixed. The most common patterns are papillary and tubulocystic. Rarely, the tumour has a reticular pattern similar to that of a yolk sac tumour. Sheets of polyhedral cells with abundant clear cytoplasm separated by a delicate fibrovascular or hyalinized stroma are characteristic of the solid pattern. The tubulocystic pattern is characterized by varying-sized tubules and cysts lined by cuboidal to flattened epithelium and occasionally hobnail cells. The papillary pattern is characterized by thick or thin papillae containing

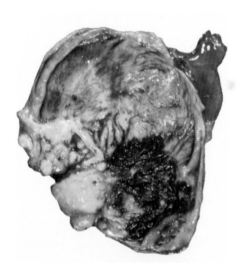

Fig. 2.41 Clear cell adenocarcinoma arising within an endometriotic cyst. The sectioned surface shows a solid tumour within a chocolate cyst.

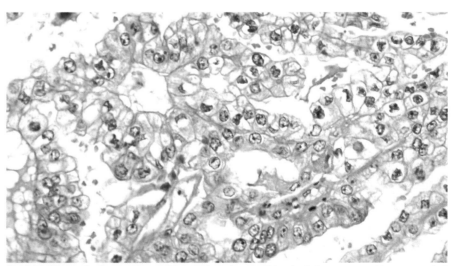

Fig. 2.42 Clear cell adenocarcinoma. The neoplasm has a solid and tubular pattern and is composed of polygonal cells with abundant cytoplasm. Most cells have clear cytoplasm, but some are eosinophilic. Nuclei are round but exhibit irregular nuclear membranes, nucleoli and abnormal chromatin patterns.

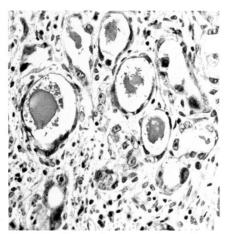

Fig. 2.43 Clear cell adenocarcinoma. Round tubules lined by flattened to highly atypical hobnail cells are present in a fibroedematous stroma (PAS-hematoxylin stain).

fibrous tissue or abundant hyaline material. The most common cell types are the clear and hobnail cells. Clear cells tend to be arranged in solid nests or masses or lining cysts, tubules and papillae, whereas hobnail cells line tubules and cysts and cover papillary structures. The clear cells tend to be rounded or polygonal with eccentric nuclei, often containing prominent nucleoli. The hobnail cells have scant cytoplasm and contain bulbous hyperchromatic nuclei that protrude into the lumens of the tubules. Flattened or cuboidal cells are also encountered. Occasionally, oxyphilic cells with abundant eosinophilic cytoplasm, which in a few instances make up the majority of the neoplasm, are observed. Signet-ring cells often contain inspissated mucinous material in the centre of a vacuole, creating what has been referred to as a "targetoid" cell. The clear cells contain abundant glycogen and may also contain some lipid. Mucin may be found, typically located in the lumens of tubules and cysts and is abundant within the cytoplasm of the signet-ring cells.

Immmunoprofile

Clear cell adenocarcinomas stain strongly and diffusely for keratins, epithelial membrane antigen, Leu M1 and B72.3. Stains for carcinoembryonic antigen are positive in 38% of cases and for CA125 (OC-125) in 50%. There have been a few reports of clear cell adenocarcinomas containing AFP. In a patient with clear cell adenocarcinoma who developed hypercalcaemia when the tumour recurred, immunostains for parathyroid hormone-related protein were strongly positive in the recurrent carcinoma but negative in the primary carcinoma {3209}.

Differential diagnosis

The differential diagnosis includes germ cell tumours, particularly yolk sac tumour, dysgerminoma and, rarely, struma ovarii, endometrioid carcinoma with secretory change and steroid cell tumours that contain prominent areas of cells with clear cytoplasm. Metastatic clear cell neoplasms from outside the female genital system are very rare.

Clinical information can be particularly helpful in the differential diagnosis as germ cell tumours occur in young women, and elevated serum alpha-feto-protein (AFP) levels are always found in patients with yolk sac tumours. Histologically, the papillary structures of clear cell carcinoma are more complex than those of yolk sac tumours and contain hyalinized cores. In contrast, yolk sac tumours display a variety of distinctive features including a prominent reticular pattern and Schiller-Duvall bodies. Negative immunostains for AFP are useful in excluding yolk sac tumours, although rare examples of AFP-containing clear cell carcinomas have been reported. Positive staining for EMA and diffuse strong positivity for cytokeratins exclude dysgerminoma. Immunostains for thyroglobulin are very useful in ruling out struma ovarii.

Endometrioid carcinomas with secretory change typically are composed of cells that are columnar with subnuclear and supranuclear vacuolization resembling early secretory endometrium. In contrast, the clear cell changes in clear cell carcinoma are more diffuse, the cells are polygonal, and they typically display the other characteristic patterns of clear cell carcinoma. A metaplastic squamous component may be seen in endometrioid carcinoma and is not observed in clear cell carcinoma. In contrast to clear cell carcinomas, steroid cell tumours of the ovary that contain prominent clear cytoplasm are smaller, well circumscribed, have low grade nuclear features and stain strongly for alpha-inhibin.

Grading

Nuclei in clear cell carcinomas range from grade 1 to grade 3, but pure grade

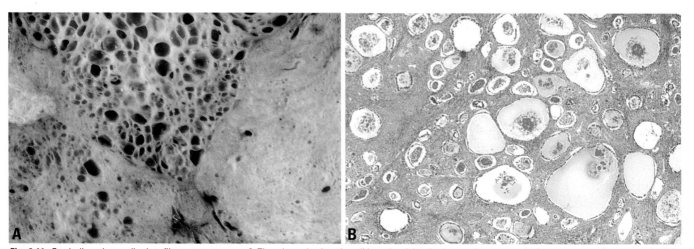

Fig. 2.44 Borderline clear cell adenofibromatous tumour. **A** Though predominantly solid on the right, the tumour is composed of numerous small cysts on the left. **B** Histologically, round glands, many of which are dilated and contain secretions, proliferate in a fibrous stroma.

1 tumours are extremely rare. Almost invariably high grade (grade 3) nuclei are identified. In view of this finding as well as the mixture of different architectural patterns, clear cell adenocarcinoma is not graded.

Prognosis and predictive factors
When controlled for stage, survival of women with clear cell adenocarcinoma may be slightly lower than that of patients with serous carcinoma. The five year survival is 69% for patients with stage I tumours, 55% for stage II, 14% for stage III and 4% for stage IV. There is no consensus in the literature about the value of pattern, cell type, mitotic index or grade as a prognostic indicator {395}.

Borderline clear cell adenofibromatous tumour

Definition
An ovarian tumour of low malignant potential composed of atypical or histologically malignant glands or cysts lined by clear or hobnail cells set in a dense fibrous stroma with an absence of stromal invasion.

Synonyms
Clear cell adenofibromatous tumour of low malignant potential, clear cell adenofibromatous tumour of borderline malignancy.

Epidemiology
Of approximately 30 cases of neoplasms classified as borderline clear cell adenofibromatous tumour, the mean age of patients was 65 years.

Macroscopy
Adenofibromas with increasing atypia including intraepithelial carcinoma have a similar appearance to adenofibromas but in addition have areas that are softer and fleshier.

Histopathology
Borderline clear cell adenofibromatous tumours include those in which the epithelium is atypical or carcinomatous without invasion. Adenofibromatous tumours in which the glands are lined by malignant epithelium are best designated as "borderline clear cell adenofibromas with intraepithelial carcinoma". They are similar to borderline adenofibromas; however, nuclear atypia is more

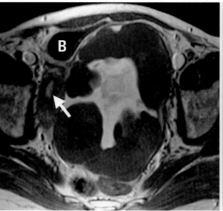
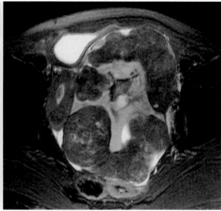

Fig. 2.45 MRI: T1-weighted image (left) and T2-weighted (right) of a borderline clear cell cystadenofibroma of the left ovary. The huge multicystic tumour fills the pelvis almost completely. The uterus with endometrial hyperplasia (arrow) is pushed to the right iliac bone, and the urinary bladder (B) is compressed.

marked with coarse chromatin clumping, prominent nucleoli and increased mitotic activity. Occasionally, minute foci of invasion can be identified, and these tumours are designated "microinvasive". The epithelium often displays stratification and budding, although true papillary structures are uncommon. Small solid masses of clear cells in the stroma raise the question of invasion.

Prognosis and predictive factors
With the exception of one case {202}, borderline clear cell adenofibromatous tumours including those with intraepithelial carcinoma and microinvasion have a benign course following removal of the ovary {583,1285,1435, 1897,2052}.

Clear cell adenofibroma

Definition
An ovarian tumour composed of histologically benign glands or cysts lined by

clear or hobnail cells set in a dense fibrous stroma.

Epidemiology
Among approximately twelve reported cases of benign clear cell adenofibroma, the mean age of patients was 45.

Macroscopy
Adenofibromas have a median diameter of 12 cm and display a smooth lobulated external surface. The sectioned surface has a fine honeycomb appearance with minute cysts embedded in a rubbery stroma.

Histopathology
Clear cell adenofibromas are characterized by tubular glands lined by one or two layers of epithelium that contains polygonal, hobnail or flattened cells. The cytoplasm may be clear, slightly granular or eosinophilic. Nuclear atypia and mitotic activity are minimal. The stroma is densely fibrous.

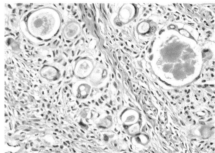

Fig. 2.46 Borderline clear cell adenofibromatous tumour. High power magnification shows simple glands with nuclear enlargement, irregular nuclear membranes and distinct nucleoli.

Fig. 2.47 Borderline clear cell tumour with microinvasion. Clear cell adenofibromatous tumour is seen on the right with the area of microinvasion on the left.

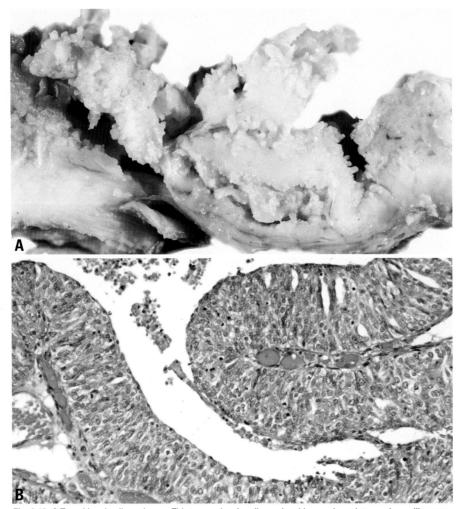

Fig. 2.48 A Transitional cell carcinoma. This tumour is primarily cystic with prominent intracystic papillary projections. **B** Papillary growth of malignant transitional epithelium with a smooth lumenal border predominates.

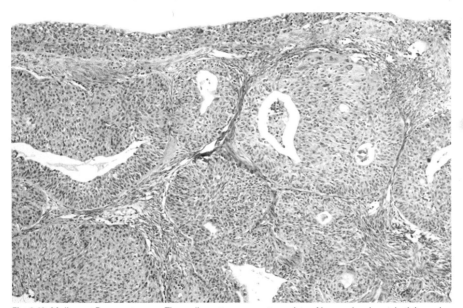

Fig. 2.49 Malignant Brenner tumour. The malignant component consists of large, closely-packed, irregular aggregates of transitional epithelial cells infiltrating the stroma. There was also an area of benign Brenner tumour (not shown).

Transitional cell tumours

Definition
Ovarian tumours composed of epithelial elements histologically resembling urothelium and its neoplasms.

Histopathology
This group of tumours includes the following:
(1) Benign Brenner tumours, distinguished by a prominent stromal component accompanying transitional cell nests.
(2) Borderline and malignant Brenner tumours in which a benign Brenner tumour component is associated with exuberantly proliferative, variably atypical but non-invasive transitional epithelium in the former and unequivocal stromal invasion in the latter.
(3) Transitional cell carcinoma in which a malignant transitional cell tumour is not associated with a benign or borderline Brenner component.

ICD-O codes
Transitional cell carcinoma (non-Brenner)	8120/3
Malignant Brenner tumour	9000/3
Borderline Brenner tumour	9000/1
Brenner tumour	9000/0

Epidemiology
Transitional cell tumours account for 1-2% of all ovarian tumours.

Transitional cell carcinoma

Definition
An ovarian tumour that is composed of epithelial elements histologically resembling malignant urothelial neoplasms and does not have a component of benign or borderline Brenner tumour.

Epidemiology
Transitional cell carcinoma is the pure or predominant element in 6% of ovarian carcinomas {2676}. The great majority of transitional cell carcinomas occur in women 50-70 years old {1110}.

Clinical features
The presentation of women with transitional cell carcinoma is the same as with other malignant ovarian tumours, abdominal pain, swelling, weight loss, and bladder or bowel symptoms {139,2676}.

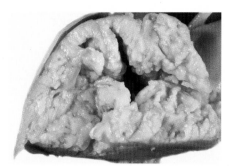

Fig. 2.50 Borderline Brenner tumour. A large, papillary, polypoid component protrudes into a cystic space.

Macroscopy

Transitional cell carcinomas are bilateral in approximately 15% of cases {139} and are macroscopically indistinguishable from other surface epithelial-stromal tumours {139,2676}.

Tumour spread and staging

At the time of diagnosis transitional cell carcinomas have spread beyond the ovary in over two-thirds of cases {2676}

Histopathology

Transitional cell carcinomas resemble those occurring in the urinary tract and lack a benign or borderline Brenner tumour component {139,2676}. Typically, they are papillary with multilayered transitional epithelium and a smooth luminal border ("papillary type"). A nested pattern characterized by malignant transitional cell nests irregularly distributed in fibrotic stroma ("malignant Brenner-like type") has been described {2464,2465}. As in urothelial carcinoma, foci of glandular and/or squamous differentiation may occur. Very commonly, transitional cell carcinoma is admixed with other epithelial cell types, primarily serous adenocarcinoma. Transitional cell carcinomas lack the prominent stromal calcification characteristic of some benign and malignant Brenner tumours.

Immunoprofile

Ovarian transitional cell carcinomas have an immunoprofile that differs from transitional cell carcinomas of the urinary tract and closely resembles that of ovarian surface epithelial-stromal tumours. Ovarian transitional cell carcinomas are consistently uroplakin, thrombomodulin and cyokeratin 13 and 20 negative and CA125 and cytokeratin 7 positive {2115, 2371}.

Grading

Transitional cell carcinomas should be graded utilizing criteria for transitional cell carcinoma of the urinary tract.

Histogenesis

The term transitional cell carcinoma is not uniformly accepted, and overlapping features with other epithelial-stromal tumours, particularly serous carcinoma, are present. It is important that strict histological criteria be applied to establish the diagnosis {2465}. Not only an architectural but also a histological resemblance to transitional epithelium is required. The frequent association with epithelial-stromal tumours of other types strongly suggests a surface epithelial origin {2465}. In addition, several immunohistochemical studies have demonstrated that the tumour lacks a urothelial phenotype {2115,2371}. Thus, the ovarian neoplasm shows histological but not immunohistochemical similarities to transitional cell carcinoma of the urinary bladder.

Prognosis and predictive factors

The overall 5-year survival rate for transitional cell carcinoma is 35%. Some, but not all, investigators have reported greater chemosensitivity and higher 5-year survival in patients whose metastases are composed purely or predominantly of transitional cell carcinoma {564, 1232,2676}.

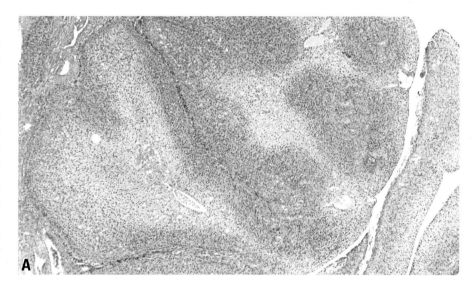

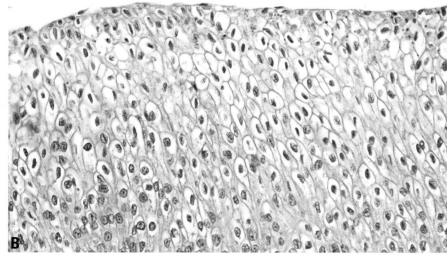

Fig. 2.51 Borderline Brenner tumour (proliferating Brenner tumour). **A** Complex undulating and papillary transitional cell epithelium protrudes into a cystic space. **B** The transitional epithelium is thick with low grade cytological features.

Malignant Brenner tumour

Definition
An ovarian tumour containing invasive transitional cell aggregates as well as benign nests of transitional epithelium set in a fibromatous stroma.

Epidemiology
The great majority of malignant Brenner tumours occur in women 50-70 years old {1110,1868,2676}. Only 5% of Brenner tumours are malignant {1110,1868}.

Clinical features
Most patients seek medical attention because of an abdominal mass or pain {139,2460,2461}. A few patients present with abnormal vaginal bleeding.

Macroscopy
Malignant Brenner tumours are typically large with a median diameter of 16-20 cm and typically have a solid component resembling benign Brenner tumour as well as cysts containing papillary or polypoid masses {2461}.

Tumour spread and staging
Malignant Brenner tumours are bilateral in 12% of cases {139,452}. About 80% of malignant Brenner tumours are stage 1 at the time of diagnosis.

Histopathology
In malignant Brenner tumours there is stromal invasion associated with a benign or borderline Brenner tumour component {139}. The invasive element is usually high grade transitional cell carcinoma or squamous cell carcinoma, although occasional tumours are composed of crowded, irregular islands of malignant transitional cells with low grade features {2460}. Glandular elements may be admixed, but pure mucinous or serous carcinomas associated with a benign Brenner tumour component should not be diagnosed as a malignant Brenner tumour. Foci of calcification are occasionally prominent.

Immunoprofile
The very small number of malignant Brenner tumours studied have exhibited a benign Brenner tumour immunoprofile in that component with a variable pattern of antigen expression in the invasive component; uroplakin immunopositivity has occurred in some {2371}.

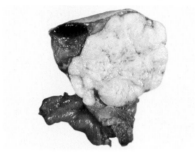

Fig. 2.52 Benign Brenner tumour. Sectioned surface is firm, lobulated and fibroma-like with a small cystic component.

Prognosis and predictive factors
When confined to the ovary, malignant Brenner tumours have an excellent prognosis. Patients with stage IA tumours have an 88% 5-year survival, and those with high stage malignant Brenner tumours have a better prognosis than stage matched transitional cell carcinomas {139}.

Borderline Brenner tumour

Synonyms
Brenner tumour of low malignant potential, proliferating Brenner tumour (for cases with low grade features).

Definition
An ovarian transitional cell tumour of low malignant potential with atypical or malignant features of the epithelium but lacking obvious stromal invasion.

Epidemiology
Only 3-5% of Brenner tumours are borderline {1110,1868}.

Tumour spread and staging
Borderline Brenner tumours are confined to the ovary and, with rare exceptions, have been unilateral {1110,1868,2461,3144}.

Clinical features
Most patients seek medical attention because of an abdominal mass or pain {139,2460,2461}. A few patients present with abnormal vaginal bleeding.

Macroscopy
Borderline Brenner tumours are typically large with a median diameter of 16-20 cm. They usually have a solid component resembling benign Brenner tumour as well as a cystic component containing a papillary or polypoid mass {2461}.

Histopathology
Borderline Brenner tumours show a greater degree of architectural complexity than benign Brenner tumours typified by branching fibrovascular papillae surfaced by transitional epithelium often protruding into cystic spaces. The transitional epithelium manifests the same spectrum of architectural and cytological features encountered in urothelial lesions of the urinary tract. By definition, there is no stromal invasion. A benign Brenner tumour component is typically present but may be small and easily overlooked. The mitotic rate is highly variable but may be brisk, and focal necrosis is common. Mucinous metaplasia may be a prominent feature. The diagnostic criteria and terminology applied to the intermediate group of transitional cell tumours is somewhat controversial {2461,2605}. Some have advocated categorizing tumours with low grade features as "proliferating" rather than borderline {2461}, and others designate those resembling grade 2 or 3 transitional cell carcinoma of the urinary tract as "borderline with intraepithelial carcinoma" {2605}.

Prognosis and predictive factors
No Brenner tumour in the intermediate category without stromal invasion has metastasized or caused the death of a patient {1110,2461}.

Benign Brenner tumour

Definition
An ovarian transitional cell tumour composed of mature urothelial-like cells arranged in solid or cystic circumscribed aggregates within a predominantly fibromatous stroma.

Epidemiology
Benign Brenner tumours account for 4-5% of benign ovarian epithelial tumours {1409,1502,1970,2865}. Most benign Brenner tumours (95%) are diagnosed in women 30-60 years old {753,905,1868, 2460,2461,2676,2685,3073,3186}.

Clinical features
The majority of patients with benign Brenner tumours are asymptomatic; over 50% of tumours are less than 2 cm and are typically discovered incidentally in ovaries removed for some other reason {753,905,2685,3073}. In only 10% of cases is the tumour larger than 10 cm;

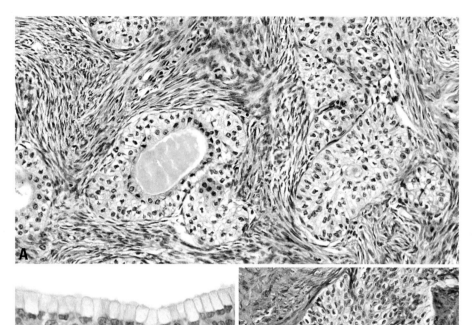

Fig. 2.53 Benign Brenner tumour. **A** One of the transitional cell nests is cystic and contains eosinophilic secretions. **B** One of the transitional cell nests contains a central lumen lined by mucinous columnar epithelium. **C** This transitional cell nest shows scattered grooved, coffee bean shaped nuclei.

such patients may present with non-specific signs and symptoms referable to a pelvic mass. Occasionally, Brenner tumours are associated with manifestations related to the elaboration of estrogens or androgens by the stromal component of the tumour.

Macroscopy
The typical benign Brenner tumour is small, often less than 2 cm, but, regardless of size, is well circumscribed with a firm, white, sometimes gritty sectioned surface due to focal or extensive calcification. Small cysts are common, and a rare tumour is predominately cystic. Brenner tumours are associated with another tumour type, usually mucinous cystadenoma, in 25% of cases

Tumour spread and staging
Only 7-8% of benign Brenner tumours are bilateral {753}

Histopathology
Benign Brenner tumours are characterized by nests and islands of transitional type epithelial cells with centrally grooved, "coffee bean" nuclei, abundant amphophilic to clear cytoplasm and distinct cell membranes growing in a dominant fibromatous stroma. The nests may be solid or exhibit central lumina containing densely eosinophilic, mucin-positive material. The lumina may be lined by transitional type cells or mucinous, ciliated or nondescript columnar cells. Variably sized cysts lined by mucinous epithelium, either pure or overlying transitional epithelium are common in benign Brenner tumours. Benign Brenner tumours with crowded transitional nests and cysts with a prominent mucinous component, sometimes with complex gland formations, are termed "metaplastic Brenner tumour" by some and not mixed epithelial tumours {2461} since the epithelial components are admixed rather than separate. Their recognition avoids confusion with borderline or malignant Brenner tumours.

Immunoprofile
Benign Brenner tumours show some urothelial differentiation evidenced by uroplakin expression, but they do not express thrombomodulin and have been immunonegative for cytokeratin 20 in most, but not all, studies {2085,2115, 2116,2371,2758}.
Benign Brenner tumours have an endocrine cell component demonstrable with immunostains for chromogranin A, serotonin and neuron specific enolase {45,2530}.

Somatic genetics
There is one report of a 12q14-21 amplification in a benign Brenner tumour {2207}.

Squamous cell lesions

Squamous cell carcinoma

Definition
Malignant ovarian tumour composed of squamous epithelial cells that is not of germ cell origin.

ICD-O code   8070/3

Epidemiology
The age of women with squamous cell carcinoma, pure or associated with endometriosis, has ranged from 23-90 years.

Macroscopy
Most squamous cell carcinomas are solid, although in some instances cystic components predominate.

Histopathology
Histologically, squamous cell carcinomas are usually high grade and show a variety of patterns including papillary or polypoid, cystic, insular, diffusely infiltrative, verruciform or sarcomatoid. They must be distinguished from endometrioid adenocarcinomas with extensive squamous differentiation and from metastatic squamous cell carcinoma from the cervix and other sites {3198}.

Histogenesis
Most squamous cell carcinomas arise from dermoid cysts and are classified in the germ cell tumour category. Less commonly, they occur in association with endometriosis {1624,1828,1973,2255, 2902}, as a component of malignant Brenner tumour {2460} or in pure form {2255} and are considered to be surface epithelial-stromal tumours. Some pure

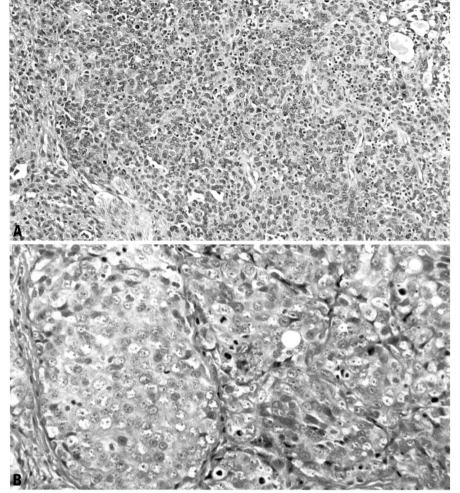

Fig. 2.54 Undifferentiated carcinoma of the ovary. **A** Sheets of tumour cells with small cystic spaces are separated by irregular fibrous septa. **B** Aggregates of undifferentiated tumour cells with pleomorphic nuclei and frequent mitotic figures are separated by thin bands of fibrous stroma.

squamous cell carcinomas have occurred in women with cervical squamous cell carcinoma in situ {1738}.

Prognosis and predictive factors
Most tumours have spread beyond the ovary at the time of presentation, and the prognosis in the small number of reported cases is poor.

Epidermoid cyst

Definition
Benign ovarian cysts lined by squamous epithelial cells that are not clearly of germ cell origin.

Histopathology
Epidermoid cysts lined by benign keratinized squamous epithelium devoid of skin appendages and unaccompanied by teratomatous elements are rare in the

ovary {823,3205}. All are small (2-46 mm) and unilateral.

Histogenesis
The presence of small epithelial cell nests resembling Walthard cell nests in the walls of epidermoid cysts suggests an epithelial rather than a teratomatous origin {3205}.

Mixed epithelial tumours

Definition
An ovarian epithelial tumour composed of an admixture of two or more of the five major cell types: serous, mucinous, endometrioid, clear cell and Brenner/transitional. The second or second and third cell types must comprise alone or together at least 10% of the tumour epithelium, or, in the case of a

mixed Brenner-mucinous cystic tumour, both components should be macroscopically visible. A mixed epithelial tumour (MET) may be benign, borderline or malignant. Endometrioid tumours with squamous differentiation and neuroendocrine tumours associated with a surface epithelial-stromal tumour are not included in this definition.

ICD-O codes
Malignant mixed epithelial tumour 8323/3
Borderline mixed epithelial tumour 8323/1
Benign mixed epithelial tumour 8323/0

Epidemiology
The reported incidence of MET varies from 0.5-4% of surface epithelial-stromal tumours. This variability is due in part to problems in developing a standardized classification.

Tumour spread and staging
Mixed epithelial borderline tumours (MEBTs) are stage I in 93% of cases and show bilateral ovarian involvement in 22% {2496}.

Histopathology
In cystadenomas the most frequent mixture is serous (ciliated) and mucinous epithelium. The mucinous epithelium should contain abundant intracytoplasmic mucin, not just apical or luminal mucin. MEBTs show papillae with detached cell clusters reminiscent of serous borderline tumours, but they generally contain a mixture of endocervical-like mucinous cells, endometrioid epithelium with focal squamous differentiation and indifferent eosinophilic epithelium. An acute inflammatory infiltrate is frequently seen. Microinvasion may be seen rarely. Mixed Brenner-mucinous tumours are usually composed of a benign, and, occasionally, a borderline Brenner component; the mucinous component may be benign, borderline or malignant. A few mucinous glands within Brenner nests or histological areas of mucinous differentiation represent mucinous metaplasia in Brenner tumours, a common finding, and are not a MET. Rarely, the tumour macroscopically contains a myriad of small cysts lined by an admixture of mucinous and transitional epithelium and the term metaplastic Brenner tumour is applied {2461}. For cystadenocarcinomas frequent combinations are serous and endometrioid,

serous and transitional cell carcinoma and endometrioid and clear cell.

Grading
The least differentiated component determines the tumour grade.

Histogenesis
Endometriosis, occasionally with atypia, is found in association with 53% of MEBT {2496} and up to 50% of mixed clear cell-endometrioid tumours {2511}. Some cases show a transition from endometriosis to neoplastic epithelium.

Somatic genetics
It is impossible to make broad statements, as studies are limited to a few cases. LOH on chromosome 17, common in serous tumours, has been found in two of five mixed endometrioid-serous tumours {959}. *PTEN* mutation, which has been associated with the endometrioid type, has also been noted in a mixed mucinous-endometrioid tumour {2075}. *KRAS* mutations, an early event in mucinous tumours, have been noted in three mixed Brenner-mucinous tumours {589}. The mucinous cystadenocarcinoma and Brenner tumour components shared amplification of 12q 14-21 in one MET, suggesting clonal relatedness {2207}.

Prognosis and predictive factors
The behaviour of MEBT is similar to that of endocervical-like mucinous borderline tumours. The dominant cell type generally dictates behaviour. An exception is mixed endometrioid and serous carcinoma, which, even when the serous component is minor, behaves more aggressively than pure endometrioid carcinoma and similarly to their serous counterpart. Mixed endometrioid and serous carcinoma may recur as serous carcinoma {2907}. This finding stresses the importance of careful sampling of an endometrioid cystadenocarcinoma to rule out a mixed serous component.

Undifferentiated carcinoma

Definition
A primary ovarian carcinoma with no differentiation or only small foci of differentiation.

ICD-O code   8020/3

Epidemiology
When applying the WHO criteria, approximately 4-5% of ovarian cancers are undifferentiated carcinoma. The frequency of undifferentiated carcinoma was 4.1% when defined as carcinomas with solid areas as the predominant component representing over 50% of the tumour {2677}.

Clinical features
In the only large series the age of the patients ranged from 39-72 (mean, 54 years) {2677}.

Macroscopy
Macroscopically, undifferentiated carcinoma does not have specific features. The tumours are predominantly solid, usually with extensive areas of necrosis.

Tumour spread and staging
According to FIGO, 6% of the patients are discovered in stage I, 3% are in stage II, 74% in stage III and 17% in stage IV; thus 91% of the tumours are discovered in stages III and IV {2677}.

Histopathology
Histologically, undifferentiated carcinoma consists of solid groups of tumour cells with numerous mitotic figures and significant cytological atypia. Areas with a spindle cell component, microcystic pattern and focal vascular invasion can be seen. It is unusual to see an undifferentiated carcinoma without any other component of müllerian carcinoma. Usually, areas of high grade serous carcinoma are present. Foci of transitional cell carcinoma can also be seen. Undifferentiated carcinoma of the ovary does not have a specific immunophenotype.

Differential diagnosis
The main differential diagnoses are granulosa cell tumour of the adult type, transitional cell carcinoma, poorly differentiated squamous cell carcinoma, small cell carcinoma and metastatic undifferentiated carcinoma.
Granulosa cell tumours may have a diffuse pattern; however, it is unusual not to have also areas with a trabecular pattern, Call-Exner bodies or areas showing sex cords. In addition, undifferentiated carci-

noma is a more anaplastic tumour with a larger number of mitotic figures.
Transitional cell carcinomas might have areas of undifferentiated tumour; however, either a trabecular pattern or large papillae are always identified in the former.
Small cell carcinoma of the hypercalcaemic type typically occurs in young women and often contains follicle-like structures. The cells of small cell carcinoma of the pulmonary type show nuclear molding and have high nuclear to cytoplasmic ratios.
Finally, metastatic undifferentiated carcinomas are uniform tumours without papillary areas.
All these differential diagnoses can usually be resolved when the tumour is well sampled, and areas with a different macroscopic appearance are submitted. Sampling will identify the different components of the tumour that are characteristic of primary ovarian lesions.

Prognosis and predictive factors
The five-year survival of patients with undifferentiated carcinoma is worse than that of ovarian serous or transitional cell carcinoma. Only 6% of these patients survive for 5 years.

Unclassified adenocarcinoma

Definition
A primary ovarian adenocarcinoma that cannot be classified as one of the specific types of müllerian adenocarcinoma because it has overlapping features or is not sufficiently differentiated. These tumours are uncommon.

ICD-O code   8140/3

Histopathology
Tumours in this category would include well or moderately differentiated tumours with overlapping features such as a mucinous tumour with cilia, or it might include a less differentiated tumour without distinctive features of one of the müllerian types of adenocarcoma.

Prognosis and predictive factors
Since this group of tumours has not yet been specifically studied, the prognosis is not known.

Sex cord-stromal tumours

F.A. Tavassoli
E. Mooney
D.J. Gersell
W.G. McCluggage
I. Konishi

S. Fujii
T. Kiyokawa
P. Schwartz
R.A. Kubik-Huch
L.M. Roth

Definition

Ovarian tumours composed of granulosa cells, theca cells, Sertoli cells, Leydig cells and fibroblasts of stromal origin, singly or in various combinations. Overall, sex cord-stromal tumours account for about 8% of ovarian neoplasms.

Granulosa-stromal cell tumours

Definition

Tumours containing granulosa cells, theca cells or stromal cells resembling fibroblasts or any combination of such cells.

Granulosa cell tumour group

Definition

A neoplasm composed of a pure or at the least a 10% population of granulosa cells often in a fibrothecomatous background. Two major subtypes are recognized, an adult and a juvenile type.

ICD-O codes

Granulosa cell tumour group
Adult granulosa cell tumour   8620/1
Juvenile granulosa cell tumour   8622/1

Epidemiology

Granulosa cell tumours account for approximately 1.5% (range, 0.6-3%) of all ovarian tumours. The neoplasm occurs in a wide age range including newborn infants and postmenopausal women. About 5% occur prior to puberty, whereas almost 60% occur after menopause {284,2588}.

Aetiology

The aetiology of these tumours is unknown. Several studies suggest that infertile women and those exposed to ovulation induction agents have an increased risk for granulosa cell tumours {2458, 2982,3125}.

Clinical features

Signs and symptoms
Granulosa cell tumours may present as an abdominal mass, with symptoms suggestive of a functioning ovarian tumour or both. About 5-15% present with symptoms suggestive of haemoperitoneum secondary to rupture of a cystic lesion {3195}. Ascites develops in about 10% of the cases. The tumour is clinically occult in 10% of the patients {829}. Granulosa cell tumours produce or store a variety of steroid hormones. When functional, most are estrogenic, but rarely androgenic activity may occur. The symptoms and clinical presentation vary depending on the patient's age and reproductive status. In prepubertal girls, granulosa cell tumours frequently induce isosexual pseudoprecocious puberty. In women of reproductive age, the tumour may be associated with a variety of menstrual disorders related to hyperoestrinism. In postmenopausal women, irregular uterine bleeding due to various types of endometrial hyperplasia or, rarely, well differentiated adenocarcinoma is the most common manifestation of hyperoestrinism. A rare unilocular thin-walled cystic variant is often androgenic when functional {1971,2059}.

Imaging
Cross sectional imaging, i.e. computed tomography and magnetic resonance imaging is of value in the surgical planning and preoperative determination of resectability of patients with granulosa cell tumours {859,1480,1728,1915,2131}. In contradistinction to epithelial ovarian tumours, granulosa cell tumours have been described as predominantly solid adnexal lesions; variable amounts of cystic components may, however, be present. Enlargement of the uterus and endometrial thickening might be seen as a result of the hormone production of the tumour {859,1480,1728,1915,2131}.

Adult granulosa cell tumour

Epidemiology

More than 95% of granulosa cell tumours are of the adult type, which occurs in middle aged to postmenopausal women.

Macroscopy

Adult granulosa cell tumours (AGCTs) are typically unilateral (95%) with an average size of 12.5 cm and are commonly encapsulated with a smooth or lobulated surface. The sectioned surface of the tumour

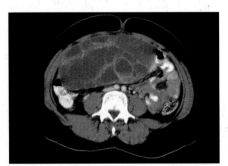

Fig. 2.55 Granulosa cell tumour. Axial contrast-enhanced computed tomography image of the pelvis shows a large, well defined, multicystic mass.

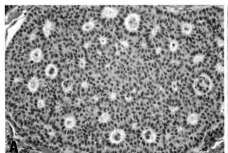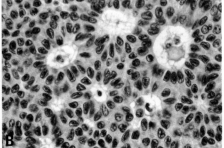

Fig. 2.56 Adult granulosa cell tumour, microfollicular pattern. **A** An aggregate of neoplastic granulosa cells contains numerous Call-Exner bodies. **B** The Call-Exner bodies contain fluid and/or pyknotic nuclei; the tumour cells have scant cytoplasm and longitudinal nuclear grooves.

is yellow to tan with a variable admixture of cystic and solid areas {906,2058}. Haemorrhage is seen in larger tumours; necrosis is focal and uncommon. A small percentage is totally cystic, either uniloculated or multiloculated {2058,2716}. A solid or cystic tumour with a combination of yellow tissue and haemorrhage is highly suggestive of a granulosa cell tumour.

Histopathology

Histologically, there is a proliferation of granulosa cells often with a stromal component of fibroblasts, theca or luteinized cells. The granulosa cells have scant cytoplasm and a round to ovoid nucleus with a longitudinal groove. The mitotic activity rarely exceeds 1-2 per 10 high power fields. When luteinized, the cells develop abundant eosinophilic or vacuolated cytoplasm, and the nuclei become round and lose their characteristic groove. The rare presence of bizarre nuclei does not have an adverse effect on the prognosis {2890,3210}. The tumour cells grow in a variety of patterns. The best known of these is the microfollicular pattern characterized by the presence of Call-Exner bodies. Others include the macrofollicular, characterized by large spaces lined by layers of granulosa cells, insular, trabecular, diffuse (sarcomatoid) and the moiré silk (watered silk) patterns. A fibrothecomatous stroma often surrounds the granulosa cells.

Immunoprofile

Granulosa cell tumours are immunoreactive for CD99, alpha-inhibin, vimentin, cytokeratin (punctate), calretinin, S-100 protein and smooth muscle actin. The tumour cells are negative for cytokeratin 7 and epithelial membrane antigen {482, 563,889,1815,2124,2379}.

Differential diagnosis

Although endometrioid carcinomas may display an abundant rosette-like arrangement of nuclei mimicking Call-Exner bodies, they often show squamous metaplasia and lack nuclear grooves. Undifferentiated carcinomas and poorly differentiated adenocarcinomas may resemble the diffuse (sarcomatoid) pattern of granulosa cell tumours. These carcinomas have abundant mitotic figures and frequently have already extended beyond the ovary at presentation.
The insular and trabecular patterns of granulosa cell tumour may be mistaken for a

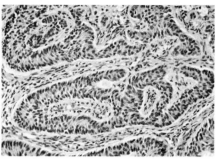

Fig. 2.57 Adult granulosa cell tumour, trabecular pattern. The granulosa cells form cords and trabeculae in a background of cellular fibrous stroma.

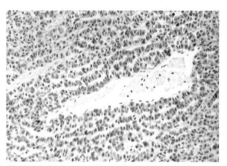

Fig. 2.59 Adult granulosa cell tumour, gyriform pattern. Immunostain for alpha-inhibin is moderately positive. The cords have a zigzag arrangement.

carcinoid and vice versa. Carcinoids have uniform round nuclei with coarse chromatin, lack nuclear grooves and show chromogranin positivity. Furthermore, primary carcinoids of the ovary are usually associated with other teratomatous elements, whereas the metastatic ones are generally multi-nodular and bilateral.
The diffuse pattern of granulosa cell tumours may be confused with a benign thecoma, particularly when there is luteinization. A reticulin stain is helpful since granulosa cells typically grow in sheets or aggregates bound by reticulin fibres, whereas thecomas contain an abundance of intercellular fibrils surrounding individual cells. The distinction

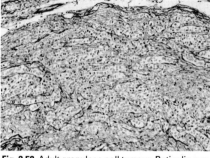

Fig. 2.58 Adult granulosa cell tumour. Reticulin surrounds the cords rather than investing individual cells (reticulin stain).

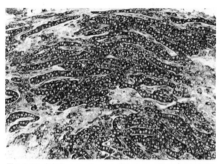

Fig. 2.60 Adult granulosa cell tumour. Immunostain for alpha-inhibin shows a diffuse, intensely positive reaction.

is important since granulosa cell tumours have an aggressive potential, whereas thecomas are with rare exceptions benign. Similarly, the presence of nuclear grooves and the absence of the characteristic vascular pattern of endometrioid stromal sarcoma distinguish AGCT from the former.

Somatic genetics

In contrast to older studies {1635,2862}, recent karyotypic and fluorescence in situ hybridization analyses have shown that trisomy and tetrasomy 12 are rarely present in granulosa cell tumours {1635, 1653,2221,2635,2862}. The few available studies have shown trisomy 14 {1043}

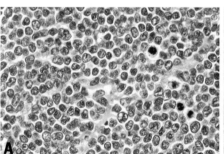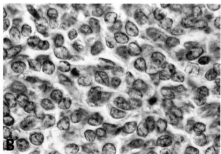

Fig. 2.61 Adult granulosa cell tumour, diffuse pattern. **A** Mitotic figures are more readily identifiable in the diffuse variant. **B** Note the presence of several nuclear grooves.

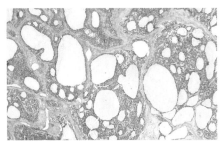

Fig. 2.62 Juvenile granulosa cell tumour. Neoplastic cell aggregates form multiple round to oval follicles containing basophilic fluid.

and structural changes in chromosome 6 with loss of 6q material {3021}.

Prognosis and predictive factors

All granulosa cell tumours have a potential for aggressive behaviour. From 10-50% of patients develop recurrences. Some recurrences of AGCT develop as late as 20-30 years following the initial diagnosis {906,2058,2786}, and long term follow-up is required.

The most important prognostic factor is the stage of the tumour {1815}. Nearly 90% of patients with granulosa cell tumour have stage I disease, however, and the prediction of tumour behaviour is most difficult in this group. Factors related to a relatively poor prognosis include age over 40 years at the time of diagnosis, large tumour size (>5cm), bilaterality, mitotic activity and atypia {906,1871, 2786}. There is, however, disagreement on the precise significance of some of these factors. Among adults, survival is adversely affected by tumour rupture.

Juvenile granulosa cell tumour

Epidemiology

Accounting for nearly 5% of all granulosa cell tumours, juvenile granulosa cell tumour (JGCT) is encountered predominantly during the first 3 decades of life {3195}.

Clinical features

In prepubertal girls, approximately 80% are associated with isosexual pseudo-precocity {277,3195,3242}.

Macroscopy

The macroscopic appearance of JGCT is not distinctive and is similar in its spectrum of appearances to the adult variant.

Tumour spread and staging

JGCT presents almost always as stage I disease; less than 5% of tumours are

bilateral, and only 2% have extraovarian spread.

Histopathology

JGCT is characterized by a nodular or diffuse cellular growth punctuated by macrofollicles of varying sizes and shapes. Their lumens contain eosinophilic or basophilic fluid. A fibrothecomatous stroma with variable luteinization and/or oedema is often evident. The typically rounded neoplastic granulosa cells have abundant eosinophilic and/or vacuolated cytoplasm; and almost all nuclei lack grooves. Mitotic figures are abundant. Cytomegaly with macronuclei, multinucleation and bizarre multilobulated nuclei is occasionally observed {2890,3210}.

Differential diagnosis
Only the entity of small cell carcinoma associated with hypercalcaemia, which

also occurs in children and young women, poses a significant diagnostic problem. The clinical presentation of JGCT with estrogenic manifestations and that of small cell carcinoma with hypercalcaemia are important clues to the precise diagnosis.

Dissemination beyond the ovary is evident in 20% of these small cell carcinomas at presentation, a feature that is most unusual for a JGCT. The presence of necrosis and more eccentric nuclei in the carcinomas are additional features that can help. The presence of mucinous epithelium in 10% of cases and clusters of larger cells in most small cell carcinomas provide further support. Finally, immunostains for alpha-inhibin are positive in granulosa cell tumours but completely negative in the carcinomas. Both tumours may be negative with a variety of epithelial markers.

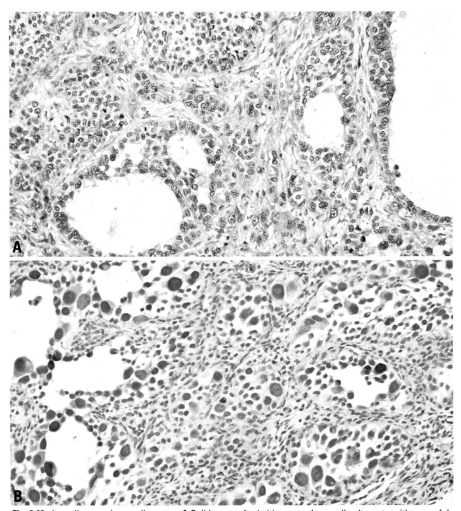

Fig. 2.63 Juvenile granulosa cell tumour. **A** Solid nests of primitive granulosa cells alternate with macrofollicles lined by the same cell population. **B** Moderate to severe atypia is sometimes evident in both the solid and the cystic areas.

Genetic susceptibility

JGCTs may present as a component of a variety of non-hereditary congenital syndromes including Ollier disease (enchondromatosis) {2857,3015} and Maffucci syndrome (enchondromatosis and haemangiomatosis) {1102,2859}. Bilateral JGCT may develop in infants with features suggestive of Goldenhar (craniofacial and skeletal abnormalities) {2306} or Potter syndrome {2468}.

Prognosis and predictive factors

Despite their more primitive histological appearance, only about 5% of JGCTs behave aggressively, and these usually do so within 3 years of presentation. The overall prognosis for JGCT is good with a 1.5% mortality associated with stage IA tumours; but it is poor in stage II or higher tumours {3195}.

Thecoma-fibroma group

Definition

Tumours forming a continuous spectrum from those composed entirely of fibroblasts and producing collagen to those containing a predominance of theca cells.

Thecoma	8600/0
Luteinized thecoma	8601/0
Fibroma, NOS	8810/0
Cellular fibroma	8810/1
Fibrosarcoma	8810/3
Stromal tumour with minor sex	
cord elements	8593/1
Sclerosing stromal tumour	8602/0

Thecoma

Definition

Thecomas are stromal tumours composed of lipid-containing cells resembling theca interna cells with a variable component of fibroblasts. Luteinized thecomas contain lutein cells in a background of thecoma or fibroma.

Epidemiology

Typical thecomas are about one-third as common as granulosa cell tumours. The great majority (84%) occur in post-menopausal women (mean age 59 years). Thecomas are rare before puberty, and only about 10% occur in women younger than 30 years {283}. The rare variant of luteinized thecoma associated

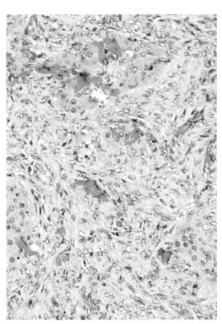

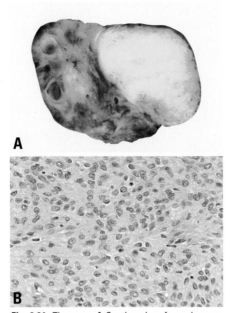

Fig. 2.64 Thecoma. **A** Sectioned surface shows a circumscribed bright yellow tumour compressing the adjacent ovary. **B** The tumour cells have abundant pale, poorly delimited cytoplasm.

Fig. 2.65 Luteinized thecoma. Nests of luteinized tumour cells with eosinophilic cytoplasm and round nucleoli occur in a background of neoplastic spindle-shaped cells.

with sclerosing peritonitis typically occurs in young women less than 30 years, only rarely occurring in older women {520}.

Clinical features

Typical thecomas may be discovered incidentally or produce non-specific signs and symptoms of a pelvic mass. Symptoms related to estrogen production including abnormal uterine bleeding occur in about 60% of patients, and about 20% of postmenopausal women with thecoma have endometrial adenocarcinoma or rarely a malignant müllerian mixed tumour or endometrial stromal sarcoma {2300}. Luteinized thecomas have a lower frequency of estrogenic manifestations than typical thecomas, and about 10% are associated with

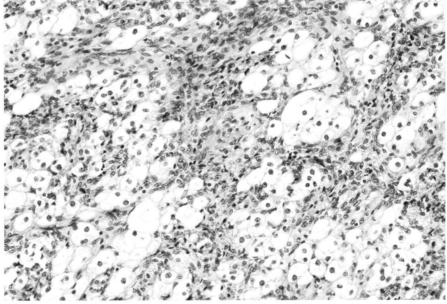

Fig. 2.66 Luteinized thecoma. There are clusters of luteinized cells with vacuolated cytoplasm dispersed among the spindle-shaped cells

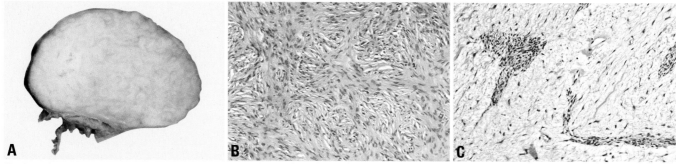

Fig. 2.67 Fibroma. **A** The sectioned surface shows a white fibrous tumour. **B** The neoplasm is composed of spindle-shaped cells with abundant collagen. **C** Oedema is striking in this fibroma associated with Meigs syndrome.

androgenic manifestations {3252}. Patients with the rare variant of luteinized thecoma associated with sclerosing peritonitis present with abdominal swelling, ascites and symptoms of bowel obstruction {520}.

Macroscopy
Thecomas may be small and non-palpable, but they usually measure 5-10 cm. The sectioned surface is typically solid and yellow, occasionally with cysts, haemorrhage or necrosis. Typical thecomas are almost invariably unilateral; only 3% are bilateral. Luteinized thecomas associated with sclerosing peritonitis are usually bilateral.

Histopathology
Typical thecomas are characterized by cells with uniform, bland, oval to spindle shaped nuclei with abundant, pale, vacuolated, lipid-rich cytoplasm. Individual cells are invested by reticulin. Mitoses are absent or rare. Rarely, the nuclei may be large or bizarre {3210}. The fibromatous component commonly contains hyaline plaques and may be calcified. Extensively calcified thecomas tend to occur in young women {3194}. Rarely, thecomas include a minor component of sex cord elements {3211}. Luteinized thecomas contain lutein cells, individually or in nests, in a background often more fibromatous than thecomatous. Oedema and microcyst formation may be striking.

Immunoprofile
Thecomas are immunoreactive for vimentin and alpha-inhibin {482,562, 1499,1816,2181,2211}.

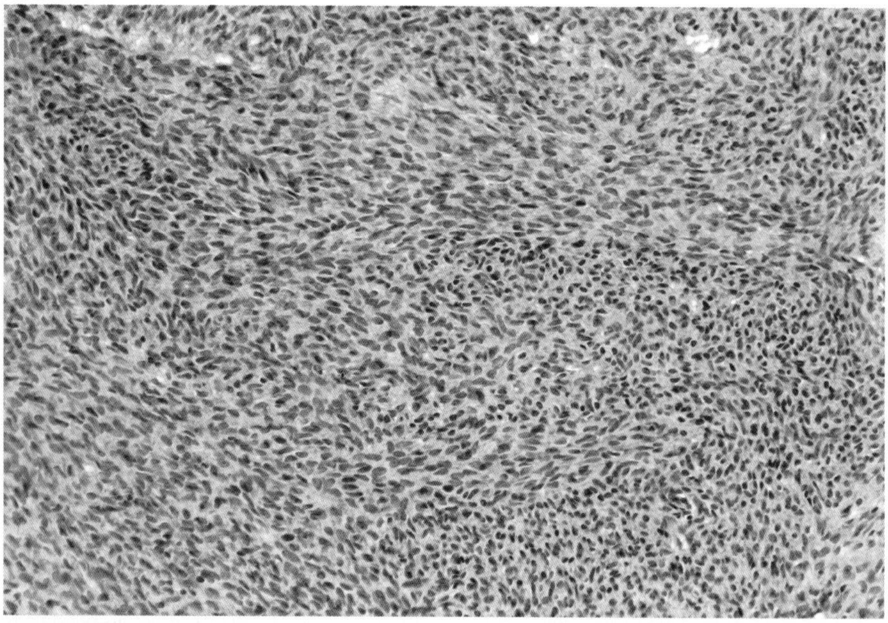

Somatic genetics
Trisomy and tetrasomy 12 have been demonstrated in tumours in the thecoma-fibroma group by karyotypic analysis and fluorescence in situ hybridization {1635,1653,2221,2635,2862}. This chromosomal abnormality is not, however, specific to tumours in this group since it has also been found in some benign and borderline epithelial tumours, as well as in occasional granulosa cell tumours {2209,2221}.

Prognosis and predictive factors
Rarely, a typical or luteinized thecoma with nuclear atypia and mitotic activity may metastasize {1819,3074,3252}, although most cases reported as "malignant thecomas" are probably fibrosarcomas or diffuse granulosa cell tumours. Patients with luteinized thecomas associated with sclerosing peritonitis may experience small bowel obstruction, and several have died of complications related to peritoneal lesions, but there has been no recurrence or metastasis of the ovarian lesion {520}.

Fibroma and cellular fibroma

Definition
Fibromas are stromal tumours composed of spindle, oval or round cells producing collagen. In cellular fibromas the cells are closely packed, collagen is scanty, and the mitotic rate is increased.

Epidemiology
Fibromas account for 4% of all ovarian tumours. They are most common in middle age (mean 48 years) {709}; less than 10% occur before age 30, and they occur only occasionally in children {328}.

Fig. 2.68 Cellular fibroma. The tumour is cellular but shows no cytological atypia and has a low mitotic rate.

Clinical features

Fibromas may be found incidentally, but when large, patients may present with non-specific signs and symptoms of a pelvic mass. Between 10-15% of fibromas over 10 cm are associated with ascites {2519}, and Meigs syndrome (ascites and pleural effusion with resolution after fibroma removal) occurs in about 1% of cases {1839}.

Macroscopy

Fibromas are hard white tumours averaging 6 cm in diameter. Oedematous tumours may be soft, and cyst formation is common. Haemorrhage and necrosis are rare outside the setting of torsion. The majority of tumours are unilateral. Only 8% are bilateral, and less than 10% show focal or diffuse calcification.

Histopathology

Fibromas are composed of spindle-shaped cells with uniform, bland nuclei and scant cytoplasm that may contain small amounts of lipid or occasionally eosinophilic droplets. The cells are arranged in fascicles or in a storiform pattern. Mitoses are absent or rare. Fibromas are generally sparsely to moderately cellular with abundant intercellular collagen, hyalinized plaques and variable degrees of oedema. The cellularity may vary from area to area. About 10% of tumours are uniformly and densely cellular (attaining the cellularity of a diffuse granulosa cell tumour) and are referred to as cellular fibromas {2289}. Cellular fibromas exhibit no more than mild cytological atypia and an average of three or less mitoses per 10 high power fields. Fibromas express vimentin and may be immunoreactive for alpha-inhibin {1816, 2211}.

Genetic susceptibility

Ovarian fibromas are common in females with the nevoid basal cell carcinoma syndrome, occurring in about 75% of patients having the syndrome referred to gynaecologists. Syndrome-related tumours are usually bilateral (75%), frequently multinodular, almost always calcified, sometimes massively, and tend to occur at a younger age, usually in children, adolescents, or young adults {1042,1354,2603}. Additional tumours may arise after local excision. The nevoid basal cell carcinoma syndrome has been reported in four

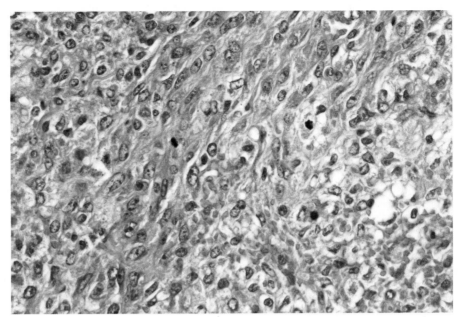

Fig. 2.69 Fibrosarcoma. Moderate to severe cytological atypia accompanied by numerous mitotic figures characterize this fibrosarcoma.

generations of a kindred lacking other stigmata of the syndrome {728,1635, 2221,2635}.

Prognosis and predictive features

Rarely, cellular fibromas recur in the pelvis or upper abdomen, often after a long interval, particularly if they were adherent or ruptured at the time of diagnosis {2289}. Very rarely, fibromatous tumours with no atypical features may spread beyond the ovary {1722}.

Fibrosarcoma

Definition

A rare fibroblastic tumour of the ovary that typically has 4 or more mitotic figures per 10 high power fields as well as significant nuclear atypia.

Epidemiology

Fibrosarcomas are the most common ovarian sarcoma, occurring at any age but most often in older women.

Macroscopy

Fibrosarcomas are large, solid tumours, commonly haemorrhagic and necrotic, and are usually unilateral.

Histopathology

Fibrosarcomas are densely cellular, spindle cell neoplasms with moderate to severe cytological atypia, a high mitotic rate (an average of 4 or more mitoses

per 10 high power fields) with atypical division figures, haemorrhage and necrosis {90,145,2289}.

Somatic genetics

Trisomy 12 as well as trisomy 8 have been reported in an ovarian fibrosarcoma {2963}.

Genetic susceptibility

Ovarian fibrosarcomas are rarely associated with Maffucci syndrome {484} and the nevoid basal cell carcinoma syndrome {1517}.

Prognosis and predictive factors

The majority of ovarian fibrosarcomas have had a malignant course.

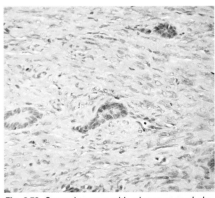

Fig. 2.70 Stromal tumour with minor sex cord elements. Rarely, fibrothecomas contain a few tubules lined by cells resembling Sertoli cells.

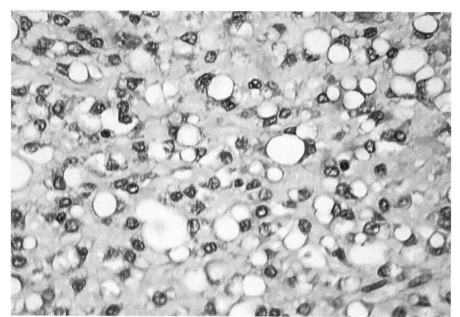

Fig. 2.71 Signet-ring stromal tumour. There is a diffuse proliferation of round cells with eccentric nuclei and a single large cytoplasmic vacuole resembling signet-ring cells.

Stromal tumour with minor sex cord elements

Definition
Stromal tumour with minor sex cord elements is a rare, fibrothecomatous tumour containing scattered sex cord elements {2605,3211}. By definition, the sex cord element must account for <10% of the composition of the tumour {2605}.

Clinical features
This tumour may occur in women of any age. It is usually hormonally inactive, but there have been several cases associated with endometrial hyperplasia or adenocarcinoma.

Macroscopy
Macroscopically, the tumour is solid, not distinguishable from thecoma or fibroma, and ranges from 1-10 cm in diameter.

Histopathology
Histological examination demonstrates the typical features of thecoma or fibroma in which sex cord structures are intermingled with the fibrothecomatous cells. Sex cord components vary in appearance between fully differentiated granulosa cells and indifferent tubular structures resembling immature Sertoli cells.

Prognosis and predictive factors
All of the reported cases are benign.

Sclerosing stromal tumour

Definition
A distinctive type of benign stromal tumour characterized by cellular pseudolobules that are composed of fibroblasts and round cells and separated by hypocellular, oedematous or collagenous tissue.

Epidemiology
This tumour accounts for 2-6% of ovarian stromal tumours, and more than 80% occur in young women in the second and third decades {433}.

Clinical features
Presenting symptoms include menstrual abnormalities or abdominal discomfort {433,1280a,1409a,1695a}. Hormonal manifestations are rare {433}, although a few tumours have been shown to produce estrogens or androgens {614, 1222,1778,2315,2964}. Virilization may occur in pregnant women {419,738, 1308}.

Macroscopy
The tumour is typically unilateral and sharply demarcated, measuring 3-17 cm in diameter. The sectioned surface is solid, grey-white with occasional yellow foci and usually contains oedematous or cystic areas.

Histopathology
Histological examination shows a characteristic pattern with pseudolobulation of the cellular areas separated by hypocellular areas of densely collage-

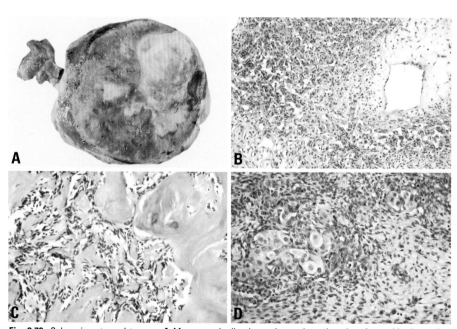

Fig. 2.72 Sclerosing stromal tumour. **A** Macroscopically, the variegated sectioned surface with alternating areas of oedema, haemorrhage and luteinization is typical. Histologically, cellular, often haemangiopericytoma-like, areas (**B**) alternate with sclerotic regions (**C**), and luteinized cell clusters (**D**).

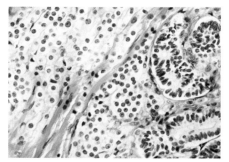

Fig. 2.73 Well differentiated Sertoli-Leydig cell tumour. The tumour shows well developed tubules lined by Sertoli cells and aggregates of Leydig cells.

nous or oedematous tissue. The cellular areas contain prominent thin-walled vessels with varying degrees of sclerosis admixed with both spindle and round cells, the latter may resemble luteinized theca cells or show perinuclear vacuolization.

Histochemical studies show the activity of steroidogenesis-related enzymes {1575,2537} and immunoreactivity for desmin and smooth muscle actin, as well as vimentin {419,1419,2512,2637}.

Prognosis and predictive factors

The tumour is benign, and there have been no recurrent cases.

Signet-ring stromal tumour

Definition

A rare stromal tumour composed of signet-ring cells that do not contain mucin, glycogen or lipid {697,2332, 2605,2811}.

Clinical findings

This tumour occurs in adults and is hormonally inactive.

Macroscopy

Macroscopically the tumours, may be both solid and cystic or uniformly solid.

Histopathology

Histological examination shows a diffuse proliferation of spindle and round cells; the latter show eccentric nuclei with a single large cytoplasmic vacuole and resemble signet-ring cells. The tumour may be composed entirely of signet-ring cells or may occur as a component of an otherwise typical fibroma. With the exception of one case {697}, nuclear atypia and mitotic figures are not present. Negative staining for mucin

distinguishes this tumour from the Krukenberg tumour. All of the reported cases are benign.

Sertoli-stromal cell tumours

Definition

Tumours containing in pure form or in various combinations Sertoli cells, cells resembling rete epithelial cells, cells resembling fibroblasts and Leydig cells in variable degrees of differentiation.

ICD-O codes

Sertoli-Leydig cell tumour group

Well differentiated	8631/0
Of intermediate differentiation	8631/1
With heterologous elements	8634/1
Poorly differentiated	8631/3
With heterologous elements	8634/3
Retiform	8633/1
With heterologous elements	8634/1
Sertoli cell tumour, NOS	8640/1

Sertoli-Leydig cell tumour group

Definition

Tumours composed of variable proportions of Sertoli cells, Leydig cells, and in

the case of intermediate and poorly differentiated neoplasms, primitive gonadal stroma and sometimes heterologous elements.

Synonym

Androblastoma.

Epidemiology

Sertoli-Leydig cell tumours (SLCTs) are rare, accounting for <0.5% of ovarian neoplasms; intermediate and poorly differentiated forms are most common. SLCTs have been reported in females from 2-75 years of age with a mean age of 23-25 years in different studies {2459, 3217,3243}.

Fig. 2.74 T1 weighted MR image of a Sertoli-Leydig cell tumour that fills the abdomen.

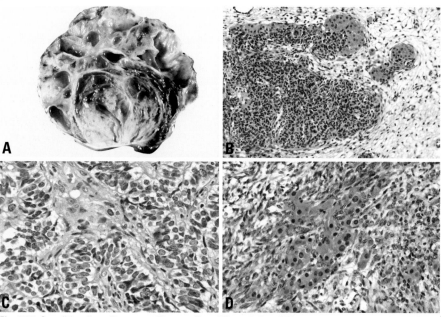

Fig. 2.75 Sertoli-Leydig cell tumour of intermediate differentiation. **A** The sectioned surface of the tumour shows solid, cystic and partly haemorrhagic areas. **B** Nests of Leydig cells are at the edge of an aggregate of Sertoli cells adjacent to an oedematous area. **C** Solid cords of Sertoli cells surround a cluster of Leydig cells in the centre of the field. **D** Leydig cells are admixed with gonadal stroma and sex cord elements.

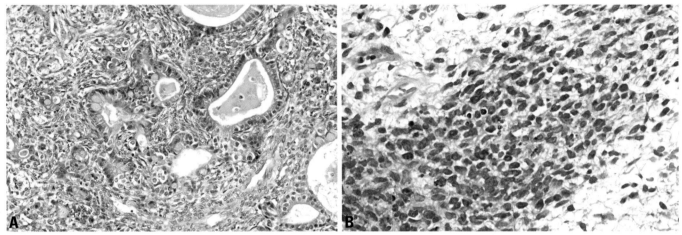

Fig. 2.76 Poorly differentiated Sertoli-Leydig cell tumour. **A** Heterologous elements consisting of mucinous glands are intimately associated with primitive gonadal stroma. **B** A nodule of primitive gonadal stroma is composed of poorly differentiated spindle-shaped cells with apoptotic bodies.

Clinical features

Signs and symptoms
One-third of patients are virilized, and others may have estrogenic manifestations. Androgenic manifestations include amenorrhea, hirsutism, breast atrophy, clitoral hypertrophy and hoarseness, whereas estrogenic effects include isosexual pseudoprecocity and menometrorrhagia. One-half of the patients have no endocrine manifestations, and the symptoms are non-specific. Patients with poorly differentiated neoplasms are slightly more likely to present with androgenic manifestations. About 10% of cases have tumour rupture or ovarian surface involvement, and 4% have ascites {3217}.

Imaging
A solid, cystic or solid and cystic mass may be identified on ultrasound, computed tomography or magnetic resonance imaging.

Macroscopy

Over 97% of SLCTs are unilateral. They may be solid, solid and cystic or, rarely, cystic. The size ranges from not detectible to 35 cm (mean 12-14 cm). Poorly differentiated tumours are larger. Solid areas are fleshy and pale yellow, pink or grey. Areas of haemorrhage and necrosis are frequent, and torsion and infarction may be seen.

Tumour spread and staging

About 2-3% of tumours have spread beyond the ovary at presentation {3217}.

Histopathology

In well differentiated SLCTs, Sertoli cells are present in open or closed tubules and lack significant nuclear atypia or mitotic activity {3216}. There is a delicate fibrous stroma in which Leydig cells may be found in small clusters.

In tumours of intermediate differentiation, cellular lobules composed of hyperchromatic spindle-shaped gonadal stromal cells with poorly defined cytoplasm are separated by oedematous stroma. These merge with cords and poorly developed tubules of Sertoli cells, some with atypia. With better differentiation of Sertoli cell elements, the distinction between the stromal and Sertoli cell components is more easily made. Leydig cells are found in clusters at the periphery of the cellular lobules or admixed with other elements. They may be vacuolated, contain lipofuscin or rarely have Reinke crystals. Mitotic figures average 5 per 10 high power fields. Mitotic figures are rare among the Leydig cells, which also lack cytological atypia.

In poorly differentiated tumours, a sarcomatoid stroma resembling primitive gonadal stroma is a dominant feature, and the lobulated arrangement of SLCT of intermediate differentiation is absent. Occasional tumours contain bizarre nuclei. The mitotic activity in the Sertoli and stromal elements is variable with a mean of over 20 per 10 high power fields.

Immunoprofile
Positivity is seen for vimentin, keratin and alpha-inhibin with differing intensity of expression between sex cord and stromal areas. Rarely, positivity for epithelial membrane antigen may be seen. Positivity for estrogen and progesterone receptors may also be seen in a minority of cases.

Grading
SLCTs are subdivided into well differentiated, intermediate and poorly differentiated forms based on the degree of tubular differentiation of the Sertoli cell component (decreasing with increasing grade) and the quantity of the primitive gonadal stroma (increasing with increasing grade). Leydig cells also decrease with increasing grade. Heterologous elements and/or a retiform pattern may be seen in all but the well differentiated variant.

Somatic genetics

Analysis of six SLCTs has shown limited, if any, loss of heterozygosity with 10 polymorphic DNA markers that have shown high rates of loss of heterozygosity in a variety of tumours. Three of these were assessed for clonality by examining the DNA methylation pattern at a polymorphic site to the androgen receptor gene. The Leydig cells in these three cases were all polyclonal in contrast to the cells from a pure Leydig cell tumour that were monoclonal. These findings suggest that the Leydig cells in SLCTs are reactive cells of ovarian stromal origin and not a neoplastic component of the tumour {1902}. Trisomy 8 was reported as the sole karyotypic abnormality in a SLCT that metastasized {1756}.

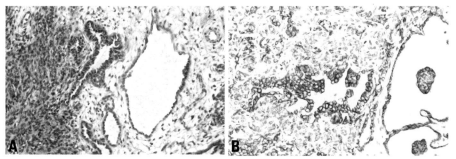
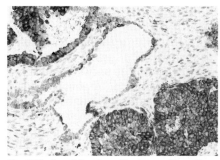

Fig. 2.77 A Retiform Sertoli-Leydig cell tumour. Note the retiform spaces surrounded by oedematous stroma at the periphery of a cellular nodule. **B** Keratin stains the retiform areas and shows limited staining of adjacent sex cord areas and stroma.

Fig. 2.78 Sertoli-Leydig cell tumour with retiform elements. The sex cord areas stain strongly for inhibin with weaker staining in retiform areas.

Genetic susceptibility

A familial occurrence of SLCTs in association with thyroid disease has been reported {1344} with occasional reports of other families since then. The thyroid abnormalities are usually adenomas or nodular goitres. Autosomal dominant inheritance with variable penetrance has been suggested as the method of genetic transmission. SLCT has been reported in association with cervical sarcoma botryoides in three cases {1026}.

Prognosis and predictive factors

The mortality from SLCTs as a group is low and is confined to those of intermediate and poor differentiation. Poor differentiation, tumour rupture and heterologous mesenchymal elements were identified as features correlating with the development of metastases {302, 2459}. In one large series none of the well differentiated tumours, 11% of those of intermediate differentiation and 59% of those that were poorly differenti-

ated behaved in a clinically malignant fashion {3217}. Presentation with stage II or higher disease is also associated with a poor outcome. However, tumours without any apparent poor prognostic factors may behave in an aggressive fashion {1903}.

Sertoli-Leydig tumour with heterologous elements

Definition

A SLCT that contains either macroscopic or histological quantities of a tissue not regarded as intrinsic to the sex cord-stromal category. Such elements include epithelial (mostly mucinous) and/or mesenchymal tissues (most commonly chondroid and rhabdomyoblastic) and tumours arising from these elements.

Clinical features

The presence of heterologous elements does not alter the presentation, but 20%

of patients have a slightly raised serum alpha-fetoprotein (AFP) due in some cases to hepatocytes as a heterologous element.

Macroscopy

Part or the entire cystic component of a SLCT may be mucinous in type; however, heterologous elements are only occasionally diagnosed macroscopically.

Histopathology

Heterologous elements are seen in approximately 20% of SLCTs. They occur only in those of intermediate or poor differentiation or in retiform tumours but are not identified in well-differentiated tumours. Heterologous mesenchymal elements occur in 5% of SLCTs and usually consist of cartilage, skeletal muscle or rhabdomyosarcoma. They may be admixed with the sex cord areas of the tumour or present as discrete areas. Both cartilage and skeletal

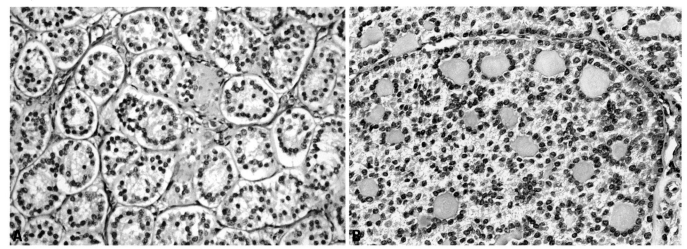

Fig. 2.79 A Sertoli cell tumour, simple tubular pattern. Note the hollow and obliterated tubules in cross section. **B** Sertoli cell tumour, complex tubular pattern. Islands of Sertoli cells are arranged around multiple round hyaline bodies.

muscle may appear cellular and of fetal type.

The mucinous epithelium is usually bland intestinal or gastric-type epithelium, but sometimes shows borderline or malignant change. Argentaffin cells, goblet cells and carcinoid may be seen. The gonadal stroma may condense around areas of mucinous epithelium, a useful clue to the diagnosis of a SLCT in a tumour that appears to be a mucinous cystadenoma. Hepatocytic differentiation may be recognized by the presence of bile plugs or an acinar arrangement of hepatocytes, but immunohistochemistry is usually necessary to distinguish hepatocytes from Leydig cells {1904}.

Immunoprofile
Variable positivity is seen in the sex cord elements for vimentin, keratin and alpha-inhibin.

The immunoprofile of the heterologous elements is what would be expected from their constituent tissues. The mucinous elements show more extensive staining for cytokeratin 7 than for cytokeratin 20. They are positive for epithelial membrane antigen and may be focally positive for chromogranin. Leydig cells are negative for pan-keratin, CAM 5.2 and AFP but show intense positivity for vimentin and alpha-inhibin. These findings distinguish them from hepatocytes. AFP may be identified in endodermal-like structures in some cases.

Prognosis and predictive factors
The small number of cases of this tumour reported make it difficult to determine the significance of individual elements. Heterologous mesenchymal elements (skeletal muscle or cartilage) or neuro-blastoma imply a poor outcome with 8 of 10 patients dead of disease {2291}. In contrast, gastrointestinal epithelium or carcinoid as the heterologous element does not have prognostic significance {3207}.

Retiform Sertoli-Leydig cell tumour and variant with retiform elements

Definition
Retiform SLCT is composed of anastomosing slit-like spaces that resemble the rete testis and comprise 90% or more of the tumour. Tumours with at least 10% but less than 90% retiform elements are classified as being of intermediate or poor differentiation and qualified "with retiform elements".

Epidemiology
Retiform tumours tend to occur in younger patients but may occur at any age {3209}. Virilization is less common in tumours with a retiform pattern.

Macroscopy
Retiform tumours may contain papillae or polypoid structures.

Histopathology
Like heterologous elements, retiform areas occur only in SLCTS of intermediate and poor differentiation {2471,3209}. They vary from slit-like spaces to areas comprising a complex microcystic pattern. Dilated spaces may be continuous with sex cord areas of the tumour. The lining cells may be flattened and non-specific or cuboidal and sertoliform. The lumens frequently contain variably inspissated eosinophilic material resembling colloid. Within the SLCT category, retiform tumours shows the highest incidence of heterologous elements {3209}.

Immunoprofile
Retiform areas stain with keratin and show moderate staining for alpha-inhibin, with a reversed pattern seen in sex cord and stromal areas of the tumour. Vimentin may show subnuclear localization in the retiform areas.

Differential diagnosis
Serous tumours, yolk sac tumours and malignant müllerian mixed tumours may resemble a retiform SLCT {3209}. The presence of primitive gonadal stroma, heterologous elements, Leydig cells and/or alpha-inhibin positivity assists in making the diagnosis.

Prognosis and predictive factors
Approximately 25% of patients with SLCTs that contain retiform elements will have an aggressive course {3209}. Many have stage II or higher disease, poor differentiation and/or heterologous elements.

Sertoli cell tumour

Definition
A neoplasm composed of Sertoli cells arranged in hollow or solid tubular formations with rare, if any, Leydig cells. Simple or complex annular tubules are dominant in those lesions that occur in association with the Peutz-Jeghers syndrome.

Epidemiology
Sertoli cell tumours are rare {2882}. Patients range in age from 2-79 years.

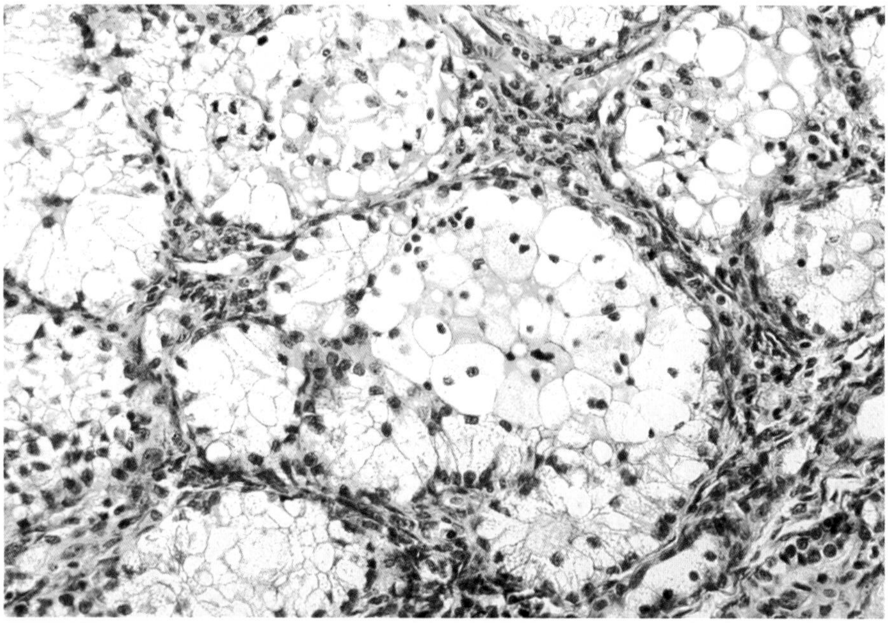

Fig. 2.80 Sertoli cell tumour, lipid-rich variant (folliculome lipidique). The Sertoli cells have abundant vacuolated cytoplasm filled with lipid.

Mean ages of 21 and 38 years and median ages of 33 and 50 years have been reported in the two largest series {2882,3215}.

Clinical features
The tumours are functional in 40-60% of cases, most often estrogenic, but occasionally androgenic or rarely both. Rarely, the tumour produces progestins. Clinical manifestations include isosexual pseudoprecocity, menometrorrhagia, amenorrhea, hirsutism, breast atrophy, clitoral hypertrophy and hoarseness. Cases with menstrual disturbances or postmenopausal bleeding may show hyperplasia or adenocarcinoma of the endometrium. A peritoneal decidual reaction may be seen. Patients with Sertoli cell tumour may have elevated levels of serum estrogen, progesterone and luteinizing hormone. Rarely, the tumour may cause hypertension due to renin production.

Macroscopy
These are unilateral neoplasms, and the ovaries are involved with equal frequency. They range in size from 1-28 cm with an average of 7-9 cm. They are well circumscribed, solid neoplasms with a smooth or lobulated external surface, a fleshy consistency and a yellow-tan sectioned surface. Areas of haemorrhage and/or cystic degeneration may be seen in larger tumours. Rare examples are totally cystic or are solid with fibrosis and ossification.

Histopathology
A variety of tubular arrangements characterize Sertoli cell tumours. The tubular pattern is either open or closed (with paired cell arrangements) and simple or complex. Simple tubules are surrounded by a basement membrane and may contain a central hyaline body. Complex tubules form multiple lumens often filled with hyaline bodies and surrounded by a thick basement membrane that may coalesce to form hyalinized areas. Diffuse and pseudopapillary patterns may be seen. In some tumours, cells distended by intracytoplasmic lipid are dominant in a pattern known as "folliculome lipidique". The Sertoli cell tumours that occur in women with the Peutz-Jeghers syndrome may have abundant eosinophilic cytoplasm, termed the oxyphilic variant {852}. The nucleus is

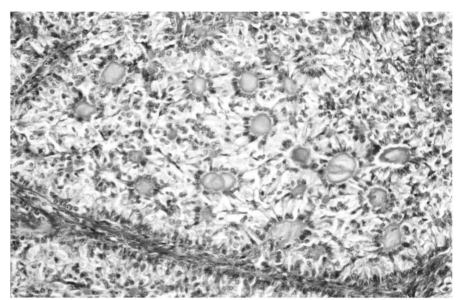

Fig. 2.81 Sex cord tumour with annular tubules in a case not associated with the Peutz-Jeghers syndrome. A complex annular tubular pattern consists of pale cells arranged around multiple hyaline bodies.

typically oval or spherical with a small nucleolus. The cytoplasm is clear or lightly vacuolated, stains for lipid are positive, and glycogen may be demonstrated. Mitotic figures are usually scanty (<1 per 10 high power fields), but >9 mitotic figures per 10 high power fields may be seen in tumours from younger women. The neoplasm may contain rare Leydig cells, but lacks the primitive gonadal stroma characteristic of Sertoli-Leydig cell tumours.

Immunoprofile
Sertoli cell tumours are variably positive for keratins, vimentin and alpha-inhibin. CD99 and calretinin are positive in about 50% of cases. The tumours are negative for epithelial membrane antigen.

Electron microscopy
A diagnostic feature of Sertoli cell tumour is the presence of Charcot-Böttcher (CB) filaments and Spangaro bodies. These bodies represent aggregates of intracytoplasmic microfilaments of varying sizeand are not present in every cell or every tumour. CB filaments have been found most frequently in the complex tubular variant, the so-called sex cord tumour with annular tubules (SCTAT).

Differential diagnosis
Sertoli cell tumours must be distinguished from struma ovarii, carcinoid

and endometrioid carcinoma (see section on endometrioid carcinoma). Phenotypic females with the androgen insensitivity syndrome (AIS) may be incorrectly diagnosed as having a Sertoli cell tumour of the ovary if the syndrome has not been diagnosed preoperatively {2498}. On the other hand, Sertoli cell tumours can occur in the testes of patients with AIS. While most are benign, rare malignant Sertoli cell tumours have been reported in this setting {3165}.

Somatic genetics
There is little information on chromosomal abnormalities in these tumours. An extra isochromosome 1q was seen in one tumour {2208}.

Genetic susceptibility
A variety of Sertoli cell phenotypes including SCTAT {2599}, oxyphilic {852} and lipid rich (folliculome lipidique) variants have been described in patients with the Peutz-Jeghers syndrome (PJS), an autosomal dominant disease with a propensity for breast, intestinal and gynaecological neoplasia.

Prognosis and predictive factors
These tumours are typically benign. In the rare forms that behave clinically in an aggressive fashion, infiltration of the ovarian stroma, extension beyond the ovary and intravascular extension may be seen. Cytological atypia and a high

mitotic rate may be present in these tumours.

Stromal-Leydig cell tumour

Definition
An ovarian stromal tumour composed of fibromatous stroma and clusters of Leydig cells containing crystals of Reinke.

Clinical features
This tumour is virilizing in approximately one-half of the cases.

Macroscopy
These extremely rare neoplasms are usually well circumscribed {302,2165,2842}. The sectioned surface has been described as lobulated with a yellow-white appearance. They may be bilateral.

Histopathology
Stromal-Leydig cell tumours have two components. Spindle-shaped or ovoid stromal cells identical to those of a fibroma or thecoma are present together with Leydig cells containing Reinke crystals {2789,3252}. Typically, in these neoplasms the fibrothecomatous element predominates with the Leydig cell component comprising small nodular aggregates.

Definitive diagnosis requires the presence of Reinke crystals, otherwise the neoplasm would be categorized as luteinized thecoma. Since Reinke crystals may be difficult to identify and since sampling errors may occur, it has been suggested that stromal-Leydig cell tumours are more common than the literature would suggest.

Prognosis and predictive factors
The clinical behaviour of stromal-Leydig cell tumours is benign, and neither clinical recurrence nor metastasis has been documented.

Sex cord-stromal tumours of mixed or unclassified cell types

Definition
Sex cord-stromal tumours that do not fall in the granulosa-stromal, Sertoli-stromal or steroid cell categories.

ICD-O codes
Sex cord tumour with annular
tubules   8623/1
  Variant associated with
  Peutz-Jeghers syndrome   8623/0
Gynandroblastoma   8632/1
Sex cord-stromal tumour, NOS 8590/1

Sex cord tumour with annular tubules

Definition
A tumour composed of sex cord (Sertoli) cells arranged in simple and complex annular tubules {2599}.

Synonym
Sertoli cell tumour, annular tubular variant.

Epidemiology
Patients with this tumour most commonly present in the third or fourth decades, but the age ranges from 4-76 years. About one-third of cases occur in women with Peutz-Jeghers syndrome (PJS). The average age of patients with PJS is in the mid-twenties and of those unassociated with PJS in the mid-thirties.

Clinical features
Nearly all women without PJS present with a palpable mass. Isosexual pseudoprecocity or other features of aberrant estrogen occurs in about 40% of cases, and, occasionally, there are progesterone effects. Those tumours that are associated with PJS are found either incidentally at autopsy or in ovaries removed as part of treatment for other gynaecological disease.

Macroscopy
These are unilateral neoplasms except for those occurring in the PJS, which are usually bilateral. PJS-associated lesions are usually macroscopically undetectable; when visible, the tumourlets are multiple and <3 cm in diameter. Bilateral lesions are present in two-thirds of women. Non-PJS cases may be up to 33 cm in diameter. The sectioned surface of the tumours is solid and yellow. Calcification or cystic degeneration may be apparent.

Histopathology
Regardless of the clinical setting, the annular tubules show Sertoli cells with pale cytoplasm and nuclei arranged antipodally around a single hyaline body (simple annular tubules) or multiple hyaline bodies (complex annular tubules). Classic tubular Sertoli cell arrangements may be admixed. In PJS lesions the annular tubules are typically widely scattered in the ovarian stroma without forming a distinct mass.

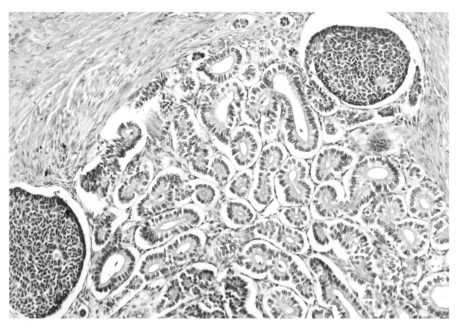

Fig. 2.82 Gynandroblastoma. Two islands of granulosa cells with Call-Exner bodies are located on either side of an aggregate of hollow tubules lined by Sertoli cells.

Tumours unassociated with PJS form masses of simple and complex tubules separated by sparse fibrous stroma. Extensive hyalinization may develop. The neoplastic cells may spill over beyond the confines of the tubules and infiltrate the surrounding stroma. Mitotic figures occasionally exceed 4 per 10 high power fields and rarely exceed 10 per 10 high power fields. Areas of well differentiated Sertoli cell tumour characterized by elongated solid tubules and/or microfollicular granulosa cell tumour are often present. Calcification of the hyaline bodies is typically found in over half of the tumours associated with PJS.

Electron microscopy
Ultrastructural assessment has shown Charcot-Böttcher filaments in several cases {2882}. While not required for diagnosis, their presence confirms the identification of the sex cord component as Sertoli cells.

Histogenesis
Although there is ultrastructural evidence supporting differentiation towards Sertoli cells in SCTAT, the histological and clinical features are sufficiently distinctive to merit its classification as a specific form of sex cord-stromal tumour.

Prognosis and predictive factors
All PJS-associated tumourlets have been benign. Up to 25% of SCTATs that occur in the absence of the PJS have been clinically malignant. Tumours with an infiltrative growth pattern and mitotic figures beyond the usual 3-4 per 10 high power fields are more likely to recur or otherwise behave aggressively. It is difficult, however, to predict the behaviour of individual cases. Some tumours produce müllerian inhibiting substance and/or alpha-inhibin, and these tumour markers may be useful in monitoring the course of disease in those cases {1091,2304}. Recurrences are often late and may be multiple. Spread through lymphatics may result in regional and distant lymph node involvement.

Somatic genetics
Germline mutations in a gene encoding serine-threonine kinase have been identified in a SCTAT associated with PJS but not in sporadic cases {548}.

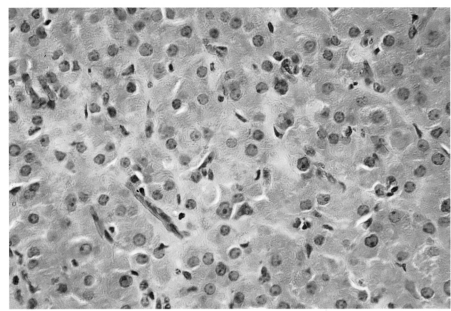
Fig. 2.83 Steroid cell tumour. The tumour is composed of large polygonal cells with eosinophilic cytoplasm containing lipofuscin pigment.

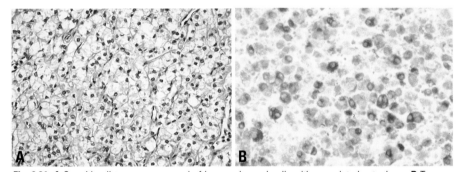
Fig. 2.84 A Steroid cell tumour composed of large polygonal cells with vacuolated cytoplasm. **B** Tumour cells show intense cytoplasmic immunoreactivity for alpha-inhibin.

Gynandroblastoma

Definition
A tumour composed of an admixture of well differentiated Sertoli cell and granulosa cell components with the second cell population comprising at least 10% of the lesion.

Clinical features
An extremely rare tumour, gynandroblastoma generally occurs in young adults, though it may be encountered in a wide age range {96,432,1820,1996}. Nearly all tumours present in stage I and may have either estrogenic or androgenic manifestations. Variable in size, they may be massive (up to 28 cm) with a predominantly solid sectioned surface showing a few cysts.

Histopathology
Well formed hollow tubules lined by Sertoli cells are generally admixed with rounded islands of granulosa cells growing in a microfollicular pattern. Variation from this typical histology with a juvenile granulosa cell pattern or an intermediate or poorly differentiated Sertoli-Leydig cell tumour with or without heterologous elements has been reported {1820}. The tumours are alpha-inhibin positive.

Prognosis and predictive factors
Almost all tumours are stage I at initial presentation and clinically benign. It is important to mention the components of the tumour in the diagnosis, in particular whether the granulosa cell component is of adult or juvenile type and also the subtype of Sertoli-Leydig cell tumour.

Unclassified sex cord-stromal tumour

Definition
Sex cord-stromal tumours in which there is no clearly predominant pattern of testicular or ovarian differentiation {2605}.

Epidemiology
They account for 5-10% of tumours in the sex cord-stromal category.

Clinical features
The tumour may be estrogenic, androgenic or non-functional {2619,2701, 3196}.

Histopathology
Histologically, the tumour cells show patterns and cell types that are intermediate between or common to granulosa-stromal cell tumours and Sertoli-stromal cell tumours.

Prognosis and predictive factors
The prognosis is similar to that of granulosa cell tumours and SLCTs of similar degrees of differentiation {2619}.

Steroid cell tumours

Definition
Tumours that are composed entirely or predominantly (greater than 90%) of cells that resemble steroid hormone-secreting cells. This category includes the stromal luteoma, steroid cell tumour, not further classified and the Leydig cell tumours that do not have another component.

ICD-O codes
Steroid cell tumour, NOS	8670/0
Well differentiated	8670/0
Malignant	8670/3
Stromal luteoma	8610/0
Leydig cell tumour	8650/0

Synonym and historical annotation
The designation "lipid cell tumour" is no longer recommended because it is inaccurate as well as nonspecific, since up to 25% of tumours in this category contain little or no lipid {2605}. The term "steroid cell tumour" has been accepted by the World Health Organization (WHO) because it reflects both the morphological features of the neoplastic cells and their propensity to secrete steroid hormones.

Steroid cell tumour, not otherwise specified

Definition
These are steroid cell tumours that cannot be classified into one of the aforementioned groups. It is probable that some of these cases represent Leydig cell tumours in which Reinke crystals cannot be identified. Some may also represent large stromal luteomas where a parenchymal location can no longer be established.

Clinical features
They are usually associated with androgenic manifestations and occasionally with estrogenic effects {1163}. Rare neoplasms have also been associated with progestogenic effects, Cushing syndrome or other paraneoplastic syndromes due to hormone secretion {3218}.

Macroscopy
These neoplasms are often large and are usually well circumscribed, often having a lobulated appearance. Occasional neoplasms are bilateral. The sectioned surface ranges from yellow to brown or black. Especially in large tumours, areas of haemorrhage and necrosis may be seen.

Histopathology
These neoplasms are usually composed of solid aggregates of cells with occasional nests or trabeculae. Tumour cells are polygonal with cytoplasm that is usually granular and eosinophilic but which may be vacuolated. Sometimes both cell types may be present. Cytoplasmic lipofuscin pigment may be identified. Nuclei may be bland, but in some cases there is considerable nuclear atypia and significant numbers of mitotic figures may be found. Areas of haemorrhage and necrosis can be present. Intracytoplasmic lipid can usually be identified with special stains and rarely may be so abundant as to result in a signet-ring appearance. Occasional tumours contain a considerable amount of fibrous stroma.

Immunoprofile
These neoplasms are usually immunoreactive to alpha-inhibin and variably with anti-cytokeratin antibodies and vimentin.

Differential diagnosis
Luteoma of pregnancy may mimic a lipid-poor or lipid-free steroid cell tumour. The former is usually discovered

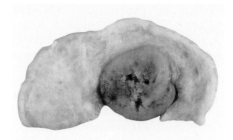

Fig. 2.85 Hilus cell tumour. Note the typical tan tumour in the hilus, well demarcated from the adjacent ovary.

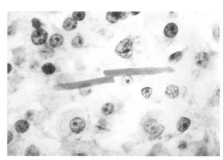

Fig. 2.86 Leydig cell tumour, non-hilus cell type. The cells are large and polygonal. Note the two large, rod-shaped crystals of Reinke.

in patients at caesarean section with a term pregnancy and typically occurs in multiparous Black patients in their third or fourth decade. Also in the differential diagnosis are oxyphilic variants of a number of other ovarian tumours, e.g. struma ovarii, clear cell carcinoma, primary or secondary malignant melanoma and carcinoid.

Prognosis and predictive factors
Approximately one-third of these neoplasms are clinically malignant, and they sometimes have extensive intra-abdominal spread at presentation. Malignant tumours are more likely to be greater than 7 cm diameter, contain areas of haemorrhage and necrosis, exhibit moderate to marked nuclear atypia and have a mitotic count of two or more per 10 high power fields. Occasionally, however, as with other endocrine neoplasms, the behaviour may be unpredictable, and tumours lacking these histological features may behave in a malignant fashion.

Stromal luteoma

Definition
Stromal luteomas are clinically benign steroid cell neoplasms of ovarian stro-

mal origin without crystals of Reinke {1164}.

Clinical features
Most occur in postmenopausal women and are associated with estrogenic effects, but occasional patients have androgenic manifestations {477}.

Macroscopy
These are usually unilateral tumours and are generally small. They are typically well circumscribed and on sectioning are usually grey-white or yellow.

Histopathology
These neoplasms are well circumscribed, are located in the ovarian stroma and are composed of a nodule of luteinized stromal cells that may be arranged diffusely or, less commonly, in nests and cords. The cytoplasm is pale or eosinophilic, the nuclei are bland, and mitoses are rare. Most cases are associated with stromal hyperthecosis in the same and/or contralateral ovary. In such cases it is arbitrary when a nodule of luteinized cells in stromal hyperthecosis is regarded as a stromal luteoma, but generally a cut-off of 1.0 cm in diameter is used. Degenerative changes may occur in stromal luteomas resulting in the formation of spaces that can simulate vessels or glandular formation. Reinke crystals are not present. Stromal luteomas usually exhibit positive immunohistochemical staining for alpha-inhibin.

Prognosis and predictive factors
All of the reported cases have behaved in a benign fashion.

Leydig cell tumours

Definition
Rare ovarian steroid cell neoplasms composed entirely or predominantly of Leydig cells that contain crystals of Reinke. In the case of larger tumours it may not be possible to determine whether the tumour arose in the ovarian parenchyma or in the hilus, and these are referred to as Leydig cell tumours not otherwise specified. Other tumours in this group include hilar cell tumours and Leydig cell tumour of non-hilar type.

Clinical features
These neoplasms typically occur in postmenopausal women {2171,2472} (average age 58 years) but may occur in young women, pregnant women {2165} or children. They are usually associated with androgenic manifestations, but occasionally produce estrogenic effects and are associated with endometrial carcinoma {1278,2455}. In single reports ovarian Leydig cell tumours have been associated with multiple endocrine neoplasia syndrome {2630} and congenital adrenal hyperplasia {1718}.

Immunoprofile
Leydig cell tumours of all types are intensely positive for alpha-inhibin and vimentin. There may be focal reactivity for keratins (CAM 5.2, AE1/AE3) with positivity for actin, CD68, desmin, epithelial membrane antigen and S-100 protein reported {2620}.

Prognosis and predictive factors
The clinical behaviour of all neoplasms in the pure Leydig cell category is benign, and neither clinical recurrence nor metastasis has been documented.

Hilus cell tumour

Definition
A Leydig cell tumour arising in the ovarian hilus separated from the medullary stroma.

Macroscopy
Hilus cell tumours are usually small, well circumscribed lesions located at the ovarian hilus and typically have a red brown to yellow appearance on sectioning. Rarely, they are bilateral {739,1718}. When they are larger, the hilar location may no longer be apparent.

Histopathology
On histological examination the lesion is well circumscribed and comprised of cells with abundant cytoplasm that usually is eosinophilic but which may be clear with abundant intracytoplasmic lipid. Lipofuscin pigment is often seen, and characteristic Reinke crystals were present in 57% of cases in the largest series {2171}. These are eosinophilic, rod-shaped inclusions. Occasionally, they are numerous, but they are often identified only after extensive searching.

PTAH histological staining or electron microscopy may facilitate their identification. Often the nuclei in Leydig cell tumours cluster with nuclear-rich areas separated by nuclear-free zones. The nuclear features are usually bland, but occasionally focal nuclear atypia may be found, an observation of no clinical significance. Mitotic figures are rare. Often, there is a background of hyperplasia of the adjacent non-neoplastic hilar cells in association with non-myelinated nerve fibres.

Although the definitive diagnosis of a hilar cell tumour requires the identification of Reinke crystals, a presumptive diagnosis can be made without crystals if the typical histological features are present in a neoplasm with a hilar location, especially if it is associated with hilus cell hyperplasia or nerve fibres {2171}.

Leydig cell tumour, non-hilar type

Definition
A Leydig cell tumour that orginates from the ovarian stroma and containing crystals of Reinke.

Epidemiology
Leydig cell tumours of non-hilar type have been reported much less often than hilus cell tumours, but their true relative frequency is unknown.

Macroscopy
These tumours are macroscopically well circumscribed and centered in the medullary region {2472}.

Histopathology
They are histologically composed of steroid cells without discernible lipid and surrounded by ovarian stroma that often shows stromal hyperthecosis. Leydig cells containing demonstrable crystals of Reinke must be identified histologically in order to make the diagnosis, and lipofuscin pigment is often present.

Histogenesis
These tumours originate from the ovarian stroma, an origin supported by the rare non-neoplastic transformation of ovarian stromal cells to Leydig cells {2789}.

Germer cell tumours

F. Nogales
A. Talerman
R.A. Kubik-Huch
F.A. Tavassoli
M. Devouassoux-Shisheboran

Definition
A heterogeneous group of tumours reflecting the capacity for multiple lines of differentiation of the main stem cell system. The great majority of these neoplasms originate at different stages of development from germ cells that colonize the ovary.

Epidemiology
Germ cell tumours account for approximately 30% of primary ovarian tumours, 95% of which are mature cystic teratomas {1409,1502}. The remaining germ cell tumours are malignant and represent approximately 3% of all ovarian cancers in Western countries but have been reported to represent up to 20% of ovarian tumours in Japanese women {1970}. The median age at presentation is 18 years {883}.

Malignant germ cell tumours are the most common ovarian cancer among children and adolescent females. Approximately 60% of ovarian tumours occurring in women under the age of 21 are of germ cell type, and up to one-third of them may be malignant {1555}.

Aetiology
The aetiology of ovarian germ cell malignancies is unknown.

Clinical features
Signs and symptoms
Pain and a mass are the common pre-

sentations in young women {2586, 2587,2903}. Teenagers who present with abdominal masses and who have never menstruated should be evaluated for the possibility of a gonadoblastoma that has undergone malignant progression. Preoperative karyotyping of such individuals can be helpful to identify underlying chromosomal abnormalities in cases of gonadoblastoma.

Imaging
The ultrasonographic appearance of dermoid cyst ranges from a predominantly solid-appearing mass due to the echogenic aspect of sebaceous material intermixed with hair to a predominantly cystic mass {2132}. Computed tomography can accurately diagnose a teratoma because of fat attenuation within the cyst, and its complex appearance with dividing septa, hypodensity, calcified structures, and the identification of the Rokitansky protuberance {1080,2132}. Radiographic studies of fetiform teratoma demonstrate portions of skull, vertebra and limb bones within the tumour {19}. There are no diagnostic findings for other germ tumours; they often have solid and cystic components.

Histopathology
Morphologically, the different tumour types present in this group replicate in a distorted, grotesque form various stages of embryonal development from early,

transient structures to mature adult tissues that in their turn may also be capable of undergoing malignant change {2248}.

Histogenesis
As for histogenesis, they are believed to be from the primordial germ cells that migrate into the gonadal ridge at 6 weeks of embryonic life {2848}. A small proportion may also arise from non-germ stem cells present in the adult female genital tract {2039}.

Primitive germ cell tumours

Definition
Tumours that contain malignant germ cell elements other than teratoma.

ICD-O codes
Dysgerminoma	9060/3
Yolk sac tumour	9071/3
Embryonal carcinoma	9070/3
Polyembryoma	9072/3
Non-gestational choriocarcinoma	9100/3
Mixed germ cell tumour	9085/3

Dysgerminoma

Definition
A tumour composed of a monotonous proliferation of primitive germ cells associated with connective tissue septa containing varying amount of lymphocytes and macrophages. Occasionally, syncytiotrophoblastic differentiation or somatic cysts occur. This tumour is identical to testicular seminoma.

Macroscopy
The usually well encapsulated tumour masses are apparently unilateral in 90% of cases. Macroscopic involvement of the contralateral ovary is apparent in 10% of cases, and in another 10% occult foci of dysgerminoma can be detected by biopsy {1929}. Tumours average 15 cm in maximal dimension and on section are solid, uniform or lobular and creamy white or light tan. Irregular areas of coag-

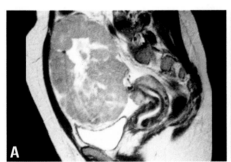
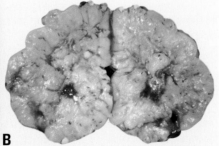

Fig. 2.87 Dysgerminoma in a 28 year old nulligravida woman. **A** Magnetic resonance image sagital view shows a 10 x 15 cm predominantly solid tumour with some central cystic changes. **B** Sectioned surface of the tumour shows a predominantly solid, multilobulated appearance with some cystic degeneration and foci of necrosis.

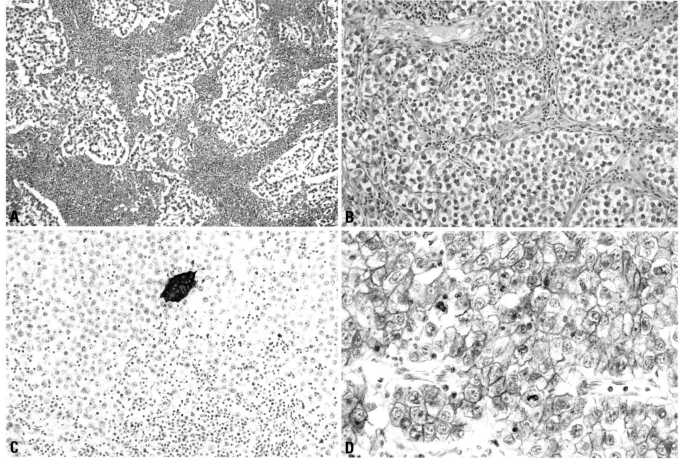

Fig. 2.88 Dysgerminoma. **A** This tumour has thick septa with an extensive chronic inflammatory reaction of granulomatous type. **B** Aggregates of tumour cells are separated by fibrous tissue septa infiltrated by lymphocytes. **C** Occasional beta-human chorionic gonadotropin-positive syncytiotrophoblasts occur. **D** The tumour cells show membranous staining for placental-like alkaline phosphatase.

ulative necrosis may be present and may be associated with cystic change or macroscopic calcification. However, the presence of minute, sandy calcifications should point towards the presence of a concomitant gonadoblastoma. Focal haemorrhagic areas may be indicative of the presence of other germ cell components, possibly containing trophoblastic tissue.

Histopathology
The proliferating germ cells have a monotonous appearance with a polygonal shape, abundant pale cytoplasm and fairly uniform nuclei. They aggregate in cords and clumps, although sometimes the lack of cohesion between cells may lead to the formation of pseudoglandular spaces. Although the stroma is usually reduced to thin perivascular sheaths, occasionally it can be abundant. It always contains variable amounts of chronic inflammatory infiltrate, mainly

composed of T lymphocytes {700} and macrophages. In fact, epithelioid granulomas are a prominent feature in a quarter of cases. Inflammation can also be present in the metastases. The mitotic rate is variable, and some tumours show anisokaryosis. Differentiation in the form of syncytiotrophoblastic cells is found in 5% of cases {3246}. In these cases, beta-human chorionic gonadotropin (β-hCG)-secreting syncytiotrophoblast originates directly from dysgerminoma cells without intervening cytotrophoblast.

Immunoprofile
Most dysgerminomas show positivity for vimentin and placental-like alkaline phosphatase (PLAP) {1660,2011}, the latter is usually found in a membranous location. An inconstant and heterogeneous cytoplasmic positivity can be found to cytoskeletal proteins such as cytokeratins (rarely), desmin, glial fibrillary acidic protein, as well as to S-100

protein and carcinoembryonic antigen (CEA). C-kit gene product (CD117) is present in dysgerminoma as it is in seminoma {2965}, further supporting the similarity to its testicular counterpart.

Precursor lesions
There is no known precursor lesion for the vast majority of dysgerminomas, except for those arising from gonadoblastoma.

Histogenesis
Some dysgerminomas may subsequently be the precursors of other primitive germ cells neoplasms such as yolk sac tumour {2185}.

Prognosis and predictive factors
Dysgerminomas respond to chemotherapy or radiotherapy. The clinical stage of the tumour is probably the only significant prognostic factor {2605}. The presence of a high mitotic index and, in some

cases, anisokaryosis has no prognostic implication The behaviour of dysgerminoma with trophoblastic differentiation is identical to the usual type, but with the advantage of having β-hCG as a serum marker.

Yolk sac tumour

Definition
Yolk sac tumours are morphologically heterogeneous, primitive teratoid neoplasms differentiating into multiple endodermal structures, ranging from the primitive gut to its derivatives of extraembryonal (secondary yolk sac vesicle) and embryonal somatic type, e.g. intestine, liver {2035}. These neoplasms have many epithelial patterns and are typically immunoreactive for alpha-fetoprotein.

Synonym and historical annotation
Since the secondary yolk sac component represents only one of its many lines of differentiation, the current nomenclature is clearly restrictive. Perhaps the term "endodermal primitive tumours" would be more accurate in defining all the possible lines of differentiation, both epithelial and mesenchymal, that occur in these neoplasms.
The term "endodermal sinus tumour", although still in use, is misleading, since the endodermal sinus is neither a structure present in human embryogenesis {1463} nor is it a constant feature of these neoplasms, as it only occurs in a minority of cases {1537}.

Macroscopy
These tumours are usually well encapsulated with an average diameter of 15 cm {1537}. The sectioned tumour surface is soft and grey-yellow with frequent areas

Table 2.05
Morphological patterns of yolk sac tumours with their equivalent types of tissue differentiation.

Site differentiated	Tissue differentiated	Histological pattern
Extraembryonal endoderm	Primitive endoderm and secondary yolk sac	Reticular Solid Endodermal sinus
	Allantois	Polyvesicular
	Murine-type (?) parietal yolk sac	Parietal
Somatic endoderm	Primitive intestine and lung (?)	Glandular
	Early liver	Hepatic

of necrosis, haemorrhage and liquefaction. Cysts can be found in the periphery forming a honeycomb appearance {2043}; rarely, they can be unicystic {522}. A relatively frequent finding is the presence of a benign cystic teratoma in the contralateral ovary {3033}.

Histopathology
Although a marked histological heterogeneity due to numerous patterns of differentiation coexisting in the same neoplasm may occur, almost invariably characteristic areas are present that allow for the correct diagnosis.
The characteristic reticular pattern formed by a loose, basophilic, myxoid stroma harbouring a meshwork of microcystic, labyrinthine spaces lined by clear or flattened epithelial cells with various degrees of atypia and cytoplasmic PAS-positive, diastase-resistant hyaline globules permits tumour identification. Irregular but constant amounts of hyaline, amorphous basement membrane material are found in relation to the epithelial cells. Both hyaline globules and the coarse aggregates of basement membrane material {2032,2979} are good histological indicators for tumour identity. Less frequently, in 13-20% of cases, papillary fibrovascular projections lined by epithelium (Schiller-Duval bodies) are found that bear a resemblance to the structures of the choriovitelline placenta of the rat, a fact that permitted the establishment of the teratoid, endodermal identity of these tumours {2896}.

Histological variants
Less common histological variants include the polyvesicular vitelline tumour, solid yolk sac tumour, parietal yolk sac

tumour, glandular types of yolk sac tumour and hepatoid yolk sac tumour.
In the polyvesicular vitelline tumour cystic, organoid change of the epithelial spaces occurs that consists of multiple dilatations lined by mesothelial-like cells that coexist with a columnar, PAS-positive epithelium {2043}.
The solid yolk sac tumour shows areas of solid epithelial sheets of cells with a characteristic abundant clear cytoplasm and numerous hyaline globules. These areas may resemble anaplastic changes of dysgerminoma or even clear cell tumours {1537} but have the distinctive immunophenotype of a yolk sac tumour.
Although exceptionally rare, parietal-type yolk sac tumours that are AFP-negative have been described {598,620}. They are analogous to the experimental murine tumour of the same name and can be identified by the massive deposition of amorphous extracellular basement membrane, a material similar to the Reichert membrane of the murine parietal yolk sac.
Differentiation into organized somatic endodermal derivatives such as endodermal type gland-like structures resembling early lung and intestine as well as liver tissue can occur in a focal fashion in as many as a third of tumours {1968, 2515,2979}. In rare instances these differentiated tissues may become the predominant elements in the tumour. Extensive differentiation of endodermal type glands characterizes the glandular variants of yolk sac tumours, which may adopt different morphological subtypes. From an embryological viewpoint the more immature type is represented by numerous dilated angular glands or papillae lined by an eosinophilic colum-

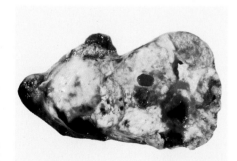

Fig. 2.89 Yolk sac tumour. Sectioned surface is predominately solid and fleshy with areas of haemorrhage, necrosis and cyst formation.

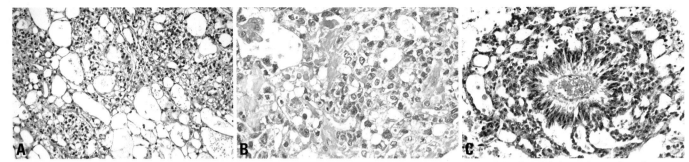

Fig. 2.90 Yolk sac tumour. **A** The reticular pattern is characterized by a loose meshwork of communicating spaces. **B** Hyaline globules and amorphous basement membrane material are present. **C** An endodermal or Schiller-Duval sinus is characteristic.

nar epithelium and surrounded by an oedematous, mesoblastic-type stroma that exhibits the characteristic appearance of early endoderm in both early differentiated intestine and the pseudoglandular phase of the embryonal lung {2038}. Indeed, similar tumours are reported in the lung itself {1968}. This gland-like aspect coupled with the presence of subnuclear vacuolization in the columnar lining mimics early secretory endometrium and endometrioid carcinoma of the ovary and, thus, was named the "endometrioid" variant {522}.

Some endometroid yolk sac tumours are highly differentiated and difficult to distinguish from grade 1 endometrioid carcinoma. Another type of glandular yolk sac tumour is composed of typical small cribriform glands resembling early intestinal differentiation. This type has been termed the intestinal-type of yolk sac tumour {533}.

Extensive differentiation into hepatic tissue is another form of somatic differentiation {2515}. In some yolk sac tumours extensive solid nodular areas of liver tissue can be found {2284} and can be so well formed that they reproduce their laminar structure complete with sinusoids and even haematopoiesis. Finally, since any immature teratoid tissue is considered to be capable of undergoing fully accomplished differentiation, it is possible that pure endodermal immature teratoma composed solely of AFP-secreting endodermal glands and mesenchyme may be closely related to yolk sac tumours {2042}.

Predominance of mesenchymal, rather than epithelial, elements with differentiation into other components such as cartilage, bone or muscle may occur as a postchemotherapeutic conversion and be responsible for the occurrence of associated sarcomas in some cases {1854}. The haematopoietic capacity of the normal secondary yolk sac may have its neoplastic counterpart in yolk sac tumours, where isolated cases of haematological disorders have been reported associated with ovarian yolk sac tumours {1782} in a similar way to those occurring in extragonadal germ cell tumours.

Immunoprofile

AFP is the characteristic marker of the epithelial component of yolk sac tumours, although it is not exclusive to them, as it can also be found in some ovarian tumours that are not of germ cell type. AFP is found as a dense granular cytoplasmic deposit and is absent in hyaline globules, which are rarely immunoreactive. A host of other substances can be found in yolk sac tumours recapitulating the complex functions of early endoderm, including those involved in haematopoiesis {1158,2011}. The usual positivity for cytokeratins may differentiate solid yolk sac tumour from dysgerminoma. CD30 is usually positive in embryonal carcinoma {736} but is only focally positive in yolk sac tumour. Leu M1, which is positive in clear cell carcinoma, is negative in yolk sac tumour. The absence of estrogen and progesterone receptors in yolk sac tumour differentiates areas of yolk sac epithelium from associated areas of true endometrioid tumour {533}.

Prognosis and predictive factors

Because numerous patterns of differenti-

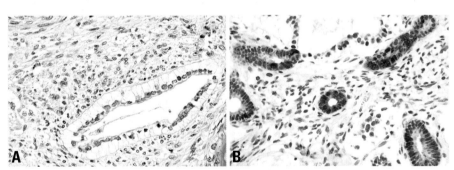

Fig. 2.91 Yolk sac tumour, glandular pattern. **A** Its glands show subnuclear vacuolization characteristic of early differentiated endoderm. **B** Marked cytoplasmic positivity for alpha-fetoprotein is seen in glandular areas.

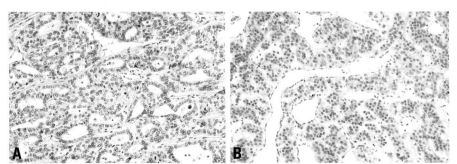

Fig. 2.92 A Yolk sac tumour, intestinal type. Note the cribriform pattern. **B** Yolk sac tumour with hepatic differentiation. The tumour is characterized by liver cell trabeculae and sinusoids.

ation may coexist in the same neoplasm, their behaviour, with some exceptions {1500}, is not conditioned by specific tumour morphology but shows a generally favourable response to chemotherapy. Although the histological appearance bears little prognostic implications, mature or well differentiated glandular forms may have an indolent course even when treated by surgery alone {1500, 2284}.

Embryonal carcinoma and polyembryoma

Definition
Embryonal carcinoma is a tumour composed of epithelial cells resembling those of the embryonic disc and growing in one or more of several patterns, glandular, tubular, papillary and solid. Polyembryoma is a rare tumour composed predomininantly of embryoid bodies resembling early embryos.

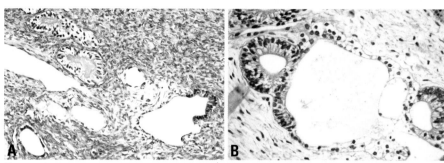

Fig. 2.93 A Yolk sac tumour. Note the polyvesicular vitelline area with biphasic lining. **B** Allantoic remnants from an aborted embryo. The allantoic remnants from an aborted embryo are identical to the polyvesicular vitelline structure shown in A.

Epidemiology
These rare tumours are the ovarian counterparts of their more frequent testicular homologues. Many are reported as a component of mixed germ cell tumours that originate from gonadoblastoma (see section on mixed germ cell-sex cord stromal tumours), arising in Y-chromosome containing dysgenetic gonads (and thus are technically "testicular"

tumours) or even in 46 XX gonads {3253}. They are multipotent stem cell tumours reproducing the primitive stages of embryonal differentiation.

Clinical features
Clinically, β-hCG stimulation may determine various hormonal manifestations such as precocious pseudopuberty in premenarchal girls and vaginal bleeding in adult women {1536}.

Histopathology
Histologically, embryonal carcinoma reveals disorganized sheets of large primitive AFP and CD30-positive cells {736,1536}, forming papillae or crevices which coexist with β-hCG positive syncytiotrophoblasts as well as early teratoid differentiation such as squamous, columnar, mucinous or ciliated epithelia. Its even more infrequent organoid variant is called polyembryoma due to a structural organization into blastocyst-like formations that resemble early presomatic embryos. These so-called embryoid bodies show embryonic disks with corresponding amniotic or primary yolk sac cavities and are surrounded by a mesoblast-like loose connective tissue. The surrounding tissues can differentiate into endodermal structures such as intestine or liver {2287} and trophoblast. However close the resemblance to normal early structures, the sequences of early embryonal development are not reproduced {1969}.

Non-gestational choriocarcinoma

Definition
A rare germ cell tumour composed of cytotrophoblast, syncytiotrophoblast and extravillous trophoblast.

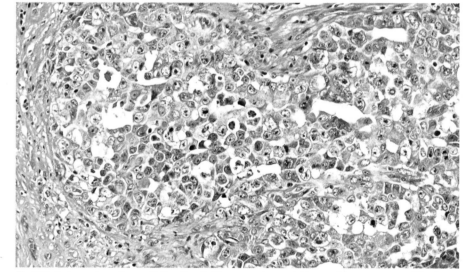

Fig. 2.94 Embryonal carcinoma. Cells with primitive-appearing nuclei form solid aggregates and line irregular gland-like spaces.

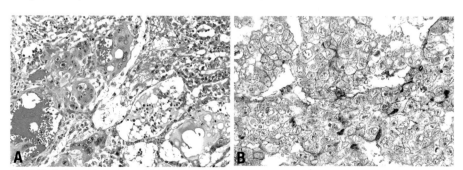

Fig. 2.95 Embryonal carcinoma. **A** Numerous syncytiotrophoblastic giant cells are typical. **B** The tumour cells show membranous staining for placental-like alkaline phosphatase.

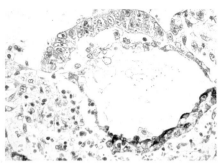

Fig. 2.96 Embryoid body in polyembryoma. Note the blastocyst-like formation consisting of an embryonic disc that is continuous with a primitive yolk sac cavity exhibiting alpha-fetoproten secretion in its distal portion.

Clinical features

Clinically, hormonal manifestations such as precocious pseudopuberty and vaginal bleeding are present in children and young adults.

Macroscopy

Macroscopically, tumours are large and haemorrhagic, and large luteinized nodules or cysts due to β-hCG stimulation may appear in the uninvolved ovarian tissue.

Histopathology

Morphologically identical to gestational choriocarcinoma, primary non-gestational choriocarcinoma is rare in pure form, differentiates as an admixture of cytotrophoblast, syncytiotrophoblast and extravillous trophoblast and is usually found associated with other germ cell components {2704}. Histologically, there are fenestrated or plexiform sheets or pseudopapillae of cytotrophoblast and extravillous trophoblast admixed with numerous syncytiotrophoblasts. Tumour can be found in blood-filled spaces and sinusoids. Vascular invasion is frequent. The immunophenotype is characteristic for each type of proliferating trophoblastic cell {1759} and includes cytokeratins, human placental lactogen and, above all, β-hCG.

Differential diagnosis

When found in a pure form in childbearing age, gestational choriocarcinoma, either primary in the ovary {3024} or metastatic {718} must be excluded. This may be accomplished by identifying paternal sequences by DNA analysis {1698,2655}.

Prognosis and predictive factors

The distinction from gestational choriocarcinoma is important since non-gestational choriocarcinoma has a less favourable prognosis and requires more aggressive chemotherapeutic treatment regimens.

Mixed germ cell tumours

Definition

Mixed germ cell tumours are composed of at least two different germ cell elements of which at least one is primitive.

Clinical features

The value of tumour markers such as β-hCG and AFP in the diagnosis and follow-up of patients with mixed germ cell tumours containing elements of choriocarcinoma or yolk sac tumour has been proven over the years {2850}. Elevated serum levels of these markers should prompt a search for different components with extensive sampling of the tumour.

Histopathology

Histologically, the most common combination of neoplastic germ cell elements found in ovarian mixed germ cell tumours is dysgerminoma and yolk sac tumour {2850}. Additional neoplastic germ cell elements, including immature or mature teratoma, embryonal carcinoma, polyembryoma and/or choriocarcinoma, may also be present. All components of a mixed germ cell tumour and their approximate proportions should be mentioned in the diagnosis.

Most ovarian embryonal carcinomas are really malignant mixed germ cell tumours, usually admixed with yolk sac tumour and showing a large or predominant component of embryonal carcinoma {2850}. Although polyembryoma may have been the predominant malignant germ cell element within the tumour, a careful review of all the published cases of ovarian polyembryoma shows that other germ cell elements were also present {2850}. Also, ovarian choriocarcinoma of germ cell origin is in the majority of cases combined with other neoplastic germ cell elements. Immunohistochemical demonstration of β-hCG and AFP is a useful diagnostic modality in this group of tumours, as is the demonstration of PLAP in a component of dysgerminoma

Prognosis and predictive factors

All elements in a malignant mixed germ cell tumour are capable of widespread metastatic dissemination. The metastases may be composed of a single neoplastic germ cell element or of various elements.

Although these tumours are highly responsive to platinum-based chemotherapy, the therapeutic regimens should be based primarily on the most malignant elements of the tumour {2850}.

Biphasic or triphasic teratomas

Definition

Tumours composed of derivatives of two or three primary germ layers (ectoderm, mesoderm, endoderm).

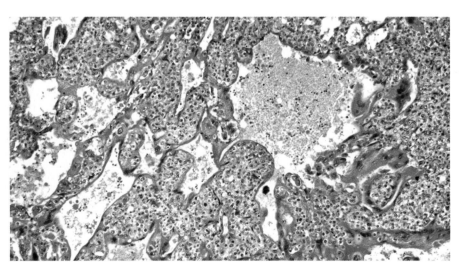

Fig. 2.97 Ovarian choriocarcinoma. A plexiform pattern is present with syncytiotrophoblasts covering clusters of smaller cytotrophoblasts.

Table 2.06
Grading of ovarian immature teratomas.

Three-tiered grading system {2060}
Grade 1 Tumours with rare foci of immature neuroepithelial tissue that occupy less than one low power field (40x) in any slide.
Grade 2 Tumours with similar elements, occupying 1 to 3 low power fields (40x) in any slide.
Grade 3 Tumours with large amount of immature neuroepithelial tissue occupying more than 3 low power fields (40x) in any slide.

Table 2.07
Management of immature teratomas according to grade of primary tumours and/or implants.

Three-tiered grading {2060}	Two-tiered grading {2072}	Stage	Combination chemotherapy
Grade 1 ovarian tumour	Low grade	Ia	Not required
Grade 2 or 3 ovarian tumour	High grade	Ia	Required
Grade 2 or 3 implants	High grade	≥ II	Required
Grade 0 implants* regardless of ovarian tumour grade		≥ II	Not required
* Those extraovarian implants that are composed of mature tissue, essentially glia.			

ICD-O codes
Immature teratoma	9080/3
Mature teratoma	9080/0
Cystic teratoma	9080/0
Dermoid cyst	9084/0

Immature teratoma

Definition
A teratoma containing a variable amount of immature, embryonal-type (generally immature neuroectodermal) tissue.

Epidemiology
Immature teratoma represents 3% of teratomas, 1% of all ovarian cancers and 20% of malignant ovarian germ cell tumours and is found either in pure form or as a component of a mixed germ cell tumour {989}. It occurs essentially during the two first decade of life (from 1-46 years; average 18) {989,1174,2060}.

Macroscopy
Immature teratoma is typically unilateral, large, variegated (6-35 cm; average, 18.5), predominantly solid, fleshy, and grey-tan and may be cystic with haemorrhage and necrosis {989,2060}.

Histopathology
Immature teratoma is composed of variable amounts of immature embryonal-type tissues, mostly in the form of neuroectodermal rosettes and tubules, admixed with mature tissue. Neuroepithelial rosettes are lined by crowded basophilic cells with numerous mitoses {2060} and may be pigmented. Immature mesenchyme in the form of loose, myxoid stroma with focal differentiation into immature cartilage, fat, osteoid and rhabdomyoblasts is often present as well {2060}. Immature endodermal structures including hepatic tissue, intestinal-type epithelium with basal

vacuolization and embryonic renal tissue resembling Wilms tumour are encountered less frequently. Immature vascular structures may occur and are sometimes prominent.

Grading
Based on the quantity of the immature neuroepithelial component, primary and metastatic ovarian immature teratomas (including peritoneal implants and lymph nodes metastases) are separately graded from 1 to 3 {2060}. More recently the possibility of using a two-tiered (low grade and high grade) grading system was suggested {2072}. Adequate sampling of the primary tumour (one block per 1 or 2 cm of tumour) and of all resected implants is crucial, as the tumour grade may vary in different implants.

Somatic genetics
Immature teratomas grades 1-2 are

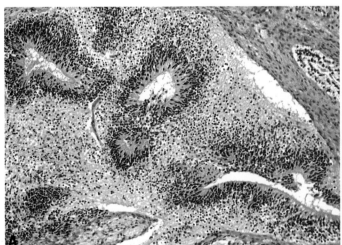
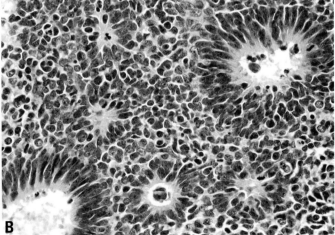

Fig. 2.98 A Immature teratoma, high grade. Neuroectodermal rosettes lie in a background of glial tissue. **B** Mitotic figures are evident within the immature neuroectodemal tissue.

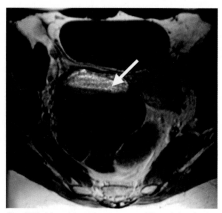

Fig. 2.99 Mature cystic teratoma. T1-weighted pre-contrast magnetic resonance image. A fat-fluid level is seen (arrow).

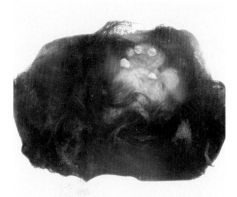

Fig. 2.100 Mature cystic teratoma with dark hair. The Rokitansky protuberance is composed of fatty tissue, bone, and teeth protuding into the lumen.

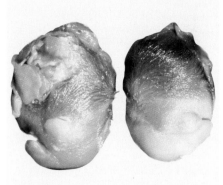

Fig. 2.101 Fetiform teratoma (homunculus). Limb buds are apparent, and there is abundant hair over the cephalic portion.

diploid in 90% of cases, whereas most (66%) of grade 3 tumours are aneuploid {165,2684}. Similarly, karyotypic abnormalities are most often seen in grade 3 tumours {165}. Immature teratomas show fewer DNA copy number changes detected by comparative genomic hybridization than other ovarian germ cell tumours and do not usually exhibit a gain of 12p or i(12p) {1518,2378}.

Prognosis and predictive factors
The stage and grade of the primary tumour and the grade of its metastases are important predictive factors. Prior to the chemotherapy era, the overall survival rate of patients with grade 1, 2 and 3 neoplasms was 82%, 63% and 30%, respectively {2060}.
The use of cisplatin-based combination chemotherapy has dramatically improved the survival rate of patients; 90-100% of those receiving this regimen remain disease-free {989}.
The tumour grade is a crucial feature that determines behaviour and type of therapy. Patients with grade 1 tumours that are stage IA and those with mature (grade 0) implants do not require adjuvant chemotherapy. Those with grade 2 or 3 tumours, including stage IA, as well as those with immature implants require combination chemotherapy. The management of patients with grade 1 implants/metastases is not well established.
A recent report from the Pediatric Oncology Group concludes that surgery alone is curative in children and adolescents with immature teratoma of any grade, reserving chemotherapy for

cases with relapse {600}. Also, in immature teratomas occurring in childhood, the presence of histological foci of yolk sac tumour rather than the grade of the immature component, per se, is the only predictor of recurrence {1174}.

Mature teratoma

Definition
A cystic or, more rarely, a solid tumour composed exclusively of mature, adult-type tissues. A cyst lined by mature tissue resembling the epidermis with its appendages is clinically designated as "dermoid cyst". Homunculus or fetiform teratoma is a rare type of mature, solid teratoma containing highly organized structures resembling a malformed fetus ("homunculus" = little man).

Epidemiology
Age
Although most mature cystic teratomas occur during the reproductive years, they have a wide age distribution, from 2-80 years (mean, 32), and 5% occur in postmenopausal women {564}. Mature solid teratoma occurs mainly in the first two decades of life {199,2922}.

Incidence
Mature cystic teratoma accounts for 27-44% of all ovarian tumours and up to 58% of the benign tumours {1502}. In addition to their pure form, dermoid cysts are found macroscopically within 25% of immature teratomas and in the ovary contralateral to a malignant primitrive germ cell tumour in 10-15% of the cases.

Clinical features
Signs and symptoms
Most mature cystic teratomas present with a mass, but at least 25% (up to 60% in some series) are discovered incidentally {546}. Symptoms such as a pelvic mass or pain are more common when the mature teratoma is solid {199,2922}.
The following complications have been described:
(1) Torsion of the pedicle occurs in 10-16% of the cases, is responsible for acute abdominal pain and may be complicated by infarction, perforation or intra-abdominal haemorrhage.
(2) Tumour rupture occurs in 1% of cases and can be spontaneous or traumatic. The spillage of the cyst contents into the peritoneum produces chemical peritonitis with granulomatous nodules mimicking tuberculosis or carcinomatosis. Rupture of mature teratoma containing neuroglial elements is thought to be responsible for gliomatosis peritonei characterized by peritoneal "implants" composed of mature glial tissue and does not affect the prognosis {2389}. However, a recent molecular study has demonstrated that these glial implants were heterozygous, whereas the associated mature ovarian teratomas were homozygous at the same microsatellite loci. This finding suggests that glial implants may arise from metaplasia of pluripotent müllerian stem cells rather than from implantation of the associated ovarian teratomas {845}. Similarly, peritoneal melanosis characterized by pigmentation of the peritoneum has been reported in cases of dermoid cysts.
(3) Infection of the tumour occurs in 1% of cases.

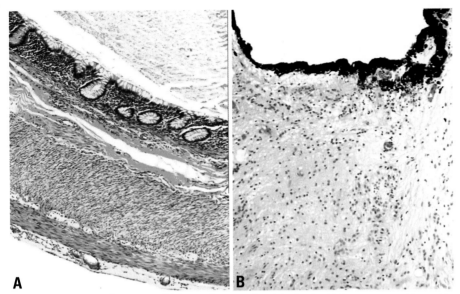

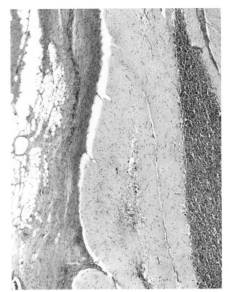

Fig. 2.102 A Mature cystic teratoma. Adult-type tissues such as intestine tend to have an organoid arrangement with two layers of smooth muscle beneath glandular mucosa. **B** Note the pigmented retinal epithelium and associated mature glial tissue.

Fig. 2.103 Mature teratoma. Note the cerebellar structures adjacent to adipose and fibrous connective tissue.

(4) Haemolytic anaemia has been reported in rare cases {1020}.

Macroscopy
Dermoid cyst is an ovoid, occasionally bilateral (8-15% of cases), cystic mass of 0.5-40 cm (average 15 cm) with a smooth external surface and is filled with sebaceous material and hair. A nodule composed of fat tissue with teeth or bone protrudes into the cyst and is termed a Rokitansky protuberance.
Mature solid teratoma is a large, solid mass with multiple cysts of varying size, a soft, cerebroid appearance and small foci of haemorrhage.

Histopathology
Mature teratomas are composed of adult-type tissue derived from two or three embryonic layers. Benign tumours such as struma ovarii, carcinoid, corticotroph cell adenoma, prolactinoma, naevus and glomus tumour may arise within a typical dermoid cyst {143, 1389,2162,2682}.

Histogenesis
The presence of Barr bodies (nuclear sex chromatin) and a 46 XX karyotype is consistent with origin through parthenogenetic development. Selective tissue microdissection and genetic analysis of mature ovarian teratomas demonstrated a genotypic difference between homozygous teratomatous tissues and heterozygous host tissue in support of their origin from a post-meiotic germ cell {1667, 3032}. Lymphoid aggregates associated with squamous or glandular epithelium within teratomas are heterozygous and derived from host tissue, whereas well differentiated thymic tissue is homozygous, suggesting capability for lymphoid differentiation {3032}.
Although multiple teratomas in the same ovary originate independently from different progenitor germ cells, they may appear histologically similar indicating the role of possible local and environmental factors in phenotypic differentiation of ovarian germ cell tumours {683}.

Prognosis and predictive factors
Dermoid cysts with histological foci (up to 21 mm²) of immature neuroepithelial tissue have an excellent prognosis {3174}. Recurrence in the form of a dermoïd cyst (3% of cases) or immature teratoma (2-2.6% of cases) in the residual ipsilateral ovary is most frequent when the initial cysts are bilateral or multiple and have ruptured {104,3174}.

Monodermal teratomas and somatic-type tumours associated with dermoid cysts

Definition
Teratomas composed exclusively or predominantly of a single type of tissue derived from one embryonic layer (ectoderm or endoderm) and adult-type tumours derived from a dermoid cyst.

ICD-O codes
Struma ovarii	9090/0
Carcinoid	8240/3
Mucinous carcinoid	8243/3
Strumal carcinoid	9091/1
Ependymoma	9391/3
Primitive neuroectodermal tumour	9473/3
Glioblastoma multiforme	9440/3
Teratoma with malignant transformation	9084/3
Malignant melanoma	8720/3
Melanocytic naevus	8720/0
Sebaceous adenoma	8410/0
Sebaceous carcinoma	8410/3
Retinal anlage tumour	9363/0

Struma ovarii

Definition
A mature teratoma composed either exclusively or predominantly of thyroid tissue. Struma ovarii may harbour changes histologically identical to thyroid adenoma, carcinoma (malignant struma ovarii) or both. Those admixed with a carcinoid (strumal carcinoid) are classified separately.

Epidemiology
Struma ovarii, the most common type of monodermal teratoma, accounts for 2.7% of all ovarian teratomas {3146} with

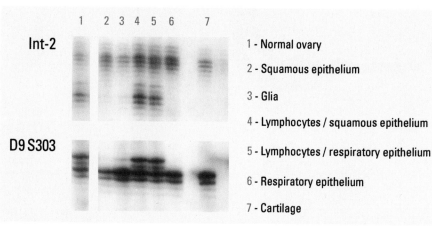

Fig. 2.104 Genetic analysis of various histological components selectively microdissected from a mature ovarian teratoma using microsatellite markers INT-2 (11q13) and D95303 (99). Teratomatous components are homozygous showing one allelic band, whereas lymphocytes associated with squamous and respiratory epithelium are heterozygous with both allelic bands, similar to host tissue (normal ovarian stroma).

1 - Normal ovary

2 - Squamous epithelium

3 - Glia

4 - Lymphocytes / squamous epithelium

5 - Lymphocytes / respiratory epithelium

6 - Respiratory epithelium

7 - Cartilage

malignant struma ovarii representing 0.01% of all ovarian tumours and 5-10% of all struma ovarii. Most patients are in their fifth decade {3146}.

Clinical features
Signs and symptoms
Patients present with a palpable abdominal mass or unusual symptoms including Meigs syndrome {983}, cervical thyroid hypertrophy and thyrotoxicosis (5% of cases) with high pelvic iodine uptake {2697}. An elevated serum level of thyroglobulin occurs in malignant struma ovarii {2412}.

Macroscopy
The tumour is unilateral and varies from 0.5-10 cm in diameter. It has a brown solid and gelatinous sectioned surface and sometimes appears as a nodule within a dermoid cyst. Entirely cystic strumas containing green gelatinous material also occur {2831}.

Histopathology
Struma ovarii is composed of normal or hyperplastic thyroid-type tissue with patterns seen in thyroid adenoma such as microfollicular, macrofollicular, trabecular and solid. Oxyphil or clear cells may be found {2832}. Cystic struma is composed of thin fibrous septa lined by flat, cuboidal cells with sparse typical thyroid follicles in the cyst wall {2831}. Immunoreactivity for thyroglobulin may be helpful in problematic cases such as cystic struma, oxyphilic or clear cell variants and a trabecular architecture that

might be indistinguishable from Sertoli-Leydig cell tumours. Criteria used for malignant changes within struma ovarii are the same as those used for a diagnosis of malignancy in the thyroid gland {677,2387}. Papillary carcinomas (85% of cases) display the characteristic ground glass nuclei. However, follicular

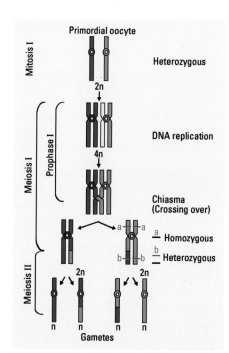

Fig. 2.105 Meiotic division. Primordial germ cells are heterozygous with all informative microsatellite markers. After the first meiotic division and crossing over between homologous chromatids, a homozygous genotype is demonstrated with microsatellite marker "a" while a heterozygous genotype is seen with microsatellite marker "b".

carcinomas are difficult to diagnose since struma ovarii generally lacks a capsule and has irregular margins. The thyroid tissue of struma may be uniformly malignant in some cases, undoubtedly arising in such cases from histological foci of normal-appearing thyroid tissue, which are not extensive enough in itself to qualify for the diagnosis of struma ovarii.

Prognosis and predictive factors
Tumours with the morphology of papillary or follicular thyroid cancer and extra-ovarian spread at presentation are probably the only lesions that deserve a designation of malignant struma, whilst the so-called "benign strumatosis", peritoneal implants composed of benign thyroid-type tissue, does not alter the prognosis. Factors increasing the likelihood of recurrences include the size, the presence of ascites or adhesions and solid architecture, whereas the mitotic rate and vascular invasion (identified in 15% of malignant strumas) are not prognostically helpful features {2387}.

Carcinoids

Definition
These tumours contain extensive components of well differentiated neuroendocrine cells and most subtypes resemble carcinoids of the gastrointestinal tract. They may occur in pure form or within a dermoid cyst, a mucinous cystic tumour or a Brenner tumour. It should be distinguished from isolated neuroendocrine cells found within some mucinous and Sertoli-Leydig cell tumours.

Epidemiology
Ovarian carcinoids account for 0.5-1.7% of all carcinoids {2743}, and the age range is 14-79 years (mean 53) {166, 2388,2390,2392}.

Clinical features
Signs and symptoms
Carcinoid syndrome is a clinical sign of insular carcinoids in 30% of patients and is rare in trabecular (13%) and strumal (3.2%) carcinoids {631,2743}. Peptide YY production by the tumour cells causes severe constipation and pain with defecation in 25% of trabecular carcinoids {2656}. Strumal carcinoids may cause symptoms of functioning thyroid tissue in 8% of cases {2390}.

Diagnostic procedures

Elevated urine 5-hydroxyindoleacetic acid (5-HIAA) and serum serotonin levels are found in patients with carcinoid syndrome {631,2388}.

Macroscopy

Primary ovarian carcinoids are unilateral and present as a firm tan nodule (less than 5 cm) protruding into a typical dermoid cyst (32-60% of tumours) or are predominantly solid with small cysts. The sectioned surface is firm, homogeneous and tan to yellow.

Histopathology

Insular carcinoid accounts for 26-53% of cases {631,2743}) and resembles midgut derivative carcinoids. It is composed of nests of round cells with uniform nuclei and abundant eosinophilic cytoplasm enclosing small red argentaffin granules at the periphery of the nests. Acinus formation and a cribriform pattern with luminal eosinophilic secretion are present {2388}.

Trabecular carcinoid accounts for 23-29% of cases {631,2743} and resembles hindgut or foregut derivative carcinoids. It exhibits wavy and anastomosing ribbons composed of columnar cells with the long axes of the cells parallel to one another and oblong nuclei with prominent nucleoli. The abundant cytoplasm is finely granular with red-orange argyrophilic granules at both poles of the nucleus {2392}.

Mucinous carcinoid accounts for only 1.5% of cases {2743} and resembles goblet cell carcinoids arising in the appendix. The well differentiated mucinous carcinoid is composed of numerous small glands lined by columnar or cuboidal cells, some of which contain intracytoplasmic mucin or have a goblet cell appearance, whilst others disclose

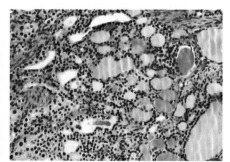

Fig. 2.106 Struma ovarii. The struma resembles a thyroid microfollicular adenoma with dystrophic nuclei.

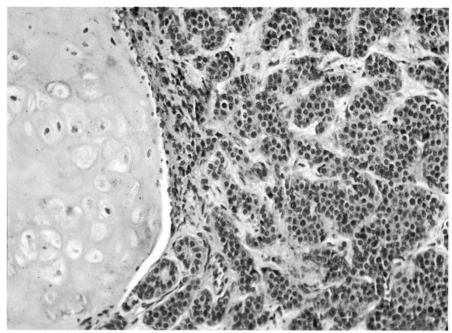

Fig. 2.107 Carcinoid arising in a teratoma. Nests and cords of carcinoid cells proliferate next to a chrondroid nodule.

orange-red neuroendocrine granules. Individual tumour cells may contain both mucin and neuroendocrine granules. Glands may be floating within pools of mucin that also dissect the surrounding fibrous stroma with isolated signet-ring cells infiltrating the stroma. Atypical mucinous carcinoid demonstrates crowded glands or a cribriform pattern. Carcinoma arising in mucinous carcinoid exhibits large islands of tumour cells or closely packed glands with high grade nuclei, numerous mitoses and necrosis {166}.

Strumal carcinoid accounts for 26-44% of cases {631,2743} and is composed of a variable proportion of thyroid tissue and carcinoid, the latter mostly having a trabecular architecture. The neuroendocrine cells invade progressively the strumal component, replacing the follicular lining cells. Glands or cysts lined by columnar epithelium with goblet cells may be found {2390}.

Carcinoids with mixed patterns (essentially insular and trabecular), are classified according to the pattern that predominates {2388}.

Immunoprofile

Carcinoids are immunoreactive to at least one of the neuroendocrine markers (chromogranin, synaptophysin, Leu-7) and various peptide hormones such as pan-

creatic polypeptide, gastrin, vasoactive intestinal peptides and glucagon {166}.

Differential diagnosis

Metastatic gastrointestinal carcinoid to the ovary should be ruled out specifically when extraovarian disease is detected. Bilateral and multinodular ovarian involvement, the absence of other teratomatous components and the persistence of the carcinoid syndrome after oophorectomy favour the diagnosis of metastasis {166,2391}.

Prognosis and predictive features

Almost all primary trabecular and strumal carcinoids occur in women with stage I disease and have an excellent outcome. The overall survival of patients with insular carcinoid is 95% at 5 years and 88% at 10 years {2388}.

Primary ovarian mucinous carcinoid, like those in the appendix, has a more aggressive behaviour with extraovarian spread and lymph node metastases. The presence of frank carcinoma within the tumour is an important prognostic factor {166}.

Neuroectodermal tumours

Definition

Tumours composed almost exclusively of neuroectodermal tissue, closely resem-

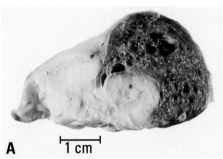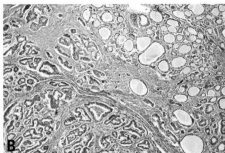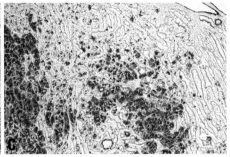

Fig. 2.108 Strumal carcinoid. **A** Sectioned surface of the ovarian tumour shows a spongy brown area reflecting the strumal component and a solid yellow region reflecting the carcinoid component. **B** The strumal and carcinoid tumour patterns are located side by side, with the struma on the right. **C** Immunoreactivity for cytokeratin 7 is present in the strumal elements but not in the carcinoid trabeculae.

bling neoplasms of the nervous system with a similar spectrum of differentiation.

Epidemiology
Less than 40 cases are reported in patients 6-69 years old (average 28), {1077,1418,1476}.

Clinical features
The tumours usually present as a pelvic mass.

Macroscopy
Tumours are unilateral and 4-20 cm in diameter, averaging 14 cm {1476}. The sectioned surface varies from solid with friable, gray-pink tissue to cystic with papillary excrescences in their inner or outer surface {1077}.

Tumour spread and staging
The majority of patients have stage II or III disease at laparotomy usually in the form of peritoneal implants {1476}.

Histopathology
These tumours are morphologically identical to their nervous system counterparts. They may be divided into three categories as follows:
(1) Well differentiated forms such as ependymoma.
(2) Poorly differentiated tumours such as primitive neurectodermal tumour (PNET), and medulloepithelioma.
(3) Anaplastic forms such as glioblastoma multiforme.
Whilst ependymomas are not found in association with teratoma, other neuroectodermal tumours in the ovary may be associated with elements of mature or immature teratoma {2605}. Cases previously reported as neuroblastoma or medulloblastoma would now most likely be classifed as PNETs since the mor-

phology of all three tumours is similar with the term medulloblastoma being reserved for cerebellar and neuroblastoma for adrenal neoplasms {1474}. Medulloepithelioma, on the other hand, has a distinctive appearance characterized by papillary, tubular or trabecular arrangements of neoplasiic neuroepithelium mimicking the embryonic neural tube {1474}.
Ependymomas and anaplastic tumours are immunoreactive for glial fibrillary acidic protein. The characteristic immunoprofile of PNETs, vimentin and MIC2 protein (CD99) positive and GFAP, cytokeratin, desmin. chromogranin, and inhibin negative, help to distinguish these tumours from small cell carcinoma and juvenile granulosa cell tumour.

Somatic genetics
Reverse transcription-polymerase chain reaction in a case of ovarian PNET led to the detection of *EWS/FLI1* chimeric transcript, originating from the characteristic t(11;22)(q24;q12) translocation of the PNET/Ewing tumour family {1418}.

Prognosis and predictive factors
Most patients with ovarian ependymomas survive despite multiple recurrences, whereas patients with PNET and anaplastic tumours have a poor outcome {1476}.

Carcinomas

Definition
A dermoid cyst in which a secondary carcinoma develops.

Epidemiology
Malignancy arising within a mature cystic teratoma is a rare complication (1-2% of cases), mostly reported in post-

menopausal women (mean 51-62 years) {1214,1429,2164}.

Clinical features
The tumour may present as a dermoid cyst or as an advanced ovarian cancer depending on tumour stage {2605}. The tumour may show adherence to surrounding pelvic structures {1214, 1429,2164}.

Macroscopy
On macroscopic examination cauliflower exophytic growth, infiltrative grey-white plaques or thickenings of the cyst wall with necrosis and haemorrhage may be seen {1214,1429,2164}.

Histopathology
The malignancy may be detectable only after histological examination, thus dermoid cysts in postmenopausal women must be adequately sampled. Any component of a mature teratoma may undergo malignant transformation. Carcinomas are the most common malignancy, with squamous cell carcinomas accounting for 80% of cases and 51% of all primary ovarian squamous cell carcinomas {1214,2255}. Adenocarcinoma is the second most common lmalignancy arising in dermoid cysts {1456}. Adenocarcinoma of intestinal type {2970}, Paget disease, adenosquamous carcinoma, transitional cell carcinoma {1456}, undifferentiated carcinoma, small cell carcinoma, basal cell carcinoma and carcinosarcoma {123} have been described {2605}. The malignant component invades other parts of the dermoid cyst and its wall.

Somatic genetics
Selective tissue microdissection and genetic analyses of malignant tumours

associated with mature teratomas showed an identical homozygous genotype for the malignant component and the mature teratomatous tissues, thus demonstrating a direct pathogenetic relationship {683}.

Prognosis and predictive features

The prognosis of squamous cell carcinoma is poor with a 15-52% overall 5-year survival and disease related death usually within 9 months. Vascular invasion is associated with a high mortality rate {1214}. Although relatively few cases have been reported, the prognosis of adenocarcinoma appears to be similar to that of squamous cell carcinoma {2970}.

Sarcomas

Sarcomas account for 8% of cases of malignancies in dermoid cysts and are more often seen in younger patients than those with squamous cell carcinoma. Cases of leiomyosarcoma, angiosarcoma {2021}, osteosarcoma {2006}, chondrosarcoma, fibrosarcoma, rhabdomyosarcoma and malignant fibrous histiocytoma have been reported {2605}.

Melanocytic tumours

Melanomas are rare, occurring much less commonly than metastatic melanoma {630}. Overall, one-half of the patients with stage I dermoid-associated melanoma are alive at 2 years {404}. Melanocytic naevi of various types may arise within a typical dermoid cyst {1544}.

Sebaceous tumours

Sebaceous tumours are specialized neoplasms arising within an ovarian dermoid cyst that resemble various forms of cutaneous sebaceous gland tumours (sebaceous adenoma, basal cell carcinoma with sebaceous differentiation, sebaceous carcinoma). The hallmark of these lesions is the presence of large numbers of mature, foamy or bubbly sebaceous cells that stain positively with oil red O in a tumour arising within a dermoid cyst {491}.

Pituitary-type tumours

Corticotroph cell adenoma and prolactinoma, respectively responsible for

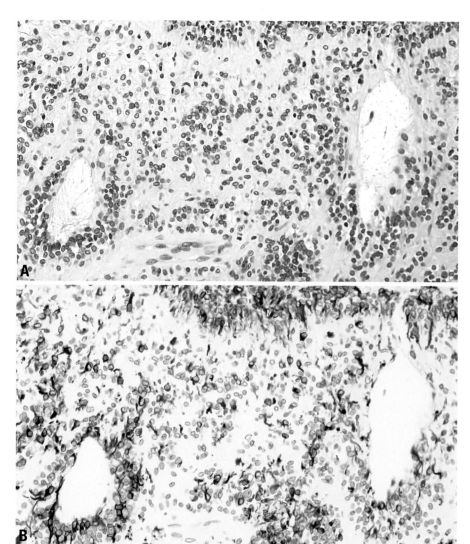

Fig. 2.109 Ependymoma of the ovary. **A** The tumour cells have uniform nuclei and form two rosettes. **B** Many tumour cells are strongly positive for glial fibrillary acidic protein with accentuated staining around the rosettes.

Cushing syndrome and hyperprolactinema with amenorrhea, may arise within a typical dermoid cyst and have a benign clinical course {143,1389,2162}.

Retinal anlage tumours

Pigmented progonoma and malignant tumours derived from retinal anlage within ovarian teratomas have macroscopically pigmented areas that correspond to solid nests, tubules and papillae composed of atypical cells with melanin-containing cytoplasm {1112,1466,2712}.

Other monodermal teratomas and related tumours

Neural cyst of the ovary lined by a single layer of ependymal cells with white matter, astrocytes and reactive glia in the underlying wall corresponds to a monodermal teratoma with unidirectional neurogenic differentiation {894}. Similarly, endodermal variants of mature teratoma lined exclusively by respiratory epithelium {508} and ovarian epidermoid cysts {823} may fall into the category of monodermal teratoma.

Mucinous cystadenomas arising within mature teratomas have a homozygous teratomatous genotype, supporting their germ cell origin {1731}. Mesodermal derived tumours such as lipoma composed of mature adipocytes with scattered benign sweat glands may occur {961}. Glomus tumour may rarely arise within a typical dermoid cyst {2682}.

Mixed germ cell-sex cord-stromal tumours

A. Talerman
P. Schwartz

This group of neoplasms is composed of a mixture of germ cell and sex cord-stromal elements. They have mainly benign clinical behaviour except in cases with a malignant germ cell component.

Gonadoblastoma

Definition
A neoplasm composed of tumour cells closely resembling dysgerminoma or seminoma, intimately admixed with sex cord derivatives resembling immature Sertoli or granulosa cells and in some cases containing stromal derivatives mimicking luteinized stromal or Leydig cells devoid of Reinke crystals.

ICD-O code
Gonadoblastoma   9073/1

Epidemiology
Gonadoblastomas typically are identified in children or young adults with one-third of the tumours being detected before the age of 15 {2598}.

Aetiology
Gonadoblastomas are frequently associated with abnormalities in the secondary sex organs {2598,2847}. In over 90% of the cases of gonadoblastoma a Y chromosome was detected {2598,2605,2849, 2850}.

Localization
Gonadoblastoma is found more often in the right gonad than in the left and is bilateral in 38% of cases {2598}. Recent reports suggest an even higher frequency of bilateral involvement {2850}.

Clinical features
Signs and symptoms
The usual patient with a gonadoblastoma is a phenotypic female who is frequently virilized {2605}. A minority may present as phenotypic males with varying degrees of feminization.
The clinical presentation of a patient with a gonadoblastoma can vary considerably depending upon whether or not a tumour mass is present, on the nature of the underlying abnormal gonads, on the development of secondary sex organs and the occasional secretion of steroid hormones {2598}. A patient with pure gonadal dysgenesis may present with a failure to develop secondary sex organs and characteristics at puberty but has a normal height, and other congenital anomalies are absent. Those with Turner syndrome have sexual immaturity, a height of less than 150 cm and one or more congenital anomalies including neonatal lymphedema, web neck, prognathism, shield-shaped chest, widely spaced nipples, cubitus valgus, congenital nevi, coarctation of the aorta, renal anomalies, short fifth metacarpal bones and others {2598}. If a germ cell malignancy develops in the dysgenetic gonad, the patient may present with lower abdominal or pelvic pain.

Macroscopy
Pure gonadoblastoma varies from a histological lesion to 8 cm, and most tumours are small, measuring only a few cm {2598,2849,2850}. When a gonadoblastoma is overgrown by dysgerminoma or other neoplastic germ cell elements, much larger tumours are encountered. The macroscopic appearance of gonadoblastoma varies depending on the presence of hyalinization and calcification and on the overgrowth by other malignant germ cell elements.

Histopathology
Histologically, gonadoblastoma is a tumour composed of two main cell types, germ cells which are similar to those present in dysgerminoma or seminoma and sex cord derivatives resembling immature Sertoli or granulosa cells. The stroma in addition may contain collections of luteinized or Leydig-like cells devoid of Reinke crystals. The tumour is arranged in collections of cellular nests surrounded by connective tissue stroma. The nests are solid, usually small, oval or round, but occasionally may be larger or elongated. The cellular nests are composed of germ cells and sex cord deriv-

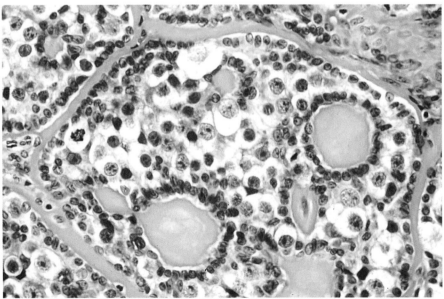

Fig. 2.110 Gonadoblastoma. The tumour consists of cellular nests(germ cells and sex cord derivatives) surrounded by connective tissue stroma. The sex cord derivatives form a coronal pattern along the periphery of the nests and also surround small round spaces containing hyaline material. A mixture of cells is present in the centre of the nests.

atives intimately admixed. The germ cells are large and round with clear or slightly granular cytoplasm and large, round, vesicular nuclei, often with prominent nucleoli, and show mitotic activity, which may be brisk. Their histological and ultra-structural appearance and histochemical reactions are similar to the germ cells of dysgerminoma or seminoma. The immature Sertoli or granulosa cells are smaller and epithelial-like. These cells are round or oval and contain dark, oval or slightly elongated carrot-shaped nuclei. They do not show mitotic activity {2598,2849, 2850}. The sex cord derivatives are arranged within the cell nests in three typical patterns as follows:
(1) Forming a coronal pattern along the periphery of the nests.
(2) Surrounding individual or collections of germ cells.
(3) Surrounding small round spaces containing amorphous, hyaline, eosinophilic, PAS-positive material resembling Call-Exner bodies.
The connective tissue stroma surrounding the cellular nests may be scant or abundant and cellular, resembling ovarian stroma, or dense and hyalinized. It may contain luteinized or Leydig-like cells devoid of Reinke crystals {2598, 2849,2850}.
Three processes, hyalinization, calcification and overgrowth by a malignant germ cell element, usually dysgerminoma, may alter the basic histological appearance of gonadoblastoma. The hyalinization occurs by coalescence of the hyaline bodies and bands of hyaline material around the nests with replacement of the cellular contents. Calcification originates in the hyaline Call-Exner-like bodies and is seen histologically in more than 80% of cases {2598}. It tends to replace the hyalinized nests forming rounded, calcified concretions. Coalescence of such concretions may lead to the calcification of the whole lesion, and the presence of smooth, rounded, calcified bodies may be the only evidence that gonadoblastoma has been present. The term "burned-out gonadoblastoma" has been applied to such lesions {2598,2849,2850}. Gonadoblastoma is overgrown by dysgerminoma in approximately 50% of cases, and in an additional 10% another malignant germ cell element is present {2598,2846, 2849,2850}. Gonadoblastoma has never been observed in metastatic lesions or

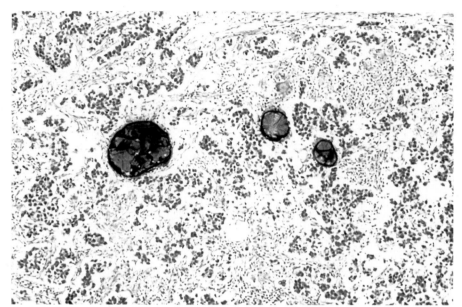

Fig. 2.111 Dysgerminoma with "burnt out" gonadoblastoma. The typical pattern of a dysgerminoma consists of aggegates of primitive germ cells separated by fibrous septa infiltrated by lymphocytes. The presence of "burnt out" gonadoblastoma is indicated by smooth, rounded, calcified bodies.

outside the gonads {2598,2849,2850}.
In most cases the gonad of origin is indeterminate because it is overgrown by the tumour. When the nature of the gonad can be identified, it is usually a streak or a testis. The contralateral gonad, when identifiable, may be either a streak or a testis, and the latter is more likely to harbour a gonadoblastoma {2598,2849, 2850}. Occasionally, gonadoblastoma may be found in otherwise normal ovaries {2077,2598,2849,2850}.

Tumour spread and staging
At the time of operation gonadoblastomas typically are bilateral, although at times they may be not macroscopically detectible in the gonad. Those that are overgrown by dysgerminoma or other malignant germ cell tumour may be much larger. If a malignant germ cell tumour develops, the potential for metastatic disease exists. Dysgerminomas typically spread by the lymphatic route, less frequently by peritoneal dissemination. Therefore, it is extremely important not only to remove both gonads but to perform surgical staging if at the time of operative consultation a malignant germ cell tumour is identified. The typical staging for a dysgerminoma or other malignant germ cell tumour includes pelvic and para-aortic lymph node sampling as well as peritoneal washings if no ascites is present {2586}.

The operation should include omentectomy, and multiple peritoneal samplings are required. For patients with spread of a malignant germ cell tumour other than dysgerminoma, aggressive cytoreduction surgery is appropriate {2586}.

Precursor lesions
Gonadoblastoma is almost invariably associated with an underlying gonadal disorder. When the disorder is identifiable, it is usually pure or mixed gonadal dysgenesis with a Y chromosome being detected in over 90% of the cases {2598, 2605}.

Prognosis and predictive factors
Clinical criteria
Patients having gonadoblastoma without dysgerminoma or other germ cell tumour are treated by surgical excision of the gonads without additional therapy. However, if dysgerminoma and/or another malignant germ cell element is present, surgical staging and postoperative combination chemotherapy, the most popular current regimen being bleomycin, etoposide and cisplatin (BEP), are required. Other regimens include etoposide and carboplatin {2586}. Dysgerminoma is exquisitely sensitive to chemotherapy, as it was previously shown to be exquisitely responsive to radiation therapy.

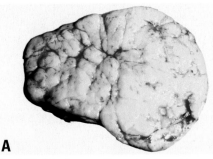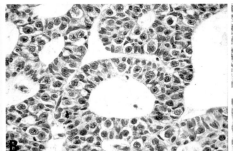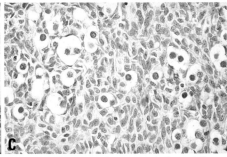

Fig. 2.112 Mixed germ cell-sex cord-stromal tumour. **A** The sectioned surface shows a lobulated, pale yellow tumour. **B** The tumour is composed of an admixture of smaller sex cord cells and larger germ cells with clear cytoplasm forming cords and trabeculae surrounded by loose oedematous connective tissue. **C** Small carrot-shaped sex cord cells are admixed with large pale germ cells in a haphazard fashion. .

Histopathological criteria

Pure gonadoblastoma may show extensive involvement of the gonad but does not behave as a malignant lesion {2598, 2849,2850}. More frequently, its germ cell component gives rise to a malignant germ cell neoplasm capable of invasion and metastases. Gonadoblastoma may sometimes undergo ablation by a process of marked hyalinization and calcification. In such cases the lesion becomes innocuous, but great care must be taken to exclude the presence of viable elements, especially of germ cell lineage.

Dysgerminoma arising within gonadoblastoma tends to metastasize less frequently and at a later stage than dysgerminoma arising de novo {2598, 2849,2850}. There is no satisfactory explanation for this phenomenon. The patients can be treated similarly to patients with pure dysgerminoma with a very high likelihood of complete cure.

Mixed germ cell-sex cord-stromal tumour

Definition

A neoplasm composed of intimately admixed germ cells and sex cord derivatives that has a different histological appearance from gonadoblastoma. Mixed germ cell-sex cord-stromal tumour also differs from gonadoblastoma by its occurrence in anatomically, phenotypically and genetically normal females {2844,2845,2847}.

Epidemiology

Mixed germ cell-sex cord-stromal tumours usually occur in infants or children under the age of 10, but have been occasionally reported in postmenarchal women {1556,2844,2852}.

Aetiology

Patients with mixed germ cell-sex cord-stromal tumour have normal gonadal development and a normal XX karyotype. The tumour is not associated with gonadal dysgenesis, and its aetiology is unknown {1556,2844,2852,3270}.

Clinical features

Patients with a mixed germ cell-sex cord-stromal tumour generally present with lower abdominal pain. In almost a fourth of the cases patients have isosexual pseudoprecocity and may have vaginal bleeding and bilateral breast development {1556,2852,3270}. Physical examination routinely reveals a large mass in the adnexal area or in the lower abdomen.

Macroscopy

This tumour, unlike gonadoblastoma, tends to be relatively large, measuring 7.5-18 cm and weighing 100-1,050 grams. Except for two reported cases, mixed germ cell-sex cord-stromal tumour is unilateral {1321,2849,2850}. The tumour is usually round or oval and is surrounded by a smooth, grey or grey-yellow capsule. In most cases it is solid, but in some cases it may be partly cystic. The sectioned surface is grey-pink or yellow to pale brown. There is no evidence of calcification. In all cases the fallopian tube, the uterus and the external genitalia are normal

Tumour spread and staging

Since mixed germ cell-sex cord-stromal tumours are less aggressive than gonadoblastoma and uncommonly bilateral, the routine evaluation of patients with a mixed germ cell-sex cord-stromal tumour can be less extensive. Although the tumours are often of considerable size, metastases have occurred in only two cases {124,1556}. If intraoperative consultation is inconclusive, it is appropriate to limit the operation to removal of the involved gonad and to await the final pathology results before performing any definitive surgery that might impair future fertility.

Histopathology

Mixed germ cell-sex cord-stromal tumour is composed of germ cells and sex cord derivatives resembling immature Sertoli or granulosa cells intimately admixed with each other. The tumour cells form four distinctive histological patterns as follows:

(1). A cord-like or trabecular pattern composed of long, narrow, ramifying cords or trabeculae that in places expand to form wider columns and larger round cellular aggregates surrounded by connective tissue stroma that varies from dense and hyalinized to loose and oedematous.

(2). A tubular pattern composed of solid tubules surrounded by fine connective tissue septa and containing peripherally located smaller epithelial-like sex cord derivatives surrounding large, round germ cells with clear or slightly granular cytoplasm and large vesicular nuclei containing prominent nucleoli.

(3). A haphazard pattern consisting of scattered collections of germ cells surrounded by sex cord derivatives, which may be very abundant.

(4). A mixed pattern showing an admixture of the three above mentioned patterns without any predominance.

The germ cells show mitotic activity and a close similarity to those of dysgerminoma, but in some cases they are better differentiated showing smaller nuclei and less marked mitotic activity. Unlike the

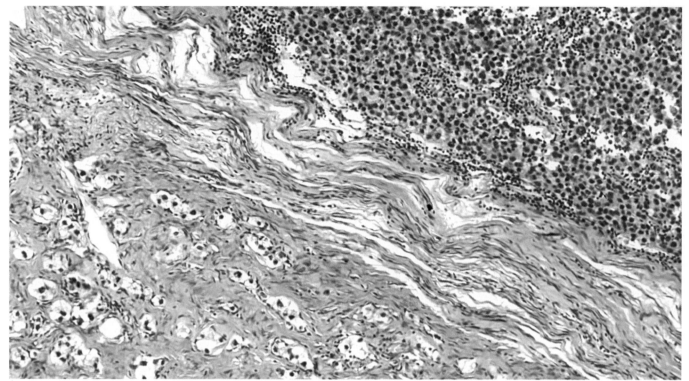

Fig. 2.113 Mixed germ cell-sex cord-stromal tumour associated with dysgerminoma. The former is composed of clusters of germ cells and small sex-cord type cells in a dense fibrous stroma. Note the dysgerminoma in the right upper portion of the field.

finding in gonadoblastoma, the sex cord derivatives also show mitotic activity {2847,2849,2850}.

The composition of a mixed germ cell-sex cord-stromal tumour varies, and in some areas the sex cord elements may predominate, whereas in others there is a predominance of germ cells. The cystic spaces seen in some tumours resemble the cystic spaces seen in cystic and retiform Sertoli cell tumours and should not be confused with cysts and papillae seen in ovarian serous tumours, which they may resemble superficially {2849, 2850}.

Although originally mixed germ cell-sex cord-stromal tumours were found to occur in pure form, it was later noted that approximately 10% of cases are associated with dysgerminoma or other malignant germ cell elements. This finding is by far less common than in gonadoblastoma.

The tumour is always found in normal ovaries, and whenever the unaffected contralateral gonad is examined, it is a normal ovary.

Genetic susceptibility
Familial clustering of these rare tumours has not been reported.

Prognosis and predictive factors
In the majority of cases the mixed germ cell-sex cord-stromal tumour occurs in pure form. Mixed germ cell-sex cord-stromal tumours are generally benign and are treated by unilateral oophorectomy. Preservation of fertility should be a priority in those patients that appear to have a unilateral mixed germ cell-sex cord-stromal tumour.

The association with other neoplastic germ cell elements is more common in postmenarchal subjects, but it may be seen in children in the first decade

{2849,2850}. One case of mixed germ cell-sex cord-stromal tumour was associated with para-aortic lymph node and abdominal metastases {1556}. Another patient developed intra-abdominal metastatic disease two years following the excision of a large ovarian tumour {124}. Both patients are well and disease free following surgery and chemotherapy. It is of interest that the tumour associated with the intra-abdominal recurrence showed an unusual histological pattern of sex cord tumour with annular tubules, but differed from the latter by the presence of numerous germ cells {124}.

In those cases with metastatic disease, aggressive surgical cytoreduction is performed, and the BEP regimen is routinely used postoperatively.

Tumours and related lesions of the rete ovarii

F. Nogales

Definition
A varied group of benign and malignant tumours and related lesions that originate from the rete ovarii, a vestigial structure present in the ovarian hilus and histologically identical to its testicular homologue.

ICD-O codes
Rete ovarii adenocarcinoma	9110/3
Rete ovarii adenoma	9110/0

Clinical features
Most lesions are incidental findings in postmenopausal patients. Sizeable cysts and tumours manifest as pelvic masses. Some cases may present with hormonal symptoms due to concomitant hilus cell hyperplasia or stromal luteinization in adenomas.

Histopathology
The rete is an unusual site for any type of pathology. In order to diagnose a lesion as originating in the rete, it must be located in the ovarian hilus and be composed of cuboidal or columnar non-ciliated cells arranged in retiform spaces. Areas of normal rete and hilus cells should be found in the vicinity of the tumour or show a transition {2495}. Dilated areas and cysts are the most frequent histological finding, but a few solid proliferative lesions have been reported.

The rete ovarii appears to be functionally related to folliculogenesis {385}. Although its embryology is not fully understood, it is likely to be mesonephric in origin. Recently, attention has been focused on its morphology and immunophenotype in order to find histogenetic relationships with neoplasms of uncertain origin such as tumours of probable wolffian origin {682} and retiform Sertoli-Leydig cell tumours {1904}, as well as to differentiate it from endometriosis {2494} and to identify new mesonephric identity markers {2110}. These studies show constant coexpression of vimentin and cytokeratin and positivity for CD10 {2110}, frequent positivity for calretinin, inhibin and CA125 and iso-lated positivity to A103 (melan-A) and epithelial membrane antigen {605,1450, 2495,2792}.

Immunoprofile
Immunohistochemically, adenomas and adenocarcinomas are positive for CAM 5.2, cytokeratin 19, CA125, CD10 and occasionally for epithelial membrane antigen and estrogen and progesterone receptors.

Adenocarcinoma
Adenocarcinoma of the rete ovarii is

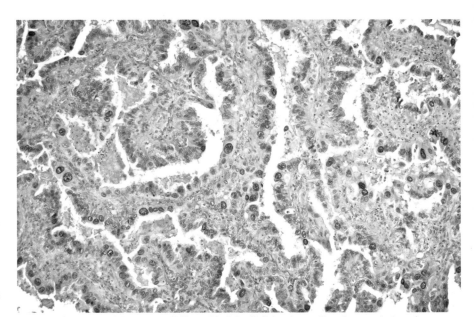

Fig. 2.114 Carcinoma of the rete ovarii. The epithelial cells lining the papillae show marked atypia.

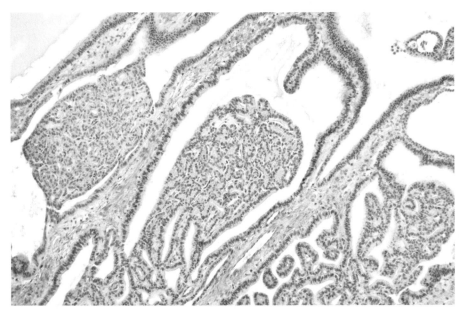

Fig. 2.115 Adenoma of the rete ovarii. Note the tubulopapillary architecture.

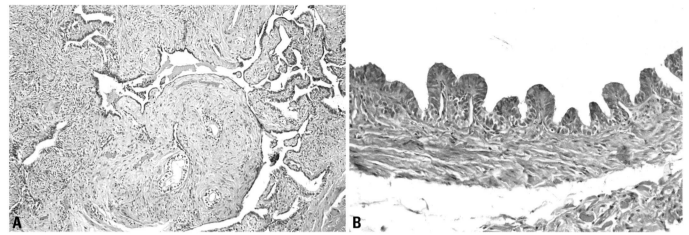

Fig. 2.116 A Adenomatous hyperplasia of the rete ovarii. Note the branching network of spaces. **B** Cyst of rete ovarii. The cyst lining has shallow infoldings.

exceptional. A bilateral tumour with a reti-form tubulopapillary histology admixed with transitional-like areas has been reported {2495}. The patient initially had stage II disease, and the tumour recurred with elevated serum levels of CA125.

Adenoma

Adenoma of the rete ovarii typically occurs as an incidental finding in middle-aged or elderly women, is located in the hilus and is well circumscribed {2495}. It is composed of closely packed elongated tubules, some of which are dilated and contain simple papillae, and may show stromal luteinization or concomitant hilus cell hyperplasia. All reported adenomas have behaved in a benign fashion.

Cystadenoma and cystadenofibroma

One cystadenofibroma and two cystadenomas of the rete ovarii, one of which was bilateral, have been reported {2040}. In both instances they originated from the rete, involved only the ovarian medulla and were tubulopapillary cystic proliferations of clear columnar cells. The stroma was densely populated by luteinized cells, which caused irregular bleeding in both postmenopausal patients. The bilateral case had on one side a non-invasive adenoma but with marked cellular atypia and pleomorphism.

Adenomatous hyperplasia

Among the proliferative lesions, adenomatous hyperplasia of the rete ovarii is similar to the same lesion in the testis {1169}. It is differentiated from adenoma only by its poorly defined margins.

Cysts

Most cysts are unilocular with an average diameter of 8.7cm {2495} and a smooth inner surface. Histologically, they show serrated contours with crevice formation. Their lining consists of a single layer of cuboidal to columnar non-ciliated cells. Their walls contain tracts of smooth muscle and foci of hilus cells, which are sometimes hyperplastic and may be responsible for some hormonal manifestations {2495}.

Miscellaneous tumours and tumour-like conditions of the ovary

L.M. Roth
A. Tsubura
M. Dietel
H. Senzaki

Definition

A group of benign and malignant ovarian tumours of diverse or uncertain origin.

ICD-O codes

Small cell carcinoma, hypercalcaemic type	8041/3
Small cell carcinoma, pulmonary type	8041/3
Large cell neuroendocrine carcinoma	8013/3
Adenoid cystic carcinoma	8200/3
Basal cell tumour	8090/1
Hepatoid carcinoma	8576/3
Malignant mesothelioma	9050/3
Gestational choriocarcinoma	9100/3
Hydatidiform mole	9100/0
Ovarian wolffian tumour	9110/1
Wilms tumour	8960/3
Paraganglioma	8693/1
Myxoma	8840/0

Small cell carcinoma, hypercalcaemic type

Definition

An undifferentiated carcinoma that is usually associated with paraendocrine hypercalcaemia and is composed primarily of small cells.

Clinical features

This neoplasm typically occurs in young women and is associated with paraendocrine hypercalcaemia in approximately two-thirds of patients {3204}. Most of the patients presented with abdominal swelling or pain related to their tumour; however, one patient had a neck exploration for presumed parathyroid disease with negative results before the ovarian tumour was discovered {3204}.

Macroscopy

The tumours are usually large and predominantly solid, pale white to gray masses. Necrosis, haemorrhage and cystic degeneration are common.

Tumour spread and staging

In approximately 50% of the patients the tumour has spread beyond the ovary at the time of initial laporatomy.

Histopathology

On histological examination the tumours typically grow diffusely, but they may form small islands, trabeculae or cords. They frequently form follicle-like spaces that almost always contain eosinophilic fluid, and nuclei show easily discernible nucleoli. Foci of either benign or malignant mucinous epithelium are present in 10-15% of the cases. Typically, the cells of the tumour contain scant cytoplasm, but in approximately one-half of cases a component of large cells with abundant eosinophilic cytoplasm and nuclei containing prominent nucleoli is present.

Immunoprofile

Small cell carcinomas generally stain for epithelial membrane antigen but not for inhibin {2376}. Variable staining of the neoplastic cells for vimentin, cytokeratin and epithelial membrane antigen is observed {46}.

Cytometric studies

Flow cytometric studies of paraffin-embedded tissue has demonstrated that the neoplastic cells are diploid {755}.

Electron microscopy

Electron microscopic examination has shown an epithelial appearance to the neoplasm consisting of small desmosomes and, in some cases, tight junctions {695}. Dilated granular endoplasmic reticulum containing amorphous material is characteristically present within the cytoplasm {695,696}. Few or no neurosecretory granules have been identified.

Differential diagnosis

Because of the young age of the patients and the presence of follicle-like spaces in the neoplasm, the differential diagnosis includes juvenile granulosa cell tumour.

Table 2.08
Comparison of small cell carcinoma of the hypercalcaemic type with juvenile granulosa cell tumour.

Small cell carcinoma, hypercalcaemic type	Juvenile granulosa cell tumour
Stage I in 50% of cases	Stage I in greater than 97% of cases
Highly malignant	Usually non-aggressive
Hypercalcaemia in two-thirds of cases	Hypercalcaemia absent
Never estrogenic	Usually estrogenic
Scant or non-specific stroma	Fibrothecomatous stroma common
Follicles often contain mucicarminophilic basophilic secretion	Follicles rarely contain mucicarminophilic basophilic secretion
Nuclei hyperchromatic	Rounded euchromatic nuclei,
Prominent nucleoli	Indistinct nucleoli
Mitoses frequent	Mitoses variable
Usually epithelial membrane antigen positive	Epithelial membrane antigen negative
Alpha-inhibin negative	Alpha-inhibin positive

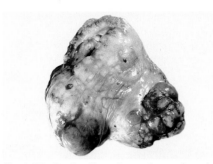

Fig. 2.117 Small cell carcinoma, hypercalcaemic type. The ovary is involved by a solid, knobby tumour that has extended through the capsule to the right.

This tumour may also be confused with adult type granulosa cell tumours, malignant lymphoma and other small cell malignant neoplasms that involve the ovary {695}. The absence of membrane immunoreactivity for MIC2 protein (CD99) serves to distinguish small cell carcinoma from primitive neuroectodermal tumour (see section on germ cell tumours).

Histogenesis
The histogenesis of small cell carcinoma has not been definitively established {755}. It has been proposed that this tumour may be a variant of a surface epithelial-stromal tumour {2376}. A study utilized a mouse xenograft model in which tumour fragments of small cell carcinoma were cultured in six subsequent generations of nude mice. The transplanted tumour morphology remained the same as that of primary tumour from the patient, and serum calcium levels were significantly higher in tumour-bearing mice compared to controls. By comparative genomic hybridization and electron microscopy the tumour appeared to be a distinct tumour entity, not related to either a germ cell tumour or epithelial ovarian cancer {3050}.

Genetic susceptibility
The neoplasm has been familial in several instances. The tumour has occurred in three sisters, in two cousins and in a mother and daughter {3204}. The familial tumours were all bilateral in contrast to the rarity of bilateral tumours in general.

Prognosis and predictive factors
In the largest series of patients approximately one-third of patients with stage IA disease were alive and free of tumour at last follow up {3204}. Almost all the patients with a stage higher than IA died of disease.

Small cell carcinoma, pulmonary type

Definition
A small cell carcinoma resembling pulmonary small cell carcinomas of neuroendocrine type.

Synonym
Small cell carcinoma of neuroendocrine type.

Clinical features
Patients typically are postmenopausal and present with pelvic or abdominal masses.

Macroscopy
The tumours are typically large and solid with a cystic component.

Histopathology
The pulmonary type resembles small cell carcinoma of the lung and is associated with a surface epithelial-stromal tumour, most often endometrioid carcinoma {761}. The neoplastic cells have nuclei with finely stippled chromatin, lack nucleoli and show molding. The cytoplasm is scant. Mitoses are numerous. The appearance varies somewhat depending on cellular preservation.

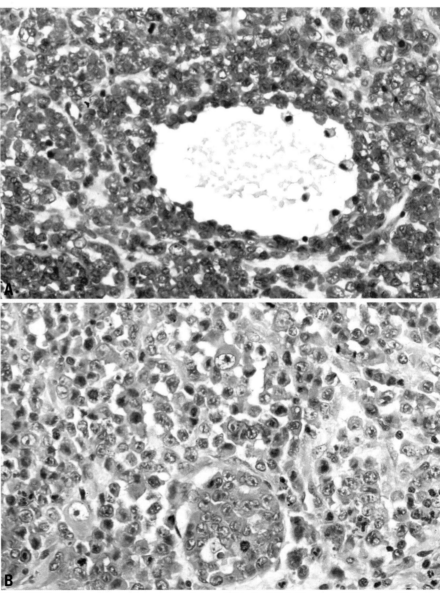

Fig. 2.118 Small cell carcinoma, hypercalcaemic type. **A** Note the follicle-like space. **B** There is a diffuse proliferation of mitotically active small cells with enlarged nuclei that contain small nucleoli.

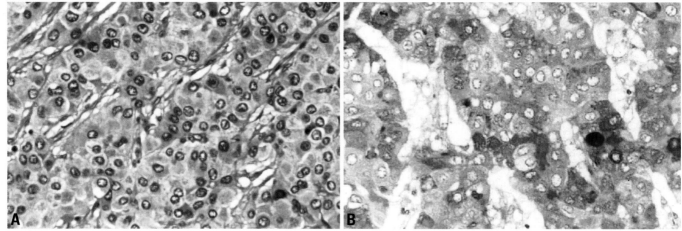

Fig. 2.119 Hepatoid carcinoma. **A** Note the trabecular pattern with thick cords of hepatoid cells. **B** Positive staining for alpha-fetoprotein is observed.

Immunoprofile
Immunohistochemical markers for neuron specific enolase are typically positive, and a minority of cases were positive for chromogranin {761}.

Cytometric studies
The majority of neoplasms are aneuploid by flow cytometry {761}.

Prognosis and predictive factors
The neoplasm is highly malignant, and the behaviour has been aggressive regardless of stage {761}.

Large cell neuroendocrine carcinoma

Definition
A malignant tumour composed of large cells that show neuroendocrine differentiation.

Synonym
Undifferentiated carcinoma of non-small cell neuroendocrine type.

Clinical features
Two series of ovarian neuroendocrine carcinomas of non-small cell type have been reported {455,756}. The patients were in the reproductive age group or beyond (mean 56 years) and presented with symptoms related to a pelvic mass in the majority of cases {756}.

Histopathology
These tumours have in all the reported cases been associated with a tumour of surface epithelial-stromal type, either benign or malignant {455,542,756}. The neuroendocrine component consisted of medium to large cells. Nuclei contained prominent nucleoli, and mitoses were frequent. The solid component stained for chromogranin, and neuropeptides were demonstrated in some cases.

Prognosis and predictive factors
This type of tumour appears to be highly aggressive; only the neuroendocrine carcinoma component was present in the metastatic sites {455}.

Hepatoid carcinoma

Definition
A primary ovarian neoplasm that histologically resembles hepatocellular carcinoma and is positive for alpha-fetoprotein.

Epidemiology
Hepatoid carcinoma of the ovary is a rare tumour; only 12 cases have been reported {1798,2629,2951}. It mainly occurs in postmenopausal women with a mean age of 59.6 years (range, 35-78 years).

Clinical features
The symptoms are not specific and are related to an ovarian mass {2629}. Elevation of serum alpha-fetoprotein (AFP) is characteristic, and CA125 is elevated in most cases.

Macroscopy
Tumours vary from 4-20 cm in maximum dimension with no distinctive macroscopic features {1798,2629,2951}. In some cases, formalin fixation reveals green-coloured areas suggestive of bile production {2629}.

Histopathology
The tumour cells are arranged in sheets, cords and trabeculae with moderate to abundant amounts of eosinophilic cytoplasm and distinctive cell borders resembling hepatocellular carcinoma. Mitoses are generally conspicuous. PAS-positive, diastase-resistant hyaline globules and Hall stain-positive bile pigment can be seen. The presence of immunoreactive AFP and protein induced by vitamin K absence or antagonist II (PIVKA-II) shows functional differentiation toward hepatocytes {1307,2629}. CA125 is positive in one-half of the tumours {2629}.

Differential diagnosis
Metastatic hepatocellular carcinoma and hepatoid yolk sac tumour must be ruled out {3197}.

Histogenesis
Tumours admixed with serous carcinoma and tumour cells positive for CA125 suggest an ovarian surface epithelial origin {1307,2610,2629}.

Prognosis and predictive factors
Clinical outcome is poor. Seven out of 12 patients died between 4 months and 5 years (mean, 19 months) after initial diagnosis, and 2 patients had a tumour recurrence after 6-7 months {1798,2629,2951}.

Tumours resembling adenoid cystic carcinoma and basal cell tumour

Definition
A group of primary ovarian tumours that histologically resemble certain tumours of the salivary glands or cutaneous basal cell carcinoma.

Clinical features

Adenoid cystic-like carcinoma presents typically as a pelvic mass or abdominal distension in postmenopausal women {758}. On the other hand, the two cases of adenoid cystic carcinoma occurred in the reproductive age group {837,3248}. Cases of basal cell carcinoma of the ovary also typically present as a pelvic mass but occur over a wide age range {758}.

Histopathology

These neoplasms histologically resemble adenoid cystic carcinoma, basal cell tumours of salivary gland or cutaneous basal cell carcinoma and occur in several forms. The adenoid cystic-like carcinomas resemble adenoid cystic carcinoma of salivary gland but lack a myoepithelial component {758}. On the other hand a myoepithelial component has been demonstrated in the cases of adenoid cystic carcinoma {837,3248}. Cribriform patterns composed of uniform small cells surrounding round lumens and cysts were typical, and luminal mucin and hyaline cylinders were common to both forms. A surface epithelial-stromal component was present in the great majority of cases of adenoid cystic-like carcinoma {758} but was absent in the cases of adenoid cystic carcinoma {837,3248}. The cases of basal cell tumour consisted of aggregates of basaloid cells with peripheral palisading {758}. Several tumours of this type had foci of squamous differentiation or gland formation, and some showed an ameloblastoma-like pattern. A case of a monomorphic adenoma of salivary gland type described as a cribriform variant of basal cell adenoma has been reported {2492}. In none of the reported cases in this group was there evidence of a teratoma or other germ cell tumour.

Immunoprofile

Actin and S-100 protein stains were both positive in the two cases of adenoid cystic carcinoma {837,3248}; however, these stains were negative in the cases of adenoid cystic-like carcinoma {758}.

Prognosis and predictive factors

The prognosis of adenoid cystic-like carcinoma is generally unfavourable and appears to depend on the degree of malignancy of the surface epithelial-stromal component. On the other hand, cases of basal cell tumour and adenoid

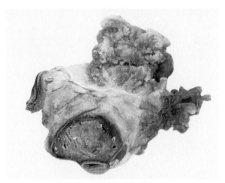

Fig. 2.120 Ovarian papillary mesothelioma. Note the papillary tumour growth on the surface and a haemorrhagic corpus luteum within the ovary.

cystic carcinoma have an excellent prognosis with relatively limited follow up.

Ovarian malignant mesothelioma

Definition

Ovarian malignant mesotheliomas (OMMs) are mesothelial tumours confined mostly or entirely to the ovarian surface and/or the ovarian hilus.

Aetiology

In the largest series there was no history of asbestos exposure {526}.

Clinical features

The clinical presentation was usually abdominal or pelvic pain or abdominal swelling and an adnexal mass on pelvic examination {526}.

Macroscopy

The tumours were typically solid and varied from 3-15 cm in maximum dimension. Most were bilateral.

Histopathology

The tumours usually involved both the serosa and the parenchyma of the ovary. The histological and immunohistochemical characteristics of the OMM are analogous to those observed in peritoneal mesotheliomas. The proliferating mesothelial tumour cells may invade and partly replace ovarian tissue and/or the hilar soft tissue.

Differential diagnosis

Just like diffuse peritoneal malignant mesotheliomas, OMMs can extensively involve one or both ovaries in a macroscopically and histologically carcinomatous growth pattern and may thus be confused with ovarian epithelial neoplasms. In this context immunohistochemical detection of thrombomodulin, calretinin, Ber-EP4 and cytokeratin 5/6 provide the most useful markers {2113}.

Prognosis and predictive factors

In the absence of sufficient follow-up data for this rare neoplasm, OMM can be assumed to have a prognosis similar to its disseminated peritoneal analogue.

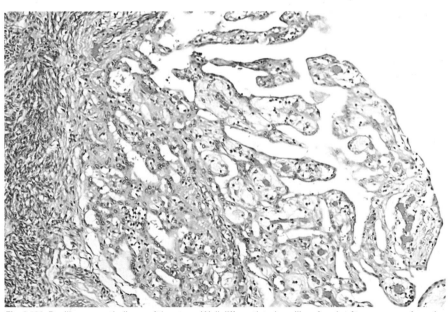

Fig. 2.121 Papillary mesothelioma of the ovary. Well differentiated papillary fronds of tumour grow from the surface of the ovary.

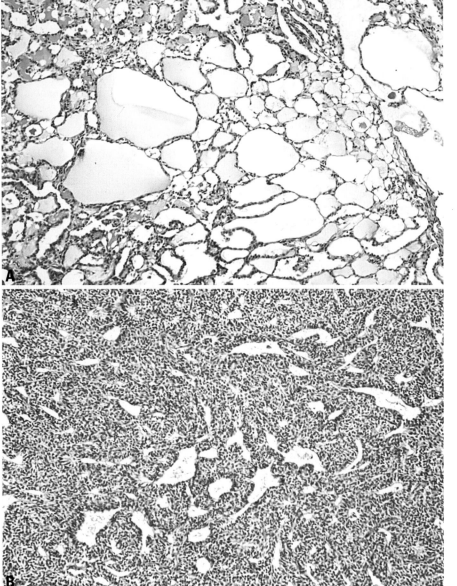

Fig. 2.122 Wolffian tumour. **A** The microcysts containing an eosinophilic material result in a sieve-like appearance. **B** The tumour cells may be spindle-shaped and form irregularly-shaped tubules simulating a retiform pattern.

Gestational choriocarcinoma

Definition
A rare tumour composed of both cytotrophoblast and syncytiotrophoblast that arises as a result of an ectopic ovarian pregnancy. No germ cell or common epithelial component is present.

Clinical features
Patients with choriocarcinoma have symptoms related to a large haemorrhagic mass that may rupture causing haematoperitoneum.

Macrosopy
Choriocarcinoma consists typically of a haemorrhagic mass.

Histopathology
The typical appearance is an admixture of syncytiotrophoblast and cytotrophoblast often arranged in a plexiform pattern {142,1317}. The specimens must be sampled extensively to rule out a germ cell, or in the older age group, a surface epithelial component. They must be distinguished from rarely reported ovarian hydatidiform moles, which have hydropic chorionic villi with cistern formation and trophoblastic proliferation.

Prognosis and predictive factors
The prognosis of gestational choriocarcinoma is more favourable than that of the nongestational type. Single agent chemotherapy with methotrexate or actinomycin D is highly effective.

Hydatidiform mole

Definition
Hydatidiform mole is an ectopic ovarian molar pregnancy. Ovarian hydatidiform moles have hydropic chorionic villi with cistern formation and trophoblastic proliferation.

Clinical features
Patients with hydatidiform mole have symptoms related to large haemorrhagic masses that may rupture causing haematoperitoneum.

Macrosopy
Hydatiform mole typically consists of a haemorrhagic mass; chorionic vesicles may be identified.

Histopathology
Hydatidiform moles show characteristic hydropic chorionic villi with cistern formation and trophoblastic proliferation {2821,3212}.

Ovarian wolffian tumour

Definition
A tumour of presumptive wolffian origin characterized by a variety of epithelial patterns.

Synonyms
Ovarian tumour of probable wolffian origin, retiform wolffian tumour.

Localization
Although more common in the broad ligament, this tumour also occurs in the ovary {1262,3212}.

Clinical features
Patients are in the reproductive age group or beyond and present with abdominal swelling or a mass {3212}. Preoperative serum oestradiol levels may be elevated and return to normal postmenopausal levels after operation {1289}.

Histopathology

This epithelial tumour may show diffuse, solid tubular, hollow tubular and sieve-like patterns, and combinations of the various patterns may occur. Cases have been reported associated with endometrial hyperplasia {1262,1289}.

Immunoprofile

The neoplasms are positive for CAM5.2, cytokeratins 7 and 19 and vimentin but are negative for cytokeratin 20, 34betaE12, B72.3, carcinoembryonic antigen, and epithelial membrane antigen {2321,2878,2926}. The neoplastic cells often express CD10 {2110} and often are weakly positive for alpha-inhibin {1499}.

Histogenesis

Cases have been reported arising within the rete ovarii {662,2878}. An immunohistochemical study based on a comparison with mesonephric remnants and paramesonephric structures supported but did not prove a mesonephric origin of these neoplasms {2926}.

Prognosis and predictive factors

These tumours typically are not aggressive; however, a significant minority of patients have had an aggressive course {3212}. The malignant cases sometimes, but not always, show nuclear atypia and increased mitotic activity.

Wilms tumour

Definition

A primary ovarian neoplasm that has the typical features of a Wilms tumour of the kidney.

Epidemiology

Several cases of pure Wilms tumour of the ovary have been reported {1303,2506}.

Clinical features

The tumour occurs in patients in the reproductive age group and beyond and presents as a rapidly growing adnexal mass.

Histopathology

They have the typical appearance of a Wilms tumour including small tubules, glomeruloid structures and blastema. No teratomatous elements were identified.

Prognosis and predictive factors

Two of the patients were living and well 10 months and 7 years postoperatively.

Paraganglioma

Definition

A unique neuroendocrine neoplasm, usually encapsulated and benign, arising in specialized neural crest cells associated with autonomic ganglia (paraganglia).

Synonym

Phaeochromocytoma.

Clinical features

A single case of a paraganglioma of the ovary in a fifteen year old girl with hypertension has been reported {832}. In addition two unpublished cases have been described {2605}.

Histopathology

The tumours consist of polygonal epithelioid cells arranged in nests separated by a fibrovascular stroma.

Immunoprofile

The tumour is positive for chromogranin. In addition, stains for S-100 protein can identify sustentacular cells {2605}.

Biochemistry

Epinephrine and norepinephrine were extracted from the tumour {832}.

Myxoma

Definition

A benign mesenchymal tumour composed of cells with bland nuclear features producing abundant basophilic intercellular ground substance.

Clinical features

Patients with ovarian myxomas present in the reproductive age group typically with an asymptomatic unilateral adnexal mass {757}.

Macrosocopy

The tumours are large, averaging 11 cm in diameter. The sectioned surface is soft, often with cystic degeneration.

Histopathology

Myxoma is a sharply demarcated tumour composed of spindle and stellate-shaped cells within an abundant, well vascularized myxoid background. Small foci of non-myxoid fibrous tissue or smooth muscle may be present. Lipoblasts are not identified. Mitoses are rare. The intercellular material stains with alcian blue and colloidal iron. Staining is prevented by pretreatment with hyaluronidase indicating that the material is hyaluronic acid.

Immunoprofile

Immunohistochemical stains show that the tumours are positive for vimentin and smooth muscle actin but negative for most other common immunohistochemical markers {567}.

Electron microscopy

Ultrastructural features of thin filaments condensed into dense bodies also support the presence of myofibroblasts {567}.

Histogenesis

Based on an immunohistochemical comparison with myxoid areas of ovarian stromal tumours, myxomas were considered to be a variant of the thecoma-fibroma group {3254}.

Prognosis and predictive factors

The tumour is practically always benign although one case diagnosed originally as myxoma had a late recurrence after 19 years {2901}. In that case the original tumour showed occasional mitotic figures (less than 1 per ten high power fields), slight atypia and occasional vacuolated cells. The recurrent neoplasm, but not the original, was aneuploid by DNA-flow cytometry {2901}.

Malignant soft tissue tumours not specific to the ovary

Pure soft tissue sarcomas of somatic type rarely occur as primary tumours of the ovary. They typically present as a rapidly enlarging adnexal mass. Their histological appearance is similar to soft tissue tumours in other locations. Among the reported cases of pure sarcomas are

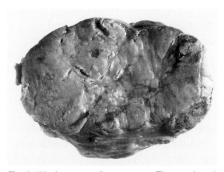

Fig. 2.123 Luteoma of pregnancy. The sectioned surface shows a nodular brown tumour.

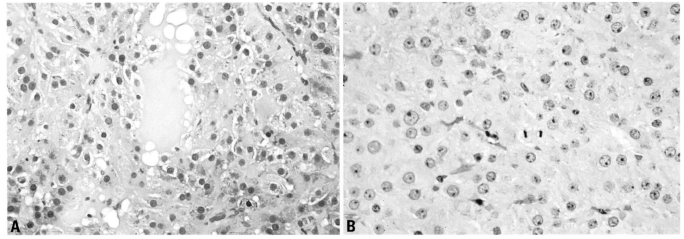

Fig. 2.124 Luteoma of pregnancy. **A** The tumour is composed of polygonal eosinophilic cells that form follicle-like spaces filled with pale fluid. **B** The tumour is composed of large polygonal eosinophilic cells that are mitotically actiive.

fibrosarcoma {1517,1867}, leiomyomyosarcoma {917,1416,1895,1983, 2037}, malignant peripheral nerve sheath tumour {2797}, lymphangiosarcoma, angiosarcoma {2021,2064}, rhabdomyosarcoma {2018}, osteosarcoma {1215} and chondrosarcoma {2851}. These tumours should be classified according to the WHO Histological Typing of Soft Tissue Tumours {3086}.

Similarly, tumours may also arise as a component of a complex ovarian tumour such as malignant müllerian mixed tumour, adenosarcoma, immature teratoma or dermoid cyst or from heterologous elements in a Sertoli-Leydig cell tumour. Rare sarcomas of various types may be associated with surface epithelial stromal tumours, particularly serous, mucinous and clear cell adenocarcinoma. These tumours must be distinguished from metastatic sarcoma to the ovary {3222}.

Benign soft tissue tumours not specific to the ovary

Of the remaining soft tissue tumours, leiomyomas and haemangiomas are most common. Occasional benign neural tumours, lipomas, lymphangiomas, chondromas, osteomas and ganglioneuromas have been reported. Their appearance is similar to soft tissue tumours in other locations. These tumours should be classified according to the World Health Organization Histological Typing of Soft Tissue Tumours {3086}.

Tumour-like conditions

Definition
Non-neoplastic conditions that can mimic an ovarian neoplasm clinically, macroscopically and/or histologically.

Luteoma of pregnancy

Definition
Single or multiple nodules composed of lutein cells with abundant eosinophilic cytoplasm that are detected at the end of a term pregnancy.

Synonym
Nodular theca-lutein hyperplasia of pregnancy.

Epidemiology
Patients with luteoma of pregnancy are typically in their third or fourth decade and multiparous, and 80% are Black {2056,2364,2788}.

Clinical features
Most patients are asymptomatic, and the tumour is usually found incidentally at term during caesarean section or postpartum tubal ligation {2788}. Exceptionally, a pelvic mass is palpable or obstructs the birth canal. Approximately 25% of patients are hirsute or show signs of virilization. Elevated levels of plasma testosterone and other androgens may be observed.

Macrosocopy
The tumours vary from not being macroscopically detectable to over 20 cm. In one series the medium diameter of the tumour was between 6-7 cm {2056}. The sectioned surface is circumscribed, solid, fleshy and red to brown. In approximately one-half of cases the lesions are multiple and at least one-third are bilateral.

Histopathology
There is a diffuse proliferation of polygonal, eosinophilic cells that contain little or no lipid {2364}. The nuclei are round and contain prominent nucleoli. Follicle-like spaces may be present. Mitotic figures may be frequent. The tumour cells were found to be positive for alpha-inhibin, CD99, cytokeratin and vimentin {2242}.

Differential diagnosis
The differential diagnosis includes lipid-poor steroid cell tumours, metastatic melanoma and corpus luteum of pregnancy. Steroid cell tumours occurring during pregnancy may present a difficult differential diagnosis; however, the typical clinical setting of luteoma of pregnancy would be an unusual presentation for a steroid cell tumour. The presence of follicle-like spaces or multiple nodules favours the diagnosis of luteoma of pregnancy. In contrast to luteoma of pregnancy, steroid cell tumours that have a high mitotic rate are likely to exhibit significant nuclear atypia. Metastatic melanoma may be multinodular and contain follicle-like spaces; however, the presence of melanin pigment in some cases and positive stains for S-100 protein and often HMB-45 and Melan A and negative stains for alpha-inhibin would confirm the diagno-

sis. Corpus luteum of pregnancy has a central cavity and a convoluted border. It is composed of granulosa-lutein and theca-lutein layers and contains hyaline or calcified bodies. Multinodularity of the tumour or bilaterality favour luteoma of pregnancy.

Histogenesis
Luteoma of pregnancy appears dependent on beta-human chorionic gonadotropin for its growth based on its clinical presentation at term and regression following the conclusion of the pregnancy.

Prognosis and predictive factors
The tumours regress after the conclusion of the pregnancy.

Uncommon tumour-like conditions associated with pregnancy

Many tumour-like conditions occur during or subsequent to a pregnancy including ovarian pregnancy, hyperreactio luteinalis, large solitary luteinized follicle cyst of pregnancy and puerperium {513}, granulosa cell proliferations of pregnancy {524}, hilus cell proliferation of pregnancy and ectopic decidua {505}.

Stromal hyperthecosis

Definition
Stromal hyperthecosis consists of hyperplastic ovarian stroma containing clusters of luteinized stromal cells.

Epidemiology
The lesion typically occurs in women in the late reproductive years and beyond.

Clinical features
The patients may present with endocrine manifestations including virilization, obesity, hypertension and decreased glucose tolerance and may have elevated levels of plasma testosterone. Bilateral ovarian enlargement is typically encountered at laparotomy .

Macrosocopy
The ovaries are typically enlarged and may measure up to 7 cm in greatest dimension {2605}. With rare exceptions, the lesion is bilateral. The sectioned surface is predominately solid and white to yellow. Multiple superficial cysts may be present in premenopausal women.

Histopathology
On histological examination hyperplastic stroma is present containing clusters of luteinized stromal cells. In premenopausal women the outer cortex may be thickened and fibrotic with luteinized follicle cysts as is observed in the polycystic ovary syndrome.

Differential diagnosis
The lesion is distinguished from the closely related condition of stromal hyperplasia by the absence of luteinized stromal cells in the latter. Polycystic ovarian disease typically occurs in younger women and is less distinctly virilizing. The ovaries are more cystic than is typically seen in stromal hyperthecosis.

Somatic genetics
Patients with acanthosis nigricans and masculinization (HAIR-AN syndrome) all had the histologic findings of pre-

menopausal hyperthecosis in their ovaries {729}.

Prognosis and predictive factors
The lesion is usually treated by oophorectomy, and the postoperative course is uneventful.

Stromal hyperplasia

Definition
A tumour-like proliferation of ovarian stromal cells without the presence of luteinized stromal cells.

Clinical features
Patients are typically menopausal or early postmenopausal. It is much less frequently estrogenic or androgenic than stromal hyperthecosis, and patients may occasionally have obesity, hypertension or abnormal glucose metabolism {2605}.

Macroscopy
Ill defined white or pale yellow nodules that sometimes coalesce are present in the cortical or medullary regions of the ovary or both. In extensive cases the ovaries may be enlarged, and the architecture replaced.

Histopathology
The medullary and to a lesser extent the cortical regions are replaced by a nodular or diffuse densely cellular proliferation of small stromal cells with scanty amounts of collagen. In advanced cases the ovarian architecture is completely replaced and follicle derivatives are not observed.

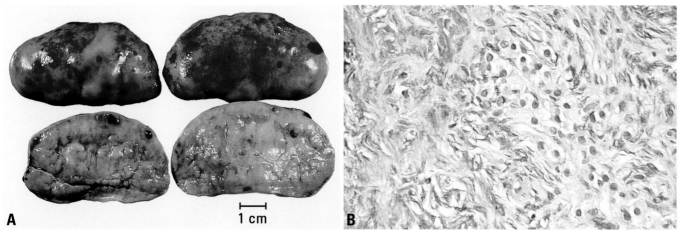

Fig. 2.125 Stromal hyperthecosis. **A** The ovaries are enlarged and solid with a smooth external surface and have a multilobulated sectioned surface with a few follicle cysts. **B** Note the clusters of luteinized stromal cells within hyperplastic ovarian stroma.

Differential diagnosis

Stromal hyperplasia is distinguished from stromal hyperthecosis by the absence of luteinized stromal cells. It is distinguished from low grade endometrial stromal sarcoma by the presence of spindle shaped rather than round or oval stromal cells and the absence of mitotic figures or spiral arterioles.

Fibromatosis

Definition

Fibromatosis is a tumour-like enlargement of one or both ovaries due to a nonneoplastic proliferation of collagen-producing ovarian stroma.

Clinical features

The patients range from 13-39 years with an average of 25. The typical presentation is menstrual irregularities, amenorrhea or, rarely, virilization {3214}.

Macroscopy

The ovaries range from 8-14 cm and have smooth or lobulated external surfaces. The sectioned surface is typically firm and grey or white, and small cysts may be apparent. About 80% of cases are bilateral.

Histopathology

There is a proliferation of spindle-shaped fibroblasts with a variable but usually large amount of collagen. Foci of luteinized stromal cells as well as oedema may be present. Ovarian architecture is maintained, and the fibrous proliferation surrounds follicle derivatives. Nests of sex cord type cells are present in some cases {384}. Most cases show diffuse involvement of the ovaries, but occasional cases are localized.

Differential diagnosis

The lesion is distinguished from fibroma in that the latter is usually unilateral and does not incorporate follicular derivatives. However, it differs from ovarian oedema in that oedema in the latter is massive and fibrous proliferation is not observed. It differs from stromal hyperplasia in that the latter does not produce abundant collagen and is usually unilateral. The sex cord type nests may superficially resemble a Brenner tumour, but the latter shows transitional cell features and replaces the ovarian architecture.

Prognosis and predictive factors

The lesion does not spread beyond the ovaries.

Massive ovarian oedema

Definition

Formation of a tumour-like enlargement of one or both ovaries by oedema fluid.

Epidemiology

The age range is 6-33 with an average of 21 years {3214}.

Clinical features

Most patients present with abdominal pain, which may be acute, and a pelvic mass. {3214}. Others may present with abnormal uterine bleeding, hirsutism or virilization. Elevated levels of plasma testosterone and other androgens may be observed. At laparotomy ovarian enlargement, which is usually unilateral, is encountered, and torsion is observed in approximately one-half of the patients.

Macrosocopy

The external surface is usually white and opaque. The ovaries range from 5-35 cm in size with an average diameter of 11 cm {3214}. The sectioned surface typically exudes watery fluid.

Histopathology

On histological examination oedematous, hypocellular ovarian stroma is present, and the ovarian architecture is preserved. The outer cortex is thickened and fibrotic. Clusters of luteinized stromal cells are present in the oedematous stroma in a minority of cases, especially those that have endocrine symptoms.

Differential diagnosis

The differential diagnosis includes an oedematous fibroma and Krukenberg

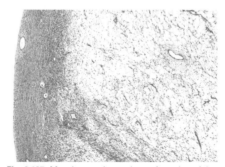

Fig. 2.127 Massive ovarian oedema. A portion of the ovarian cortex remains around an oedematous ovary.

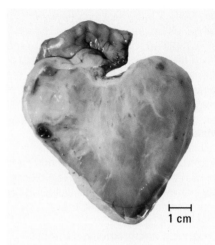

Fig. 2.126 Massive ovarian oedema. The sectioned surface of the ovary was moist and exuded watery fluid.

tumour. The diffuse nature of the process and the preservation of ovarian architecture are unlike an oedematous fibroma, which is likely to be a circumscribed mass. The distinction from Krukenberg tumour is based on the absence of signet-ring cells and the typically unilateral mass, whereas Krukenberg tumours are bilateral in the vast majority of cases. It is important for the pathologist to recognize this lesion at the time of intraoperative consultation so that fertility may be maintained in these young patients.

Histogenesis

In many cases the oedema is due to partial torsion of the ovary insufficient to cause necrosis {1390,2463}.

Prognosis and predictive factors

The lesion is usually treated by oophorectomy, and the postoperative course in uneventful.

Other tumour-like conditions

A wide variety of other conditions can, on occasion, mimic an ovarian neoplasm. Those not associated with pregnancy include follicle cyst, corpus luteum cyst, ovarian remnant syndrome, polycystic ovarian disease, hilus cell hyperplasia, simple cyst, idiopathic calcification, uterus-like adnexal mass {48}, spenic-gonadal fusion, endometriosis and a variety of infections.

Lymphomas and leukaemias

L.M. Roth
R. Vang

Malignant lymphoma

Definition
A malignant lymphoproliferative neoplasm that may be primary or secondary.

Epidemiology
Although unusual, ovarian involvement is more frequent than that of other sites in the female genital tract {1588}. The peak incidence of ovarian involvement by lymphoma is in the fourth and fifth decades, although it may occur at any age. Ovarian involvement by lymphoma may either be primary or secondary; however, the latter is much more common.

Clinical features
Lymphoma rarely presents clinically as an ovarian mass, and in most cases it is only one component of an intra-abdominal or generalized lymphoma {483}. An exception is Burkitt lymphoma, which may account for about one-half of the cases of malignant ovarian neoplasms in childhood in endemic areas {2605}. In such cases involvement of one or both ovaries is second in frequency only to jaw involvement.

Macroscopy
Lymphoma is bilateral in approximately one-half of the cases. The tumours are large and typically have an intact capsule. The sectioned surfaces are typically white, tan or grey-pink and occasionally contain foci of haemorrhage or necrosis.

Tumour spread and staging
Ovarian involvement by lymphoma is rare and is associated with simultaneous involvement of the ipsilateral tube in 25% of the cases {2119}.

Histopathology
The histological appearance of ovarian lymphomas is similar to that observed at other sites; however, the neoplastic cells tend to proliferate in cords, islands and trabeculae with occasional follicle-like spaces or alveoli and often have a sclerotic stroma {2605}. In some cases ovarian follicular structures may be spared, but in others the entire ovarian architecture is obliterated.

Almost any type of lymphoma may occur in the ovary; however, the most common are diffuse large B-cell, Burkitt and follicular lymphomas {1900,2119}.

Differential diagnosis
Dysgerminoma is the most important and perhaps the most difficult differential diagnosis of ovarian lymphoma, particularly of the large B-cell type, which it may mimic both macroscopically and histologically {2605,3226}. Careful attention to the appearance of the cell nuclei and immunohistochemical stains for lymphoid markers and placental-like alkaline phosphatase are important in reaching the correct diagnosis. Other tumours that may be confused with lymphoma include granulocytic sarcoma, undifferentiated carcinoma, small carcinoma of the hypercalcaemic type and metastatic breast carcinoma {2605,3226}.

Prognosis and predictive factors
Almost one-half (47%) of the patients with lymphoma who presented with ovarian involvement were alive at their last follow up with a median survival of 5 years {1900}.

Leukaemia

Definition
A malignant haematopoetic neoplasm that may be primary or secondary.

Epidemiology
Ovarian involvement by leukaemia may either be primary or secondary; however, the latter is much more common {428}. A series of primary granulocytic sarcomas of the female genital tract including 7 cases of the ovary was reported {2099}.

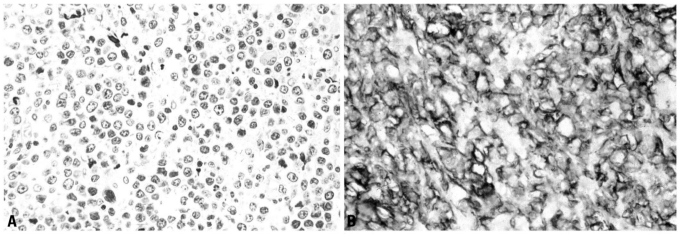

Fig. 2.128 Diffuse large B-cell lymphoma of ovary. **A** Intermediate-power magnification shows a diffuse growth pattern. Nuclei are medium-sized to large and polymorphic. **B** Immunohistochemical stain is positive for CD20.

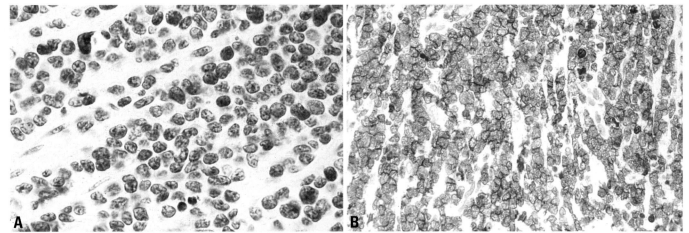

Fig. 2.129 Precursor T-cell lymphoblastic lymphoma of ovary. **A** High power magnification shows small to medium-sized cells with scant cytoplasm, round nuclei and fine chromatin. **B** Immunohistochemical stain is positive for CD99.

Clinical features
Rarely, a patient presents with an ovarian granulocytic sarcoma with or without haematological evidence of acute myeloid leukaemia {2099}. Cases of acute lymphoblastic leukaemia, mostly in children and teenagers, are known to recur in the ovaries during haematological remission.

Macroscopy
The ovarian tumours are usually large and may be either unilateral or bilateral. They are typically solid, soft, and white, yellow or red-brown; occasionally, they may be green, and such tumours have been designated as a "chloroma" {2605}.

Histopathology
Granulocytic sarcomas have a predominantly diffuse growth pattern, but sometimes a cord-like or pseudoacinar arrangement of the tumour cells is present focally {2099}. They are usually composed of cells with finely dispersed nuclear chromatin and abundant cyto-plasm that may be deeply eosinophilic. The identification of eosinophilic myelo-cytes is helpful in establishing the diagnosis; however, they are not always present.

Differential diagnosis
The most important differential diagnosis is malignant lymphoma. Histochemical stains for chloracetate esterase or immunohistochemical stains for myelo-proxidase, CD68 and CD43 will establish the diagnosis in almost all cases {2099}.

Plasmacytoma

Definition
A clonal proliferation of plasma cells that is cytologically and immunophenotypi-cally identical to plasma cell myeloma but manifests a localized growth pattern.

Histopathology
The tumour cells may be mature or immature. The mature type has eccentric nuclei with clumped chromatin, low nuclear to cytoplasmic ratios, abundant cytoplasm and a prominent perinuclear hof. The immature form is pleomorphic with frequent multinucleated cells.

Clinical findings
Ovarian plasmacytoma is a rare tumour that may present clinically with a unilater-al adnexal mass. The 7 reported patients were 12-63 years old {782}.

Macroscopy
The tumours were large, and the sectioned surface was white, pale yellow or grey.

Prognosis and predictive factors
One patient developed multiple myeloma 2 years after removal of the tumour.

Secondary tumours of the ovary

J. Prat
P. Morice

Definition

Malignant tumours that metastasize to the ovary from extraovarian primary neoplasms. Tumours that extend to the ovary directly from adjacent organs or tissues are also included in this category. However, most ovarian carcinomas associated with uterine cancers of similar histological type are independent primary neoplasms. General features of ovarian metastasis include: bilaterality, small multinodular surface tumours, extensive extraovarian spread, unusual patterns of dissemination, unusual histological features, blood vessel and lymphatic invasion and a desmoplastic reaction.

Synonym

Metastatic tumours.

The term Krukenberg tumour refers to a metastatic mucinous/signet-ring cell adenocarcinoma of the ovaries which typically originates from primary tumours of the G.I. tract, most often colon and stomach.

Epidemiology

Metastatic tumours to the ovary are common and occur in approximately 30% of women dying of cancer. Approximately 6-7% of all adnexal masses found during physical examination are actually metastatic ovarian tumours, frequently unsuspected by gynaecologists {1587, 2605,2980}. The metastasis often masquerades as a primary ovarian tumour

and may even be the initial manifestation of the patient's cancer. Pathologists also tend to mistake metastatic tumours for primary ovarian neoplasms even after histological examination. Carcinomas of the colon, stomach, breast and endometrium as well as lymphomas and leukaemias account for the vast majority of cases {3226}. Ovarian metastases are associated with breast cancer in 32-38% of cases, with colorectal cancer in 28-35% of cases and with tumours of the genital tract (endometrium, uterine cervix, vagina, vulva) in 16% of cases. In recent years attention has been drawn to mucinous tumours of the appendix, pancreas and biliary tract that often spread to the ovary and closely simulate ovarian mucinous borderline tumours or carcinomas {590,1848,2406,3199,3200}.

Aetiology

The routes of tumour spread to the ovary are variable. Lymphatic and haematogenous metastasis to the ovaries is the most common form of dissemination {1587,2605,2980}. Direct extension is also a common manner of spread from adjacent tumours of the fallopian tube, uterus and colorectum {3226}. Transtubal spread provides an explanation for some surface ovarian implants from uterine cancers. Neoplasms may also reach the ovary by the transperitoneal route from abdominal organs, such as the appendix {3199}. Embolic spread often produces

Table 2.09
Metastatic tumours to the ovary.

Clues to the diagnosis
1 - Bilaterality (mucinous and endometrioid-like)
2 - Small, superficial, multinodular tumours
3 - Vascular invasion
4 - Desmoplastic reaction
5 - Extensive, unusual extraovarian spread
6 - Unusual clinical history

multiple nodules within the substance of the ovary and commonly is accompanied by prominent intravascular nests of tumour in the ovarian hilum, mesovarium and mesosalpinx.

Clinical features

Signs and symptoms
Ovarian metastases can be discovered in patients during follow-up after treatment of a primary tumour, seredipitously diagnosed during a surgical procedure for treatment of an abdominal tumour or fortuitously found at autopsy. The circumstances leading to the discovery of these metastatic lesions depends on the site of the primary tumour {951,1802}. Ovarian metastasis was detected before the breast cancer in only 1.5% of cases

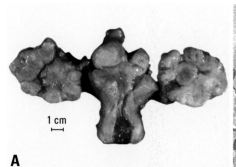

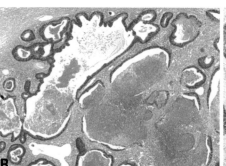

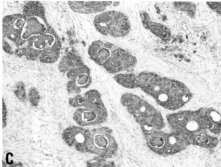

Fig. 2.130 Metastatic colonic adenocarcinoma of the ovaries. **A** The ovaries are replaced by bilateral, multinodular metastases. Note the additional leiomyomas of the corpus uteri (centre). **B** This tumour shows a garland-like glandular pattern with focal segmental necrosis of glands and luminal necrotic debris. **C** Immunohistochemical stain for carcinoembryonic antigen is strongly positive.

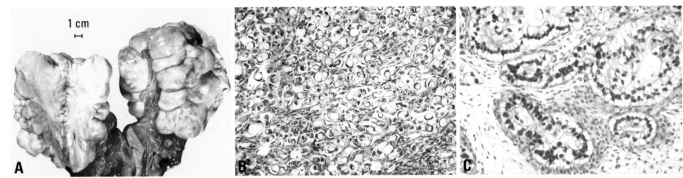

Fig. 2.131 Krukenberg tumour. **A** Note the bilateral nodular ovarian masses of solid yellow-white tissue. **B** Histology shows the typical features of metastatic gastric carcinoma consisting of signet-ring cells within a fibrous stroma. **C** Tubular variant. This mucin-secreting adenocarcinoma resembles a primary ovarian clear cell adenocarcinoma.

{951}. In patients with a gastrointestinal cancer, the ovarian malignant growth was discovered before, or more frequently, at the same time as the gastrointestinal primary {2232}. In 35% of patients with a Krukenberg tumour, the diagnosis of the digestive primary preceded the diagnosis of the ovarian metastasis {1933,2545}. When a patient presents with abdominopelvic symptoms leading to suspicion of an ovarian tumour, the symptoms are non-specific and similar to those of ovarian cancer, i.e. pelvic masses, ascites or bleeding {1598,2545}. Eighty percent of patients with a Krukenberg tumour had bilateral ovarian metastases, and 73% of patients with ovarian metastases from breast carcinoma had extraovarian metastases {951,2545}.

Imaging
Several studies have evaluated radiological findings in patients with a Krukenberg tumour {1094,1460}. When imaging features were compared, patients with a Krukenberg tumour more frequently had a solid mass with an intratumour cyst, whereas primary ovarian growths were predominantly cystic {1460}. Magnetic resonance (MR) imaging seems to be more specific than computed tomography scan. Identification of hypointense solid components in an ovarian mass on T2-weighted MR images seems to be characteristic of a Krukenberg lesion, but this aspect is not specific {1094}.

Macroscopy
Ovarian metastases are bilateral tumours in approximately 70% of cases {2605}.

They grow as superficial or parenchymatous solid nodules or, not uncommonly, as cysts. The size of ovarian metastases is variable even from one side to the other. The ovaries may be only slightly enlarged or measure 10 cm or more.

Site of origin
The frequencies of various sites of origin of secondary ovarian tumours differ among different countries according to the incidence of various cancers therein. Colonic adenocarcinoma probably accounts for most metastatic ovarian tumours that cause errors in diagnosis {1587,2605,3226}. Frequently, the ovarian metastases and the primary tumour are discovered synchronously, or the intestinal tumour has been resected months or years previously.

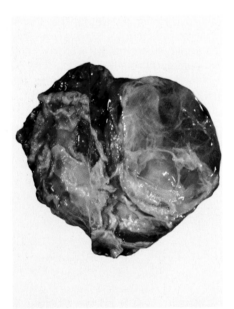

Fig. 2.132 Metastatic adenocarcinoma of colon. Note the solid and cystic mucinous appearance.

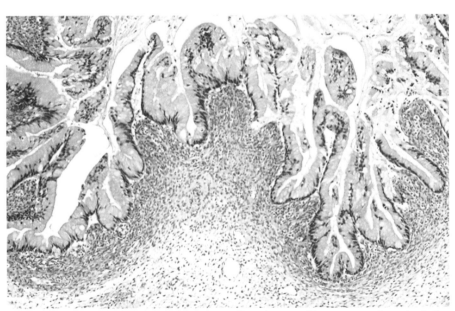

Fig. 2.133 Metastatic adenocarcinoma of pancreas. Note the resemblance to a mucinous borderline tumour.

Occasionally, the colonic adenocarcinoma is found several months to years after resection of the ovarian metastases. Rectal or sigmoid colon cancer accounts for 75% of the metastatic colon tumours to the ovary {1587,2605,3226}. The primary tumour can also be located in the pancreas, biliary tract or the appendix {590,1848,2406,3199,3200}.

The Krukenberg tumour is almost always secondary to a gastric carcinoma but may occasionally originate in the intestine, appendix, breast or other sites {367,2605,3226}. Rarely, breast cancer metastatic to the ovary presents clinically as an ovarian mass. A much higher percentage of cases of lobular carcinoma of the breast, including those of signet-ring cell type, metastasizes to the ovary than does ductal carcinoma {1142}. A wide variety of other tumours may metastasize to the ovary.

Histopathology

The identification of surface implants, multinodularity and intravascular tumour emboli are extremely helpful histological clues in the recognition of secondary ovarian tumours that spread through the abdominal cavity and tubal lumen. The histological appearance of the metastases is variable, depending on the nature of the primary tumour.

Differential diagnosis

Sometimes, metastases resemble primary ovarian tumours {2605,2980,3226}. Metastatic colonic adenocarcinoma to the ovary may be confused with primary endometrioid or mucinous carcinoma depending on whether the colonic carcinoma is predominantly mucinous or non-mucinous. Features that help to distinguish colon cancer from endometrioid carcinoma include luminal necrotic debris, focal segmental necrosis of the glands, occasional presence of goblet cells and the absence of müllerian features (squamous differentiation, an adenofibromatous component or association with endometriosis). Also the nuclei lining the glands of metastatic colon carcinoma exhibit a higher degree of atypia than those of endometrioid carcinoma. Metastatic tumours may also closely resemble primary mucinous ovarian tumours. The former may be moderately differentiated or so well differentiated that they can be mistaken for mucinous borderline or less often benign ovarian

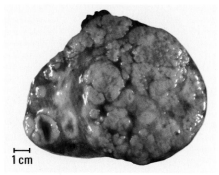

Fig. 2.134 Metastatic lobular carcinoma of the breast. Sectioned surface shows a solid, multinodular tumour.

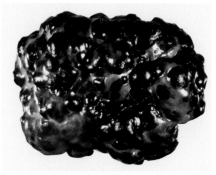

Fig. 2.135 Metastatic malignant melanoma. The ovary is replaced by a multinodular nodular black tumour.

tumours. Metastatic mucinous tumours to the ovary can originate in the large intestine, pancreas, biliary tract or the appendix. Features supportive of the diagnosis of a metastasis include bilaterality, histological surface involvement by epithelial cells (surface implants), irregular infiltrative growth with desmoplasia, single cell invasion, signet-ring cells, vascular invasion, coexistence of benign-appearing mucinous areas with foci showing a high mitotic rate and nuclear hyperchromasia and histological surface mucin {1614}.

Immunostains for cytokeratin 7 and 20 should be used with caution and along with thorough consideration of all clinical information keeping in mind that no tumour shows absolute consistency in its staining with these markers {2183}.

Krukenberg tumours must be distin-

guished from primary and other metastatic ovarian tumours including clear cell adenocarcinoma, mucinous (goblet cell) carcinoid and a variety of ovarian tumours that contain signet-ring-like cells filled with non-mucinous material. Ovarian clear cell adenocarcinoma may have a signet-ring cell component that simulates a Krukenberg tumour; however, the identification of a characteristic tubulocystic pattern, hobnail cells, stromal hyalinization and eosinophilic secretion are helpful in establishing the diagnosis. Mucinous carcinoid, either primary or metastatic, may contain large areas of signet-ring cells; however, teratomatous elements other than carcinoid are usually present in the former.

The tubular variant of Krukenberg tumour, sometimes associated with stro-

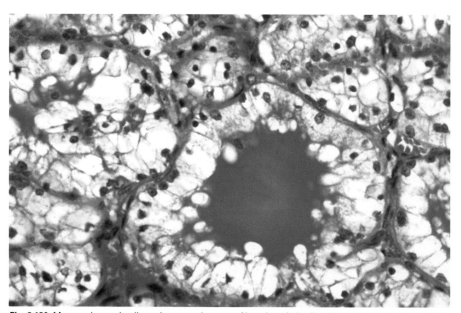

Fig. 2.136 Metastatic renal cell carcinoma to the ovary. Note the tubules lined by cells with abundant clear cytoplasm.

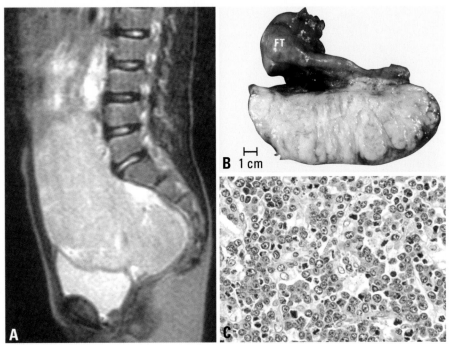

Fig. 2.137 Burkitt-like lymphoma. **A** T2 weighted sagital computed tomography scan from an 8-year old girl shows a large pelvic mass. **B** Sagital section of the ovarian tumour shows a homogeneous, pale surface. Notice the enlargement of the fallopian tube (FT). **C** A starry-sky pattern is apparent (B5 fixation).

mal luteinization, can be confused with a Sertoli-Leydig cell tumour. Positive mucicarmine and PAS-stains with diastase digestion are of great value in establishing the diagnosis of a Krukenberg tumour. Occasional Krukenberg tumours may closely resemble fibromas on macroscopic examination and may contain relatively few signet-ring cells. Bilaterality and positive mucin stains facilitate the differential diagnosis.

Distinction between a transitional cell carcinoma of the urinary tract metastatic to the ovary and a primary transitional cell carcinoma may be difficult {2100,3220}. Clinical information may be necessary to resolve the issue.

Renal cell carcinoma rarely metastasizes to the ovaries; however, when it does, it must be distinguished from a primary clear cell carcinoma. The metastatic tumour usually shows a sinusoidal vascular pattern, a homogenous clear cell pattern without hobnail cells, the absence of hyalinized papillae and the absence of mucin {3226}.

A *metastatic carcinoid* can be confused with a primary carcinoid, granulosa cell tumour, Sertoli-Leydig cell tumour, Brenner tumour, adenofibroma or endometrioid carcinoma {2605,3226}. Bilaterality and extraovarian extension are important features of metastatic carcinoid.

In the ovary, *metastatic malignant melanoma* may be confused with primary malignant melanoma; the latter is unilateral and usually associated with a dermoid cyst. When a melanoma is composed predominantly of large cells, it may resemble steroid cell lesions such as steroid cell tumour or luteoma of pregnancy; when it is composed predominantly of small cells it may be confused with a variety of other tumours characterized by small cells {3223}. Positive stains for melanin, S-100 protein, melan A, and/or HMB-45 should establish the diagnosis of melanoma.

Sarcomas may metastasize to the ovary from the uterus or extragenital sites and may occasionally be discovered before the primary tumour {3222}. Metastatic low grade endometrial stromal sarcoma

(ESS) may simulate a primary ovarian sex cord-stromal tumour. Features helpful in their distinction include the presence of extraovarian disease, bilaterality and the characteristic content of spiral arterioles in metastatic low grade ESS. Metastatic epithelioid leiomyosarcoma may have an appearance that simulates the solid tubular pattern of a Sertoli cell tumour.

Although *lymphoma and leukaemia* can involve the ovaries simulating various primary tumours, they rarely present clinically as an ovarian mass. In countries where Burkitt lymphoma is endemic, however, it accounts for approximately half the cases of malignant ovarian tumours in childhood. Dysgerminoma is one of the most common and difficult differential diagnoses. The appearance of the cell nuclei is very important. Immunohistochemistry for lymphoid markers and placental alkaline phosphatase are helpful. Carcinoid, granulosa cell tumour or small cell carcinoma can also resemble lymphoma. In patients with acute myeloid leukaemia, ovarian involvement in the form of granulocytic sarcoma ("chloroma") may rarely constitute the initial clinical presentation of the disease. Histological examination reveals a diffuse growth pattern with a prominent "single file" arrangement of the tumour cells. Myeloid differentiation can be demonstrated by the chloroacetate esterase stain. Immunoperoxidase stains for lysozyme, CD68, and LCA are also helpful.

Recognition of the secondary nature of an ovarian tumour depends on a complete clinical history, a careful operative search for a primary extraovarian tumour, and accurate evaluation of the macroscopic and histological features of the ovarian tumour. In rare cases the primary tumour is not found until several years after resection of the ovarian metastases {2605,3226}.

Prognosis and predictive factors
Ovarian metastases often represent a late disseminated stage of the disease in which other haematogenous metastases are also found. The prognosis is, therefore, poor.

Peritoneal tumours

S.C. Mok
J.O. Schorge
W.R. Welch
M.R. Hendrickson
R.L. Kempson

Definition

Rare neoplasms with primary manifestation in the abdominal cavity in the absence of a visceral site of origin. Both malignant and benign tumours may occur.

ICD-O code

Peritoneal mesothelioma	9050/3
Multicystic mesothelioma	9055/1
Adenomatoid tumour	9054/0
Desmoplastic small round cell tumour	8806/3
Primary peritoneal carcinoma	8461/3
Primary peritoneal borderline tumour	8463/1

Clinical features

Signs and symptoms
Patients with malignant peritoneal tumours typically present with non-specific manifestations including abdominal discomfort and distension, digestive disturbances and ascites. Less frequently, a palpable mass or pelvic pain may be evident. Benign peritoneal tumours are usually asymptomatic.

Tumour spread and staging

Malignant peritoneal tumours spread primarily by exfoliation of cancer cells from the primary site of origin. Lymphatic and haematogenous dissemination also com-

monly occurs. However, some tumours have been shown to arise from separate intra-abdominal sites and are believed to have a multifocal origin {2576 The staging involves a combination of radiological and operative findings, but these tumours do not have individual staging systems given their relative infrequency. Most malignant tumours are confined to the abdominal cavity at initial presentation. Benign peritoneal tumours do not metastasize and present as an isolated lesion, often detected at the time of operation for another indication.

Mesothelial tumours

Definition

Benign or malignant mesothelial tumours that arise within the peritoneum.

Peritoneal malignant mesothelioma

Definition

Malignant mesothelial tumours that arise within the peritoneum. Epithelial mesotheliomas may be divided into diffuse, well differentiated papillary and deciduoid types. A less common variant is the sarcomatous mesothelioma, which includes the desmoplastic type.

Epidemiology

Age and sex distribution
Patients with diffuse mesotheliomas are on average 50 years old {1443}, and those with well differentiated papillary tumours are 58 {383}.

Incidence and mortality
Primary neoplasms of the peritoneum are rare compared to the wide variety of benign and malignant peritoneal müllerian proliferations that women develop. Two clinically benign to low grade proliferations, multicystic mesothelioma and well differentiated papillary mesothelioma are more common than diffuse malignant mesothelioma, and the latter is vastly less common than primary or secondary extraovarian serous carcinoma.

Aetiology

Well differentiated papillary, diffuse epithelial and deciduoid mesotheliomas appear clinically related to asbestos exposure in some cases {383,2633}.

Clinical features

The most common presenting features are ascites and abdominal pain {1443}.

Macroscopy

The tumour typically consists of multiple nodules measuring <1.5 cm in greatest

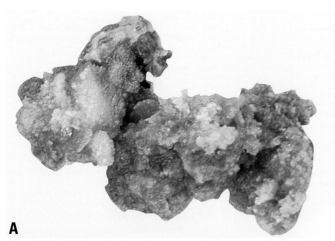

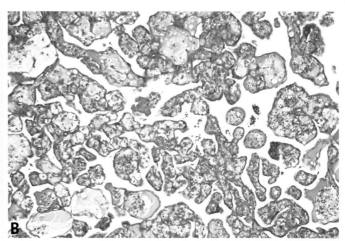

Fig. 2.138 Well differentiated papillary mesothelioma of the peritoneum. **A** Note the distinct papillary architecture of this peritoneal tumour. **B** Papillae with fibrous connective tissue cores are lined by a single layer of uniform mesothelial cells.

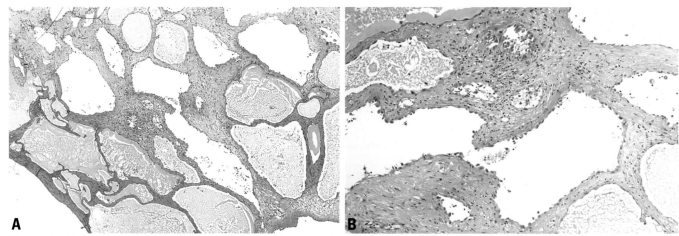

Fig. 2.139 Multicystic peritoneal mesothelioma. **A** Note the multiple cysts lined by mesothelial cells within a fibrous stroma. **B** Irregular cysts are lined by a single layer of cuboidal mesothelial cells.

dimension {1443}. The serosal surfaces have an appearance indistinguishable from the more common peritoneal carcinomatosis or extraovarian carcinoma.

Histopathology

Well differentiated papillary and diffuse malignant mesotheliomas are the most common types. Diffuse and well differentiated papillary mesotheliomas typically are composed of characteristic uniform cells with abundant eosinophilic cytoplasm. Another variant of epithelial mesothelioma is the deciduoid type that simulates an exuberant ectopic decidual reaction {2633}. Sarcomatous mesotheliomas, including the desmoplastic type, also occur but are relatively less common than in the pleura {493}.

All well differentiated papillary meostheliomas have, at least focally, a conspicuous well developed papillary architecture or a tubulopapillary pattern. A single layer of uniform, cuboidal or flattened mesothelial cells with bland nuclear features lines the papillae and tubules. Mitoses are rare. Occasionally, mild cytological atypia is present. Extensive fibrosis associated with irregularity of the glandular elements is common, and such areas may be confused with invasive foci of malignant mesothelioma or adenocarcinoma. Psammoma bodies are present in some cases.

Differential diagnosis

The most reliable indicator of malignancy in these tumours is invasion of fat or of organ walls; however, in small biopsies invasion may be difficult to assess {493}. In the peritoneal cavity entrapment of

benign cells in organizing granulation tissue or between fat lobules is frequent and confusing {493}.

Diffuse peritoneal malignant mesotheliomas may macroscopically and histologically show a carcinomatous growth pattern and thus may be confused with primary peritoneal serous papillary neoplasms. In this context immunohistochemical detection of calretinin in the nuclei and Ber-EP4 were the most useful markers, whereas other mesothelial markers had too low a sensitivity for practical use {2113}. Well differentiated papillary mesothelioma lacks the stratification, complex papillae and the mixed cell population of low grade serous neoplasms and lacks the stratification, cytological atypia and mitotic figures of serous carcinoma. Similarly, it lacks the cytological atypia of diffuse malignant mesothelioma and in some instances is localized within the peritoneum. The absence of a history of a prior operation or reactive changes elsewhere and the formation of convincing papillae distinguish well differentiated papillary mesothelioma from mesothelial hyperplasia.

Prognosis and predictive factors

The diffuse epithelial mesotheliomas are typically highly aggressive; however, unlike pleural mesotheliomas, a sizeable number of tumours are relatively indolent {1443}. No morphological features were found to separate the favourable and unfavourable group of these tumours. The well differentiated papillary type is often localized and has a relatively favourable outcome {383,1027} compared to the diffuse peritoneal type.

Multicystic mesothelioma

Definition

A multiloculated cystic mesothelial tumour that typically has an indolent course. In a few instances multiple recurrences occur, and the disease may progress to diffuse malignant mesothelioma {1039}.

Synonym

Multilocular peritoneal inclusion cyst.

Epidemiology

The tumour most frequently occurs in young to middle aged women.

Clinical findings

Patients typically present with an abdominal or pelvic mass associated with chronic pain. Occasional tumours are found incidentally at laparotomy.

Aetiology

An association with asbestos exposure has not been reported.

Macroscopy

Typically, the lesion is a large multicystic mass that may be solitary but is more commonly either diffuse or multifocal and consists of multiple, translucent, grape-like clusters of fluid filled cysts delimited by fibrous bands. The individual cysts are usually less than 1.0 cm in diameter but may be up to 20 cm.

Tumour spread and staging

The tumour affects chiefly the pelvic peritoneum, particularly the cul-de-sac, uterus and rectum, and there may be an

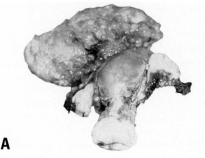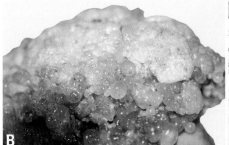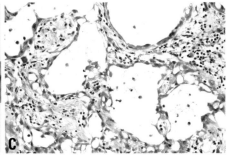

Fig. 2.140 Cystic adenomatoid mesothelioma. **A** The tumour emanates from the uterus. **B** The lesion shows numerous cysts and vesicles in the extrauterine component. **C** Even in the more solid areas of the extrauterine tumour, small cysts dominated microscopically.

abdominal or retroperitoneal component. It grows along the serosa as multiple translucent, fluid-filled cysts. Occasionally, the cysts are solitary or form a free floating mass.

Histopathology

The tumour is made up of multiple cysts lined by one to several layers of flattened or cuboidal mesothelial cells embedded in a delicate fibrovascular stroma {3087}. The lesions typically do not have atypia or significant mitotic activity; however, the occasional presence of cytological atypia may lead to a misdiagnosis of malignancy. Hobnail-shaped cells, foci of mesothelial hyperplasia and, less frequently, squamous metaplasia may be seen. Fibrous septa are usually prominent and may occasionally produce foci with the appearance of an adenomatoid tumour. The stroma may show marked inflammatory change that make it difficult to recognize the nature of the lesion.

Differential diagnosis
The chief differential diagnostic consideration is malignant mesothelioma. Attention to the macroscopic appearance, i.e. multiple cysts rather than solid plaque-like necrotic masses and the usual absence of cytological atypia are sufficient to avoid the error in most cases. Cystic lymphangioma may mimic a multicystic peritoneal mesothelioma, but the cells lining the former do not express keratin.

Histogenesis

The majority of investigators consider this entity to be an unusual type of mesothelial neoplasm that has a tendency to recur locally and may rarely transform into a conventional mesothelioma and show aggressive behaviour {1039,3087}. Some investigators, however, consider the lesion to be a non-neoplastic reactive mesothelial proliferation {2456}. A case termed cystic adenoma-

toid mesothelioma showed a transition from a uterine adenomatoid tumour and is illustrated above.

Prognosis and predictive factors

These tumours have an indolent course, but approximately one-half of cases recur at intervals ranging from 1-27 years {1410,2456}. There are rare instances of multiple recurrences and of transformation into a conventional malignant mesothelioma {1039,3087}. In the largest series 8% of patients with adequate follow up died of tumour {3087}.

Adenomatoid tumour

Definition

A benign tumour of the peritoneum originating from mesothelium and forming gland-like structures.

Synonym

Benign mesothelioma.

Epidemiology

Peritoneal origin of this neoplasm is very rare {571}.

Macroscopy

Lesions are usually solitary, less than 2 cm in diameter and have a white-grey appearance.

Histopathology

Histologically, multiple, small, slit-like or ovoid spaces are lined by a single layer of low cuboidal or flattened epithelial-like cells. Although adenomatoid tumours can be confused with carcinomas, nuclear atypia is absent or minimal, and mitotic figures are infrequent. Notably, adenomatoid tumours have no significant intracellular mucin, as might be found in neoplasms of müllerian origin. Clinically, they are asymptomatic, and

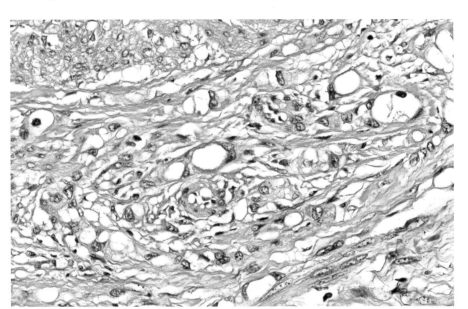

Fig. 2.141 Adenomatoid tumour. Note the small tubules with prominent vacuolization.

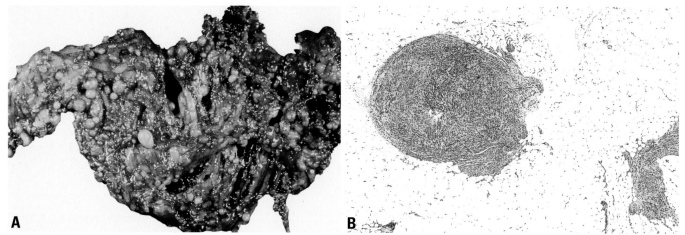

Fig. 2.142 Leiomyomatosis peritonealis disseminata. **A** There are numerous small nodules dispersed throughout the omental surfaces. **B** One of multiple nodules composed of uniform smooth muscle cells in the peritoneum is illustrated.

rarely, if ever, do they recur after adequate excision {506}.

Smooth muscle tumour

Leiomyomatosis peritonealis disseminata

Definition
A benign entity in which numerous small nodules composed of smooth muscle are present in the peritoneal cavity.

Synonym
Diffuse peritoneal leiomyomatosis.

Epidemiology
This condition is rare and occurs in women predominantly in their late reproductive years.

Clinical findings
With few exceptions the patients are asymptomatic. The tumours are found incidentally at the time of laparotomy for a leiomyomatous uterus or during caesarean section. At the time of operation the surgeon is likely to be alarmed since this entity may be macroscopically indistinguishable from diffuse carcinomatosis of the peritoneum. Intraoperative consultation is required to establish the diagnosis.

Macroscopy
The tumour typically consists of numerous small, grey-white nodules.

Histopathology
The tumours consist of multiple nodules of well differentiated smooth muscle

arranged in an intersecting pattern. Cases may occur in conjunction with endometriosis or muticystic mesothelioma, and a single case was associated with both conditions {3268}.

Prognosis and predictive factors
The tumours may regress spontaneously, and conservative management is appropriate.

Tumour of uncertain origin

Desmoplastic small round cell tumour

Definition
A malignant peritoneal tumour of uncertain origin that shows divergent differentiation and is typically composed of nodules of small cells surrounded by a prominent desmoplastic stroma.

ICD-O code   8806/3

Epidemiology
Desmoplastic small cell tumour (DSRCT) is an extremely rare malignancy that has a strong male predilection and occurs most commonly in adolescents and young adults (mean age 19 years) {984}.

Histopathology
Histologically, DSRCT consists of sharply circumscribed aggregates of small epithelioid cells separated by fibrous stroma. The tumour cells typically are uniform with scanty cytoplasm, have indistinct cell borders, and small to medium-sized, round, oval or spindle-shaped hyperchro-

matic nuclei. Mitotic figures are numerous. Immunohistochemistry indicates simultaneous divergent expression within the tumour including reactivity for epithelial (keratin, epithelial membrane antigen), neural (neuron-specific enolase) and muscle/mesenchymal (desmin) markers {984}.

Histogenesis
These tumours are malignant neoplasms of uncertain histogenesis. Their location primarily in the peritoneum suggests a possible histogenetic relationship with mesothelium. The distinctive immunophenotype suggests multilineage {984,1038}.

Somatic genetics
DSRCT has a characteristic reciprocal chromosome translocation t(11;22)(p13; q12) which results in the fusion of the Ewing tumour (*EWS*) gene and the Wilms tumour (*WT1*) gene {900,903}. The resultant chimeric *EWS-WT1* transcript produces a tumour-specific fusion protein that turns the *WT1* tumour suppressor gene into a dominant oncogene {2340}. As a result, cytogenetic analysis can be helpful in excluding the diagnosis of other round cell tumours.

Genetic susceptibility
No familial clustering has been described.

Prognosis and predictive factors
Clinical criteria
Multimodality therapy with induction chemotherapy, aggressive surgical debulking and external beam radiotherapy is advocated for the initial treatment of DSRCT. However, the prognosis is over-

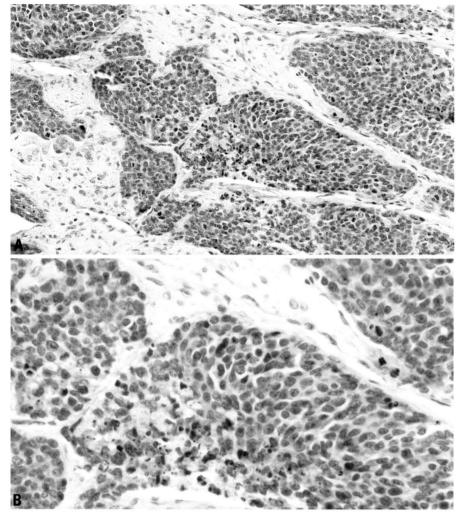

Fig. 2.143 Desmoplastic small round cell tumour of the peritoneum. **A** Irregular islands of tumour cells are separated by fibrous stroma. **B** The tumour cells are small and round with high nuclear to cytoplasmic ratios.

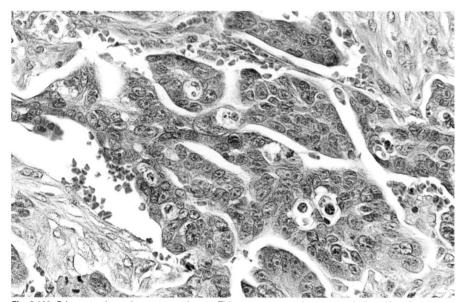

Fig. 2.144 Primary peritoneal serous carcinoma. This serous tumour is composed of papillary fronds and gland-like spaces.

whelmingly poor {1038,1547,2310}.

Histopathological criteria
Although the detection rate of micrometastases in bone marrow and body fluids has recently been shown to be higher with reverse transcriptase polymerase chain reaction of the *EWS-WT1* fusion transcript, the clinical significance of molecularly-detectable micrometastases of DSRCT remains unknown {128}.

Primary epithelial tumours of müllerian type

Definition
Primary epithelial tumours of the peritoneum that resemble malignant ovarian surface epithelial-stromal tumours.

Primary peritoneal carcinoma

Definition
A variety of extraovarian neoplasms that histologically resemble surface-epithelial-stromal tumours of ovarian origin.

Epidemiology
Primary peritoneal carcinoma (PPC) occurs almost exclusively in women with a median age of 62 years. The lifetime risk is estimated to be 1 case per 500 women, since approximately 15% of "typical" epithelial ovarian cancers are actually PPCs {2575,2576}.

Histopathology
Histological and immunohistochemical examination of PPC is virtually indistinguishable from epithelial ovarian carcinoma. The most common histological variant is serous adenocarcinoma, but clear cell, mucinous, transitional cell and squamous cell carcinomas have all been reported to originate from the peritoneum. Rare cases of primary psammocarcinoma of the peritoneum have been described {1001}. The following are required to meet the criteria for PPC:
(1). Both ovaries must be normal in size or enlarged by a benign process.
(2). The involvement in the extraovarian sites must be greater than the involvement on the surface of either ovary
(3). The ovarian tumour involvement must be either non-existent, confined to ovarian surface epithelium without stromal invasion, or involving the cortical stroma with

tumour size less than 5 x 5 mm {2575}.

Histogenesis

PPC is believed to develop de novo from the peritoneal lining of the pelvis and abdomen {2575}. It may develop in a woman years after having bilateral oophorectomy {2262}. Some cases have been shown to originate from multiple peritoneal sites, supporting the hypothesis that cells derived from the coelomic epithelium may independently undergo malignant transformation {1954,2575,2576}.

Somatic genetics

PPC exhibits a distinct pattern of chromosomal allelic loss compared to epithelial ovarian cancer {176,421,1259}. Overexpression of the *TP53*, *EGFR*, *ERBB2*, *ERBB3*, and *ERBB4* genes has been reported, in addition to loss of normal *WT1* expression {2574,2575}. *TP53* gene mutations commonly occur in PPC, but *KRAS* mutations are very infrequent {965,2575}. PPC *BRCA1* mutation carriers have a higher incidence of *TP53* mutations, are less likely to exhibit *ERBB2* overexpression, and are more likely to have a multifocal disease origin {2575}. This unique molecular pathogenesis of *BRCA*-related PPC is believed to affect the ability of current methods to reliably prevent or detect this disease prior to metastasis {1402}.

Genetic susceptibility

Germline *BRCA1* mutations occur in PPC with a frequency comparable to the *BRCA1* mutation rate in ovarian cancer. Although the penetrance is unknown, PPC should be considered a possible phenotype of the familial breast and ovarian cancer syndrome {175}. The multifocal disease origin is thought to explain why PPC has been a common cause of detection failures in familial ovarian cancer screening programs. Screening strategies for these women cannot rely on ultrasonography and CA125 testing to detect early disease {1402}.

Prognosis and predictive factors

The staging, treatment and prognosis of PPC are similar to those of epithelial ovarian cancer. Optimal surgical cytoreduction for histological grade 1 and 2

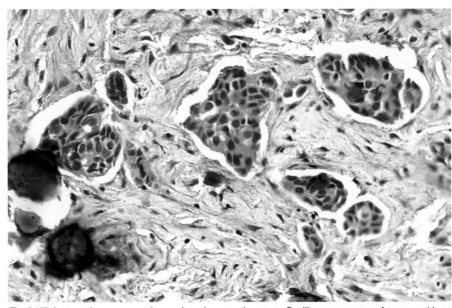

Fig. 2.145 Low grade serous carcinoma, invasive growth pattern. Papillary aggregates of tumour without connective tissue cores are present within retraction spaces surrounded by myxoid fibrous tissue. Note several calcified psammoma bodies on the left.

lesions are associated with longer median survival {2575}. Carboplatin or cisplatin in conjunction with paclitaxel is the current first-line recommended chemotherapy {1436}. The clinical behaviour of psammocarcinoma more closely resembles that of serous borderline tumours than that of serous carcinomas of the usual type. Patients with psammocarcinoma follow a protracted course and have a relatively favourable prognosis {1001}.

Primary peritoneal borderline tumours

Definition

A variety of extraovarian neoplasms that histologically resemble borderline surface epithelial-stromal tumours of ovarian origin. By definition minimal or no ovarian surface involvement is present.

Epidemiology

The age in the two largest series has ranged from 16-67 years with a mean of 32 years.

Clinical features

Infertility and abdominal pain are the most common presenting complaints {204}. Occasional patients present with

an abdominal mass. At operation the peritoneal lesions may be focal or diffuse. They commonly appear as miliary granules and may be mistaken for peritoneal carcinomatosis.

Histopathology

The vast majority of cases are serous in type. The histological appearance is similar to that of non-invasive peritoneal implants of epithelial or desmoplastic type {278}. Psammoma bodies are a prominent feature.

Prognosis and predictive factors

The usual treatment is hysterectomy, bilateral salpingo-oophorectomy and omentectomy. Younger patients who desire to maintain fertility may be treated conservatively {278}. The prognosis is excellent. Occasional tumour recurrences with bowel obstruction have been described. Rarely, the patient may develop an invasive low grade serous carcinoma of the peritoneum. Rare deaths due to tumour have been reported.

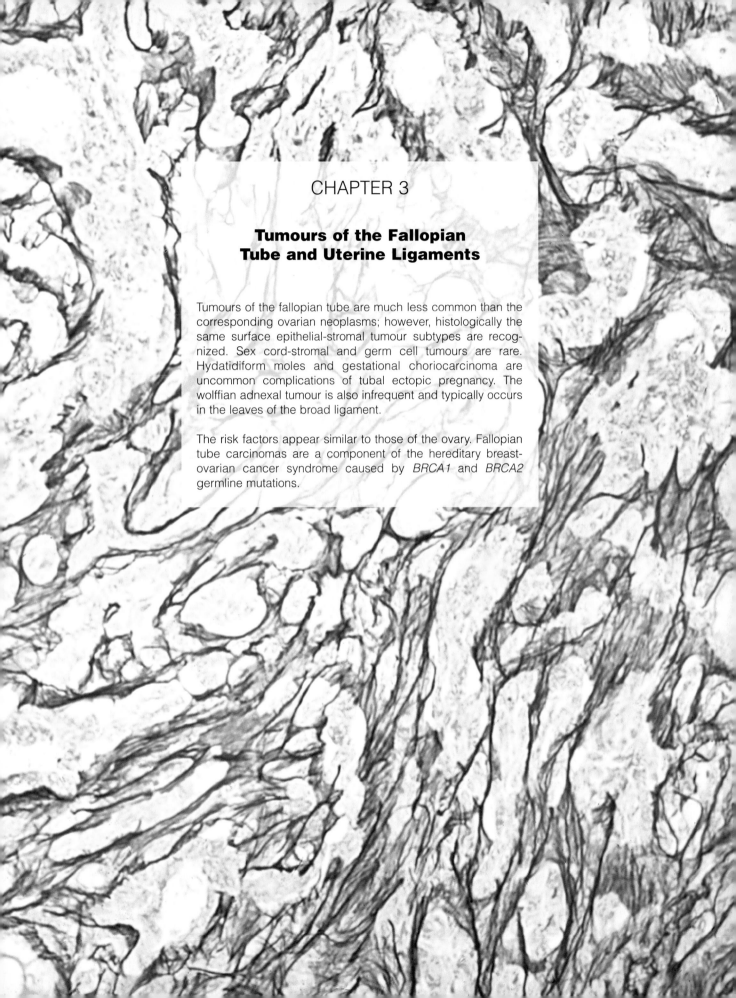

CHAPTER 3

Tumours of the Fallopian Tube and Uterine Ligaments

Tumours of the fallopian tube are much less common than the corresponding ovarian neoplasms; however, histologically the same surface epithelial-stromal tumour subtypes are recognized. Sex cord-stromal and germ cell tumours are rare. Hydatidiform moles and gestational choriocarcinoma are uncommon complications of tubal ectopic pregnancy. The wolffian adnexal tumour is also infrequent and typically occurs in the leaves of the broad ligament.

The risk factors appear similar to those of the ovary. Fallopian tube carcinomas are a component of the hereditary breast-ovarian cancer syndrome caused by *BRCA1* and *BRCA2* germline mutations.

WHO histological classification of tumours of the fallopian tube

Epithelial tumours
Malignant
    Serous adenocarcinoma   8441/3[1]
    Mucinous adenocarcinoma   8480/3
    Endometrioid adenocarcinoma   8380/3
    Clear cell adenocarcinoma   8310/3
    Transitional cell carcinoma   8120/3
    Squamous cell carcinoma   8070/3
    Undifferentiated carcinoma   8020/3
    Others
Borderline tumour (of low malignant potential)
    Serous borderline tumour   8442/1
    Mucinous borderline tumour   8472/1
    Endometrioid borderline tumour   8380/1
    Others
Carcinoma in situ (specify type)
Benign tumours
    Papilloma (specify type)
    Cystadenoma (specify type)
    Adenofibroma (specify type)
    Cystadenofibroma (specify type)
    Metaplastic papillary tumour
    Endometrioid polyp
    Others
Tumour-like epithelial lesions
    Tubal epithelial hyperplasia
    Salpingitis isthmica nodosa
    Endosalpingiosis

Mixed epithelial-mesenchymal tumours
    Malignant müllerian mixed tumour   8950/3
    (carcinosarcoma; metaplastic carcinoma)
    Adenosarcoma   8933/3

Soft tissue tumours
    Leiomyosarcoma   8890/3
    Leiomyoma   8890/0
    Others

Mesothelial tumours
    Adenomatoid tumour   9054/0

Germ cell tumours
    Teratoma
        Mature   9080/0
        Immature   9080/3
    Others

Trophoblastic disease
    Choriocarcinoma   9100/3
    Placental site trophoblastic tumour   9104/1
    Hydatidiform mole   9100/0
    Placental site nodule
    Others

Lymphoid and haematopoetic tumours
    Malignant lymphoma
    Leukaemia

Secondary tumours

---

[1] Morphology code of the International Classification of Diseases for Oncology (ICD-O) {921} and the Systematized Nomenclature of Medicine (http://snomed.org). Behaviour is coded /0 for benign tumours, /3 for malignant tumours, and /1 for borderline or uncertain behaviour.

WHO histological classification of tumours of the broad ligament and other uterine ligaments

Epithelial tumours of müllerian type
Serous adenocarcinoma   8460/3
Endometrioid adenocarcinoma   8380/3
Mucinous adenocarcinoma   8480/3
Clear cell adenocarcinoma   8310/3
Borderline tumour (of low malignant potential), (specify type)
Adenoma and cystadenoma (specify type)

Miscellaneous tumours
Wolffian adnexal tumour   9110/1
Ependymona   9391/3

Papillary cystadenoma (with von-Hippel-Lindau disease)   8450/0
Uterus-like mass
Adenosarcoma   8933/3
Others

Mesenchymal tumours
Malignant
Benign

Secondary tumours

---

[1] Morphology code of the International Classification of Diseases for Oncology (ICD-O) {921} and the Systematized Nomenclature of Medicine (http://snomed.org). Behaviour is coded /0 for benign tumours, /3 for malignant tumours, and /1 for borderline or uncertain behaviour.

TNM and FIGO classification of carcinomas of the fallopian tube

TNM and FIGO classification [1,2]

T – Primary Tumour

TNM Categories	FIGO Stages	
TX		Primary tumour cannot be assessed
T0		No evidence of primary tumour
Tis	0	Carcinoma in situ (preinvasive carcinoma)
T1	I	Tumour confined to fallopian tube(s)
T1a	IA	Tumour limited to one tube, without penetrating the serosal surface
T1b	IB	Tumour limited to both tubes, without penetrating the serosal surface
T1c	IC	Tumour limited to one or both tube(s) with extension onto or through the tubal serosa, or with malignant cells in ascites or peritoneal washings
T2	II	Tumour involves one or both fallopian tube(s) with pelvic extension
T2a	IIA	Extension and/or metastasis to uterus and/or ovaries
T2b	IIB	Extension to other pelvic structures
T2c	IIC	Pelvic extension (2a or 2b) with malignant cells in ascites or peritoneal washings
T3 and/or N1	III	Tumour involves one or both fallopian tube(s) with peritoneal implants outside the pelvis and/or positive regional lymph nodes
T3a	IIIA	Microscopic peritoneal metastasis outside the pelvis
T3b	IIIB	Macroscopic peritoneal metastasis outside the pelvis 2 cm or less in greatest dimension
T3c and/or N1	IIIC	Peritoneal metastasis more than 2 cm in greatest dimension and/or positive regional lymph nodes

M1   IV   Distant metastasis (excludes peritoneal metastasis)

Note: Liver capsule metastasis is T3/stage III, liver parenchymal metastasis, M1/stage IV. Pleural effusion must have positive cytology for M1/stage IV.

N – Regional Lymph Nodes [3]

NX	Regional lymph nodes cannot be assessed
N0	No regional lymph node metastasis
N1	Regional lymph node metastasis

M – Distant Metastasis

MX	Distant metastasis cannot be assessed
M0	No distant metastasis
M1	Distant metastasis

Stage Grouping

Stage 0	Tis	N0	M0
Stage IA	T1a	N0	M0
Stage IB	T1b	N0	M0
Stage IC	T1c	N0	M0
Stage IIA	T2a	N0	M0
Stage IIB	T2b	N0	M0
Stage IIC	T2c	N0	M0
Stage IIIA	T3a	N0	M0
Stage IIIB	T3b	N0	M0
Stage IIIC	T3c	N0	M0
	Any T	N1	M0
Stage IV	Any T	Any N	M1

[1] {51,2976}.
[2] A help desk for specific questions about the TNM classification is available at http://tnm.uicc.org.
[3] The regional lymph nodes are the hypogastric (obturator), common iliac, external iliac, lateral sacral, para-aortic, and inguinal nodes.

Tumours of the fallopian tube

I. Alvarado-Cabrero
A. Cheung
R. Caduff

Malignant epithelial tumours

Definition
A malignant epithelial tumour of the tubal mucosa, usually with glandular differentiation. In order to be considered a primary carcinoma of the fallopian tube, the tumour must be located macroscopically within the tube or its fimbriated end, and the uterus and ovary must either not contain carcinoma or, if they do, it must be clearly different from the fallopian tube lesion.

ICD-O codes
Serous adenocarcinoma   8441/3
Mucinous adenocarcinoma   8480/3
Endometrioid adenocarcinoma   8380/3
Clear cell adenocarcinoma   8310/3
Transitional cell carcinoma   8120/3
Undifferentiated carcinoma   8020/3

Epidemiology
Primary fallopian tube carcinomas are rare, amounting to 0.3-1.1% of gynaecological malignancies {158}. The risk factors appear similar to those of epithelial ovarian cancer. Adenocarcinoma is the most frequent tumour of the fallopian tube {2566}.

Macroscopy
On macroscopic examination, the tube shows abnormal dilatation or nodular thickening resembling a hydrosalpinx or haematosalpinx and contains a dominant localized tumour mass. When found in the proximal part of the tube, the

tumour may protrude through the fimbriated end. On the sectioned surface the adenocarcinoma usually consists of soft, grey-brown, villous or polypoid tissue.

Tumour spread and staging
The tumour spread is very similar to that of ovarian carcinoma and involves adjacent organs, the peritoneum and regional lymph nodes. Involvement of the adjacent ovary may make it difficult to determine whether the tumour is primary in the tube or ovary. When the origin remains unclear, the tumour is classified as tubo-ovarian carcinoma {1256}.
Surgical staging is performed according to the FIGO classification system {51,2976}.

Histopathology
All carcinoma subtypes documented in the ovaries have been identified in the fallopian tube. Serous carcinoma is the most common cellular subtype. In one series of 151 cases, 80% of the tumours were serous {158}. In other large series, about half of these carcinomas were serous, one-fourth endometrioid, one-fifth transitional cell or undifferentiated and the remainder of other cell types {75}.

Serous adenocarcinoma

Most serous carcinomas of the tube are invasive tumours with a high histological grade. In one series 50% of the cases were grade 3 {75}. Occasional serous

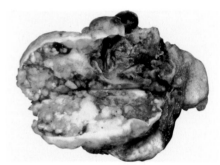

Fig. 3.01 Carcinoma of the fallopian tube. The sectioned surface shows a dilated fallopian tube filled with papillary tumour exhibiting foci of haemorrhage.

carcinomas have an extensive inflammatory cell infiltration that may simulate a salpingitis of non-tuberculous type {472}.

Mucinous adenocarcinoma

These tumours are extremely rare and often are associated with other mucinous neoplasms of the female genital tract {2617}. Reported cases have been predominantly in situ mucinous carcinomas {2450}. A case of synchronous, trifocal mucinous papillary adenocarcinoma involving the uterine cervix and both fallopian tubes has been reported {1316}. We are only aware of a single case of an invasive mucinous adenocarcinoma. The histological appearance of these tumours resembles that of ovarian mucinous carcinomas, and goblet cells may be prominent.

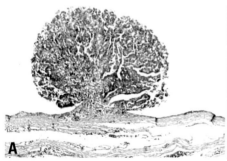
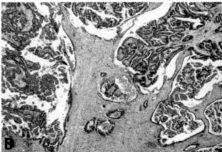
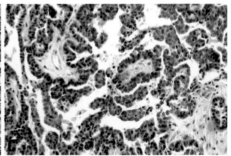

Fig. 3.02 Serous papillary adenocarcinoma of the fallopian tube. **A** Pedunculated papillary tumour arises from the wall of the tube. There is no invasion of the muscular wall. **B** Note the well differentiated papillary fronds. **C** This papillary tumour shows prominent budding from the primary papillae. The nuclei show stratification and atypia.

Endometrioid adenocarcinoma

Endometrioid carcinomas of the tube are characteristically non-invasive or only superficially invasive and have a generally favourable prognosis {1985}. The typical variant is the most common form of endometrioid carcinoma encountered in the tube. By definition these tumours closely resemble their uterine counterparts. Endometrioid carcinomas with a prominent spindle-shaped epithelial cell component {2942} or with the glands lined exclusively by oxyphilic cells {2258} also occur in the tube. An unusual form of endometrioid carcinoma resembling the patterns seen in the wolffian adnexal tumour has been found relatively often in the fallopian tube {641,1985}. These tumours are characterized by a prominent pattern of small, closely packed cells punctured by numerous glandular spaces, a large number of which contain a dense colloid-like secretion. The finding of areas with the typical appearance of endometrioid carcinoma enables one to make the correct diagnosis.

Clear cell adenocarcinoma

These neoplasms constitute 2-10% of all fallopian tube carcinomas {75,1181a, 3031}. The majority of the reported cases have shown a tubulocystic pattern varying from flattened cuboidal epithelium to an irregular pattern with prominent hobnail and clear cells. A papillary pattern featuring the hobnail type of epithelium lining fibrovascular stalks has also been described {3031}.

Transitional cell carcinoma

These carcinomas are rare in the female genital tract but occur relatively more often than in the ovary {2676}. The fre-

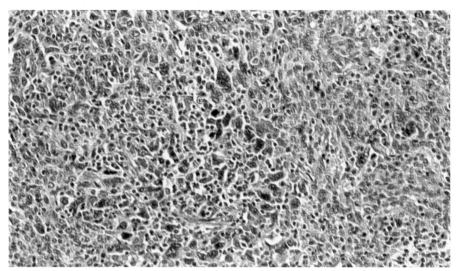

Fig. 3.03 Undifferentiated carcinoma of the fallopian tube. Note the sheets of cells with scattered tumour giant cells.

quency of transitional cell carcinoma of the fallopian tube in previous reports has varied from 11-43% {75,2974}. Transitional cell metaplasia of the epithelium has been suggested as a possible source of tubal carcinoma of the same cell type {750}.

Undifferentiated carcinoma

These carcinomas fail to show evidence of either glandular or squamous differentiation. The tumour displays a diffuse growth pattern composed of sheets of small cells resembling those of small cell carcinoma of the lung. These densely cellular tumours may have a relatively conspicuous myxoid matrix. Some tumours have large epithelial cells arranged in nests surrounded by a dense lymphocytic infiltrate resembling a lymphoepithelioma-like carcinoma. Extensive tumours areas consisting predominantly of multinucleated giant cells may also be present {75}.

Hormone-producing carcinoma

Ectopic beta-human chorionic gonadotropin (β-hCG) production has been reported in two women with serous or undifferentiated carcinoma of the tube {75,399}. Each of the tumours contained syncytiotrophoblast-like cells, many of which stained positively for β-hCG. Unusual reported cases include a renin-producing tumour {3234} and an alpha-fetoprotein producing carcinoma that had a hepatoid appearance {111}.

Miscellaneous epithelial tumours

Rare examples of unusual neoplasms arising in the tube include cases of squamous cell {290,470,1747}, adenosquamous, glassy cell {75,1191} and lymphoepithelioma-like carcinoma {75}.

Genetic susceptibility
The discovery of the *BRCA1* cancer predisposition gene in 1994 and the *BRCA2*

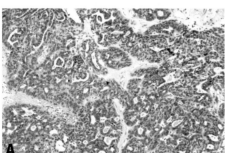
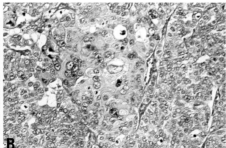
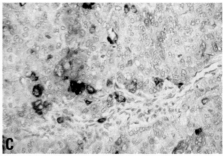

Fig. 3.04 Carcinoma of the fallopian tube. **A** The poorly differentiated tumour shows papillary fronds and gland-like spaces. **B** Note the syncytiotrophoblast-like multinucleated tumour giant cells in the centre. **C** The syncytiotrophoblast-like giant cells stain positively for beta-human chorionic gonadotropin (β-hCG).

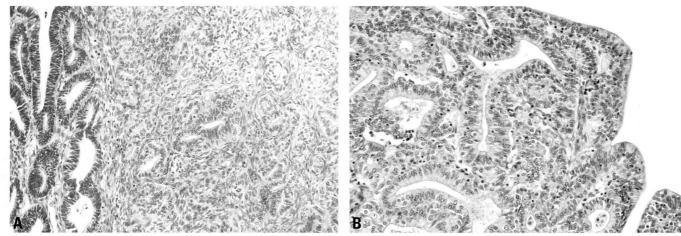

Fig. 3.05 Endometrioid carcinoma of the fallopian tube. **A** Closely packed tubules of endometrioid carcinoma are present adjacent to a focus of endometriosis composed of larger glands present on the left. **B** The tumour forms closely packed glands lined by pseudostratified epithelium.

cancer predisposition gene in 1995 has allowed the identification of a group of women who are at a greatly increased risk of developing breast and ovarian cancer {8,499}. Two previous series in which 5% and 11% respectively of patients with tubal cancer also had breast carcinoma suggest an association between breast cancer and tubal carcinoma {75,2225}. Recently, several high-risk "breast-ovarian cancer families" with *BRCA1* mutations and fallopian tube cancer have been reported. Additionally, a family history of fallopian tube cancer was found to be predictive of the presence of a *BRCA1* mutation in a panel of 26 Canadian "breast-ovarian cancer families" {2939}. A slightly increased risk of ovarian cancer and of early-onset breast cancer was found in the first-degree relatives of the fallopian tube cancer cases {144}. Thus, fallopian tube carcinoma should be considered to be a clinical component of the hereditary breast-ovarian cancer syndrome and may be associated with *BRCA1* and *BRCA2* mutations. See Chapter 8.

Prognosis and predictive factors
The surgical stage is an independent prognostic factor {75,158} and is critical for determining whether adjuvant therapy is appropriate. Stage I carcinomas that occur in the tubal fimbriae appear to have a worse prognosis than stage I tubal carcinomas that are nonfimbrial {74}.

Borderline epithelial tumours

Borderline epithelial tumours of the fallopian tube are rare and include cases of serous, mucinous and endometrioid types {74}. Borderline serous tumours involve the tube, including its fimbriated portion, and have histological features similar to those of the ovary {74,1421, 3257}. Mucinous tumours are sometimes associated with mucinous metaplasia of the fallopian tube or the Peutz-Jeghers syndrome {1806,2617}. Patients that have multiple organ involvement or pseudomyxoma peritonei may have a metastatic lesion to the tube, and in all cases the appendix needs to be ruled out as a source.

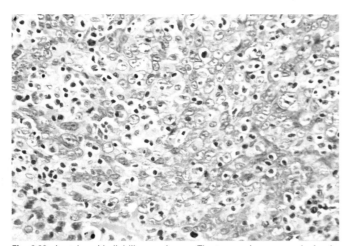

Fig. 3.06 Lymphoepithelial-like carcinoma. The tumour is composed of pale epithelial cells with large vesicular nuclei and prominent nucleoli. Note the lymphocytic infiltration.

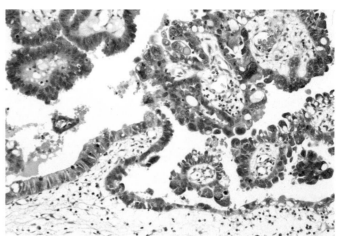

Fig. 3.07 Serous borderline tumour. The tumour consists of papillae with connective tissue cores lined by epithelium showing cellular stratification and tufting, resembling its ovarian counterpart.

Two examples of adenofibroma of borderline malignancy have been reported {74,3257}. One of the tumours appeared in a pregnant woman and on ultrasound was interpreted as an ectopic pregnancy; the other was detected incidentally during an elective tubal ligation. Both neoplasms were located at the fimbriated end of the fallopian tube. One tumour was of serous type and the other endometrioid.

Although relatively few cases of tubal borderline tumours have had long term follow up, the prognosis appears favourable, and it has been suggested that they can be managed conservatively {3257}.

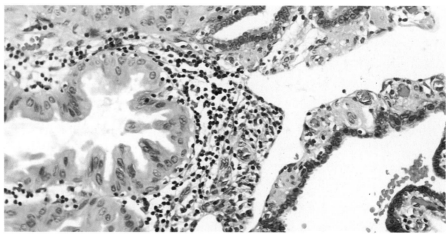
Fig. 3.08 Metaplastic papillary tumour. The tumour is composed of variably sized papillae showing a proliferation of atypical epithelial cells with cellular budding and abundant eosinophilic cytoplasm.

Carcinoma in situ

Rare cases of tubal intraepithelial carcinoma have been reported, and one of these occurred after tamoxifen therapy of breast carcinoma {2747}. With the exception of one case in which a small papillary tumour was found {1875}, the tumours are not detectable on macroscopic examination.

They are characterized by replacement of the tubal epithelium by malignant glandular epithelial cells with pleomorphic nuclei {178,2835}. Florid epithelial proliferation, sometimes even with a cribriform or sieve-like pattern, may occur in association with salpingitis and should not be mistaken for carcinoma in situ {472}.

Benign epithelial tumours

Polypoid adenofibromas, papillomas, benign serous cystadenoma and endometrioid tumours are rarely found in the fallopian tube, including the fimbria {74,1615}. They may be complicated by torsion, especially during pregnancy.

Papilloma and cystadenoma

Serous papilloma and cystadenoma are uncommon lesions of the fallopian tube. Papillomas may be intramural or involve the fimbriated end {74}. Papillomas typically are loosely attached to the tubal mucosa and consist of delicate branching fibrovascular stalks lined by epithelial cells that are indifferent in appearance or resemble those of the fallopian tube lining. The lesion may cause tubal obstruc-

tion {1012,1407}. Cystadenomas are similar but lack papillary features {74}. Mucinous cystadenomas also have been reported {2617}.

Adenofibroma and cystadenofibroma

Fallopian tube adenofibromas and cystadenofibromas are rare. About fifteen examples of these tumours have been documented {74,3257}. The age range is from the third to the eight decade with a mean age of 49 years. Most women are asymptomatic, and the majority of the tumours are incidental findings at the time of an operation for another gynaecological disorder {3257}. The neoplasm presents as a round, solitary mass (average 0.5-3 cm) that is either intraluminal or attached to the fimbriated end or the serosal surface and may have a smooth or papillary surface. In one case the tumour was bilateral {451}.

Histologically, two components are present, a connective tissue stroma without nuclear pleomorphism or mitoses and papillary structures on the surface or tubal structures lined by epithelial cells. The epithelial cell type has been serous in most of the cases but occasionally may be endometrioid {647}.

Metaplastic papillary tumour

Metaplastic papillary tumour is an uncommon lesion that typically occurs as an incidental histological finding in segments of fallopian tube removed during the postpartum period for sterilization {187,1425,2504}. Only rare lesions occur

in women who were not recently pregnant. The intraluminal tumour usually involves part of the mucosal circumference and is composed of variable sized papillae covered by atypical epithelial cells that superficially resemble a serous borderline tumour. The epithelial lining shows cellular budding and the presence of abundant eosinophilic cytoplasm in most of the tumour cells. Some of the cells may contain intracellular mucin, and extracelluar mucin may be abundant. Mitotic figures are rarely observed.

Endometrioid polyp

Endometrial (adenomatous) polyps occur in the interstitial portion of the fallopian tube {1170,1180}. They are commonly found in radiographic studies of infertile patients. They may obstruct the lumen and result in infertility or tubal pregnancy. They are often attached to the tubal epithelium by a broad base and, thus, macroscopically resemble intrauterine endometrial polyps. They may be occasionally associated with ectopic endometrial epithelium elsewhere in the tube {342}.

Tumour-like epithelial lesions

Definition
Proliferations of the tubal mucosa that simulate neoplasms.

Tubal epithelial hyperplasia

Pseudocarcinomatous hyperplasia in chronic salpingitis may mimic adenocar-

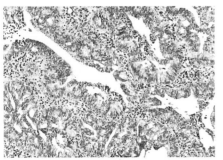

Fig. 3.09 Prominent mucosal hyperplasia. A glandular proliferation producing a cribriform pattern simulates a neoplastic process within the plicae of the fallopian tube.

cinoma histologically because of the pseudoglandular and cribriform permeation of the tubal wall by hyperplastic epithelium and the florid mesothelial hyperplasia {472}. The typically young age of the patients, the presence of marked chronic inflammation, the absence of a macroscopically detected tumour or solid epithelial proliferation, the mildness of the nuclear atypia and the paucity of mitotic figures facilitate the differential diagnosis.

Recently, atypical hyperplasia of the fallopian tube has been observed in patients on tamoxifen therapy for breast cancer {2244}.

Salpingitis isthmica nodosa

Salpingitis isthmica nodosa is a manifestation of tubal diverticulosis and is associated with female infertility and ectopic pregnancy {1064}. These nodules in the isthmus are composed of hypertrophic myosalpinx and glandular spaces lined by tubal epithelium.

Endosalpingiosis

Endosalpingiosis is the benign transformation of the mesothelium into tubal epithelium with ciliated and secretory cells. Psammoma bodies and atypical changes may be found {2919}. Endosalpingiosis is distinguished from endometriosis by the absence of endometrial stroma since tubal type epithelium can also occur occasionally in endometriosis. Endosalpingiosis occurs in the peritoneum and may involve the serosal surfaces of the uterus and its adnexa.

Endosalpingiosis may either present as pelvic pain or may be discovered as an incidental finding {659,1591}. Rarely, endosalpingiosis can present clinically as a cystic mass and can be confused with a neoplasm on macroscopic examination {518a}.

Mixed epithelial and mesenchymal tumours

Definition
Neoplasms composed of an admixture of neoplastic epithelial and mesenchymal elements. Each of these components may be either benign or malignant.

ICD-O codes
Malignant müllerian mixed tumour 8950/3
Adenosarcoma 8933/3

Malignant müllerian mixed tumour

As a group, these malignancies are uncommon. The fallopian tube is the least common site for malignant müllerian mixed tumours in the female genital system, accounting for less than 4% of the reported cases {1124}. Patients are almost always postmenopausal (mean age, 57 years) and usually present with abdominal pain, atypical genital bleeding or abdominal distension {1124,1284}. The histological appearance of these tumours resembles that of ovarian malignant müllerian mixed tumour. The prognosis is poor {1124,1284,3079}.

Adenosarcoma
This tumour is exceedingly uncommon. Only one well documented case that arose in the fimbriated end of the tube and recurred on the pelvic wall has been reported {1036}. Another example of a tubal tumour of this type was characterized by marked adenoacanthotic atypia of its epithelial component {2605}.

Gestational trophoblastic disease

Definition
A heterogeneous group of gestational and neoplastic conditions arising from trophoblast, including molar gestations and trophoblastic tumours.

ICD-O codes
Choriocarcinoma 9100/3
Placental site trophoblastic tumour 9104/1
Hydatidiform mole 9100/0

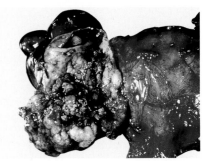

Fig. 3.10 Malignant müllerian mixed tumour of fallopian tube. The fallopian tube is distended and distorted by a multinodular tumour mass that has extended through the serosa.

Choriocarcinoma

Tubal choriocarcinomas account for approximately 4% of all choriocarcinomas {660}. Most of the cases are discovered by chance during an ectopic pregnancy, but about 40% present with an enlarging adnexal mass {2078}. Histological examination shows typical features of gestational choriocarcinoma. In the older literature before the advent of modern chemotherapy, choriocarcinomas associated with ectopic pregnancy were frequently very aggressive, and 75% showed metastases at the time of diagnosis. The response to modern chemotherapy generally has been encouraging {1717,1953}.

Placental site trophoblastic tumour

This neoplasm is composed predominantly of intermediate trophoblast. It is generally benign but occasionally may be highly malignant {1540}. To date, only one case of tubal placental site trophoblastic tumour has been reported {2810}.

Hydatidiform mole

Approximately thirty tubal hydatidiform moles have been reported {1999}; however, only four valid examples of this lesion were accepted in 1981 {2078}. Those authors concluded that the remaining "moles" were actually ectopic pregnancies with villous hydrops. This tumour usually occurs as an isolated growth, but it may be associated with an intrauterine pregnancy {1048}. The histological appearance may be that of a complete, partial or invasive mole with clear

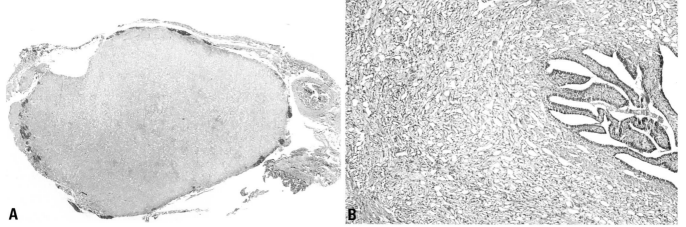

Fig. 3.11 Adenomatoid tumour. **A** The wall of the fallopian tube contains a solid mass. Note the uninvolved cross section of the tube on the right. **B** Variably shaped small cystic spaces and tubule-like structures proliferate in the wall of the tube. The mucosa is on the right.

evidence of trophoblastic proliferation in addition to hydropic swelling of the villi.

Placental site nodule

Placental site nodule is an asymptomatic non-neoplastic proliferation of intermediate trophoblast from a previous gestation that failed to involute. This lesion has recently been reported to occur at the site of an ectopic gestation; two were located in the fallopian tube and one in the broad ligament in direct contact with the tube {391,1514}.

Other tumours

Adenomatoid tumour

ICD-O code   9054/0

The adenomatoid tumour is the most frequent type of benign tubal tumour and usually is found as an incidental finding in a middle-aged or elderly woman {1290}. It typically appears as a grey, white or yellow nodular swelling measuring 1-2 cm in diameter located beneath the tubal serosa The tumour may be large enough to displace the tubal lumen eccentrically {2787}. Rare examples are bilateral {3230}. It originates from the mesothelium and is composed of gland-like structures lined by flat to cuboidal cells {2787}.

Germ cell tumours

To date only about 50 teratomas of the tube have been reported {1242,3051, 3189}. Many of them were found incidentally, measuring 1-2 cm in diameter, and none has been diagnosed preoperatively. The patients have the risk factors for ectopic pregnancy such as prior salpingitis and tubal occlusion {1953}. A malignant mixed germ cell tumour has been reported {1652}.

Soft tissue tumours

Primary sarcomas of the fallopian tube are exceedingly rare; approximately 37 cases have been reported in the literature in more than 100 years {1322}. The clinical signs and symptoms are usually non-specific and include lower abdominal pain and pelvic pressure. The age at diagnosis varies from 21-70 years with a median of 47 years.
Leiomyosarcoma is the most common type and may arise from the tube or broad ligament {1322}. Other reported fallopian tube or broad ligament malignancies include chondrosarcoma {2245}, embryonal rhabdomyosarcoma {361}, myxoid liposarcoma {2708} and Ewing tumour {1692}. The prognosis is poor, although several long-term survivors have been reported {1322}.

Malignant lymphoma and leukaemia

Tubal involvement by lymphoma is rare and is associated almost invariably with simultaneous involvement of the ipsilateral ovary {2119}. In one large series more than 25% of patients with ovarian lymphoma had tubal involvement, most often by Burkitt or Burkitt-like (small non-cleaved cell) lymphoma or diffuse large-cell lymphoma {2119}. One example of an apparent primary malignant lymphoma of the fallopian tube has been observed {2605}. The tube may also be infiltrated in cases of leukaemia {428}.

Secondary tumours

Metastatic tumours involving the tube usually are the result of secondary spread from carcinomas of the ovary or endometrium {3145}. In most cases, the spread is by direct extension. In one study 89% of secondary carcinomas in the tube were of ovarian origin, and the remainder originated in the endometrium. Blood-borne metastases from breast carcinomas or other extrapelvic tumours may also occur {862,3145}. The authors are aware of a case of adenocarcinoma of the gallbladder metastatic to the fallopian tube {862}.

Tumours of the uterine ligaments

S.F. Lax
R. Vang
F.A. Tavassoli

Definition

Benign and malignant tumours that arise in the broad ligament and other uterine ligaments.

ICD-O codes

Serous adenocarcinoma	8460/3
Endometrioid adenocarcinoma	8380/3
Mucinous adenocarcinoma	8480/3
Clear cell adenocarcinoma	8310/3
Wolffian adnexal tumour	9110/1
Ependymoma	9391/3
Papillary cystadenoma (with von Hippel-Lindau disease)	8450/0
Adenosarcoma	8933/3

Epithelial tumours of müllerian type

Definition

Epithelial tumours of müllerian type are the most frequent neoplasms of the broad and other ligaments {2919}. In general, tumours of every müllerian cell type and of every degree of malignancy can occur in this location but are infrequent compared to their occurrence in the ovary. The criteria for malignancy and for the borderline category are the same as described for müllerian type epithelial tumours occurring in the ovary and the peritoneum.

Carcinomas

Less than 20 cases have been reported, of which most were of serous, endometrioid and clear cell types {127a,604a, 715a,1481a,1850a,2402a,2775a,2912a}. An association with endometriosis was observed in some endometrioid and clear cell carcinomas. The age of the patients ranged from 28-70 years. The tumours were cystic, solid or mixed, and their diameter ranged from 4.5-13 cm. All carcinomas were unilateral, but some had spread beyond the broad ligament. Due to the small number of cases and limited follow-up in many of the cases, the prognosis of these tumours cannot be established.

Borderline tumours

More than 30 cases, mostly serous cystic tumours (age range 19-67 years; mean age 33 years) have been reported {73,127,434,606,740,1341,1702,2626}. One mucinous tumour has been reported {1342}. The tumours measured 1-13 cm in greatest diameter, were unilateral, clearly separated from the ovary and confined to the broad ligament.

Benign tumours

Serous cystadenoma is the most common type {962}. As in the ovary, the distinction

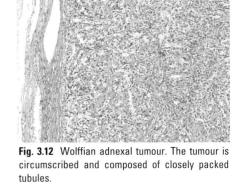

Fig. 3.12 Wolffian adnexal tumour. The tumour is circumscribed and composed of closely packed tubules.

from non-neoplastic serous cysts is ill defined. A suggested distinction is that serous cystadenomas have a thick wall composed of cellular stroma resembling ovarian stroma and lack folds and plicae in contrast to the histology of serous cysts {1236,1335}. Several Brenner tumours ranging from 1-16 cm in diameter have occurred {1120}, and they may be associated with serous or mucinous cystadenomas {169,1628,2302,3040}.

Wolffian adnexal tumour

Definition

A tumour of presumptive wolffian origin characterized by a variety of epithelial patterns.

Synonyms

Retiform wolffian adenoma, retiform wolffian adenocarcinoma.

Sites of involvement

Wolffian tumours occur mainly within the leaves of the broad ligament but may appear as pedunculated lesions arising from it. Less than 50 examples have been described that are predominantely located within the area where mesonephric remnants are distributed. They occur mainly in the broad ligament but also in the mesosalpinx, the serosa of the fallopian tube, the ovary and the retroperitoneum {637,670,682,1400, 2653,2877,2926,3212}.

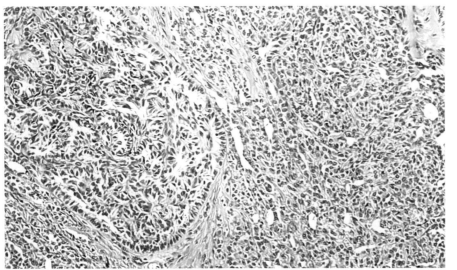

Fig. 3.13 Wolffian adnexal tumour. The tumour is composed of crowded tubules.

Clinical features

Patients range in age from 15-81 years, and most present with a unilateral adnexal mass. Ultrasound studies may show an ill defined mass {637}.

Macroscopy

These predominantly solid tumours range from 0.5-18 cm in diameter. The sectioned surface may contain variably sized cysts and is yellow-tan to grey-white {2877}. The tumour is firm to rubbery and occasionally may have areas of haemorrhage and necrosis.

Tumour spread and staging

Tumour implants may be present at the time of diagnosis and indicate an aggressive tumour {637,2653}.

Histopathology

The tumour shows a variable admixture of diffuse, solid and sieve-like cystic areas, with the solid pattern dominating in the majority of cases. The diffuse, solid areas show a compact proliferation of ovoid to spindle-shaped cells reflecting closed tubules bound by a basement membrane and separated by variable amounts of fibrous stroma or none at all. The round to ovoid nuclei may show indentations. The hollow tubules have a retiform or sertoliform appearance. When the closed tubules dominate, the lesion resembles a mesenchymal tumour; a PAS or reticulin stain helps unmask the tubular pattern. The cells lining the tubules are cuboidal to low columnar with a minimal amount of eosinophilic cytoplasm and round to spindle-shaped, uniform nuclei. Sieve-like areas display clusters of variably sized cysts lined by attenuated cells. Most cases do not show atypia or mitotic figures.

Immunoprofile

The tumour cells are positive for most cytokeratins and vimentin and are often positive for calretinin (91%), inhibin (68%) and CD10 {2110}. They are usually negative for epithelial membrane antigen, estrogen receptor (ER) and progesterone receptor (PR) and are negative for cytokeratin 20, 34betaE12 and glutathione S-transferase {682,2926}.

Cytometry

The ploidy of a metastatic tumour was assessed and found to be diploid {2653}.

Electron microscopy

At the ultrastructural level, the tubules are surrounded by basal lamina and lined by cells with complex interdigitations, desmosomes and/or tight junctions and a few microvilli along the luminal border; no cilia are identifiable {670}. The cytoplasmic organelles are not distinctive and include lysosomes, a small amount of smooth endoplasmic reticulum and a few lipid droplets.

Differential diagnosis

The main tumours in the differential diagnosis are Sertoli cell tumour, Sertoli-Leydig cell tumour, and well differentiated endometrioid carcinoma. The presence of a sieve-like pattern and the absence of Leydig cells help distinguish wolffian tumours from all these lesions. The absence of immunoreactivity with either ER or PR also would distinguish wolffian tumours from well differentiated endometrioid carcinomas; the latter are invariably positive for ER and PR; however, positive immunostaining does not exclude the possibility of a wolffian tumour {682}.

Prognosis and predictive factors

The tumour stage as well as cytological atypia and frequent mitotic figures are important predictors of aggressive behaviour. Careful follow-up of all women with wolffian adnexal tumours is prudent {637,2653}.

Most wolffian adnexal tumours are benign and adequately treated by unilateral salpingo-oophorectomy. About 10% either recur or metastasize. Recurrences and metastases to the lungs and liver have been reported within 1 year or as late as 8 years after diagnosis {637,2653}. The metastatic tumour often has more atypia compared to the primary. Some aggressive tumours have had no significant atypia or mitotic activity in either the primary or the metastatic lesion {2653}.

Ependymoma

Definition

Tumours closely resembling neoplasms of the central nervous system that show ependymal differentiation.

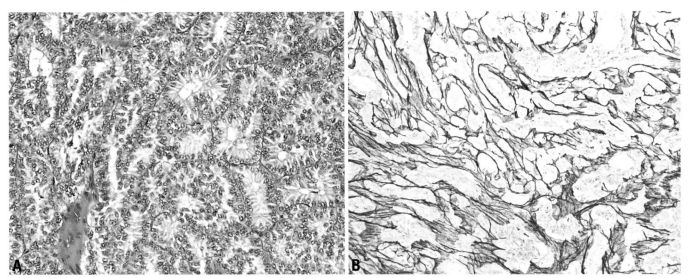

Fig. 3.14 Wolffian adnexal tumour. **A** The pattern of closely packed tubules simulates a Sertoli cell tumour. **B** Reticulin stain accentuates the tubular pattern.

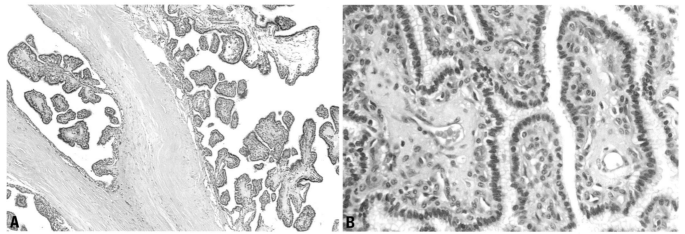

Fig. 3.15 Papillary cystadenoma associated with VHL. **A** A cystic lesion with multiple papillary excrescences is characteristic. **B** The papillae are lined by a single layer of cuboidal to low columnar cells with bland nuclei; there is no atypia or notable mitotic activity.

Localization

Only four ependymomas have been described in the uterine ligaments, three in the broad ligament and one in the uterosacral ligament {208,727,1068}.

Clinical features

Patients were 13-48 years of age with a mean of 38 years and presented with a mass associated with lower quadrant tenderness.

Macroscopy

The tumours are solid or multicystic, soft in consistency and vary from 1 cm to massive in size. The sectioned surface shows haemorrhage and necrosis in the larger tumours.

Histopathology

The lesions are characterized by papillae lined by flat to columnar ciliated cells with central to apical, round to elongated nuclei that protrude into cystic spaces. In more cellular solid areas, the cells form true perivascular ependymal rosettes and pseudorosettes. Mitotic figures may be few or numerous. A few psammoma bodies and small nodules of mature cartilage may be present.

At the ultrastructural level the cells have cilia, blepharoplasts and intermediate filaments {208,727}.

Differential diagnosis

The papillary architecture and psammoma bodies closely resemble serous papillary carcinoma. The ependymal cells are immunoreactive for glial fibrillary acidic protein, however, helping to distin-

guish the two lesions. The cells are also positive for cytokeratin and vimentin.

Prognosis and predictive factors

These are malignant tumours capable of spread beyond the ligaments {208,727, 1068}. Two of the reported cases had spread beyond the broad or uterosacral ligament at presentation, whilst a third had two recurrences over a 24 year period.

Papillary cystadenoma associated with von Hippel-Lindau disease

Definition

A benign tumour of mesonephric origin that occurs in women with von Hippel-Lindau (VHL) disease.

Clinical features

Reported in women 20-46 years of age, one case was not only bilateral but also the first manifestation of the disease; the remaining three were unilateral {939,949, 988,1505}.

Imaging

Ultrasonography shows a sonolucent mass containing an echogenic region {1505}. By computed tomography the lesion appears as an adnexal mass with both water attenuation and soft tissue attenuation areas and curvilinear calcification {939}.

Macroscopy

The tumours are up to 4 cm in diameter and cystic with polypoid papillary protrusions.

Histopathology

Histologically, the lesion is characterized by a complex, arborizing, papillary architecture. Generally, a single layer of non-ciliated cuboidal cells with vacuolated to lightly eosinophilic cytoplasm and bland round nuclei line the papillae {939, 949,988,1505}. The papillary stalks vary from cellular to oedematous and hyalinized. Atypia and necrosis are absent, and mitotic figures are rare to absent. The cells contain glycogen but not mucinous material. A prominent basement membrane is evident beneath the epithelial cells. The cyst wall is fibrous and may have small bundles of smooth muscle or focal calcification.

Genetic susceptibility

VHL disease is an autosomal dominant disorder with inherited susceptibility to a variety of benign and malignant neoplasms including haemangioblastomas of the retina and central nervous system, renal cell carcinoma, pancreatic microcystic adenomas and a variety of other cysts, adenomas and congenital abnormalities. Papillary cystadenomas of mesonephric origin are rare VHL-associated lesions that occur more often in the epididymis but also rarely in the retroperitoneum and broad ligament in women; only four examples of the latter have been documented.

Genetics

The tumour suppressor gene responsible for VHL disease has been mapped to chromosome 3p25 and subsequently identified. Genetic studies on a variety of

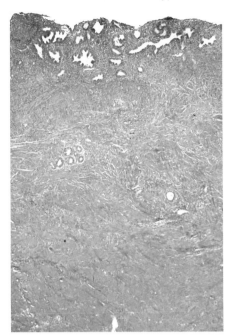

Fig. 3.16 Uterus-like mass. The cystic mass resembles the uterus and is composed of a layer of endometrium consisting of glands and stroma overlying smooth muscle.

tumours from patients with VHL disease have demonstrated loss of heterozygosity at chromosome 3p within the VHL gene region. Two papillary cystadenomas (one from broad ligament, the other retroperitoneal) were studied by polymerase chain reaction and single-strand conformation polymorphism with four polymorphic markers spanning the VHL gene locus (D3S1038, D3S1110, D3S2452, 104/105) {2640}. Both tumours showed loss of heterozygosity at one or more of the markers providing evidence that somatic loss of the VHL gene is responsible for the genesis of these papillary cystadenomas {2640}.

Prognosis and predictive features
All lesions reported so far have been benign.

Uterus-like mass

Definition
A tumour-like lesion composed of endometrial tissue and smooth muscle, histologically resembling the uterus.

Clinical features
Patients present with a pelvic mass. Most arise within the ovary, but extrauterine

cases have been described. Cases reported in the uterosacral and broad ligaments have occurred in women under 50 years of age {48}.

Macroscopy
The lesions form a cystic mass.

Histopathology
The inner lining consists of benign endometrial glands and endometrial stroma with an arrangement resembling endometrium. The outer layer of the cyst wall consists of thickened smooth muscle bundles appearing similar to myometrium.

Immunoprofile
Lesions may express ER and PR in the endometrial and myometrial components.

Differential diagnosis
"Endomyometriosis" is likely the same entity as uterine-like mass. "Endometriosis with smooth muscle metaplasia" is histologically related to uterus-like mass, if not the same. Adenomyoma is distinguished from uterus-like mass by lacking the uterus-like organization. A uterus-like mass lacks the classic features of endometrioid carcinoma and extrauterine adenosarcoma.

Genetics
A deletion on the short arm of chromosome 2 has been identified.

Prognosis and predictive factors
Benign behaviour would be expected.

Adenosarcoma

A single case of a high grade adenosarcoma arising from the round ligament was reported {1396}.

Mesenchymal tumours

Mesenchymal tumours originating from the broad and other ligaments are rare. Almost any kind of malignant or benign mesenchymal tumour may occur.

Malignant tumours
Sarcomas are extremely rare, the most frequent being leiomyosarcoma, {465, 689,1192,1608,1630,2210} for which the same diagnostic criteria should be applied as for its uterine counterpart.

Approximately 10 cases have been reported, and the prognosis is poor. Other sarcomas reported include endometrioid stromal sarcoma arising in endometriosis {2220}, embryonal rhabdomyosarcoma (occurring in children and having a poor prognosis) {991}, alveolar rhabdomyosarcoma (in an adult) {558}, mixed mesenchymal sarcoma {2822}, myxoid liposarcoma {2708} and alveolar soft part sarcoma {2017}.

Benign tumours
The most common tumours are leiomyomas and lipomas {340,962}. It is often difficult to determine the site of origin of leiomyomas within the broad ligament. It has been suggested that leiomyomas be designated as ligamentous only if clearly separated from the myometrium. A leiomyoma of the broad ligament was imitated by Dracunculosis {70}. Lipomas are usually small and located within the mesosalpinx {847} and may be mixed with leiomyomas. Cases of other mesenchymal tumours of the broad and round ligament have been reported including two benign mesenchymomas {2069}, neurofibromas, schwannomas {246,1047,2910} and a fibroma with heterotopic bone formation {2899}. Massive ascites and bilateral pleural effusion has been described in association with broad ligament leiomyoma and with paraovarian fibroma (pseudo-Meigs syndrome) {357,364, 992}.

Miscellaneous tumours

A variety of miscellaneous tumours have been described. Many of them are of ovarian type, such as germ cell and sex cord-stromal tumours. Although the question of origin from accessory ovarian tissue may be raised, in most cases no pre-existing ovarian tissue is identified. Mature teratomas, in particular dermoid cysts, occurred bilaterally within accessory ovaries of the broad ligament {941}. A dermoid cyst containing pituitary tissue occurred in the uterosacral ligament {1179}. A yolk sac tumour was found in the broad ligament {1270}.
Other reported cases included granulosa cell tumours, but some of these were in fact wolffian adnexal tumours {962,1427,2347,2997}. Several broad ligament tumours of the thecoma-fibroma group, some of which had estro-

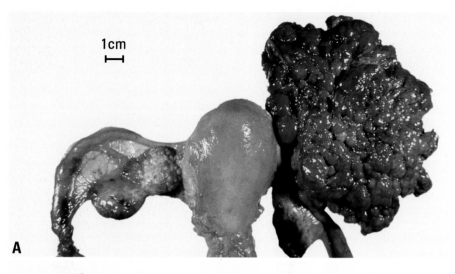

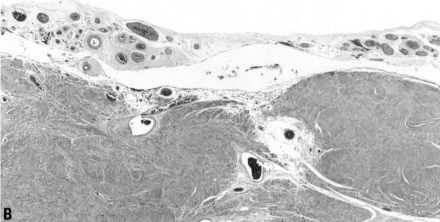

Fig. 3.17 Cotyledonoid dissecting leiomyoma. **A** Viewed posteriorly, an exophytic, congested, multinodular mass resembling placental tissue arises from the right cornual region of the uterus and extends laterally. **B** In the extrauterine component, a cotyledonoid process composed of smooth muscle is covered by connective tissue containing congested vessels.

genic effects, have been reported. Several cases of steroid cell tumour with possible origin from accessory ovaries or adrenocortical remnants have been described {38,2462,2538,2996}. Three phaeochromocytomas, two that caused hypertension and elevated vanillylmandelic acid levels and one non-functional tumour {54,58,122}, and a carcinoid {1325} have been described.

Secondary tumours

Any type of malignant tumour originating from the uterus, its adnexae, other sites within the abdomen or from any other organ of the body may spread to the uterine ligaments by direct extension, lymphatics or blood vessels. In particular, intravenous leiomyomatosis {523, 1122,1940,2051}, diffuse uterine leiomyomatosis {2394} and endometrial stromal sarcoma from the uterus may present as a mass within the broad ligament. Although it is far more common to spread to the broad ligament from the uterus, intravenous leiomyoma may exceptionally arise in the broad ligament {1154}. Cotyledonoid dissecting leiomyoma, the Sternberg tumour, is an unusual benign uterine smooth muscle neoplasm that spreads to the broad ligament {2470}. It is characterized by dissecting growth within the uterus, degenerative changes and a rich vascular component but does not have intravascular extension.

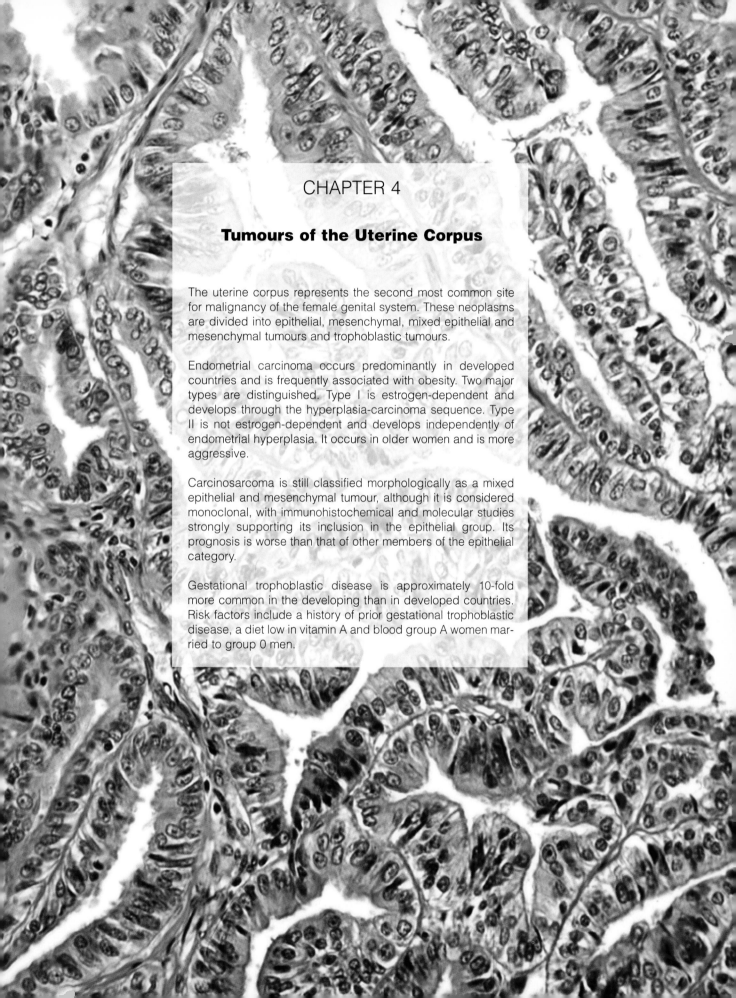

CHAPTER 4

Tumours of the Uterine Corpus

The uterine corpus represents the second most common site for malignancy of the female genital system. These neoplasms are divided into epithelial, mesenchymal, mixed epithelial and mesenchymal tumours and trophoblastic tumours.

Endometrial carcinoma occurs predominantly in developed countries and is frequently associated with obesity. Two major types are distinguished. Type I is estrogen-dependent and develops through the hyperplasia-carcinoma sequence. Type II is not estrogen-dependent and develops independently of endometrial hyperplasia. It occurs in older women and is more aggressive.

Carcinosarcoma is still classified morphologically as a mixed epithelial and mesenchymal tumour, although it is considered monoclonal, with immunohistochemical and molecular studies strongly supporting its inclusion in the epithelial group. Its prognosis is worse than that of other members of the epithelial category.

Gestational trophoblastic disease is approximately 10-fold more common in the developing than in developed countries. Risk factors include a history of prior gestational trophoblastic disease, a diet low in vitamin A and blood group A women married to group 0 men.

WHO histological classification of tumours of the uterine corpus

Epithelial tumours and related lesions

Endometrial carcinoma

Endometrioid adenocarcinoma	8380/3
Variant with squamous differentiation	8570/3
Villoglandular variant	8262/3
Secretory variant	8382/3
Ciliated cell variant	8383/3
Mucinous adenocarcinoma	8480/3
Serous adenocarcinoma	8441/3
Clear cell adenocarcinoma	8310/3
Mixed cell adenocarcinoma	8323/3
Squamous cell carcinoma	8070/3
Transitional cell carcinoma	8120/3
Small cell carcinoma	8041/3
Undifferentiated carcinoma	8020/3
Others	

Endometrial hyperplasia
    Nonatypical hyperplasia
        Simple
        Complex (adenomatous)
    Atypical hyperplasia
        Simple
        Complex
Endometrial polyp
Tamoxifen-related lesions

Mesenchymal tumours

Endometrial stromal and related tumours

Endometrial stromal sarcoma, low grade	8931/3
Endometrial stromal nodule	8930/0
Undifferentiated endometrial sarcoma	8930/3

Smooth muscle tumours

Leiomyosarcoma	8890/3
Epithelioid variant	8891/3
Myxoid variant	8896/3
Smooth muscle tumour of uncertain malignant potential	8897/1
Leiomyoma, not otherwise specified	8890/0
Histological variants	
Mitotically active variant	
Cellular variant	8892/0
Haemorrhagic cellular variant	
Epithelioid variant	8891/0
Myxoid	8896/0
Atypical variant	8893/0
Lipoleiomyoma variant	8890/0
Growth pattern variants	
Diffuse leiomyomatosis	8890/1
Dissectiing leiomyoma	
Intravenous leiomyomatosis	8890/1
Metastasizing leiomyoma	8898/1

Miscellaneous mesenchymal tumours

Mixed endometrial stromal and smooth muscle tumour	
Perivascular epithelioid cell tumour	
Adenomatoid tumour	9054/0
Other malignant mesenchymal tumours	
Other benign mesenchymal tumours	

Mixed epithelial and mesenchymal tumours

Carcinosarcoma (malignant müllerian mixed tumour; metaplastic carcinoma)	8980/3
Adenosarcoma	8933/3
Carcinofibroma	8934/3
Adenofibroma	9013/0
Adenomyoma	8932/0
Atypical polypoid variant	8932/0

Gestational trophoblastic disease

Trophoblastic neoplasms

Choriocarcinoma	9100/3
Placental site trophoblastic tumour	9104/1
Epithelioid trophoblastic tumour	9105/3

Molar pregnancies

Hydatidiform mole	9100/0
Complete	9100/0
Partial	9103/0
Invasive	9100/1
Metastatic	9100/1

Non-neoplastic, non-molar trophoblastic lesions
    Placental site nodule and plaque
    Exaggerated placental site

Miscellaneous tumours

    Sex cord-like tumours
    Neuroectodermal tumours
    Melanotic paraganglioma
    Tumours of germ cell type
    Others

Lymphoid and haematopoetic tumours

    Malignant lymphoma (specify type)
    Leukaemia (specify type)

Secondary tumours

---

[1] Morphology code of the International Classification of Diseases for Oncology (ICD-O) {921} and the Systematized Nomenclature of Medicine (http://snomed.org). Behaviour is coded /0 for benign tumours, /3 for malignant tumours, and /1 for borderline or uncertain behaviour.

TNM and FIGO classification of non-trophoblastic tumours of the uterine corpus

TNM and FIGO classification[1,2,3]

T – Primary Tumour

TNM Categories	FIGO Stages	
TX		Primary tumour cannot be assessed
T0		No evidence of primary tumour
Tis	0	Carcinoma in situ (preinvasive carcinoma)
T1	I*	Tumour confined to corpus uteri
T1a	IA	Tumour limited to endometrium
T1b	IB	Tumour invades less than one half of myometrium
T1c	IC	Tumour invades one half or more of myometrium
T2	II	Tumour invades cervix but does not extend beyond uterus
T2a	IIA	Endocervical glandular involvement only
T2b	IIB	Cervical stromal invasion
T3 and/or N1	III	Local and/or regional spread as specified in T3a, b, N1, and FIGO IIIA, B, C below
T3a	IIIA	Tumour involves serosa and/or adnexa (direct extension or metastasis) and/or cancer cells in ascites or peritoneal washings
T3b	IIIB	Vaginal involvement (direct extension or metastasis)
N1	IIIC	Metastasis to pelvic and/or para-aortic lymph nodes
T4	IVA	Tumour invades bladder mucosa and/or bowel mucosa

Note: The presence of bullous edema is not sufficient evidence to classify a tumour as T4.

M1	IVB	Distant metastasis (*excluding* metastasis to vagina, pelvic serosa, or adnexa)

Note: * FIGO recommends that Stage I patients given primary radiation therapy can be clinically classified as follows:
Stage I: Tumour confined to corpus uteri
Stage IA: Length of uterine cavity 8cm or less
Stage IB: Length of uterine cavity more than 8cm

N – Regional Lymph Nodes[4]

NX	Regional lymph nodes cannot be assessed
N0	No regional lymph node metastasis
N1	Regional lymph node metastasis

M – Distant Metastasis

MX	Distant metastasis cannot be assessed
M0	No distant metastasis
M1	Distant metastasis

Stage Grouping

Stage 0	Tis	N0	M0
Stage IA	T1a	N0	M0
Stage IB	T1b	N0	M0
Stage IC	T1c	N0	M0
Stage IIA	T2a	N0	M0
Stage IIB	T2b	N0	M0
Stage IIIA	T3a	N0	M0
Stage IIIB	T3b	N0	M0
Stage IIIC	T1, T2, T3	N1	M0
Stage IVA	T4	Any N	M0
Stage IVB	Any T	Any N	M1

[1] {51,2976}.
[2] A help desk for specific questions about the TNM classification is available at http://tnm.uicc.org.
[3] The classification applies to carcinomas and malignant mixed mesodermal tumours.
[4] The regional lymph nodes are the pelvic (hypogastric [obturator, internal iliac], common and external iliac, parametrial, and sacral) and the para-aortic nodes.

TNM and FIGO classification of gestational trophoblastic tumours

TNM and FIGO classification[1,2,3]

T–Primary Tumour

TM Categories	FIGO Stages*	
TX		Primary tumour cannot be assessed
T0		No evidence of primary tumour
T1	I	Tumour confined to uterus
T2	II	Tumour extends to other genital structures: vagina, ovary, broad ligament, fallopian tube by metastasis or direct extension
M1a	III	Metastasis to lung(s)
M1b	IV	Other distant metastasis

Note: *Stages I to IV are subdivided into A and B according to the prognostic score

M – Distant Metastasis

MX	Metastasis cannot be assessed
M0	No distant metastasis
M1	Distant metastasis
M1a	Metastasis to lung(s)
M1b	Other distant metastasis

Note: Genital metastasis (vagina, ovary, broad ligament, fallopian tube) is classified T2. Any involvement of non-genital structures, whether by direct invasion or metastasis is described using the M classification.

Stage grouping

Stage	T	M	Risk Category
I	T1	M0	Unknown
IA	T1	M0	Low
IB	T1	M0	High
II	T2	M0	Unknown
IIA	T2	M0	Low
IIB	T2	M0	High
III	Any T	M1a	Unknown
IIIA	Any T	M1a	Low
IIIB	Any T	M1a	High
IV	Any T	M1b	Unknown
IVA	Any T	M1b	Low
IVB	Any T	M1b	High

Prognostic score

Prognostic Factor	0	1	2	4
Age	<40	≥ 40		
Antecedent pregnancy	Hydatidiform mole	Abortion	Term pregnancy	
Months from index pregnancy	<4	4-<7	7-12	>12
Pretreatment serum β-hCG (IU/ml)	$< 10^3$	$10^3 - <10^4$	$10^4 - <10^5$	$\geq 10^5$
Largest tumour size, including uterus	<3 cm	3-<5 cm	≥ 5 cm	
Site of metastasis	Lung	Spleen, kidney	Gastrointestinal tract	Liver, brain
Number of metastases		1-4	5-8	>8
Previous failed chemotherapy			Single drug	2 or more drugs

Risk Categories: Total prognostic score 7 or less = low risk; Total score 8 or more = high risk

---

[1] {51,2976}
[2] A help desk for specific questions about the TNM classification is available at http://tnm.uicc.org
[3] The classification applies to choriocarcinoma (9100/3), invasive hydatidiform mole (9100/1), and placental site trophoblastic tumour (9104/1).

Epithelial tumours and related lesions

S.G. Silverberg
R.J. Kurman
F. Nogales

G.L. Mutter
R.A. Kubik-Huch
F.A. Tavassoli

Endometrial carcinoma

Definition
A primary malignant epithelial tumour, usually with glandular differentiation, arising in the endometrium that has the potential to invade into the myometrium and to spread to distant sites.

ICD-O codes

Endometrioid adenocarcinoma	8380/3
Variant with squamous differentiation	8570/3
Villoglandular variant	8262/3
Secretory variant	8382/3
Ciliated cell variant	8383/3
Mucinous adenocarcinoma	8480/3
Serous adenocarcinoma	8441/3
Clear cell adenocarcinoma	8310/3
Mixed adenocarcinoma	8323/3
Squamous cell carcinoma	8070/3
Transitional cell carcinoma	8120/3
Small cell carcinoma	8041/3
Undifferentiated carcinoma	8020/3

Epidemology
Endometrial carcinoma is the most common malignant tumour of the female genital system in developed countries, where estrogen-dependent neoplasms account for 80-85% of cases and the non-estrogen dependent tumours make up the remaining 10-15% of cases. The estrogen-dependent tumours are low grade, i.e. well or moderately differentiated and predominantly of endometrioid type. Patients with this form of endometrial cancer frequently are obese, diabetic, nulliparous, hypertensive or have a late menopause. Obesity is an independent risk factor {388}, and in Western Europe, is associated with up to 40% of endometrial cancer {241a}. On the other hand, patients with a large number of births, old age at first birth, a long birth period and a short premenopausal delivery-free period have a reduced risk of postmenopausal endometrial cancer, emphasizing the protective role of progesterone in the hormonal background of this disease {1212}.

In contrast, the non-estrogen dependent type occurs in older postmenopausal women; the tumours are high grade and consist predominantly of histological subtypes such as serous or clear cell as well as other carcinomas that have high grade nuclear features. They lack an association with exogenous or endogenous hyperoestrinism or with endometrial hyperplasia and have an aggressive behaviour {497,2005,2646}.

Pathogenesis
Endometrial cancer is made up of a biologically and histologically diverse group of neoplasms that are characterized by a different pathogenesis. Estrogen-dependent tumours (type I) are low grade and frequently associated with endometrial hyperplasias, in particular atypical hyperplasia. Unopposed estrogenic stimulation is the driving force behind this group of tumours. It may be the result of anovulatory cycles that occur in young women with the polycystic ovary syndrome or due to normally occurring anovulatory cycles at the time of menopause. The iatrogenic use of unopposed estrogens as hormone replacement therapy in older women also is a predisposing factor for the development of endometrial cancer. The second type (type II) of endometrial cancer appears less related to sustained estrogen stimulation.

Clinical features
Signs and symptoms
Although endometrial carcinoma and related lesions can be incidental findings in specimens submitted to the pathologist for other reasons (for example, endometrial biopsy for infertility or hysterectomy for uterine prolapse), in the great majority of cases they present clinically with abnormal uterine bleeding. Since most of these lesions are seen in postmenopausal women, the most common presentation is postmenopausal bleeding, but earlier in life the usual clinical finding is menometrorrhagia {1104}. The most common type of endometrial carcinoma, endometrioid adenocarcinoma, may be manifested by such clinical findings as obesity, infertility and late menopause, since it is often related either to exogenous estrogen

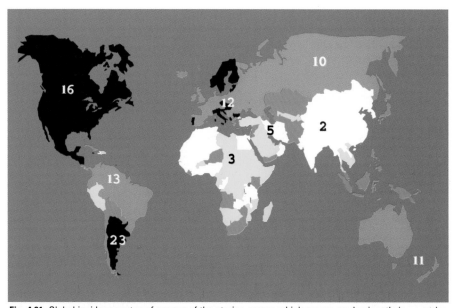

Fig. 4.01 Global incidence rates of cancer of the uterine corpus which occurs predominantly in countries with advanced economies and a Western lifestyle. Age-standardized rates (ASR) per 100,000 population and year. From Globocan 2000 {846}.

administration or to endogenous hyperoestrinism {2276,2648,2805}. Endometrial hyperplasia and atypical hyperplasia have similar clinical associations.

Imaging
Transvaginal ultrasound (US) is the imaging technique of choice for the assessment of the endometrium in symptomatic patients, e.g. in cases of postmenopausal bleeding {133}. In postmenopausal women without hormonal replacement an endometrial thickness of 5 mm is regarded as the upper normal limit {133,2650}. The presence of endometrial thickening on ultrasound or cross sectional imaging is, however, a nonspecific finding. It may be due to endometrial hyperplasia, polyps or carcinoma. The final diagnosis usually needs to be determined by endometrial sampling {133}.

Whereas currently magnetic resonance imaging (MRI) has no established role in screening for endometrial pathology, it is regarded as the best imaging technique for preoperative staging of endometrial carcinoma proven by endometrial sampling. MRI was shown to be superior to computed tomography (CT) in this regard {1135}. It is especially useful for patients with suspected advanced disease, for those with associated uterine pathology, such as leiomyomas, and for those with histological subtypes that signify a worse prognosis {916,1136}.

Macroscopy
Endometrial carcinoma usually arises in the uterine corpus, but some cases originate in the lower uterine segment, and recent studies suggest that the latter may

have different clinical and histological features {1323,3067}. Regardless of the histological type, the macroscopic appearance of endometrial carcinoma is generally that of a single dominant mass, usually occurring in an enlarged uterus, although occasionally the uterus is small or the tumour presents as a diffuse thickening of most of the endometrial surface, particularly in the serous type. Endometrial carcinoma is seen more frequently on the posterior than on the anterior wall {2691}.
The typical carcinoma is exophytic and has a shaggy, frequently ulcerated surface beneath which a soft or firm white tumour may extend shallowly or deeply into the underlying myometrium. In advanced cases the tumour may penetrate the serosa or extend into the cervix. An estimate of the extent of tumour may be requested preoperatively or operatively in order to determine the extent of the surgical procedure to be performed {594}. In occasional cases no tumour may be visible macroscopically, with carcinoma identified only at histological examination.

Tumour spread and staging
The staging of uterine tumours is by the TNM/FIGO classification {51,2976}.

Endometrioid adenocarcinoma

Definition
A primary endometrial adenocarcinoma containing glands resembling those of the normal endometrium.

Histopathology
All but a few rare endometrial carcinomas are adenocarcinomas, and the most

common of these is the endometrioid type {2691}. Endometrioid adenocarcinoma represents a spectrum of histological differentiation from a very well differentiated carcinoma difficult to distinguish from atypical complex hyperplasia to minimally differentiated tumours that can be confused not only with undifferentiated carcinoma but with various sarcomas as well. A highly characteristic feature of endometrioid adenocarcinoma is the presence of at least some glandular or villoglandular structures lined by simple to pseudostratified columnar cells that have their long axes arranged perpendicular to the basement membrane with at least somewhat elongated nuclei that are also polarized in the same direction. As the glandular differentiation decreases and is replaced by solid nests and sheets of cells, the tumour is classified as less well differentiated (higher grade). Deep myometrial invasion and lymph node metastases are both more frequent in higher grade carcinomas, and survival rates are correspondingly lower {574, 1359}. It should be noted that:
(1). Only those cells which are considered to be of glandular type are considered in the grading schema, so that solid nests of cells showing squamous or morular differentiation do not increase the tumour grade.
(2). Bizarre nuclear atypia should raise the grade by one, e.g. from 1 to 2 or 2 to 3.
(3). It should be emphasized that the presence of bizarre nuclei occurring in even a predominantly glandular tumour may indicate serous or clear cell rather than endometrioid differentiation {2691}. The distinction of very well differentiated

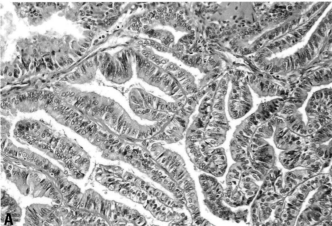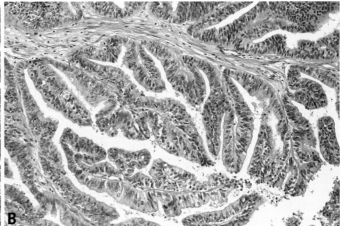

Fig. 4.02 Well differentiated endometrioid adenocarcinoma. **A** Invasion is indicated by back to back glands, complex folds and stromal disappearance. **B** The neoplastic glands are lined by columnar cells with relatively uniform nuclei; note the altered stroma in the top of the field.

endometrioid adenocarcinoma from atypical complex hyperplasia is best provided by stromal disappearance between adjacent glands, i.e. confluent, cribriform or villoglandular patterns {1433,1689,2688,2691}. Other features that may be helpful include a stromal desmoplastic response and/or tumour necrosis. Stromal foam cells may be associated with adenocarcinoma or its precursors.

Variants of endometrioid adenocarcinoma

Endometrial proliferations may exhibit a variety of differentiated epithelial types including squamous/morules, mucinous, ciliated, cleared or eosinophilic cells, and architectural variations including papillary formations. These cell types are often called metaplasias and may be encountered in benign, premalignant and malignant epithelia. When prominent in a carcinoma the neoplasm is termed a "special variant" carcinoma.

Variant with squamous differentiation
From 20-50% or more of endometrioid adenocarcinomas contain varying amounts of neoplastic epithelium showing squamous differentiation. Although the distinction between endometrioid adenocarcinoma with and without squamous differentiation is not clinically important, the recognition of squamous differentiation is nevertheless essential because the squamous or morular elements should not be considered a part of the solid component that increases the grade of an endometrioid carcinoma.
The criteria for squamous differentiation {2691} are as follows:
(1) Keratinization demonstrated with standard staining techniques.
(2) Intercellular bridges and/or
(3) Three or more of the following four criteria:
(a) Sheet-like growth without gland formation or palisading.
(b) Sharp cell margins.
(c) Eosinophilic and thick or glassy cytoplasm.
(d) A decreased nuclear to cytoplasmic ratio as compared with foci elsewhere in the same tumour.

Villoglandular variant
This type is the next most commonly encountered endometrioid adenocarcinoma variant and is usually seen involv-

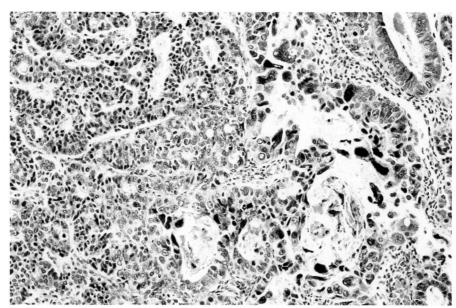

Fig. 4.03 Endometrioid adenocarcinoma. The bizarre nuclear atypia raises the tumour grade but should also prompt consideration of a serous adenocarcinoma.

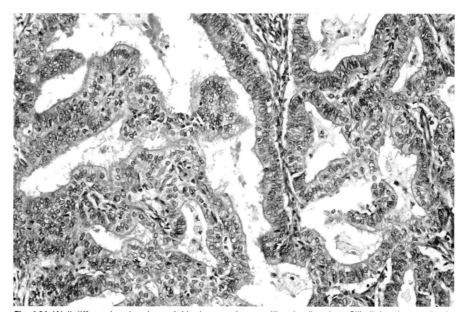

Fig. 4.04 Well differentiated endometrioid adenocarcinoma, ciliated cell variant. Cilia lining the neoplastic glands are prominent.

ing part of a low grade endometrioid carcinoma but not the entire tumour. In this pattern numerous villous fronds are seen, but their central cores are delicate, and cells with the usual cytological features (including stratification perpendicular to the basement membrane) line the villi. These features are in contrast to the more complex papillary architecture and high grade nuclear features that are typical of serous and clear cell adenocarcinomas growing in a papillary pattern.

Secretory variant
Occasional endometrioid adenocarcinomas are composed of glands lined by epithelium with voluminous, usually subnuclear, glycogen vacuoles reminiscent of early secretory endometrium. These tumours have minimal nuclear atypia and are diagnosable as carcinoma only by virtue of a confluent, cribriform or villoglandular pattern. As with the other variants, this pattern may be seen as the only one in an endometrioid adenocarci-

Table 4.01
Grading of type I (endometrioid and mucinous) endometrial adenocarcinoma.

> – Grade 1: ≤ 5% non-squamous, non-morular growth pattern
> – Grade 2: 6-50% non-squamous, non-morular growth pattern
> – Grade 3: > 50% non-squamous, non-morular growth pattern
>
> Note: Squamous/morular components are excluded from grading. Bizarre nuclear atypia should raise the grade by one (i.e. from 1 to 2 or 2 to 3) but may also signify type II differentiation.

noma or may coexist with the usual endometrioid pattern within a single tumour.

Ciliated cell variant

Although occasional ciliated cells may be seen in many endometrioid adenocarcinomas, the diagnosis of the ciliated cell variant is made only when ciliated cells line the majority of the malignant glands. Defined in this manner, this is a rare variant, and the glands often have a strong resemblance to tubal epithelium.

Mucinous adenocarcinoma

Definition

A primary adenocarcinoma of the endometrium in which most of the tumour cells contain prominent intracytoplasmic mucin.

Epidemiology

Mucinous adenocarcinoma comprises up to 9% of all cases of surgical stage I endometrial carcinoma {2454}. However, in most published series it is a relatively rare type of endometrial carcinoma {1842}.

Histopathology

Both endometrioid and clear cell adenocarcinomas may have large amounts of intraluminal mucin, but only mucinous adenocarcinoma contains the mucin within the cytoplasm. The mucin is usually easily visible with hematoxylin and eosin staining but may also be demonstrated with a mucicarmine or other mucin stain.

Variants

Some mucinous adenocarcinomas have a microglandular pattern and may be difficult to distinguish from microglandular hyperplasia of the endocervix in a biopsy specimen {2066}. These neoplasms have been reported as microglandular carcinomas {3224,3241}. Rare mucinous adenocarcinomas of the endometrium may show intestinal differentiation, containing numerous goblet cells.

Differential diagnosis

The main differential diagnosis of the usual endometrial mucinous adenocarcinoma is with a primary mucinous adenocarcinoma of the endocervix. The distinction may be particularly difficult in a biopsy or curettage specimen but is crucial for therapy and may have to be resolved by clinical and imaging studies. Some studies have claimed that immunohistochemistry is useful in determining the site of origin of an adenocarcinoma in such a specimen, with endometrial carcinomas being vimentin and estrogen receptor-positive and carcinoembryonic antigen-negative and the opposite findings for endocervical adenocarcinomas {3180}. Others have found, however, that this distinction is based more on differentiation (endometrioid vs. mucinous) than on site of origin {1393}.

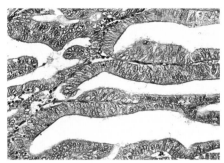

Fig. 4.05 Well differentiated endometrioid adenocarcinoma, villoglandular variant. Villous fronds have delicate central cores and are lined by cells with stratified nuclei.

Grading

Mucinous adenocarcinomas are theoretically graded in the same way as endometrioid adenocarcinomas, but in practice almost all of them are grade 1.

Prognosis and predictive factors

The prognosis appears to be similar to that of other low grade endometrial adenocarcinomas and thus is generally favourable.

Serous adenocarcinoma

Definition and historical annotation

A primary adenocarcinoma of the endometrium characterized by a complex pattern of papillae with cellular budding and not infrequently containing psammoma bodies.

Although long recognized as a common type of adenocarcinoma of the ovary, serous adenocarcinoma was first characterized as a common endometrial tumour in the early 1980s {1186,1590}.

Clinical features

Serous carcinoma typifies the so-called type II endometrial carcinoma, which dif-

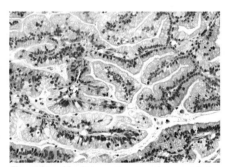

Fig. 4.06 Mucinous adenocarcinoma of the endometrium. All of the tumour cells in this field contain voluminous intracytoplasmic mucin.

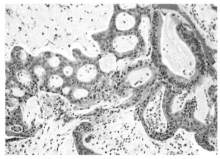

Fig. 4.07 Microglandular carcinoma. Atypia, mitoses and the endometrial location distinguish this tumour from endocervical microglandular hyperplasia.

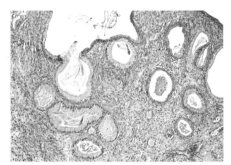

Fig. 4.08 Mucinous metaplasia. Mucinous glands are prominent, however, glandular crowding or atypia is not present.

fers from the prototypical type I endometrioid adenocarcinoma by its lack of association with exogenous or endogenous hyperoestrinism, its lack of association with endometrial hyperplasia and its aggressive behaviour {497, 2005,2646}.

Histopathology

Serous adenocarcinoma is usually, but not always, characterized by a papillary architecture with the papillae having broad fibrovascular cores, secondary and even tertiary papillary processes and prominent sloughing of the cells. The cells and nuclei are generally rounded rather than columnar and lack a perpendicular orientation to the basement membrane. The nuclei are typically poorly differentiated, are often apically rather than basally situated and usually have large, brightly eosinophilic macronucleoli. Mitoses, often atypical and bizarre, and multinucleated cells are commonly present, as are solid cell nests and foci of necrosis. Psammoma bodies are found in about 30% of cases and may be numerous. When the tumour grows in a glandular pattern, the glands are generally complex and "labyrinthine." Serous carcinoma is considered a high grade carcinoma by definition and is not graded.

Precursor lesions

A putative precursor of serous adenocarcinoma is serous endometrial intraepithelial carcinoma, which has also been called endometrial carcinoma in situ and surface serous carcinoma {79,975,2764, 3256}. This lesion is characterized by a noninvasive replacement of benign (most commonly atrophic) endometrial surface and glandular epithelium by highly malignant cells that resemble those of invasive serous carcinoma. Serous endometrial intraepithelial carcinoma has been proposed as the precursor or in situ phase of serous carcinoma, and in most reported studies it has co-existed with invasive serous and, occasionally, clear cell, adenocarcinoma. Clinically, serous endometrial intraepithelial carcinoma has a significance very similar to that of invasive serous adenocarcinoma since it can also be associated with disseminated disease outside the uterus (usually in the peritoneal cavity) even in the absence of invasive carcinoma in the endometrium {79,160,975,2764,3105,3256}.

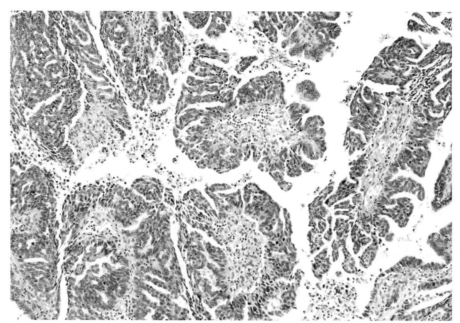

Fig. 4.09 Serous adenocarcinoma of the endometrium. Broad papillary stalks are covered by secondary micropapillae with considerable exfoliation of tumour cells.

Prognosis and predictive factors

This tumour has a tendency to develop deep myometrial invasion and extensive lymphatic invasion, and patients commonly present with extrauterine spread at the time of diagnosis. However, even in the absence of a large or deeply invasive tumour extrauterine spread is common, as are recurrence and a fatal outcome {160,1370,3105}.

Clear cell adenocarcinoma

Definition

An adenocarcinoma composed mainly of clear or hobnail cells arranged in solid, tubulocystic or papillary patterns or a combination of these patterns.

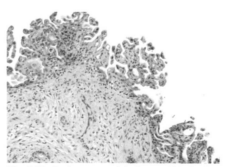

Fig. 4.10 Surface syncytial change. This benign papillary syncytial proliferation is distinguished from serous adenocarcinoma by the lack of atypia.

Epidemiology

The other major type II carcinoma of the endometrium is clear cell adenocarcinoma. It is less common than serous carcinoma (1-5%, as opposed to 5-10% of all endometrial carcinomas) but occurs in the same, predominantly older, patient population.

Tumour spread and staging

Similar to serous adenocarcinoma, patients with clear cell adenocarcinoma are frequently diagnosed in advanced clinical stages.

Histopathology

Histologically, clear, glycogen-filled cells and hobnail cells that project individually into lumens and papillary spaces characterize the typical clear cell adenocarcinoma. Unlike similarly glycogen-rich secretory endometrioid adenocarcinomas, clear cell adenocarcinoma contains large, highly pleomorphic nuclei, often with bizarre and multinucleated forms. The architectural growth pattern may be tubular, papillary, tubulocystic or solid and most frequently consists of a mixture of two or more of these patterns. Although psammoma bodies are present in approximately one-third of serous adenocarcinomas, they are rarely seen in clear cell adenocarcinomas. Occasionally, the tumour cells have granular

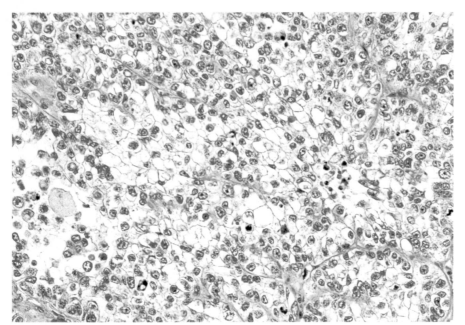

Fig. 4.11 Clear cell adenocarcinoma of the endometrium. The tumour has a predominantly solid pattern with occasional poorly formed tubules. The cytoplasm is clear, and cell walls are distinct.

eosinophilic (oncocytic) cytoplasm rather than the more characteristic clear cytoplasm {2258,2678}. This cell type may comprise the entire tumour and make it difficult to recognize as a clear cell adenocarcinoma. Endometrial clear cell adenocarcinomas are not graded.

Serous endometrial intraepithelial carcinoma may also be seen in association with clear cell adenocarcinoma, and the associated benign endometrium is generally atrophic rather than hyperplastic.

Prognosis and predictive factors

Patients with clear cell adenocarcinoma are frequently diagnosed in advanced clinical stages, and, thus, have a poor prognosis {24,400,1595,3003}. On the other hand, clear cell adenocarcinoma limited to the uterine corpus has a considerably better prognosis than serous adenocarcinoma of the same stage.

Mixed adenocarcinoma

Definition

Mixed adenocarcinoma is a tumour composed of an admixture of a type I (endometrioid carcinoma, including its variants, or mucinous carcinoma) and a type II carcinoma (serous or clear cell) in which the minor type must comprise at least 10% of the total volume of the tumour. The percentage of the minor component should be stated in the

pathology report. It is generally accepted that 25% or more of a type II tumour implies a poor prognosis, although the significance of lesser proportions is not well understood {2646,2691}.

Squamous cell carcinoma

Definition

A primary carcinoma of the endometrium composed of squamous cells of varying degrees of differentiation.

Epidemiology

Squamous cell carcinoma of the endometrium is uncommon; only about seventy cases have been reported {2397}.

Clinical features

Squamous cell carcinoma of the endometrium usually occurs in postmenopausal women and is often associated with cervical stenosis and pyometra.

Histopathology

Its histological appearance is essentially identical to that of squamous cell carcinoma of the cervix and similarly includes a rare verrucous variant {2654}.

Differential diagnosis

The much more common situation of a cervical squamous cell carcinoma extending into the endometrium must be exclud-

ed. Predominantly squamous differentiation of an endometrioid adenocarcinoma must also be excluded before making the diagnosis of primary pure squamous cell carcinoma of the endometrium.

Prognosis and predictive factors

The prognosis of most squamous cell carcinomas of the endometrium is rather poor, although the verrucous variant may be more favourable.

Transitional cell carcinoma

Definition

A carcinoma in which 90% or more is composed of cells resembling urothelial transitional cells. Lesser quantities of transitional cell differentiation would qualify the tumour as a mixed carcinoma with transitional cell differentiation.

Epidemiology

Transitional cell differentiation in endometrial carcinomas is extremely uncommon with fewer than 15 cases reported {1554,1669}. Among patients with known racial origin, 50% are non-White (African, Hispanic, or Asian). The median age is 61.6 years (range 41-83 years).

Clinical features

The main complaint at presentation is uterine bleeding.

Macroscopy

The tumours are often polypoid or papillary with a mean size of 3.5 cm. Infiltration of the myometrium is apparent in some cases.

Histopathology

The transitional cell component is often grade 2 or 3 and assumes a papillary configuration. It is always admixed with another type of carcinoma, most often endometrioid, but it may be clear cell or serous. HPV-associated koilocytotic changes occur rarely. Only the transitional cell component invades the myometrum deeply {1669}. All endometrial transitional cell carcinomas are negative for cytokeratin 20 (CK20), but half are positive for cytokeratin 7 (CK7) {1554,1669}.

Differential diagnosis

The differential diagnosis includes metastatic transitional cell carcinoma from the ovary and bladder. Unlike primary endometrial tumours, those metastatic to the endometrium are pure transitional cell tumours. The CK7 positive, CK20 negative immunoprofile also supports müllerian rather than urothelial differentiation.

Somatic genetics

Human papillomavirus (HPV) type 16 has been detected in 22% of cases studied; however, the results were negative for types 6, 11, 18, 31 and 33 in all cases assessed {1554,1672}. These findings suggest that HPV may play an aetiologic role in at least some cases.

Prognostic and predictive factors

Although information on prognostic factors is limited on these rare tumours, several women who have survived have had low stage (stage I) disease. At least two cases with extrauterine extension of the disease to either the adnexa or ovarian hilus have survived over 5 years following radiation therapy suggesting that these tumours may have a more favourable response to radiation therapy than other stage II endometrial carcinomas.

Small cell carcinoma

Definition

An endometrial carcinoma resembling small cell carcinoma of the lung.

Epidemiology

Small cell carcinoma of neuroendocrine type is an uncommon tumour of the endometrium that comprises less than 1% of all carcinomas.

Histopathology

The histological appearance is similar to that of small cell carcinoma in other organs. Small cell carcinomas are positive for cytokeratin and mostly positive for neuroendocrine markers, whereas one-half are positive for vimentin.

Prognosis and predictive factors

In contrast to small cell carcinoma elsewhere in the female genital tract, the prognosis is far better in stage I disease with a 5-year survival of about 60% {23, 1271}.

Undifferentiated carcinoma

Undifferentiated carcinomas are those lacking any evidence of differentiation.

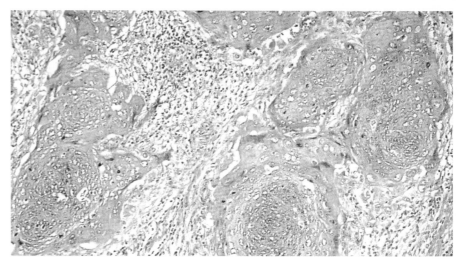

Fig. 4.12 Squamous cell carcinoma of the endometrium. This invasive tumour forms well differentiated squamous pearls. Note the reactive stroma with inflammatory cells.

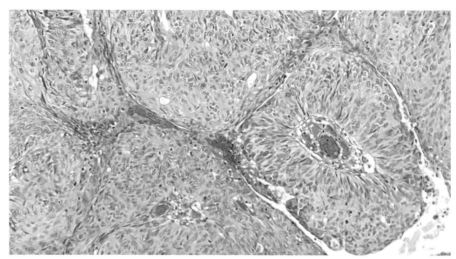

Fig. 4.13 Transitional cell carcinoma. The neoplasm forms papillae lined by low grade stratified transitional type epithelium.

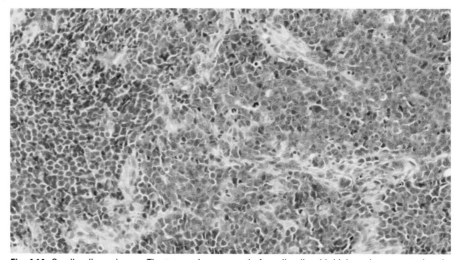

Fig. 4.14 Small cell carcinoma. The tumour is composed of small cells with high nuclear to cytoplasmic ratios.

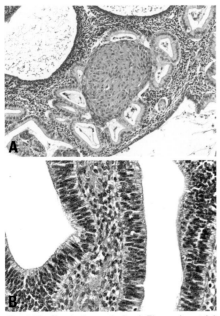

Fig. 4.15 Simple hyperplasia. **A** The endometrial glands vary from dilated to compact and are bridged by a large squamous morule. **B** Note the pseudostratified columnar epithelium with elongated nuclei lacking atypia.

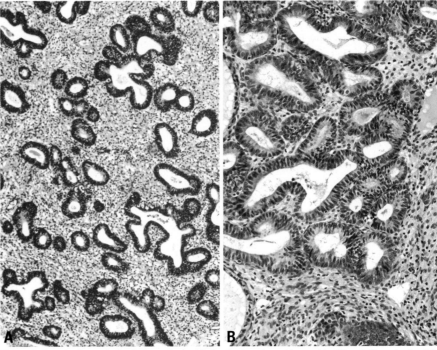

Fig. 4.16 Complex hyperplasia. **A** The endometrial glands show branching and budding. **B** There is glandular crowding; however, cytological atypia is absent.

Rare types of endometrial carcinoma

Almost every type of carcinoma reported elsewhere has been described in at least a single case report as primary in the endometrium.

Histopathology
These tumours are histologically (and usually clinically, if enough cases are available for analysis) identical to their more common counterparts in other organs. They include adenoid cystic carcinoma {985}, glassy cell carcinoma {1103} and mesonephric carcinoma {2110}. Oncocytic/oxyphilic carcinoma is thought by some to be a variant of clear

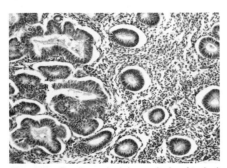

Fig. 4.17 Focal atypical hyperplasia. Atypical hyperplasia is seen on the left and a cyclic endometrium on the right.

cell carcinoma, whereas others consider it to be a separate tumour.

Endometrial hyperplasia

Definition
A spectrum of morphologic alterations ranging from benign changes, caused by an abnormal hormonal environment, to premalignant disease.

Criteria for histological typing
The endometrial hyperplasias are classified by their degree of architectural complexity as simple or complex (adenomatous) and by their cytological (nuclear) features as hyperplasia or atypical hyperplasia.

The endometrium is uniquely endowed throughout the female reproductive lifespan with a complex regular cycle of periodic proliferation, differentiation, breakdown and regeneration. This high cellular turnover, conditioned by ovarian hormones and growth factors, has many opportunities for losing its regulatory controls. Endometrial hyperplasia encompasses conditions that range from benign estrogen-dependent proliferations of glands and stroma to monoclonal outgrowths of genetically altered glands.

The high degree of morphological variability of endometrial proliferations even within the same sample is responsible for the difficulty in defining consistent and clinically meaningful diagnostic criteria {240,3135}. A further complication is fragmentation and scantiness of many aspiration biopsies. Nevertheless, histological interpretation remains the most accessible, albeit somewhat subjective, method of evaluating endometrial hyperplasias.

WHO classification
Many classifications had been proposed prior to 1994 when the World Health Organization (WHO) adopted its current

Table 4.02
World Health Organization classification of endometrial hyperplasia {2602}.

Hyperplasias (typical)
Simple hyperplasia without atypia
Complex hyperplasia without atypia (adenomatous without atypia)

Atypical hyperplasias
Simple atypical hyperplasia
Complex atypical hyperplasia (adenomatous with atypia)

schema {1535,2602}. Although this classification has been widely applied, its reproducibility is somewhat disappointing {240,1433}, and molecular data with direct implications for histological diagnosis were unavailable at the time of the 1994 classification {1956}. Nevertheless, it remains the best available classification and has been adopted in this new edition.

Endometrial hyperplasias are assumed to evolve as a progressive spectrum of endometrial glandular alterations divided into four separate categories by architecture and cytology. The vast majority of endometrial hyperplasias mimic proliferative endometria, but rare examples demonstrate secretory features. The entire spectrum of metaplastic changes may be observed in hyperplastic endometria.

Hyperplasias without atypia

Hyperplasias without atypia represent the exaggerated proliferative response to an unopposed estrogenic stimulus; the endometrium responds in a diffuse manner with a balanced increase of both glands and stroma. In simple hyperplasia the glands are tubular although frequently cystic or angular, and some even show minor epithelial budding. The lining is pseudostratified with cells displaying regular, elongated nuclei lacking atypia. In complex (adenomatous) hyperplasia the glands display extensive complicated architectural changes represented by irregular epithelial budding into both lumina and stroma and a typical cytology with pseudostratified but uniform, elongated and polarized glandular nuclei; squamous epithelial morules can be present. There is most often a shift in the gland to stroma ratio in favour of the glands.

Atypical hyperplasias

The main feature which differentiates this category from the previous one is the atypical cytology of the glandular lining as represented by loss of axial polarity, unusual nuclear shapes that are often rounded, irregularity in the nuclear membranes, prominent nucleoli and cleared or dense chromatin. Atypia occurs nearly always focally.

Simple atypical hyperplasia features atypical glandular cytology superimposed on the architecture of simple hyperplasia. This pattern is extremely unusual. The frequently found complex atypical (adenomatous with atypia) hyperplasia is a lesion characterized by an increased glandular complexity with irregular outgrowths and cytological atypia. There may be associated foci of non-endometrioid differentiation such as squamous morules. Due to the expansion and crowding of glands, the interglandular stroma is diminished but remains present. Characteristic features of adenocarcinoma are absent.

The assessment of cytological atypia is the key problem in assigning individual cases to one of the four different WHO categories. Definitions of cytological atypia are difficult to apply in the endometrium because nuclear cytological changes occur frequently in hormonal imbalance, benign regeneration and metaplasia {1619,2033}. Paradoxically, atypical hyperplasia may exhibit more atypical features than adenocarcinoma {2688}, and some grade 1 invasive endometrioid carcinomas have an extremely bland cytology. Perhaps, it would be more appropriate to consider cytological changes in the context of overall glandular architecture. Indeed, architectural focality of the lesion is so closely linked with atypia that possibly they are inseparable. In this way, atypia is best observed by comparison with adjoining normal glands.

Caveat: sampling problems

The focal nature of atypical endometrial hyperplasias may allow young women to maintain fertility, but has the disadvantage of possible underdiagnosis due to incomplete sampling. The problem is greatest in scanty fragmented specimens, something commonly encountered in routine office biopsies. Clearly, this situation is responsible for the false negative biopsies during follow up.

Hysteroscopic direction may assist in targeting a macroscopically apparent localized lesion but is not a common practice in most settings.

Contemporary approach to endometrial hyperplasia

Poor reproducibility of the 1994 WHO hyperplasia schema {240,1433} has led to a proposal to reduce the number of diagnostic classes {240}. New concepts of pathogenesis have been incorporated into an integrated genetic, histomorphometric and clinical outcome model of

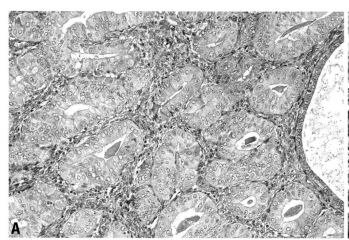
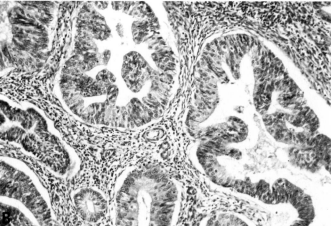

Fig. 4.18 Complex atypical hyperplasia. **A** There is glandular crowding with eosinophilic cytoplasm and nuclear enlargement, loss of polarity and prominent nucleoli. On the right is a residual, non-atypical cystic gland. **B** The glands are tortuous with epithelial tufts (reflecting abnormal polarity) protruding into the lumens and show cytological atypia.

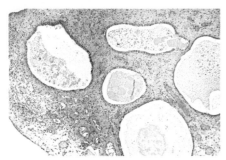

Fig. 4.19 Endometrial polyp. The glands are cystic and contain mucoid material, the stroma is fibrous, and the vessels are prominent.

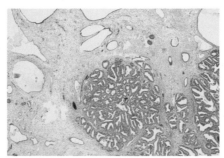

Fig. 4.20 Endometrial polyp with complex hyperplasia. Note the foci of crowded, convoluted glands in an atrophic endometrial polyp.

premalignant disease {1956,1958} (see section on genetics of endometrial carcinoma and precursor lesions). The clinical relevance of the model, however, has yet to be established.

Endometrial polyp

Definition
A benign nodular protrusion above the endometrial surface consisting of endometrial glands and stroma that is typically at least focally fibrous and contains thick-walled blood vessels.

Histopathology
Histologically, they are pedunculated or sessile lesions with a fibrous stroma in which characteristic thick-walled, tortuous, dilated blood vessels are found. The glandular component is patchily distributed and shows dilated, occasionally crowded glands lined with an atrophic epithelium, although rarely cyclic activity may be observed. Rare cases of atypical

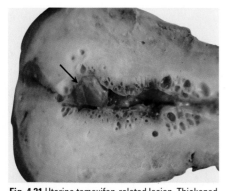

Fig. 4.21 Uterine tamoxifen-related lesion. Thickened myometrium in a 69 year old patient with subendometrial cysts and a polyp (arrow).

stromal cells have been documented in endometrial polyps {2834}, similar to those seen in polyps of the lower female genital system. Polyps can be differentiated from polypoid hyperplasias due to the distinctive stromal and vascular features of the former. Atypical hyperplasias and malignant tumours including adenocarcinomas of endometrioid and other types such as serous, as well as sarcomas and mixed tumours {2675} can be found arising in polyps.

Somatic genetics
Endometrial polyps constitute benign monoclonal proliferations of mesenchyme {891} and frequently show karyotypic abnormalities of chromosomal regions 6p21 and 12q15 {2854}, sites in which the *HMGIC* and *HMGIY* genes are located.

Prognosis and predictive factors
Polyp resection or polypectomy are the treatments of choice with few recurrences reported {2928}.

Tamoxifen-related lesions

Definition
Lesions that develop in the endometrium in patients undergoing long term tamoxifen therapy.

Epidemiology
Patients undergoing long term tamoxifen treatment often have enlarged uteri and frequently show endometrial cysts; up to 25% have endometrial polyps {531}.

Macroscopy
Tamoxifen-related polyps differ from non-iatrogenic endometrial polyps in that they

are larger, sessile with a wide implantation base in the fundus and frequently show a honeycomb appearance.

Histopathology
Histologically, the differential features with normal endometrial polyps include the bizarre stellate shape of glands and the frequent epithelial (mucinous, ciliated, eosinophilic, microglandular) and stromal (smooth muscle) metaplasias {665,1437,2558}. There is often a periglandular stromal condensation (cambium layer). Malignant transformation occurs in up to 3% of cases, and endometrioid adenocarcinoma is the most frequent type. However, other types of malignant neoplasm such as serous carcinoma and carcinosarcoma may develop in this setting.

Somatic genetics
Despite these histological differences, the cytogenetic profile of tamoxifen-related polyps is identical to non-iatrogenic polyps {609}.

Genetics of endometrial carcinoma and precancer

Genotype and histotype
Endometrial adenocarcinoma is characterized by the abrogation of *PTEN* or *TP53* tumour suppressor pathways, respectively, for the endometrioid (type I) and non-endometrioid (type II, including serous and clear cell types) clinicopathological subgroups {2647}. Deletion and/or mutation of the *PTEN* and *TP53* genes themselves are early events with widespread distribution in advanced tumours and a presence in the earliest

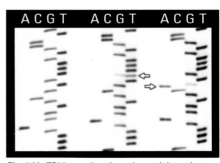

Fig. 4.22 *TP53* mutations in endometrial carcinoma. Left: Wild type sequence in an endometrioid carcinoma: Exon 8 mutations in two serous carcinomas (arrows). Middle: GTT > TTT; Val > Phe (codon 274). Right: CGT > CAT; Arg > His (codon 273).

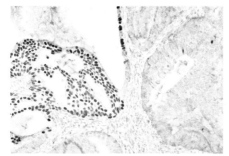

Fig. 4.23 Endometrioid adenocarcinoma (type I). Note the focal accumulation of mutant TP53 protein within a *TP53* wild-type carcinoma.

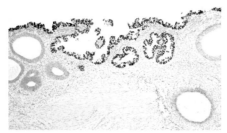

Fig. 4.24 Serous intraepithelial carcinoma (type II) expresses TP53 mutant protein.

Table 4.03
Altered gene function in sporadic endometrioid (type I) and non-endometrioid (type II) endometrial adenocarcinoma.

Gene	Alteration	Type I	Type II	References
TP53	Immunoreactivity (mutant)	5-10%	80-90%	{228,2647}
PTEN	No immunoreactivity	55%	11%	{1957}
KRAS	Activation by mutation	13-26	0-10%	{228,1512,1594,1787}
Beta-catenin	Immunoreactivity (mutant)	25-38%	rare	{1787}
MLH1	Microsatellite instability / epigenetic silencing	17%	5%	{799,826,1594}
P27	Low immunoreactivity	68-81%	76%	{2562}
Cyclin D1	High immunoreactivity	41-56%	19%	{2562}
P16	Low immunoreactivity	20-34%	10%	{2562}
Rb	Low immunoreactivity	3-4%	10%	{2562}
Bcl-2	Low immunoreactivity	65%	67%	{1512}
Bax	Low immunoreactivity	48%	43%	{1512}
Receptors				
ER and PR	Positive immunoreactivity	70-73%	19-24%	{1512}

ER = Estrogen receptor
PR = Progesterone receptor

detectable premalignant (type I) {1959} or non-invasive malignant (type II) phases of tumourigenesis {2647,2863}. A comprehensive model of sequential genetic damage has not been formulated for endometrial cancer despite a growing number of candidate genes.

PTEN checks cell division and enables apoptosis through an Akt-dependent mechanism. Functional consequences of *PTEN* mutation may be modulated in part by the hormonal environment, as *PTEN* is expressed only during the estrogen-driven proliferative phase of the endometrium {1957}. The use of PTEN immunohistochemistry as a tool for diagnosis of clinically relevant neoplastic endometrial disease is limited by the fact that one-third to one-half of type I cancers continue to express PTEN protein, and loss of *PTEN* function occurs as an early event that may precede cytological and architectural changes {1959}.

TP53 is the prototypical tumour suppressor gene capable of inducing a stable growth arrest or programmed cell death. Mutant protein accumulates in nuclei, where it can be readily demonstrated by immunohistochemistry in most serous (type II) adenocarcinomas {228}. Staining for TP53 is not routinely indicated, but the association of positive stain-ing with a poor clinical outcome may be informative in suboptimal, scanty or fragmented specimens.

Molecular delineation of premalignant disease
Type I cancers begin as monoclonal outgrowths of genetically altered premalignant cells, and many bear genetic stigmata of microsatellite instability, *KRAS* mutation and loss of *PTEN* function that are conserved in subsequent cancer {1642,1956}. The earliest molecular changes, including *PTEN*, are detectable at a stage before glands have under-gone any change in morphology {1959}. The accumulation of genetic damage is thought to cause emergence of histologically evident monoclonal lesions. Further elaboration of the histopathology of endometrial precancers has been accomplished through correlative histomorphometric analysis of genetically ascertained premalignant lesions {1958}. Because these lesions were initially defined by molecular methods, their diagnostic criteria differ from those of atypical endometrial hyperplasia. They have been designated endometrial intraepithelial neoplasia ("EIN") {1955},

Table 4.04
Essential diagnostic criteria of endometrial intraepithelial neoplasia (EIN).

EIN Criterion	Comments
1. Architecture	Gland area exceeds that of stroma, usually in a localized region.
2. Cytological alterations	Cytology differs between architecturally crowded focus and background.
3. Size >1 mm	Maximum linear dimension should exceed 1 mm. Smaller lesions have unknown natural history.
4. Exclude benign mimics and cancer	

and many examples with correlative genotypes and morphometry can be seen online at www.endometrium.org.

Endometrial intraepithelial neoplasia (EIN)
This lesion is defined as the histopathological presentation of premalignant endometrial disease as identified by integrated molecular genetic, histomorphometric and clinical outcome data. Tissue morphometry (D-Score {153} predictive of cancer outcome) and genetic studies are cross validating in that these methodologically independent techniques provide concordant identification of EIN lesions when applied to a common pool of study material {1958}. The EIN scheme partitions endometrial proliferations into different therapeutic groups. Distinctive diagnostic categories include:
(1) Benign architectural changes of unopposed estrogens (endometrial hyperplasia).
(2) EIN.
(3) Well differentiated adenocarcinoma.

The histological changes produced by unopposed estrogens (non-atypical hyperplasias) are quite unlike localizing EIN lesions. The latter originate focally through monoclonal outgrowth of a mutant epithelial clone with altered cytology and architecture. Computerized morphometric analysis, which quantifies specific architectural patterns associated with increased clinical cancer risk {154}, objectively defined the morphology of monoclonal EIN lesions. Because of differing diagnostic criteria, only 79% of atypical endometrial hyperplasias translate to EIN, and approximately a third of all EIN diagnoses are garnered from non-atypical hyperplasia categories.

Genetic susceptibility
The overwhelming majority of endometrial cancers are sporadic, but they may rarely present as a manifestation of multicancer familial syndromes. Examples include hereditary nonpolyposis colon cancer (HNPCC), caused by mutation of DNA mismatch repair genes that produce constitutive microsatellite instability {799} and Cowden syndrome in patients with germline *PTEN* inactivation {1957}.

Prognosis and predictive factors
In addition to tumour type and, for type I adenocarcinomas, tumour grade, other histological and non-histological determinations influence the prognosis of endometrial carcinoma. The most important of these is the surgical stage, which in 1988 replaced the clinical staging system that had been in use for many years {2642}. The extent of surgical staging performed is based in part on the medical condition of the patient and in part on the preoperative or intraoperative assessment of tumour risk factors such as type and grade, depth of myometrial invasion and extension to involve the cervix {2692,2714}.
Myometrial invasion is thus an important issue, both as a prognostic factor in its own right and as a determinant of the extent of staging and of subsequent therapy in cases treated by hysterectomy. FIGO divides stage I tumours into IA (limited to the endometrium), IB (invasion of less than half of the myometrium), and IC (invasion of more than half of the myometrium), {51,2976}. Some oncologists, however, make treatment decisions based on thirds (inner, mid, outer) of myometrial invasion or distance in millimetres (mm) from the serosal surface. Thus, the pathologist can best satisfy the desires for all of this information by reporting the maximal depth of tumour invasion from the endomyometrial junction and the thickness of the myometrium at that point (e.g. 7 mm tumour invasion into a 15 mm thick myometrium) {2686}. True myometrial invasion must be distinguished from carcinomatous extension (not invasion) into pre-existing "tongues"

of endometrium penetrating the myometrium or into foci (sometimes deep-seated) of adenomyosis {2652, 2688}. It should also be noted that tumour extension to the uterine serosa raises the stage to IIIA. Vascular or lymphatic space invasion is an unfavourable prognostic factor that should be reported {78}. Perivascular lymphocytic infiltrates may be the first clue to vascular invasion and, thus, should prompt deeper levels within the suspect block and/or the submission of more tissue sections for histological examination.
It is also important to evaluate cervical involvement in the hysterectomy specimen since extension to the cervix raises the stage to II. The distinction between stage IIA and IIB is based on whether the extension involves the endocervical surface and/or underlying glands only or invades the cervical stroma. One should be aware that an adenocarcinoma involving glands only might be an entirely separate adenocarcinoma in situ primary in the endocervix.
Non-histological factors may also play a role in determining the prognosis of endometrial carcinoma. It is unclear at the present time, however, what the cost/benefit ratio of performing additional studies might be since the prognosis and treatment are currently based on the combination of tumour type, grade, where appropriate, and extent, as discussed above. Nevertheless, patients with carcinomas of intermediate prognosis, such as stage I well differentiated endometrioid adenocarcinoma with focal deep myometrial invasion might benefit from additional information including such factors as tumour ploidy {1349,1441}, hormone receptor status {575,1441}, tumour suppressor genes {1309,1449}, oncogenes {1205,1449}, proliferation markers {966,1449,2012} and morphometry {2751}. Which, if any, of these or other studies will prove to be most useful is problematic at this time.

Mesenchymal tumours and related lesions

M.R. Hendrickson
F.A. Tavassoli
R.L. Kempson
W.G. McCluggage
U. Haller
R.A. Kubik-Huch

Definition

Uterine mesenchymal tumours are derived from the mesenchyme of the corpus consisting of endometrial stroma, smooth muscle and blood vessels or admixtures of these. Rarely, these tumours may show mesenchymal differentiation that is foreign to the uterus.

Epidemiology

The most common malignant mesenchymal tumours of the uterine corpus are leiomyosarcoma and endometrial stromal tumours, and both are more frequent in Black than in White women {1139, 1729}.

Clinical features

Signs and symptoms

The most common presentation for mesenchymal tumours is uterine enlargement, abnormal uterine bleeding or pelvic pain.

Imaging

Non-invasive imaging, usually by ultrasound, but occasionally by magnetic resonance imaging (MRI), can be utilized in selected cases to distinguish between a solid ovarian tumour and a pedunculated leiomyoma or to distinguish leiomyomas from adenomyosis. On MRI leiomyomas present as well delineated lesions of low signal intensity on T1 and T2-weighted images. They may, however, undergo degenerative changes resulting in various, non-specific MRI appearances {1947,2971}. On MRI the presence of a large, heterogeneous mass with irregular contours should raise concern for sarcoma.

Endometrial stromal and related tumours

Definition and historical annotation

Endometrial mesenchymal tumours in their better-differentiated forms are composed of cells resembling those of proliferative phase endometrial stroma. Numerous thin-walled small arteriolar type (plexiform) vessels are characteristically present.

Endometrial stromal sarcomas (ESS) have been traditionally divided into low and high grade types based on mitotic count. However, since high grade endometrial sarcomas lack specific differentiation and bear no histological resemblance to endometrial stroma, it has been proposed that they be designated undifferentiated endometrial or uterine sarcoma {811}. In this classification the distinction between low grade ESS and undifferentiated endometrial sarcoma is not made on the basis of mitotic count but on features such as nuclear pleomorphism and necrosis.

ICD-O codes

Endometrial stromal sarcoma,
  low grade   8931/3
Endometrial stromal nodule   8930/0
Undifferentiated endometrial
  sarcoma   8930/3

Histopathology

Endometrial stromal tumours are composed of cells resembling those of proliferative endometrial stroma and are far less frequent than smooth muscle tumours. Endometrial stromal tumours are subdivided into benign and malignant groups based on the type of tumour margin {1432,2054,2097,2883}.

Those with pushing margins are benign stromal nodules, whereas those with infiltrating margins qualify as stromal sarcomas. There is general agreement on the morphologic definition of typical cases of both low grade ESS and undifferentiated endometrial sarcoma. Characteristically, low grade ESS, a clinically indolent neoplasm, features a plexiform vasculature, minimal cytological atypia and infrequent mitotic figures. The usual undifferentiated sarcoma, a highly aggressive neoplasm, lacks a plexiform vasculature, features substantial cytological atypia and has frequent and often atypical mitotic figures. However, there is no valid evidence that the isolated finding of a mitotic index of 10 or more per 10 high power fields is an adverse prognostic finding in a neoplasm that is otherwise a typical low grade ESS. A small minority of cases share features of low grade ESS and undifferentiated sarcoma, and their classification is controversial.

Immunoprofile

The neoplastic cells of both the stromal nodule and low grade ESS are immunoreactive for vimentin, CD10

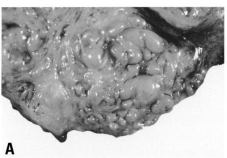
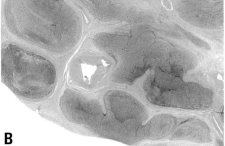
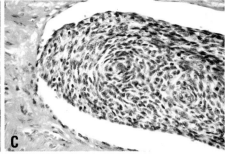

Fig. 4.25 Low grade endometrial stromal sarcoma (ESS). **A** Worm-like, soft, yellow masses focally replace the myometrium. **B** The myometrium is extensively infiltrated by basophilic islands of low grade ESS. **C** A tongue of low grade ESS protrudes into a vascular space.

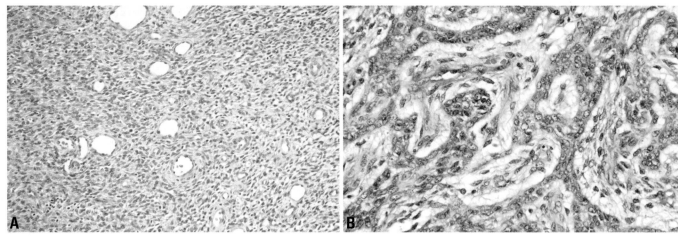

Fig. 4.26 Low grade endometrial stromal sarcoma (ESS). **A** There is a proliferation of endometrial stromal cells lacking atypia around spiral arteriole-like blood vessels. **B** Note a sex cord-like pattern in a low grade ESS.

{486,1821} and at least focally for actin {914}. They are usually, but not always {914}, negative for desmin and h-caldesmon {2065,2101,2488}. Low grade ESS is almost always positive for both estrogen and progesterone receptors. {1411,2350,2502}. Rarely, low grade endometrial stromal tumours, particularly those with areas displaying a sex cord pattern, may be positive for alpha-inhibin {1521}, CD99 {167} and cytokeratin {29}. The sex cord areas may also be immunoreactive for desmin, whereas the surrounding endometrial stromal cells are not {678,1661}.

Somatic genetics

Fusion of two zinc finger genes (*JAZF1* and *JJAZ1*) by translocation t(7;17) is present in most low grade endometrial stromal tumours {1189,1252,1503}. Endometrial stromal nodules and low grade ESSs are typically diploid with a low S-phase fraction {292,1220}.

Prognosis and predictive factors

The histological distinction between undifferentiated endometrial sarcoma and low grade ESS has important implications regarding prognosis {2601} Low grade ESSs are indolent tumours with a propensity for local recurrence, usually many years after hysterectomy. Distant metastases are less common. In contrast, undifferentiated endometrial sarcomas are highly aggressive tumours with the majority of patients presenting with extrauterine disease at the time of diagnosis and dying within two years of diagnosis {232,811}.

Endometrial stromal sarcoma, low grade

Definition

This tumour fits the definition of endometrial stromal tumour presented above and is distinguished from the stromal nodule on the basis of myometrial infiltration and/or vascular space invasion.

Epidemiology

Low grade ESS is a rare tumour of the uterus accounting for only 0.2% of all genital tract malignant neoplasms {645, 1509,1745}. In general low grade ESSs affect younger women than other uterine malignancies; studies have demonstrated that the mean age ranges from 42-58 years, and 10-25% of patients are premenopausal {437,645}.

Clinical features

The clinical features have been discussed above.

Macroscopy

Low grade ESS may present as a solitary, well delineated and predominantly intramural mass, but extensive permeation of the myometrium is more common, with extension to the serosa in approximately half of the cases. The sectioned surface appears yellow to tan, and the tumour has a softer consistency than the usual leiomyoma. Cystic and myxoid degeneration as well as necrosis and haemorrhage are seen occasionally.

Localization

Metastases are rarely detected prior to the diagnosis of the primary lesion {29,684,3222}. Extrauterine extension is present in up to a third of the women with low grade ESS at the time of hysterectomy. The extension may appear as worm-like plugs of tumour within the vessels of the broad ligament and adnexa.

Histopathology

Low grade ESS is usually a densely cellular tumour composed of uniform, oval to spindle-shaped cells of endometrial stromal-type; by definition significant atypia and pleomorphism are absent. Although most tumours are paucimitotic, mitotic rates of 10 or more per 10 high power fields can be encountered, and a high mitotic index does not in itself alter the diagnosis. A rich network of delicate small arterioles resembling the spiral arterioles of the late secretory endometrium supports the proliferating cells. Cells with foamy cytoplasm (tumour cells, foamy histiocytes, or both) are prominent in some cases. Endometrial type glands occur in 11-40% of endometrial stromal tumours {516,1343,2054}. Sex cord-like structures may also be found {511}. Myxoid and fibrous change may occur focally or diffusely {2054,2102}. Perivascular hyalinization and a stellate pattern of hyalinization occur in some cases. Reticulin stains usually reveal a dense network of fibrils surrounding individual cells or small groups of cells. Necrosis is typically absent or inconspicuous.

Focal smooth muscle differentiation (spindle or epithelioid) or cells with differentiation that is ambiguous between stromal and smooth muscle cells may develop in endometrial stromal tumours; these areas are limited to less than 30% of the tumour. When the smooth muscle component comprises 30% or more of the tumour, the lesion is designated as a mixed endometrial stromal and smooth muscle tumour. Focal rhabdoid differentiation has been described in one case {1813}.

The differential diagnosis includes stromal nodule, intravenous leiomyomatosis, adenomyosis with sparse glands and adenosarcoma. In a biopsy or curettage specimen it is often impossible to distinguish low grade ESS from a stromal nodule, a non-neoplastic stromal proliferation or a highly cellular leiomyoma.

Histogenesis

Extrauterine primary endometrioid stromal sarcomas occur and often arise from endometriosis {280}.

Prognosis and predictive factors

Low grade ESS is characterized by indolent growth and late recurrences; up to one-half of patients develop one or more pelvic or abdominal recurrences. The median interval to recurrence is 3-5 years but may exceed 20 years. Pulmonary metastases occur in 10% of stage I tumours {1311}.

The 5-year survival rate for low grade ESS ranges from 67% {2048} to nearly 100% with late metastases and a rela-tively long-term survival despite tumour dissemination {437,811,2263}. The surgical stage is the best predictor of recurrence and survival for ESSs {300,437}.

Both recurrent and metastatic ESSs may remain localized for long periods and are amenable to successful treatment by resection, radiation therapy, progestin therapy or a combination thereof {300,1750,3089}.

Conservative management has been advocated for some patients with low grade ESS {1677}. In some studies that have utilized progestin therapy, 100% survival rates have been achieved even for patients with stage III tumours {2263}.

Endometrial stromal nodule

Definition

A benign endometrial stromal tumour characterized by a well delineated, expansive margin and composed of neoplastic cells that resemble proliferative phase endometrial stromal cells supported by a large number of small, thin-walled arteriolar-type vessels.

Clinical features

Women with a stromal nodule range in age from 23-75 years with a median of 47 years {292,437,2098,2101,2102,2883}. About one-third of the women are post-menopausal. Two-thirds of the women present with abnormal uterine bleeding and menorrhagia. Pelvic and abdominal pain occur less frequently.

Macroscopy

The tumour is characteristically a solitary, well delineated, round or oval, fleshy nodule with a yellow to tan sectioned surface. The median tumour diameter is 4.0 cm (range 0.8-15 cm) {2883}. About two-thirds are purely intramural without any apparent connections to the endometrium, 18% of the lesions are polypoid, and others involve both the endometrium and myometrium.

Histopathology

The histological appearance is identical to that described above for low grade ESS except for the absence of infiltrative margins {292,437,2097,2098,2101,2102,2883}. Rare, focal marginal irregularity in the form of finger-like projections that do not exceed 3 mm is acceptable. Smooth and skeletal muscle along with sex cord differentiation may be present focally {1685}.

The differential diagnosis includes low grade ESS and highly cellular leiomyoma. The presence of at least focal typical neoplastic smooth muscle bundles, large, thick walled vessels and strong immunoreactivity with desmin and h-caldesmon and the absence of reactivity with CD10 help distinguish a highly cellular leiomyoma from a stromal nodule.

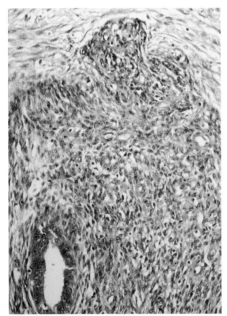

Fig. 4.27 Low grade endometrial stromal sarcoma (ESS). Myoinvasive low grade ESS that shows endometrial glandular differentiation. The myometrium is seen above.

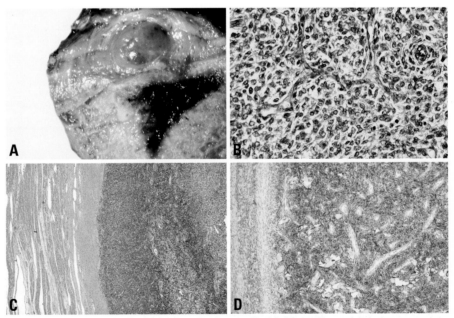

Fig. 4.28 Endometrial stromal nodule. **A** Note the circumscribed, bulging, yellow nodule in the myometrium. **B** Cytologically bland ovoid cells without discernible cytoplasm proliferate in a plexiform pattern and are supported by small arterioles. **C** The circumscribed myometrial nodule is composed of closely packed cells. **D** The tumour cells are strongly immunoreactive for CD10.

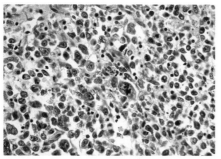

Fig. 4.29 Undifferentiated endometrial sarcoma. Atypical tumour cells show no resemblance to normal endometrial stromal cells. Note the presence of an abnormal mitotic figure.

Prognosis and predictive factors

Endometrial stromal nodules are benign {437,2101,2883}. A hysterectomy may be required if the lesion has not been completely excised.

Undifferentiated endometrial sarcoma

Definition

A high grade endometrial sarcoma that lacks specific differentiation and bears no histological resemblance to endometrial stroma.

Synonym

Undifferentiated uterine sarcoma.

Macroscopy

Macroscopically, undifferentiated uterine sarcomas are characterized by one or more polypoid, fleshy, grey to yellow endometrial masses and often show prominent haemorrhage and necrosis.

Histopathology

Histologically, undifferentiated endometrial sarcomas show marked cellular atypia and abundant mitotic activity, often including atypical forms. They lack the typical growth pattern and vascularity of low grade ESS {651,811} and displace the myometrium in contrast to the infiltrative pattern of low grade ESS. They resemble the sarcomatous component of a carcinosarcoma, and the possibility of carcinosarcoma and other specific sarcomas should be excluded with adequate sampling.

These sarcomas are most often aneuploid with an S-phase fraction greater than 10% {292} and negative for estrogen and progesterone receptors.

Prognosis and predictives factors

These tumours are aggressive, and death occurs from tumour dissemination within three years after hysterectomy in most cases.

Smooth muscle tumours

Definition

Benign or malignant neoplasms composed of cells demonstrating smooth muscle differentiation.

ICD-O codes

Leiomyosarcoma, NOS	8890/3
Epithelioid variant	8891/3
Myxoid variant	8896/3
Smooth muscle tumour of uncertain malignant potential	8897/1
Leiomyoma, NOS	8890/0
Leiomyoma, histological variants	
Cellular leiomyoma	8892/0
Epithelioid leiomyoma	8891/0
Myxoid leiomyoma	8896/0
Atypical leiomyoma	8893/0

Table 4.05
Diagnostic criteria for leiomyosarcoma.

	Standard smooth muscle differentiation	Epithelioid differentiation	Myxoid differentiation
Histology	Fascicles of cigar-shaped spindled cells with scanty to abundant eosinophilic cytoplasm	Rounded cells with central nuclei and clear to eosinophilic cytoplasm	Spindle-shaped cells set within an abundant myxoid matrix
Criteria for leiomyosarcoma	Any coagulative tumour cell necrosis In the absence of tumour cell necrosis the diagnosis requires diffuse, moderate to severe cytological atypia and a mitotic index of ≥ 10mf/10hpf. When the mitotic index is less than 10mf/10hpf, the chance of recurrence is low (less than a 2-3%) and the tempo of recurrence is slow. This group is labelled "atypical leiomyoma with low risk of recurrence".	Any coagulative tumour cell necrosis In the absence of tumour cell necrosis the diagnosis requires diffuse, moderate to severe cytological atypia and a mitotic index of ≥ 5mf/10hpf	Any coagulative tumour cell necrosis In the absence of tumour cell necrosis, the diagnosis requires diffuse, moderate to severe cytological atypia and a mitotic index of ≥ 5mf/10hpf
Comments	In the absence of coagulative tumour cell necrosis and significant atypia a high mitotic index is compatible with a benign clinical course. When the mitotic index exceeds 15 mf/10hpf the term "mitotically active leiomyoma with limited experience" can be used The category "leiomyoma with limited experience" is also used for smooth muscle neoplasms that have focal moderate to severe atypia	Focal epithelioid differentiation may be mimicked by cross-sectioned fascicles of standard smooth muscle	The very common perinodular hydropic degeneration should not be included in this group

mf/10hpf = mitotic figure(s) per 10 high power fields. See ref. {211} for discussion of mitosis counting techniques.

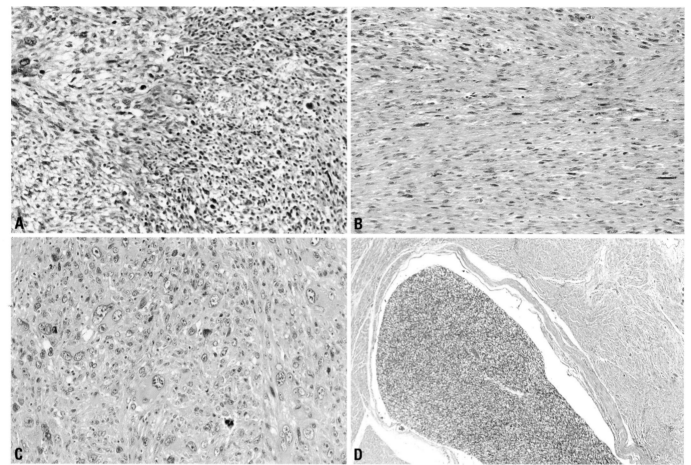

Fig. 4.30 Leiomyosarcoma. **A** This tumour exhibits typical coagulative tumour cell necrosis on the right. This pattern of necrosis features an abrupt transition from viable tumour cells to necrotic tumour cells without intervening collagen or granulation tissue. **B** This tumour has a low level of atypia. This degree of atypia should prompt careful search for more diagnostic features. **C** A high level of atypia and apotosis is apparent in this tumour. **D** Leiomyosarcoma with intravascular tumour growth. The differential diagnosis includes intravenous leiomyomatosis, low grade endometrial stroma sarcoma (ESS) and leiomyosarcoma with vascular invasion. High power showed a poorly differentiated neoplasm with marked cytologic atypia and a high mitotic index. These are not features of low grade ESS or intravenous leiomyomatosis.

Lipoleiomyoma	8890/0
Leiomyoma, growth pattern variants	
Diffuse leiomyomatosis	8890/1
Intravenous leiomyomatosis	8890/1
Benign metastasizing leiomyoma	8898/1

Leiomyosarcoma

Definition
A malignant neoplasm composed of cells demonstrating smooth muscle differentiation.

Epidemiology
Leiomyosarcoma represents the most common pure uterine sarcoma and comprises slightly over 1% of all uterine malignancies {1139}. The incidence of leiomyosarcoma is reported to be 0.3-0.4/100,000 women per year {1139}. Leiomyosarcoma arises nearly exclusively in adults. The median age of patients with leiomyosarcoma was 50-55 years in larger studies {947,1745}, and 15% of the patients were younger than 40 years. The risk factors for endometrial carcinomas such as nulliparity, obesity, diabetes mellitus and hypertension are not known to relate to leiomyosarcoma.

Clinical features
Leiomyosarcomas localized to the uterus and leiomyomas produce similar symptoms. Although a rapid increase in the size of the uterus after menopause may raise the possibility of leiomyosarcoma, in fact sarcoma is not more prevalent (less than 0.5%) in women with "rapidly growing" leiomyomas {1622,2187}.

Leiomyosarcoma may spread locally, regionally or by haematogenous dissemination. This fact of natural history has implications for both diagnosis and management. Local and regional extension may produce an abdominal or pelvic mass and gastrointestinal or urinary tract symptoms. Haematogenous dissemination is most often to the lungs. Leiomyosarcoma is only infrequently diagnosed on endometrial samplings {1622}.

Macroscopy
Leiomyosarcomas are characteristically solitary intramural masses and are usually not associated with leiomyomas. Leiomyosarcomas average 8.0 cm in diameter and are fleshy with poorly defined margins. Zones of haemorrhage and necrosis characteristically interrupt their grey-yellow or pink sectioned surface.

Histopathology

The usual leiomyosarcoma is a cellular tumour composed of fascicles of spindle-shaped cells that possess abundant eosinophilic cytoplasm. Typically, the nuclei are fusiform, usually have rounded ends and are hyperchromatic with coarse chromatin and prominent nucleoli. Tumour cell necrosis is typically prominent but need not be present. The mitotic index usually exceeds 15 figures per 10 high power fields. Vascular invasion is identified in up to 25% of leiomyosarcomas. Giant cells resembling osteoclasts occasionally are present in otherwise typical leiomyosarcomas, and, rarely, xanthoma cells may be prominent {1058,1776}.

A diagnosis of leiomyosarcoma should be made with great caution in women less than 30 years of age and only after exclusion of exposure to Leuprolide, which sometimes induces a pattern of necrosis identical to coagulative tumour cell necrosis {664}.

Epithelioid variant

Epithelioid leiomyosarcomas combine an "epithelioid" phenotype with the usual features of malignancy, i.e. high cellularity, cytological atypia, tumour cell necrosis and a high mitotic rate {130,1538, 2292}. Specifically, epithelioid differentiation denotes tumour cells that have a rounded configuration with eosinophilic to clear cytoplasm. When the cytoplasm is totally clear the label "clear cell" is used. Most malignant epithelioid smooth muscle tumours are of the leiomyoblastoma type, although clear cell leiomyosarcoma has been reported.

Myxoid variant

Myxoid leiomyosarcoma is a large, gelatinous neoplasm that often appears to be circumscribed on macroscopic examina-

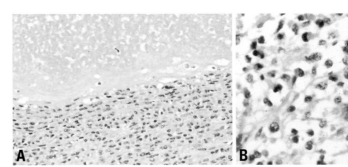

Fig. 4.31 Epithelioid leiomyosarcoma. **A** Tumour cell necrosis is present in the upper half of the field adjacent to highly pleomorphic cells. **B** The tumour cells exhibit nuclear pleomorphism, and mitotic figures are easily found.

tion {131,1465}. The smooth muscle cells are widely separated by myxoid material. The characteristic low cellularity largely accounts for the presence of only a few mitotic figures per 10 high power fields in most myxoid leiomyosarcomas. In almost all instances myxoid leiomyosarcomas show cellular pleomorphism and nuclear enlargement. They commonly show myometrial and, sometimes, vascular invasion.

Prognosis and predictive factors

Leiomyosarcoma is a highly malignant neoplasm {1745,2096}. The variation in survival rates reported historically is largely the result of the use of different criteria for its diagnosis. Overall 5-year survival rates range from 15-25% {185,231,377,812,1585,3005,3109}. The 5-year survival rate is 40-70% in stage I and II tumours {291,947,1381,1585, 1765,1797,2045,2049,2200,3139}. Premenopausal women have a more favourable outcome in some series {947, 1381,1585,1797,3005,3139} but not in others {185,1148}. Most recurrences are detected within 2 years {231,377,1148, 1381}.

The prognosis of leiomyosarcoma depends chiefly upon the extent of

spread. For tumours confined to the uterine corpus, some investigators have found that the size of the neoplasm is an important prognostic factor {812,1364, 2049} with the best demarcation occurring at 5 cm. Several recent series, including the large Gynecologic Oncology Group study of early stage leiomyosarcoma, have found the mitotic index to be of prognostic significance {811,947,1585,1745}, whereas others have not {812}. The utility of grading leiomyosarcomas is controversial, and no universally accepted grading system exists. Pathologists should comment on the presence or absence of extrauterine extension and/or vascular space involvement, the maximum tumour diameter and the mitotic index.

Smooth muscle tumour of uncertain malignant potential

Definition

A smooth muscle tumour that cannot be diagnosed reliably as benign or malignant on the basis of generally applied criteria.

Histopathology

This category of smooth muscle tumour of uncertain malignant potential should

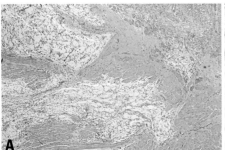
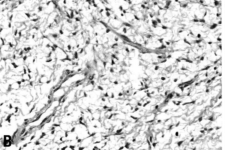
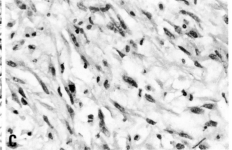

Fig. 4.32 Myxoid leiomyosarcoma. **A** A paucicellular myxoid neoplasm infiltrates the myometrium. **B** Relatively bland spindle-shaped tumour cells are widely spaced in a myxoid matrix containing a delicate vasculature. **C** Nuclear pleomorphism and mitotic figures, although few in number, can be found.

be used sparingly and is reserved for smooth muscle neoplasms whose appearance is ambiguous for some reason, and the relevant diagnostic possibilities differ in their clinical implications {211}. Examples include cases in which the subtype of smooth muscle differentiation is in doubt, i.e. standard smooth muscle, epithelioid or myxoid, and application of the competing classification rules would lead to different clinical predictions. On other occasions the assessment of a diagnostic feature, e.g. the type of necrosis or the interpretation of mitotic figures, is ambiguous, and the competing alternative interpretations would lead to different clinical predictions.

Leiomyoma

Definition
A benign neoplasm composed of smooth muscle cells with a variable amount of fibrous stroma.

Macroscopy
Leiomyomas are typically multiple, spherical and firm. The sectioned surface is white to tan and has a whorled trabecular texture. Leiomyomas bulge above the surrounding myometrium from which they are easily shelled out. Submucosal leiomyomas distort the overlying endometrium, and, as they enlarge, they may bulge into the endometrial cavity and produce bleeding. Rare examples become pedunculated and prolapse through the cervix. Intramural leiomyomas are the most common. Subserosal leiomyomas can become pedunculated, and on torsion with necrosis of the pedicle the leiomyoma may lose its connection with the uterus. Very rarely, some become attached to another pelvic structure (parasitic leiomyoma). The appearance of a leiomyoma often is altered by degenerative changes. Submucosal leiomyomas frequently are ulcerated and haemorrhagic. Haemorrhage and necrosis are observed in some leiomyomas, particularly in large ones in women who are pregnant or who are undergoing high-dose progestin therapy. Dark red areas represent haemorrhage and sharply demarcated yellow areas reflect necrosis. The damaged smooth muscle is replaced eventually by firm white or translucent collagenous tissue. Cystic degeneration also occurs, and some leiomyomas become extensively calcified.

Histopathology
Most leiomyomas are composed of easily recognized smooth muscle featuring whorled, anastomosing fascicles of uniform, fusiform cells. Characteristically, the spindle-shaped cells have indistinct borders and abundant, often fibrillar, eosinophilic cytoplasm. Sometimes, particularly in cellular leiomyomas, the cytoplasm is sparse, and the fascicular arrangement of the cells may be muted.

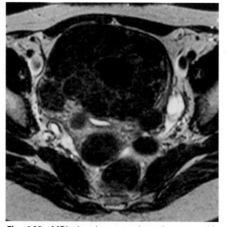

Fig. 4.33 MRI showing an enlarged uterus with multiple leiomyomas.

Table 4.06
Definition of terms used in the diagnosis of uterine smooth muscle neoplasms.

Term	Definition or comment
Necrosis	Death of a portion of tissue
Coagulative tumour cell necrosis	Abrupt transition from viable tumour to necrotic tumour, ghost outlines of cells usual, haemorrhage and inflammation uncommon.
Hyaline necrosis	Intervening zone of collagen or granulation tissue between nonviable and viable tumour, haemorrhage common, cellular outlines often not visible.
Atypia	Assessed at scanning power
Diffuse vs. focal	Cells diffusely present in most fields examined vs. scattered widely spaced aggregates of cells
None to mild	
Moderate to severe	Pleomorphic type: Nuclear pleomorphism appreciated at scanning power Uniform type: Cells lack pleomorphism but exhibit uniform but marked nuclear chromatin abnormalities
Mitotic index	Expressed in mitotic figures per 10 high power fields in the mitotically most active areas
	Only unequivocal mitotic figures are counted {211}

Nuclei are elongated with blunt or tapered ends and have finely dispersed chromatin and small nucleoli. Mitotic figures usually are infrequent.

Most leiomyomas are more cellular than the surrounding myometrium. Leiomyomas lacking increased cellularity are identified by their nodular circumscription and by the disorderly arrangement of the smooth muscle fascicles within them, out of alignment with the surrounding myometrium.

Degenerative changes are common in leiomyomas. Hyaline fibrosis, oedema and, on occasion, marked hydropic change can be present {525}. Haemorrhage, necrosis, oedema, myxoid change, hypercellular foci and cellular hypertrophy occur in leiomyomas in women who are pregnant or taking progestins. Not infrequently, there is increased mitotic activity near the areas of necrosis.

On the other hand, the coagulative tumour cell necrosis common in leiomyosarcoma is not associated very often with acute inflammation and haemorrhage. Progestational agents are associated with a slight increase in mitotic activity, but not to the level observed in a leiomyosarcoma. In addition, the mitotic figures seen in conjunction with inflammatory necrosis have a normal histologi-

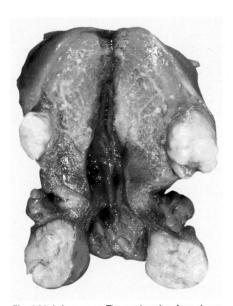

Fig. 4.34 Leiomyomas. The sectioned surface shows typical circumscribed, rubbery, white nodules.

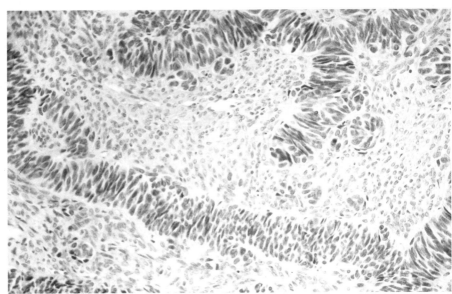

Fig. 4.35 Epithelioid leiomyoma with sex cord-like features. The presence of smooth muscle rules out an endometrial stromal or pure sex cord-like tumour.

cal appearance. The margins of most leiomyomas are histogically circumscribed, but occasional benign tumours demonstrate interdigitation with the surrounding myometrium, which may rarely be extensive.

Immunoprofile
Smooth muscle neoplasms react with antibodies to muscle-specific actin, alpha-smooth muscle actin, desmin and h-caldesmon. Anomalous expression of cytokeratin immunoreactivity is observed frequently both in the myometrium and in smooth muscle tumours, the extent and intensity of reactivity depending on the antibodies used and the fixation of the specimen. Epithelial membrane antigen is negative in smooth muscle tumours. CD10 reactivity may focally be present.

Histological variants
Most subtypes of leiomyoma are chiefly of interest in that they mimic malignancy in one or more aspects.

Mitotically active leiomyoma
Mitotically active leiomyomas occur most often in premenopausal women. They have the typical macroscopic and histological appearances of a leiomyoma with the exception that they usually have 5 or more mitotic figures per 10 high power fields {211,2293}. Occasionally, these smooth muscle tumours contain >15 mitotic figures per 10 high power fields,

in which case the term mitotically active leiomyoma with limited experience is used. The clinical evolution is benign, even if the neoplasm is treated by myomectomy. It is imperative that this diagnosis not be used for neoplasms that exhibit moderate to severe nuclear atypia, contain abnormal mitotic figures or demonstrate zones of coagulative tumour cell necrosis.

Cellular leiomyoma
Cellular leiomyoma accounts for less than 5% of leiomyomas, and by definition their cellularity is "significantly" greater than that of the surrounding myometrium {211,2101}. The isolated occurrence of hypercellularity may suggest a diagnosis of leiomyosarcoma, but cellular leiomyomas lack tumour cell necrosis and moderate to severe atypia and have infre-

quent mitotic figures. A cellular leiomyoma comprised of small cells with scanty cytoplasm can be confused with an endometrial stromal tumour. This problem becomes particularly difficult with what has been termed the highly cellular leiomyoma.

Haemorrhagic cellular leiomyoma and hormone induced changes
A haemorrhagic cellular or "apoplectic" leiomyoma is a form of cellular leiomyoma that is found mainly in women who are taking oral contraceptives or who either are pregnant or are postpartum {1960,2050}. Macroscopic examination reveals multiple stellate haemorrhagic areas. Coagulative tumour cell necrosis is generally absent. Normal mitotic figures are present and are usually confined to a narrow zone of granulation

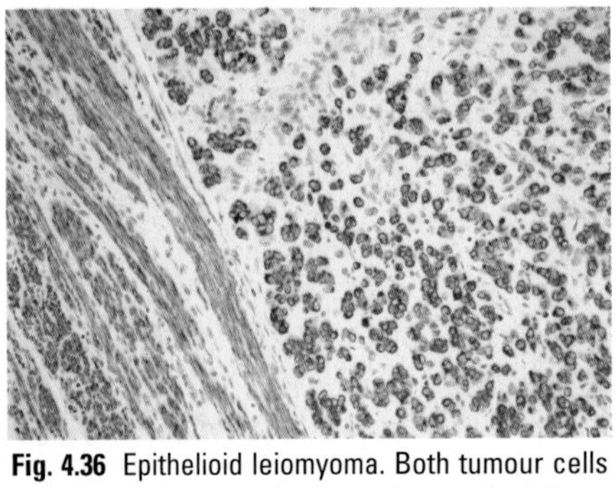

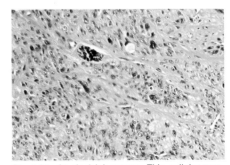

Fig. 4.36 Epithelioid leiomyoma. Both tumour cells on the right and normal myometrium on the left are immunoreactive for desmin.

Fig. 4.37 Atypical leiomyoma. This cellular neoplasm exhibits nuclear pleomorphism but no mitotic figures or tumour cell necrosis.

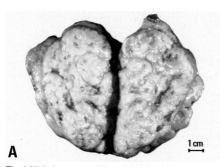
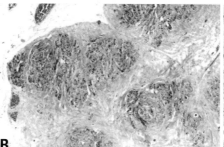
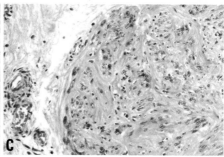

Fig. 4.38 Leiomyoma with perinodular hydropic degeneration. **A** Sectioned surface shows a lobulated neoplasm. **B** Nodules of smooth muscle are delimited by oedematous bands of collagen in which are suspended large calibre vessels. **C** The tumour is composed of uniform spindle-shaped smooth muscle cells.

tissue in relation to areas of haemorrhage.

Epithelioid leiomyoma

Epithelioid leiomyomas are composed of epithelial-like cells {130,1538,2292}. They are yellow or grey and may contain visible areas of haemorrhage and necrosis. They tend to be softer than the usual leiomyoma, and most are solitary. Histologically, the epithelioid cells are round or polygonal, they are arranged in clusters or cords, and their nuclei are round, relatively large and centrally positioned. There are three basic subtypes of epithelioid leiomyoma: leiomyoblastoma, clear cell leiomyoma and plexiform leiomyoma. Mixtures of the various patterns are common, hence the designation "epithelioid" for all of them.

Small tumours without cytological atypia, tumour cell necrosis or an elevated mitotic index can be safely regarded as benign. Plexiform tumourlets invariably are benign. Epithelioid leiomyomas with circumscribed margins, extensive hyalinization and a predominance of clear cells generally are benign. The behaviour of epithelioid leiomyomas with two or more of the following features is not well established:
(1). Large size (greater than 6 cm).
(2). Moderate mitotic activity (2-4 mitotic figures per 10 high power fields),
(3) Moderate to severe cytological atypia
(4) Necrosis

Such tumours should be classified in the uncertain malignant potential category, and careful follow-up is warranted. Neoplasms with 5 or more mitotic figures per 10 high power fields metastasize with sufficient frequency that all should be regarded as epithelioid leiomyosarcoma.

Myxoid leiomyoma

Myxoid leiomyomas are benign smooth muscle tumours in which myxoid material separates the tumour cells {131,1465}. They are soft and translucent. Histologically, abundant amorphous myxoid material is present between the smooth muscle cells. The margins of a myxoid leiomyoma are circumscribed, and neither cytological atypia nor mitotic figures are present.

Atypical leiomyoma (pleomorphic, bizarre or symplastic leiomyoma)

When unassociated with either coagulative tumour cell necrosis or a mitotic index in excess of 10 mitotic figures per 10 high power fields, cytological atypia, even when severe, is an unreliable criterion for identifying clinically malignant uterine smooth muscle tumours. These atypical cells have enlarged hyperchromatic nuclei with prominent chromatin clumping (often smudged). Large cytoplasmic pseudonuclear inclusions often are present. The atypical cells may be distributed throughout the leiomyoma (diffuse) or they may be present focally (possibly, multifocally). When the atypia is at most multifocal and the neoplasm has been completely sampled, such tumours are designated "atypical leiomyoma with minimal, if any, recurrence

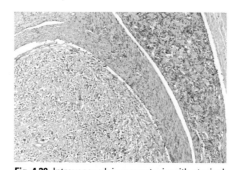

Fig. 4.39 Intravenous leiomyomatosis with atypical (symplastic and epithelioid) features. Note the tumour plugs in myometrial vessels at the lower left and mid-right.

potential." Such lesions have behaved benignly except for a single reported case.

Lipoleiomyoma

Scattered adipocytes in an otherwise typical leiomyoma are a relatively common finding; a leiomyoma that contains a striking number of these cells is called a lipoleiomyoma {2357,2671}.

Growth pattern variants

Growth pattern variants may produce unusual clinical, macroscopic and/or histological features.

Diffuse leiomyomatosis

Diffuse leiomyomatosis is an unusual condition in which numerous small smooth muscle nodules produce symmetrical, sometimes substantial, enlargement of the uterus {518}. The hyperplastic smooth muscle nodules range from histological to 3 cm in size, but most are less than 1 cm in diameter. They are composed of uniform, bland, spindle-shaped smooth muscle cells and are less circumscribed than leiomyomas. The clinical course may be complicated by haemorrhage, but the condition is benign.

Dissecting leiomyoma

Dissecting leiomyoma refers to a benign smooth muscle proliferation with a border marked by the dissection of compressive tongues of smooth muscle into the surrounding myometrium and, occasionally, into the broad ligament and pelvis {2469}. This pattern of infiltration may also be seen in intravenous leiomyomatosis. When oedema and congestion are prominent, a uterine dissecting leiomyoma with extrauterine extension may resemble placental tissue; hence the name cotyledonoid dissecting leiomyoma {2470}.

Intravenous leiomyomatosis

Intravenous leiomyomatosis is a very rare smooth muscle tumour featuring nodular masses and cords of histologically benign smooth muscle growing within venous channels outside the confines of a leiomyoma {1928,2051}. Intravenous leiomyomatosis should be distinguished from the common vascular intrusion within the confines of a leiomyoma. Macroscopically, Intravenous leiomyomatosis consists of a complex, coiled or nodular myometrial growth often with convoluted, worm-like extensions into the uterine veins in the broad ligament or into other pelvic veins. On occasion, the growth extends into the vena cava, and sometimes it extends into the right heart. Histologically, tumour is found within venous channels that are lined by endothelium. The histological appearance is highly variable, even within the same tumour. The cellular composition of some examples of intravenous leiomyomatosis is similar to a leiomyoma, but most contain prominent zones of fibrosis or hyalinization. Smooth muscle cells may be inconspicuous and difficult to identify. Any variant smooth muscle histology, i.e. cellular, atypical, epithelioid or lipoleiomyomatous, may be encountered in intravenous leiomyomatosis.

Benign metastasizing leiomyoma

Benign metastasizing leiomyoma is an ill-defined clinicopathological condition which features "metastatic" histologically benign smooth muscle tumour deposits in the lung, lymph nodes or abdomen that appear to be derived from a benign uterine leiomyoma {798,2923}. Reports of this condition often are difficult to evaluate. Almost all cases of benign metastasizing leiomyoma occur in women who have a history of pelvic surgery. The primary neoplasm, typically removed years

before the extrauterine deposits are detected, often has been inadequately studied. Most examples of "benign metastasizing leiomyoma," however, appear to be either a primary benign smooth muscle lesion of the lung in a woman with a history of uterine leiomyoma or pulmonary metastases from a histologically non-informative smooth muscle neoplasm of the uterus. The findings of a recent cytogenetic study were most consistent with a monoclonal origin of both uterine and pulmonary tumours and the interpretation that the pulmonary tumours were metastatic {2923}. The hormone dependence of this proliferation is suggested by the finding of estrogen and progesterone receptors in metastatic deposits and the regression of tumour during pregnancy, after the menopause and after oophorectomy.

Somatic genetics

Uterine leiomyomas often have chromosomal abnormalities detectable by cytogenetic analysis, most frequently involving the *HMGIC* (12q15) and *HMGIY* (6p21) genes {2204a}.

Miscellaneous mesenchymal tumours

Definition

A diverse group of mesenchymal tumours of the uterus that do not show predominantly smooth muscle or stromal differentiation.

Mixed endometrial stromal and smooth muscle tumour

Definition and historical annotation

These neoplasms, previously designated stromomyoma, are composed of an admixture of endometrial stromal and

smooth muscle elements {1448,2098, 2550,2860}. Small areas of smooth muscle differentiation are commonly seen in otherwise typical endometrial stromal neoplasms and vice versa, but a minimum of 30% of the minor component is recommended for the designation of mixed endometrial stromal-smooth muscle neoplasm {2098}.

Macroscopy

These neoplasms may have a predominant intramural, submucosal or subserosal location. Some have been described as well circumscribed, whereas others have been multinodular or have had infiltrating margins. Some neoplasms contain areas with a whorled appearance admixed with tan foci that are softer than typical leiomyomas {2098}.

Histopathology

A population of small cells with round to ovoid nuclei and inconspicuous cytoplasm characterizes the endometrial stromal component. Numerous small arterioles are a characteristic feature. The endometrial stromal component usually exhibits minimal cytological atypia, and the mitotic rate is variable. Areas exhibiting sex cord-like differentiation and perivascular hyalinization may be present in the endometrial stromal component {2098}. A case has been described with an associated glandular component consisting of benign endometrial glands surrounded by endometrial stroma {1812}.

The smooth muscle component is usually benign in appearance and is often arranged in nodules with a prominent central area of hyalinization creating a starburst appearance. However, in some cases the smooth muscle component may exhibit any one or a combination of

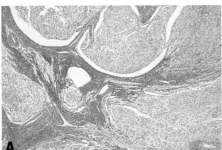
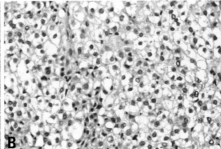
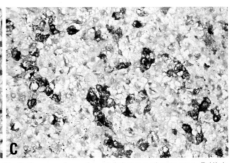

Fig. 4.40 Perivascular epithelioid cell tumour. **A** Low power image shows a "tongue-like" growth pattern, similar to low grade endometrial stromal sarcoma. **B** High power image shows epithelioid cells with clear to pale granular cytoplasm without significant atypia or mitotic figures. **C** HMB-45 stain is positive.

cytological atypia, tumour cell necrosis and conspicuous mitotic activity.

The smooth muscle component is positive for desmin and alpha-smooth muscle actin. However, there may be positivity of the endometrial stromal component with these antibodies, and they cannot be used to reliably distinguish between endometrial stroma and smooth muscle. Studies have shown that markers such as CD10 that stain endometrial stroma but are focally positive in many smooth muscle neoplasms and h-caldesmon and calponin that stain smooth muscle may be of value in distinguishing the two components {44,486,1821,2065}. Sex cord-like areas may exhibit immunohistochemical staining with alpha-inhibin and other sex cord-stromal markers {1521, 1808}.

Prognosis and predictive factors
The limited literature on these rare neoplasms suggests that they should be evaluated and reported in the same way as endometrial stromal neoplasms; i.e. malignant if there is vascular or myometrial invasion, benign otherwise {2098, 2311}.

Perivascular epithelioid cell tumour

Definition
A tumour composed predominantly or exclusively of HMB-45-positive perivascular epithelioid cells with eosinophilic granular cytoplasm. It is a member of a family of lesions thought to be composed, at least in part, of perivascular epithelioid cells. Other members of this group include some forms of angiomyolipoma and lymphangioleiomyomatosis, as well as clear cell 'sugar' tumour.

Synonym
PEComa.

Epidemiology
The age of patients ranged from 40-75 years with a mean of 54 {2998}.

Clinical features
Most patients present with abnormal uterine bleeding.

Macroscopy
A mass is present in the uterine corpus.

Histopathology
The tumours are divided into two groups {2998}. The first demonstrates a tongue-

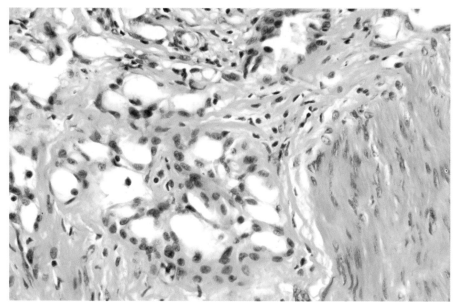

Fig. 4.41 Uterine adenomatoid tumour. The tumour is composed of tubules lined by bland cuboidal cells within the myometrium.

like growth pattern similar to that seen in low grade ESS. These tumours are composed of cells that have abundant clear to eosinophilic pale granular cytoplasm and stain diffusely for HMB-45 and also variably express muscle markers. The second group is composed of epithelioid cells with less prominent clear cell features and a smaller number of cells that are HMB-45 positive. These tumours exhibit more extensive muscle marker expression and a lesser degree of tongue-like growth than the first group.

Genetic susceptibility
One-half of the patients in the second group had pelvic lymph nodes involved by lymphangioleiomyomatosis, and one-fourth had tuberous sclerosis.

Prognosis and predictive factors
Hysterectomy is the usual treatment. Some uterine cases have exhibited aggressive behaviour. Uterine perivascular epithelioid cell tumour should be considered of uncertain malignant potential until long-term outcome data for a larger number of patients become available {2998}.

Adenomatoid tumour

Definition
A benign tumour of the uterine serosa and myometrium originating from mesothelium and forming gland-like structures.

ICD-O code   9054/0

Clinical features
They are usually an incidental finding in a hysterectomy specimen. Occasionally, they may be multiple or associated with a similar lesion in the fallopian tube.

Macroscopy
Macroscopically, adenomatoid tumours may resemble leiomyomas, being well circumscribed intramural masses. However, in many cases they are less well defined and of softer consistency. They may occur anywhere within the myometrium but are often located towards the serosal surface.

Histopathology
On low power examination adenomatoid tumour is usually composed of multiple small, often slit-like, interconnecting spaces within the myometrium. On higher power these are composed of tubules lined by a single layer of cells that may be cuboidal or attenuated. The lesion often has an infiltrative appearance. Sometimes the spaces are dilated resulting in a cystic pattern that was confused with lymphangioma in the past, and in other cases a more solid growth pattern is apparent. There is little nuclear atypia or mitotic activity, and there is no stromal desmoplastic response. Occasional tumours may exhibit signet-ring cell histology, focally or diffusely, which may

cause obvious diagnostic problems. Sometimes a papillary pattern may be apparent. Ultrastructural examination shows the long slender microvilli characteristic of mesothelial cells.

Immunoprofile
Immunohistochemical positivity with anti-cytokeratin antibodies and anti-mesothelial antibodies, such as HBME1 and calretinin, is usual. This finding may be useful in the distinction between adenomatoid tumour and lymphangioma. There is no reactivity with Ber-EP4, helping to exclude a carcinoma in those cases that have signet-ring cell morphology {211, 2101,2123}.

Histogenesis
The histogenesis has been debated in the past, but immunohistochemical and ultrastructural studies have shown these neoplasms to be of mesothelial origin. When located within the uterus {654, 2041,2311,2768,2924}, they are probably derived from the serosal mesothelium.

Prognosis and predictive factors
Adenomatoid tumours are invariably benign with no risk of recurrence or metastasis.

Rare mesenchymal tumours

Definition
A variety of mesenchymal tumours, both malignant and benign, occurring within the uterus that are not endometrial stromal, smooth muscle or mesothelial in type. These are rare and are identical histologically to their counterparts arising in more usual sites.

Malignant tumours
In cases of malignancy the neoplasm should be extensively sampled in order to exclude sarcomatous overgrowth in a MMMT or an adenosarcoma. The most common of these neoplasms to arise in the uterus is *rhabdomyosarcoma* {716, 1149,1814,2112}. The latter is usually of embryonal type in young females and of pleomorphic type in the middle aged or elderly. Occasional cases of uterine alveolar rhabdomyosarcoma have also been described {475}. Occasional residual entrapped benign endometrial glands may be present, especially towards the surface of these neoplasms. That finding should not be taken as evidence of an adenosarcoma. Other malignant mesenchymal neoplasms described in the uterus include *malignant fibrous histiocytoma* {1404}, *angiosarcoma* (including the epithelioid variant) {2551,2853}, *liposarcoma* {180}, *osteosarcoma* {784, 1137,1844}, *chondrosarcoma* {1489}, *alveolar soft part sarcoma* {2319}, *Ewing tumour*, *malignant peripheral nerve sheath tumour*, *malignant pigmented neuroectodermal tumour of infancy* {2580} and *peripheral primitive neuroectodermal tumour* {638,1894,2017}. In general, these are all bulky neoplasms, frequently high stage at presentation, and the histology is similar to their counterparts elsewhere. Immunohistochemical studies may assist in establishing a definitive diagnosis.

Haemangiopericytoma has also been described in the uterus, but it is likely that most of the reported cases represent vascular endometrial stromal neoplasms {2693}.

Malignant rhabdoid tumours have also been described {948,1255}. Since a rhabdoid component may rarely be found in an otherwise typical endometrial stromal neoplasm {1813}, it is possible that some rhabdoid tumours represent an unusual histological variant of an endometrial stromal or some other neoplasm. As with other extrarenal rhabdoid tumours, the uterine neoplasm may represent a peculiar histological growth pattern that may be found in a variety of neoplasms; therefore, extensive sampling should be undertaken to exclude a diagnosis of rhabdoid differentiation in another more common neoplasm. Only when other elements are not identified should a diagnosis of uterine malignant rhabdoid tumour be considered.

Benign tumours
Benign tumours include lipoma, haemangioma, lymphangioma and rhabdomyoma {466,686}. Occasional uterine myxomas have been described in Carney syndrome {2654}. Before diagnosing these entities, a lipoleiomyoma should be excluded in the case of lipoma, a vascular leiomyoma in the case of haemangioma, an adenomatoid tumour in the case of lymphangioma and a myxoid smooth muscle neoplasm in the case of myxoma. A single case of postoperative spindle cell nodule of the endometrium that occurred following a uterine curettage has been described {504}.

Mixed epithelial and mesenchymal tumours

W.G. McCluggage
U. Haller
R.J. Kurman
R.A. Kubik-Huch

Definition
Tumours of the uterine corpus composed of an epithelial and a mesenchymal component.

ICD-O codes
Carcinosarcoma	8980/3
Adenosarcoma	8933/3
Carcinofibroma	8934/3
Adenofibroma	9013/0
Adenomyoma	8932/0
Atypical polypoid variant	8932/0

Carcinosarcoma

Definition
A neoplasm composed of an admixture of malignant epithelial and mesenchymal components.

Synonyms
Malignant müllerian mixed tumour, malignant mesodermal mixed tumour, metaplastic carcinoma.

These tumours are still classified as "mixed" by convention, although there is increasing evidence that they are monoclonal and should be considered subsets of endometrial carcinoma.

Epidemiology
Carcinosarcoma is the most common neoplasm of this group {703}. Carcinosarcomas usually occur in elderly postmenopausal women, although occasional cases may occur in younger women and rarely even in young girls. The median age of patients presenting with carcinosarcoma is 65 years, higher than that of patients with leiomyosarcoma {813,1745}. Less than 5% of patients are younger than 50 years.

Aetiology
An occasional case is secondary to prior pelvic irradiation. In recent years an association between long term tamoxifen therapy and the development of uterine carcinosarcoma has been suggested {813,1811,2947}.

Clinical features
Signs and symptoms
Vaginal bleeding is the most frequent presenting symptom of patients with carcinosarcoma, followed by an abdominal mass and pelvic pain {703}. Carcinosarcomas may be polypoid and may prolapse through the cervix to present as an upper vaginal mass. The most important diagnostic method is uterine curettage, but in 25% of cases the diagnosis is made following hysterectomy {2965}.

Imaging
Magnetic resonance imaging (MRI) of women with a typical carcinosarcoma usually shows an enlarged uterus with a widened endometrial cavity and evidence of deep myometrial invasion. Whereas a carcinosarcoma cannot be distinguished from endometrial carcinoma by means of MRI, the presence of a large tumour with extensive myometrial invasion as well as the presence of ovarian or intraperitoneal metastases should raise suspicion {1060,2838}.

Macroscopy
At the time of presentation uterine carcinosarcomas are usually polypoid, bulky, necrotic and haemorrhagic neoplasms that fill the endometrial cavity and deeply invade the myometrium, often extending beyond the uterus. If cartilage or bone forms a significant portion of the neoplasm, the neoplasm may have a hard consistency. Occasionally, these neoplasms may arise within a benign endometrial polyp.

Tumour spread and staging
Intra-abdominal and retroperitoneal nodal metastases are frequent {1745}.

Histopathology
The malignant epithelial element is usually glandular, although rarely it may be non-glandular, most commonly consisting of squamous or undifferentiated carcinoma. The glandular component may be either endometrioid or non-endometrioid, such as serous or clear cell in type. The sarcomatous elements may be either homologous or heterologous. In homologous neoplasms the mesenchymal component usually consists of undifferentiated sarcoma, leiomyosarcoma or endometrial stromal sarcoma and is usually, although not always, high grade. Heterologous mesenchymal elements most commonly consist of malignant cartilage or malignant skeletal muscle in the

Table 4.07
Nomenclature of mixed epithelial and mesenchymal tumours defined by phenotypes of epithelial and mesenchymal components.

	Benign epithelium	Malignant epithelium
Benign mesenchyme	Adenofibroma Adenomyoma (including atypical)	Carcinofibroma
Malignant mesenchyme	Adenosarcoma	Carcinosarcoma

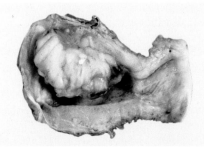

Fig. 4.42 Carcinosarcoma. Sagittal section of the uterus shows a solid, polypoid tumour within the fundus.

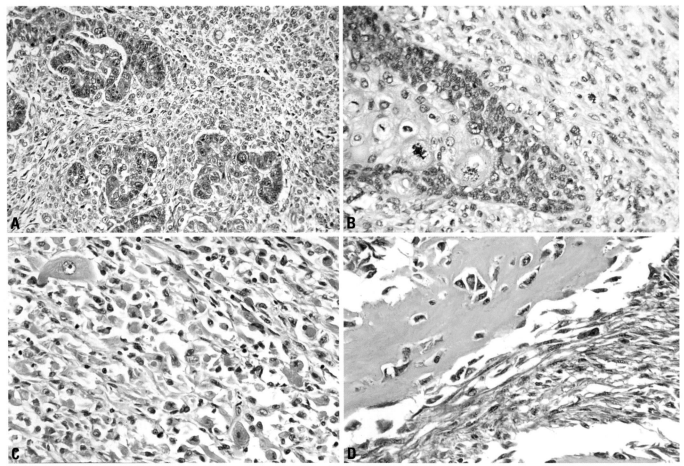

Fig. 4.43 Carcinosarcoma. **A** A biphasic tumour is composed of poorly differentiated malignant glands and sarcomatous elements. **B** A biphasic tumour is composed of a solid aggregate of malignant epithelium with central squamous differentiation and sarcomatous elements. Mitoses are frequent. **C** High power image shows a mesenchymal component resembling rhabdomyosarcoma. **D** High power image shows a mesenchymal component resembling osteosarcoma.

form of rhabdomyoblasts, although other elements such as osteosarcoma and liposarcoma may rarely occur.

In general, both carcinomatous and sarcomatous elements are easily identifiable, although in some cases one or other element may form a minor component that may be only identified following extensive sampling of the neoplasm. Any uterine neoplasm composed of high grade sarcoma, especially when heterologous elements are present, should be extensively sampled in order to rule out a carcinosarcoma or sarcomatous overgrowth in an adenosarcoma. In most instances the two elements are sharply demarcated, but in some they appear to merge with transitional forms between the two elements. Eosinophilic hyaline inclusions are commonly seen, especially in the sarcomatous elements {2359}.

Occasionally, a carcinosarcoma may be identified in an otherwise benign endometrial polyp. A uterine carcinosar-

coma with a component of yolk sac tumour has been described in a patient with an elevated serum alpha-fetoprotein level {2665}. Occasional tumours with a rhabdoid phenotype {190} or a malignant neuroectodermal component {931} have also been described. Occasional uterine carcinosarcomas of mesonephric origin have been reported {3171}. Other unusual histological features include melanocytic {77} and neuroendocrine differentiation {537}.

Immunoprofile

In general, the epithelial elements are immunoreactive with anti-cytokeratin antibodies and the mesenchymal elements with vimentin. The mesenchymal elements often show focal staining with anti-cytokeratin antibodies supporting an epithelial origin of this component. The usual concordance of TP53 stains between the epithelial and mesenchymal components supports a common mono-

clonal origin for both elements {1796, 2827}. Desmin, myoD1, myoglobin and sarcomeric actin staining may highlight a rhabdomyosarcomatous mesenchymal component. Cartilaginous elements usually stain with S-100 protein.

Histogenesis

It should be noted that clinical, immunohistochemical, ultrastructural and molecular studies have all suggested that carcinosarcomas are really metaplastic carcinomas in which the mesenchymal component retains at least some epithelial features in the vast majority of cases {1809}. Though still classified as "mixed" by convention, these tumours are perhaps better considered subsets of endometrial carcinoma and certainly should not be grouped histogenetically or clinically with uterine sarcomas {1810}. On the other hand, the tumours other than carcinosarcoma in this group are considered to be true mixed tumours.

Prognosis and predictive factors

The clinical course of uterine carcinosarcoma is generally aggressive with a poor overall prognosis, considerably worse than that of a poorly differentiated endometrial carcinoma. The pattern of spread is generally similar to that of high grade endometrial carcinoma, and deep myometrial invasion and extrauterine spread are often observed at the time of presentation. The clinical staging is the same as that for endometrial carcinoma. Some studies have found no independent prognostic factors other than tumour stage, whereas others have found that the characteristics of the epithelial component such as high grade carcinoma, including serous or clear cell components, are associated with a worse prognosis {2692}. Previously, it was thought that the presence of heterologous mesenchymal components indicated a worse outcome; however, recent larger studies have suggested that the histological features of the mesenchymal component bear no relationship to the overall prognosis {2692}.

The biological behaviour of uterine carcinosarcomas is more akin to high grade endometrial carcinomas than to uterine sarcomas {282,2692}. Carcinosarcomas primarily spread via lymphatics, whereas pure uterine sarcomas commonly spread haematogenously. Detailed studies of uterine carcinosarcoma have shown that metastatic foci and foci within lymphatic or vascular spaces are commonly carcinomatous with pure sarcomatous elements being rare {282,2692,2767}.

Although the tumour stage is the most important prognostic factor, recurrences may be encountered even in those rare cases lacking myometrial infiltration. However, tumours confined to an otherwise benign polyp appear to have a somewhat better outcome {188,1382}.

Adenosarcoma

Definition

Adenosarcoma is a biphasic neoplasm containing a benign epithelial component and a sarcomatous mesenchymal component.

Epidemiology

Adenosarcoma occurs in women of all ages, ranging from 15-90 years with a median age at diagnosis of 58. Adenosarcomas have been reported in women undergoing tamoxifen therapy for breast cancer {509} and occasionally after prior pelvic radiation {515}. There is no association of adenosarcoma with obesity or hypertension.

Clinical features

Typical symptoms of patients with adenosarcoma are abnormal vaginal bleeding, an enlarged uterus and tissue protruding from the external os. The tumour may not be correctly diagnosed as adenosarcoma until re-excision of a recurrent polypoid lesion {515}.

Macroscopy

Adenosarcomas typically grow as exophytic polypoid masses that extend into the uterine cavity. Rarely, they may arise in the myometrium, presumably from adenomyosis. Although the tumour is usually a single polypoid mass, it sometimes may present as multiple papillary masses. On sectioning, the surface is tan brown with foci of haemorrhage and necrosis. Small cysts are frequently present. Most adenosarcomas do not invade the myometrium.

Histopathology

Under low magnification a leaf-like pattern closely resembling phyllodes tumour of the breast is observed. Isolated glands, often dilated and compressed into thin slits, are dispersed throughout the mesenchymal component. Characte- ristically, there is stromal condensation surrounding the glands and clefts. It is in these areas where the greatest degree of stromal atypia and mitotic activity is present. By definition the epithelium is benign and may show focal metaplastic changes. The mesenchymal component of an adenosarcoma is generally a low grade homologous stromal sarcoma containing varying amounts of fibrous tissue and smooth muscle. Mesenchymal mitotic figures, usually stated to be more than one per 10 high power fields, are required in the hypercellular cuffs. Cytological atypia is typically only mild, but is occasionally moderate. Sex cord-like components resembling those in endometrial stromal sarcomas are found in less than 10% of adenosarcomas. Heterologous components consisting of striated muscle (most commonly), cartilage, fat and other components are present in approximately 10-15% of tumours The diagnosis of sarcomatous overgrowth is made if the pure

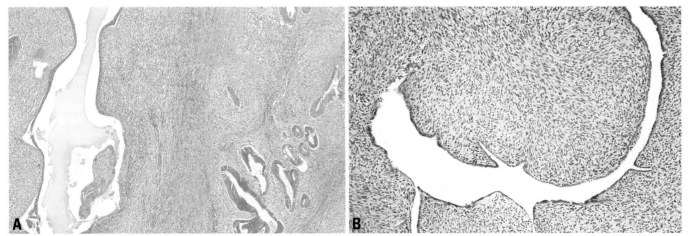

Fig. 4.44 Adenosarcoma. **A** The tumour is composed of tubular and convoluted, cleft-like glands of endometrioid type surrounded by a cuff of cellular mesenchyme. **B** A polypoid structure compresses a glandular lumen producing a leaf-like pattern similar to that of a mammary phyllodes tumour. The epithelial component is cytologically bland, and the mesenchymal component is cellular and fibromatous without significant nuclear atypia but contained abundant mitoses.

sarcomatous component, usually of high grade, occupies 25% or more of the total tumour volume.

Immunoprofile

As might be expected, the epithelial component reacts with a broad spectrum of antibodies to cytokeratins. The mesenchymal component usually reacts focally with antibodies to CD10. Variable degrees of staining for smooth muscle markers, desmin and caldesmon, can also be observed.

Differential diagnosis

The differential diagnosis includes adenofibroma and in children sarcoma botryoides (embryonal rhabdomyosarcoma).

Prognosis and predictive factors

Adenosarcoma is considered a low grade neoplasm but recurs in approximately 25-40% of cases, typically in the pelvis or vagina, and distant metastasis has been reported in 5% of cases {515}. The metastases almost always are composed of a sarcomatous element only, but rarely epithelium has been reported. Factors in the primary tumour that are predictive of a poor outcome are extrauterine spread, deep myometrial invasion into the outer half of the myometrium and sarcomatous overgrowth. Vascular invasion is usually not identified but, if present, is a poor risk factor. Rhabdomyosarcomatous differentiation was an adverse prognostic factor in one series {1388}. There appears to be no correlation between the prognosis and the level of mitotic activity. Long-term follow-up is necessary because recurrences may manifest after many years. Most tumour deaths occur more than five years after the diagnosis.

Carcinofibroma

Definition

A neoplasm composed of an admixture of a malignant epithelial element and a benign mesenchymal component.

Epidemiology

These are extremely uncommon neoplasms with few cases reported in the literature {1286,2228,2916}.

Histopathology

In one case the epithelial component was clear cell in type {2228}. The mesenchymal component is usually fibrous, although occasional cases with a heterologous mesenchymal component have been described and have been designated as carcinomesenchymoma {459}.

Prognosis and predictive factors

The behaviour is not well established since so few cases have been reported but would be expected to depend on the stage, depth of myometrial invasion and histological subtype of the epithelial component.

Adenofibroma

Definition

A biphasic uterine neoplasm composed of benign epithelial and mesenchymal components.

Epidemiology

Uterine adenofibroma is an uncommon neoplasm, much less frequent than adenosarcoma, which occurs most often in postmenopausal patients but also in younger women. {3245}. Occasional cases have been associated with tamoxifen therapy {1258}.

Macroscopy

Adenofibromas usually present as polypoid lesions, commonly have a fibrous consistency on sectioning, and sometimes contain dilated cystic spaces.

Histopathology

Adenofibromas have a papillary or club-like growth pattern. They are composed of benign epithelial and mesenchymal components, the epithelial component forming a lining on the underlying mesenchymal core. Cleft-like spaces are often present. The epithelial component may be endometrioid or ciliated in type but often is non-descript cuboidal or columnar. Rarely, there are foci of squamous metaplasia. The mesenchyme is usually of a non-specific fibroblastic type, although rarely it may contain endometrial stromal or smooth muscle components. Stromal atypia, mitotic activity and periglandular cuffing are absent or inconspicuous. Rarely, adipose tissue or skeletal muscle components are present, and such lesions have been designated lipoadenofibroma or adenomyofibroma {1239,2711}.

Differential diagnosis

If there is a stromal mitotic count of >1 mitosis per 10 high power fields, marked stromal hypercellularity with periglandular cuffing and/or more than mild stromal atypia, a diagnosis of low grade adenosarcoma should be made.

Prognosis and predictive factors

Adenofibromas are benign lesions, although they may recur following "polypectomy" {2625}. Occasional

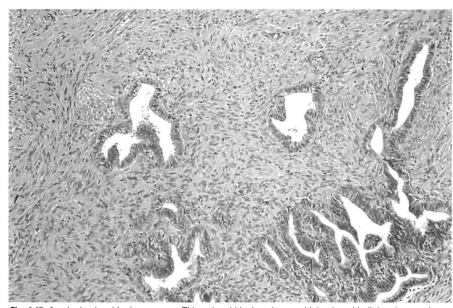

Fig. 4.45 Atypical polypoid adenomyoma. This polypoid lesion shows a biphasic epithelial and stromal proliferation. The glandular component consists of endometrioid glands with a variable degree of complexity, whereas the mesenchymal component is myofibromatous and cytologically bland.

tumours may superficially invade the myometrium, but metastases have not been reported. Invasion of myometrial veins has also been described {514}. Occasional cases have been focally involved by adenocarcinoma, but the association is probably incidental {1873}.

Adenomyoma including atypical polypoid adenomyoma

Definition
A lesion composed of benign epithelial (usually endometrial glands) and mesenchymal components in which the mesenchymal component is fibromyomatous Atypical polypoid adenomyoma is a variant of adenomyoma in which the glandular component exhibits architectural complexity with or without cytological atypia.

Epidemiology
Adenomyoma may occur at any age, whereas atypical polypoid adenomyoma characteristically occurs in premenopausal women {1690,1801,3228}.

Macroscopy
Adenomyomas and atypical polypoid adenomyomas usually are polypoid submucosal lesions but may rarely be intramural or subserosal {1002}. They have a firm sectioned surface. Atypical polypoid adenomyoma usually involves the lower uterine segment or upper endocervix.

Histopathology
Adenomyoma is composed of an admixture of benign endometrial glands (there may be minor foci of tubal, mucinous or squamous epithelium) with minimal cytological atypia and architectural complexity embedded in a benign fibromyomatous mesenchyme. Often endometrial type stroma surrounds the endometrial glandular component, and the former is in turn surrounded by smooth muscle {1002}.

Atypical polypoid adenomyoma
In atypical polypoid adenomyoma the glands characteristically show marked architectural complexity; there is no endometrial type stroma around the distorted glands. There is often also cytological atypia that varies from mild to marked. Foci may be present that architecturally resemble well differentiated adenocarcinoma, and such tumours have been designated "atypical polypoid adenomyoma of low malignant potential" {1690}. Extensive squamous or morular metaplasia of the glandular elements, with or without central necrosis, is a common finding. The mesenchymal component is composed of swirling and interlacing fascicles of benign smooth muscle.

Differential diagnosis
It should be noted that many simple endometrial polyps contain a minor component of smooth muscle within the stroma; however, this finding alone is not sufficient for the diagnosis of adenomyoma. The designation adenomyoma has also been used for a localized adenomyosis that forms a discrete mass, but such usage is confusing and not recommended.

Differentiation from a well differentiated endometrioid adenocarcinoma invading the myometrium may be difficult, especially on a curettage or biopsy specimen. However, the usual lack of pronounced cellular atypia and the absence of a stromal desmoplastic response would be against a diagnosis of adenocarcinoma. Additional features against a diagnosis of carcinoma are the usual youth of the patient and the presence of normal endometrial fragments in the sample.

Genetic susceptibility
Atypical polypoid adenomyomas may occur in women with Turner syndrome {517}.

Prognosis and predictive factors
Adenomyoma is generally cured by simple polypectomy, but if associated with myometrial adenomyosis, symptoms may persist. Atypical polypoid adenomyoma may recur, especially following incomplete removal. In addition, superficial myometrial infiltration is often identified in hysterectomy specimens, a finding that may be more common in those cases with marked glandular architectural complexity {1690}. A small number of cases are associated with an underlying endometrioid adenocarcinoma with a transition zone between the two components {1882, 2813}.

Gestational trophoblastic disease

D.R. Genest
R.S. Berkowitz
R.A. Fisher
E.S. Newlands
M. Fehr

Definition

A heterogeneous group of gestational and neoplastic conditions arising from trophoblast, including molar gestations and trophoblastic tumours.

Epidemiology

Gestational trophoblastic disease (GTD) varies widely among various populations with figures as high as 1 in 120 pregnancies in some areas of Asia and South America compared to 0.6-1.1 per 1000 in the United States {1162}. The incidence of hydatidiform moles is greater in women older than 40 years {161} and is also increased in those younger than 20 years. Patients who have had prior GTD are more at risk of having a second GTD after subsequent pregnancies. Other risk factors include: a diet low in vitamin A, lower socioeconomic status and blood group A women married to group 0 men {161,162,244,363}.

Aetiology

Hydatiform moles arise from abnormal conceptions. Partial moles result from diandric triploidy, whereas complete moles result from diandry (fertilization of an empty ovum). Up to 50% of choriocarcinomas and 15% of placental site trophoblastic tumours follow complete moles.

Table 4.08
The U.S. National Institutes of Health staging classification for gestational trophoblastic disease (GTD).

I Benign GTD
    A. Complete hydatidiform mole
    B. Partial hydatidiform mole
II Malignant GTD
    A. Non-metastatic GTD
    B. Metastatic GTD
        1. Good prognosis:
           absence of any risk factor
        2. Poor prognosis:
           presence of any risk factor
             a. Duration of GTD >4months
             b. Pre-therapy serum
                β-hCG>40,000 mIU/mL
             c. Brain or liver metastasis
             d. GTD after term gestation
             e. Failed prior chemotherapy
                for GTD

Clinical features

Signs and symptoms

A complete molar pregnancy usually presents with first trimester bleeding, a uterus larger than expected for gestational age and the absence of fetal parts on ultrasound in association with a markedly elevated beta-human chorionic gonadotropin (β-hCG) level {568}. Other signs include hyperemesis, toxaemia during the first or second trimester, theca lutein cysts and hyperthyroidism. Patients with partial molar gestations usually present as spontaneous abortions, sometimes with increased β-hCG levels. GTD should always be considered when a patient has continued vaginal bleeding following delivery or abortion.

Imaging

A characteristic pattern of multiple vesicles (snowstorm pattern) is commonly seen with complete molar pregnancy. The diagnosis of partial molar pregnancy by ultrasonography is more difficult.

Tumour spread and staging

Choriocarcinoma spreads haematogenously and may involve the lung (57-80%), vagina (30%), pelvis (20%), brain (17%), and liver (10%) {168,243}. Since β-hCG titres accurately reflect the clinical disease, histological verification is not required for diagnosis. Staging should be based on history, clinical examination and appropriate laboratory and radiological studies.

Metastatic GTD is also categorized by the WHO scoring system as low, medium, and high risk {51,2976}. The individual scores for each prognostic factor are added together to obtain a total score. A total prognostic score less than or equal to 4 is considered low risk, a total score of 5-7 is considered middle risk, and a total score of 8 or greater is considered high risk. (See TNM and FIGO classification of gestational trophoblastic tumours at the beginning of the chapter).

Somatic genetics

Overexpression of TP53 protein may be associated with more aggressive behaviour in gestational trophoblastic disease since it is more commonly observed in complete moles and choriocarcinoma {937,1616,2307}, but TP53 mutations are uncommon {471}. Overexpression of the p21 gene has also been detected in complete moles and choriocarcinoma {469}. No correlation between p21 and TP53 expression has been detected in gestational trophoblastic disease.

Both complete mole and choriocarcinoma exhibit overexpression of several growth factors including c-Myc, epidermal growth factors receptor (EGFR), c-erbB-2, Rb, mdm2, and bcl-2 as compared to normal placenta and partial mole {938,2966}. Expression of c-fms protein does not differ between normal placenta and gestational trophoblastic diseases {938}. In one study strong immunostaining of c-erbB-3 and epidermal growth factor receptor in extravillous trophoblast of complete mole was significantly correlated with the development of persistent gestational trophoblastic tumour {2966}. The molecular pathogenesis of gestational trophoblastic diseases may involve these and potentially other growth-regulatory factors.

Prognosis and predictive factors

Major adverse prognostic variables for GTD are:

(1) Age >39
(2) Prior term pregnancy
(3) Interval from antecedent pregnancy of >12 months
(4) β-hCG >105 IU/litre
(5) Tumour mass >5cm
(6) Disease in liver and brain
(7) Failure of 2 or more prior chemotherapies

The above factors are included in a prognostic score (see the TNM and FIGO classification of gestational trophoblastic tumours at the beginning of the chapter). The patients are separated into low risk and high risk groups for different treatments {1123,3111}.

The prognosis of patients with low risk disease is very close to 100% survival, whilst patients with high risk disease have a survival of 85-95%, depending on the number of patients with ultra high riskdisease in the patient population.

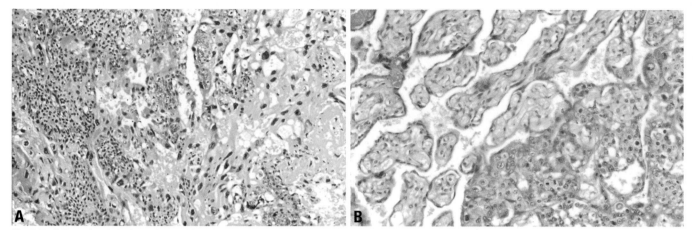

Fig. 4.46 **A** Gestational choriocarcinoma. Note the plexiform pattern with triphasic differentiation into cytotrophoblast, syncytiotrophoblast and intermediate trophoblast and marked cytological atypia. **B** Intraplacental choriocarcinoma. There is a distinct interface between malignant biphasic trophoblast in the maternal intervillous space seen on the lower right and mature chorionic villi on the left.

Trophoblastic tumours

Definition
Neoplasms derived from trophoblast.

ICD-O codes
Choriocarcinoma   9100/3
Placental site trophoblastic tumour 9104/1
Epithelioid trophoblastic tumour   9105/3

Gestational choriocarcinoma

Definition
A malignant neoplasm composed of large sheets of biphasic, markedly atypical trophoblast without chorionic villi.

Clinical features
Gestational choriocarcinoma may occur subsequent to a molar pregnancy (50%

of instances), an abortion (25%), a normal gestation (22.5%) or an ectopic pregnancy (2.5%) {1203}.
In rare cases an intraplacental choriocarcinoma is diagnosed immediately following pregnancy from placental pathological examination {343,722,907,1923}.

Histopathology
Choriocarcinoma consists of an admixture of syncytiotrophoblast, cytotrophoblast and intermediate trophoblast as single cells and clusters of cells with prominent haemorrhage, necrosis and vascular invasion {775a,1593,1801a, 1802a,2011,2024a,2077a}. Choriocarcinoma does not possess tumour stroma or vessels; correspondingly, the diagnostic viable tumour is located at the periphery of haemorrhagic foci.
Extraordinarily, choriocarcinomas have

developed and been diagnosed as intraplacental tumours {112,343,722,907, 1562,1923,2103}.

Immunoprofile
All trophoblastic cell types are strongly immunoreactive for cytokeratins {640}. In addition, the syncytiotrophoblast is strongly immunoreactive for β-hCG and weakly immunoreactive for human placental lactogen (hPL); intermediate trophoblast shows the opposite immunoprofile {935}.

Differential diagnosis
The differential diagnosis of choriocarcinoma in endometrial curettings includes previllous trophoblast from an early gestation, persistent molar tissue following hydatidiform mole, placental site trophoblastic tumour, epithelioid tro-

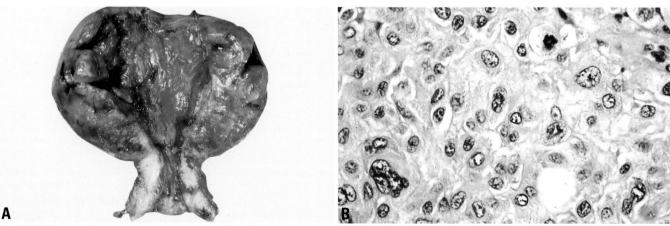

Fig. 4.47 **A** Placental site trophoblastic tumour. Coronal section shows the neoplasm diffusely infiltrating the uterine wall. **B** Tumour cells show marked cytological atypia and numerous mitotic figures.

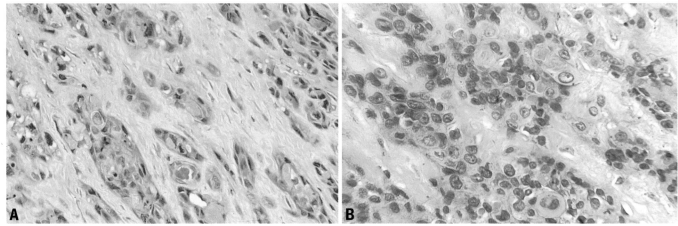

Fig. 4.48 Epithelioid trophoblastic tumour. **A** Neoplastic aggregates are better defined than in placental site trophoblastic tumour and may resemble carcinoma. **B** Groups of tumour cells, occasionally with clear cytoplasm, are separated by a hyaline stroma.

phoblastic tumour and undifferentiated carcinoma.

Somatic genetics

Recent studies using cDNA microarray analysis have demonstrated decreased expression of heat shock protein-27 in choriocarcinoma, a finding which has been associated with chemotherapy responsiveness in other cancers {3014}.

Placental site trophoblastic tumour

Definition

A monophasic neoplasm composed of intermediate trophoblast and cytotrophoblast without a significant component of syncytiotrophoblast.

Histopathology

The tumour cells are medium to large sized and mononuclear or multinucleated with mild to marked nuclear atypia, prominent nucleoli, eosinophilic to clear cytoplasm, scattered mitoses and occasional intranuclear inclusions {746,747, 842,861,933,1018,1019,1177,1237, 1511,1540,1543,1589,2967,3202,3227}. They permeate the myometrium and vessels in a manner reminiscent of the implantation site trophoblast.

Differential diagnosis

The differential diagnosis of placental site trophoblastic tumour includes placental site nodule, exaggerated implantation site, epithelioid leiomyosarcoma, epithelioid trophoblastic tumour and poorly differentiated carcinoma. Extensive sampling and immunohisto-

chemistry for keratin, β-hCG and hPL are helpful in distinguishing among the above lesions {2658,2659}.

Somatic genetics

A Y-chromosomal locus and/or new (paternal) alleles not present in adjacent normal uterine tissue was demonstrated in all cases of placental site trophoblastic tumour studied confirming the placental origin of these neoplasms {2747}.

Prognosis and predictive factors

Placental site trophoblastic tumours are rare, and their biological behaviour is variable. The major prognostic variable is a long interval from the last known antecedent pregnancy. All patient deaths from placental site trophoblastic tumour in the Charing Cross series occurred when the interval from the last known pregnancy was greater than 4 years. An elevated mitotic index predicts a poor outcome {842}.

Epithelioid trophoblastic tumour

Definition

A tumour composed of a monomorphic population of intermediate trophoblastic cells closely resembling those of the chorion laeve (membranous chorion).

Histopathology

The epithelioid trophoblastic tumour is a relatively uncommon, recently described neoplasm that differs from the placental site trophoblastic tumour in that the tumour cells of the epithelioid trophoblastic tumour are smaller and less pleomorphic and grow in a nodular as

opposed to a diffusely infiltrative pattern. Because they are frequently found in the cervix, they may be confused with hyalinizing squamous cell carcinomas. Epithelioid trophoblastic tumours are focally immunoreactive for placental-like alkaline phosphatase (PLAP) and hPL but strongly and diffusely immunoreactive for E-cadherin and epidermal growth factor receptor {2658}.

Somatic genetics

A Y-chromosomal locus and/or new (paternal) alleles not present in adjacent normal uterine tissue was demonstrated in all cases of epithelioid trophoblastic tumour studied confirming the placental origin of this neoplasm {2747}.

Prognosis and predictive factors

Based on available data, the behaviour of epithelioid trophoblastic tumour resembles that of placental site trophoblastic tumour.

Hydatidiform mole

Definition

An abnormal placenta with villous hydrops and variable degrees of trophoblastic proliferation.

ICD-O codes

Hydatidiform mole, NOS	9100/0
Complete	9100/0
Partial	9103/0
Invasive	9100/1

Complete hydatidiform mole

Definition

A hydatidiform mole involving most of the

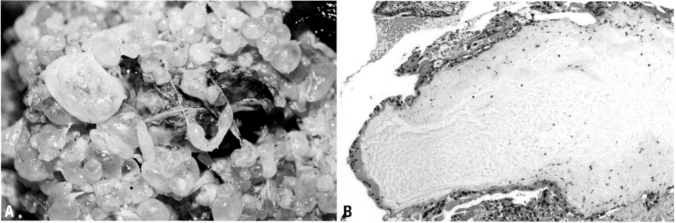

Fig. 4.49 A Classic complete hydatidiform mole. Note the dilated chorionic villi with the typical "bunch of grapes" appearance. **B** This molar villus is cavitated with circumferential trophoblastic hyperplasia and atypia.

chorionic villi and typically having a diploid karyotype.

Histopathology

The villous hydrops of a complete mole is characterized by extensive cavitation. The trophoblastic proliferation differs from normal villi by its circumferential distribution, hyperplasia and cytological atypia {978,1203}. Intermediate trophoblast of the molar implantation site characteristically displays marked cytologic atypia {1901}. A gestational sac, amnion, umbilical cord and fetal tissue are not found {481}. It has recently been suggested that villous stromal nuclear negative staining for the paternally imprinted gene product p57 may be diagnostically useful for confirming the diagnosis of a complete mole {425}. The extent of trophoblastic atypia and

hyperplasia do not correlate with the behaviour in complete mole {776,978}. In the past most complete hydatidiform moles were diagnosed early in the second trimester at an average gestational age of 14 weeks {1924}. Currently, with the widespread use of routine ultrasonography in pregnancy, complete moles are diagnosed between 8 and 12 weeks of gestational age {1924}. Moles diagnosed at this "early" stage differ histologically from moles diagnosed in the second trimester {1426,1924}. Although villous cavitation may be minimal in an "early" mole, other characteristic villous stromal features are present, including hypercellularity and a myxoid basophilic stroma (resembling that of a myxoid fibroadenoma). In addition, unusual villous shapes with complex bulbous protrusions ("cauliflower-

like" villi) and trophoblastic atypia are present.

Somatic genetics

Complete and partial molar pregnancies have distinctly different cytogenetic origins. Complete moles generally have a 46,XX karyotype, and the molar chromosomes are completely of paternal origin {1385}. Most complete moles appear to arise from an anuclear empty ovum fertilized by a (23X) haploid sperm that then replicates its own chromosomes {3172}. Whereas most complete moles have a 46,XX chromosomal pattern, about 10% of complete moles have a 46,XY karyotype {2197}. The 46,XY complete mole arises from fertilization of an anuclear empty egg by two sperm. While all chromosomes in a complete mole are entirely of paternal

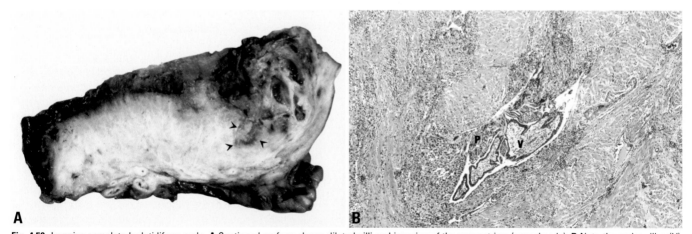

Fig. 4.50 Invasive complete hydatidiform mole. **A** Sectioned surface shows dilated villi and invasion of the myometrium (arrowheads). **B** Note the molar villus (V) within a myometrial vein showing a fibroedematous core surrounded by hyperplastic trophoblastic proliferation (P).

origin, the mitochondrial DNA is of maternal origin {146}.

Partial hydatidiform mole

Definition
A hydatidiform mole having two populations of chorionic villi, one of normal size and the other hydropic, with focal trophoblastic proliferation. The lesion typically has a triploid karyotype.

Histopathology
Histologically, partial moles are characterized by the concurrence of four features {977,1319,1593,2170,2348,2365, 2828,2829}:
(1) Two populations of villi, one hydropic and one "normal";
(2) Minimal trophoblastic hyperplasia involving syncytiotrophoblast.
(3) Enlarged cavitated villi.
(4) Other villi with scalloped borders, often containing trophoblastic inclusions. Stromal blood vessels often contain nucleated fetal red blood cells; other evidence suggesting fetal development is common, including portions of the chorionic sac wall, amnion, umbilical cord and embryonic/fetal tissue.
The differential diagnosis of partial hyda-

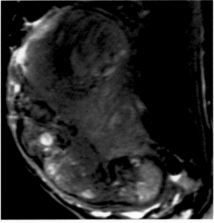

Fig. 4.51 MRI of hydatidiform mole adjacent to a normal fetus in a twin pregnancy.

tidiform mole includes:
(1) Complete mole.
(2) Hydropic abortus.
(3) Several rare sporadic genetic syndromes with focal placental hydrops and a fetus, such as the Beckwith-Weidemann syndrome {1558} and placental angiomatous malformation {2522}, which collectively have been termed "placental mesenchymal dysplasia" {1337}.
In instances in which the histological diagnosis is uncertain, cytogenetic

analysis or flow cytometry may be of assistance {549,882,933,1485,1557-1563,2170}.

Somatic genetics
In contrast to complete moles, partial moles generally have a triploid karyotype that results from fertilization of an apparently normal ovum by two sperm {2828}. The reported incidence of triploidy in partial moles varies from 90-93% respectively {1560,1593}. When fetuses are identified with partial moles, they usually have stigmata of triploidy including multiple congenital anomalies and growth retardation.

Invasive hydatidiform mole

Definition
Invasive hydatidiform mole is defined as villi of hydatidiform mole within the myometrium or its vascular spaces.

Histopathology
Most invasive moles follow complete hydatidiform mole and have the characteristic histological appearance of that lesion. Rare examples of invasive partial mole have also been described {33, 942,1065,2841,3131}. A hysterectomy is usually required for the histological diagnosis.

Metastatic hydatidiform mole

Definition
Metastatic hydatidiform mole is defined as extrauterine molar villi within blood vessels or tissues, most commonly the vagina or the lung.

Non-neoplastic, non-molar trophoblastic lesions

Placental site nodule or plaque

The placental site nodule or plaque {1260,3203} is a well circumscribed lesion with abundant hyalinized stroma infiltrated by scattered, degenerated-appearing intermediate trophoblastic cells; these cells show no significant cytological atypia, but rare mitoses may be present.

Exaggerated placental site

The exaggerated implantation site represents a non-neoplastic exaggeration of the normal implantation process, usually found concurrently with immature villi.

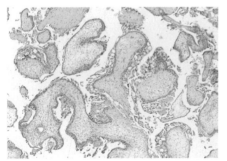

Fig. 4.52 "Early" complete mole. Some villi have toe-like bulbous protrusions. Trophoblastic proliferation and cavitation are minimal. The stroma is hypercellular and myxoid.

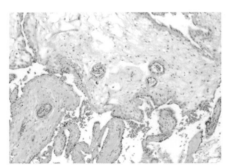

Fig. 4.53 Partial hydatidiform mole. There are two populations of villi; the larger is markedly irregular with scattered cavitation, numerous trophoblastic inclusions and minimal hyperplasia.

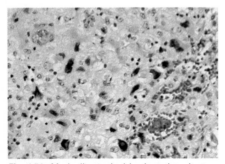

Fig. 4.54 Markedly atypical implantation site trophoblast in a case of early hydatidiform mole.

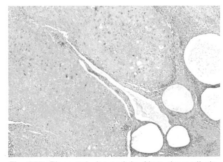

Fig. 4.55 Placental site nodule. Note the well circumscribed eosinophilic endomyometrial nodules.

Sex cord-like, neuroectodermal and neuroendocrine tumours, lymphomas and leukaemias

F. Nogales
F.A. Tavassoli

Sex cord-like tumours

Definition
Tumours of the uterine corpus that closely resemble some true ovarian sex cord tumours.

Epidemiology
Among these rare tumours the most numerous are the sex cord-like tumours {511}, which closely resemble some true ovarian sex cord tumours.

Histopathology
These are diagnosed only when they are not found within otherwise classical endometrial stromal or smooth muscle tumours. Histologically, sex cord elements are represented by trabecular ribbons and nodules or isolated cells with luteinized or foamy cytoplasm that are histologically and immunohistochemically identical to ovarian steroid-producing cells, being strongly positive for alpha-inhibin, calretinin and CD99 {167, 1521,1808}. They may be capable of hormone-secreting activity {2034}. They have a prominent epithelial component that can be tubular, retiform {3247} or glomeruloid. They also show frequent positivity for cytokeratins, vimentin, smooth muscle actin and, occasionally, epithelial membrane antigen (EMA) {930}.

Neuroectodermal tumours

Definition
A variety of tumours of the uterine corpus that show neuroectodermal differentiation.

Epidemiology
Different types of neuroectodermal tumours are found in the uterus. When pure, they usually present in young patients {1188}; however, when mixed with carcinoma or carcinosarcoma they are usually found in older women {638, 931,2710}. Recently, peripheral primitive neuroectodermal tumour/Ewing tumour has been reported in both young {1597} and postmenopausal patients {2710}.

Histopathology
Well differentiated variants with an appearance similar to low grade astrocytoma {3201} should be differentiated from non-neoplastic fetal parts implanted in the endometrium following abortion. Most often, the tumour cells differentiate into neuroblastic, neuroepithelial, glial and neuronal elements {1188}. Peripheral primitive neuroectodermal tumour/Ewing tumour shows a characteristic immunophenotype positive for neuron-specific enolase, vimentin and CD99 as well as the presence of *EWS/FLI-1* fusion transcripts.

Prognosis and predictive factors
All neuroectodermal tumours except the well differentiated astrocytic forms behave in a highly malignant fashion.

Melanotic paraganglioma

Definition
A tumour morphologically identical to paraganglioma, but functionally producing mainly melanin pigment instead of neuroendocrine granules.

Epidemiology
Only two examples of melanotic paraganglioma have been described in the uterus in women 31 and 46 years of age {2866}.

Macroscopy
Both were incidental findings in uteri removed for unrelated benign lesions. The larger lesion was 1.5 cm and appeared as a black pigmented lesion on macroscopic examination; the other was a histological finding.

Histopathology
Both lesions were well circumscribed and composed of large nests of round or angulated polygonal cells with abundant clear or granular pale eosinophilic cytoplasm. Both cases had psammoma bodies, and large amounts of coarse melanin

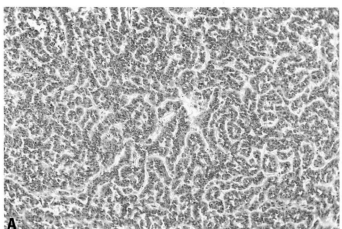
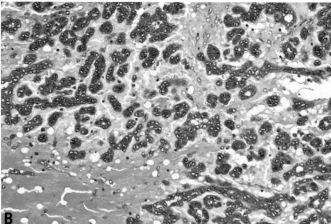

Fig. 4.56 Sex cord-like tumour. **A** Trabecular pattern is prominent. **B** The neoplasm shows a cord-like pattern.

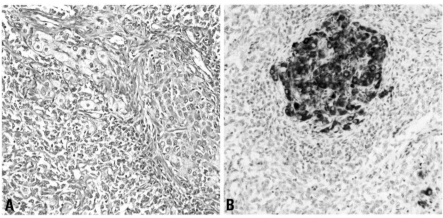

Fig. 4.57 Sex cord-like tumour. **A** Several nodules composed of luteinized cells with ample eosinophilic to vacuolated cytoplasm are present. **B** The nodule of luteinized cells stains positively for alpha-inhibin.

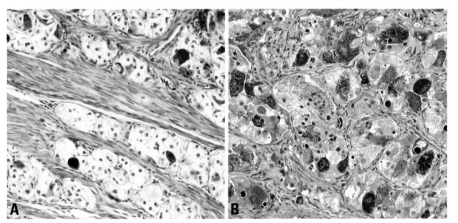

Fig. 4.58 Melanotic paraganglioma. **A** Note the nests of polyhedral cells with abundant clear cytoplasm. **B** Tumour cells have uniform nuclei and contain coarse melanin pigment.

granules were present in many cells. The large cells do not stain with S-100 protein. At the ultrastructural level intracellular melanosomes and premelanosomes abound, and a few neuroendocrine granules are present; the cells lack microvilli or dendritic processes.

Prognosis and predictive factors
Both women were free of any recurrences at 2.2 and 3.2 years after the discovery of the tumour {2866}.

Lymphomas and leukaemias

Definition
A malignant lymphoproliferative or haematopoetic neoplasm that may be primary or secondary.

Clinical findings
The patients typically present with vaginal bleeding {2354}.

Tumour spread and staging
Most lymphomas and leukaemias that involve the uterine corpus are a manifestation of disseminated disease. On rare occasions the corpus is the first known site of a malignant lymphoma.

Histopathology
The majority of cases are of the large B cell type {114}. Lymphomas of the uterine corpus must be distinguished from an atypical lymphoma-like inflammatory lesion of the endometrium. The latter is characterized by a massive infiltrate of lymphoid cells, some of which are immature. The presence of other inflammatory cells including plasma cells and neutrophils within the infiltrate and the typical absence of myometrial invasion or a macroscopic mass are helpful in the differential diagnosis {851}. Cases of uterine leiomyoma massively infiltrated by lymphocytes may also mimic a lymphoma {488}.

Rare tumours

Definition
A variety of benign or malignant tumours of the uterine corpus that are not otherwise categorized.

Histopathology
Germ cell tumours such as teratomas and yolk sac tumours can develop in the endometrium, either in a pure form {398, 2196,2763,2836} or associated with endometrioid tumours {103,2665}. Extrarenal Wilms tumours (nephroblastomas) have also been reported in the uterus {1783,1934}. Their histological appearance is similar to that of the tumours occurring in other sites.

Secondary tumours of the uterine corpus

V. Abeler
U. Haller

Definition
Tumours of the uterine corpus that originate from, but are discontinuous with, a primary extrauterine tumour or a tumour in the cervix or elsewhere in the uterus.

Clinical features
Signs and symptoms
The mean age of patients with extragenital tumour metastasis to the uterus is 60 years. Patients have abnormal uterine bleeding since most neoplasms metastatic to the uterus infiltrate the endometrium diffusely.

Imaging
Imaging studies are non-specific {1240, 1282,1576,3184}.

Macroscopy
Metastases may appear as solitary or multiple tumours or be diffusely infiltrating.

Histopathology
The majority of metastases to the uterus are confined to the myometrium. However, approximately one-third involve the endometrium and thus can be detected in biopsy specimens {1529}. Metastatic carcinoma within the endometrium and/or myometrium characteristically infiltrates as single cells, cord or glands. The appearance is particularly striking in lobular carcinoma of the breast, which usually retains its single-file pattern, and with metastatic signet-ring cell carcinoma of the stomach or colon. Metastatic colon carcinoma of the usual type may form large tumour masses and can mimic an endometrial carcinoma of mucinous or endometrioid type.

Metastatic carcinoma in the endometrium should be suspected if one or more of the following features are present {1539}.

(1) A tumour with an unusual macroscopic or histological pattern for primary endometrial carcinoma.
(2) Diffuse replacement by tumour of endometrial stroma with sparing of occasional normal endometrial glands.
(3) Lack of premalignant changes in endometrial glands.
(4) Lack of tumour necrosis

For specific identification of certain primary tumours immunohistochemical studies are frequently required.

Origin and histogenesis
In most instances the primary tumour is well known, or disseminated disease is clinical evident. Occasionally, a tumour diagnosed by curettage or hysterectomy represents the first sign of an extrauterine primary tumour.

Secondary tumours of the uterine corpus can be divided into two major groups: tumours of the genital and extragenital organs. Neoplasms of neighbouring organs such as cervix, fallopian tubes, ovaries, bladder and rectum can metastasize to the uterine corpus via lymphatics or blood vessels but mostly represent local direct extension.

Haematogenous or lymphatic uterine metastases from any extragenital primary tumour may occur but are extremely rare. Reported primary tumours include carcinomas of the breast, stomach, colon, pancreas, gallbladder, lung, urinary bladder and thyroid and melanoma {192,1452,1455,1529,1531, 1620,1720}. Mammary lobular carcinoma, gastric signet-ring cell carcinoma and colonic carcinoma are the most frequently reported extragenital primary tumours {1529,1531}.

Prognosis and predictive factors
When uterine metastases are present, the patient usually has widely disseminated disease. However, in one series the average survival was 20 months after the diagnosis of uterine metastases. The reason for this relatively favourable outcome might be the predominance of cases of metastatic breast carcinoma {1529}.

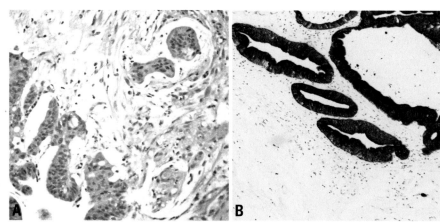

Fig. 4.59 Metastatic colon carcinoma to the myometrium. **A** Note the tumour cells in lymphatic vessels in the right upper portion of the field with a plexiform pattern on the left. **B** The neoplastic glands are positive for cytokeratin 20.

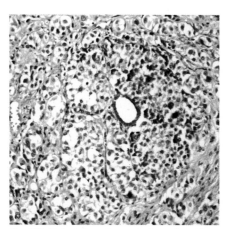

Fig. 4.60 Metastatic melanoma to the endometrium. Tumour cells containing melanin pigment surround an atrophic endometrial gland.

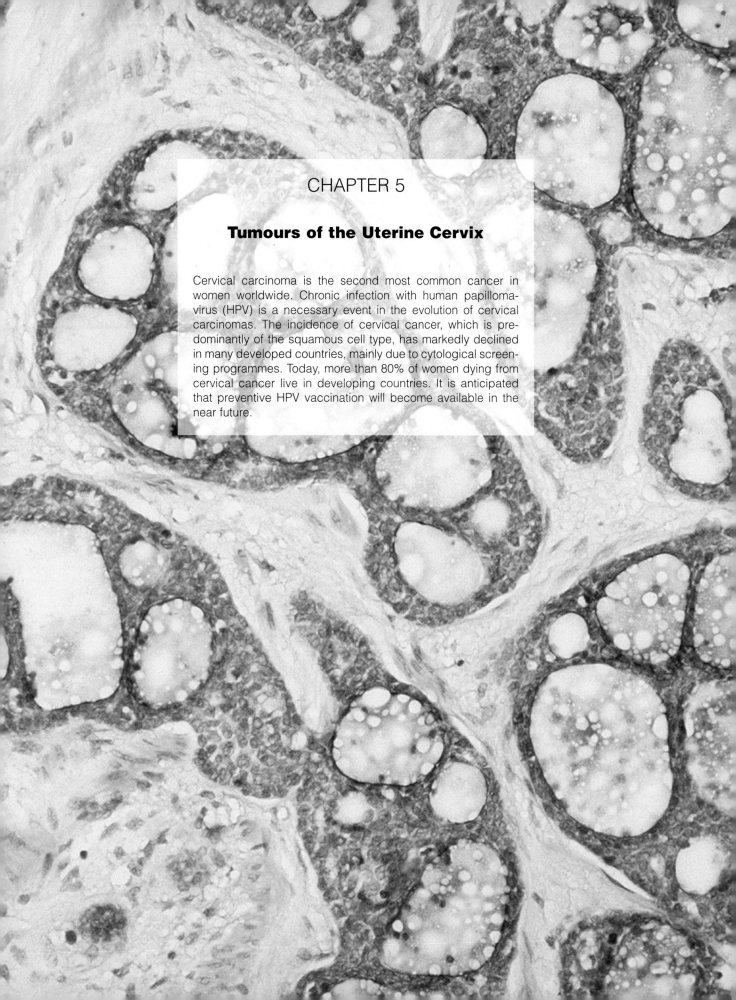

CHAPTER 5

Tumours of the Uterine Cervix

Cervical carcinoma is the second most common cancer in women worldwide. Chronic infection with human papillomavirus (HPV) is a necessary event in the evolution of cervical carcinomas. The incidence of cervical cancer, which is predominantly of the squamous cell type, has markedly declined in many developed countries, mainly due to cytological screening programmes. Today, more than 80% of women dying from cervical cancer live in developing countries. It is anticipated that preventive HPV vaccination will become available in the near future.

WHO histological classification of tumours of the uterine cervix

Epithelial tumours

Squamous tumours and precursors

Squamous cell carcinoma, not otherwise specified	8070/3
Keratinizing	8071/3
Non-keratinizing	8072/3
Basaloid	8083/3
Verrucous	8051/3
Warty	8051/3
Papillary	8052/3
Lymphoepithelioma-like	8082/3
Squamotransitional	8120/3
Early invasive (microinvasive) squamous cell carcinoma	8076/3

Squamous intraepithelial neoplasia

Cervical intraepithelial neoplasia (CIN) 3 /	8077/2
squamous cell carcinoma in situ	8070/2

Benign squamous cell lesions

Condyloma acuminatum	
Squamous papilloma	8052/0
Fibroepithelial polyp	

Glandular tumours and precursors

Adenocarcinoma	8140/3
Mucinous adenocarcinoma	8480/3
Endocervical	8482/3
Intestinal	8144/3
Signet-ring cell	8490/3
Minimal deviation	8480/3
Villoglandular	8262/3
Endometrioid adenocarcinoma	8380/3
Clear cell adenocarcinoma	8310/3
Serous adenocarcinoma	8441/3
Mesonephric adenocarcinoma	9110/3
Early invasive adenocarcinoma	8140/3
Adenocarcinoma in situ	8140/2
Glandular dysplasia	

Benign glandular lesions

Müllerian papilloma	
Endocervical polyp	

Other epithelial tumours

Adenosquamous carcinoma	8560/3
Glassy cell carcinoma variant	8015/3
Adenoid cystic carcinoma	8200/3
Adenoid basal carcinoma	8098/3

Neuroendocrine tumours

Carcinoid	8240/3
Atypical carcinoid	8249/3
Small cell carcinoma	8041/3
Large cell neuroendocrine carcinoma	8013/3
Undifferentiated carcinoma	8020/3

Mesenchymal tumours and tumour-like conditions

Leiomyosarcoma	8890/3
Endometrioid stromal sarcoma, low grade	8931/3
Undifferentiated endocervical sarcoma	8805/3
Sarcoma botryoides	8910/3
Alveolar soft part sarcoma	9581/3
Angiosarcoma	9120/3
Malignant peripheral nerve sheath tumour	9540/3
Leiomyoma	8890/0
Genital rhabdomyoma	8905/0
Postoperative spindle cell nodule	

Mixed epithelial and mesenchymal tumours

Carcinosarcoma (malignant müllerian mixed tumour;	
metaplastic carcinoma)	8980/3
Adenosarcoma	8933/3
Wilms tumour	8960/3
Adenofibroma	9013/0
Adenomyoma	8932/0

Melanocytic tumours

Malignant melanoma	8720/3
Blue naevus	8780/0

Miscellaneous tumours

Tumours of germ cell type

Yolk sac tumour	9071/3
Dermoid cyst	9084/0
Mature cystic teratoma	9080/0

Lymphoid and haematopoetic tumours

Malignant lymphoma (specify type)	
Leukaemia (specify type)	

Secondary tumours

---

[1] Morphology code of the International Classification of Diseases for Oncology (ICD-O) {921} and the Systematized Nomenclature of Medicine (http://snomed.org). Behaviour is coded /0 for benign tumours, /2 for in situ carcinomas and grade 3 intraepithelial neoplasia, /3 for malignant tumours, and /1 for borderline or uncertain behaviour.

[2] Intraepithelial neoplasia does not have a generic code in ICD-O. ICD-O codes are only available for lesions categorized as squamous intraepithelial neoplasia grade 3 (e.g. cervical intraepithelial neoplasia 3) = 8077/2, squamous cell carcinoma in situ = 8070/2, glandular intraepithelial neoplasia grade 3 = 8148/2 and adenocarcinoma in situ = 8140/2.

TNM and FIGO classification of carcinomas of the uterine cervix

TNM classification[1,2]

T – Primary Tumour

TNM Categories	FIGO Stages	
TX		Primary tumour cannot be assessed
T0		No evidence of primary tumour
Tis	0	Carcinoma in situ (preinvasive carcinoma)
T1	I	Cervical carcinoma confined to uterus (extension to corpus should be disregarded)
T1a	IA	Invasive carcinoma diagnosed only by microscopy. All macroscopically visible lesions - even with superficial invasion - are T1b/Stage IB
T1a1	IA1	Stromal invasion no greater than 3.0 mm in depth and 7.0 mm or less in horizontal spread
T1a2	IA2	Stromal invasion more than 3.0 mm and not more than 5.0 mm with a horizontal spread 7.0 mm or less

Note: The depth of invasion should not be more than 5 mm taken from the base of the epithelium, either surface or glandular, from which it originates. The depth of invasion is defined as the measurement of the tumour from the epithelial-stromal junction of the adjacent most superficial epithelial papilla to the deepest point of invasion. Vascular space involvement, venous or lymphatic, does not affect classification.

TNM	FIGO	
T1b	IB	Clinically visible lesion confined to the cervix or microscopic lesion greater than T1a2/IA2
T1b1	IB1	Clinically visible lesion 4.0 cm or less in greatest dimension
T1b2	IB2	Clinically visible lesion more than 4 cm in greatest dimension
T2	II	Tumour invades beyond uterus but not to pelvic wall or to lower third of the vagina
T2a	IIA	Without parametrial invasion
T2b	IIB	With parametrial invasion
T3	III	Tumour extends to pelvic wall, involves lower third of vagina, or causes hydronephrosis or non-functioning kidney
T3a	IIIA	Tumour involves lower third of vagina, no extension to pelvic wall
T3b	IIIB	Tumour extends to pelvic wall or causes hydronephrosis or non-functioning kidney
T4	IVA	Tumour invades mucosa of bladder or rectum or extends beyond true pelvis

Note: The presence of bullous oedema is not sufficient to classify a tumour as T4.

M1	IVB	Distant metastasis

N – Regional Lymph Nodes[3]

NX	Regional lymph nodes cannot be assessed
N0	No regional lymph node metastasis
N1	Regional lymph node metastasis

M – Distant Metastasis

MX	Distant metastasis cannot be assessed
M0	No distant metastasis
M1	Distant metastasis

Stage Grouping

Stage 0	Tis	N0	M0
Stage IA	T1a	N0	M0
Stage IA1	T1a1	N0	M0
Stage IA2	T1a2	N0	M0
Stage IB	T1b	N0	M0
Stage IB1	T1b1	N0	M0
Stage IB2	T1b2	N0	M0
Stage IIA	T2a	N0	M0
Stage IIB	T2b	N0	M0
Stage IIIA	T3a	N0	M0
Stage IIIB	T1, T2, T3a	N1	M0
	T3b	Any N	M0
Stage IVA	T4	Any N	M0
Stage IVB	Any T	Any N	M1

---

[1] {51,2976}.
[2] A help desk for specific questions about the TNM classification is available at http://tnm.uicc.org.
[3] The regional lymph nodes are the paracervical, parametrial, hypogastric (internal iliac, obturator), common and external iliac, presacral, and lateral sacral nodes.

Epithelial tumours

M. Wells   J.M. Nesland
A.G. Östör   A.K. Goodman
C.P. Crum   R. Sankaranarayanan
S. Franceschi   A.G. Hanselaar
M. Tommasino   J. Albores-Saavedra

This section covers the entire spectrum of invasive squamous and glandular carcinomas and their intraepithelial precursor lesions that originate for the most part from the transformation zone of the cervix. In addition, benign epithelial tumours are described which are not considered precursors of invasive cancer.

Epidemiology

In 1990 cervical cancer comprised 10% of cancers in women for a total of approximately 470,000 cancer cases world-wide {846}, representing the third most common cancer in females and the most common cancer in Sub-Saharan Africa, Central America, South Central Asia and Melanesia. Approximately 230,000 women die annually from cervical cancer, and over 190,000 of those are from developing countries. Zimbabwe and India stand out not only for their high incidence but also for an unfavourable incidence to mortality ratio. Some relatively high-incidence countries can also be found in Eastern and Central Europe {1638}.

The incidence of cervical cancer has been declining in the last three or four decades in most developed countries predominantly due to the introduction of cervical screening programmes. Other reasons include a decrease in parity {1943} and improved living conditions {226}. In women under 45 years of age, however, mortality rates are levelling off or increasing in several countries {226}. Stable or, in some instances, upward mortality trends in high-risk populations in Latin America {2395} and Eastern Europe {1638} are especially disturbing. Finally, adenocarcinoma of the cervix, which accounts for 10-15% of all cervical cancers, has shown an increased incidence in the last three decades {3028}.

Aetiology

Sexually transmitted virus, human papillomavirus (HPV), is the major aetiological factor, as shown by:
(1) the identification of HPV DNA in most cervical cancer biopsy specimens worldwide {3044};

(2) relative risks (RRs) for cervical squamous cell and adenocarcinoma of greater than 70 for several high-risk HPV types in case-control studies {1199, 1293};
(3) RRs of approximately 10 for women with HPV infection in cohort studies {3143}.

Several host and environmental factors contribute, however, to enhance the probability of HPV persistence and progression to cervical neoplasia. Immune impairment, whether due to immunosuppressive treatments {274} or human immunodeficiency (HIV) infection {913, 920}, increases the risk of cervical intraepithelial neoplasia (CIN) and invasive cancer of the cervix 5 to 10-fold. Among HPV-DNA positive women long-term use of oral contraceptives {1911}, high parity {1943}, tobacco smoking {3164} and certain sexually transmitted infections, such as Chlamydia trachomatis {2733}, are associated with a RR between 2 and 4.

HPV-induced carcinogenesis

The products of two early genes, *E6* and *E7*, have been shown to play a major role in HPV-mediated cervical carcinogenesis This has been established by three different lines of evidence:
(1) The first indication came from the analysis of HPV-infected cells, which showed that viral DNA is randomly integrated in the genome of the majority of cervical carcinomas. Integration leads to disruption of several viral genes with preservation of only the *E6* and *E7* genes, which are actively transcribed.
(2) The discovery that E6 and E7 proteins are able to induce cellular transformation in vitro confirmed their oncogenic role. Immortalized rodent fibroblasts can be fully transformed by expression of HPV 16 E6 or E7 protein. These rodent cells acquire the ability to grow in an anchorage-independent manner and are tumorigenic when injected in nude mice. In addition, HPV 16 E6 and E7 are able to immortalize primary human keratinocytes, the natural host cell of the virus. In agreement with the in vitro assays, transgenic mice co-expressing both viral genes exhibit epidermal hyperplasia and various tumours.
(3) Finally, biochemical studies have clarified the mechanism of action of E6

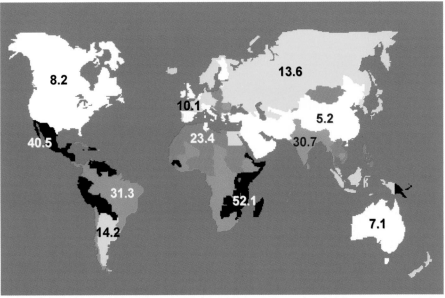

Fig. 5.01 Global burden of cervical cancer. Age-standardized incidence rates (ASR) per 100,000 population and year. From Globocan 2000 {846}.

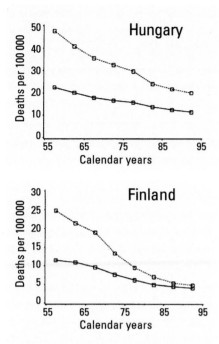

Fig. 5.02 A marked decrease in the mortality of uterine cancer (cervix and corpus) has been achieved in many countries. Upper curves: age group 35-64 years. Lower curves: all age groups combined. From F. Levi et al. {1637}.

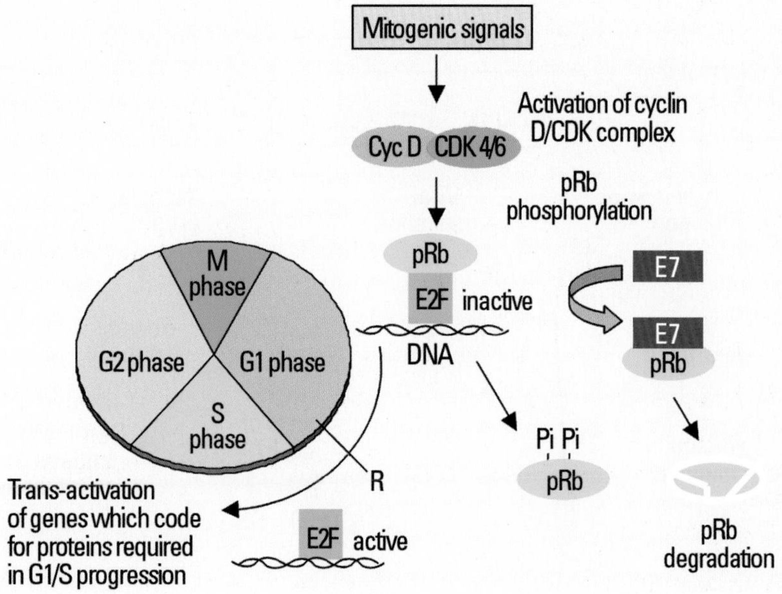

Fig. 5.03 Deregulation of the restriction point (R) by HPV16 *E7*. In quiescent cells, pRb is present in a hypophosphorylated form and is associated with transcription factors, e.g. members of the E2F family, inhibiting their transcriptional activity. When quiescent cells are exposed to mitogenic signals, G1 specific cyclin D/CDK complexes are activated and phosphorylate pRb in mid-G1 phase, causing release of active E2F and progression through the restriction point (R). E7 binding to pRb mimics its phosphorylation. Thus, E7 expressing cells can enter S phase in the absence of a mitogenic signal. From M. Tommasino {2938a}.

and E7. The viral oncoproteins are able to form stable complexes with cellular proteins and alter, or completely neutralize, their normal functions.

The best understood interactions of E6 and E7 with cellular proteins are those involving the tumor suppressor proteins TP53 and pRb, respectively. Both interactions lead to a rapid degradation of the cellular proteins via the ubiquitin pathway. The major role of TP53 is to safeguard the integrity of the genome by inducing cell cycle arrest or apoptosis, while pRb plays a key role in controlling the correct G1/S transition acting at the restriction point (R) of the cell cycle. Therefore, loss of TP53 and pRb functions results in abrogation of apoptosis and in unscheduled proliferation. Both events greatly increase the probability of HPV-infected cells evolving towards malignancy.

Clinical features
Signs and symptoms
Early invasive cancers can be asymptomatic. As the tumour grows and becomes exophytic, vaginal bleeding and discharge are the two most common

symptoms. With lateral growth into the parametrium, the ureters become obstructed. If both ureters are obstructed, the patient presents with anuria and

uraemia. Pelvic sidewall involvement can cause sciatic pain and, less commonly, lymphoedema of the lower extremities. Anterior tumour growth in advanced

Table 5.01
Risk factors for cervical cancer: HPV infection vs. persistence and malignant transformation.

Risk factor	HPV infection	HPV persistence and transformation	Reference
Multiple sex partners	+	n.e.	{320}
Partner's multiple partners	+	n.e.	{320}
Poor hygiene	+	n.e.	{193}
Absence of male circumcision	+	+	{423}
Immunodeficiency, HIV	+	+	{920}
High parity	n.e.	+	{1944}
Oral contraceptives	n.e.	+	{1911}
Smoking	n.e.	+	{2826}
STDs other than HPV	n.e.	+	{108,2734}
Poor nutritional status	n.e.	+	{2324}

STDs = Sexually transmitted diseases (especially *C. trachomatis*).
n.e. = No evidence for being a risk factor at this time.

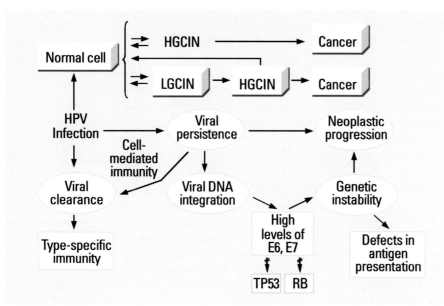

Fig. 5.04 Mechanisms of human papillomavirus (HPV) carcinogenesis. LG = Low grade, HG = High grade, CIN = Cervical intraepithelial neoplasia, RB = Retinoblastoma gene.

stage disease causes urinary frequency, bladder pain and haematuria. Direct extension into the bladder may cause urinary retention from bladder outlet obstruction and eventually a vesicovaginal fistula. Posterior extension leads to low back pain, tenesmus and rectovaginal fistula.

On examination cervical cancer may appear as a red, friable, exophytic or ulcerated lesion. Rectovaginal palpation can detect induration or nodularity of the parametria in advanced lesions.

Colposcopy

The colposcope is a noninvasive binocular instrument with a magnification of 6 to 40-fold designed to examine the cervix. The area of the cervix where the transformation of columnar to metaplastic squamous epithelium occurs is known as the transformation zone. Since most cervical neoplasia arises in the transformation zone, the relevant colposcopic signs are observed within its limits. Whenever the transformation zone is not seen in its entirety, the colposcopy is termed "unsatisfactory".

Colposcopy involves the application of 4-5% acetic acid on the cervix and is based on the colour and margin of the aceto-white epithelium, the surface contour, the arrangement of the blood vessels and iodine staining. Abnormal colposcopic findings include leukoplakia, aceto-white epithelium, punctation and mosaic and atypical vessels {372,417, 2705}. White keratotic lesions apparent before the application of acetic acid are termed "leukoplakia".

Aceto-white epithelium, which appears only after contact with acetic acid, is most marked with cervical intraepithelial neoplasia (CIN) and early invasive cancer. Significant lesions are sharply delineated, densely opaque and persist for several minutes. Glandular lesions produce more subtle changes {3159}.

Fine or coarse stippling within aceto-white epithelium produced by the end-on view of finger-like intraepithelial capillaries is called punctation. A mosaic pattern arises when the stromal ridges containing the blood vessels subdivide the aceto-white epithelium into blocks of varying size and shape. Atypical tortuous vessels with bizarre irregular branches showing gross variation in calibre are suggestive of early invasive disease. Cervical neoplasia fails to stain deeply with iodine due to the lack of glycogen.

Variations in quality and quantity of the above atypical appearances help in differentiating cervical neoplasia from physiological, benign, infective, inflammatory and reactive changes in the cervix. Colposcopy and histopathology are complementary to the diagnosis and management of CIN.

Tumour spread and staging

Cervical cancer is the only gynaecological cancer that is clinically staged by physical examination, chest X-ray, intravenous pyelogram, cystoscopy and proctoscopy. The staging of cervical tumours is by the TNM/FIGO classification {51,2976}.

One-half of early invasive foci originate from the surface epithelium {2349}. The uterine corpus is commonly involved as the tumour expands. Ovarian metastasis is rare, occurring more frequently in bulky cancers and in adenocarcinomas as compared to squamous cell cancers {1914,1966}. Clinically undetected parametrial spread is identified by histological examination in 31-63% of stage IB

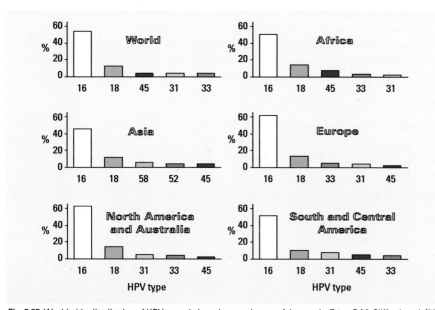

Fig. 5.05 Worldwide distribution of HPV types in invasive carcinoma of the cervix. From G.M. Clifford et al. {528}.

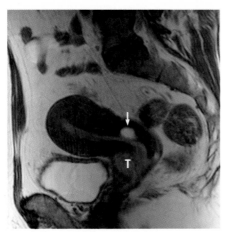

Fig. 5.06 Sagittal T2-weighted MRI of a cervical carcinoma (T). This projection facilitates preoperative staging. The arrow indicates the presence of ovula Nabothi.

and 58% of stage IIA patients {221}. Cervical cancers spread along fascial planes. As the parametria are invaded, the incidence of pelvic node involvement increases to 36% {221}. All para-aortic nodal metastases are associated with pelvic node metastasis; 11.5% of stage IB, 26.7% of stage IIA and 40% of stage IIB cancers had pelvic node involvement and 2.1%, 0% and 7.2% of these had para-aortic node involvement respectively {2514}. In contrast to the orderly lymphatic spread of cervical cancers, lung and brain metastases reflect haematogenous spread and are an aberrant behaviour that cannot be predicted by stage of disease {1737}.

Precursor lesions
Precursor lesions of squamous cell carcinoma and adenocarcinoma are well defined with the exception of low grade cervical glandular intraepithelial neoplasia, i.e. glandular dysplasia or glandular atypia.

Somatic genetics
TP53
Inactivation of *TP53* appears to play a key role in the development of cervical carcinoma {1178,2911} either because binding with the E6 protein of oncogenic HPV types inactivates it or because it undergoes mutation. Patterns of TP53 immunoreactivity suggest also that *TP53* inactivation is important in the progression from intraepithelial to invasive neoplasia {1659,2004,2954}. TP53 reactivity has been demonstrated in both in situ

and invasive adenocarcinoma {495, 1807}. *TP53* gene alterations are rare in minimal deviation adenocarcinoma {2937} and are not found in villoglandular adenocarcinomas {1363}.

Loss of heterozygosity
Loss of heterozygosity (LOH) has been detected in multiple chromosomal regions in CIN (3p, 5p, 5q, 6p, 6q, 11q, 13q, 17q), invasive carcinoma (3p, 6p, 6q, 11q, 17p, 18q) and lymph node metastases from cervical carcinomas (3p, 6p, 11q, 17p, 18q, X) {263,666, 1119,1444,1445,1584,1706,1712}. These changes accumulate in a fashion that parallels the progression of cervical carcinoma and indicate the stepwise nature of cervical carcinogenesis. Chromosomal instability is probably an early event. At least two tumour suppressor genes on 6p related to invasive cervical carcinoma have been demonstrated in 50% of cases of low grade CIN and in 90% of cases of high grade CIN {447}.

FHIT gene
Recent studies have found that abnormalities of the *FHIT* (fragile histidine triad) gene, including loss of heterozygosity, homozygous deletions and aberrant transcripts, are common in cervical carcinomas, implicating this gene in cervical carcinogenesis {1938,2807,3187}. *FHIT* abnormalities have been observed

in various histological types of cervical carcinomas {2616}.
FHIT gene abnormalities have been found in both CIN and invasive carcinoma, but the incidence did not increase with progression to invasion or with advancing clinical stage {1964}. By contrast, another group {3188} found aberrations of *FHIT* to be more common in invasive carcinomas than in CIN suggesting that *FHIT* gene inactivation occurred as a late event in cervical carcinogenesis, after the tumour had acquired an invasive character

Monoclonality
The finding that early invasive carcinoma is monoclonal supports the view that monoclonality is not a late event due to clonal competition or selection {1086}. Nearly all cases of high grade CIN have been found to be monoclonal, whilst only a small proportion of low grade CIN are monoclonal {489,789,2184}.
Recurrent chromosome aberrations have been demonstrated in both invasive cervical squamous carcinoma and high grade CIN, there being a consistent chromosome gain at 3q and deletions at 3p {1208,1469}.

Genetic susceptibility
Few studies have addressed familial clustering in cervical carcinoma {743, 2230}, the largest report being based on

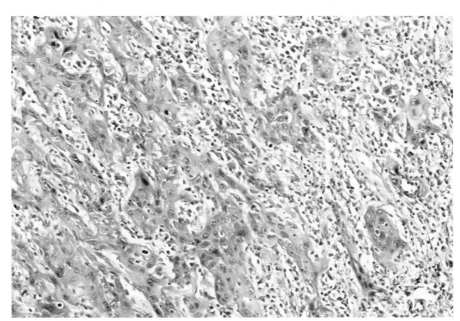

Fig. 5.07 Squamous cell carcinoma, non-keratinizing type. The tumour has a tentacular, or "finger-like" infiltrative pattern.

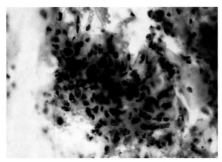

Fig. 5.08 Keratinizing squamous cell carcinoma. Note the partly spindle-shaped cells with eosinophilic cytoplasm and hyperchromatic nuclei.

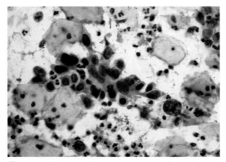

Fig. 5.09 Non-keratinizing squamous cell carcinoma. There is a syncytium with anisokaryosis, irregular distributed coarsely chromatin and nucleoli.

the Swedish Family-Cancer Database {1184}. The relative risk when the mother or a daughter was affected by cervical cancer was 2. An aggregation of tobacco-related cancers and cancers linked with HPV and immunosuppression was found in such families. Thus, familial predisposition for cervical cancer is likely to imply genes which modulate immune response, e.g. human leukocyte antigen (HLA) haplotypes {2524} and/or shared sexual or lifestyle factors in family members.

Prognosis and predictive factors
Clinical criteria
The clinical factors that influence prognosis in invasive cervical cancer are age, stage of disease, volume, lymphatic spread and vascular invasion {370,663, 673,818,970,1506,2525,2672,2782}. In a large series of cervical cancer patients treated by radiation therapy, the frequency of distant metastases (most frequently to the lung, abdominal cavity, liver and gastrointestinal tract) was shown to increase with increasing stage of disease from 3% in stage IA to 75% in stage IVA {818}.

Radiotherapy and surgery produce similar results for early invasive cancer (stages IB and IIA). More advanced lesions (IIB to IV) are treated with a combination of external radiotherapy and intracavitary radiation. Randomized phase III trials have shown a significant overall and disease free survival advantage for cisplatin-based therapy given concurrently with radiotherapy {1063, 2908}. A significant benefit of chemoradiation on both local (odds ratio 0.61) and distant recurrence (odds ratio 0.57) has been observed. The absolute benefit with combined therapy on overall survival was 16%. Based on this evidence, concurrent chemotherapy with radiothera-

py is emerging as the new standard of care for advanced cervical cancer.

Histopathological criteria
Among histopathological variables based on histological findings and not included in the staging system for cervical cancer {1532}, the grading of tumours does not seem to be a strong predictive factor {3233}. In non-squamous cell carcinomas the only histological type of cervical cancer of prognostic significance is small cell carcinoma {68}. There is some evidence that women with adenocarcinoma and adenosquamous carcinoma have a poorer prognosis than those with squamous cell carcinoma after adjustment for stage {2314}.

Genetic predictive factors
TP53. The prognostic value of TP53 immunoreactivity in cervical carcinoma is controversial. Some have found no association between p53 overexpression or the presence of mutant p53 protein and clinical outcome {1267,2251}, whilst others have reported that TP53 expression identifies a subset of cervical carcinomas with a poor prognosis {2969}.
c-erbB. Frequent amplification of c-erbB-2 has been documented in cervical carcinoma {2634}, and c-erbB-2 immunostaining has been found to be significantly associated with poor survival and was considered to be a marker of high risk disease {1998}. Additionally, c-erbB-2 immunostaining was found to be an important prognostic factor for predicting tumour recurrence in cervical carcinomas treated by radiotherapy {1967, 2026}. On the other hand, overexpression of c-erbB-3 oncoprotein in squamous, adenosquamous and adenocarcinomas of the cervix showed no association with clinical outcome {1267}

c-myc. c-myc amplification has been demonstrated in CIN and invasive cervical carcinoma {110,666,2004} suggesting that it is important in early cervical carcinogenesis. Moreover, c-myc overexpression correlates with high risk HPV-positive neoplasia and with cellular proliferation {666}. It has been claimed that an increased level of *c-myc* transcripts is strongly indicative of a poor prognosis in early stage cervical carcinoma {1314} but not in late stage disease {2823}.

Squamous tumours and precursors

Definition
Primary squamous epithelial tumours of the uterine cervix, either benign or malignant.

ICD-O codes
Squamous cell carcinoma	8070/3
Keratinizing	8071/3
Non-keratinizing	8072/3
Basaloid	8083/3
Verrucous	8051/3
Warty	8051/3
Papillary	8052/3
Lymphoepithelioma-like	8082/3
Squamotransitional cell	8120/3
Microinvasive squamous cell carcinoma	8076/3
Cervical intraepithelial neoplasia 3	8077/2
squamous cell carcinoma in situ	8070/2
Squamous papilloma	8052/0

Squamous cell carcinoma

Definition
An invasive carcinoma composed of squamous cells of varying degrees of differentiation.

Macroscopy
Macroscopically, squamous cell carcinoma may be either predominantly exophytic, in which case it grows out from the surface, often as a papillary or polypoid excrescence, or else it may be mainly endophytic, such that it infiltrates into the surrounding structures without much surface growth.

Histopathology

There have been few recent developments in the histological diagnosis of frankly invasive squamous cell carcinoma of the cervix {362,1201}. They vary in their pattern of growth, cell type and degree of differentiation. Most carcinomas infiltrate as networks of anastomosing bands with intervening stroma and appear as irregular islands, sometimes rounded, but more usually angular and spiked. Often, particularly in small tumours, CIN may be found on the surface and at the edge of the invasive tumour, and, occasionally, difficulty may be encountered in distinguishing between invasive islands and CIN involving crypts. Similarly, invasion cannot be excluded when neoplastic squamous epithelium shows features of CIN 2 or 3 but underlying stroma is not present.

A number of histological grading systems have been proposed that depend upon the type and degree of differentiation of the predominant cell {2794}. A simpler classification is a modification of the four grades of Broders {350} and subdivides the tumours into well differentiated (keratinizing), moderately differentiated and poorly differentiated types. Approximately 60% are moderately differentiated, and the remaining tumours are evenly distributed between the well and poorly differentiated groups.

A simple two-tiered classification is recommended, keratinizing and non-keratinizing, to avoid nosological confusion with small cell carcinoma, a term that should be reserved for tumours of neuroendocrine type.

The cervical stroma separating the islands of invasive carcinoma is usually infiltrated by a variety of cell types, mainly lymphocytes and plasma cells. A markedly eosinophilic stromal response {262} or a foreign body type giant cell reaction is occasionally seen.

A variety of histological types of squamous cell carcinoma have been described.

Keratinizing

These tumours contain keratin pearls composed of circular whorls of squamous cells with central nests of keratin. Intercellular bridges, keratohyaline granules and cytoplasmic keratinization are usually observed. The nuclei are usually large and hyperchromatic with coarse chromatin. Mitotic figures are not fre-

quent and are usually seen in the less-well differentiated cells at the periphery of the invasive masses.

In cytological preparations the cells usually have bizarre shapes with mostly eosinophilic cytoplasm and large, irregular, hyperchromatic nuclei. Necrotic debris is present.

Non-keratinizing

These tumours are composed of generally recognizable polygonal squamous cells that may have individual cell keratinization and intercellular bridges, but keratin pearls are absent. Cellular and nuclear pleomorphism is more obvious than in the well differentiated tumours, and mitotic figures are usually numerous. In cytological preparations the cells are solitary or arranged in syncytia and show anisokaryosis. The nuclei are relatively large with unevenly distributed, coarsely granular chromatin and may have irregular nucleoli

Basaloid

Basaloid squamous cell carcinoma is composed of nests of immature, basal type squamous cells with scanty cytoplasm that resemble closely the cells of squamous carcinoma in situ of the cervix. Some keratinization may be evident in the centres of the nests, but keratin pearls are rarely present. In the vulva this tumour has been associated with HPV infections, predominantly type 16 {1541,2936}.

This underrecognized variant of squamous cell carcinoma is an aggressive tumour with basaloid features {1057}. This tumour along with adenoid cystic carcinoma is at one end of the spectrum of basaloid tumours of the cervix. At the opposite end are low grade lesions such as adenoid basal carcinoma. To avoid confusion in the diagnosis of a cervical tumour with basaloid features, the term "basaloid carcinoma" should be avoided {1057}.

Verrucous

Verrucous carcinoma is a highly differentiated squamous cell carcinoma that has a hyperkeratotic, undulating, warty surface and invades the underlying stroma in the form of bulbous pegs with a pushing border. The tumour cells have abundant cytoplasm, and their nuclei show minimal atypia. Features of HPV infection are not evident. Verrucous carcinomas

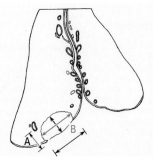

Fig. 5.10 Schematic representation of the FIGO definition of stage 1A carcinoma of the cervix. A: Depth of invasion no greater than 5 mm; B: Horizontal spread 7 mm or less.

have a tendency to recur locally after excision but do not metastasize. They are distinguished from condyloma by their broad papillae that lack fibrovascular cores and the absence of koilocytosis. Verrucous carcinoma is distinguished from the more common types of squamous cell carcinoma in that it shows no more than minimal nuclear atypia.

Warty

This lesion is defined as a squamous cell carcinoma with a warty surface and cellular features of HPV infection {720, 1541,2936}. High risk HPV-DNA is typically detected {2936}. It is also referred to as condylomatous squamous cell carcinoma.

Papillary

This is a tumour in which thin or broad papillae with connective tissue stroma are covered by epithelium showing the features of CIN. Whilst a superficial biopsy may not reveal evidence of invasion, the underlying tumour is usually a typical squamous cell carcinoma {345,2333}. Such tumours are positive for HPV type 16. Papillary squamous cell carcinoma differs from warty squamous carcinoma by the inconspicuous keratinization and lack of cellular features of HPV infection and from transitional cell carcinoma by its squamous cell differentiation {345}.

Lymphoepithelioma-like

Histologically, lymphoepithelioma-like carcinoma is strikingly similar to the nasopharyngeal tumour of the same name. It is composed of poorly defined islands of undifferentiated cells in a background intensely infiltrated by lym-

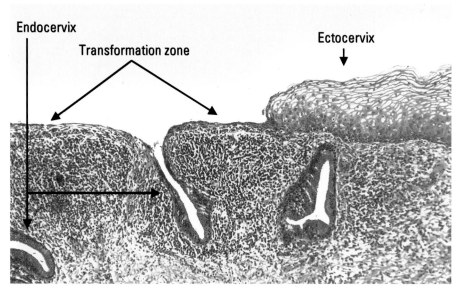

Fig. 5.11 Transformation zone of the cervix. Photomicrograph of the early (immature) cervical transformation zone consisting of a thin layer of basal cells between the ectocervical and endocervical mucosa.

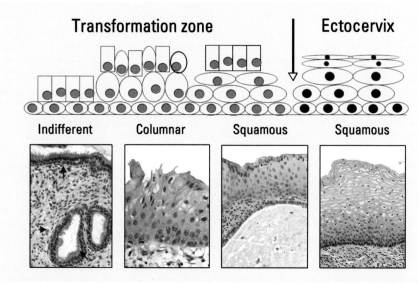

Fig. 5.12 Transformation zone of the cervix. Schematic of the transformation zone (upper) illustrating the range of differentiation beyond the original squamocolumnar junction (vertical arrow). This area supports (from left to right) reserve cells that are indifferent (yet uncommitted, arrows) or committed to squamous and columnar differentiation as depicted in the photomicrographs below.

phocytes. The tumour cells have uniform, vesicular nuclei with prominent nucleoli and moderate amounts of slightly eosinophilic cytoplasm. The cell borders are indistinct, often imparting a syncytial-like appearance to the groups. Immunohistochemistry identifies cytokeratins within the tumour cells and T-cell markers in the majority of the lymphocytes. The presence of an intense chronic inflammatory reaction in a tumour indicates a cell-mediated immune reaction, and some evidence suggests that lymphoep-

ithelioma-like carcinoma of the cervix may have a favourable prognosis. Using the polymerase chain reaction to examine frozen tissue from a lymphoepithelioma-like carcinoma of the cervix, Epstein-Barr virus (EBV) genomic material was not identified in a case from the United States {3084}. On the other hand EBV DNA was identified in 11 of 15 lymphoepithelioma-like carcinomas from Taïwan, whereas HPV DNA was uncommon (3 of 15) suggesting that EBV may play a role in the aetiology of this tumour

in their Asian population {2957}. It is of note that EBV was not identified in a case analysed from Spain {1696}. Thus, if EBV plays a role in the genesis of this tumour, it exhibits geographical variation.

Squamotransitional carcinoma
Rare transitional cell carcinomas of the cervix have been described that are apparently indistinguishable from their counterpart in the urinary bladder. They may occur in a pure form or may contain malignant squamous elements {56,66, 1488}. Such tumours demonstrate papillary architecture with fibrovascular cores lined by a multilayered, atypical epithelium resembling CIN 3. The detection of HPV type 16 and the presence of allelic losses at chromosome 3p with the infrequent involvement of chromosome 9 suggest that these tumours are more closely related to cervical squamous cell carcinomas than to primary urothelial tumours {1672,1742}. Furthermore, these tumours are more likely to express cytokeratin 7 than 20, which suggests only a histological, rather than an immunophenotypic, resemblance to transitional epithelium {1488}. There is no evidence that this tumour is related to transitional cell metaplasia {1140,3085}, an infrequently occurring somewhat controversial entity in the cervix.

Early invasive squamous cell carcinoma

Definition
A squamous cell carcinoma with early stromal invasion, the extent of which has not been precisely defined, and a low risk of local lymph node metastasis.

Synonym
Microinvasive squamous cell carcinoma.

Histopathology
Certain features of high grade CIN increase the likelihood of identifying early invasion. These include:
(1) Extensive CIN 3,
(2) Widespread, expansile and deep extension into endocervical crypts.
(3) Luminal necrosis and intraepithelial squamous maturation {57}.
The first sign of invasion is referred to as early stromal invasion; this is an unmeasurable lesion less than 1 mm in depth that can be managed in the same way as high grade CIN. The focus of early

stromal invasion often appears to be better differentiated than the overlying CIN. Early stromal invasion is encompassed in the term microinvasive carcinoma.

The criteria for the diagnosis of microinvasive carcinoma were historically based on the depth of invasion, and the ascribed upper limit has varied in the literature from 3 to 5 mm. Microinvasive carcinoma now equates most closely to FIGO stage IA, the definition of which includes both the depth and horizontal dimension of the tumour. The current FIGO staging is controversial because it does not recognize early stromal invasion as a separate entity {371}. Whether microinvasive carcinoma should include FIGO Stage IA2 because there is a significantly increased risk of local lymph node metastasis between 3 and 5 mm depth of invasion has also been questioned. Pooled data indicate that a maximum depth of invasion of 3 mm or less is associated with a risk of lymph node metastasis of <1% and a risk of an invasive recurrence of 0.9%. On the other hand, invasion of 3.1-5.0 mm is associated with an overall risk of lymph node metastases of 2% and a recurrence rate of 4% {2138}. Microinvasive squamous cell carcinoma is usually associated with stromal oedema and a stromal desmoplastic and lymphocytic response, features that aid in its distinction from crypt involvement by CIN. Immunohistochemical stains for CD31 and CD34 may aid in the recognition of lymphatic vascular space involvement.

Preclinical invasive carcinomas of the cervix with dimensions greater than those acceptable as stage IA carcinoma should be designated by the histopathologist simply as stage IB carcinomas.

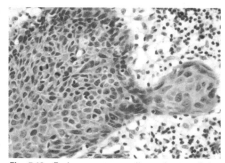

Fig. 5.13 Early squamous cell carcinoma of the cervix. Early stromal invasion is indicated by a bud of more mature squamous cells extending from a focus of in situ carcinoma.

Table 5.02
Classification of HPV-associated intraepithelial lesions of the cervix.

Term	HPV risk category	Comparison of classification systems		
		Two-tiered CIN	Dysplasia/CIS	SIL
Exophytic condyloma	Low risk	——	——	LGSIL
Squamous papilloma	Low risk	——	——	LGSIL
Flat condyloma	Low and high risk	——	——	LGSIL
CIN 1	Low and high risk	Low grade CIN	Mild dysplasia	LGSIL
CIN 2	High risk	High grade CIN	Moderate dysplasia	HGSIL
CIN 3	High risk	High grade CIN	Severe dysplasia/CIS	HGSIL

CIN = Cervical intraepithelial neoplasia
SIL = Squamous intraepithelial lesion
CIS = Carcinoma in situ

LG = Low grade
HG = High grade

"Finger-like" or "confluent" patterns of stromal invasion are of questionable clinical significance and probably are a reflection of a greater depth of stromal invasion.

Cervical intraepithelial neoplasia

Definition
The spectrum of CIN representing the precursor lesions of cervical squamous cell carcinoma {2368}.

Synonyms
Dysplasia/carcinoma-in-situ, squamous intraepithelial lesion.

Epidemiology
The risk of CIN is closely linked to the number of sexual partners and to HPV exposure. It is highest in early reproductive life {1160}. HPV is detected in as many as 39% of adolescents in a single screening visit {2451}, and 20% of women under age 19 in a sexually transmitted disease clinic developed CIN 2 or 3 {1513}. The strong association between HPV 16 and high grade CIN coupled with follow-up studies suggests that infections by this virus induce a high grade lesion over a relatively short period of time {586,1513,1699}. The risk of CIN drops substantially in the fourth and fifth decades, coinciding with a sharp reduction in frequency of HPV attributed to the development of immunity to HPV and

elimination of the virus from the genital tract in most women. Other factors influencing risk include immunological, such as HIV infection, and other host factors, including coincident cervical infections and HLA status.

Aetiology
At puberty there is a change in the anatomical relationships of the lower part of the cervix composed of squamous epithelium, an original squamocolumnar junction and endocervical columnar epithelium. There is eversion of the columnar epithelium, which undergoes squamous metaplasia through a sequence of reserve cell hyperplasia, immature squamous metaplasia and mature squamous metaplasia with the formation of a new squamocolumnar junction. These histological changes are entirely physiological. However, it is this epithelium of the cervical transformation zone that is particularly susceptible to oncogenic stimuli.

In the last 25 years "flat" and exophytic condylomata of the cervix and CIN have been linked by an association with HPVs, many of them weakly or strongly associated with cancer (intermediate and high risk HPVs) {586,737,1014,1841,2305}. Although some HPVs are not associated with cervical cancer (low risk HPVs), the majority are associated with high risk HPVs {1699}. High risk HPV infection may present histologically as CIN 1, although certain infections, such as HPV type 16, have a strong association with high grade CIN lesions {587,1088,1699, 1878,3127}. CIN represents the preinvasive counterpart of invasive cervical squamous cell carcinoma, and there is now abundant evidence for its malignant potential. However, there is no inevitability about neoplastic progression; such lesions may regress, remain phenotypically stable or progress {2137}.

Histopathology

Conventionally, these are subjectively divided into three grades: CIN 1, 2 and 3, though the histological features represent a diagnostic continuum. Increasing-ly, there is a tendency to use a two-tiered classification of low and high grade CIN that equates to CIN 1 and CIN 2 and 3 respectively. These precursors may also be referred to as low and high grade squamous intraepithelial lesion (SIL) {2177}. Because of the inherent difficulty in distinguishing pure HPV infection from unequivocal CIN 1 in flat, non-condylomatous epithelium (sometimes confusingly referred to as flat condyloma), HPV infection alone is included in the low grade SIL category, a terminology that has been more widely accepted by cytopathologists {1612}. The relationship of the varying terminology is shown in Table 5.1.

Cervical intraepithelial neoplasia 1

Maturation is present in the upper two-thirds of the epithelium, and the superficial cells contain variable but usually mild atypia, which may include viral cytopathic effect (koilocytosis). Nuclear abnormalities are present throughout but are slight. Mitotic figures are present in the basal third and are not numerous. Abnormal forms are rare.

Cervical intraepithelial neoplasia 2

Maturation is present in the upper half of the epithelium, and nuclear atypia is conspicuous in both the upper and lower epithelial layers. Mitotic figures are generally confined to the basal two-thirds of the epithelium. Abnormal forms may be seen.

Cervical intraepithelial neoplasia 3

Maturation (including surface keratinization) may be absent or confined to the superficial third of the epithelium. Nuclear abnormalities are marked throughout most or all of the thickness of the epithelium. Mitotic figures may be numerous and are found at all levels of the epithelium. Abnormal mitoses are frequent.

Growth fraction

HPVs, particularly high risk HPVs, are associated with alterations in the cell cycle. Therefore, cell cycle biomarkers may be useful in distinguishing non-diagnostic atypia from CIN. Expression of a generic cell cycle proliferation marker (Ki-67) is typically confined to the suprabasal cells of the lower third of the normal epithelium. The presence of Ki-67 positive cells in the upper epithelial layers occurs in HPV infection, which induces cell cycle activity in these cells {1881,2356}. P16^{ink4}, a cyclin-dependent kinase inhibitor, is a promising marker of CIN {1422,2527}.

Differential diagnosis

Transitional cell metaplasia is a benign condition that may be mistaken for high grade CIN. After the menopause immature squamous mucosa may exhibit histological features resembling transitional epithelium {1140,3085}.

Related lesions

CIN is usually associated with the cytopathic effects of HPV infection, which include koilocytosis, dyskeratosis and multinucleation. Koilocytosis is characterized by karyomegaly, nuclear enlargement with binucleation, irregularities in the nuclear membrane and hyperchromasia {1508}. Atypical reserve cell hyperplasia and atypical immature squamous metaplasia may be regarded as variants of CIN, though grading of such lesions may be difficult {979,2179}.

Cytopathology

In cytology the grading of CIN is largely based on nuclear characteristics. The number of abnormal cells and the relative nuclear area increase with the severity of the lesion.

In CIN 1 the cells show a slightly enlarged nucleus (less than one-third of the total area of the cell), some aniso-karyosis, finely granular and evenly distributed chromatin and mild hyperchromasia. The cytoplasmic borders are well defined.

In CIN 2 the cells and nuclei vary in size and shape. The nuclear to cytoplasmic ratio is increased (nucleus less than half of cell area). Nuclear chromatin is moderately hyperchromatic and shows some irregular distribution.

In CIN 3 the nuclear to cytoplasmic ratio is high (nucleus at least two-thirds of cell area). Nuclei are hyperchromatic with coarsely granular and irregularly distributed chromatin.

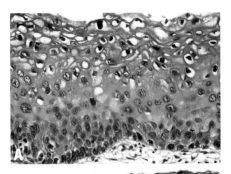

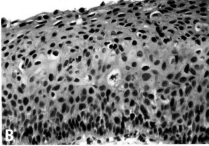

Fig. 5.14 A Cervical intraepithelial neoplasia (CIN 1). The upper two-thirds of the epithelium show maturation and focal koilocytosis. There is mild atypia throughout. **B** CIN 2. Nuclear abnormalities are more striking than in CIN 1, and mitoses are seen (centre). The upper third of the epithelium shows maturation.

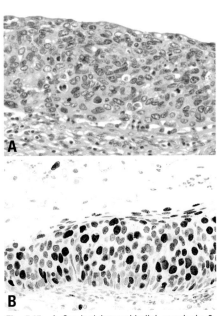

Fig. 5.15 A Cervical intraepithelial neoplasia 3. Squamous epithelium consists entirely of atypical basaloid cells. Note the moderate nuclear polymorphism, coarse chromatin and mitotic figures in the upper half of the epithelium. **B** Ki-67 staining shows proliferation in all cell layers.

Cells typical of carcinoma in situ are arranged singly or in syncytial aggregates (indistinct cell borders and overlapping nuclei). Cytoplasm is scarce or absent; nuclei are round to oval.

Prognosis and predictive factors

Systematic reviews of randomized controlled trials in subjects who underwent cryotherapy, laser ablation, loop electro-surgical excision procedure (LEEP) or surgical conization for the treatment of CIN of any grade reveal no substantial differences in outcome {1777,2068, 2299}.

Benign squamous cell lesions

Condyloma acuminatum

Definition

A benign tumour characterized by papillary fronds containing fibrovascular cores and lined by stratified squamous epithelium with evidence of HPV infection, usually in the form of koilocytosis.

Aetiology

The exophytic condyloma is strongly associated with HPV types 6 and 11 {3057}.

Histopathology

These lesions exhibit acanthosis, papillomatosis and koilocytosis. The latter is characterized by karyomegaly, nuclear enlargement with binucleation, irregularities in the nuclear membrane and hyperchromasia. These lesions closely resemble vulvar condylomas {585}.

Squamous papilloma

Definition

A benign tumour composed of a single papillary frond in which mature squamous epithelium without atypia or koilocytosis lines a fibrovascular stalk.

Epidemiology

Lesions with a histological appearance similar to squamous papillomas of the vagina and vulva are rare in the cervix.

Aetiology

There is no evidence that squamous papilloma as defined above is or is not related to human papillomavirus.

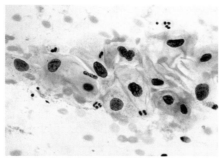

Fig. 5.16 Cervical intraepithelial neoplasia 1. Cells have well defined cell borders, slightly enlarged nuclei and some anisokaryosis.

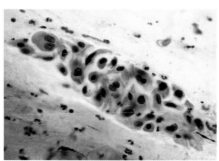

Fig. 5.18 Cervical intraepithelial neoplasia 2. Cells and nuclei vary in size and shape; nuclear chromatin is hyperchromatic and irregularly distributed.

Macroscopy

The squamous papilloma is usually solitary, arising on the ectocervix or at the squamocolumnar junction.

Histopathology

Histological examination shows a single papillary frond composed of mature squamous epithelium without atypia or koilocytosis lining a fibrovascular stalk.

Differential diagnosis

Squamous papilloma is distinguished from condyloma by the absence of complex branching papillae and koilocytes. However, it is important to note that there may be a time during the evolution of condylomas when koilocytes are not easily identifiable.

Squamous papilloma also should be distinguished from papillary immature metaplasia of the cervix, which is characterized by slender filiform papillae and also does not have koilocytosis {3057}. In the latter condition the squamous epithelium is less mature with higher nuclear to cytoplasmic ratios but lacks nuclear atypia. Papillary immature metaplasia has been associated with HPV types 6 or 11 {3057}.

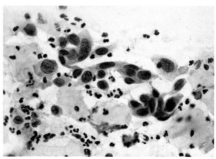

Fig. 5.17 Cervical intraepithelial neoplasia 3. Cells have increased nuclear to cytoplasmic ratios, anisokaryosis and coarsely granular chromatin.

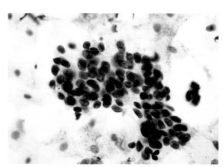

Fig. 5.19 Cervical intraepithelial neoplasia 3 (carcinoma in situ). The syncytial aggregate of round to oval nuclei which have coarsely granular chromatin.

Fibroepithelial polyp

Definition

A polyp lined by squamous epithelium that contains a central core of fibrous tissue in which stellate cells with tapering cytoplasmic processes and irregularly shaped thin-walled vessels are prominent features.

Synonym

Stromal polyp.

Aetiology

Unlike condyloma, fibroepithelial polyps rarely contain HPV nucleic acids {1837}, and, thus, are not related to HPV infection.

Clinical features

This lesion can occur at any age but has a predilection for pregnant women.

Macroscopy

These are polypoid lesions and are usually solitary.

Histopathology

These polypoid lesions are characterized by a prominent fibrovascular stroma covered by squamous epithelium {380}. Unlike squamous papilloma, they do not show acanthosis or a papillary architecture. Bizarre stromal cells, marked hypercellularity and elevated mitotic counts including atypical forms have been described that can lead to an erroneous diagnosis of sarcoma {2067}.

Glandular tumours and precursors

ICD-O codes

Adenocarcinoma, NOS	8140/3
Mucinous adenocarcinoma	8480/3
Endocervical	8482/3
Intestinal	8144/3
Signet-ring cell	8490/3
Minimal deviation	8480/3
Villoglandular	8262/3
Endometrioid adenocarcinoma	8380/3
Clear cell adenocarcinoma	8310/3
Serous adenocarcinoma	8441/3
Mesonephric adenocarcinoma	9110/3
Early invasive adenocarcinoma	8140/3
Adenocarcinoma in situ	8140/2

Adenocarcinoma

Definition
A carcinoma that shows glandular differentiation.

Clinical features
About one-half of all adenocarcinomas are exophytic, polypoid or papillary masses. Others are nodular with diffuse enlargement or ulceration of the cervix. Deep infiltration of the wall produces a barrel-shaped cervix. Approximately 15% of patients have no visible lesion.

Histopathology
Immunohistochemistry may be useful to distinguish between benign and malignant conditions of the cervix, to discriminate between the various subtypes and to separate primary endocervical from primary endometrial tumours. The tumour that is estrogen receptor positive, vimentin positive and carcinoembryonic antigen negative is almost certainly of endometrial origin, whilst an endocervical source is very likely for the tumour that is estrogen receptor negative, vimentin negative and carcinoembryonic antigen positive {424,1822}. A moderate to high Ki-67 proliferation index also points towards endocervical neoplasia {495}. It is equally important to recognize that none of these stains are needed in the majority of cases, where the clinical evidence and history are entirely adequate. Carcinoembryonic antigen is usually negative in benign mimics, such as microglandular hyperplasia {2780}. In contrast to normal endocervical epithelium, some of the cells of a minimal deviation adenocarcinoma are reactive for serotonin and gastrointestinal tract-pancreatic peptide hormones and uniformly lack immunoreactivity for estrogen and progesterone receptors and CA125.

Mucinous adenocarcinoma

Definition
An adenocarcinoma in which at least some of the cells contain a moderate to large amount of intracytoplasmic mucin.

Endocervical
The endocervical type accounts for 70% of cervical adenocarcinomas, and the tumour cells resemble those of the endocervix. Most tumours are well to moderately differentiated. The glandular elements are arranged in a complex pattern. Papillae may project into the gland lumens and from the surface. At times a cribriform arrangement is observed. A microglandular pattern resembling microglandular hyperplasia of the cervix {3224} and a microcystic variant are rarely seen {2856}. The stroma may be desmoplastic. The cells are typically stratified with basal nuclei and abundant pale granular cytoplasm that stains positively for mucin. They show considerable nuclear atypia with variation in nuclear size, coarsely clumped chromatin and prominent nucleoli. Mitoses are usually numerous. Large amounts of mucin may be found in the stroma forming mucin lakes or pools in the so-called colloid carcinoma {1646,2975}. In poorly differentiated tumours the cells contain less cytoplasm but usually still form recognizable glandular structures. Co-existent CIN occurs in up to 40% of cases {1739}, and adenocarcinoma in situ is also common. Synchronous mucinous tumours may be found elsewhere in the female genital tract {1392,3219}.

In cytological preparations the cells are arranged in crowded cell aggregates with overlapping nuclei. Gland openings, rosettes, strips with palisading and pseudostratification and cell balls may be seen. The cytoplasm is vacuolated. The nuclei are round, oval or "cigar" shaped and vary in size. The nuclear chromatin is coarse and unevenly distributed with clearing, and nucleoli are present.

Intestinal variant
These tumours resemble adenocarcinoma of the large intestine. Intestinal-type change may be found diffusely or only focally within a mucinous tumour. They frequently contain goblet cells and less commonly endocrine and Paneth cells.

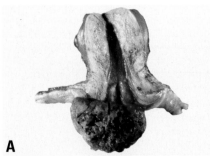
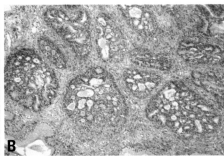
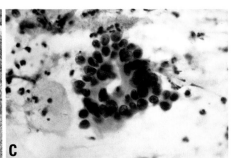

Fig. 5.20 Adenocarcinoma. **A** A large, polypoid, exophytic tumour arises from the cervix with focal cystic change and necrosis. **B** A cribriform pattern along with other features may indicate an invasive, rather than an in situ, neoplastic glandular process. **C** Endocervical variant. Atypical cells with enlarged nuclei, coarsely granular cleared chromatin and nucleoli form a gland opening.

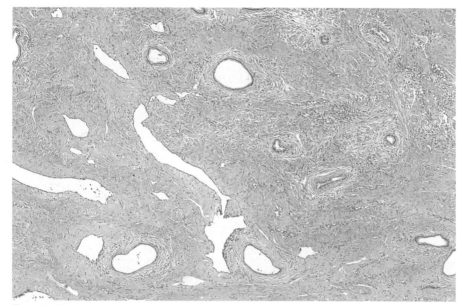

Fig. 5.21 Minimal deviation adenocarcinoma of the cervix. Irregular claw-shaped glands infiltrate the stroma.

Signet-ring cell variant

Primary signet-ring cell adenocarcinoma is rare in pure form {1157,1799,1893, 3013}. Signet-ring cells occur more commonly as a focal finding in poorly differentiated mucinous adenocarcinomas and adenosquamous carcinomas. The differential diagnosis includes metastatic tumours {908,1434} or rare squamous cell carcinomas with signet-ring-like cells that are mucin negative {1533}.

Minimal deviation variant

This is a rare highly differentiated mucinous adenocarcinoma in which most of the glands are impossible to distinguish from normal. Adenoma malignum is a synonym.

Histopathology. Most of the glands are lined by deceptively bland, mucin-rich columnar cells with basal nuclei. In the majority of cases, however, occasional glands display moderate nuclear atypia, are angulated or elicit a desmoplastic stromal reaction. The most reliable criteria are the haphazard arrangement of the glands that extend beyond the depth of those of the normal endocervix and the presence of occasional mitoses, which are uncommon in the normal endocervical epithelium. Vascular and perineural involvement is frequent. Transmural and/or parametrial and/or myometrial spread is seen in 40% of cases {1004, 1391}. Because the depth of penetration of the glands is a key histological feature,

the diagnosis cannot be made in punch biopsies in most cases. Minimal deviation adenocarcinoma should be differentiated from the benign conditions of diffuse laminar endocervical glandular hyperplasia {1362}, lobular endocervical glandular hyperplasia {2061}, endocervicosis {3193} and adenomyoma of endocervical type {1005}. An endometrioid variant of minimal deviation adenocarcinoma has also been described {1391, 1972,3225}.

Somatic genetics. The genetic locus for the putative tumour suppressor gene is in the region of chromosome 19p 13.3 {1610}. Somatic mutations of the *STK11* gene, the gene responsible for the Peutz-Jeghers syndrome, are characteristic of minimal deviation adenocarcinoma {1397}. They were found in 55% of patients with minimal deviation adenocarcinoma and in only 5% of other types of mucinous adenocarcinoma of the cervix.

Genetic susceptibility. These tumours are more likely than any other type of cervical adenocarcinoma to precede or develop coincidentally with ovarian neoplasia, the most common being mucinous adenocarcinoma and sex cord tumour with annular tubules {2769}. The latter is associated with the Peutz-Jeghers syndrome in 17% of cases {453}. A germline mutation of *STK11* was detected in one patient with Peutz-Jeghers syndrome

who had a mucinous adenocarcinoma of the cervix {1397}.

Villoglandular variant

These have a frond-like pattern resembling villoglandular adenoma of the colon. The tumours generally occur in young women. A possible link to oral contraceptives has been suggested.

The epithelium is generally moderately to well differentiated. One or several layers of columnar cells, some of which contain mucin, usually line the papillae and glands. If intracellular mucin is not demonstrable, the tumour may be regarded as the endometrioid variant. Scattered mitoses are characteristic. Invasion may be absent or minimal at the base; rare neoplasms, however, invade deeply. The invasive portion is typically composed of elongated branching glands separated by fibrous stroma. The non-invasive tumours may, in fact, be examples of papillary adenocarcinoma in situ. Associated CIN and/or adenocarcinoma in situ are common. Lymph node metastases are rare {1366,1387,1391}.

Endometrioid adenocarcinoma

These adenocarcinomas account for up to 30% of cervical adenocarcinomas and have the histological features of an

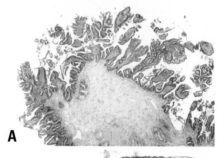

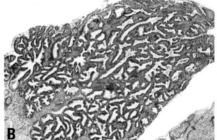

Fig. 5.22 Well differentiated villoglandular adenocarcinoma. **A** In the absence of frank invasion, the alternative diagnosis would be papillary adenocarcinoma in situ. **B** The villoglandular growth pattern is prominent.

endometrioid adenocarcinoma of the endometrium; however, squamous elements are less common. Little or no intracellular mucin is present. A distinction from an endocervical type adenocarcinoma is only possible in well differentiated lesions. This neoplasm must be distinguished from one extending into the cervix from the endometrium.

Clear cell adenocarcinoma

An adenocarcinoma that is composed mainly of clear or hobnail cells arranged in solid, tubulocystic or papillary patterns or a combination.

This rare tumour is histologically similar to clear cell adenocarcinoma of the ovary, endometrium and vagina, where they are more common. Although well known because of its association with in utero exposure to diethylstilbestrol (DES) in young women, its peak frequency is at present in the postmenopausal group. Genomic instability has been suggested as a mechanism of DES-related carcinogenesis {330}.

Serous adenocarcinoma

A complex pattern of papillae with cellular budding and the frequent presence of psammoma bodies characterize serous adenocarcinoma. Before a diagnosis of primary serous adenocarcinoma of the cervix can be made, spread from the endometrium, ovaries or peritoneum should be excluded. These rare cervical tumours are histologically identical to their ovarian counterparts {565}. A single case was familial. The patient, identical twin sister and mother all had serous tumours of the genital tract {1398}.

Mesonephric adenocarcinoma

These adenocarcinomas arise from mesonephric remnants and are most often located in the lateral to posterior wall of the cervix but may involve the cervix circumferentially. Among the 20 reported examples, the patients ranged in age from 33-74 years with a median age of about 52 years. Whereas they often present as exophytic lesions, they may remain completely intramural simply expanding the cervical wall. Histologically, they are commonly characterized by tubular glands lined by mucin-free cuboidal epithelium containing eosino-

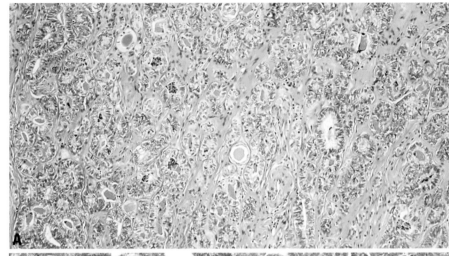
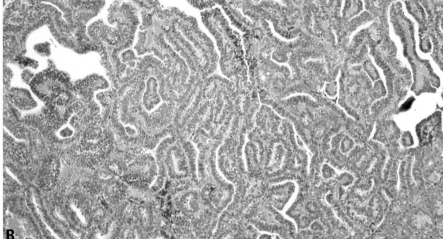
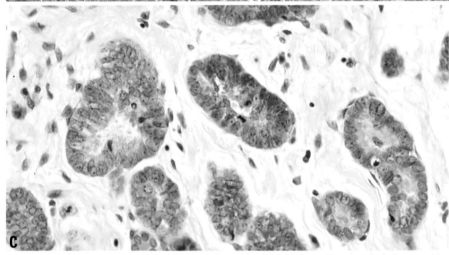

Fig. 5.23 Mesonephric adenocarcinoma. **A** In some areas of the tumour, the proliferation of tubules resembles the diffuse pattern of mesonephric hyperplasia with intraluminal colloid-like secretions. **B** Other areas contain a more complex growth pattern with early formation of papillary structures (same case as in A). **C** The tubules exhibit nuclear atypia and mitotic figures.

philic, hyaline secretion in their lumens in its well differentiated areas or larger glands showing endometrioid differentiation {521}, but other patterns including solid, papillary, ductal and a retiform arrangement may develop. A vast majority arise in a background of mesonephric remnant hyperplasia {850,2036,2679}.

The tubular variant is distinguished from focal, florid and diffuse hyperplasia of mesonephric remnants by the presence of cytologic atypia, mitotic activity and the focal presence of intraluminal nuclear debris instead of the colloid-like secretion typical of mesonephric remnants {2679}.

Mesonephric adenocarcinomas are immunoreactive for epithelial markers (AE1/3, cytokeratin 1, Cam5.2, cytokeratin 7 and epithelial membrane antigen) in 100% of cases, for calretinin (88%), and vimentin (70%). The absence of immunoreactivity with estrogen and progesterone receptor helps to distinguish the endometrioid variant from endometrioid adenocarcinoma {2679}. Positive immunoreactivity for CD10 may be another helpful feature {2110}. The behaviour of the lesions and prognosis are stage dependent.

Early invasive adenocarcinoma

Definition
Early invasive adenocarcinoma refers to a glandular neoplasm in which the extent of stromal invasion is so minimal that the risk of local lymph node metastasis is negligible.

Synonym
"Microinvasive" adenocarcinoma.

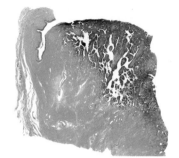

Fig. 5.24 Early invasive adenocarcinoma, mounted section.

Tumour spread and staging
Adenocarcinomas of the cervix exist in early and frankly invasive forms {1611, 2139}. The entity of "early invasive" or "microinvasive" carcinoma is controversial. The current, 1995 FIGO staging, omits specific reference to glandular lesions in stage IA {1300}. In addition, there are practical problems in identifying microinvasive adenocarcinoma histologically (see below). Nevertheless, it is recommended that the FIGO classification be adopted.

Histopathology
The sine qua non of microinvasive adenocarcinoma is stromal invasion. There may be marked glandular irregularity with effacement of the normal glandular architecture, the tumour extending beyond the deepest normal crypt. Cribri-form, papillary or solid patterns may be present.

There may be a stromal response in the form of oedema, chronic inflammatory infiltrate or a desmoplastic reaction. Lymphatic capillary-like space involvement is helpful in confirming invasion. Having established the presence of invasion, the depth of invasion and the width of the tumour must be measured. In most cases the depth is measured from the surface rather than the point of origin, which is hard to establish in some cases. Thus, tumour thickness, rather than "depth of invasion", is measured. The width is the greatest diameter of the neoplasm measured parallel to the surface; the measurement should be done by calibrated optics.

Prognosis and predictive factors
The prognosis of microinvasive adenocarcinoma (FIGO Stage 1A), as defined above, is excellent and essentially the same as that of its squamous counterpart {768,2143,2573,2732,3076}.

Adenocarcinoma in situ

Definition
A lesion in which normally situated glands are partly or wholly replaced by cytologically malignant epithelium; in the former case the border is characteristically sharp.

Histopathology
The epithelium is usually devoid of intracellular mucin and may resemble endo-

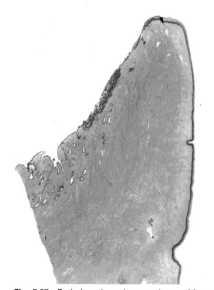

Fig. 5.25 Early invasive adenocarcinoma. Mounted section shows that its horizontal spread is much greater than the depth of invasion.

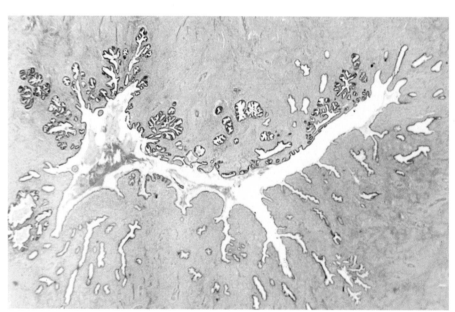

Fig. 5.26 Extensive adenocarcinoma in situ. Note that the neoplastic glands conform to the configuration of normal crypts and do not extend beyond them, and there is no stromal reaction.

metrial epithelium. In some cases the glands are lined by intestinal epithelium containing goblet, neuroendocrine and Paneth cells. The neoplastic glands conform to the expected location of normal endocervical glands and do not extend beyond the deepest normal crypt. A cribriform pattern is common. The epithelium is usually stratified with the long axes of the cells perpendicular to the base. The elongated, pleomorphic and hyperchromatic nuclei are basal in position.

Mitoses are common and are disposed on the luminal side {2142}. Apoptosis is prominent {279}. The neoplastic epithelium may affect the surface, where it is often single layered, but more commonly is found in the crypts. These features help to explain the frequent failure of its colposcopic detection. The cell types, in order of frequency, are endocervical, endometrioid and intestinal. A putative tubal variant has also recently been described {2559}. Although the stroma may be intensely inflamed, there is no desmoplastic reaction. Adenocarcinoma in situ is associated with CIN in at least 50% of cases and is immunoreactive for carcinoembryonic antigen in 80% of cases.

Prognosis and predictive factors
Evidence supporting the precancerous potential of adenocarcinoma in situ includes its occurrence 10-15 years earlier than its invasive counterparts, its common association with microinvasive or invasive adenocarcinoma, its histological similarity to invasive adenocarcinoma and the frequent occurrence of high-risk HPV types. The transformation of adenocarcinoma in situ into invasive adenocarcinoma over time has also been documented on rare occasions {1224,2076}. Although the treatment of adenocarcinoma in situ is controversial, increasing evidence is available that conservative therapy, such as conization only, is safe and effective in selected cases {1870,2140}

Glandular dysplasia

Definition
A glandular lesion characterized by significant nuclear abnormalities that are more striking than those in glandular atypia but fall short of the criteria for adenocarcinoma in situ.

Histopathology
The nuclei are not cytologically malignant, and mitoses are less numerous than in adenocarcinoma in situ. Nuclear hyperchromasia and enlargement identify the involved glands, and pseudostratification of cells is prominent. Cribriform and papillary formations are usually absent.

The concept that glandular dysplasia forms a biological spectrum of cervical glandular intraepithelial neoplasia remains unproven {420,1032,1534}.

Glandular dysplasia must be distinguished from glandular atypia. The latter is an atypical glandular epithelial alteration which does not fulfil the criteria for glandular dysplasia or adenocarcinoma in situ and which may be associated with inflammation or irradiation.

Benign glandular lesions

Müllerian papilloma

Definition
A rare, benign, papillary tumour composed of a complex arborizing fibrovascular core covered by a mantle of single or double-layered mucinous epithelium that may undergo squamous metaplasia.

Clinical features
Müllerian papilloma occurs almost exclusively in children typically between 2 and 5 years of age (range 1-9 years), who present with bleeding, discharge or a friable, polypoid to papillary, unifocal or multifocal mass, usually less than 2 cm in greatest dimension.

Histopathology
These tumours consist of multiple small polypoid projections composed of fibrous stroma and lined by simple epithelium. Occasional cells may have a hobnail appearance simulating clear cell adenocarcinoma; however, no clear cells, atypia or mitoses are present. The stroma is often inflamed and rarely contains psammoma bodies.

Prognosis and predictive factors
Occasional cases recur {2736}. (See chapter on the vagina).

Endocervical polyp

Definition
An intraluminal protrusion composed of bland endocervical glands and a fibrovascular stroma.

Epidemiology
These are very common lesions that rarely are of concern clinically and are easy to diagnose histologically.

Clinical features
In 75% of cases they are asymptomatic. The rest present with bleeding (especially post-coital) and/or discharge.

Macroscopy
The great majority are less than 1 cm and single {15}.

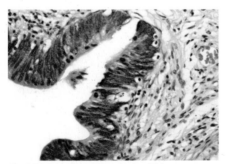

Fig. 5.27 Adenocarcinoma in situ. High power magnification shows pseudostratified nuclei and a marked degree of apoptosis.

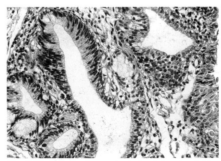

Fig. 5.28 High grade cervical glandular dysplasia. The histological features are not of sufficient severity to be regarded as adenocarcinoma in situ.

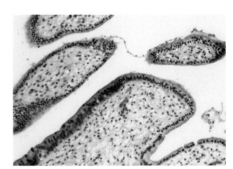

Fig. 5.29 Glandular dysplasia involving endocervical papillae.

Histopathology

Endocervical polyps are usually covered by cuboidal and/or columnar epithelium that often shows atypical regenerative changes that may be mistaken cytologically for malignancy. Polyps are often composed of large retention cysts distended by mucus and covered by normal metaplastic squamous epithelium. Ulceration is uncommon, but the stroma is often inflamed.

The presence of bizarre stromal atypia, atypical mitoses or stromal hypercellularity may lead to an unwarranted diagnosis of sarcoma {2067}. Other benign alterations within polyps that may be mistaken for malignancy include florid immature squamous metaplasia, papillary hyperplasia, microglandular hyperplasia and decidual reaction {2930}.

Prognosis and predictive factors

Polyps occasionally recur, even after complete excision.

Uncommon carcinomas and neuroendocrine tumours

Definition

Epithelial tumours of the uterine cervix other than those of squamous or glandular types.

ICD-O-codes

Adenosquamous carcinoma	8560/3
Glassy cell variant	8015/3
Adenoid cystic carcinoma	8200/3
Adenoid basal carcinoma	8098/3
Neuroendocrine tumours	
Carcinoid	8240/3
Atypical carcinoid	8249/3
Small cell carcinoma	8041/3
Large cell neuroendocrine carcinoma	8013/3
Undifferentiated carcinoma	8020/3

Adenosquamous carcinoma

Definition

A carcinoma composed of a mixture of malignant glandular and squamous epithelial elements.

Histopathology

Both elements show atypical features. Scattered mucin-producing cells in an otherwise ordinary looking squamous cell

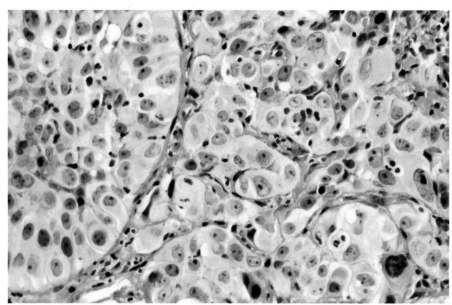

Fig. 5.30 Glassy cell carcinoma. Note the ground glass appearance of the cytoplasm and the well defined cytoplamic membranes.

carcinoma have been referred to as mucoepidermoid carcinoma. As there is no convincing evidence that such tumours behave differently, routine mucin staining of squamous cell carcinomas is not recommended, and the former term should no longer be employed. Poorly differentiated tumours resembling poorly differentiated squamous cell carcinoma but with many mucin-producing cells and lacking keratinization or intercellular bridges should be diagnosed as poorly differentiated adenocarcinoma.

Glassy cell carcinoma variant

Glassy cell carcinoma is a poorly differentiated variant of adenosquamous carcinoma and accounts for 1-2% of all cervical carcinomas. The tumour occurs in young women, grows rapidly, develops frequent distant metastases and responds poorly to radiotherapy; however, chemotherapy may be promising {1863}. The tumour cells lack estrogen and progesterone receptors {132}. Usually, no preinvasive lesion is seen. The tumour cells are large

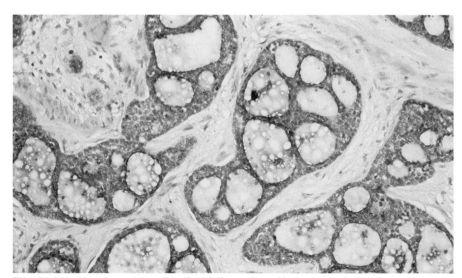

Fig. 5.31 Adenoid cystic carcinoma. Note the cribriform pattern with abundant luminal mucin.

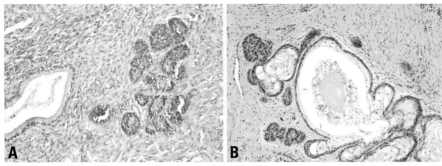

Fig. 5.32 Adenoid basal carcinoma. **A** Clusters of basaloid cells show mature central squamous differentiation. **B** Note small clusters of basaloid cells adjacent to cystic glands.

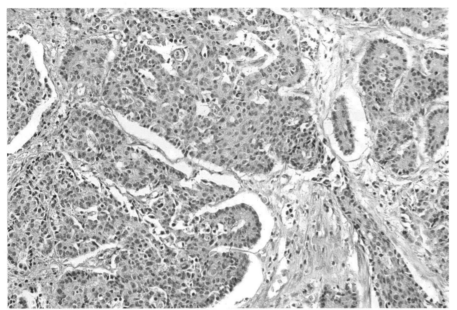

Fig. 5.33 Atypical carcinoid. Islands of tumour cells with moderate nuclear atypia are surrounded by fibrous stroma.

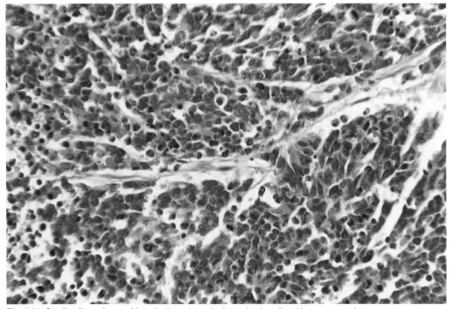

Fig. 5.34 Small cell carcinoma. Note the loosely packed neoplastic cells with scant cytoplasm.

with distinct cell borders and a ground-glass cytoplasm. A prominent eosinophilic infiltration in the stroma helps to separate the tumour from non-keratinizing squamous cell carcinoma {1701}.

Prognosis and predictive factors
The prognosis of adenosquamous carcinoma remains uncertain {68}.

Adenoid cystic carcinoma

Definition
A carcinoma of the cervix that resembles adenoid cystic carcinoma of salivary gland origin.

Epidemiology
Most of the patients are over 60 years of age, and there is a high proportion of Black women {849}.

Clinical features
The majority of patients present with postmenopausal bleeding and have a mass on pelvic examination {849}.

Histopathology
This rare tumour of the cervix has a histological appearance similar to its counterpart in salivary glands. The characteristic cystic spaces are filled with a slightly eosinophilic hyaline material or basophilic mucin and are surrounded by palisaded epithelial cells {849}. In contrast to adenoid cystic carcinoma of salivary gland, the cervical carcinomas show greater nuclear pleomorphism, a high mitotic rate and necrosis {849}. A solid variant has been described {65}. Immunostains for basement membrane components such as collagen type IV and laminin are strongly positive {1918}. In contrast to an earlier study {849}, the majority of the tumours stained for S-100 protein and HHF35 suggesting myoepithelial differentiation {1059}.
The differential diagnosis includes small cell carcinoma, adenoid basal carcinoma and non-keratinizing squamous cell carcinoma.

Histogenesis
This tumour, basaloid squamous cell carcinoma and adenoid basal carcinoma are part of a morphological and biological spectrum of basaloid cervical neoplasms, and a putative reserve cell origin has been suggested {1059}. Circumstantial evidence suggests that adenoid

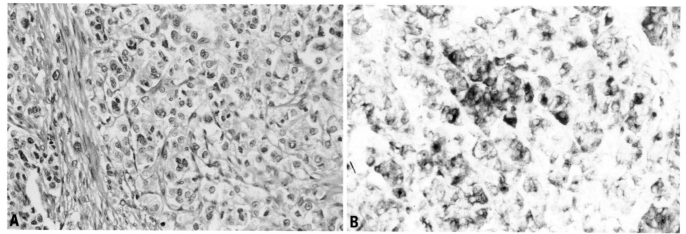

Fig. 5.35 Large cell neuroendocrine carcinoma. **A** The tumour is composed of large cells with pleomorphic nuclei and frequent mitotic figures. **B** Note the strong cytoplasmic immunoreactivity for chromogranin A.

basal carcinoma may be a precursor of adenoid cystic carcinoma {1059}.

Prognosis and predictive factors

The tumours frequently recur locally or metastasize to distant organs and have an unfavourable prognosis.

Adenoid basal carcinoma

Definition

A cervical carcinoma in which rounded, generally well differentiated nests of basaloid cells show focal gland formation or sometimes central squamous differentiation.

Epidemiology

Adenoid basal carcinoma is a rare tumour. The patients are usually more than 50 years old.

Clinical findings

Patients are usually asymptomatic and without a clinically detectable abnormality of the cervix. The tumour is often discovered as an incidental finding.

Histopathology

The histological appearance shows small nests of basaloid cells, almost always beneath and often arising from CIN or small invasive squamous cell carcinomas {849}. The cells are small with scanty cytoplasm and are arranged in cords and nests with focal glandular or squamous differentiation. There is frequently associated CIN {332,849}. The differential diagnosis includes other small cell tumours {2280}.

Histogenesis

This tumour, basaloid squamous cell carcinoma and adenoid cystic carcinoma are part of a morphological and biological spectrum of basaloid cervical neoplasms and a putative reserve cell origin has been suggested {1059}.

Prognosis and predictive factors

The tumour is low grade and rarely metastasizes.

Neuroendocrine tumours

The group of neuroendocrine tumours includes carcinoid, atypical carcinoid, large cell neuroendocrine carcinoma and small cell carcinoma {63,2803}.
Neuroendocrine differentiation is demonstrated with pan-neuroendocrine markers such as chromogranin A, synaptophysin and neuron specific enolase. A variety of peptides and hormones are also present, such as calcitonin, gastrin, serotonin, substance P, vasoactive intestinal peptide, pancreatic polypeptide, somatostatin and adrenocorticotrophic hormone {22}, but their clinical significance is limited {2612}.

Carcinoid

Generally benign, carcinoids have the same characteristic organoid appearance as observed in other sites. The degree of nuclear atypia and mitotic activity are important in the differential diagnosis between typical and atypical carcinoids.

Atypical carcinoid

An atypical carcinoid is a carcinoid with cytologic atypia that exhibits increased mitotic activity (5-10 per high power field) and contains foci of necrosis {63}.

Small cell carcinoma

Small cell carcinomas account for 1-6% of cervical carcinomas {22}. Squamous or glandular differentiation may be present {22,248, 830,1761,2219}. The 5-year survival rate is reported to be 14-39% {22,248,2803}.

Large cell neuroendocrine carcinoma

Large cell neuroendocrine carcinoma is a rare tumour that often has focal adenocarcinomatous differentiation {592a, 1521a, 2361a}. The tumour cells have abundant cytoplasm, large nuclei and prominent nucleoli. Mitoses are frequent. The differential diagnosis includes non-neuroendocrine undifferentiated carcinoma, adenocarcinoma with neuroendocrine features, metastatic neuroendocrine carcinoma and undifferentiated sarcoma. The tumours are aggressive and appear to have a similar outcome to small cell carcinoma {1006}.

Undifferentiated carcinoma

Undifferentiated carcinoma is a carcinoma lacking specific differentiation. The differential diagnosis includes poorly differentiated squamous cell carcinoma, adenocarcinoma, glassy cell carcinoma and large cell neuroendocrine carcinoma.

Mesenchymal tumours

M.L. Carcangiu

Definition
A variety of rare benign and malignant mesenchymal tumours that arise in the uterine cervix and which exhibit smooth muscle, skeletal muscle, vascular, peripheral nerve and other types of mesenchymal tissue differentiation. Smooth muscle tumours are the most common.

Malignant mesenchymal tumours

ICD-O codes
Leiomyosarcoma	8890/3
Endometrioid stromal sarcoma, low grade	8931/3
Undifferentiated endocervical sarcoma	8805/3
Sarcoma botryoides	8910/3
Alveolar soft part sarcoma	9581/3
Angiosarcoma	9120/3
Malignant peripheral nerve sheath tumour	9540/3

Epidemiology
Sarcomas are extremely rare. Of 6,549 malignant tumours arising in the uterine cervix reported in the United States in a 5 year period (1973-1977), only 36 (0.5%) were sarcomas {3191}. Leiomyosarcoma is the most common primary sarcoma, although less than thirty cases have been described in the literature {25,212, 543,912,927,1045,1058,1405,2473}. About 100 cases of sarcoma botryoides of the cervix have been reported {170, 333,642,1041,1898,3250}. Fifteen cases of undifferentiated endocervical sarcoma {20,25,1324}, ten cases of alveolar soft part sarcoma and six of malignant peripheral nerve sheath tumour primary in the uterine cervix are on record {21,892, 901,1056,1375,1424,1504,1916,2017, 2507,2721}. All the other types of mesenchymal tumours have been case reports. Cervical mesenchymal tumours affect adult patients with the exception of sarcoma botryoides, which usually occurs in children and young women (mean age 18 years) {642}. The prognosis of cervical sarcomas as a group is poor with the exception of sarcoma botyroides.

Clinical features
Most patients with these cervical tumours present with vaginal bleeding or discharge. Large tumours may compress adjacent organs or, if polypoid, protrude through the cervical os into the vagina. Less frequently, the passing of tissue through the vagina is the presenting symptom.

At operation sarcomas may be seen to infiltrate the entire thickness of the cervical wall. Pelvic recurrences or regional lymph node metastases are the most common late events.

Leiomyosarcoma

Definition
A malignant tumour composed of smooth muscle cells.

Clinical features
Leiomyosarcoma presents as a mass replacing and expanding the cervix or as a polypoid growth.

Macrosocopy
The tumours have a soft and fleshy consistency and often contain areas of necrosis or haemorrhage. The rare myxoid variant of leiomyosarcoma has a typical gelatinous appearance.

Histopathology
Leiomyosarcomas show hypercellular interlacing fascicles of large spindle-shaped or round cells with diffuse moderate to marked nuclear atypia, a high mitotic rate, atypical mitoses, single or multiple prominent nucleoli and tumour cell necrosis. Infiltrative borders and vascular invasion are also frequently seen. Cervical epithelioid leiomyosarcoma, and one case each of myxoid and xanthomatous cervical leiomyosarcoma

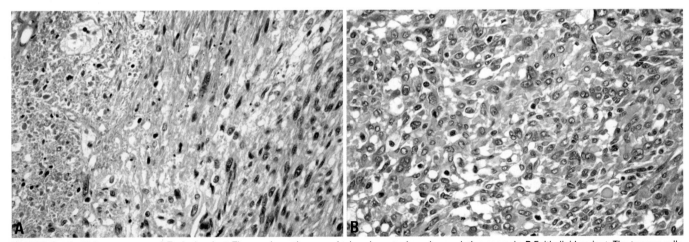

Fig. 5.36 Cervical leiomyosarcoma. **A** Typical variant. The neoplasm shows marked nuclear atypia and coagulative necrosis. **B** Epithelioid variant. The tumour cells are round and uniform.

have been reported {543,912,927,1045, 1058}.

Differential diagnosis
The criteria used in the distinction from leiomyoma are the same as those for smooth muscle tumours of the uterine corpus. At least two of three features (marked nuclear atypia, a mitotic rate higher than 10 mitoses per 10 high power fields and tumour necrosis) are required for the diagnosis of leiomyosarcoma {211}. For epithelioid leiomyosarcoma a mitotic count higher than 5 mitoses per 10 high power fields is considered diagnostic of malignancy. A low mitotic count is typical of the myxoid variant {912}. Antibodies to smooth muscle actin and/or desmin may be used to demonstrate smooth muscle differentiation in these tumours.

Leiomyosarcoma should be differentiated from postoperative spindle cell nodule {1420}. The latter is mitotically active and may infiltrate the underlying tissue. The distinction from leiomyosarcoma or other malignant spindle cell tumour depends to a large extent on the history of a recent operation at the same site.

Endometrioid stromal sarcoma, low grade

Definition
A sarcoma arising outside of the fundus composed of cells resembling endometrial stromal cells.

Epidemiology
Very rarely, tumours with the features of low grade endometrial stromal sarcoma arise in the cervix {295,437}.

Histopathology
This tumour may arise from cervical endometriosis and must be distinguished from stromal endometriosis and primary endometrial stromal sarcoma that has invaded the cervix. The term undifferentiated endocervical sarcoma is preferred for high grade lesions.

Undifferentiated endocervical sarcoma

Definition
An endocervical sarcoma lacking endometrial stromal or other specific differentiation {20,1324}.

Histopathology
Tumours described in the literature as undifferentiated endocervical sarcoma are characterized by a polypoid or infiltrative cervical growth similar to that exhibited by malignant peripheral nerve sheath tumours arising in the uterine cervix {25,1424}.

The tumour is composed of spindle or stellate-shaped cells with scanty cytoplasm, ill defined cell borders and oval hyperchromatic nuclei arranged in a sheet-like, fasciculated or storiform pattern {25}. The prominent vascular pattern typical of endometrioid stromal sarcoma is not a characteristic of these tumours, and the stromal proliferation tends to encircle the endocervical glands creating a focal resemblance to adenosarcoma. Nuclear atypia and markedly increased mitotic activity are seen in all cases, as well as areas of haemorrhage, necrosis and myxoid degeneration.

Sarcoma botryoides

Definition
A tumour composed of cells with small, round, oval or spindle-shaped nuclei, some of which show evidence of differentiation towards skeletal muscle cells.

Synonym
Embryonal rhabdomyosarcoma.

Macroscopy
Embryonal rhabdomyosarcoma usually grows in a polypoid fashion. The grape-like type of growth classically exhibited by vaginal sarcoma botryoides is only rarely seen in cervical tumours. The polypoid masses have a glistening translucent surface and a soft consistency and may be pedunculated or sessile. Their size ranges from 2-10 cm {642}. The sectioned surface of the tumour appears smooth and myxoid with small haemorrhagic areas.

Histopathology
The histological features are described in the section on the vagina. Islands of mature neoplastic cartilage are more frequently seen in cervical than in vaginal tumours {642}.

Somatic genetics
In one case of sarcoma botryoides chromosomal analysis has demonstrated deletion of the short arm of chromosome 1,

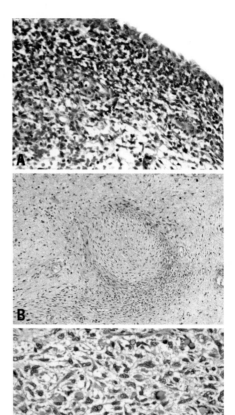

Fig. 5.37 Cervical sarcoma botryoides. **A** The subepithelial cambium layer is prominent. **B** Note the focus of neoplastic cartilage. **C** Tumour cells with eosinophilic cytoplasm exhibit myoblastic differentiation.

and trisomies 13 and 18 {2156}, and in another a point mutation in exon 6 of *TP53* was found, but no *KRAS* point mutations at codons 12,13 and 61 were detected {2627}.

Genetic susceptibility
An association between ovarian Sertoli-Leydig tumour and cervical sarcoma botryoides has been described {1026}

Prognosis and predictive factors
The use of neoadjuvant chemotherapy allows a more conservative approach for these neoplasms {170,1041,3250}.

Alveolar soft part sarcoma

Definition
A sarcoma characterized by solid and alveolar groups of large epithelial-like cells with granular, eosinophilic cytoplasm.

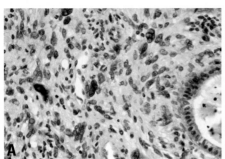
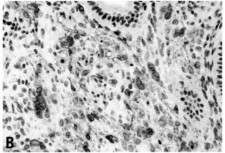

Fig. 5.38 Malignant peripheral nerve sheath tumour (MPNST). **A** Atypical tumour cells are adjacent to an endocervical gland in a MPNST presenting as an endocervical polyp. **B** Tumour cells are positive for S-100 protein.

Macroscopy

These appear macroscopically as a polyp or an intramural nodule measuring less than 5 cm and have a friable or solid consistency.

Histopathology

They are histologically similar to their counterparts in other sites. Most of the tumours exhibit an alveolar architecture, where nests of tumour cells with central loss of cellular cohesion are supported by thin-walled, sinusoidal vascular spaces. A solid pattern of growth may also be present. The tumour cells have an abundant eosino-philic cytoplasm, large nuclei, prominent nucleoli and contain PAS-positive, diastase-resistant, rod-shaped crystals {1056}. A predominantly clear cytoplasm may characterize some neoplasms, and some cells may exhibit prominent nuclear atypia. Electron microscopy shows characteristic intracytoplasmic crystals, electron-dense secretory granules, numerous mitochondria, prominent endoplasmic reticulum, glycogen and a well developed Golgi apparatus {1937}.

Prognosis and predictive factors

Alveolar soft part sarcomas of the female genital tract, including those primary in the uterine cervix, appear to have a better prognosis than their counterpart in other sites {2017}.

Angiosarcoma

Definition

A malignant tumour the cells of which variably recapitulate the morphologic features of endothelium.
The macroscopic appearance of angiosarcoma is similar to that in other sites forming a haemorrhagic, partially cystic or necrotic mass {2551}, and the neoplastic cells are immunoreactive for CD31, CD34, and factor VIII-related antigen {2551}.

Malignant peripheral nerve sheath tumour

Definition

A malignant tumour showing nerve sheath differentiation.

Histopathology

Cervical malignant peripheral nerve sheath tumour (MPNST) is similar to MPNST arising in other sites including the occurrence of less common variants such as epithelioid and melanocytic types {2721}. The tumour is composed of fascicles of atypical spindle cells invading the cervical stroma and surrounding endocervical glands with a pattern reminiscent of adenosarcoma. Myxoid paucicellular areas are characteristically intermixed with others with a dense cellularity {1375}. Mitoses are common. The tumour cells are positive for S-100 protein and vimentin and negative for HMB-45, smooth muscle actin, desmin and myogenin {1424}.

Other malignant tumours

Other malignant mesenchymal tumours include alveolar rhabdomyosarcoma {781}, liposarcoma {2840,3016}, osteosarcoma {289,588} and malignant fibrous histiocytoma {308}.

Benign mesenchymal tumours and tumour-like lesions

Definition

Benign mesenchymal tumours and tumour-like lesions that arise in the uterine cervix.

ICD-O codes
Leiomyoma 8890/0
Genital rhabdomyoma 8905/0

Leiomyoma

Definition

A benign tumour composed of smooth muscle cells.

Epidemiology

Leiomyoma is the most common benign mesenchymal tumour of the cervix. It has been estimated that less than 2% of all uteri contain cervical leiomyomas, and that about 8% of uterine leiomyomas are primary in the cervix {2020,2925}.

Histopathology

Cervical leiomyoma is histologically identical to those that occur in the uterine corpus.

Genital rhabdomyoma

Definition

A rare benign tumour of the lower female genital tract composed of mature striated muscle cells separated by varying amounts of fibrous stroma.

Clinical features

Cervical rhabdomyoma presenting as a polypoid lesion has been rarely reported {690}.

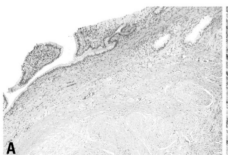
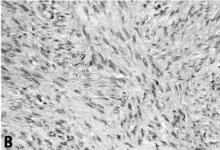

Fig. 5.39 Cervical leiomyoma. **A** Note the endocervical glandular mucosa overlying a leiomyoma. **B** The tumour is composed of interlacing fascicles of uniform spindle-shaped cells.

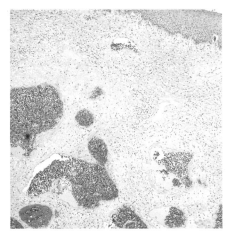

Fig. 5.40 Venous haemangioma. Vascular channels of variable size occupy the cervical stroma. Note a portion of the ectocervical squamous epithelium in the right upper corner of the field.

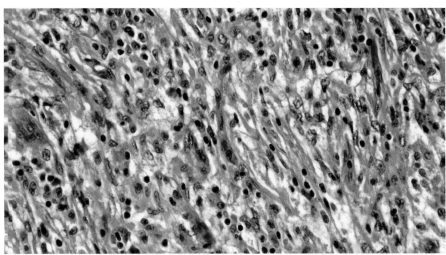

Fig. 5.41 Postoperative spindle cell nodule. The lesion is composed of spindle-shaped mesenchymal and inflammatory cells..

Histopathology
The tumour is composed of rhabdomyoblasts with small, uniform nuclei dispersed in a myxoid and oedematous stroma. The typical cambium layer of sarcoma botryoides is absent {690}.

Postoperative spindle cell nodule

Definition
A localized, non-neoplastic reactive lesion composed of closely packed proliferating spindle cells and capillaries simulating a leiomyosarcoma occurring at the site of a recent excision.

Clinical features
The lesion develops at the site of a recent operation several weeks to several months postoperatively {1420,2020}.

Histopathology
The lesion is composed of closely packed, mitotically active, spindle-shaped mesenchymal cells and capillaries often with an accompaniment of inflammatory cells, and may infiltrate the underlying tissue.

Differential diagnosis
Postoperative spindle cell sarcoma may closely resemble a leiomyosarcoma or other malignant spindle cell tumours, but the history of a recent operation at the same site facilitates its diagnosis.

Other benign tumours

Rare examples of cervical lipoma {334,1910}, haemangioma {47,629}, glomus tumour {64}, localized neurofibromatosis {381,986}, schwannoma {1093}, pigmented melanocytic schwannoma {2900}, granular cell tumour {553,952, 1101}, ganglioneuroma {858} and paraganglioma {3229} have been reported.

Mixed epithelial and mesenchymal tumours

W.G. McCluggage
R.A. Kubik-Huch

Definition

Tumours composed of an admixture of neoplastic epithelial and mesenchymal elements. Each of these components may be either benign or malignant.

ICD-O codes

Carcinosarcoma	8980/3
Adenosarcoma	8933/3
Wilms tumour	8960/3
Adenofibroma	9013/0
Adenomyoma	8932/0

Epidemiology

These neoplasms are much less common than their counterparts in the uterine corpus. They may occur in any age group, but carcinosarcomas most commonly involve elderly postmenopausal women {527,1060}.

Clinical features

The presenting symptom is usually abnormal uterine bleeding. In some cases, especially in cases of carcinosarcoma, a friable mass may extrude from the vaginal introitus. The tumour may be identified following an abnormal cervical smear.

Carcinosarcoma

Definition

A neoplasm composed of an admixture of malignant epithelial and mesenchymal elements.

Synonyms

Malignant müllerian mixed tumour, malignant mesodemal mixed tumour, metaplastic carcinoma.

Epidemiology

Carcinosarcomas most commonly involve elderly postmenopausal women {527,1060}. These neoplasms are much less common than their counterparts in the uterine body.

Aetiology

An occasional case of cervical carcinosarcoma has been associated with prior radiation treatment. HPV infection, especially HPV 16, has been found in the epithelial and mesenchymal components suggesting a role in the evolution of these neoplasms {1060}.

Histopathology

The histological features are similar to its counterpart in the uterine corpus. However, the epithelial elements are more commonly non-glandular in type and include squamous (keratinizing, non-keratinizing or basaloid), adenoid cystic, adenoid basal or undifferentiated carcinoma {527,1060,1757,1785,3177}. Adjacent severe dysplasia of the squamous epithelium has also been described. Mesonephric adenocarcinomas of the cervix with a malignant spindle cell component have been reported, representing an unusual subtype of cervical carcinosarcoma {521}. Before diagnosing a cervical carcinosarcoma, extension from a primary uterine corpus neoplasm should be excluded {960, 3245}.

Prognosis and predictive factors

Cervical carcinosarcomas are aggressive neoplasms, and treatment is usually radical hysterectomy followed by chemotherapy and/or radiotherapy. The prognosis may be better in small tumours with a polypoid appearance. Although aggressive, these neoplasms appear to be more often confined to the uterus compared to their counterparts in the corpus and may have a better prognosis {527,1060}.

Adenosarcoma

Definition

A neoplasm composed of an admixture of benign epithelial and malignant mesenchymal elements.

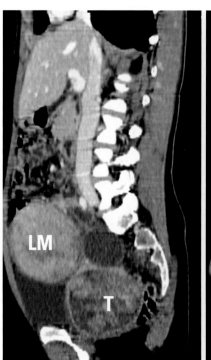
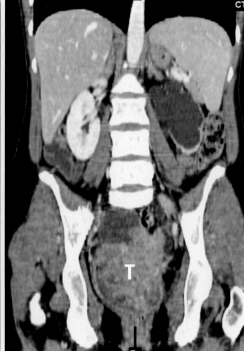

Fig. 5.42 CT scans of malignant mullerian tumour (T) of the cervix, extensively involving uterine corpus. On the sagittal image (left) note a large leiomyoma (LM) of the uterine fundus. The coronal reconstruction (right) shows the large extension of the tumour (T). Note the hydronephrosis of the left kidney.

Epidemiology

Cervical adenosarcomas are much less common than their counterparts in the uterine corpus.

Histopathology

The histological features are similar to its counterpart in the corpus. However, the epithelium is more likely to be squamous or mucinous. Adenosarcomas may or may not invade the underlying cervical stroma.

Prognosis and predictive factors

Because these neoplasms are rare, management is individualized. The therapy is usually simple hysterectomy, and radiation may be considered for deeply invasive neoplasms. They may recur following conservative therapy by simple excision or polypectomy. The prognostic features are not well established The prognosis is much better than that of cervical carcinosarcoma {848}.

Wilms tumour

Definition

A malignant tumor showing blastema and primitive glomerular and tubular differentiation resembling Wilms tumour of the kidney.

Epidemiology

Occasional cases of Wilms tumour arising within the cervix have been described, usually in adolescents {155, 215,1302}.

Macroscopy

Macroscopically, these neoplasms are composed of polypoid masses that protrude through the vagina.

Histopathology

Histologically, the classic triphasic pattern of epithelial, mesenchymal and blastemal elements may be present.

Prognosis and predictive factors

In two cases prolonged survival has been reported following local excision and chemotherapy {155,206,215,1302}.

Adenofibroma

Definition

A mixed neoplasm composed of benign epithelial and mesenchymal components.

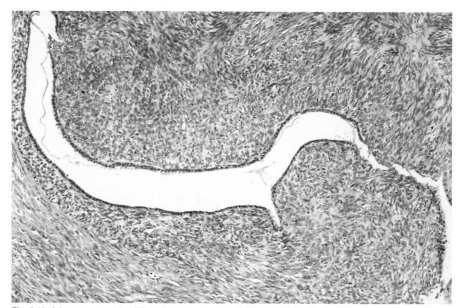

Fig. 5.43 Adenosarcoma. Leaf-like glands are surrounded by a cuff of cellular mesenchyme.

Epidemiology

These are uncommon in the cervix and are more commonly found within the uterine body {3245}.

Macroscopy

Cervical adenofibromas are polypoid neoplasms that usually protrude into the endocervical canal. On sectioning small cystic spaces may be identified.

Histopathology

Histologically, adenofibroma is a benign papillary neoplasm composed of fronds lined by benign epithelium that is usually glandular in type. The epithelium may be cuboidal, columnar, attenuated, ciliated or mucinous.

Occasionally, benign squamous epithelium may be present. The mesenchymal component shows little mitotic activity and is usually composed of non-specific fibrous tissue. The main differential diagnosis is a low grade adenosarcoma; the latter, however, exhibits malignant mesenchymal features including hypercellularity with condensation around glands, nuclear atypia and increased mitotic activity.

Prognosis and predictive factors

The therapy is usually local excision or simple hysterectomy.

Local excision is usually curative, although recurrence may follow incomplete removal.

Adenomyoma

Definition

A tumour composed of a benign glandular component and a benign mesenchymal component composed exclusively or predominantly of smooth muscle. These tumours are rare within the cervix. A variant is the atypical polypoid adenomyoma.

Macroscopy

Cervical adenomyomas are usually polypoid lesions with a firm sectioned surface. In some cases small cystic areas may be seen that may contain abundant mucin. Rare tumours are entirely intramural.

Histopathology

Three variants of cervical adenomyoma have been described, the endocervical type, the endometrial type and atypical polypoid adenomyoma.

Endocervical type

The endocervical type, which may be confused with minimal deviation adenocarcinoma, is composed largely of endocervical mucinous glands surrounded by a mesenchymal component consisting predominantly of smooth muscle {1005}. The glands are lined by tall mucin-secreting cells and are typically irregularly shaped with papillary infoldings. Occasionally, tubal-type epithelium or endometrial-type glands surrounded by endometrial-type stroma are focally pres-

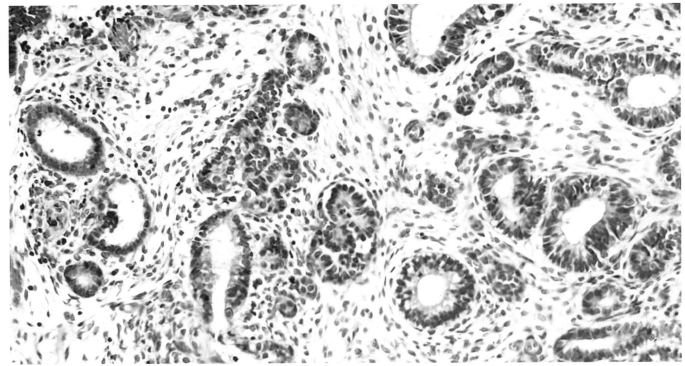

Fig. 5.44 Wilms tumour. The tumour is composed of primitive tubules set in a background of renal blastema.

ent. Both the epithelial and smooth muscle components are uniformly bland without any significant mitotic activity. Differentiating features from minimal deviation adenocarcinoma include the well circumscribed nature of adenomyoma and the absence of a desmoplastic stromal reaction or focal atypia {1005}.

Endometrial type

Another variant of cervical adenomyoma is similar to that found within the corpus {1002}. It is composed of endometrial-type glands surrounded by endometrial-type stroma that is, in turn, surrounded by smooth muscle that predominates. The glands and stroma are bland. Minor foci of tubal, mucinous or squamous epithelium may be found. These adenomyomas may or may not be associated with uterine adenomyosis. The most likely differential diagnoses are atypical polypoid adenomyoma and low grade adenosarcoma.

Atypical polypoid adenomyoma

In atypical polypoid adenomyoma the glandular component exhibits architectural complexity that is usually marked. It is similar to the corresponding tumour within the uterine corpus and usually involves the lower uterine segment or upper endocervix (see chapter on uterine corpus).

Prognosis and predictive factors

Simple polypectomy or local excision cures most cervical adenomyomas. However, recurrences have been described following local excision, and residual tumour may be found at hysterectomy.

Melanotic, germ cell, lymphoid and secondary tumours of the cervix

C.B. Gilks
S. Carinelli

Definition

A variety of primary benign or malignant tumours of the uterine cervix that are not otherwise categorized as well as secondary tumours.

ICD-O codes

Malignant melanoma	8720/3
Blue naevus	8780/0
Yolk sac tumour	9071/3
Dermoid cyst	9084/0
Mature cystic teratoma	9080/0

Malignant melanoma

Definition

A malignant tumour of melanocytic origin.

Epidemiology

Malignant melanoma of the cervix is considerably less common than vulvar or vaginal melanoma with fewer than 30 well documented cases reported {396, 667,940}. All occurred in adults, and approximately one-half had spread beyond the cervix at the time of presentation {396}.

Clinical features

These tumours commonly present with abnormal vaginal bleeding.

Malignant melanomas are typically described as polypoid or fungating, pigmented masses. However, they may be amelanotic and non-specific in appearance.

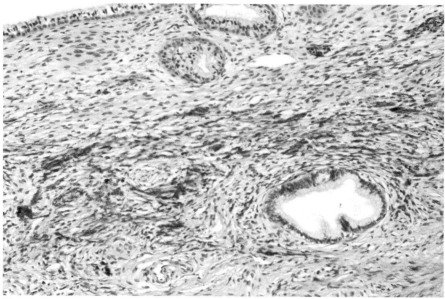

Fig. 5.45 Blue naevus of the cervix. Note the aggregates of heavily pigmented dendritic melanocytes within the endocervical stroma.

Tumour spread and staging

Spread to the vagina is often present at the time of presentation {396}.

Histopathology

A junctional component was reported in approximately 50% of cases. In tumours lacking a junctional component, exclusion of the possibility of metastatic melanoma to the cervix requires clinical correlation. The histological appearance of cervical melanomas is noteworthy for the frequent presence of spindle-shaped cells. Desmoplastic and clear cell variants have also been reported {940, 1306}. The immunophenotype of cervical melanoma is indistinguishable from that of other sites.

Prognosis and predictive factors

The prognosis for patients with cervical melanoma is dismal, with only two reports of patients surviving more than 5 years {1360,2893}.

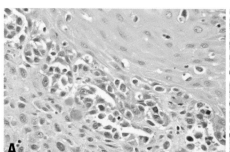
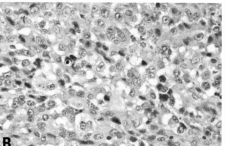
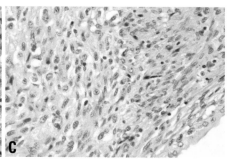

Fig. 5.46 Malignant melanoma of the cervix. **A** The tumour shows junctional growth and transepidermal migration. **B** This tumour is composed of large epithelioid cells with pleomorphic nuclei in association with melanin pigment. **C** Note the spindle cell growth pattern of malignant melanocytes.

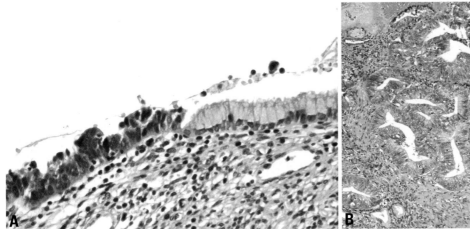

Fig. 5.47 Implant of endometrial carcinoma. **A** Non-invasive implant. To the right is the mucinous epithelium of the endocervix; to the left the epithelium has been replaced by malignant epithelium of endometrioid type. **B** Invasive implant. Note the aggregates of well differentiated endometrioid carcinoma in the stroma that do not conform to the pattern of endocervical glands.

Blue naevus

Definition
A naevus composed of dendritic melanocytes that are typically heavily pigmented.

Clinical features
Benign pigmented lesions are asymptomatic and are typically incidental findings in hysterectomy specimens {2972, 2973}. As most blue naevi occur in the endocervical canal, they are not visible colposcopically {2972,2973}. Occasional examples are visible as pigmented macules on the ectocervix with a smooth overlying mucosa {1744}.

Histopathology
Blue naevi are recognized histologically by the presence of poorly circumscribed collections of heavily pigmented, bland, spindle-shaped cells with fine dendritic processes in the superficial cervical stroma. They are most commonly located under the endocervical epithelium, but examples that involved the ectocervix have been reported {1744}.

Differential diagnosis
The differential diagnosis includes other benign melanocytic lesions. In contrast to the frequency with which blue naevi are encountered, the cervical equivalent of common junctional, compound or intradermal naevi of skin is vanishingly rare in the cervix, with no convincing examples reported. Benign melanosis {3182} and lentigos {2568} of the ectocervical squamous mucosa are, however, occasionally encountered.

Yolk sac tumour

Definition
A primitive malignant germ cell tumour characterized by a variety of distinctive histological patterns, some of which recapitulate phases in the development of the normal yolk sac.

Synonym
Endodermal sinus tumour.

Epidemiology
The cervix is the second most common site in the lower female genital tract for yolk sac tumour after the vagina. It may be difficult or impossible to determine the primary site (vagina vs. cervix) in some cases {557}.

Clinical features
These tumours commonly present with abnormal vaginal bleeding. Yolk sac tumours are polypoid, friable masses, protruding into the vagina {557}.

Histopathology
The histological features are the same as for vaginal yolk sac tumours {557,3213}.

Prognosis and predictive factors
The prognosis for patients with cervicovaginal yolk sac tumours is good with modern chemotherapy {1794}.

Dermoid cyst

Definition
A mature teratoma characterized by a predominance of one or a few cysts lined by epidermis accompanied by its appendages.

Synonym
Mature cystic teratoma.

Clinical features
Cervical teratomas appear as smooth cervical polyps that may be pedunculated {1451}.

Histopathology
The histological appearance is indistinguishable from mature teratomas at other sites. Glial and squamous epithelial elements are common, but a wide range of mature tissue types have been reported {1451}.

Differential diagnosis
The differential diagnosis includes benign glial polyp of the cervix, a polypoid mass of mature glial tissue in women of reproductive age that is probably closely related to the cervical dermoid cyst. The former is thought to most probably arise from implantation of fetal tissue {1069,1711,2396}.

Histogenesis
It has been proposed that these are not true neoplasms but are implanted fetal tissues {2968}; molecular studies to determine whether the cells of cervical teratomas are genetically identical to the host and, thus, neoplastic rather than fetal in origin have not been performed.

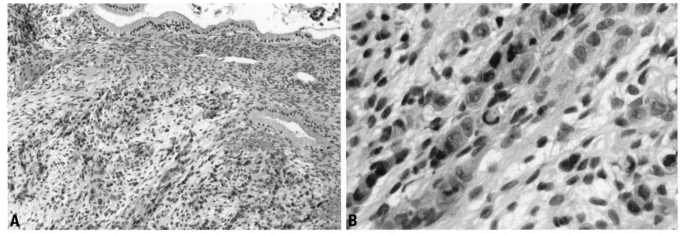

Fig. 5.48 Metastatic gastric carcinoma to the uterine cervix. **A** Solid aggregates of metastatic carcinoma occur within the endocervical stroma. Note the surface endocervical mucinous epithelial lining and the endocervical glands in the upper portion of the field. **B** Note the cords of highly pleomorphic neoplastic cells within the endocervical stroma.

Lymphoma and leukaemia

Definition
A malignant lymphoproliferative or haematopoetic neoplasm that may be primary or secondary.

Epidemiology
Involvement of the cervix by lymphoma or leukaemia may rarely be primary but is more commonly part of systemic disease with no specific symptoms referable to the cervix {1145}.

Clinical features
With cervical involvement by lymphoma or leukaemia the cervix appears enlarged and barrel-shaped, although polypoid or nodular masses may be seen {1145,2457,3000}. For the histological description see chapter on the vagina.

Secondary tumours

Definition
Tumours of the uterine cervix that originate outside the cervix.

Incidence and origin
The majority of clinically significant secondary tumours of the cervix originate in the female genital system (endometrium ovary, vagina and fallopian tube in that order) {1625,1939}. Endometrial carcinoma presents with stage II disease in 12% of patients {576}. Secondary cervical involvement is more common with high grade endometrial carcinoma, including serous carcinoma {576}. Extragenital pri-

mary sites include the breast, stomach and large bowel {1625,2608}. Cervical involvement by an extragenital tumour is almost always associated with disseminated disease and rapid progression to death. In occasional cases, however, cervical involvement may be the only evidence of disease at presentation or the first sign of recurrence {1087,1625,1802, 2892}.

Clinical features
The most common symptom of secondary cervical tumour is abnormal bleeding {1625,1939,2608}. Malignant cells may be detected on cervical cytologic preparations {1087}. On examination there are usually no abnormalities of the cervix {1939}. Occasionally, the cervix may appear enlarged, nodular or distorted, tumour may protrude from the os, or the cervix may be abnormally firm on palpation {1625,1802,2608,3179}.
Secondary cervical involvement by endometrial carcinoma may present as raised nodules of tumour in the endocervical canal and have a similar appearance to the primary endometrial tumour. In most cases of stage II endometrial carcinoma, however, no clinical abnormality is evident {2608}.

Histopathology
Secondary involvement of the cervix by endometrial carcinoma may be superficial with replacement of normal cervical epithelium by neoplastic cells of endometrial carcinoma (Stage IIA) or tumour may invade the underlying stroma (Stage IIB). The assessment of possi-

ble invasion into the cervical stroma poses the same problems in cases of secondary involvement of the cervix by endometrial carcinoma as for primary cervical adenocarcinoma. The cervical tumour may be either discontinuous or contiguous with the dominant endometrial tumour {2608}. Metastases of endometrial carcinoma to the cervix by lymphatic spread are less common than superficial mucosal implants and are present in only 6% of stage II endometrial carcinomas {2608}. The distinction of primary cervical adenocarcinoma from secondary involvement may be difficult or impossible in a small biopsy, as the different histological subtypes of adenocarcinoma seen in the female genital tract are not site-specific. Metastases from extragenital primary tumours may be suspected based on the submucosal location of tumour cells with a normal overlying cervical epithelium. Widespread lymphatic dissemination is also suggestive of a secondary origin. In the case of metastatic lobular carcinoma of the breast or diffuse gastric carcinoma, small nests, cords and individual cells infiltrate the cervical stroma, an appearance not characteristic of primary cervical adenocarcinoma.

CHAPTER 6

Tumours of the Vagina

Although the incidence rate of vaginal intraepithelial neoplasia is increasing, that of squamous cell carcinoma is decreasing, reflecting earlier detection and more successful treatment. Human papillomavirus infection is a risk factor for both vaginal intraepithelial neoplasia and squamous cell carcinoma.

In past decades, clear cell adenocarcinoma occurred in young women, about two-thirds of whom had been exposed transplacentally to diethylstilbestrol. At that time, it was the the most important glandular lesion of the vagina and the second most common epithelial malignancy. The precursor lesion appears to be atypical adenosis.

The most important non-epithelial tumours are malignant melanoma and sarcoma botyoides.

WHO histological classification of tumours of the vagina

Epithelial tumours
Squamous tumours and precursors
    Squamous cell carcinoma, not otherwise specified   8070/3
        Keratinizing   8071/3
        Non-keratinizing   8072/3
        Basaloid   8083/3
        Verrucous   8051/3
        Warty   8051/3
    Squamous intraepithelial neoplasia
        Vaginal intraepithelial neoplasia 3 /   8077/2
        squamous cell carcinoma in situ   8070/2
    Benign squamous lesions
        Condyloma acuminatum
        Squamous papilloma (vaginal micropapillomatosis)   8052/0
        Fibroepithelial polyp
Glandular tumours
    Clear cell adenocarcinoma   8310/3
    Endometrioid adenocarcinoma   8380/3
    Mucinous adenocarcinoma   8480/3
    Mesonephric adenocarcinoma   9110/3
    Müllerian papilloma
    Adenoma, not otherwise specified   8140/0
        Tubular   8211/0
        Tubulovillous   8263/0
        Villous   8261/0
Other epithelial tumours
    Adenosquamous carcinoma   8560/3
    Adenoid cystic carcinoma   8200/3
    Adenoid basal carcinoma   8098/3
    Carcinoid   8240/3
    Small cell carcinoma   8041/3
    Undifferentiated carcinoma   8020/3

Mesenchymal tumours and tumour-like conditions
    Sarcoma botryoides   8910/3

    Leiomyosarcoma   8890/3
    Endometrioid stromal sarcoma, low grade   8931/3
    Undifferentiated vaginal sarcoma   8805/3
    Leiomyoma   8890/0
    Genital rhabdomyoma   8905/0
    Deep angiomyxoma   8841/1
    Postoperative spindle cell nodule

Mixed epithelial and mesenchymal tumours
    Carcinosarcoma (malignant müllerian mixed tumour;
    metaplastic carcinoma)   8980/3
    Adenosarcoma   8933/3
    Malignant mixed tumour resembling synovial sarcoma   8940/3
    Benign mixed tumour   8940/0

Melanocytic tumours
    Malignant melanoma   8720/3
    Blue naevus   8780/0
    Melanocytic naevus   8720/0

Miscellaneous tumours
Tumours of germ cell type
    Yolk sac tumour   9071/3
    Dermoid cyst   9084/0
Others
    Peripheral primitive neuroectodermal tumour /   9364/3
    Ewing tumour   9260/3
    Adenomatoid tumour   9054/0

Lymphoid and haematopoetic tumours
    Malignant lymphoma (specify type)
    Leukaemia (specify type)

Secondary tumours

---

[1] Morphology code of the International Classification of Diseases for Oncology (ICD-O) {921} and the Systematized Nomenclature of Medicine (http://snomed.org). Behaviour is coded /0 for benign tumours, /2 for in situ carcinomas and grade 3 intraepithelial neoplasia, /3 for malignant tumours, and /1 for borderline or uncertain behaviour.
[2] Intraepithelial neoplasia does not have a generic code in ICD-O. ICD-O codes are only available for lesions categorized as squamous intraepithelial neoplasia grade 3 (e.g. vaginal intraepithelial neoplasia/VAIN grade 3) = 8077/2; squamous cell carcinoma in situ = 8070/2.

TNM and FIGO classification of carcinomas of the vagina

TNM and FIGO classification[1,2]

T – Primary Tumour

TNM Categories	FIGO Stages	
TX		Primary tumour cannot be assessed
T0		No evidence of primary tumour
Tis	0	Carcinoma in situ (preinvasive carcinoma)
T1	I	Tumour confined to vagina
T2	II	Tumour invades paravaginal tissues but does not extend to pelvic wall
T3	III	Tumour extends to pelvic wall
T4	IVA	Tumour invades *mucosa* of bladder or rectum, and/or extends beyond the true pelvis

Note: The presence of bullous oedema is not sufficient evidence to classify a tumour as T4.

M1	IVB	Distant metastasis

N – Regional Lymph Nodes[3]

NX	Regional lymph nodes cannot be assessed
N0	No regional lymph node metastasis
N1	Regional lymph node metastasis

M – Distant Metastasis

MX	Distant metastasis cannot be assessed
M0	No distant metastasis
M1	Distant metastasis

Stage Grouping

Stage 0	Tis	N0	M0
Stage I	T1	N0	M0
Stage II	T2	N0	M0
Stage III	T3	N0	M0
	T1, T2, T3	N1	M0
Stage IVA	T4	N0	M0
Stage IVB	Any T	Any N	M1

---

[1] {51,2976}.
[2] A help desk for specific questions about the TNM classification is available at http://tnm.uicc.org.
[3] The regional lymph nodes are: Upper two-thirds of vagina: the pelvic nodes including obturator, internal iliac (hypogastric), external iliac, and pelvic nodes, NOS. Lower third of vagina: the inguinal and femoral nodes.

Epithelial tumours

E.S. Andersen
J. Paavonen
M. Murnaghan
A.G. Östör

A.G. Hanselaar
C. Bergeron
S.P. Dobbs

Squamous tumours

Definition
Primary squamous epithelial tumours of the vagina are the most frequent neoplasms at this site. They occur in all age groups but preferentially in the elderly. Vaginal intraepithelial neoplasia (VAIN) is considered a typical, though not obligatory, precursor lesion of squamous cell carcinoma.

ICD-O codes
Squamous cell carcinoma   8070/3
Vaginal intraepithelial neoplasia
  (VAIN), grade 3   8077/2
  Squamous cell carcinoma in situ 8070/2
Squamous papilloma   8052/0

Squamous cell carcinoma

Definition
An invasive carcinoma composed of squamous cells of varying degrees of differentiation. According to the International Federation of Gynaecology and Obstetrics (FIGO), a tumour of the vagina involving the uterine cervix or the vulva should be classified as a primary cervical or vulvar cancer, respectively. Additionally, before the diagnosis of a primary vaginal carcinoma can be established, a 5-10 year disease free interval is required to rule out recurrent disease in those patients with a prior preinvasive or invasive cervical or vulvar neoplasm.

Epidemiology
Squamous cell carcinoma comprises up to 85% of vaginal carcinomas and accounts for 1-2% of all malignant tumours of the female genital tract {634, 1193}. The mean age of patients is about 60 years.

Aetiology
In squamous cell carcinoma persistent infection with high-risk human papillomavirus (HPV) is probably a major aetiological factor. The same risk factors are observed as for vaginal intraepithelial neoplasia (VAIN), i.e. previous preinvasive or invasive disease of the lower genital tract, immunosuppression and prior pelvic irradiation {303}. The development of VAIN and eventual progression to invasive disease is most likely, though the progression rate is unknown {347}.

Prior pelvic irradiation is a predisposing factor for vaginal squamous carcinoma {303,748,3075}. Simultaneous or prior preinvasive or invasive disease elsewhere in the lower genital tract is observed in up to 30% of cases {220,2227,2480}.

Clinical features
Signs and symptoms
The commonest symptom is a bloody vaginal discharge. Nearly 75% of patients present with painless bleeding, urinary tract symptoms or postcoital bleeding; however, the patient may be completely asymptomatic. Pelvic pain and dysuria usually signify advanced disease {2499}. Most cases occur in the upper third of the vagina and are located on the posterior wall {2265}.

Imaging
Magnetic resonance imaging (MRI) of the pelvis can be used to image vaginal tumours as well as to assess whether pelvic or inguinal lymphadenopathy is present. The MRI appearance, however, is not specific, and inflammatory changes and congestion of the vagina may mimic vaginal carcinoma {439}.

Exfoliative cytology
Occasionally, cancer cells of vaginal origin may be observed in cervical smears.

Macroscopy
Tumours may be exophytic, ulcerative or annular and constricting. The lesions vary in size from being undetectable to greater than 10 cm. They may be polypoid, sessile, indurated, ulcerated or fun-

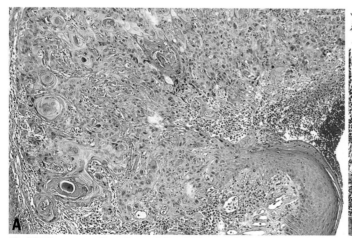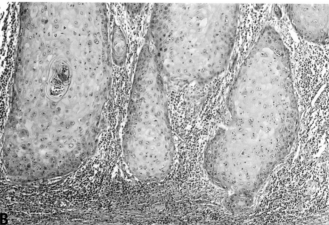

Fig. 6.01 Squamous cell carcinoma. **A** Keratinizing type. Carcinoma arises from the surface epithelium and forms several keratin pearls. **B** Non-keratinizing type. The neoplasm forms prominent squamous pearls with little keratinization.

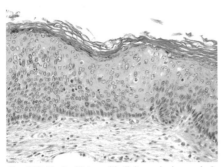

Fig. 6.02 Vaginal intraepithelial neoplasia, grade 2. Nuclear features of intraepithelial neoplasia are evident in the lower two-thirds of the squamous epithelium with overlying parakeratosis.

Table 6.01
Terminology of premalignant vaginal squamous epithelial lesions.

Classification	Synonyms	
Vaginal intraepithelial neoplasia, grade 1	Mild dysplasia	Low grade VAIN
Vaginal intraepithelial neoplasia, grade 2	Moderate dysplasia	High grade VAIN
Vaginal intraepithelial neoplasia, grade 3	Severe dysplasia and carcinoma in situ	High grade VAIN
VAIN = vaginal intraepithelial neoplasia		

gating and may be found anywhere within the vagina. Squamous cell carcinoma, the commonest vaginal carcinoma, is ulcerative in half of cases, exophytic in a third and annular and constricting in the remainder.

Tumour spread and staging
Squamous cell carcinoma spreads predominantly laterally to the paravaginal and parametrial tissues when located in the lower and upper vagina, respectively. Tumours also invade lymphatics, metastasizing to regional lymph nodes and eventually distant sites including the lungs, liver and brain. The staging of vaginal tumours is by the TNM/FIGO classification {51,2976}. Approximately 25% of patients present with stage I disease, one-third with stage II disease and 40% with stage III or IV disease {220,748, 1245,1524,2301,2480}.

Histopathology
Vaginal squamous cell carcinoma has the same histological characteristics as such tumours in other sites. Most cases are moderately differentiated and non-keratinizing {2301}. Rarely, the tumours have spindle-cell features {2778}. Warty carcinoma is another variant of vaginal squamous cell carcinoma {2339}. The tumour is papillary with hyperkeratotic epithelium. Nuclear enlargement and koilocytosis with hyperchromasia, wrinkling of the nuclear membrane and multinucleation are typical changes {1541, 2936}. Verrucous carcinoma has a papillary growth pattern with pushing borders and bulbous pegs of acanthotic epithelium with little or no atypia and surface maturation in the form of parakeratosis and hyperkeratosis. For a more detailed discussion of the subtypes of squamous cell carcinoma see chapter 5 or 7.

Prognosis and predictive factors
Radiation is the preferred treatment for most cases of vaginal carcinoma {1524, 2217,2981}. In Stage I disease located in the upper part of the vagina, a radical hysterectomy, pelvic lymphadenectomy and partial vaginectomy may be considered {55,171}. Otherwise, radiation therapy given as intracavitary therapy, interstitial implants and/or external pelvic/inguinal radiation, often in combination, is the most frequently adopted modality {1524,2217}. In tumours of the middle or lower third of the vagina the external radiation field should include the inguinal and femoral lymph nodes.
The clinical stage is the most significant prognostic factor {220,748,1245,1524, 2301,2480}. Recurrences are typically local and usually happen within 2 years of treatment. The five-year survival rates are 70% for stage I, 45% for stage II, 30% for stage III and 15% for stage IV. The overall 5-year survival is about 42% {220,748,1245,1524,2301,2480}.
Tumour localization, grade or keratinization or patient age has not been demonstrated to have prognostic significance.

Vaginal intraepithelial neoplasia

Definition
A premalignant lesion of the vaginal squamous epithelium that can develop primarily in the vagina or as an extension from the cervix. VAIN is often a manifestation of the so-called lower genital tract neoplastic syndrome. Histologically, VAIN is defined in the same way as cervical intraepithelial neoplasia (CIN).

Synonyms
Dysplasia/carcinoma in situ, squamous intraepithelial lesion.

Epidemiology
VAIN is much less common than CIN, though its true incidence is unknown. There is some evidence that the incidence of VAIN has increased in recent decades, particularly among young and immunosuppressed women. The mean age for patients with VAIN is approximately 50 years. The majority of VAIN cases occur in women who have had a prior hysterectomy or who have a history of cervical or vulvar neoplasia {1626, 2403}.

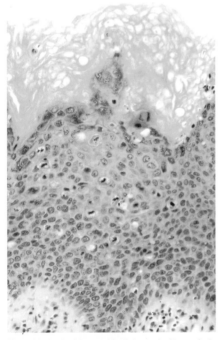

Fig. 6.03 Vaginal intraepithelial neoplasia, grade 3. The upper portion of the epithelium is covered by hyperkeratosis. The remaining cells are characterized by nuclear enlargement and pleomorphism.

Aetiology

The fact that both VAIN and vaginal carcinoma are much less common than cervical neoplasia has been explained by the absence of a vulnerable transformation zone in the vagina. VAIN is associated with HPV infection in most cases. At least 15 different HPV types have been identified in VAIN. As in the cervix, VAIN 2 and VAIN 3 are associated with high-risk HPV types, of which type 16 is the most frequent. Mixed HPV types have also been identified in multifocal VAIN lesions and also in a single lesion {239, 2565}. In VAIN 1 a mixture of low and high-risk HPV types can be detected.

Clinical features

Signs and symptoms

VAIN may be isolated but is more commonly multifocal {710,1626}. Isolated lesions are mainly detected in the upper one-third of the vagina and in the vaginal vault after hysterectomy. VAIN is asymptomatic and cannot be diagnosed by the naked eye.

Colposcopy

VAIN may be suspected by a cervicovaginal cytology preparation, but the diagnosis can only be made by a colposcopically directed biopsy. If the colposcopy of the cervix is normal after an abnormal cytological smear, a careful colposcopic examination of all the vaginal epithelium should be performed. VAIN lesions are always iodine-negative. The presence of punctation on a sharply demarcated aceto-white area is the single most reliable colposcopic feature suggestive of VAIN {2565}.

Histopathology

The histopathology of VAIN is similar to that of CIN. Many VAIN 3 lesions also

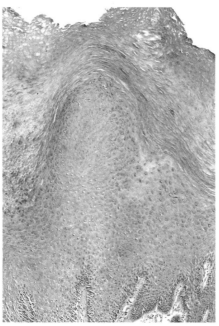

Fig. 6.04 Condyloma acuminatum. Papillomatosis, acanthosis and hyperkeratosis are associated with a few koilocytes in the superficial layers.

show hyperkeratosis. The so-called "flat condyloma" shows koilocytosis in the superficial layers of the epithelium with normal or only hyperplastic basal layers without nuclear atypia.However, the distinction between flat condyloma and VAIN 1 with koilocytosis is not always possible. Other differential diagnoses of VAIN include atrophy, squamous atypia and transitional cell metaplasia {3085} as well as immature squamous metaplasia in women with adenosis. A distinction is made based on the nuclear features of the epithelium.

The relationship of the VAIN terminology to that of dysplasia and carcinoma in situ of the vagina is shown in Table 6.01.

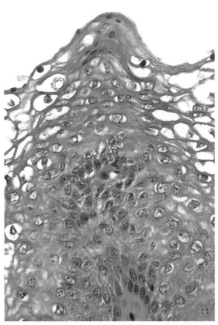

Fig. 6.05 Spiked condyloma. Papillomatosis is associated with HPV-infected cells with a clear cytoplasm (koilocytes).

Prognosis and predictive factors

The natural history of VAIN has been less extensively studied than that of CIN. In one study 23 patients with a mean age of 41 years were followed for at least 3 years with no treatment {49}. One-half of the VAIN lesions were multifocal. Progression to invasive vaginal carcinoma occurred in only 2 cases, and VAIN persisted in 3 additional cases. Thus, VAIN spontaneously regressed in 78% of cases. A retrospective review of 121 women with VAIN showed that the recurrence rate was 33% {710}. Progression to invasive vaginal cancer occurred in 2%. In another study of 94 patients with VAIN, the progression rate to cancer was 5% {2674}.

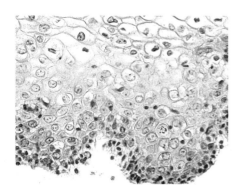

Fig. 6.06 Vaginal intraepithelial neoplasia, grade 1. Note the koilocytosis and the slightly thickened and disorganized basal layers.

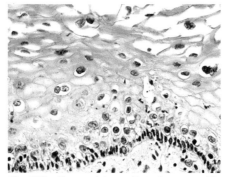

Fig. 6.07 Flat condyloma. Note the cytopathic effects of human papilomavirus (koilocytosis) with a normal basal layer of the squamous epithelium.

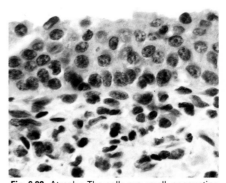

Fig. 6.08 Atrophy. The cells are small, accounting for the nuclear crowding. Nuclei are uniform with discernible nucleoli. Mitoses are not detectable.

High grade VAIN appears to be an important precursor of invasive cancer; progression occurred in 8% of cases of high grade VAIN despite the fact that most of the patients were treated, whereas low grade VAIN regressed in 88% of women without treatment {2403}.

Condyloma acuminatum

Definition
A benign neoplasm characterized by papillary fronds containing fibrovascular cores and lined by stratified squamous epithelium with evidence of HPV infection, usually in the form of koilocytosis.

Epidemiology
Condylomas are sexually transmitted. There is strong evidence that their incidence has increased since the 1960s. The incidence is much higher in women than in men. They often occur on the mucosal epithelium of the vagina. However, because condylomas are often subclinical and not reported, their true incidence remains unknown.

Aetiology
Non-oncogenic HPV types 6 and 11 are found in the majority of condylomas {1837}. Patients with visible condylomas can be simultaneously infected by other HPV types (mixed HPV infection).

Clinical features
Signs and symptoms
Vaginal lesions are easily overlooked during a speculum examination. Vaginal condylomas present in the same way as those on the vulva and the cervix {1070, 2144}. They can be single or multiple. Condylomas can cover most of the vaginal mucosa and extend to the cervix and may be small or large. Most commonly, they occur adjacent to the introitus and in the vaginal fornices. Condylomas can be papular or macular. The latter has been also called "flat condyloma", noncondylomatous wart virus infection or subclinical papillomavirus infection.

Colposcopy
Typical exophytic condylomas show digitate projections with vascularized cores producing loop-like patterns or punctation {1070,2144}. The application of acetic acid augments the diagnosis of vaginal condylomas. Micropapillary vaginal condylomas may be diffuse and may completely cover the vagina. This manifestation is known as condylomatous vaginitis. Reverse punctation can be seen by colposcopy after acetic acid application. Spiked condylomas appear as small and elongated white spikes focally or diffusely distributed on the vaginal wall {1070, 2144}.

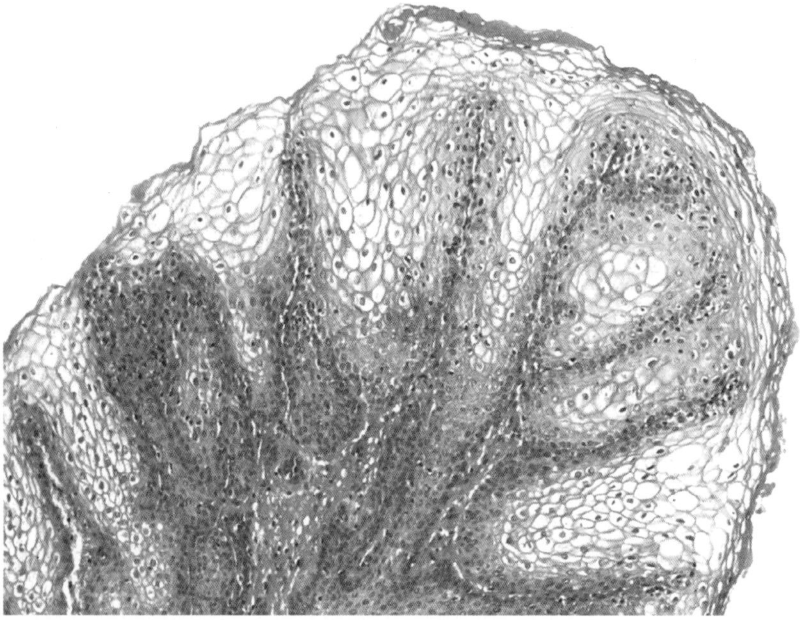

Histopathology
Condyloma acuminatum has a complex, arborizing architecture with hyperkeratosis, parakeratosis, acanthosis and papillomatosis as well as the typical cytopathic effects of HPV. It can be distinguished by clinical examination alone from vaginal micropapillomatosis, which has no significant relationship with HPV infection and is believed by some to be a normal anatomical variant of the lower genital tract {967}. The latter also lacks the histological features of condyloma.

Squamous papilloma

Definition
A benign papillary tumour in which squamous epithelium without atypia or koilocytosis lines a fibrovascular stalk.

Synonyms
Vaginal micropapillomatosis, squamous papillomatosis.
These terms are applicable when numerous lesions are present.

Epidemiology
Squamous papillomas do not appear to be sexually transmitted.

Aetiology
Based on in situ hybridization studies using the polymerase chain reaction, vaginal micropapillary lesions appear unrelated to human papillomavirus {967}, and their aetiology is unknown.

Clinical features
Squamous papillomas may be single or multiple. When numerous, they occur near the hymenal ring and are referred to as vaginal micropapillomatosis. The lesions are usually asymptomatic but may be associated with vulvar burning or dyspareunia. They may be difficult to distinguish from condyloma by inspection. However, on colposcopic and histological examination papilloma is composed of a single papillary frond with a central fibrovascular. core.

Histopathology
In squamous papilloma the squamous epithelium covers a central fibrovascular core and shows acanthosis but lacks koilocytosis. It has a smooth surface and lacks significant vascular structures. It lacks the complex arborizing architecture and koilocytes of condylomas.

Fig. 6.09 Squamous papilloma. The fibrovascular core is covered by squamous epithelium with a smooth surface that lacks koilocytosis but shows acanthosis and papillomatosis.

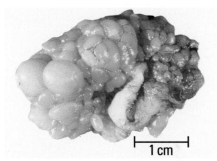

Fig. 6.10 Fibroepithelial polyp. A multilobulated polypoid lesion arises from the vaginal wall.

However, it is important to note that there may be a time during the evolution of condylomas when koilocytes are not easily identifiable.

Fibroepithelial polyp

Definition
A polyp lined by squamous epithelium that contains a central core of fibrous tissue in which stellate cells with tapering cytoplasmic processes and irregularly shaped thin-walled vessels are prominent features.

Synonym
Stromal polyp.

Clinical features
This lesion can occur at any age but has a predilection for pregnant women.

Macroscopy
These are polypoid lesions, usually solitary.

Histopathology
These polypoid lesions are characterized by a prominent fibrovascular stroma covered by squamous epithelium {380}. They lack epithelial acanthosis and papillary architecture. Bizarre stromal cells, marked hypercellularity and elevated mitotic counts including atypical forms have been described that can lead to an erroneous diagnosis of sarcoma botryoides, but a cambium layer and rhabdomyoblasts are absent, and mitotic activity is typically low {2067}.

Glandular tumours and their precursors

ICD-O codes
Adenocarcinoma, NOS	8140/3
Clear cell adenocarcinoma	8310/3
Endometrioid adenocarcinoma	8380/3
Mucinous adenocarcinoma	8480/3
Mesonephric adenocarcinoma	9110/3
Adenoma, NOS	8140/0
Tubular	8211/0
Tubulovillous	8263/0
Villous	8261/0

Clear cell adenocarcinoma

Definition
An invasive neoplasm with an epithelial component that contains one or more cell types, most commonly clear cells and hobnail cells, but flat and/or eosinophilic cells may, on occasion, predominate.

Epidemiology
The occurrence of cases of vaginal clear cell adenocarcinoma associated with in utero exposure to diethylstilbestrol (DES) was responsible for an increase in incidence of adenocarcinoma in young women from the 1970s {1194}. In the early 1970s the peak incidence of clear cell adenocarcinoma was around 19 years, the youngest patient being 8 years. With the ageing of the DES-exposed cohort, the peak incidence has been shifting towards an older age group.

Aetiology
DES was prescribed for threatened or repeated abortions from the 1940s to the early 1970s. Millions of women were exposed in utero to this and related drugs in several countries, including the United States, France and the Netherlands {2946}. DES is a teratogen and causes a variety of congenital abnormalities of the lower genital tract in about 30% of the female offspring {1883}. The absolute risk of clear cell adenocarcinoma of the vagina or cervix is estimated at 1:1000 {1843}. About two-thirds of the cases of clear cell adenocarcinoma occurring in individuals under the age of 40 are linked to transplacental DES exposure. DES inhibits the development of urogenital sinus-derived squamous epithelium that is destined to become vaginal epithelium and normally grows up to the junction of the ectocervix and endocervix, replacing the pre-existing müllerian-derived columnar epithelium. The embryonic müllerian epithelium that is not replaced persists and develops into adenosis. Adenosis is found immediately adjacent to the tumour in over 90% of cases and is thought to be the precursor of clear cell adenocarcinoma. The rarity of clear cell adenocarcinoma in the exposed population suggests that DES is an incomplete carcinogen or that susceptibility factors are necessary for it to produce neoplastic transformation. Genetic factors and hormonal disruption by environmental toxins are implicated. A maternal history of prior spontaneous abortion increases the risk of clear cell adenocarcinoma {2161}. Endogenous estrogens probably also play a role,

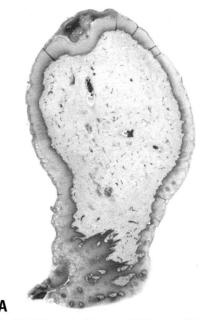
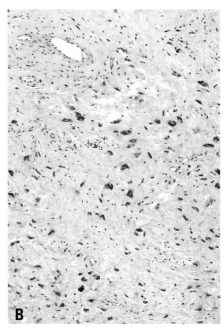

A   **B**

Fig. 6.11 Fibroepithelial polyp. **A** This polypoid lesion is composed of stroma and covered by squamous epthelium. **B** The stroma contains scattered bizarre multinucleated giant cells.

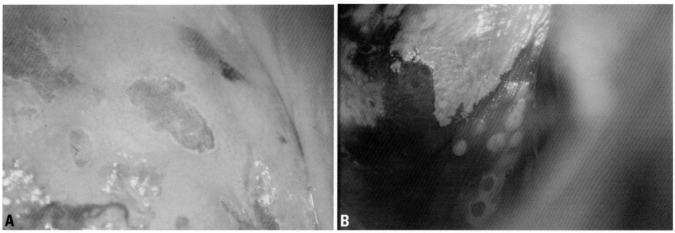

Fig. 6.12 Adenosis of the vagina. **A** By colposcopy red granular areas of adenosis are apparent. **B** Colposcopy after iodine application. The areas of adenosis do not stain.

since most cases of clear cell adenocarcinoma are first detected around the time of puberty.

Localization
Whilst any part of the vagina may be involved, clear cell adenocarcinoma most often arises from its upper part. A primary vaginal clear cell adenocarcinoma may also involve the cervix. According to FIGO criteria about two-thirds of clear cell adenocarcinomas after DES exposure are classified as tumours of the vagina and one-third of the cervix {1131}. In non-DES exposed young women and post-menopausal women this ratio is reversed.

Clinical features
Vaginal bleeding, discharge and dyspareunia are the most common symptoms, but women may be asymptomatic. Abnormal cytologic findings may lead to detection, but care must be taken to sample the vagina as well as the cervix since cervical smears are relatively insensitive for the detection of clear cell adenocarcinoma {1132}.

Clear cell adenocarcinomas typically are polypoid, nodular, or papillary but may also be flat or ulcerated. Some clear cell adenocarcinomas are confined to the superficial stroma and may remain undetected for a long time {1131,2386}. Such small tumours may be invisible on macroscopic or even colposcopic examination and are only detected by palpation or when tumour cells are shed through the mucosa and detected by exfoliative cytology. Large tumours may be up to 10 cm in diameter.

Histopathology
Clear cell adenocarcinoma of the vagina has an appearance similar to those arising in the cervix, endometrium and ovary. Clear cell adenocarcinomas may show several growth patterns; the most common pattern is tubulocystic, but it also may be solid or mixed. A papillary growth pattern is seldom predominant. The main cell types are clear cells and hobnail cells. The appearance of the clear cells is due to the presence of abundant intracytoplasmic glycogen. Hobnail cells are characterized by inconspicuous cytoplasm and a bulbous nucleus that protrudes into glandular lumens. The tumour cells may also be flat with bland nuclei and scant cytoplasm in cystic areas or have granular eosinophilic cytoplasm without glycogen. The nuclei vary considerably in appearance. They may be significantly enlarged with multiple irregular nucleoli in clear and hobnail cells, or they may have fine chromatin and inconspicuous nucleoli in flat cells. The num-

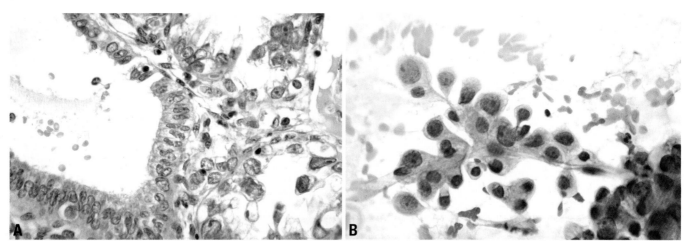

Fig. 6.13 Clear cell adenocarcinoma. **A** Note the neoplastic tubules lined by hobnail cells on the right and adenosis of the tuboendometrial type on the left. **B** Cytological preparation shows hobnail cells with anisonucleosis, unevenly distributed chromatin, nucleoli and vacuolated cytoplasm.

ber of mitoses varies but is usually less than 10 per 10 high power fields. Psammoma and intracellular hyaline bodies may occasionally be encountered.

Cytopathology
In cytological preparations the malignant cells may occur singly or in clusters and resemble large endocervical or endometrial cells. Typically, the nuclei are large with one or more prominent nucleoli. Nuclei may be bizarre. The bland cytological features of tumours that show only mild nuclear atypia may, however, hamper cytological detection.

Prognosis and predictive factors
Clear cell adenocarcinoma may be treated by radical hysterectomy, vaginectomy and lymphadenectomy or by external beam or local radiotherapy. The tumour spreads primarily by local invasion and lymphatic metastases and has a recurrence rate of 25%. The incidence of lymph node disease increases dramatically with tumour invasion beyond 3 mm in depth. Lymph node metastases occur in 16% of patients with stage I disease and 50% of those with stage II disease. Haematogenous metastasis to distant organs occurs mainly to the lungs. The 5-year survival of patients with tumours of all stages is approximately 80% and is close to 100% for patients with stage I tumours. Most recurrences occur within 3 years. Long disease-free intervals of more than 20 years have been observed. Factors associated with a favourable prognosis are: low stage, small tumour size, a tubulocystic pattern, low mitotic activity and mild nuclear atypia.

Adenosis

Definition
Adenosis is the presence of glandular epithelium in the vagina and is thought to be the result of the persistence of embryonic müllerian epithelium.

Epidemiology
Adenosis has been reported to occur in approximately 30% of women after in utero exposure to DES. Congenital adenosis may be present in up to 8% of unexposed women. Adenosis has been described after laser vaporization or intravaginal application of 5-fluorouracil {730}.

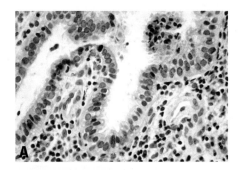
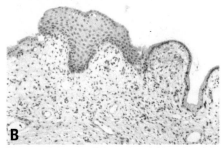

Fig. 6.14 Adenosis of the vagina. **A** Note the tubo-endometrioid type glands. **B** On the surface within adenosis is a focus of squamous metaplasia .

Localization
The most frequent site of involvement is the anterior upper third of the vagina.

Clinical features
Signs and symptoms
Adenosis is usually asymptomatic. Some women present with a mucous discharge, bleeding or dyspareunia.. Adenosis may spontaneously regress at the surface and be replaced by metaplastic squamous epithelium, particularly with increasing age. Because of the risk of development of clear cell adenocarcinoma within the vaginal wall, palpation, colposcopic examination and cytological smears are necessary to monitor patients with adenosis.

Colposcopy
Areas of adenosis and associated squamous metaplasia may be visible colposcopically and by iodine staining {2046}. Adenosis may be occult or may present as cysts or as a diffusely red granular area.

Cytology
Cytology can be helpful in the diagnostic evaluation of DES-exposed women (see below). It may serve a dual purpose, as a means for detection of adenocarcinoma or as a follow-up procedure after treatment of the lesion.

Fig. 6.15 Submucosal atypical adenosis of the vagina. Note the nuclear enlargement and atypia in the glands.

Adenosis can be detected on cytological examination by the finding of columnar or metaplastic squamous cells in scrapes of the middle and upper third of the vagina. However, similar findings may occur in non-DES-exposed women as a result of contamination of the vaginal specimen by columnar or metaplastic squamous cells from the cervix.

Histopathology
Adenosis is characterized by the presence in the vagina of columnar epithelium resembling mucinous epithelium of the endocervix (mucinous type) and/or the endometrium or the fallopian tube (tuboendometrial type). Adenosis may be found on the surface or deeper in the stroma. Mixtures of the various types of adenosis may be encountered. Squamous metaplasia may occur as a result of healing.

Atypical adenosis

Definition
Atypical adenosis is the presence of atypical glandular epithelium in the vagina. It is reported to be a precursor lesion of clear cell adenocarcinoma.

Histopathology
Atypical adenosis occurs in the tuboendometrial type of adenosis and is a fre-

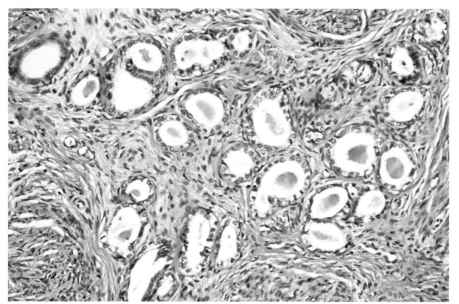

Fig. 6.16 Mesonephric remnants. The wall of the vagina contains clusters of uniform dilated tubules with luminal hyaline material.

quent finding immediately adjacent to clear cell adenocarcinoma. The atypical glands tend to be more complex than those of mucinous adenosis and are lined by cells with enlarged, atypical, pleomorphic, hyperchromatic nuclei that contain prominent nucleoli. Mitotic figures are infrequent, and hobnail cells may be present.

Differential diagnosis
A distinction from clear cell adenocarcinoma may be difficult if the atypical adenosis shows a pseudoinfiltrative pattern of small glands. Conversely, clear cell adenocarcinoma displaying a tubulocystic pattern may be erroneously interpreted as adenosis. However, unlike tubulocystic clear cell adenocarcinoma with bland flattened cells, atypical adenosis is composed of cuboidal or columnar epithelium.

Prognosis and predictive factors
Management may be local excision or follow-up {2609}.

Endometrioid adenocarcinoma

Only a few primary endometrioid adenocarcinomas of the vagina have been reported. The histological appearance resembles that of the much more common endometrioid adenocarcinoma of the endometrium. A few cases have been described in association with adenosis as well as cases arising in vaginal endometriosis {1155,3251}.

Mucinous adenocarcinoma

Primary mucinous adenocarcinoma of the vagina is rare. Only a few cases have been reported {745}. Like the other non-clear cell adenocarcinomas of the vagina, this type of tumour is predominantely reported in peri-menopausal women. Histologically, the tumour may resemble typical endocervical or intestinal adenocarcinomas of the cervix {909}. Due to its rarity, little is known about its aetiology and behaviour. A relationship to vaginal adenosis has been described {3168}, suggesting a müllerian origin. An unusual variant of mucinous adenocarcinoma has been described in neovaginas {1218,1941}.

Mesonephric adenocarcinoma

Mesonephric (Gartner) duct remnants are mostly situated deep in the lateral walls of the vagina. Only a few cases of carcinoma arising from mesonephric remnants in the vagina have been reported, and none since 1973. These tumours are composed of well-formed tubules lined by atypical, mitotically-active, cuboidal to columnar epithelium that resemble mesonephric duct remnants. Unlike clear cell adenocarcinoma, mesonephric carcinoma does not contain clear or hobnail cells, intracellular mucin or glycogen, and the tubules are often surrounded by a basement membrane.

Müllerian papilloma

Müllerian papilloma may arise in the vagina of infants and young women {2977} (see also chapter on the cervix). A few examples have arisen in the wall of the vagina {1817}. Occasional local recurrences have been reported {1719}, and in one instance repeated removal of recurrent müllerian papillomas was necessary {708}. The origin of the tumour is not clear, although reports support a müllerian origin {1719}.

Tubular, tubulovillous and villous adenoma

Definition
Benign glandular tumours with enteric differentiation {494}.

Clinical features
Patients may be premenopausal or postmenopausal. Clinical examination may reveal a polypoid mass.

Histopathology
The adenomas are histologically similar to colonic types and have been subclassified as tubular, tubulovillous or villous. The epithelium is stratified and contains columnar cells with mucin. The nuclei are oval to elongated and dysplastic. Adenocarcinoma arising from a vaginal adenoma has been reported {1935}.

Differential diagnosis
Aside from endometriosis and prolapsed fallopian tube, the most important lesions in the differential diagnosis are metastatic carcinoma and extension or recurrence of endometrial or endocervical adenocarcinoma. An adenoma is generally polypoid and lacks invasive borders, marked architectural complexity or high grade cytological features.

Uncommon epithelial tumours

Definition
Primary epithelial tumours of the vagina other than those of squamous or glandular type. These tumours are described in more detail in the chapter on the cervix.

ICD-O codes

Adenosquamous carcinoma	8560/3
Adenoid cystic carcinoma	8200/3
Adenoid basal carcinoma	8098/3
Carcinoid	8240/3
Small cell carcinoma	8041/3
Undifferentiated carcinoma	8020/3

Adenosquamous carcinoma

A carcinoma composed of a mixture of malignant glandular and squamous epithelial elements {2360}.

Adenoid cystic carcinoma

An adenocarcinoma which resembles adenoid cystic carcinoma of salivary gland origin but usually lacks the myoepithelial cell component of the latter {2781}.

Adenoid basal carcinoma

A carcinoma with rounded, generally well differentiated nests of basaloid cells showing focal gland formation; central squamous differentiation may be present as well {1906,1986}.

Carcinoid

A tumour resembling carcinoids of the gastrointestinal tract and lung {936}.

Small cell carcinoma

A carcinoma of neuroendocrine type that resembles small cell carcinomas of the lung {1371,1869,1877,2281}.

Undifferentiated carcinoma

A carcinoma that is not of the small cell type and lacks evidence of glandular, squamous, neuroendocrine or other types of differentiation.

Mesenchymal tumours

Vaginal sarcomas

Definition
Malignant mesenchymal tumours that arise in the vagina.

ICD-O codes
Sarcoma botryoides	8910/3
Leiomyosarcoma	8890/3
Endometrioid stromal sarcoma, low grade	8931/3
Undifferentiated vaginal sarcoma	8805/3

Epidemiology
Sarcomas are rare and comprise <2% of all malignant vaginal neoplasms {633}.

Aetiology
There are virtually no clues to the pathogenesis of this group of tumours.

Clinical features
Signs and symptoms
Malignant tumours usually present with bleeding and/or discharge and a mass and are usually readily detected by clinical examination. Occasional cases are detected by an abnormal cytological examination. Some sarcomas, however, are asymptomatic, and the diagnosis is, therefore, delayed.

Imaging
The extent of tumour spread may be determined by transvaginal ultrasound.

Tumour spread and staging
Vaginal sarcomas spread by direct extension and by metastasis; the latter occurs both by lymphatic and haematogenous routes. The tumour initially grows into the vaginal wall and soft tissue of the pelvis, bladder or rectum. The staging of vaginal sarcomas in adults utilizes the TNM/FIGO classification {51,2976}.

Sarcoma botryoides

Definition
A malignant mesenchymal tumour composed of small, round or oval to spindle-

shaped cells, some of which show evidence of striated muscle differentiation.

Synonym
Embryonal rhabdomyosarcoma.

Epidemiology
Sarcoma botryoides (Greek bothryos: grapes) is the most common vaginal sarcoma and occurs almost exclusively in children and infants <5 years of age (mean 1.8 years) {633}, although occasional cases are encountered in young adults or even postmenopausal women. At least two cases of sarcoma botryoides have been described in pregnancy {2709}.

Clinical features
These tumours present typically as a vaginal mass that on clinical and macroscopic examination appears soft, oedematous and nodular, papillary, polypoid or grape-like, often protruding through the introitus.

Macroscopy
The tumours vary from 0.2-12 cm in maximum dimension and may be covered by an intact mucosa or be ulcerated and bleeding. The sectioned surface displays grey to red areas of myxomatous change and haemorrhage.

Tumour spread and staging
In children the Intergroup Rhabdomyosarcoma Study group clinical classi-

fication is used, which is based on the combined features of extent of disease, resectability and histological evaluation of margins of excision {99}.

Histopathology
The neoplasm is composed of cells with round to oval or spindle-shaped nuclei and eosinophilic cytoplasm that may show differentiation towards striated muscle cells. Typically, there is a dense cambium layer composed of closely packed cells with small hyperchromatic nuclei immediately subjacent to the squamous epithelium that may be invaded. The nuclei have an open chromatin pattern and inconspicuous nucleoli. The central portion of the polypoid mass is typically hypocellular, oedematous or myxomatous. The mitotic rate is high. Rhabdo-myoblasts (strap cells), which may be sparse, may be found in any of the patterns. Their recognition may be facilitated by immunohistochemical staining with antibodies directed against actin, desmin or myoglobin. Although the first two antibodies are more sensitive than myoglobin, they are not specific for skeletal muscle differentiation. Ultrastructural examination may reveal characteristic features of rhabdomyoblastic differentiation, such as thick and thin filaments with Z-band material.

Differential diagnosis
The distinction from a benign fibroepithelial polyp with bizarre nuclei is important.

Table 6.02
Clinical classification of vaginal sarcoma botyroides / rhabdomyosarcoma {99}.

I	Complete surgical resection
IIa	Excision, margin positive
IIb	Excision, lymph nodes positive
IIIa	Biopsy only
IIIb	Partial surgical excision (gross disease present)
IV	Metastatic disease

302 Tumours of the vagina

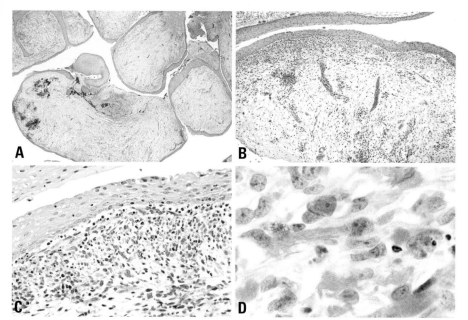

Fig. 6.17 Sarcoma botryoides. **A** Polypoid masses of tumour are covered by squamous epithelium. **B** A subepithelial cambium layer overlies oedematous tissue. **C** Higher magnification of the cellular subepithelial cambium layer. **D** The positive immunostain for desmin confirms the myoblastic differentiation. Note the nuclear pleomorphism.

The clinical setting, the characteristic low power appearance, the absence of a cambium layer and striated cells and a typically low mitotic index establish the correct diagnosis of a fibroepithelial polyp {2055,2067,2141}.

Genetic susceptibility
One instance of sarcoma botryoides has been reported in a child with multiple congenital abnormalities and bilateral nephroblastomas suggesting a possible genetic defect {1965}.

Prognosis and predictive factors
The prognosis of sarcoma botryoides in the past was poor, but an 85% 3-year survival rate has recently been achieved with wide local excision and combination chemotherapy. Second malignancies in long-term survivors of vaginal embryonal rhabdomyosarcoma have not been reported to date.

Leiomyosarcoma

Definition
A malignant tumour composed of smooth muscle cells.

Epidemiology
Although leiomyosarcoma is the most common vaginal sarcoma in the adult and the second most common vaginal sarcoma, only approximately 50 cases have been reported {599}. They accounted for only 5 of 60 cases in the only large series of vaginal smooth muscle tumours {2879}.

Macroscopy
Macroscopically, they are sometimes multilobulated and form masses from 3-5 cm. The sectioned surface has a pink-grey, "fish-flesh" appearance with scattered foci of haemorrhage, myxoid change or necrosis. The overlying mucosa may be ulcerated.

Histopathology
Histologically, they are identical to their counterparts elsewhere. It may be difficult to predict the behaviour of some smooth muscle tumours. Currently, it is recommended that vaginal smooth muscle tumours that are larger than 3 cm in diameter and have 5 or more mitoses per 10 high-power fields, moderate or marked cytological atypia and infiltrating margins be regarded as leiomyosarcoma {2879}. An epithelioid variant with a myxoid stroma has also been described {456}. As in the uterus, occasional sarcomas arise from leiomyomas {1682}.

Differential diagnosis
Leiomyosarcomas should be differentiated from the benign condition of post-operative spindle cell nodule {2861}. The latter is a localized non-neoplastic lesion composed of closely packed spindle-shaped cells and capillaries occurring several weeks to several months postoperatively in the region of an excision. It may closely resemble a leiomyosarcoma, but the history of a recent operation at the same site facilitates its diagnosis.

Prognosis and predictive factors
Leiomyosarcomas are treated primarily by radical surgical excision (vaginectomy, hysterectomy and pelvic lymphadenectomy). In the only large series of 60 smooth muscle tumours, both benign and malignant, only 5 neoplasms recurred, and in one of these, a tumour with an infiltrative margin, the patient died of lung metastases {2879}.

Endometrioid stromal sarcoma, low grade

Definition
A sarcoma with an infiltrating pattern that in its well differentiated form resembles normal endometrial stromal cells.

Histopathology
Low grade endometrioid stromal sarcomas have been rarely encountered in the vagina and resemble their counterparts in the endometrium. In two cases the tumours appear to have arisen from endometriosis {245}. Before concluding that such a neoplasm is primary in the vagina, an origin within the uterus should be excluded {633,1051,2226}. The term undifferentiated vaginal sarcoma is preferred for the high grade lesions.

Undifferentiated vaginal sarcoma

Definition
A sarcoma with an infiltrating pattern composed of small spindle-shaped cells lacking specific features.

Histopathology
Undifferentiated vaginal sarcomas are rare, polypoid or diffusely infiltrating lesions. Spindle to stellate cells with scanty cytoplasm are arranged in sheet-like, fascicular or storiform patterns. The cells exhibit various degrees of nuclear pleomorphism and hyperchromasia. The mitotic index is ≥10 per 10 high power fields.

Prognosis and predicitive factors

Death from recurrent or metastatic tumour has occurred within 2 years of treatment in about 50% of patients {20, 3236}.

Rare malignant mesenchymal tumours

Rare examples of malignant schwannoma {633}, fibrosarcoma {2160}, malignant fibrous histiocytoma {3078}, angiosarcoma {1804,2298,2931}, alveolar soft part sarcoma {402}, synovial sarcoma {2095}, malignant peripheral nerve sheath tumour {2226} and unclassifiable sarcoma {633} have all been described in the vagina, but they do not exhibit unique clinical or morphological features.

Benign mesenchymal neoplasms

Of the benign tumours only leiomyomas are relatively common.

ICD-O codes

Leiomyoma	8890/0
Genital rhabdomyoma	8905/0
Deep angiomyxoma	8841/1

Clinical features

Most benign tumours are asymptomatic, but depending on their size and position they may cause pain, bleeding, dyspareunia and urinary or rectal symptoms.

Leiomyoma

Definition

A benign neoplasm composed of smooth muscle cells having a variable amount of fibrous stroma.

Epidemiology

Approximately 300 cases of vaginal leiomyoma have been reported. Although the age at presentation ranges from 19-72 years, they typically occur during reproductive life (mean age 44 years) {2879}. Leiomyomas of the vagina are not related to those of the uterus, either in frequency or in racial distribution, the White to Black ratio for uterine and vaginal leiomyomas being 1:3 and 4:1 respectively {222}.

Aetiology

There are virtually no clues to the pathogenesis of this group of tumours. Rare leiomyomas may recur in one or more pregnancies suggesting hormone dependency {2501}.

Histopathology

Vaginal leiomyomas resemble their uterine counterparts. A case of bizarre (symplastic) leiomyoma has been described {264}.

Histogenesis

The histogenesis of smooth muscle tumours is not clear, but myoepithelial cells such as are found in smooth muscle cells of venules or of the vaginal muscularis and myofibroblasts have all been implicated.

Prognosis and predictive factors

Nearly all are treated by local excision {1682,2486,2523}. An occasional tumour, especially if large, may recur {685,1682}.

Genital rhabdomyoma

Definition

An uncommon benign tumour of the lower female genital tract showing skeletal muscle differentiation.

Epidemiology

About 20 cases have been reported {1313,2812}.

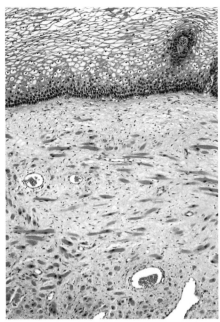

Fig. 6.18 Genital rhabdomyoma. The tumour is composed of individual mature rhabdomyoblasts separated by abundant connective tissue stroma.

Clinical features

These tumours occur in middle age women (range 30-48 years) and present as a well defined, solitary mass with the clinical appearance of a benign vaginal polyp {1397}.

Macroscopy

Genital rhabdomyomas are solitary, nodular or polypoid, ranging in size from

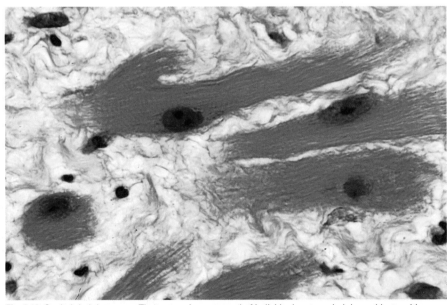

Fig. 6.19 Genital rhabdomyoma. The tumour is composed of individual mature rhabdomyoblasts with cross striations in the cytoplasm and bland nuclei without mitotic activity.

1-11 cm. They may arise anywhere in the vagina, and some protrude into the lumen. The overlying mucosa is usually intact since the tumour arises in the wall. The texture is rubbery and the sectioned surface is grey and glassy.

Histopathology
They are composed of mature, bland rhabdomyoblasts that are oval or strap-shaped with obvious cross striations in the cytoplasm. Mitotic activity and nuclear pleomorphism are absent. Abundant connective tissue stroma surrounds individual muscle cells. Rhabdo-myoma should not be confused with sarcoma botryoides.

Prognosis and predictive factors
No recurrences have been reported after complete local excision.

Deep angiomyxoma

Definition
A locally infiltrative tumour with a predilection for the pelvic and perineal regions and a tendency for local recurrence composed of fibroblasts, myofibroblasts and numerous, characteristically thick-walled, blood vessels embedded in an abundant myxoid matrix.

Synonym
Aggressive angiomyxoma.

Clinical features
Most patients present with a large, slowly growing, painless mass in the pelviperineal region that may give rise to pressure effects on the adjacent urogenital or anorectal tracts. Imaging studies often show the mass to be substantially larger than clinically suspected.

Macroscopy
Macroscopically, the tumour is lobulated but poorly circumscribed due to finger-like extensions into the surrounding tissue. The neoplasm is grey-pink or red-tan and rubbery or gelatinous.

Tumour spread and staging
Deep angiomyxoma is a locally infiltrative but non-metastasizing neoplasm that occurs for the most part during the reproductive years. At least two cases have been reported within the vagina, an uncommon site for this neoplasm {81, 496}.

Histopathology
The tumour is of low to moderate cellularity and is composed of small, uniform, spindle-shaped to stellate cells with poorly defined, pale eosinophilic cytoplasm and bland, often vesicular nuclei. An abundant myxoid matrix contains a variable number of rounded, medium-sized to large vessels that possess thickened focally hyalinized walls. A characteristic feature is the presence of loosely organized islands of myoid cells around the larger nerve segments and vessels {3086}. The neoplasm is positive for desmin in almost all cases, whereas stains for S-100 protein are consistently negative {1431,2082}.

Prognosis and predictive factors
The treatment for this locally aggressive but non-metastasizing neoplasm is primarily surgical with close attention to margins. Approximately 30% of tumours recur locally.

Postoperative spindle cell nodule

Definition
A non-neoplastic localized lesion composed of closely packed proliferating spindle cells and capillaries simulating a leiomyosarcoma.

Clinical features
The lesion develops at the site of a recent operation several weeks to several months postoperatively {2861}.

Histopathology
The lesion is composed of closely packed, mitotically active, spindle-shaped mesenchymal cells and capillaries often with an accompaniment of inflammatory cells.

Differential diagnosis
The history of a recent operation at the same site serves to distinguish this lesion from leiomyosarcoma. Postoperative spindle cell nodule may closely resemble a leiomyosarcoma or other spindle cell sarcoma, but the history of a recent operation at the same site facilitates its diagnosis.

Mixed epithelial and mesenchymal tumours

S.G. Silverberg

Definition
Tumours in which both an epithelial and a mesenchymal component can be histologically identified as integral neoplastic components.

ICD-O codes
Carcinosarcoma	8980/3
Adenosarcoma	8933/3
Malignant mixed tumour	8940/3
Benign mixed tumour	8940/0

Epidemiology
These mixed tumours are among the rarest of vaginal primary tumours, which are themselves uncommon primary tumours of the female genital tract. No mixed tumours were found among 753 primary vaginal tumours compiled from ten reports in the literature {2714}. The U.S. National Cancer Data Base Report on Cancer of the Vagina {577} includes only 25 "complex mixed or stromal tumours" among 4,885 submitted cases of vaginal cancer. As expected, there are no epidemiological data available on mixed tumours {2226}.

Aetiology
The aetiology of the tumours in this group that are more often primary in the endometrium, i.e. carcinosarcoma and adenosarcoma is discussed in the chapter on the uterine corpus of this publication. The aetiology of vaginal malignant mixed tumour is essentially unknown.

Carcinosarcoma

Definition
A tumour with malignant epithelial and mesenchymal components. Before the diagnosis of a primary vaginal tumour is made, extension from elsewhere in the female genital tract must be excluded.

Synonyms
Malignant müllerian mixed tumour, malignant mesodermal mixed tumour, metaplastic carcinoma.

Clinical features
These tumours present clinically as a palpable vaginal mass. Carcinosarcomas usually bleed and may occur years after therapeutic irradiation for some

other lesion {2226,2714}. Imaging studies have not been reported for any of these lesions.

Macroscopy
Carcinosarcomas in their rare primary vaginal manifestations are identical in macroscopic appearance to their far more common endometrial counterparts. Although primary vaginal tumours of this sort are exophytic lesions, carcinosarcomas are more likely to be metastases from the endometrium or elsewhere in the female genital tract and may be deeper in the wall.

Tumour spread and staging
Staging and spread of these malignant tumours are identical to those of primary vaginal carcinomas {2714}

Histopathology
Primary vaginal carcinosarcoma is histologically identical to its endometrial counterpart. A vaginal metastasis from an endometrial or other primary carcinosarcoma may contain only the carcinomatous or rarely the sarcomatous component {1388,2692}.

Prognosis and predictive factors
Most women with primary vaginal carcinosarcomas have rapidly developed metastases and died.

Adenosarcoma

Definition
A mixed tumour composed of a benign or atypical epithelial component of müllerian type and a malignant appearing mesenchymal component.

Clinical features
Adenosarcoma presents clinically as a palpable vaginal mass.

Macroscopy
Although primary vaginal adenosarcoma is typically an exophytic lesion, adenosarcomas are more likely to be metastases from the endometrium or

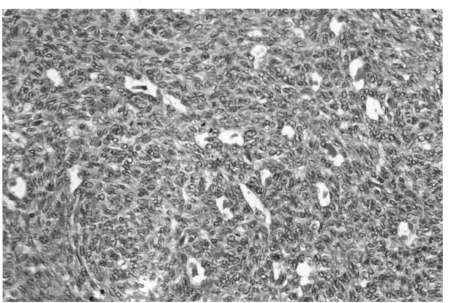

Fig. 6.20 Malignant mixed tumour of the vagina. The cellular tumour is composed of sheets of oval to spindle-shaped cells with occasional gland-like formations and mitotic figures.

elsewhere in the female genital tract and may be deeper in the wall.

Histopathology
Primary vaginal adenosarcoma is histologically identical to its endometrial counterpart. Metastatic adenosarcoma generally consists of the sarcoma alone {2692}

Prognosis and predictive factors
Adenosarcomas of the vagina are not reported in enough numbers or detail to establish their prognosis.

Malignant mixed tumour resembling synovial sarcoma

Definition
An extremely rare biphasic malignant tumour resembling synovial sarcoma and containing gland-like structures lined by flattened epithelial-appearing cells and a highly cellular mesenchymal component. There is no evidence of müllerian differentiation.

Clinical features
The two reported cases of mixed tumour resembling synovial sarcoma presented as polypoid masses in the lateral fornix in women of ages 24 and 33.

Histopathology
The mixed tumour resembling synovial sarcoma, as its name suggests, is composed of gland-like structures lined by round to flattened epithelial-appearing cells embedded in a spindle cell matrix. In one reported case electron microscopic study suggested synovial-like differentiation {2095}, whilst in another, a possible origin from mesonephric rests was proposed {2652}.

Prognosis and predictive factors
Follow-up was too short to establish the clinical malignancy and survival rates of the two malignant mixed tumours resembling synovial sarcoma reported in the literature.

Benign mixed tumour

Definition
A well circumscribed benign tumour histologically resembling the mixed tumour of salivary glands with a predominant mesenchymal-appearing component and epithelial cells of squamous or glandular type.

Synonym
Spindle cell epithelioma.

Clinical features
The benign mixed tumour is usually asymptomatic, typically is a well-demarcated submucosal mass and has a predilection for the hymenal region {335, 2714}.
It tends to occur in young to middle-aged women, with a mean age of 40.5 in the largest series reported {335}.

Macroscopy
Benign mixed tumours are circumscribed, grey to white, soft to rubbery masses, usually measuring from 1-6 cm {335,2714}

Histopathology
The spindle cell component predominates histologically and lacks atypia or significant mitotic activity. Randomly interspersed are nests of benign-appearing squamous cells and, less frequently, glands lined by low cuboidal to columnar epithelium commonly demonstrating squamous metaplasia. Hyaline globular aggregates of stromal matrix are also frequently seen.

Immunoprofile
In an immunohistochemical study of a large series of cases, the spindle cells were strongly keratin-immunoreactive in 90% cases {335}. They showed only minimal expression for smooth muscle actin and were uniformly negative for S-100 protein, glial fibrillary acidic protein and factor VIII-related antigen {335,2717}. The tumours coexpressed CD34, CD99 and Bcl-2 {2717}.

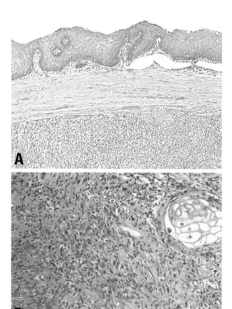

Fig. 6.21 Benign mixed tumour. **A** Low power magnification shows circumscription without involvement of the overlying squamous epithelium. **B** Note the squamous nest within a spindle cell proliferation.

Histogenesis
The only benign vaginal tumour classically designated as a mixed tumour because of its histological resemblance to the benign mixed tumour (pleomorphic adenoma) of salivary glands has been renamed spindle cell epithelioma because of immunohistochemical and ultrastructural evidence suggesting purely epithelial differentiation {335}.
Unlike mixed tumours of salivary glands, these vaginal tumours show no immunohistochemical or ultrastructural features of myoepithelial cells {2717}. Origin from a primitive/progenitor cell population has been postulated {2717}.

Prognosis and predictive factors
The benign mixed tumour has never metastasized in reports of over forty cases; however, local recurrences have been noted.

Melanotic, neuroectodermal, lymphoid and secondary tumours

R. Vang
F.A. Tavassoli
E.S. Andersen

Melanocytic tumours

Definition
A tumour composed of melanocytes, either benign or malignant.

ICD-O codes
Malignant melanoma	8720/3
Blue naevus	8780/0
Melanocytic naevus	8720/0

Malignant melanoma

Definition
A tumour composed of malignant melanocytes.

Epidemiology
Malignant melanoma is a rare but very aggressive tumour of the vagina. Patients have an average age of 60 years and most are White {492}.

Clinical features
They typically present with vaginal bleeding, and some may have inguinal lymphadenopathy. The more common loca-

tions are in the lower third of the vagina and on the anterior vaginal wall.

Macroscopy
The lesions are pigmented and usually 2-3 cm in size.

Histopathology
The lesions are invasive and may display ulceration. Most have a lentiginous growth pattern, but junctional nests can be seen. In-situ or pagetoid growth is not typical. The cells are epithelioid or spindle-shaped and may contain melanin pigment. There is brisk mitotic activity. Tumour cells express S-100 protein, melan A and HMB-45.

Differential diagnosis
As "atypical" or dysplastic melanocytic lesions of the vagina have not been evaluated, histological separation of "borderline" melanocytic lesions from melanoma is not always possible. Nests of epithelioid cells raise the possibility of a poorly differentiated carcinoma. Spindle cell differentiation may create confusion with sarcomas.

Prognostic and predictive factors
Clinical criteria
Patients have been treated by a combination of surgery, radiation and chemotherapy. The prognosis is poor with a 5-year survival rate of 21% and a mean survival time of 15 months {314}.

Histopathological criteria
Assessment of Clark levels, as is done for melanomas of skin, is not possible given the lack of normal cutaneous anatomical landmarks. Most tumours have a significant thickness, but even a thin melanoma does not necessarily portend a favourable prognosis. One study found that mitotic activity correlates better with the clinical outcome than the depth of invasion {314}.

Blue naevus

Definition
A proliferation of subepithelial dendritic melanocytes.

Clinical features
Though rare, both common and cellular variants of blue naevus have been reported in the vagina {2400,2929}. The common variant typically presents as a blue-black macule and the cellular variant as a nodule.

Histopathology
Classic blue naevi contain melanocytes with elongated dendritic processes and heavy cytoplasmic pigmentation. Cellular

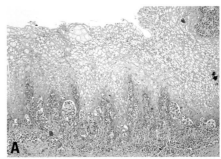
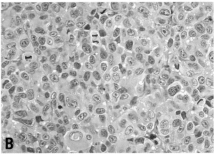
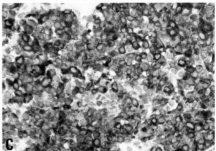

Fig. 6.23 Melanoma of the vagina. **A** Note the prominent junctional component. **B** The tumour cells are epithelioid with abundant eosinophilic cytoplasm, large pleomorphic nuclei, prominent nucleoli, intranuclear inclusions and mitotic figures. **C** Immunostain shows diffuse, strong expression for melan A.

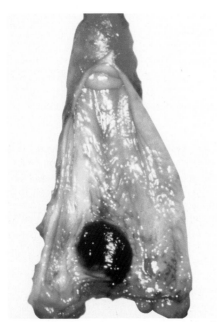

Fig. 6.22 Melanoma of the lower anterior vaginal wall. Note the large, polypoid heavily pigmented tumour.

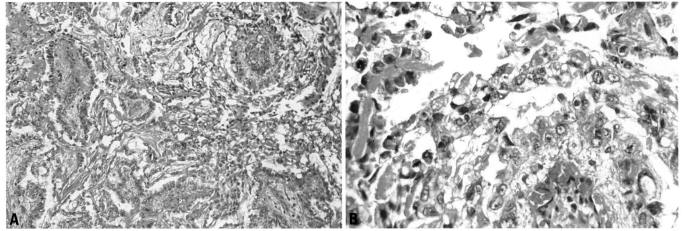

Fig. 6.24 Yolk sac tumour. **A** The tumour has a labryinthine pattern with occasional Schiller-Duvall bodies. **B** Papillary cores and labryinthine structures are lined by primitive cuboidal cells with cytoplasmic vacuolization and rare hyaline globules.

variants have a biphasic composition with areas similar to common blue naevus admixed with round nodules. The cells are arranged in nests and short fascicles with a whorled pattern and are plump and spindle-shaped with oval bland nuclei and pale cytoplasm.

Differential diagnosis

The common variant should not pose a diagnostic problem. The cellular variant may cause confusion with melanoma and smooth muscle tumours. Nuclear atypia and numerous mitotic figures would favour melanoma. Well defined interlacing fascicles, large thick-walled blood vessels, immunohistochemical positivity for muscle markers and negativity for S-100 protein should assist in making the diagnosis of a smooth muscle tumour.

Melanocytic naevus

Definition

Melanocytic nevi are defined as proliferation of nests of naevus cells.

Clinical features

Melanocytic nevi of the vagina are thought to be similar to their counterparts in the skin {1539}.

Yolk sac tumour

Definition

A primitive malignant germ cell tumour characterized by a variety of distinctive histological patterns, some of which recapitulate phases in the development of the normal yolk sac.

ICD-O code 9071/3

Synonym

Endodermal sinus tumour.

Clinical features

Patients are usually under 3 years of age. Vaginal bleeding and discharge are the most common symptoms. Serum levels of alpha-fetoprotein may be elevated. A polypoid friable mass is seen on clinical examination with a mean size of 3 cm.

Histopathology

Vaginal cases resemble their ovarian counterparts.

Differential diagnosis

Although sarcoma botryoides may be simulated clinically, the histological features resolve any confusion. Clear cell and endometrioid carcinomas may create difficulty in histological separation.

Prognosis and predictive factors

Combined surgery and chemotherapy may provide a favourable outcome. A disease-free survival of up to 23 years is possible {557}.

Peripheral primitive neuroectodermal tumour / Ewing tumour

Definition

Tumours of uncertain lineage within the small round blue cell family of tumours.

ICD-O code

Peripheral primitive
   neuroectodermal tumour / 9364/3

Ewing tumour 9260/3

Clinical features

Peripheral primitive neuroectodermal tumour/Ewing tumour (PNET/ET) is rare within the vagina {3002}. A reported case occurred in a 35-year-old woman who presented with a vaginal mass.

Histopathology

Histological features are similar to PNET/ET in non-vaginal sites. Typically, PNET/ET grows as a diffuse sheet of uniform small cells with scant pale cytoplasm and an intermediate to high nuclear to cytoplasmic ratio. The nuclei are round with evenly dispersed chromatin. Mitotic figures may be numerous, and rosettes may be seen.

Immunoprofile

Expression of CD99 would be expected in almost all cases.

Differential diagnosis

PNET/ET should not be mistaken for rhabdomyosarcoma, non-Hodgkin lymphoma (NHL), melanoma, small cell carcinoma or endometrial stromal sarcoma because of differences in prognosis and treatment. A broad immunohistochemical panel and, if need be, molecular studies, performed on paraffin-embedded tissue should assist in making the correct diagnosis.

Molecular genetics

Identification of the *EWS/FLI1* fusion transcript derived from the t(11;22)(q24;q12) chromosomal translocation by the

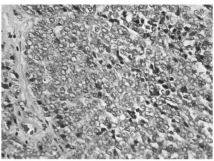

Fig. 6.25 Peripheral primitive neuroectodermal tumour. Note the sheets of small to medium sized cells with round, pale nuclei, minimal cytoplasm and high nuclear to cytoplasmic ratios.

reverse transcriptase-polymerase chain reaction and Southern blot hybridization would confirm the diagnosis.

Prognosis and predictive factors
The experience with PNET/ET of the vagina is limited, but patients with localized tumours in soft tissue sites can potentially be cured with a combination of surgery, chemotherapy and radiation therapy.

Dermoid cyst

Definition
A cystic tumour composed of more than one germ cell layer in which all elements are mature.

ICD-O code
Dermoid cyst   9084/0
Mature cystic teratoma   9080/0

Synonym
Mature cystic teratoma.

Macroscopy and histopathology
These resemble the same tumour in the ovary.

Adenomatoid tumour

ICD-O code   9054/0

A single case occurring in a 47-year-old woman has been reported {1697}.

Lymphoid and haematopoetic tumours

Definition
Tumours of the lymphoid and haematopoetic systems as well as secondary tumours of the vagina.

Lymphoma

Definition
Tumours with lymphoid differentiation arising as either primary (localized) or secondary (disseminated) disease.

Clinical features
Lymphomas of the vagina are predominantly of the non-Hodgkin's type {3001}. Patients with primary NHL have a mean age of 42 years, usually present with vaginal bleeding and have a mass on clinical examination. Patients with secondary NHL have a mean age of 65 years, present with vaginal bleeding and usually have a history of NHL.

Histopathology
Almost all NHLs primary in the vagina are diffuse large B-cell lymphomas

Table 6.03
Immunohistochemical and cytogenetic profile of various small cell tumours of the vagina.*

Immunohistochemical or molecular markers	Peripheral primitive neuroectodermal tumour/Ewing tumour	Rhabdomyosarcoma	B-cell non-Hodgkin lymphoma	Melanoma	Small cell carcinoma	Endometrial stromal sarcoma
Cytokeratin	+/-	+/-	-	-	+	+/-
Muscle specific actin/ desmin	-	+	-	-	-	+/-
Chromogranin/ synaptophysin	+/-	-	-	-	+/-	-
S-100 protein	+/-	-	-	+	-	-
HMB-45	-	-	-	+	-	-
Leukocyte common antigen/ CD20	-	-	+	-	-	-
CD10	-	-	+/-	-	-	+
CD99	+	+/-	+/-	-	-	-
t(11;22)	+	-	-	-	-	-
t(2;13)/ t(1;13)	-	+/-	-	-	-	-
Monoclonal immunoglobulin heavy chain gene rearrangement	-	-	+/-	-	-	-

Key: +/-, variable rate of positivity; *, Not all markers have been thoroughly tested for each tumour, but expected results are listed.

growing in sheets. Some may have sclerosis. The neoplastic cells are large with round nuclei, vesicular chromatin and nucleoli. Secondary cases are usually diffuse large B-cell lymphomas and are histologically similar to the primary cases.

Immunoprofile
Almost all NHLs of the vagina (primary or secondary) are of B-cell lineage and typically express CD20.

Differential diagnosis
The main lesions in the differential diagnosis of NHL include granulocytic sarcoma and other haematological malignancies, carcinoma, melanoma and small round blue cell tumours such as rhabdomyosarcoma. Knowledge of the age, previous history of NHL or leukaemia, and the immunoprofile (keratin, CD20, CD3, CD43, myeloperoxidase, S-100 protein, desmin and other muscle markers) should help establish the correct diagnosis.

Somatic genetics
Southern blot analysis and polymerase chain reaction (PCR) can demonstrate monoclonal immunoglobulin heavy chain gene rearrangements in vaginal NHL. In-situ hybridization has not confirmed the presence of human papillomavirus DNA or Epstein-Barr virus (EBV) RNA {2999}; however, EBV DNA has been found by PCR {2718}.

Prognosis and predictive factors
Vaginal NHL is usually treated by chemotherapy and radiation. The determination of the Ann Arbor stage is prognostically important for vaginal NHL. Patients with low stage tumours (stages IE and IIE) have a longer disease-free survival than those with high-stage disease have (stages IIIE and IV).

Leukaemia

Definition
A malignant haematopoetic neoplasm that may be primary or secondary.

Synonym
Granulocytic sarcoma.

Epidemiology
Vaginal involvement by leukaemia may either be primary or secondary; however, the latter is much more common {428}.

Clinical features
Leukaemia of the vagina is rare but is usually of the myeloid type (granulocytic sarcoma or "chloroma") {2099}. Patients are elderly, have a mass on clinical examination and may have other evidence of acute myeloid leukaemia.

Histopathology
A series of primary granulocytic sarcomas of the female genital tract including 3 cases of the vagina was reported {2099}. Granulocytic sarcomas are usually composed of cells with finely dispersed nuclear chromatin and abundant cytoplasm that may be deeply eosinophilic. The identification of eosinophilic myelocytes is helpful in establishing the diagnosis; however, they are not always present. The tumours are positive for chloroacetate esterase.

Immunoprofile
Granulocytic sarcomas express lysozyme, myeloperoxidase, CD43 and CD68. Staining for CD45 may be seen, but the tumour cells are negative for CD20 and CD3.

Differential diagnosis
The most important differential diagnosis is malignant lymphoma. Enzyme histochemical stains for chloracetate esterase or immunohistochemical stains for myeleproxidase, CD68 and CD43 will establish the diagnosis in almost all cases {2099}.

Prognosis and predictive factors
Granulocytic sarcoma of the vagina appears to behave in an aggressive fashion. Although experience is limited, the few reported granulocytic sarcomas of the vagina have also been treated with chemotherapy or radiation.

Secondary tumours

Definition
Tumours of the vagina that originate outside the vagina.

Incidence and origin
Metastatic tumours are more frequent than primary malignant tumours of the vagina. Tumours may spread by direct extension, most commonly from the cervix or vulva, vascular and lymphatic dissemination or by implantation. Metastatic adenocarcinomas originate from the endometrium, colon, rectum and, more rarely, the breast. Transitional cell carcinoma metastatic from the urethra and the bladder and renal cell carcinomas have been reported. In the past vaginal metastases were reported in up to 50% of cases of uterine choriocarcinoma.

Clinical features
The primary tumour is often clinically evident or has previously been treated. The most significant symptom is abnormal vaginal bleeding. Vaginal cytology may aid detection. A biopsy is contraindicated in metastatic trophoblastic disease due to the risk of excessive bleeding.

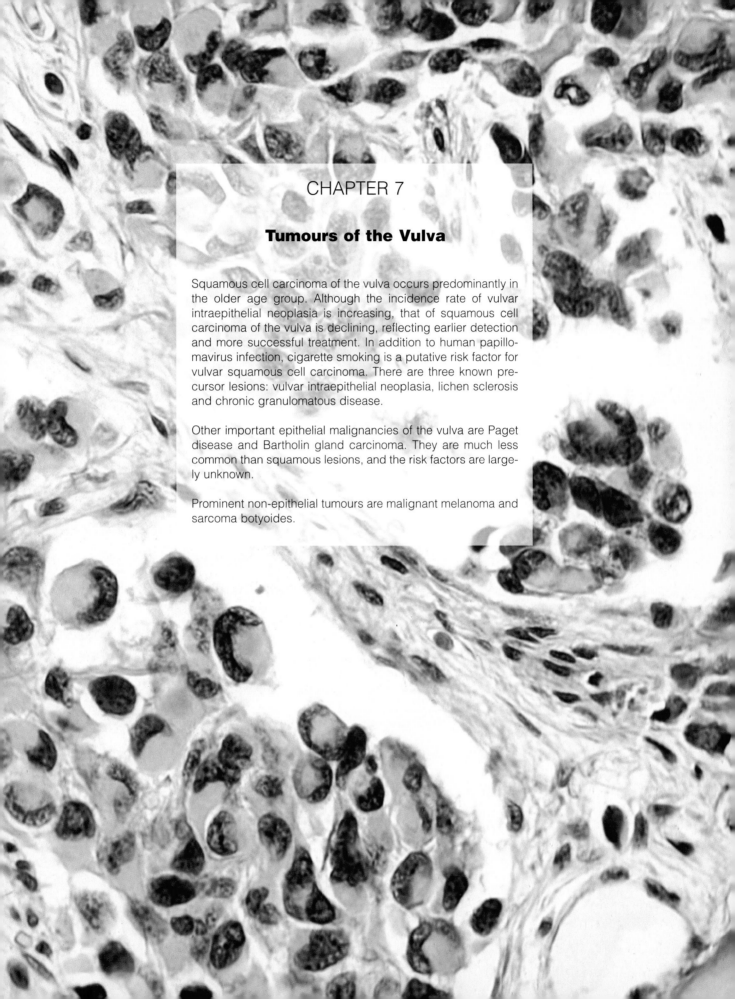

CHAPTER 7

Tumours of the Vulva

Squamous cell carcinoma of the vulva occurs predominantly in the older age group. Although the incidence rate of vulvar intraepithelial neoplasia is increasing, that of squamous cell carcinoma of the vulva is declining, reflecting earlier detection and more successful treatment. In addition to human papillomavirus infection, cigarette smoking is a putative risk factor for vulvar squamous cell carcinoma. There are three known precursor lesions: vulvar intraepithelial neoplasia, lichen sclerosis and chronic granulomatous disease.

Other important epithelial malignancies of the vulva are Paget disease and Bartholin gland carcinoma. They are much less common than squamous lesions, and the risk factors are largely unknown.

Prominent non-epithelial tumours are malignant melanoma and sarcoma botyoides.

WHO histological classification of tumours of the vulva

Epithelial tumours
Squamous and related tumours and precursors
    Squamous cell carcinoma, not otherwise specified   8070/3
        Keratinizing   8071/3
        Non-keratinizing   8072/3
        Basaloid   8083/3
        Warty   8051/3
        Verrucous   8051/3
        Keratoacanthoma-like
        Variant with tumour giant cells
        Others
    Basal cell carcinoma   8090/3
    Squamous intraepithelial neoplasia
        Vulvar intraepithelial neoplasia (VIN) 3 /   8077/2
        squamous cell carcinoma in situ   8070/2
    Benign squamous lesions
        Condyloma acuminatum
        Vestibular papilloma (micropapillomatosis)   8052/0
        Fibroepithelial polyp
        Seborrheic and inverted follicular keratosis
        Keratoacanthoma
Glandular tumours
    Paget disease   8542/3
    Bartholin gland tumours
        Adenocarcinoma   8140/3
        Squamous cell carcinoma   8070/3
        Adenoid cystic carcinoma   8200/3
        Adenosquamous carcinoma   8560/3
        Transitional cell carcinoma   8120/3
        Small cell carcinoma   8041/3
        Adenoma   8140/0
        Adenomyoma   8932/0
        Others
    Tumours arising from specialized anogenital
    mammary-like glands
        Adenocarcinoma of mammary gland type   8500/3
        Papillary hidradenoma   8405/0
        Others
    Adenocarcinoma of Skene gland origin   8140/3
    Adenocarcinomas of other types   8140/3
    Adenoma of minor vestibular glands   8140/0
    Mixed tumour of the vulva   8940/0

Tumours of skin appendage origin
    Malignant sweat gland tumours   8400/3
    Sebaceous carcinoma   8410/3
    Syringoma   8407/0
    Nodular hidradenoma   8402/0
    Trichoepithelioma   8100/0
    Trichilemmoma   8102/0
    Others

Soft tissue tumours
    Sarcoma botryoides   8910/3
    Leiomyosarcoma   8890/3
    Proximal epithelioid sarcoma   8804/3
    Alveolar soft part sarcoma   9581/3
    Liposarcoma   8850/3
    Dermatofibrosarcoma protuberans   8832/3
    Deep angiomyxoma   8841/1
    Superficial angiomyxoma   8841/0
    Angiomyofibroblastoma   8826/0
    Cellular angiofibroma   9160/0
    Leiomyoma   8890/0
    Granular cell tumour   9580/0
    Others

Melanocytic tumours
    Malignant melanoma   8720/3
    Congenital melanocytic naevus   8761/0
    Acquired melanocytic naevus   8720/0
    Blue naevus   8780/0
    Atypical melanocytic naevus of the genital type   8720/0
    Dysplastic melanocytic naevus   8727/0

Miscellaneous tumours
    Yolk sac tumour   9071/3
    Merkel cell tumour   8247/3
    Peripheral primitive neuroectodermal tumour /   9364/3
    Ewing tumour   9260/3

Haematopoetic and lymphoid tumours
    Malignant lymphoma (specify type)
    Leukaemia (specify type)

Secondary tumours

---

[1] Morphology code of the International Classification of Diseases for Oncology (ICD-O) {921} and the Systematized Nomenclature of Medicine (http://snomed.org). Behaviour is coded /0 for benign tumours, /2 for in situ carcinomas and grade 3 intraepithelial neoplasia, /3 for malignant tumours, and /1 for borderline or uncertain behaviour.
[2] Intraepithelial neoplasia does not have a generic code in ICD-O. ICD-O codes are only available for lesions categorized as squamous intraepithelial neoplasia grade 3 (e.g. intraepithelial neoplasia/VIN grade 3) = 8077/2; squamous cell carcinoma in situ 8070/2.

TNM classification of carcinomas of the vulva

TNM Classification[1,2]

T – Primary Tumour

TX   Primary tumour cannot be assessed
T0   No evidence of primary tumour
Tis Carcinoma in situ (preinvasive carcinoma)

T1   Tumour confined to vulva or vulva and perineum, 2 cm or less in greatest dimension
T1a Tumour confined to vulva or vulva and perineum, 2 cm or less in greatest dimension and with stromal invasion no greater than 1 mm
T1b Tumour confined to vulva or vulva and perineum, 2 cm or less in greatest dimension and with stromal invasion greater than 1 mm

T2   Tumour confined to vulva or vulva and perineum, more than 2 cm in greatest dimension

T3   Tumour invades any of the following: lower urethra, vagina, anus

T4   Tumour invades any of the following: bladder mucosa, rectal mucosa, upper urethra; or is fixed to pubic bone

Note: The depth of invasion is defined as the measurement of the tumour from the epithelial-stromal junction of the adjacent most superficial dermal papilla to the deepest point of invasion.

N – Regional Lymph Nodes[3]
NX   Regional lymph nodes cannot be assessed
N0   No regional lymph node metastasis
N1   Unilateral regional lymph node metastasis
N2   Bilateral regional lymph node metastasis

M – Distant Metastasis
MX   Distant metastasis cannot be assessed
M0   No distant metastasis
M1   Distant metastasis (including pelvic lymph node metastasis)

Stage Grouping (TNM and FIGO)

Stage	T	N	M
Stage 0	Tis	N0	M0
Stage I	T1	N0	M0
Stage IA	T1a	N0	M0
Stage IB	T1b	N0	M0
Stage II	T2	N0	M0
Stage III	T1, T2	N1	M0
	T3	N0, N1	M0
Stage IVA	T1, T2, T3	N2	M0
	T4	Any N	M0
Stage IVB	Any T	Any N	M1

---

[1] {51,2976}.
[2] A help desk for specific questions about the TNM classification is available at http://tnm.uicc.org.
[3] The regional lymph nodes are the femoral and inguinal nodes.

Epithelial tumours

E.J. Wilkinson
M.R. Teixeira

Squamous tumours

Definition
Malignant or benign epithelial tumours composed primarily of squamous cells.

ICD-O codes
Squamous cell carcinoma	8070/3
Keratinizing	8071/3
Non-keratinizing	8072/3
Basaloid	8083/3
Warty	8051/3
Verrucous	8051/3
Basal cell carcinoma	8090/3
Vulvar intraepithelial neoplasia (VIN), grade 3 /	8077/2
squamous cell carcinoma in situ	8070/2
Vestibular papilloma	8052/0

Squamous cell carcinoma

Definition
An invasive carcinoma composed of squamous cells of varying degrees of differentiation.

Epidemiology
Squamous cell carcinoma is the most common malignant tumour of the vulva. Primary squamous cell carcinoma of the vulva occurs more frequently in the older age group; the reported incidence rates are 1:100,000 in younger women and 20 in 100,000 in the elderly {2804}.

Table 7.01
Currently recognized precursors of vulvar squamous cell carcinoma.

(1) Vulvar intraepithelial neoplasia (VIN) and associated human papillomavirus (HPV) infection.
(2) The simplex (differentiated) type of VIN not associated with HPV infection {1621,3175}.
(3) Lichen sclerosus {1621} with associated squamous cell hyperplasia {403}.
(4) Chronic granulomatous vulvar disease such as granuloma inguinale {2628}.

Aetiology
In addition to human papillomavirus (HPV), cigarette smoking is a risk factor for vulvar carcinoma {611}. However, the specific aetiology of most vulvar epithelial tumours is unknown. The carcinomas associated with HPV include warty and basaloid carcinomas with the corresponding intraepithelial precursor lesions {584,1106,1541,2180,2936}. Verrucous carcinoma is associated with HPV, usually of type 6 or 11. In some cases there is no recognized precursor lesion. Squamous cell hyperplasia per se is apparently not a precursor of vulvar squamous cell carcinoma {1461}.

There are currently four recognized precursor of vulvar carcinoma (See table 7.1). Vulvar intraepithelial neoplasia (VIN) of the simpex (differentiated) type is usually associated with lichen sclerosus. The latter is also considered to be a precursor of keratinizing squamous cell carcinoma and is not HPV associated {3175}. In the retrospective evaluation of vulvectomy specimens from women with vulvar squamous cell carcinoma, the frequency of identifying associated lichen sclerosus ranges from 15-40%, the higher rate being observed in deeply invasive carcinomas {403,1621,3240}. The lifetime risk of squamous cell carcinoma arising in vulvar lichen sclerosus is unknown but may exceed 6% {403,1621,1824,2369, 2606}. The squamous cell carcinomas associated with lichen sclerosus involving the vulva are usually of the keratinizing type.

Localization
Vulvar squamous cell carcinoma is usually solitary and is found most commonly on the labia minora or majora; the clitoris is the primary site in approximately 10% of cases.

Clinical features
Signs and symptoms
Squamous cell carcinoma may present as an ulcer, nodule, macule or pedunculated mass. Symptoms may be similar to those seen with VIN, although in more advanced cases discharge, bleeding, pain, odour or self-palpation of a mass may bring the patient to the physician.

Imaging
Imaging studies are generally not applicable for the detection of vulvar tumours. When the regional lymph nodes are clinically suspicious, imaging studies, including computed tomography or magnetic resonance, are employed, where available, to evaluate pelvic and para-aortic lymph nodes. Dye and technetium-99m labelled colloid have been used to detect inguino-femoral sentinel lymph nodes {646}.

Colposcopy
Colposcopic examination employing topically applied 3% acetic acid to enhance visualization of lesions and photographic recording of vulvar lesions may be of value in clinical management and follow-up {3124}

Exfoliative and aspiration cytology
Although exfoliative cytology has been applied to the evaluation of primary tumours of the vulva, this practice is not commonly used, and directed biopsy of identified lesions is the most effective method of primary diagnosis.

Fine needle aspiration cytology is of value in assessing suspicious lymph nodes or subcutaneous nodules {1283}.

Macroscopy
Most vulvar squamous carcinomas are solitary. The tumours may be nodular, verruciform or ulcerated with raised firm edges.

Tumour spread and staging
The staging of vulvar tumours is by the TNM/FIGO classification {51,2976}.

Superficially invasive vulvar carcinoma, stage 1A as defined by FIGO, is a single focus of squamous cell carcinoma having a diameter of 2 cm or less and a depth of invasion of 1 mm or less. The definition includes cases that have capillary-like space involvement by tumour. The term "microinvasive carcinoma" is not recommended.

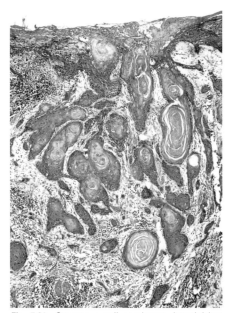

Fig. 7.01 Squamous cell carcinoma, keratinizing type. Keratin pearls are prominent. Invasion is confluent with a desmoplastic stromal response.

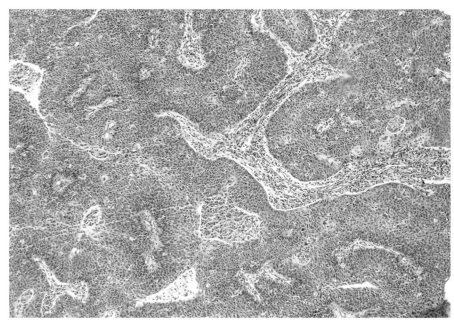

Fig. 7.02 Squamous cell carcinoma, basaloid type. Irregular aggregates of poorly differentiated squamous cells without keratinization infiltrate the stroma in the form of interconnecting columns. The tumour is composed of poorly differentiated basaloid type cells.

Histopathology

Squamous cell carcinoma is an invasive neoplasm composed of squamous cells of varying degrees of differentiation. Several morphological variants have been described:

Keratinizing

Keratinizing squamous cell carcinoma contains keratin pearls.

Non-keratinizing

Non-keratinizing squamous cell carcinoma does not form appreciable keratin; it may contain small numbers of individually keratinized cells but lacks keratin pearls. Rarely, the tumour is composed predominantly of spindle-shaped cells {2529}. In some cases the carcinoma may have a sarcoma-like stroma {2778}.

Basaloid

Basaloid squamous cell carcinoma is composed of nests of immature, basal type squamous cells with scanty cytoplasm that resemble closely the cells of squamous carcinoma in situ of the cervix. Some keratinization may be evident in the centres of the nests, but keratin pearls are rarely present. This tumour may be associated with HPV infections, predominantly type 16 {1541, 2936}.

Warty

Warty (condylomatous) squamous cell carcinoma has a warty surface and cellular features of HPV infection {720, 1541,2936}.

Verrucous

Verrucous carcinoma is a highly differentiated squamous cell carcinoma that has a hyperkeratinized, undulating, warty surface and invades the underlying stroma in the form of bulbous pegs with a pushing border.

Verrucous carcinoma accounts for 1-2% of all vulvar carcinomas and has little or no metastatic potential. The cellular features include minimal nuclear atypia and abundant eosinophilic cytoplasm. Mitotic figures are rare and, when present, are typical. There is usually a prominent chronic inflammatory cell infiltrate in the stroma. HPV, especially type 6, has been identified in a number of cases. Giant condyloma (Buschke-Lowenstein tumour) is considered by some to be synonymous with verrucous carcinoma {100, 348,1336,1501}.

Keratoacanthoma-like

These tumours, often referred to as keratoacanthoma, may arise on the hair-bearing skin of the vulva. They are rapidly growing but are usually self-limited. Histologically, they consist of a central crater filled with a glassy squamous epithelial proliferation in which horny masses of keratin are pushed upward, while tongues of squamous epithelium invade the dermis. Metastasis of so-called keratoacanthoma has been described {1227}. Complete excision with a clear histological margin is the recommended treatment.

Variant with tumour giant cells

Squamous cell carcinoma with a prominent tumour giant cell component is a highly aggressive neoplasm that can be confused with malignant melanoma {3122}.

Tumour measurements

It is recommended that the following features should be included in the pathology report {2601,3119}:
(1) Depth of invasion (mm).
(2) Tumour thickness.
(3) Method of measurement of depth of invasion and thickness of the tumour.
(4) Presence or absence of vascular space involvement by tumour.
(5) Diameter of the tumour, including the clinically measured diameter, if available. In the event that invasion is equivocal

even with additional sectioning, it is recommended that invasion should not be diagnosed {3119}.

The following criteria apply to the measurement of vulvar squamous cell carcinoma:
(1) Thickness: measurement from the surface, or the granular layer if keratinized, to the deepest point of invasion.
(2) Depth of invasion: measurement from the epithelial-stromal junction of the adjacent most superficial dermal papillae to the deepest point of invasion.

The preferred measurement is the depth of invasion, as defined above.

Somatic genetics
Cytogenetic data exist on 11 squamous cell carcinomas of the vulva {2897,3156}. The most common karyotypic changes are loss of 3p, 8p, 22q, Xp, 10q and 18q and gain of 3q and 11q21. There is an inverse correlation between histological differentiation and karyotypic complexity. Furthermore, a comparative genomic hybridization study of 10 cases revealed losses of 4p, 3p, and 5q and gains of 3q and 8p {1338}. Loss of 10q and 18q seems to be particularly associated with a poor prognosis in squamous cell carcinoma {2897,3156}. On the other hand, the only cytogenetically analysed squamous cell carcinoma in situ of the vulva (VIN 3) had a rearrangement of 11p as the sole anomaly {2818}.

TP53 mutation or HPV can independently lead to cell cycle disruption relevant to vulvar squamous cell carcinogenesis. Besides mutational inactivation, *TP53* can be inactivated through binding of HPV protein E6. *PTEN* is another gene that is frequently mutated in carcinomas of the vulva {1234}. Both *TP53* and *PTEN* mutations have also been detected in VIN, indicating that they are early events in vulvar carcinogenesis {1234,1866}. High frequencies of allelic imbalance have been detected at 1q, 2q, 3p, 5q, 8p, 8q, 10p, 10q, 11p, 11q, 15q, 17p, 18q, 21q and 22q, most of these irrespective of HPV status {2256}. This finding suggests that despite a different pathogenesis both HPV-positive and HPV-negative vulvar squamous cell carcinomas share several genetic changes during their progression.

Prognosis and predictive factors
Risk factors for recurrence include advanced stage, tumour diameter >2.5 cm, multifocality, capillary-like space involvement, associated VIN 2 or VIN 3 and involved margins of resection {1235,2004}. The extent of lymph node involvement and mode of treatment may also influence survival {721}. Patients whose tumours have a "spray" or finger-like pattern of invasion have a poorer survival than those with a "pushing" pattern {1235}.

For patients with stage 1A carcinoma, the therapy is usually local excision with at least a 1-cm margin of normal tissue {3, 1428}. Inguinofemoral lymph node dissection is usually unnecessary {247,373,374,1105, 1428}. The risk of recurrence in stage 1A cases is very low, with 5 and 10-year recurrence-free tumour specific survivals of 100% and 94.7%, respectively {1732}. Late recurrence or "reoccurrence" of a second squamous carcinoma in another site within the vulva is rare but can occur, and therefore long-term follow-up is warranted.

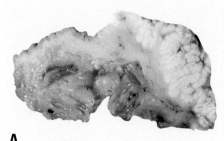
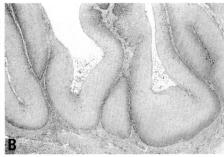

Fig. 7.03 Verrucous carcinoma. **A** The characteristic exophytic and endophytic growth pattern is evident in the sectioned surface of the tumour on the right side of the field. **B** The tumour is composed of well differentiated squamous epithelium with an undulating surface, minimal cytological atypia and a pushing border.

For tumours greater than stage 1A partial or total deep vulvectomy with ipsilateral or bilateral inguino-femoral lymph node resection may be required. If superficial lymph nodes contain tumour, radiotherapy to the deep pelvic nodes or chemoradiation may be necessary {360,373, 1749,2783}.

Basal cell carcinoma

Definition
An infiltrating tumour composed predominantly of cells resembling the basal cells of the epidermis.

Clinical features
This tumour presents as a slow growing, locally invasive, but rarely metastasizing lesion in the vulva {218,833,1872, 2260}.

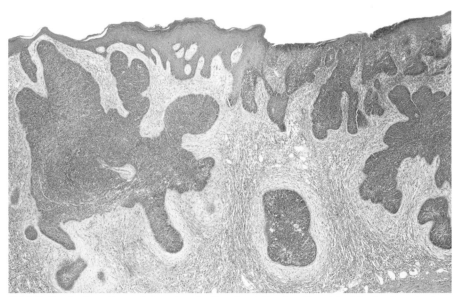

Fig. 7.04 Basal cell carcinoma. Aggregates of uniform basaloid cells with peripherial palisading arise from the basal layer of the overlying squamous epithelium and infiltrate the stroma.

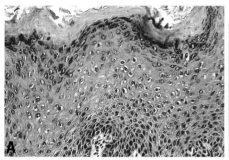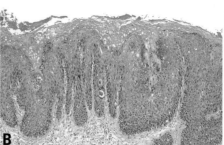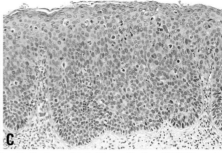

Fig. 7.05 Vulvar intraepithelial neoplasia (VIN). **A** VIN 1. Hyperkeratosis is prominent. Nuclear crowding is confined to the lower third of the epithelium. **B** VIN 3, warty type (severe displasia). Beneath a hyperkeratotic surface the epithelial cells are crowded and show minimal maturation. **C** VIN 3 (carcinoma in situ, basaloid type). Nearly the entire epithelium is composed of closely packed basaloid cells.

Histopathology

The tumour is composed of aggregates of uniform basal cells with peripheral palisading. Squamous cell differentiation may occur at the centre of the tumour nests. Tumours containing gland-like structures are referred to as "adenoid basal cell carcinoma" {1850}. Those containing infiltrating malignant-appearing squamous cells may be diagnosed as metatypical basal cell carcinoma or basosquamous carcinoma. Immunohistochemical findings reflect these histological subtypes {183}. Basal cell carcinoma has been reported in association with vulvar Paget disease {1084}.

Histogenesis

This tumour is derived from the basal cells of the epidermis or hair follicles.

Prognosis and predictive factors

Basal cell carcinoma of the vulva is usually treated by local excision; however, groin metastases have been reported {1017}.

Vulvar intraepithelial neoplasia

Definition

An intraepithelial lesion of the vulvar squamous epithelium characterized by disordered maturation and nuclear abnormalities, i.e. loss of polarity, pleomorphism, coarse chromatin, irregularities of the nuclear membrane and mitotic figures, including atypical forms.

Synonym

Dysplasia/carcinoma in situ.

Epidemiology

The incidence of VIN, unlike that of vulvar carcinoma, has been increasing over the past 20 years, especially in women of

reproductive age, with the highest frequency reported in women 20-35 years old {538,1312,2804}.

Aetiology

VIN is predominately of the warty or basaloid types, and both are associated with HPV, most commonly type 16 {1106, 1197,1663,2936}. Women with HPV-related vulvar disease have an increased risk of associated cervical intraepithelial neoplasia (CIN) {2766}. Women infected with human immunodeficiency virus (HIV) have a high frequency of HPV infection of the lower genital tract and associated CIN and/or VIN {2766}.

Clinical features

Women with VIN may present with vulvar pruritus or irritation or may observe the lesions and seek medical assistance {919}. VIN is typically a macular or papular lesion or lesions, which in approximately one-half of the cases are white or aceto-white. Approximately one-quarter of VIN lesions are pigmented. VIN is multifocal in approximately two-thirds of the cases. The remaining patients usually present as a solitary lesion, a more common finding in older women {431}. Large confluent lesions are uncommon {919, 3123}.

Tumour spread and staging

Up to one-fifth of the women presenting with VIN are found to have an associated squamous cell carcinoma {431,1197, 1272}. In most cases these squamous cell carcinomas are superficially invasive.

Histopathology

The epithelial cells are typically crowded, and acanthosis may be present. A prominent granular layer may be associated

with parakeratosis, hyperkeratosis or both. Involvement of skin appendages is seen in over one-third of the cases, which in hairy skin may be as deep as 2.7 mm. Skin appendage involvement should not be misinterpreted as invasion {219,2636}. There may be associated HPV changes. The term "bowenoid papulosis" should not be used as a histological diagnosis (see below).

The grading of HPV-related VIN is similar to that used in the cervix. The simplex type of VIN (carcinoma in situ, simplex

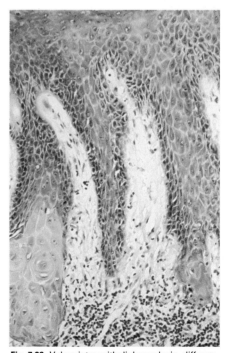

Fig. 7.06 Vulvar intraepithelial neoplasia, differentiated (simplex) type. The atypia is confined to the basal and parabasal layers. The squamous cells have nuclear abnormalities with prominent eosinophilic abortive pearl formations in the deeper portions of the epithelium. The presence of paradoxical maturation abutting on the epithelial-stromal junction is suggestive of impending invasion.

type) is a highly differentiated lesion resembling well differentiated squamous cell carcinoma in which the atypia is most prominent in or confined to the basal and parabasal layers of the epithelium, where the cells have abundant cytoplasm and form pearls and the nuclei are relatively uniform in size and contain coarse chromatin and prominent nucleoli {3175}.

Somatic genetics
The only cytogenetically analysed case of VIN 3 (squamous cell carcinoma in situ) of the vulva had a rearrangement of 11p as the sole anomaly {2818}.
Genomic deletions have been demonstrated in the simplex (differentiated) form of VIN and its subsequent squamous carcinoma unrelated to HPV infection {1663}. These also express TP53 {1824,3175}.

Prognosis and predictive factors
VIN is usually treated by local excision. Laser or other ablative procedure may also have a role {1197,1369,3124}. Spontaneous regression of VIN 2 and 3 in younger women with papular pigmented lesions is recognized, and such lesions are referred to clinically as

bowenoid papulosis by some investigators {1369}. The recurrence of VIN is well recognized, especially in women who are heavy cigarette smokers or positive for HIV.

Condyloma acuminatum

Definition
A benign neoplasm characterized by papillary fronds containing fibrovascular cores and lined by stratified squamous epithelium with evidence of HPV infection, usually in the form of koilocytosis.

Tumour spread and staging
Co-infection of the vulva and cervix is well recognized {1528}. Vulvar carcinoma in young women has been associated with genital condyloma {2945}.

Histopathology
The lesions are typically multiple and papillomatous or papular. The epithelium is acanthotic with parabasal hyperplasia and koilocytosis in the upper portion. Hyperkeratosis and parakeratosis are usual, and binucleated and multinucleated keratinocytes are often present. The rete ridges are elongated and thickened. A chronic inflammatory infiltrate is usual-

ly present within the underlying connective tissue.
HPV infection in the vulvar epithelium is expressed in three broad categories:
(1) Fully expressed, with morphological features of HPV infection, as seen in condyloma acuminatum
(2) Minimally expressed, with only mild morphological changes, e.g. koilocytosis
(3) Latent, in which no characteristic morphological changes are seen, although HPV can be detected with the use of molecular techniques {1013}.

Vestibular papilloma

Definition
A benign papillary tumour with a squamous epithelial mucosal surface that overlies a delicate fibrovascular stalk.

Synonyms
Micropapillomatosis labialis, vestibular micropapillomatosis.
These terms are applicable when numerous lesions are present.

Clinical features
The lesions may be solitary but frequently are multiple, often occurring in clusters near the hymenal ring, resulting in a condition referred to as vestibular papillomatosis or micropapillomatosis or micropapillomatosis labialis {238,644, 980,1930,2277}. They are less than 6 mm in height. Unlike condylomas, they do not typically respond to podophyllin and/or interferon {2277}.

Histopathology
These lesions have papillary architecture and a smooth surface without acanthosis or koilocytotic atypia. They lack the complex arborizing architecture of condyloma.

Aetiology
The great majority of studies of vestibular micropapillomatosis as defined above have demonstrated no relationship of these lesions to HPV {238,644,1856, 2118,2277}.

Fibroepithelial polyp

Definition
A polypoid lesion covered by squamous epithelium and containing a central core of fibrous tissue in which stellate cells with tapering cytoplasmic processes and

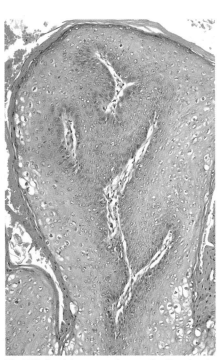

Fig. 7.07 Condyloma acuminatum. Papillary fronds with fibrovascular cores are lined by squamous epithelium with hyperkeratosis, acanthosis and koilocytosis.

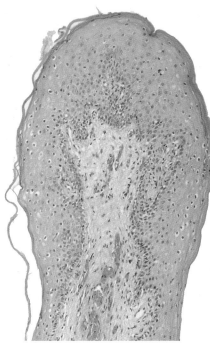

Fig. 7.08 Vestibular papilloma. Smooth surfaced squamous epithelium without acanthosis or koilocytotic atypia lines a delicate fibrovascular stalk.

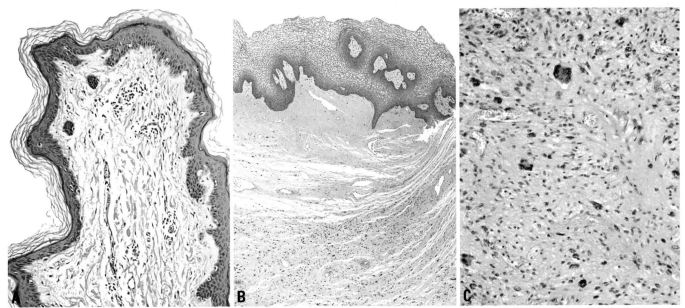

Fig. 7.09 Fibroepithelial polyp of the vulva. **A** The central core of fibrous tissue contains thin-walled vessels. The epithelium is not acanthotic. **B** Stratified squamous epithelium covers dense fibrous stroma. **C** Note the scattered bizarre multinucleated giant cells in the stroma.

irregularly shaped thin-walled vessels are prominent features.

Histopathology
These polypoid lesions are characterized by a prominent fibrovascular stroma covered by squamous epithelium without evidence of koilocytosis. In contrast to vulvar condylomas, fibroepithelial polyps do not show epithelial acanthosis or papillary architecture. Bizarre stromal cells have been described in these polyps that do not influence behaviour {416}.

Aetiology
In contrast to condylomas, fibroepithelial polyps appear unrelated to HPV infection and rarely contain HPV nucleic acids {1837}.

Prognosis and predictive factors
Although benign, the lesion may recur if incompletely excised {2141}.

Seborrheic keratosis and inverted follicular keratosis

Definition
A benign tumour characterized by proliferation of the basal cells of the squamous epithelium with acanthosis, hyperkeratosis and the formation of keratin-filled pseudohorn cysts. Some cases may have an incidental HPV infection {3263}. Inverted follicular keratosis is a seborrheic keratosis of follicular origin and con-

tains prominent squamous eddies. An inverted follicular keratosis of the vulva has been reported that may have been related to close shaving {2467}.

Keratoacanthoma

This rare squamoproliferative lesion commonly occurs on sun-exposed skin. It is thought to arise from follicular epithelium and was originally considered to be benign. It has a central keratin-filled crater and focal infiltration at its dermal interface. In some instances the lesion regresses spontaneously {2361}. Two cases have been described in the vulva {997}. At present the lesion originally described as keratoacanthoma is generally accepted as a well differentiated squamous cell carcinoma, keratoacanthoma type {1227}, and the latter diagnosis is recommended (see section on squamous cell carcinoma).

Glandular tumours

ICD-O codes
Paget disease	8542/3
Bartholin gland tumours	
Adenocarcinoma	8140/3
Squamous cell carcinoma	8070/3
Adenoid cystic carcinoma	8200/3
Adenosquamous carcinoma	8560/3
Small cell carcinoma	8041/3
Transitional cell carcinoma	8120/3

Adenoma	8140/0
Adenomyoma	8932/0
Papillary hidradenoma	8405/0
Adenocarcinoma of Skene gland origin	8140/3
Adenoma of minor vestibular glands	8140/0
Mixed tumour of the vulva	8940/0

Vulvar Paget disease

Definition
An intraepithelial neoplasm of cutaneous origin expressing apocrine or eccrine glandular-like features and characterized by distinctive large cells with prominent cytoplasm referred to as Paget cells. It may also be derived from an underlying skin appendage adenocarcinoma or anorectal or urothelial carcinoma {3121}.

Epidemiology
Primary cutaneous Paget disease is an uncommon neoplasm, usually of postmenopausal White women. In approximately 10-20% of women with vulvar Paget disease, there is an invasive component or an underlying skin appendage adenocarcinoma {825,3121}.

Clinical features
Paget disease typically presents as a symptomatic red, eczematoid lesion that may clinically resemble a dermatosis {1028,3121,3267}. Paget disease that is related to anorectal adenocarcinoma

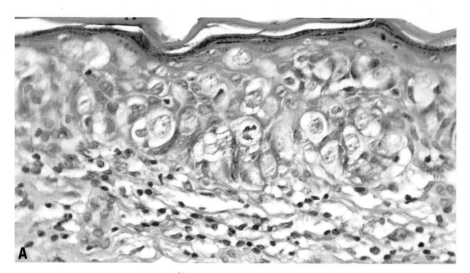

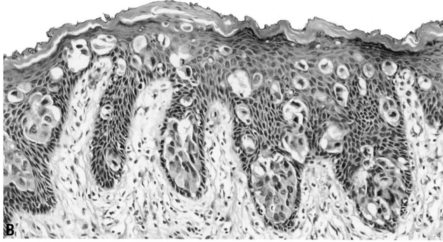

Fig. 7.10 Paget disease of the vulva. **A** Paget disease of cutaneous origin. Clusters of large pale Paget cells with atypical nuclei are present within the epidermis. A mitotic figure is evident. **B** Paget disease of urothelial origin. Clusters of large pale cells resembling transitional cell carcinoma involve predominantly the parabasal area of the epidermis with sparing of the basal layer.

clinically involves the perianal mucosa and skin, as well as the adjacent vulva.

Histopathology
The Paget cell of cutaneous origin is typically a large, round cell with a large nucleus and prominent nucleolus. The cytoplasm is pale on routine hematoxylin and eosin stain, is often vacuolated and stains with mucicarmine. The cytoplasm contains PAS-positive material that is resistant to diastase. The Paget cells may also express CA125 and Her-2/neu but do not express estrogen receptor {573,3119,3121}.
Paget disease that is related to urothelial neoplasia contains cells with the morphological features of high grade urothelial neoplasms {1746,3121}. It may histo-

logically resemble primary cutaneous Paget disease, though it has a different immunohistochemical profile.

Somatic genetics
Three cytogenetically abnormal clones were detected in Paget disease of the vulva {2897}, a finding consistent with the view that this disease may arise multicentrically from pluripotent stem cells within the epidermis. DNA aneuploidy in Paget disease is associated with an increased risk of recurrence {2553}.

Bartholin gland carcinoma

Definition
Primary carcinoma of diverse cell types located at the site of the Bartholin gland.

Clinical features
Bartholin gland carcinoma occurs predominantly in women over 50 years of age and presents as an enlargement in the Bartholin gland area that may clinically resemble a Bartholin duct cyst.

Tumour spread and staging
Approximately 20% of cases are associated with ipsilateral inguinofemoral lymph node metastases at presentation {556,1634,3108}.

Histopathology
The tumour is typically solid and deeply infiltrative. A transition from an adjacent Bartholin gland to tumour is of value in identifying its origin. Various types of carcinoma have been described.

Adenocarcinoma
Adenocarcinoma accounts for approximately 40% of Bartholin gland tumours {556,1634}. Adenocarcinomas may be mucinous, papillary or mucoepidermoid in type. They are usually carcinoembryonic antigen immunoreactive.

Squamous cell carcinoma
This tumour accounts for approximately 40% of Bartholin gland tumours and is composed of neoplastic squamous cells.

Adenoid cystic carcinoma
Adenoid cystic carcinoma accounts for approximately 15% of Bartholin gland tumours {556,675}. It is composed typically of rounded islands of uniform malignant epithelial cells with a cribriform pattern. A hyaline stroma may form cylinders separating rows of tumour cells. The intraluminal material is basement membrane-like rather than a secretion, supporting a squamous rather than glandular origin.
The cytogenetic analysis of an adenoid cystic carcinoma of Bartholin gland revealed a complex karyotype involving chromosomes 1, 4, 6, 11, 14 and 22 {1457}.

Adenosquamous carcinoma
Adenosquamous carcinoma accounts for approximately 5% of Bartholin gland tumours. It is composed of neoplastic mucin-containing glandular and neoplastic squamous cells.

Transitional cell carcinoma
Transitional cell carcinoma is a rare tumour of Bartholin gland composed of

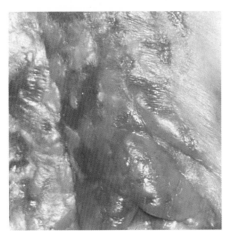

Fig. 7.11 Paget disease of the vulva. Note the red, eczematous appearance.

Table 7.02
Immunohistochemical findings of Paget disease.

Type of Paget disease	CK-7	CK 20	GCDFP-15	CEA	UP-III
Primary skin neoplasm	+	-	+	+	-
Related to anorectal carcinoma	+	+	-	+	-
Related to urothelial carcinoma	+	(+)	-	-	+

Abbreviations for antibodies used as follows:
CK = cytokeratin; CEA = carcinoembryonic antigen; GCDFP-15 = gross cystic disease fluid protein-15; UP-III = uroplakin III {2088,3121}.

neoplastic urothelial-type cells, occasionally with a minor component of glandular or squamous cells.

Small cell carcinoma
This rare highly malignant neoplasm is composed of small neuroendocrine cells with scant cytoplasm and numerous mitotic figures {1361}.

Benign neoplasms of Bartholin gland

Adenoma and adenomyoma
Bartholin gland adenoma is a rare benign tumour of Bartholin gland characterized by small clustered closely packed glands and tubules lined by columnar to cuboidal epithelium with colloid-like secretion arranged in a lobular pattern and contiguous with identifiable Bartholin gland elements. Bartholin gland adenoma has been reported in association with adenoid cystic carcinoma {1487}. Bartholin gland nodular hyperplasia can be distinguished from adenoma by the preservation of the nor-

mal duct-acinar relationships present in hyperplasia. Bartholin gland adenomyoma has a fibromuscular stromal element that is immunoreactive for smooth muscle actin and desmin as well as a lobular glandular architecture with glands lined by columnar mucin-secreting epithelial cells adjacent to tubules {1487}.

Tumours arising from specialized anogenital mammary-like glands

Definition
Malignant and benign tumours, usually of glandular type and resembling neoplasms of the breast, may arise in specialized anogenital mammary-like glands. These glands and the tumours that arise from them are usually identified in or adjacent to the intralabial sulcus. Adenocarcinoma with morphological features of breast carcinoma has been reported as a primary vulvar tumour {687}. Such tumours are currently thought to arise from the specialized anogenital glands and not from ectopic breast tissue {2991,2992}. The papillary

hidradenoma is an example of a benign neoplasm {2991,2992}. Intraductal adenocarcinoma of mammary-type within a hidradenoma has been reported {2212}.

Papillary hidradenoma
Definition
A benign tumour composed of epithelial secretory cells and underlying myoepithelial cells lining complex branching papillae with delicate fibrovascular stalks.

Epidemiology
This tumour is rare in the vulva but is the most common benign glandular neoplasm at this site.

Clinical features
It usually presents as an asymptomatic mass within or adjacent to the intralabial sulcus and may cause bleeding resembling carcinoma if the gland prolapses and/or ulcerates.

Histopathology
The tumour is distinctly circumscribed and composed of complex papillae and

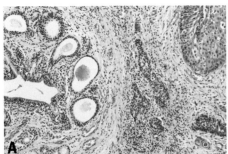
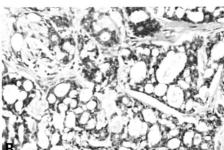
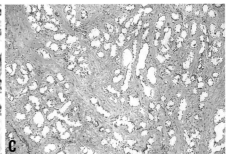

Fig. 7.12 Bartholin gland neoplasms. **A** Squamous cell carcinoma. Aggregates of neoplastic squamous cells infiltrate Bartholin gland seen on the left. **B** Adenoid cystic carcinoma. Note the cribriform pattern with the lumens containing basophilic mucin. **C** Bartholin gland adenoma. A nodule is composed of clustered glands lined by mucinous epithelium.

glandular elements surrounded by fibrous tissue. Relatively uniform columnar epithelial secretory cells with underlying myoepithelial cells cover the glands and papillary stalks.

Adenocarcinoma of Skene gland origin

An adenocarcinoma of Skene gland with associated metastasis has been reported {2726}. Skene gland is the female homologue of the male prostate, and the tumour expresses prostate antigens by immunohistochemistry {2726}. A carcinoma of Skene duct origin was associated with systemic coagulopathy {2895}.

Adenocarcinomas of other types

These tumours may arise from endometriosis or ectopic cloacal tissue {307,3126,3237}.

Adenoma of minor vestibular glands

Adenoma of minor vestibular glands is a rare benign tumour composed of clusters of small glands lined by mucin-secreting columnar epithelial cells arranged in a lobular pattern without intervening Bartholin duct elements. It is usually an incidental finding measuring 1-2 mm in diameter, although one example was as large as 10 mm. Nodular hyperplasia of the minor vestibular glands may also occur {141,2295}

Mixed tumour of the vulva

Definition
A benign epithelial tumour composed of epithelial cells arranged in tubules or nests mixed with a fibrous stromal component that may include chondroid, osseous and myxoid elements.

Synonyms
Pleomorphic adenoma, chondroid syringoma.

Clinical features
Mixed tumour of the vulva usually presents as a subcutaneous nodule involving the labum majus and/or the Bartholin gland area.

Histopathology
The histological features are similar to those of mixed tumours of salivary glands. The tumour with its stromal-like elements is believed to arise from pluripotential myoepithelial cells that are present in Bartholin gland, sweat glands and the specialized anogenital (mammary-like) glands of the vulva {2410}.

Prognosis and predictive factors
Although these tumours are considered benign, insufficient cases of vulvar mixed tumours have been reported to determine their natural history at this site. The tumour may recur locally. A carcinoma arising in a mixed tumour has been described {2117}. Complete local excision with free margins is the recommended therapy for the primary tumour as well as for local recurrences.

Tumours of skin appendage origin

Definition
Benign or malignant tumours differentiating towards hair follicles or sweat or sebaceous glands.

ICD-O codes
Malignant sweat gland tumour	8400/3
Sebaceous carcinoma	8410/3
Syringoma	8407/0
Nodular hidradenoma	8402/0
Trichoepithelioma	8100/0
Trichilemmoma	8102/0

Malignant sweat gland tumours

Vulvar malignant sweat gland tumours include eccrine adenocarcinoma, porocarcinoma, clear cell hidradenocarcinoma, and apocrine adenocarcinoma, the last of which may be associated with Paget disease {3112}.

Sebaceous carcinoma

Vulvar sebaceous carcinoma resembles its cutaneous counterpart. It is a malignant tumour composed of cords and nests of basaloid appearing neoplastic glandular elements with cellular features of sebaceous epithelium. The tumour may be associated with neoplastic sebaceous cells present in pagetoid nests within the parabasal component of the overlying epithelium and in larger clusters near the epithelial surface {405,795}. Sebaceous carcinoma of the vulva may be associated with VIN {1318}.

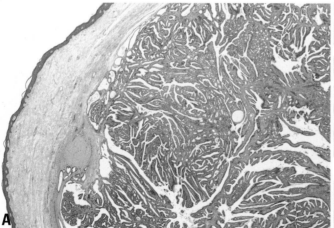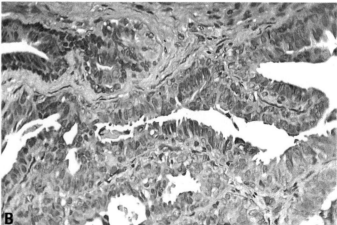

Fig. 7.13 Papillary hidradenoma of the vulva. **A** Note the circumscribed tumour composed of complex branching papillae. **B** The epithelial lining is composed of a double layer of cells, an inner layer of secretory cells and an outer layer of myoepithelial cells.

Syringoma

Definition
A benign epithelial tumour believed to arise from eccrine ducts that is composed of small and relatively uniform epithelial-lined tubules and cysts within a densely fibrous dermis.

Clinical findings
It presents as asymptomatic or pruritic papules that are small, clustered and non-pigmented and involve the deeper skin layers of the labia majora. The nodules are often bilateral {415}.

Histopathology
Histologically, small epithelial cysts and dilated duct-like spaces lined by two rows of cells, an inner epithelial and an outer myoepithelial, are seen. The ductular structures typically form comma-like shapes. The tumour lacks a clearly defined capsule or margin; the dermis surrounding the neoplastic ducts has a fibrotic appearance.

Nodular hidradenoma

Definition
Nodular hidradenoma is an infrequent benign tumour of sweat gland origin composed of epithelial cells with clear cytoplasm arranged in lobules and nests.

Synonym
Clear cell hidradenoma.

Histopathology
It is composed of epithelial cells with clear cytoplasm arranged in lobules and nests {1950}.

Prognosis and predictive factors
Complete local excision is considered adequate therapy.

Trichoepithelioma

Definition
A benign tumour composed of complex interconnected nests of basaloid cells that form small "horn cysts" (cysts containing keratin).

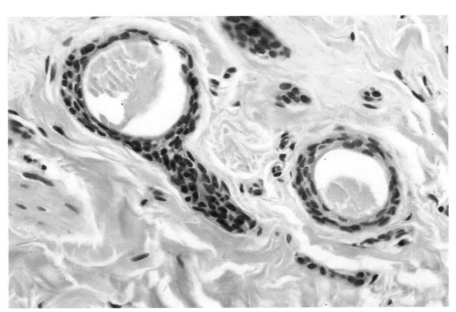

Fig. 7.14 Syringoma of the vulva. The tumour is composed of well differentiated ductal elements of eccrine type consisting of irregular, sometimes comma-shaped, cord-like and tubular structures that infiltrate the dermis.

Clinical features
On clinical examination single or multiple cutaneous nodules with overlying skin abnormalities are identified.

Histopathology
Nests of cells form small keratin-containing cysts. The neoplastic epithelial cells are monomorphic without nuclear hyperchromasia or atypia. The tumour has a defined dermal interface and lacks an infiltrative appearance. Rupture of the keratin-containing cysts may result in a granulomatous reaction with foreign body giant cells. Hair follicles may be identified in some cases.

Histogenesis
The tumour is considered to be of follicular origin {478}.

Prognosis and predictive factors
The treatment is complete local excision.

Trichilemmoma

Definition
A benign epithelial tumour composed of relatively uniform epithelial cells with pale-staining cytoplasm that may have some nuclear pleomorphism. It is thought to arise from the proliferation of outer root sheath epithelial cells of the hair follicle.

Synonym
Proliferating trichilemmal tumour.

Clinical findings
Clinically, these tumours have been reported in the dermis of the labium majus, presenting as a slow-growing solid mass {140}.

Histopathology
The tumour has a lobulated appearance with a dermal pushing border that may show no connection with the overlying epithelium. The cells show peripheral palisading and increased clear cytoplasm as they stratify toward the centre. Amorphous keratin is present in the lumens, although no granular layer is formed. Calcification may occur.

Uncommon vulvar skin appendage tumours

Proliferating trichilemmal cysts (pilar tumours) {2329}, trichoblastic fibroma {1003} and apocrine cystadenoma {1021} have been described on the vulva. A local excision is therapeutic.

Mesenchymal tumours

R.L. Kempson
M.R.Teixeira
M.R. Hendrickson

Definition
A variety of benign and malignant soft tissue tumours that occur in the vulva.

Malignant soft tissue tumours

Definition
Malignant soft tissue tumours that arise in the vulva.

ICD-O codes

Sarcoma botryoides	8910/3
Leiomyosarcoma	8890/3
Proximal-type epithelioid sarcoma	8804/3
Alveolar soft part sarcoma	9581/3
Liposarcoma	8850/3
Dermatofibrosarcoma protuberans	8832/3

Sarcoma botryoides

Definition
A malignant neoplasm exhibiting striated muscle differentiation that occurs almost exclusively in children younger than 10 years of age {555,558,2002}.

Synonym
Embryonal rhabdomyosarcoma.

Clinical features
In girls the neoplasm typically arises from the labial or perineal area and presents with bleeding and ulceration. The neoplasm usually presents as a solid vulvar mass; the distinctive "bunch of grapes" appearance is more characteristic of vaginal primaries.

Tumour spread and staging
When both the vulva and vagina are involved, the tumour is regarded as vaginal for staging purposes.

Histopathology
For the typical histological features of sarcoma botryoides see the chapter on the vagina. Vulvar rhabdomyosarcoma sometimes exhibits an alveolar pattern, usually a focal finding, but occasionally diffuse. In this pattern tumour cells grow in loosely cohesive nests separated by fibrous septa. Towards the centre of the nests, the cells show loss of cohesion and float freely within a space, whilst the cells at the periphery are adherent to the septa, a pattern that simulates pulmonary alveoli. The tumour cell cytoplasm stains with a variety of muscle markers including actin, myosin, desmin, myogenin and myoD-1.

Prognosis and predictive factors
The prognosis depends both upon the clinical stage and the histological type {99}. An alveolar histology, even when focal, is an unfavourable prognostic feature, whereas classic botryoid embryonal rhabdomyosarcoma is associated with a greater than 90% survival {558}.

Leiomyosarcoma

Definition
A rare malignant neoplasm showing smooth muscle differentiation.

Clinical features
These neoplasms occur in adults in any part of the vulva and present as a rapidly enlarging mass, sometimes with pain.

Histopathology
Most reported cases are high grade neoplasms with the usual features of necrosis, infiltrative margins, cytological atypia and mitotic indices in excess of 10 mitotic figures per 10 high power fields. Problematic tumours are those with no necrosis and a low mitotic index {2880}.

Differential diagnosis
Leiomyosarcoma should be differentiated from postoperative spindle cell nodule {1397}. The latter is mitotically active and may infiltrate the underlying tissue. The distinction from leiomyosarcoma or other malignant spindle cell tumours depends to a large extent on the history of a recent operation at the same site {1762}.

Proximal-type epithelioid sarcoma

Definition
A malignant tumour histologically similar to epithelioid sarcoma of soft parts.

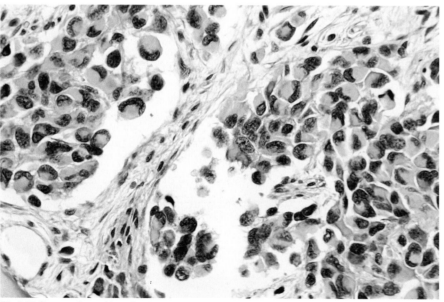

Fig. 7.15 Sarcoma botryoides, alveolar type. The tumour cells grow in loosely cohesive nests separated by fibrous septa that simulate pulmonary alveoli.

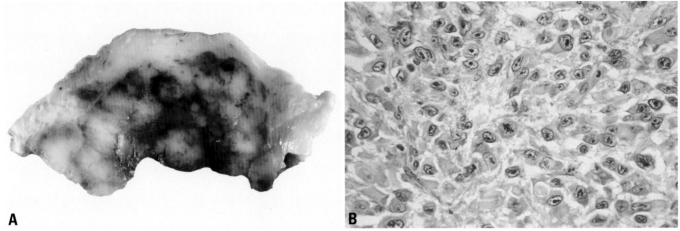

Fig. 7.16 Epithelioid sarcoma of the vulva. **A** The tumour forms a multinodular mass beneath the skin with areas of haemorrhage. **B** The neoplasm is composed of large epithelioid cells with pleomorphic nuclei, prominent nucleoli and frequent mitotic figures.

Synonym
Malignant rhabdoid tumour, adult type.

Histopathology
This tumour, which has histological and immunological features similar to epithelioid sarcoma of the extremities, has a predilection for the vulva {1078}. The growth pattern is frequently nodular, and the tumour cells are large with abundant amphophilic cytoplasm. The nuclei are either large and pleomorphic with small nucleoli or vesicular with prominent nucleoli. Keratin and vimentin stains are positive in essentially all tumours, and CD34 is positive in approximately one-half of the cases.

Prognosis and predictive factors
Frequent recurrences and a high incidence of metastasis mark the clinical course.

Alveolar soft part sarcoma

Definition
A sarcoma characterized by solid and alveolar groups of large epithelial-like cells with granular, eosinophilic cytoplasm.

Histopathology
The rare cases of alveolar soft part sarcoma reported in the vulva have the same distinctive histology as those neoplasms occurring in more conventional soft tissue locations {2639}. The tumour is composed of large uniform cells with abundant granular to vacuolated eosinophilic cytoplasm; the cells are compartmentalized into packets by thin-walled often sinusoidal vessels. Most of the tumours contain characteristic intracytoplasmic PAS-positive, diastase resistent, rod-shaped crystals.

Liposarcoma

Liposarcomas are extremely rare in this location {354,2062}. Both atypical lipomatous tumours (well differentiated liposarcomas) and myxoid liposarcomas have been reported.

Dermatofibrosarcoma protuberans

Dermatofibrosarcoma protuberans is a highly recurrent low grade cutaneous sarcoma that is usually located on the trunk. Although rare, more than 10 cases have been reported in the vulva, and in one such case a supernumerary ring chromosome with the characteristic *COL1A1/PDGFB* fusion gene was found {3004}.

Benign soft tissue tumours

Definition
Benign soft tissue tumours that arise in the vulva.

ICD-O codes
Deep angiomyxoma	8841/1
Superficial angiomyxoma	8841/0
Angiomyofibroblastoma	8826/0
Cellular angiofibroma	9160/0
Leiomyoma	8890/0
Granular cell tumour	9580/0

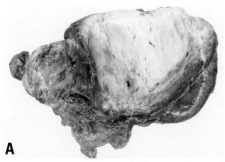
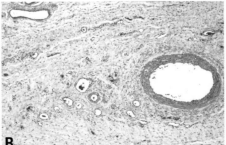
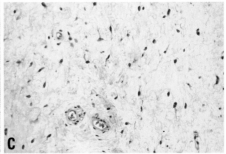

Fig. 7.17 Deep angiomyxoma. **A** The tumour forms a large bulging mass with a pale myxoid surface. **B** The neoplasm contains vessels of variable calibre, some of which are thick-walled. **C** The tumour is sparsely cellular and composed of uniform stellate cells set in a myxoid matrix.

Table 7.03
Differential diagnosis of myxoid soft tissue lesions of the vulva.

	Sarcoma botryoides	Deep angiomyxoma	Angiomyofibro-blastoma	Superficial angiomyxoma	Fibroepithelial polyp
Age at presentation	Pre-pubertal	Reproductive years	Reproductive years	Reproductive years	Reproductive years
Size, site and macroscopic configuration	Polypoid, exophytic or mass	Often larger than 5 cm, never exophytic	Subcutaneous, less than 5 cm	Small, dermal lobulated, superficial	Small, subepithelial, exophytic
Margins	Infiltrative	Infiltrative	Compressive		Poorly circumscribed
Cellularity and cells	Largely paucicellular with a variably pronounced cambium layer Spindle shaped cells including rhabdomyoblasts in the myxoid zones	Paucicellular Cytologically bland, stellate	More cellular than DA Perivascular concentration of cells is usual. Cytologically bland Plasmacytoid or epithelioid cells may be prominent.		Bland spindle cells in addition to enlarged, pleomorphic stromal cells with smudged chromatin
Vessels	Inconspicuous	Medium calibre, thick-walled vessels; pinwheel collagen	Smaller vessels than DA Perivascular concentration of stromal cells	Elongated thin-walled vessels	
Matrix		Paucicellular, myxoid			
Mitotic index	Usually easily found	Rare	Rare	Rare	Rare
Immunohistochemistry	Actin and desmin positive. Myogenin and myoD positive.	Actin, desmin and vimentin positive.	Strongly desmin positive. Minority of cells in occasional cases show positivity for either smooth muscle actin or panmuscle actin (HHF35). Negative for S-100 protein, keratin, fast myosin and myoglobin.	Desmin negative	Often desmin positive
Associated findings				Stromal neutrophils When multiple, consider Carney syndrome	Overlying epithelium may demonstrate intraepithelial neoplasia
Clinical course	Fully malignant neoplasm Alveolar histology adverse prognostic factor	Local recurrence common; never metastasizes	Does not recur Occasional lesions have hybrid features of DA and AMFB and should be treated as DA		Benign, no recurrences

Abbreviations: DA = Deep angiomyxoma; AMFB = Angiomyofibroblastoma

Deep angiomyxoma

Definition
A locally infiltrative tumour composed of fibroblasts, myofibroblasts and numerous, characteristically thick-walled, blood vessels embedded in an abundant myxoid matrix.

Synonym
Aggressive angiomyxoma.

Clinical features
Most patients present with a relatively large, often greater than 10 cm, slowly growing, painless mass in the pelviperineal region that may give rise to pressure effects on the adjacent urogenital or anorectal tracts. Imaging studies often show the mass to be substantially larger than clinically suspected.

Macroscopy
Macroscopically, the tumour is lobulated but poorly circumscribed due to finger-like extensions into the surrounding tissue. The neoplasm is grey-pink or tan and rubbery or gelatinous.

Tumour spread and staging
Deep angiomyxoma is a locally infiltrative but non-metastasizing neoplasm that occurs during the reproductive years {198,853,2779}.

Histopathology
The constituent cells of this paucicellular neoplasm are small, uniform, spindle-shaped to stellate with poorly defined, pale eosinophilic cytoplasm and bland, often vesicular nuclei. The abundant myxoid matrix contains a variable number of rounded medium-sized to large vessels that possess thickened focally hyalinized walls. Multinucleated cells may be present, and occasionally there is morphological overlap with angiomyo-fibroblastoma (see below). Actin and desmin stains are positive in almost all cases, whereas S-100 protein is consistently negative {1431,2082}.

Differential diagnosis
The differential diagnosis includes angiomyofibroblastoma, fibroepithelial polyp (so-called pseudosarcoma botryoides) and superficial angiomyxoma {1054,2063}.
Other less common lesions that may enter the differential diagnosis are:
(1) Myxoid neurofibroma, which has more buckled or wavy nuclei and whose cells are S-100 protein positive.
(2) Low grade myxofibrosarcoma, which has thin–walled curvilinear vessels, shows more nuclear atypia and is essentially always desmin negative.
(3) Myxoid liposarcoma, which contains delicate arborizing vessels and small lipoblasts.
(4) Cellular angiofibroma, which is well circumscribed.

Somatic genetics
A single case of vulvar deep angiomyxoma showed a loss of one X chromosome as the only cytogenetic aberration, a chromosomal change that is uncommon in this neoplasm {1438}.

Prognosis and predictive factors
The treatment for this locally aggressive but non-metastasizing proliferation is primarily surgical with close attention to margins. Approximately 30% of patients develop one or more local recurrences.

Superficial angiomyxoma

Definition
A multilobulated, dermal or subcutaneous lesion composed of fibroblasts and thin-walled vessels in a myxoid matrix that occurs in adults.

Clinical features
The tumour occurs as a subcutaneous mass during the reproductive years.

Histopathology
Scattered multinucleated fibroblasts are often seen {389,854}. There is no cytological atypia or pleomorphism, but scattered mitoses may be found. The stroma generally contains an inconspicuous mixed inflammatory infiltrate that is notable for the presence of neutrophils despite the absence of ulceration or necrosis. Up to one-third contain an epithelial component, usually squamous epithelium.

Prognosis and predictive factors
Approximately one-third of the lesions recur locally in a non–destructive fashion, usually as a consequence of an incomplete or marginal excision. Less than 5% of cases recur repeatedly.

Angiomyofibroblastoma

Definition
A benign, non-recurring, well circumscribed, myofibroblastic lesion composed of spindle-shaped to round cells

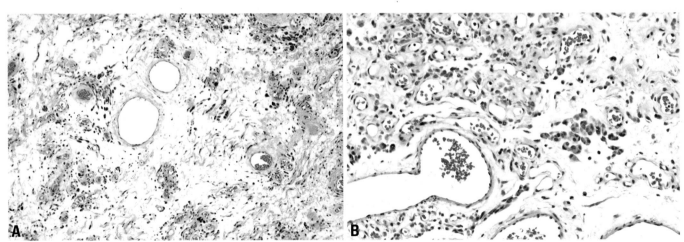

Fig. 7.18 Angiomyofibroblastoma. **A** Alternating hypercellular and hypocellular areas are associated with a prominent vascular pattern. **B** Binucleate and trinucleate tumour cells are common, and some cells have a plasmacytoid appearance.

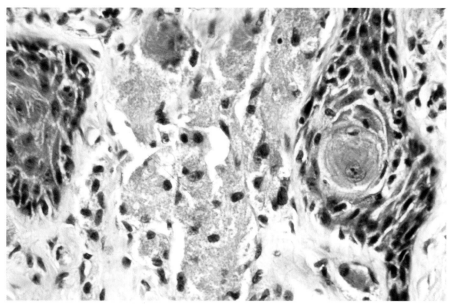

Fig. 7.19 Granular cell tumour of the vulva. The neoplasm is composed of cells with abundant granular cytoplasm and small uniform nuclei between pegs of proliferative squamous epithelium.

that tend to concentrate around vessels {890,1054,2019,2082}.

Clinical features
Angiomyofibroblastoma occurs in the reproductive years and usually presents as a slowly growing, painless, well circumscribed, subcutaneous mass measuring less than 5 cm in maximum diameter.

Macroscopy
Macroscopically, a narrow fibrous pseudocapsule delimits these tumours.

Histopathology
At low power angiomyofibroblastoma shows alternating hypercellular and hypocellular areas associated with a prominent vascular pattern throughout. Binucleate or multinucleate tumour cells are common, and some cells have denser, more hyaline cytoplasm, imparting a plasmacytoid appearance. Mitoses are very infrequent. The constituent cells are desmin positive. The major differential diagnostic considerations are deep angiomyxoma and fibroepithelial polyp.

Cellular angiofibroma

Definition
A recently described distinctive benign mesenchymal tumour composed of bland spindle-shaped cells admixed with numerous hyalinized blood vessels.

Clinical features
The tumour typically presents as a circumscribed solid rubbery vulvar mass in middle-aged women.

Histopathology
Cellular angiofibroma is usually a well circumscribed cellular lesion that is composed of bland spindle-shaped cells interspersed with medium to small blood vessels, which typically have thick hyalinized walls {597,1818,2063}. Mature adipocytes, especially around the periphery of the lesion, are a characteristic feature.
Cellular angiofibroma is vimentin-positive and desmin-negative, an immunoprofile that differentiates this tumour from deep angiomyxoma and angiomyofibroblastoma.

Prognosis and predictive factors
A local recurrence following excision has been described in a single case {1818}.

Leiomyoma
These benign neoplasms do not differ macroscopically or histologically from leiomyomas encountered elsewhere in the female genital tract and are treated by simple excision. Problematic smooth muscle neoplasms are those that are greater than 7.0 cm in greatest dimension, have infiltrative margins and a mitotic index in excess of 5 per 10 high power fields {2880} (see section on leiomyosarcoma).

Granular cell tumour

Definition
A tumour composed of cells with uniform central nuclei and abundant granular, slightly basophilic cytoplasm.

Histopathology
These have the same appearance as in other more common sites. A proliferation of cells with small uniform nuclei and abundant, granular, slightly basophilic cytoplasm diffusely involves the superficial connective tissue {2554}. The tumour cells are uniformly S-100 protein positive. Of particular importance in the vulva is the tendency for the overlying squamous epithelium to undergo pseudoepitheliomatous hyperplasia and simulate a well differentiated squamous carcinoma {3138}. Malignant varieties are rare and show high cellularity, nuclear pleomorphism, tumour cell necrosis and frequent mitotic figures {824}.

Other benign tumours and tumour-like conditions
Other benign tumours and tumour-like conditions that occur in the vulva include lipoma, haemangioma, angiokeratoma, pyogenic granuloma (lobular capillary haemangioma), lymphangioma, neurofibroma, schwannoma, glomus tumour, rhabdomyoma and post-operative spindle cell nodule {1762}. The histological features are similar to their appearance in more common sites.

Melanocytic tumours

E.J. Wilkinson
M.R. Teixeira

Malignant melanomas account for 2-10% of vulvar malignancies {2316} and occur predominantly in elderly White women. A variety of naevi that must be distinguished from melanoma also occur in the vulva.

ICD-O codes

Malignant melanoma	8720/3
Congenital melanocytic naevus	8761/0
Acquired melanocytic naevus	8720/0
Blue naevus	8780/0
Atypical melanocytic naevus of the genital type	8720/0
Dysplastic melanocytic naevus	8727/0

Malignant melanoma

Definition
A malignant tumour of melanocytic origin.

Clinical features
Signs and symptoms
Symptoms include vulvar bleeding, pruritus and dysuria. Although vulvar malignant melanoma usually presents as a pigmented mass, 27% are non-pigmented {2320}. Satellite cutaneous nodules occur in 20% of cases {2320}. Melanoma may arise in a prior benign or atypical appearing melanocytic lesion. {1912, 3151}. The majority present as a nodule or polypoid mass. Approximately 5% are ulcerated {2320}. They occur with nearly equal frequency in the labia majora, labia minora or clitoris.

Imaging
Radiological, magnetic resonance imaging and/or radiolabelled isotope scan studies may be used to assess tumour that is present outside the vulva.

Histopathology
Three histological types of melanoma are identified: superficial spreading, nodular and mucosal/acral lentiginous {216, 1355,2261,2864}. Approximately 25% of the cases are unclassifiable {2320}. Melanomas may be composed of epithelioid, spindle, dendritic, nevoid or mixed cell types. The epithelioid cells contain abundant eosinophilic cytoplasm, large nuclei and prominent nucleoli. The dendritic cells have tapering cytoplasmic extensions resembling nerve cells and show moderate nuclear pleomorphism. Spindle-shaped cells have smaller, oval nuclei and may be arranged in sheets or bundles. Certain cell types may predominate within a given tumour. The amount of melanin within the tumour cells is highly variable, and cells may contain no melanin.

Both mucosal/acral lentiginous and superficial spreading melanomas can be entirely intraepithelial. When invasive, both histological types have vertical and radial growth phases, the vertical growth component representing the invasive focus of tumour. Nodular melanomas display predominately a vertical growth phase. Atypical melanocytes characteristic of melanoma in situ usually can be identified within the epithelium adjacent to mucosal/acral lentiginous and superficial spreading melanomas.

Superficial spreading melanomas have malignant melanocytic cells within the area of invasion that are typically large with relatively uniform nuclei and prominent nucleoli, similar to the adjacent intraepithelial melanoma. The intraepithelial component is considered to be the radial growth portion of the tumour.

Nodular melanomas may have a small neoplastic intraepithelial component adjacent to the invasive tumour and are generally not considered to have a significant radial growth phase. The cells of nodular melanomas may be epithelioid or spindle-shaped. These tumours are typically deeply invasive.

Mucosal/acral lentiginous melanomas are most common within the vulvar vestibule, including the clitoris. They are characterized by spindle-shaped neoplastic melanocytes within the junctional zone involving the adjacent superficial stroma in a diffuse pattern. The spindle-shaped cells are relatively uniform, lacking significant nuclear pleomorphism. Within the stroma the tumour is usually associated with a desmoplastic response.

There is some variation in the reported frequency of melanoma types involving the vulva; however, in a large series of 198 cases mucosal/acral lentiginous melanoma comprised 52% of the cases, nodular melanoma 20% and superficial

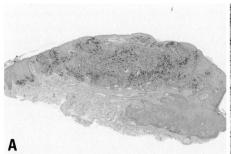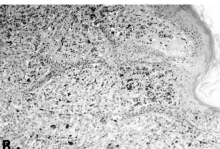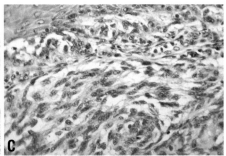

Fig. 7.20 Malignant melanoma of the vulva. **A** Low power micrograph of a heavily pigmented melanoma. **B** The neoplastic cells involve the epithelium and the junctional areas as well as the adjacent dermis. Note the large, pleomorphic nuclei with prominent nucleoli. Some cells contain melanin. **C** This neoplasm is composed of spindle-shaped cells with elongated nuclei resembling a spindle cell sarcoma.

Table 7.04
Clark levels of cutaneous melanoma {3120}.

Level I	Melanoma in situ
Level II	Superficial papillary dermis
Level III	Fills and expands papillary dermis
Level IV	Reticular dermis
Level V	Deeper than reticular dermis into fat or other deeper tissue

spreading melanoma 4%, with the remainder of the cases being unclassifiable {2320,3120}.

Immunoprofile
Melanomas usually are immunoreactive for S-100 protein, HMB-45 and Melan A {3119}. Unlike some tumours of epithelial origin, including Paget disease, they are not immunoreactive for AE1/3, cytokeratins 7 and 20, epithelial membrane antigen, carcinoembryonic antigen or gross cystic disease fluid protein-15 {3120}.

Somatic genetics
The only two malignant melanomas of the vulva so far karyotyped showed trisomy 20 and del(18)(p11), respectively {2897}.

Prognosis and predictive factors
Clinical criteria
Treatment for a vulvar melanoma with a thickness of 0.75 mm or less is usually a wide local excision with a 1-cm circumferential margin and a 1-2 cm deep margin. Melanomas with a thickness of 1-4 mm require a 2 cm circumferential margin and a deep margin of at least 1-2 cm {2949}. Melanomas with a thickness greater than 4 mm are usually treated by radical vulvectomy {2950}. Depending on the tumour size, bilateral inguino-femoral lymphadenectomy may also be performed {1912,2261,2864, 3151}.

Histopathological criteria
Clark levels and Breslow thickness measurements are used to assess cutaneous vulvar melanomas.
Breslow thickness measurements for cutaneous malignant melanoma require measurement from the deep border of the granular layer of the overlying epithelium to the deepest point of tumour invasion. If a melanoma is less than 0.76 mm

in thickness, it has little or no metastatic potential {1694,3120}.
Survival following a diagnosis of vulvar melanoma is adversely influenced by numerous factors including a tumour thickness exceeding 2 mm, a tumour interpreted as Clark level IV or greater, a mitotic count within the tumour exceeding 10 mitoses per square mm, surface ulceration of the tumour and advanced tumour stage {3120}.

Congenital melanocytic naevus

The congenital melanocytic naevus is a benign tumour of melanocytes that is present at birth. Tumours may be small or involve a large area.

Acquired melanocytic naevus

The acquired melanocytic naevus appears in childhood and continues to grow with increasing age. This lesion may be junctional, i.e. at the epidermal-dermal junction, intradermal or compound (junctional and intradermal).

Blue naevus
The blue naevus is located entirely within the dermis and is composed of spindle-shaped or dendritic melanocytes that are typically heavily pigmented. A subtype known as the cellular blue naevus has a low potential for metastasis.

Atypical melanocytic naevus of the genital type

Definition
One type of atypical melanocytic proliferation in the genital area that forms a distinctive clinicopathological entity that can be distinguished from melanoma and dysplastic naevus.

Synonym
Atypical vulvar naevus.

Clinical features
The atypical melanocytic naevus of the genital type occurs primarily in young women of reproductive age. Unlike the dysplastic naevus, it is not associated with dysplastic naevi in other sites.
Vulvar naevi can be influenced by hormonal changes and may appear more active or atypical during pregnancy.

Histopathology
The atypical melanocytic naevus of the genital type has junctional melanocytic nests that are variably sized and include some atypical superficial melanocytes, These lesions lack significant atypia or mitotic activity in the deeper dermal melanocytes and do not involve skin appendages. In addition the lesion is small, well circumscribed and lacks pagetoid spread or necrosis {31,498}.

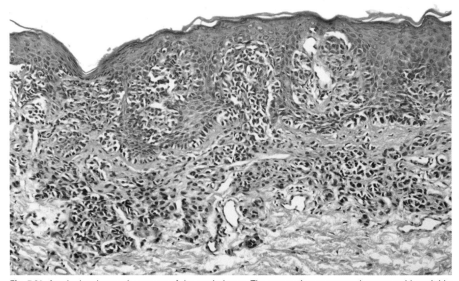

Fig. 7.21 Atypical melanocytic naevus of the genital type. The tumour is a compound naevus with variably sized melanocytic nests and atypia confined to the superficial melanocytes..

Dysplastic melanocytic naevus

Definition
A naevus that exhibits slight to moderate nuclear atypia that occurs only in the cells in the superficial portion.

Clinical features
These naevi occur predominantly in young women of reproductive age and present as elevated pigmented lesions with irregular borders typically exceeding 0.5 cm in diameter. Dysplastic naevi are rare on the vulva and may be associated with similar naevi elsewhere on the trunk and extremities.

Histopathology
They are composed of large epithelioid or spindle-shaped naevus cells with nuclear pleomorphism and prominent nucleoli. The atypical naevus cells are clustered in irregularly spaced junctional nests and involve hair shafts and the ducts of sweat glands and other skin appendages {31,498}. The dysplastic naevus may be compound or junctional. Features that distinguish a dysplastic naevus from malignant melanoma include symmetrical growth evident on full cross-section and the predominance of atypical cells in the superficial cellular component of the naevus. Limited pagetoid spread of single melanocytes with minimal or no involvement of the upper one-third of the epithelium may also be seen {31,498,2362}.

Genetic susceptibility
These vulvar naevi may occur in patients with the dysplastic naevus syndrome.

Germ cell, neuroectodermal, lymphoid and secondary tumours

E.J. Wilkinson

Definition
Primary tumours of the vulva that are not epithelial, mesenchymal or melanocytic in type, as well as secondary tumours.

ICD-O codes
Yolk sac tumour	9071/3
Merkel cell tumour	8247/3
Peripheral primitive neuroectodermal tumour/	9364/3
Ewing tumour	9260/3

Yolk sac tumour

Definition
A primitive malignant germ cell tumour characterized by a variety of distinctive histological patterns, some of which recapitulate phases in the development of the normal yolk sac.

Synonym
Endodermal sinus tumour.

Epidemiology
Yolk sac tumour is rare in the vulva and has been reported primarily in children and young women {888}.

Histopathology
For the histological features see the chapter on the ovary.

Prognosis and predictive factors
Vulvar yolk sac tumour is treated by local wide excision and chemotherapy, which is usually platinum-based {888}.

Merkel cell tumour

Definition
A malignant tumour composed of small neuroendocrine type cells of the lower epidermis.

Synonym
Neuroendocrine carcinoma of the skin.

Epidemiology
Merkel cell tumours are rare in the vulva and aggressive {324,554,996}.

Histopathology
The neoplastic cells have scanty cytoplasm and nuclei with finely stippled chromatin. Glandular and squamous differentiation has been reported {2607}.

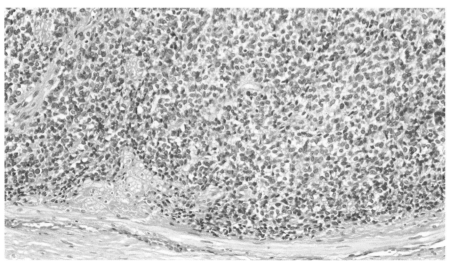

Fig. 7.22 A highly cellular peripheral primitive neuroectodermal tumour of vulva in an 18 year old.

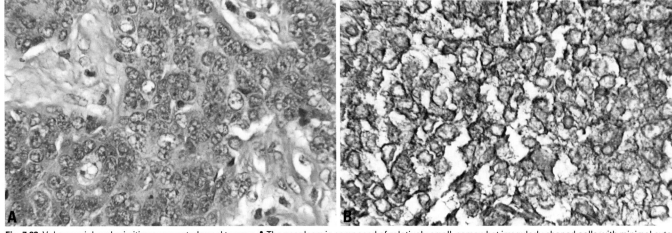

Fig. 7.23 Vulvar peripheral primitive neuroectodermal tumour. **A** The neoplasm is composed of relatively small, somewhat irregularly shaped cells with minimal cytoplasm. The nuclei are pleomorphic with granular chromatin and occasional small nucleoli. **B** Intense immunoreactivity for MIC 2 (CD99) is evident.

Immunohistochemical stains for cytokeratin demonstrate a distinctive perinuclear globular cytoplasmic pattern, and markers of neuroendocrine differentiation are usually positive {1209}. Electron microscopic examination demonstrates intermediate filaments in a globular paranuclear arrangement and dense core granules {554,996,1209}.

Histogenesis
These neoplasms are derived from small, neuroendocrine cells of the lower epidermis.

Peripheral primitive neuroectodermal tumour / Ewing tumour

Definition
An embryonal tumour arising outside of the central nervous system composed of undifferentiated or poorly differentiated neuroepithelial cells.

Clinical features
This is a rare primary tumour of the vulva that has been in reported in children and adult women of reproductive age {2839, 3002} and presents as a subcutaneous mass.

Histopathology
It is circumscribed but not encapsulated and composed of relatively small cells with minimal cytoplasm and ill defined cell borders. The nuclei are hyperchromatic with finely granular chromatin. Small nucleoli are evident. The mitotic count is variable, with an average of 3 per 10 high power fields reported {3002}. The tumour is usually multilobulated but is variable in appearance with solid areas, sinusoidal-appearing areas with cystic spaces containing eosinophilic proteineaceous material and Homer Wright rosettes {2839,3002}.

The tumour cells are immunoreactive for CD99 and vimentin and may be reactive for synaptophysin. Pan-cytokeratin may be focally positive in some cases. Dense core neurosecretory granules are not identified by electron microscopy.

Somatic genetics
A vulvar peripheral primitive neuroectodermal tumour/Ewing tumour has been shown to express the *EWS/FLI1* chimeric transcript due to the chromosome translocation t(11;22)(q24;q12), which is pathognomonic for this tumour type and is present in approximately 90% of tumours of this type {3002}.

Malignant lymphoma

Definition
A malignant lymphoproliferative neoplasm that may be primary or secondary.

Clinical features
This is a rare neoplasm that presents as a vulvar mass {1279,2266,3002}.

Histopathology
In the largest series two-thirds of the cases were diffuse large B-cell lymphomas {3002}.

Prognosis and predictive factors
Malignant lymphoma of the vulva is usually an aggressive disease {3002}.

Leukaemia

Definition
A malignant haematopoetic neoplasm that may be primary or secondary.

Clinical features
Rarely, granulocytic sarcoma presents as a vulvar mass {1583}

Histopathology
See chapters on the cervix and vagina.

Secondary tumours of the vulva

Definition
Tumours of the vulva that originate outside the vulva.

Incidence and origin
The vulva is a rare site of secondary involvement by tumour. Tumours may involve the vulva by lymphatic spread or contiguous growth. The primary site of a secondary tumour of the vulva is most commonly the cervix, followed by the endometrium or ovary. Occasionally, breast carcinoma, renal cell carcinoma, gastric carcinoma, lung carcinoma, and, rarely, gestational choriocarcinoma, malignant melanoma or neuroblastoma spread to the vulva. Vaginal, urethral, urinary bladder and anorectal carcinomas may extend directly into the vulva {1631, 1802,3121}.

CHAPTER 8

Inherited Tumour Syndromes

Inherited cancer susceptibility is now recognized as a significant risk for cancer of the breast and female genitals organs. For many inherited tumour syndromes, the underlying germline mutations have been identified. This allows genetic testing and counseling of at risk family members and to estimate the associated disease burden. The genetic basis involves mutational inactivation of tumour supressor and DNA repair genes. Such germline mutations follow a mendelian inheritance pattern and usually confer substantial cancer risks, with breast and ovary as most frequent target organs. Additional familial aggregations have been observed but the responsible genes have not yet been identified and may involve multigenic traits.

Familial aggregation of cancers of the breast and female genital organs

D. Goldgar
M.R. Stratton

Evidence of familial aggregation of breast, ovarian, and other tumours of the female genital organs derived from anecdotal observation of large families and from systematic analyses of cancer incidence in relatives of cancer cases. Although there are a number of potential measures of familial aggregation, the most commonly used is the familial relative risk (FRR) or standardized incidence rate (SIR). This is defined as the ratio of the incidence of disease among relatives of an individual with disease compared with the incidence in the population as a whole. The FRR is most often estimated through comparison of family history data between cases and controls, with the resulting odds ratio used as an estimator of the familial risk. Using genealogical resources linked to cancer registries has a number of advantages; the number of cases is usually large compared to case-control studies and, more importantly, all cancers found among relatives are confirmed in the cancer registry.

Breast cancer

Evidence that women with a positive family history of breast cancer are at increased risk for developing the disease has been accumulating for over 50 years; virtually every study has found significantly elevated relative risks to female relatives of breast cancer patients. Most studies have found relative risks between 2 and 3 for first-degree relatives of breast cancer patients selected without regard to age at diagnosis or laterality. A recent review of 74 published studies {2238} calculated familial relative risks of 2.1 (95% CI 2.0, 2.2) for breast cancer in any first degree relative, 2.3 for a sister affected, and 2.0 for an affected mother, and a relative risk of 3.6 if an individual had both a mother and sister affected. For individuals with a first degree relative diagnosed with breast cancer under age 50, the relative risk to develop breast cancer before age 50 was 3.3 (CI 2.8, 3.9).

In a population-based study of familial cancer using the Utah Population Database, Goldgar et al. {1029} studied the incidence of breast and other cancers among 49 202 first-degree relatives of 5559 breast cancer probands diagnosed before age 80. This study estimated a relative risk of 1.8 in first degree relatives of these breast cancer probands. When restricted to early-onset cancer (diagnosed before age 50), the relative risk of breast cancer among first-degree relatives increased to 2.6 and the risk for early-onset breast cancer among these relatives was 3.7 (95% CI. 2.8–4.6). The Swedish family cancer database {715} contains >9.6 million individuals, with data on nearly 700,000 invasive cancers and consists of individuals born in Sweden after 1934 and their parents. Analyzing cancers diagnosed between the years 1958 to 1996, the standardized incidence ratio for breast cancer was 1.85 (95% CI 1.74–1.96) for having an affected mother, 1.98 (1.79–2.18) for having an affected sister, and 2.4 (1.72–3.23) if both mother and sister were affected. Other studies found larger familial effects among relatives of young bilateral probands compared with young probands with unilateral breast cancer {700,1246,2129}.

The issue of relationship of histology to familial breast cancer is less clear {375, 500,1724,2441,2989}. Some studies found that lobular carcinoma is more often associated with a positive family history {791} while others {1566} observed that cases with tubular carcinoma were more frequently associated with a positive family history. Multi-centricity was also found to be positively associated with family history {1564}. Occurrence of breast cancer in a male conveys a two to three fold increased risk of breast cancer in female relatives {94,2449}.

Ovarian cancer

In a population-based case-control study of families of 493 ovarian cancer cases and 2465 controls, Schildkraut and Thompson {2557} reported an odds ratio for ovarian cancer in first degree relatives of 3.6 (95% CI 1.8–7.1). A comprehensive study of first-degree relatives of 883 ovarian cancer probands from the Utah Population Database estimated a relative risk of 2.1 (1.0–3.4) for ovarian cancer in the relatives {1029}. Analysis of the Swedish family cancer database {715} found a standardized incidence ratio for ovarian cancer of 2.81 (95% CI 2.21–3.51) for having an affected mother, 1.94 (0.99–3.41) for having an affected sister, and 25.5 (6.6–66.0) if both mother and sister were affected. A meta-analysis of all case-control and cohort studies published before 1998 estimates the risk to first degree relatives at 3.1, with a 95%CI of 2.6-3.7 {2801}.

Endometrial cancer

Gruber and Thompson {1071} in a study of first-degree relatives of 455 cases of primary epithelial carcinoma of the endometrium and 3216 controls, report an odds ratio (OR) of 2.8 (CI 1.9 – 4.2) for having one or more relatives affected with endometrial cancer. In a similar size study (726 cases and 2123 controls) Parrazini et al. {2173} found a smaller effect, with an OR of 1.5 (CI 1.0–2.3). This may partly be explained by the fact that in the former study, cases were restricted to ages 20-54, while in the latter, the median age at diagnosis was 61. A Danish case-control study of 237 cases of endometrial cancer diagnosed under age 50 and 538 population controls reported an OR for family history of 2.1 (1.1–3.8). In contrast to most other sites, the two registry/geneaology based studies of endometrial cancer produced conflicting results, with the Utah study finding a FRR of 1.32 and the Swedish family cancer database reporting a SIR of 2.85. The reason for this discrepancy is unclear, but may to some extent reflect differences in the age distribution of the two populations.

Cervical cancer

In the Utah Population Database {1029}, a FRR to first degree relatives of 999 cervical cancer cases of 1.74 was obtained (95% CI 1.03-2.53) while in the Swedish family cancer database {715}, a slightly higher risk of 1.93 (1.52-2.42) in mothers of invasive cervical cancer cases and 2.39 (1.59-3.46) in sisters. Unlike many other cancers, there did not appear to be a significant effect of age at diagnosis in familial risk of cervical cancer, although the risks to mothers did depend on the number of affected daughters. In this study, significant familial aggregation was also found for in situ carcinoma of the cervix (FRR 1.79, (1.75-1.84).

Multiple cancer sites

In most but not all studies, a familial association between cancers of the breast and ovary have been found, particularly when the breast cancer cases have been diagnosed at a young age. Undoubtedly, the majority of the association between breast and ovarian cancer detected in these population studies is due to the *BRCA1* gene, which is known to be involved in a large proportion of extended kindreds with clearly inherited susceptibility to breast and ovarian cancer. It is likely that some of the discrepant results are linked to the frequency of *BRCA1* deleterious alleles in the respective populations in these studies.

For breast cancer, the most consistent finding has been a small (FRR/SIR ~ 1.2) but highly significant familial association with prostate cancer. Other sites found to be associated in at least two studies with breast cancer in the familial context have been thyroid cancer and other endocrine-related tumours.

For endometrial cancer, there is a familial association with colorectal cancer which is consistently found in a number of studies with statistically significant OR/SIRs ranging from from 1.3 to 1.9. Some, but not all studies have also reported associations with ovarian cancer, particularly among relatives of younger patients.

The strongest and most consistent familial association between cervical and other sites is for lung cancer with statistically significant SIRs of 1.8 and 1.64 found in the Swedish FCDB and the Utah UPDB, respectively. Other cancers with possible associations in both studies are

Table 8.01
Specific inherited syndromes involving cancers of the breast and female genital organs.

Syndrome	MIM	Gene	Location	Associated sites / tumours
BRCA1 syndrome	113705	*BRCA1*	17q	Breast, ovary, colon, liver, endometrium, cervix, fallopian tube, peritoneum
BRCA2 syndrome	600185	*BRCA2*	13q	Breast (female and male), ovary, fallopian tube, prostate, pancreas, gallbladder, stomach, melanoma
Li-Fraumeni	151623	*TP53*	17p	Breast, sarcoma, brain, adrenal, leukaemia
Cowden	158350	*PTEN*	10q	Skin, thyroid, breast, cerebellum, colon
HNPCC	114500	*MLH1* *MSH2* *MSH6*	3p 2p 2p	Colon, endometrium, small intestine, ovary, ureter/renal pelvis, hepatobiliary tract, brain, skin
Muir Torre	158320	*MLH1* *MSH2*	3p 2p	HNPCC sites plus sebaceous glands
Peutz-Jeghers	175200	*STK11*	19p	Small intestine, ovary, cervix, testis, pancreas, breast
Ataxia Telangiectasia	208900	*ATM*	11q	Breast (heterozygotes)

lip/skin (SIR 2.4 and 1.83) and bladder cancer (SIR=1.6), though the latter was not statistically significant in the UPDB study.

In addition to this statistical and observational evidence for the role of genetic factors in the development of these cancers, a number of specific genes have been identified. Of these, the most important in terms of both risk and frequency are the breast cancer susceptibility loci *BRCA1* and *BRCA2*, and the mismatch repair genes *MSH2*, *MLH1*, and *MSH6* in the context of the hereditary non-polyposis colorectal cancer (HNPCC).

Search for additional genes

While some of the familial clustering may be due to shared environmental factors, it seems likely that a number of additional loci remain to be identified for cancers of the breast and female genital tract. Some studies have shown that only about one-fifth of the familial aggregation of breast

cancer is attributable to the *BRCA1* and *BRCA2* genes {107,592,2230} and that these genes only explain less than half of all high risk site-specific breast cancer families {898,2631}. Whether the remaining familial aggregation is due to additional moderate to high risk loci or to the combined effects of a number of more common, but lower risk, susceptibility alleles is unknown {2236}. In contrast, it appears that almost all of the familial clustering in ovarian cancer can be ascribed to the effects of the *BRCA1/2* and HNPCC loci {2802}. Although no systematic studies have been done for endometrial cancer, it is also likely that the HNPCC loci account for a substantial fraction of familial aggregation in this cancer as well.

BRCA1 syndrome

D. Goldgar   R.H.M. Verheijen
R. Eeles   C. Szabo
D. Easton   A.N. Monteiro
S.R. Lakhani   P. Devilee
S.Piver   S. Narod
J.M. Piek   E.H. Meijers-Heijboer
P.J. van Diest   N. Sodha

Definition

Inherited tumour syndrome with autosomal dominant trait and markedly increased susceptibility to breast and ovarian tumours, due to germline mutations in the *BRCA1* gene. Additional organ sites include colon, liver, endometrium, cervix, fallopian tube, and peritoneum.

MIM No.   113705 {1835}

Synonyms

Breast cancer 1, early onset breast ovarian cancer syndrome.

Incidence

The prevalence of *BRCA1* mutations in most Caucasian populations is estimated to be 1 in 883 {897}. However, in certain populations, this is higher, e.g. 1% in Ashkenazi Jews {3065}. Using recombination techniques, *BRCA1* mutations have been dated to the early Roman times {1997}. De novo mutations are rare.

Diagnostic criteria

A definitive diagnosis is only possible by genetic testing. *BRCA1* mutations are common in certain populations and in families with numerous early onset breast cancer cases (≥4 cases of breast cancer at <60 years) or in those with ovarian cancer at any age in addition to early onset breast cancer. The chance of a mutation in either *BRCA1* or *BRCA2* is lower (<30%) when only two or three breast cancer cases are present in a family. The main difference between *BRCA1* and *BRCA2* is the increased risk of male breast cancer in *BRCA2*. The American Society of Clinical Oncology (ASCO) guidelines suggest offering testing at a probability of mutation of >10% but many other countries will only offer testing to those with a chance >30% because of the need to concentrate resources.

Breast tumours

Penetrance

Analyses of worldwide data submitted to the Breast Cancer Linkage Consortium (BCLC) have provided general estimates of penetrance {8}. Estimates for specific populations have shown that the Ashkenazim have a lower than average lifetime breast cancer penetrance of about 50-60% {3065}. Population based studies in UK breast cancer patients also revealed a lower penetrance and indicate that the presence of a mutation within a familial breast cancer cluster does confer a higher penetrance {2230}. This may be due to an association with other genes or epidemiological factors that are present in the family. There are also reports of variable penetrance dependent on the position of the mutation within the *BRCA1* gene {2914}.

Clinical features

Breast cancer in *BRCA1* mutation carriers occurs more often at a younger age, typically before age 40 {1687}. It tends to progress directly to invasive disease without a precancerous DCIS component {8,1574}. Accordingly, there appears to be a lower chance of early detection by mammographic screening and a higher proportion of invasive cancers {1025}. There is an almost linear increase in the lifetime risk of contralateral breast cancer from the age of 35 years, reaching a level of 64% by the age of 80 {742}.

Pathology

Certain morphological types of breast cancer, including medullary carcinoma, tubular carcinoma, lobular carcinoma in situ, and invasive lobular carcinoma, have been reported more commonly in patients with a positive family history of breast cancer {191,1566,1684,1724, 2441}.

Patients with *BRCA1* germline mutations have an excess of medullary or atypical medullary carcinoma compared to controls {8,764,1767}. Tumours in *BRCA1* mutation carriers are generally of a higher grade than their sporadic counterparts {8,764,1767}. Ductal carcinoma in situ (DCIS) adjacent to invasive cancer is observed less frequently while the frequency of lobular neoplasia in situ is similar in both groups {8}. However, in a multifactorial analysis of the BCLC database, the only features significantly associated with *BRCA1* were total mitotic count, continuous pushing margins, and lymphocytic infiltrate. All other features, including the diagnosis of medullary and atypical medullary carcinoma, were not found to be significant {1572}.

BRCA1-associated tumours are more likely to be estrogen (ER) and progesterone receptor (PgR) negative {766, 1352,1574,2121}. Data on *ERBB2* are limited but *BRCA1*-linked tumours are more likely to be negative than controls {1352,1574}. *BRCA1*-linked tumours show a higher frequency of *TP53* mutations and p53 expression than sporadic breast cancer {580,581,765,1574}. *BRCA1*-associated tumours show very low expression of Cyclin D1 in both the invasive and in situ components {2122}. The absence of Cyclin D1 in these tumours could be an additional evidence

Table 8.02
Probability of *BRCA1/2* mutation in women with breast/ovarian cancer.

Chance of mutation	Clinical criteria
<10%	Single breast cancer / ovarian cancer case at <40 years in non Ashkenazim
10-30%	2-3 female breast cancers <60 years (no ovarian / male breast cancer)
30%	One female breast cancer <60 and one ovarian cancer
	Female breast cancer <40 in Ashkenazi
>60%	Four cases of female breast cancer at <60 years
	≥2 cases female breast cancer <60 and ovarian cancer any age
	≥2 cases female breast cancer <60 and male breast cancer any age

From R.A. Eeles {749}.

of hormone independence of *BRCA1*-associated breast cancers.

Prognosis and prognostic factors
Studies on the prognosis of breast cancer associated with *BRCA1* range from poorer prognosis, to no difference, to a better prognosis {441}. There is a potential survival bias since at least one patient in each family must have survived in order to have blood taken for gene testing. The most optimal studies are therefore those which have taken this into consideration, either by discounting the proband in a family who has presented for testing {3022} or by testing specific founder mutations in archival tumour tissue material from all cases in a specific population (for example, see Foulkes et al. {904}).

Ovarian tumours

Age distribution and penetrance
About 7-10% of ovarian carcinomas are due to inherited *BRCA1* (or *BRCA2*) mutations; as these are on autosomes, they can be inherited from either the mother or the father. Although ovarian cancer can occur earlier in *BRCA1* (and indeed *BRCA2*) carriers, the presence of an older onset ovarian cancer still can indicate an underlying mutation in either of these genes. The penetrance for ovarian cancer in *BRCA1* mutation carriers is shown in Fig. 8.02; it starts to rise at an earlier age than the curve for *BRCA2*, which starts to rise at about 50 years. The penetrance is 44-60% by age 70. This is markedly higher than the lifetime risk of 1.8% (1 in 55) for sporadic ovarian cancer in women living in developed countries.

Clinical features
In a retrospective cohort study of Jewish subjects, women with advanced-stage ovarian cancer and a *BRCA1* or *BRCA2* founder mutation had a longer survival than women with non-hereditary ovarian cancer (P = 0.004) and a longer median time to recurrence (14 months versus 7 months) (P< 0.001) {329}.
BRCA1/2 heterozygotes had higher response rates to primary therapy compared with patients who had sporadic disease (P = 0.01), and those with advance-stage disease had improved survival compared with patients who had advanced stage sporadic carcinoma {422}.

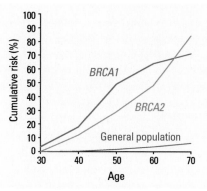

Fig. 8.01 The breast cancer penetrance of *BRCA1* and *BRCA2* from the BCLC data.

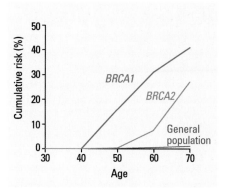

Fig. 8.02 The ovarian cancer penetrance of *BRCA1* and *BRCA2* from the BCLC data.

Pathology
In patients with *BRCA1* germline mutations, epithelial tumours (carcinomas) are the most common histological diagnosis. All subtypes of malignant epithelial ovarian neoplasms have been reported, including the very rare entity of malignant transitional cell carcinoma {3102}. Interobserver variation in typing of ovarian carcinoma is likely to account, at least in part, for the different results reported to date {572,1716,2513}. Some studies indicate that papillary serous adenocarcinoma is the predominant ovarian cancer that occurs in familial ovarian cancer syndromes {229,2479,

2800} while others report that they occur with similar frequency in *BRCA1/2* mutation carriers and sporadic cases {329, 2239,3102}. The large majority of studies have shown mucinous carcinoma to be under-represented in *BCRA1* mutation carriers {50,229,1974,2239,2479,2800, 3102}.
The frequency of endometrioid and clear cell carcinoma occurring in *BRCA1* mutation carriers is similar to that of sporadic cases {50,229,1353,2239,2479, 2800,3102,3272}.
The current data suggest that germline mutations in *BRCA1/2* genes do not pre-

Table 8.03
Lifetime cancer risks of *BRCA1* carriers.

Cancer site	Relative risk (95% CI)	Cumulative risk by age 70, % (95% CI)
Breast	Age-dependent	87
Ovary	Age-dependent	44
Colon	4.11 (2.36-7.15) {896} 2.03 (1.45-2.85) {2915}[1]	-
Cervix	3.72 (2.26-6.10)	3.57 (3.16-4.04)
Uterus	2.65 (1.69-4.16)	2.47 (2.02-3.04)
Pancreas	2.26 (1.26-4.06)	1.2 (0.9-1.7)
Prostate	3.33 (1.78-6.20) {896} 1.82 (1.01-3.29) {2915}[2]	2.64 (1.95-3.57) (Europe) 7.67 (4.77-12.20) (North America)
All cancers[3] – male	0.95 (0.81-1.12)	16.89 (14.52-19.81)
All cancers[3] – female	2.30 (1.93-2.75)	23.27 (21.73-24.89)

From D. Ford et al. {896} and D. Thompson et al. {2915}.
[1] When considered together with rectal cancer, the relative risk was no longer significantly elevated above 1.0; no excess risk was noted among men.
[2] For men under the age of 65.
[3] All cancers other than nonmelanoma skin cancer, breast cancer, or ovarian cancer.

dispose individuals to the development of borderline neoplasms {1044,1704}. However, occasional invasive {2479, 3272} and borderline {50} mucinous neoplasms have been reported.

Stromal tumours and malignant germ cell ovarian neoplasms appear not to be associated with BRCA1/2 germline mutations. However, several families in which more than one relative had been diagnosed with a malignant ovarian germ cell tumour have been published {2790}. Single cases of dysgerminoma {3103} and transitional cell ovarian carcinoma {3101} have been observed in BRCA1 carriers with a family history of breast and ovarian cancer. The development of these lesions may be unrelated to the germline BRCA1 mutations in these cases.

The first report on BRCA1-associated ovarian carcinoma found that overall the tumours were of higher grade and higher stage than their historic age-matched controls {2479}. These findings have been largely reproduced by a number of other groups {50,229,2239,3102,3272}. In contrast, Berchuck et al. {229} found that although the BRCA1 cases in their study were all of advanced stage (III/IV), they were half as likely to be as poorly differentiated as cases without mutations. Johannsson et al. {1353} did not identify a difference in grade between the ovarian cancers in their BRCA1 mutation carriers and the control population-based cancer registry group.

Prognosis and prognostic factors
The majority of BRCA1 ovarian cancers are serous cystadenocarcinomas which have a poor prognosis generally if diagnosed when they have spread outside the ovary. Studies of ovarian cancer occurring in BRCA1 carriers have reported a somewhat better prognosis {213}, but it is uncertain whether this is because of the bias in carrier detection in this population or whether they are more sensitive to treatment. If the latter were true, this would refer to platinum treatments as these data have been reported prior to the use of taxanes.

Tumours of the fallopian tube
Definition
Hereditary fallopian tube carcinoma arises from epithelium overlying the lamina propria of the endosalpinx in women at high hereditary risk to develop ovarian

carcinoma, typically due to loss of the wild-type allele of BRCA1 or BRCA2. The tumour has to fulfill the clinical and histological criteria for tubal carcinoma {1256} as well as clinical genetic criteria shown in Table 8.02.

Incidence
From 1997 to 2002, a total of 15 hereditary breast/ovarian family related tubal tumours have been reported in literature. In 8 cases a BRCA1 mutation was detected. However, the true incidence of both hereditary and sporadic tubal carcinoma is probably much higher. This is caused by the fact that primary tubal tumours are often mistaken for primary ovarian carcinomas {3150}. Moreover, some primary ovarian carcinomas might actually derive from inclusion cysts lined by tubal epithelial cells included into the ovarian stroma {2247}.

Age distribution
In general the age of onset is younger in hereditary cases when compared to sporadic cases.

Diagnostic criteria
The criteria of Hu et. al. {1256} as modified by Sedlis {2614} and Yoonessi {3185} are applied to differentiate hereditary tubal carcinomas from ovarian- and endometrial-carcinoma. These criteria require that: a) the main tumour is in the fallopian tube and arises from the endosalpinx, b) the histological features resemble a tubal pattern, c) if the tubal wall is involved, the transition between malignant and benign tubal epithelium should be detectable, d) the fallopian tube contains more tumour than the ovary or endometrium.

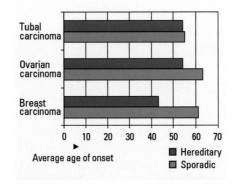

Fig. 8.03 Average age of onset of BRCA1 and BRCA2 related carcinomas.

Table 8.04
BRCA1 mutation status in relation to histopathology of 200 malignant ovarian epithelial tumours.

Histologic type	BRCA1-negative families		BRCA1-positive families	
Serous	80	(59%)	44	(67%)
Mucinous	12	(9%)*	0	(0%)*
Endometrioid	10	(7%)	5	(8%)
Clear cell	13	(10%)	3	(4%)
Undifferentiated	10	(7%)	9	(14%)
MMMT[a]	3	(2%)	1	(2%)
Transitional cell	2	(2%)	1	(2%)
Mixed[b]	5	(4%)	2	(3%)
Total	135	(100%)	65	(100%)

Excludes borderline tumours.
Adapted from B.A. Werness et al. {3102}.
[a] Malignant müllerian mixed tumour.
[b] > 10% minor histologic type.
* P = 0.01 for the difference in prevalence between BRCA1-positive and BRCA1-negative families.

Clinical features
Symptoms and signs. To date, there is no indication that clinical hereditary tubal carcinoma features are different from those of its sporadic counterpart. In addition to occasional abdominal discomfort, the classical triad of symptoms include: (i) prominent watery vaginal discharge, (ii) pelvic pain and (iii) a pelvic mass {158}. Cervical cytology reveals adenocarcinomatous cells in approximately 10% of patients {3185}.

Tumour marker. As in ovarian carcinoma, elevation of serum CA125 levels are found in approximately 80% of cases {1173}.

Imaging. CT/MRI are inconclusive with respect to the differential diagnosis of tubal or ovarian carcinomas. However, these techniques can be helpful in determining the extent of disease. Likewise, ultrasonography can not distinguish tubal from ovarian disease {2720}.

Histopathology and grading
Serous papillary carcinoma is the most common form of hereditary tubal carcinoma.

Grading is of limited value in these tumours and, if used, is based on the papillary architecture, nuclear atypia and mitotic activity. Grade I cancers show papillary growth with well differentiated columnar cells and low mitotic rate. Grade II cancers are papillary with evident gland formation with intermediately differentiated cells with moderate mitotic activity. Grade III shows solid growth with loss of papillae and a medullary/glandular pattern. The cells are poorly differentiated and the mitotic activity is high.

Immunohistochemistry. Being predominantly of serous papillary type, hereditary tubal carcinomas are positive for cytokeratins 7 and 8, MUC1, CEA, OVTL3, OV632, CA125, and negative or showing only low expression for cytokeratin 20, CEA and vimentin. Also, p53 is often expressed, and cyclins E and A and Ki67 show a varying number of proliferating cells, whereas staining for ERBB2 and cyclin D1 is usually negative. Steroid receptor content varies. In the rare clear cell cancers, p21 is highly expressed.

Seeding and metastasis
Hereditary tubal carcinomas presumably spread like their sporadic counterparts. Empirical data are available to date point to a mode of spread similar to ovarian cancer.

Prognosis
The five-year survival rate of 30% in sporadic cases varies with stage {158,3185}, but not with grade. The survival rate of hereditary tubal carcinomas has yet to be established since only small numbers of patients have been reported and most patients have still not completed their 5-year follow-up.

Other tumours
BRCA1 predominantly predisposes to female breast cancer and ovarian cancer. Unlike *BRCA2*, it is not thought to predispose to male breast cancer. A few families with male breast cancer and a *BRCA1* mutation have been described, but these may be within the numbers expected by chance. A study of causes of mortality by Ford et al. {896} reported an increased risk of colon cancer and prostate cancer. However, a reanalysis {2914} has shown a small pancreatic cancer excess, as is seen in *BRCA2* carriers and an excess of prostate cancer risk only at age <60 years. The excess of colonic cancer was counteracted by a deficit of rectal cancer. See Table 8.03 for details on risk estimates.

Genetics
Chromosomal location and gene structure
The *BRCA1* gene is located on chromosome 17q21 {1109}. The 24 exons of the *BRCA1* gene (22 coding exons; alternative 5'UTR exons, 1a & 1b) span an 81-kb chromosomal region, that has an unusually high density of Alu repetitive DNA (41.5%) {1864,2735}. A partial pseudogene (*BRCA1Ψ*) consisting of a tandem duplication of exons 1a, 1b and 2 lies 44.5kb upstream of *BRCA1* {356,2303}. Exon 11 of *BRCA1* (3.4 kb) encodes 61% of the 1863 amino acid protein. The amino-terminal RING finger domain and the carboxy-terminal BRCT repeats {316} of BRCA1 are highly conserved among vertebrates {2825}, while the rest of the protein bears little homology to other known genes.

Gene expression
Several alternatively spliced transcripts have been described for the *BRCA1* gene, the most prevalent of these lead to in-frame deletions of exon 11 (*BRCA1-Δ11*). Both full length and Δ11 transcripts are ubiquitously expressed. The 100- and 97-kDa Δ11 protein isoforms lack the nuclear localization signal and are cytoplasmic {1864,2904}. However, the full-length 220-kDa protein is predominantly observed in the nucleus. Its expression and phosphorylation is cell-cycle dependent, commencing in G1 and reaching maximal levels by early S-phase. BRCA1 colocalizes with the BRCA2 and Rad51 proteins in discrete foci during S-phase. DNA damage leads to hyperphosphorylation of BRCA1, dispersal of the BRCA1/BRCA2/Rad51 nuclear foci, and their relocalization to PCNA-containing DNA replication structures. In meiotic cells, BRCA1, BRCA2 and Rad51 colocalize on the axial elements of developing synaptonemal complexes {450,2594,2596}. A large protein complex consisting of other tumour suppressor and DNA repair proteins, known as BASC (BRCA1-associated genome surveillance complex) has been identified. Among these, partial colocalization of BRCA1 with Rad50, MRE11 and BLM in nuclear foci analogous to those observed with BRCA2 and Rad51 has been demonstrated {3054}. In addition to its interactions with BRCA2, Rad51, and BASC, the BRCA1 protein has been shown to form complexes with a number of other proteins involved in diverse cellular functions, including DNA repair, transcription, chromatin remodeling, and protein ubiquination (reviewed in {3018}). During mouse embryonic development, *Brca1* exhibits a dynamic expression

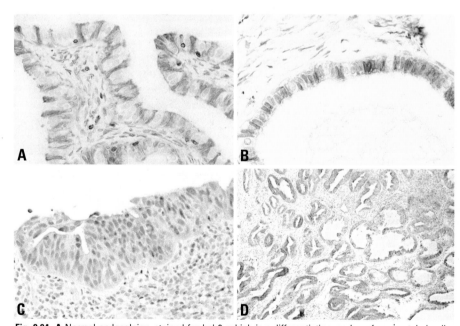

Fig. 8.04 A Normal endosalpinx, stained for bcl-2, which is a differentiation marker of serous tubal cells. **B** Tubal cell-lined inclusion cyst in the ovary stained for bcl-2. **C** Dysplastic lesion in a fallopian tube of a *BRCA1* mutation carrier, stained for p53. **D** Serous adenocarcinoma of the fallopian tube stained for bcl-2 (note: not all serous carcinomas are bcl-positive).

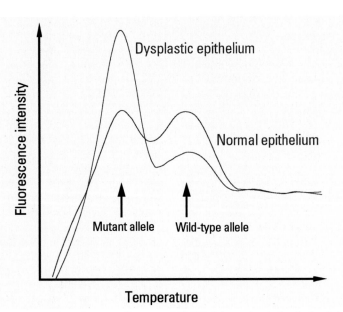

Fig. 8.05 To assess whether wild-type and/or mutated *BRCA1* alleles are lost in dysplastic tubal epithelium of a *BRCA1* mutation carrier, light-cycler polymerase chain reaction (PCR) melting curve analysis is performed. This technique utilizes the properties of probes to anneal less stringent to mutated DNA than to wild-type DNA, resulting in a lower denaturation temperature for mutated DNA. Two peaks, indicating different denaturing temperatures, are detected in non-dysplastic epithelium, indicating the presence of both wild-type and mutated *BRCA1* DNA. One clear peak at the melting temperature for the mutated *BRCA1* DNA in the dysplastic epithelium indicates loss of wild-type *BRCA1* DNA. From J.M. Piek et al. {2246}.

pattern, which parallels *Brca2* expression in that the highest expression levels occur in epithelial tissues undergoing concurrent proliferation and differentiation. In adult mice, *Brca1* and *Brca2* expression is induced during mammary gland ductal proliferation, morphogenesis and differentiation occuring at puberty and again during proliferation of the mammary epithelium during pregnancy {1582,1769,2323}.

Consistent with its role as a tumour-suppressor gene, the wild-type allele of *BRCA1* is lost in the majority of tumours of individuals with inherited mutations, presumably leading to absence of normal protein {560}. In sporadic cancer, BRCA1 protein expression is absent or reduced in the majority of high grade breast carcinomas and sporadic ovarian tumours {2493,3130}. Although few somatic mutations in the *BRCA1* coding sequence have been identified {1846}, somatic inactivation of protein expression may occur through several mechanisms, including gross chromosomal rearrangements – approximately 50% of primary breast tumours show loss of heterozygosity of chromosome 17q21 {559, 1134}, or epigenetic inactivation of expression, such as promoter hypermethylation {426}.

Gene function

The BRCT domain of BRCA1 is a protein-protein interaction module found in proteins involved in DNA repair and cell cycle control {316}. The RING domain mediates the interaction with BARD1 and the dimer displays ubiquitin ligase (E3) activity {159}. The physiologic substrates of this activity remain unknown although the Fanconi anaemia D2 protein is a likely candidate {958}. The integrity of the RING and BRCT domains is indispensable for the functions of BRCA1 as demonstrated by the presence of cancer-associated mutations in these regions.

A number of different mutations have been introduced into mouse *Brca1*, all resulting in embryos with γ-irradiation hypersensitivity and genetic instability. Mice with a conditional mutation of *Brca1* in the mammary gland developed tumorigenesis associated with genetic instability, providing an important link to human disease {3167}. Interestingly, mouse cells lacking Brca1 are deficient in repair of chromosomal double-strand breaks (DSB) by homologous recombination {1931}. Taken together, these results suggest a role for BRCA1 in the DNA damage response.

Expression of wild type but not disease-associated *BRCA1* alleles in *BRCA1*-

deficient human cells restores resistance to DNA-damaging agents {2595} and several BRCA1-containing complexes involved in DNA repair have been identified. These include S-phase nuclear foci containing BRCA2 and Rad51 {450}, the hRad50-hMre11-NBS1[p95] (R/M/N) complex, involved in a wide variety of DNA repair processes {3258}, and the BASC complex which contains ATM, the BLM helicase, mismatch repair proteins MSH2, MSH6, MLH1 and the R/M/N complex {3054}. DNA damaging agents induce BRCA1 hyperphosphorylation, which is likely to modulate the association of BRCA1 with these different protein complexes {2597}. These biochemical approaches corroborate the notion that BRCA1 participates in the cellular response to promote DNA break recognition and repair, as shown in Fig. 8.08.

The involvement of BRCA1 in a variety of DNA repair processes suggests that it may be an upstream effector common to various responses to DNA damage {3018}. In line with the idea of *BRCA1*'s pleiotropic role, it also acts as a negative regulator of cell growth. Ectopic expression of BRCA1 causes cell cycle arrest at G1 via the induction of the cdk inhibitor p21[Waf1/CiP1] {2745}. Conversely, inhibition of *BRCA1* expression with antisense oligonucleotides results in the accelerated growth of mammary epithelial cell lines {2917}. Also, BRCA1 seems to be required for efficient radiation-induced G2/M and S-phase checkpoints pointing to a broad involvement of BRCA1 in checkpoint control {3166,3178}.

Several lines of evidence suggest that one of the molecular functions of BRCA1 is the regulation of transcription. The BRCA1 C-terminus acts as a transactivation domain and germline mutations found in *BRCA1* abolish this activity {1899}. BRCA1 can be copurified with RNA polymerase II and upon replication blockage, a novel complex containing BRCA1 and BARD1 is formed, suggesting that BRCA1 protein redistributes to different complexes in response to replication stress {476,2593}. BRCA1 also associates and, in some cases, modulates the activity of several proteins involved in the regulation of gene expression such as transcription factors, coactivators, corepressors and chromatin remodeling complexes {297,1247, 1899,3255}. A recent exciting development, of yet unknown physiologic significance, was the discovery of direct DNA binding by BRCA1 in vitro which may be important for its function in transcription and DNA repair {2198}.

Putative BRCA1 transcriptional target genes identified so far play a role in some aspect of the DNA damage response. BRCA1 induces the transactivation of p21^WAF1/CiP1 in p53-dependent and independent manners, insuring a potent cell cycle arrest, reinforcing the connection between cell cycle checkpoint control and transcription regulation {2130,2745}. Experiments using cDNA arrays identified the DNA-damage-responsive gene GADD45 as a major target of BRCA1-mediated transcription {1138,1727}. These results, coupled with studies showing that disruption of p53 partially rescues embryonic lethality in Brca1^-/- mouse, link the p53 pathway and BRCA1 function {1108,1710}. Importantly, the majority of tumours derived from BRCA1-linked patients or from Brca1^-/- mice present mutations in p53 {581,3167}.

Mutation spectrum

Germline mutations in BRCA1 have been detected in 15-20% of clinic-based breast cancer families, and in 40-50% of breast-ovarian cancer families {2657, 3023}. Mutations occur throughout the entire coding region, and hence the mutation spectrum has taught us relatively little about the gene's function. The majority of the mutations are predicted to lead to a prematurely truncated protein when translated. In conjunction with the observed loss of the wildtype allele in tumours arising in mutation carriers {560}, this indicates that inactivation of the gene is an important step in tumorigenesis. Despite the strong variability in mutations detected in families, founder effects have led to some mutations being very prevalent in certain populations of defined geographical or ethnic background. An example is the 185delAG mutation, which is present in approximately 1% of all individuals of Ashkenazi Jewish descent {1151}. As a result, mutation spectra may vary according to ethnic background of the sampled population {2824}. In some populations, specific large interstitial deletions or insertions, which are difficult to detect by conventional PCR-based mutation scanning technologies, have been observed to be particularly frequent. They may comprise between 10 and 20% of the total mutation spectrum {944,1229}.

In recent years, an increasing number of missense changes are being detected in BRCA1, of which the clinical significance is uncertain. These already comprise up to 40% of all known sequence changes in BRCA1. The Breast Cancer Information Core (BIC) maintains a website providing a central repository for information regarding mutations and polymorphisms {http://research.nhgri.nih.gov/bic/}.

Genotype-phenotype correlations

Initially, the breast and ovarian cancer cancer risks conferred by mutations in BRCA1 were estimated from BRCA1-linked, multiple-case families (see Figs. 8.01 and 8.02) {896,898}. More recently, estimates from specific populations have come up with lower estimates {106,3065}. This could point to 1) the existence of mutation-specific risks (because different populations have different mutation spectra, the overall cancer risks would differ), 2) the existence of genetic variants in other genes, particularly prevalent in certain populations, which might modify the BRCA1-related cancer risks, 3) population-specific differences in environmental risk modifiers.

BRCA1 mutation position

One report observed a significant correlation between the location of the mutation in the gene and the ratio of breast to ovarian cancer incidence within each family {974}, suggesting a transition in risk such that mutations in the 3' third of the gene were associated with a lower proportion of ovarian cancer. It wasn't clear, however, whether this was due to higher breast cancer risks, or lower ovarian cancer risks. A much larger study of 356 BRCA1-linked families {2914} found the breast cancer risk associated with mutations in the central region to be significantly lower than for other mutations (relative risk, 0.71), and the ovarian cancer risk associated with mutations 3' to nucleotide 4191 to be significantly reduced relative to the rest of the gene (relative risk, 0.81). Recent work suggests that the risk to ovarian cancer might also be influenced by genetic variation in the wildtype BRCA1 copy in BRCA1 carriers {1009}.

Genetic risk modifiers

One study showed that the risk for ovarian cancer was 2.11 times greater for BRCA1 carriers harbouring one or two rare HRAS1 alleles, compared to carriers with only common alleles (P = 0.015). Susceptibility to breast cancer did not appear to be affected by the presence of rare HRAS1 alleles {2240}. Likewise, a length-variation of the polyglutamine repeats in the estrogen receptor co-activator NCOA3 and the androgen receptor influences breast cancer risk in carriers of BRCA1 and BRCA2 {2342,2345}. The variant progesterone receptor allele named PROGINS was associated with an odds ratio of 2.4 for ovarian cancer among 214 BRCA1/2 carriers with no past exposure to oral contraceptives, compared to women without ovarian cancer and with no PROGINS allele {2487}.

These results support the hypothesis that pathways involving endocrine signalling may have a substantial effect on BRCA1/2-associated cancer risk. Genetic variation in the genes constituting the DNA repair pathways might also be involved. A C/G polymorphism in the 5' untranslated region of RAD51 was found to modify both breast and ovarian

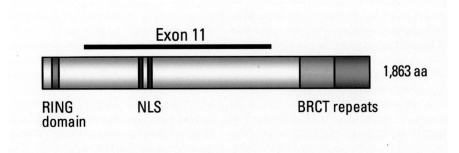

Fig. 8.06 Functional domains in BRCA1. The RING domain contains a C3HC4 motif that interacts with other proteins. NLS = nuclear localization signal. BRCT = BRCA1-related C-terminal. The proportion encoded by exon 11 is indicated.

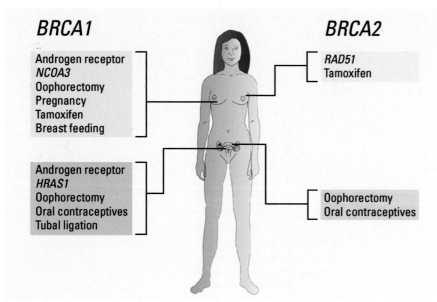

BRCA1

Androgen receptor
NCOA3
Oophorectomy
Pregnancy
Tamoxifen
Breast feeding

Androgen receptor
HRAS1
Oophorectomy
Oral contraceptives
Tubal ligation

BRCA2

RAD51
Tamoxifen

Oophorectomy
Oral contraceptives

Fig. 8.07 Factors that modify risk of breast or ovarian cancer. Most of these proposed factors are based on results of a single study and require confirmation. From S.A. Narod {1975}.

cancer risk, initially only in carriers of BRCA2 {1328,1644,3053}.

Hormonal factors as risk modifiers
Oral contraceptives
Because of the observed protective effects of oophorectomy and tamoxifen, it is of concern that supplemental estrogen, in the form of oral contraceptives or hormone replacement therapy, may increase the risk of breast cancer. In the Oxford overview analysis, current use of birth control pills was associated with a relative risk of 1.2 {539}. However, in a recent large American case-control study, no adverse effect was noted {2607}. In a large international case-control study of oral contraceptives and hereditary breast cancer {1977} a mild increase in risk was seen among BRCA1 carriers (relative risk 1.2) but not among BRCA2 carriers (relative risk 0.89). The overall result was not significant, but risk increases were found for women who first took a contraceptive before age 30, for women who developed breast cancer before age 40, for women with five or more years of pill use, and for women who first took an oral contraceptive prior to 1975. It appears that short-term use of modern contraceptives poses no increase in risk, but further studies are needed in this regard. No studies have been conducted yet regarding whether or not HRT increases the risk of breast cancer in BRCA1/2 mutation carriers.

It is important to establish whether oral contraceptives are hazardous to the breast, because their use has been proposed as a preventive measure against ovarian cancer. A protective effect of oral contraceptives on ovarian cancer risk has been observed in three case-control studies of BRCA1/2 mutation carriers {1976,1979,1980} but there has been one conflicting report {1886}. In a recent study of 232 ovarian cancer cases and 232 controls, oral contraceptive use was associated with a 56% reduction in the risk of ovarian cancer (p = 0.002) {1976}. Tubal ligation has been found to be protective against ovarian cancer in the general population {1126} and among BRCA1 mutation carriers {1980}. An adjusted relative risk of 0.39 was reported for tubal ligation and subsequent ovarian cancer (a risk reduction of 61%). The mechanism of risk reduction is unclear.

Pregnancy
Hormonal levels rise dramatically during pregnancy and two groups found pregnancy to be a risk factor for early breast cancer in BRCA1/2 mutation carriers. Johannsson et al. reported ten pregnancy-related breast cancers in 37 BRCA1/2 mutation carriers, versus the expected 3.7 {1351}. Jernstrom et al. reported that the risk of breast cancer increased with each pregnancy in BRCA1/2 carriers before the age of 40 {1348}. This was

found for BRCA1 and BRCA2 mutation carriers, but was only significant for the former group. In the general population, pregnancy offers protection against breast cancer after the age of 40, but appears to increase the risk for very early-onset breast cancer {227}. This is consistent with the hypothesis that the ovarian hormones produced during pregnancy are mitogenic, and accelerate the growth of existing tumours. During pregnancy breast differentiation occurs and thereafter the population of susceptible cells is reduced. This may explain why pregnancy prevents breast cancers at a later age. In the general population, only a small proportion of breast cancers occur before age 40, and pregnancy confers an overall advantage. Early-onset breast cancers are typical among BRCA1 mutation carriers, however, and a high proportion of cancers occur before age 40. A case-control study of breast-feeding and breast cancer in BRCA1/2 mutation carriers reported a protective effect in women with BRCA1 mutations, but not with BRCA2 mutations {1347}. BRCA1 mutation carriers who breast-fed for more than one year were 40% less likely to have breast cancer than those who breast-fed for a shorter period (p = 0.01). The observed protective effect among BRCA1 carriers was greater than that observed for members of the general population {224}.

Prognosis and preventive options
The overall life expectancy of unaffected women with a BRCA1 or BRCA2 mutation clearly is decreased due to their high risk of developing breast cancer and ovarian cancer, in particular at young ages. The overall mortality from breast and ovarian cancer within 10 years of diagnosis of cancer is still significant, 40% and 60% respectively.

Currently the following avenues are being explored to improve the prognosis of women with a BRCA1 or BRCA2 mutation, all aiming for either early detection or prevention of breast cancer and/or ovarian cancer: i) regular surveillance, ii) prophylactic surgery, and iii) chemoprevention.

Preventive surveillance
No evidence exists that regular breast surveillance using mammography leads to earlier detection of cancers in mutation carriers {1442}. Preliminary results on

breast surveillance using MRI suggest that there is an increased frequency of early detection of tumours, but definite conclusions cannot yet be made {1875, 2835}. Also, no evidence exists that regular ovarian surveillance detects ovarian cancer at curable stages.

Prophylactic surgery
Prophylactic bilateral mastectomy lowers the risk of breast cancer in mutation carriers by more than 90%, also on the long-term {178,1407}. Prophylactic bilateral salpingo-oophorectomy prevents ovarian cancer, though a minimum long-term risk of 4% of peritoneal cancer remains after this procedure {2344}.

The incidence of breast cancer in *BRCA1* carriers is maximal in the age group 40 to 55 and then declines slightly thereafter {1978}. This observation suggests that ovarian hormones may have a promoting role in breast carcinogenesis. In support of this, oophorectomy has been found to be protective against breast cancer in *BRCA1/2* mutation carriers in several studies {1976,2504}. Rebbeck et al. compared the breast cancer risk in a historical cohort of *BRCA1* mutation carriers, some of whom had undergone an oophorectomy and some of whom had both ovaries intact {2343,2344}. The estimated relative risk of breast cancer associated with oophorectomy was approximately one-half. This was confirmed in a case-control study {763} and in a prospective follow-up study of 170 women {1413}. Among *BRCA1* mutation carriers; the risk of breast cancer among women who had an oophorectomy was decreased by 61% (odds ratio 0.39; 95% CI 0.20 to 0.75). These studies suggest that oophorectomy might be used as a strategy to decrease the risk of breast cancer among *BRCA1* mutation carriers. However, in young women the procedure is associated with acute and long-term side effects.

Members of a *BRCA1*-linked family are at risk also to develop tubal carcinoma {3271}. Piek et al. studied prophylactically removed fallopian tubes of 12 women with a predisposition for ovarian cancer, in 7 of whom a *BRCA1* mutation was detected {2246}. Six showed dysplasia, including one case of severe dysplasia. Five harboured hyperplastic lesions, and in one woman no histological aberrations were found. Therefore, it is recommended to perform a complete adnexectomy in women harbouring a *BRCA1* mutation. Whether an abdominal hysterectomy should be performed to dissect the intra-uterine part of the tube, is still in debate. However, most studies indicate that tubal carcinomas in fact predominantly arise in distal parts of the tube.

The interest of women with a *BRCA1* or *BRCA2* mutation in the various options differs greatly between countries {1425}, and may also change over time when the efficacy of surveillance, chemoprevention, or treatment improves. However, at present in some countries up to 50-60% of unaffected women chose to have prophylactic bilateral mastectomy, and 65% prophylactic bilateral salpingo-oophorectomy {1012,2285}.

Chemoprevention
Tamoxifen is an anti-estrogenic drug that is routinely used in the treatment of estrogen-receptor positive breast cancer that has also been demonstrated to be of value in reducing the risk of primary invasive and pre-malignant breast cancer in high risk women {865,1464,1976} and of contralateral breast cancer in unselected women {10}. Narod, et al. {1976} studied tamoxifen and contralateral breast cancer in a case-control study of *BRCA1* and *BRCA2* mutation carriers. Tamoxifen use was equivalent to a 62% risk reduction in *BRCA1* carriers. A reduction in risk of contralateral cancer was also seen with oophorectomy and chemotherapy. This result implies that the combination of tamoxifen and oophorectomy may be more effective than either treatment alone, and that the two prevention strategies may be complementary. Until more definitive guidlines are established, the interest in participation in chemoprevention trials is likely to remain small {2285}.

Table 8.05
Effects of modifying factors on breast and ovarian cancer risk.

	Breast cancer		Ovarian cancer	
	BRCA1	*BRCA2*	*BRCA1*	*BRCA2*
Genetic factors				
Androgen receptor	↓↑	?	↓↑	?
NCOA3	↑	?	?	?
RAD51	−	↑	?	?
HRAS1	?	?	↑	?
Lifestyle factors				
Oophorectomy	↓	↓?	↓	↓
Mastectomy	↓	↓	−	−
Tubal ligation	−	−	↓	↓?
Pregnancy*	↑	↑?	?	?
Breastfeeding	↓	↑?	?	?
Oral contraceptives	↑?	↑?	↓	↓
Tamoxifen	↓	↓	−	−
Hormone-replacement therapy	?	?	?	?

↑? = suggested increase in cancer risk, but uncertain
↓? = suggested decrease in cancer risk, but uncertain
↑ = significant increase in cancer risk
↓ = significant decrease in cancer risk
? = not studied
− = no modifying effect seen

From S.A. Narod {1975}.
* The pregnancy effect was seen for early-onset (40 years) breast cancer only.

BRCA2 syndrome

R. Eeles
S. Piver
S.R. Lakhani
J.M. Piek
A. Ashworth

P. Devilee
S. Narod
E.H. Meijers-Heijboer
A.R. Venkitaraman

Definition
Inherited tumour syndrome with autosomal dominant trait and markedly increased susceptibility to early onset breast cancer and an additional risk for the development of male breast cancer and, less frequently, pancreatic and ovarian cancer. Occasionally, carriers of a *BRCA2* germline mutation present with skin melanoma, gall bladder and bile duct tumours, and cancer of the fallopian tube.

MIM No.   600185 {1835}

Synonyms
Site specific early onset breast cancer syndrome, breast cancer 2, FANCD1.

Incidence
The *BRCA2* syndrome is generally uncommon (about 1 in 1000 individuals), but in certain populations, it is more prevalent. For example, a specific mutation (6174delT) is present in 1.5% of the Ashkenazim and another (999del5) in 0.6% of Icelanders, due to founder effects {2382,2921}.

Diagnostic criteria
BRCA2 mutations are more often present in families with multiple female breast cancer (>4 cases of early onset at <60 years) and male breast cancer. The risk of ovarian cancer is lower than in *BRCA1* families. The definitive diagnosis relies on the identification of a *BRCA2* germline mutation.

Breast tumours
Penetrance and age distribution
Analyses of the worldwide data submitted to the Breast Cancer Linkage Consortium (BCLC) studies have been used to provide general estimates of penetrance (see Fig. 8.01) {8}. Population based studies of mutations in breast cancer patients from the UK have shown a lower penetrance than the BCLC, indicating that the presence of a mutation within a familial breast cancer cluster does confer a higher penetrance {2230}. This may be due to association with other genes or exposure and lifestyle factors that are present in the family. Specific estimates for different populations have shown that the Ashkenazim have a somewhat lower lifetime breast cancer penetrance of about 50-60% {3065}. There are also reports of variable penetrance, dependent upon mutation position {2914}. There is an increased risk of contralateral breast cancer of about 56% lifetime after a diagnosis of a first breast primary. Breast cancer in *BRCA2* carriers occurs more often at younger ages than in the general population, but at older ages than in *BRCA1* carriers.

Pathology
Although lobular and tubulo-lobular carcinoma has been reported to be associated with *BRCA2* germline mutation in one study {1767}, this has not been confirmed in a larger study and no specific histological type is thought to be associated with *BRCA2* {8,1572}. In a multifactorial analysis, the only factors found to be significant for *BRCA2* were tubule score, fewer mitoses and continuous pushing margins. All other features were not found to be significant {1572}. *BRCA2* tumours are overall higher grade than sporadic cancers {8,43,1767}. Ductal carcinoma in situ (DCIS) is observed less frequently in *BRCA1* cases than in controls, but this is not the case for *BRCA2*. Lobular carcinoma in situ shows no difference between the groups {8}.
Invasive lobular carcinoma clearly does have a familial association and a trend has been identified in familial breast cancer not linked to *BRCA1* or *BRCA2* (i.e. BRCAX) {1571}.
BRCA2 tumours are similar to sporadic cancers in steroid receptor (ER, PgR) expression {766,1574,2121}. Data on ERBB2 are limited but *BRCA1* and *BRCA2* tumours are more likely to be negative than controls {1574}. *BRCA2* tumours do not show a higher frequency

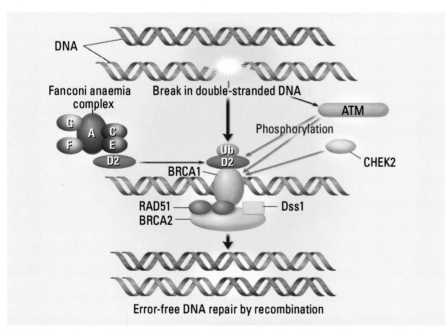

Fig. 8.08 Several genes (*ATM, CHEK2, BRCA1* and *BRCA2*) whose inactivation predisposes people to breast and other cancers participate in the error-free repair of breaks in double-stranded DNA by homologous recombination. Genes for another chromosome instability disorder named Fanconi anaemia have been connected to this DNA repair pathway. Ub denotes mono-ubiquitin. From A.R. Venkitaraman {3019}.

of TP53 mutation and p53 expression compared to sporadic breast cancer {580,581,1574}.

Prognosis and prognostic factors
Since the breast cancers associated with BRCA2 mutations are more often estrogen receptor positive and are associated with DCIS, they would be expected to have a better prognosis. The most systematic study to investigate prognosis has analysed the survival of Ashkenazi women with breast cancer who have mutations as tested from paraffin-stored tissue. This is possible because they have a single 6174delT founder mutation. There was no difference in survival between carriers and non-carriers {441}.

Risk modifiers and prevention
The preventive effect of oophorectomy and tamoxifen, mastectomy, and the possible hazard associated with oral contraceptives are similar in both BRCA syndromes have been dealt with in the preceding section on BRCA1.

Ovarian tumours

Penetrance and age distribution
About 7-10% of ovarian carcinomas are due to inherited BRCA1 or BRCA2 mutations; as these are on autosomes, they can be inherited from either the mother or the father. Although ovarian cancer can occur earlier in BRCA1 and indeed BRCA2 carriers, the presence of an older onset ovarian cancer still can indicate an underlying mutation in either of these genes. The penetrance of ovarian cancer in BRCA2 carriers is shown in Fig. 8.02; the risk of developing ovarian cancer by age 70 in BRCA2 families is approximately 27% {898}. It should be noted that the penetrance curve starts to rise later than for BRCA1 which could have implications for the timing of prophylactic oophorectomy.

Pathology
Compared with the information on the pathology of BRCA1-associated ovarian cancers, little is reported on BRCA2 mutation-related ovarian tumours. The paucity of information is accounted for by the low incidence of this disease compared with that of BRCA1-linked cases {329,973}. Some recent studies indicate that the histological phenotype of these ovarian neoplasms is similar to that of BRCA1-associated carcinomas

and are predominantly of papillary serous type {329,2239,3272}. A single case of an ovarian malignant mixed müllerian tumour (carcinosarcoma), has been reported as occurring in a BCRA2 mutation carrier {2748}.

The data on grade are similar to those of BRCA1 ovarian cancers with an association with higher grade but limited numbers in study and interobserver variation {329,2239,2479,3102,3272} in the scoring of grade should be taken into account when considering the evidence There are no data to support a role of BRCA2 in borderline ovarian lesions {1044,1704} nor are there germ cell or sex cord stromal tumours.

Prevention by oral contraceptives
Although it has been long known that oral contraceptives can decrease the risk of developing ovarian cancer in the general population {2}, recently there is evidence that this may also be true for hereditary ovarian cancer {1976,1979,1980}. See the preceding section on BRCA1 syndrome for further details.

Prognosis and prognostic factors
In a retrospective cohort study, women with BRCA1 or BRCA2 founder mutation advanced-stage ovarian cancer had a longer survival compared with women with non-hereditary ovarian cancer (P = 0.004) and a longer median time to recurrence (14 months versus 7 months) (P< 0.001) {329}.
Studies of ovarian cancer occurring in BRCA2 carriers have reported a better prognosis {329}, but it is uncertain whether this is because of the bias in carrier detection in this population or whether they are more sensitive to treatment. If the latter is true, this would be platinum treatments as these data are prior to the use of taxanes.

Tumours of the fallopian tube
Hereditary fallopian tube carcinoma arises from epithelium overlying the lamina propria of the endosalpinx in women at high hereditary risk to develop ovarian carcinoma. Loss of the wild-type breast cancer 1 or 2 gene (BRCA1/2) allele is most likely pivotal in carcinogenesis of these tumours. To be unequivocally identified, the tumour has to fulfill the clinical and histological criteria for tubal carcinoma {1256} as well as clinical genetic criteria.

Incidence
From 1997 to 2002, a total of 15 hereditary breast/ovarian family related tubal tumours have been reported in literature. In 4 cases, a BRCA2 mutation was detected. However, the true incidence of hereditary tubal carcinoma is probably much higher, as is suggested for its sporadic counterpart. This is caused by the fact that primary tubal tumours are often mistaken for primary ovarian carcinomas {3150}. Moreover, some primary ovarian carcinomas might actually derive from inclusion cysts lined by tubal epithelial cells included into the ovarian stroma {2247}.

Age distribution
In general the age of onset is younger in hereditary cases when compared to sporadic cases.

Diagnostic criteria
The criteria of Hu et. al. {1256} as modified by Sedlis {2614} and Yoonessi {3185} are applied to differentiate hereditary tubal carcinomas from ovarian and endometrial carcinoma. These criteria require that: (i) the main tumour is in the fallopian tube and arises from the endosalpinx, (ii) the histological features resemble a tubal pattern, (iii) if the tubal wall is involved, the transition between malignant and benign tubal epithelium should be detectable, (iv) the fallopian tube contains more tumour than the ovary or endometrium.

Clinical features

Symptoms and signs. To date, there is no indication that clinical hereditary tubal carcinoma features are different from those of its sporadic counterpart; abdominal discomfort is more or less common, but an atypical complaint. The classical but rare triad of symptoms include: (i) prominent watery vaginal discharge, (ii) pelvic pain and (iii) pelvic mass {158}. It has been reported that approximately 10% of patients will have adenocarcinomatous cells in cervical cytology {3185}.

Tumour markers. As in ovarian carcinoma elevation of serum CA125 levels can be found in approximately 80% of cases {1173}.

Imaging. CT / MRI are inconclusive with respect to the differential diagnosis of tubal or ovarian carcinomas. However, these techniques can be helpful in determining the extent of disease. Likewise, ultrasonography can not distinguish tubal from ovarian disease {2720}.

Pathology

Histopathology and grading. Serous papillary carcinoma is the most common form of hereditary tubal carcinoma. Grading is of limited value in these tumours and, if used, is based on the papillary architecture, nuclear atypia and mitotic activity. Grade I cancers show papillary growth with well differentiated columnar cells and low mitotic rate. Grade II cancers are papillary with evident gland formation with intermediately differentiated cells with moderate mitotic activity. Grade III shows solid growth with loss of papillae and a medullary/glandular pattern. The cells are poorly differentiated and the mitotic activity is high.

Immunoprofile. Being predominantly of serous papillary type, hereditary tubal carcinomas are positive for cytokeratins 7 and 8, MUC1, CEA, OVTL3, OV632, CA125, and negative or showing only low expression for cytokeratin 20, CEA and vimentin. Also, p53 is often expressed, and cyclins E and A and Ki67 show a varying number of proliferating cells, whereas staining for HER-2/neu and cyclin D1 is usually negative. Steroid receptor content varies. In the rare clear cell cancers, p21 is highly expressed.

Seeding and metastasis
Hereditary tubal carcinomas presumably spread like their sporadic counterparts. However, only empirical data are available to date, pointing to a mode of spread similar to ovarian cancer.

Survival
The five-year survival rate of 30% in sporadic cases varies with stage {158,3185}, but not with grade. The survival rate of hereditary tubal carcinomas has yet to be established since only small numbers of patients have been reported and most patients have still not completed their 5-year follow-up.

Prophylactic interventions
In one study, 30 women with either a documented deleterious *BRCA1* or *BRCA2* mutation or a suggestive family history

Table 8.06
Cancer risks of *BRCA2* carriers.

Cancer site or type	Relative risk (95% CI)	Cumulative Risk By Age 70, % (95% CI)
Breast (female)	Age-dependent	84 (43 – 95)
Breast (male)	150	6.3 (1.4 – 25.6)
Ovary	Age-dependent	27 (0 – 47)
Gall bladder and bile ducts	4.97 (1.50 – 16.5)	-
Prostate	4.65 (3.48 – 6.22)	7.5 (5.7 – 9.3)
Prostate before age 65	7.33 (4.66 – 11.52)	-
Pancreas[1]	3.51 (1.87 – 6.58)	Males: 2.1 (1.2 – 3.0)) Females: 1.5 (0.9 – 2.1)
Stomach[1]	2.59 (1.46 - 4.61)	-
Malignant melanoma[1]	2.58 (1.28 – 5.17)	-
All cancers[2]	2.45 (2.15 – 2.78)	-

From D. Ford et al. 1998 {898}, D.F. Easton et al. 1997 {744} and the Breast Cancer Linkage Consortium 1999 {11}.
[1] Relative risks were slightly higher for individuals aged 65 or under.
[2] All cancers other than nonmelanoma skin cancer, breast cancer, or ovarian cancer.

underwent prophylactic oophorectomy {1617}. Five of these (17%) were found to have clinically occult malignancy, 3 of which involved a primary fallopian tube malignancy. Three of the five were known *BRCA1* mutation carriers, one had a documented *BRCA2* mutation. Therefore, it is recommended to perform a complete adnexectomy in women carrying a *BRCA1* or a *BRCA2* mutation. Whether an abdominal hysterectomy should be performed to dissect the intra-uterine part of the tube, is still in debate. However, most studies indicate that tubal carcinomas in fact predominantly arise in distal parts of the tube.

Other tumours
BRCA2 confers an increased risk of ovarian cancer, but not as high as that for BRCA1. Statistically significant increases in risk were observed for a number of other tumour types, including prostate, pancreatic and stomach cancer. The risk for prostate cancer is probably not sufficiently high to cause an appreciable fraction of early-onset prostate cancer cases. The risk for male breast cancer, although the hallmark of *BRCA2* mutations, is based on only four observed cases and hence is very imprecise.

Genetics
Chromosomal location and gene structure
BRCA2 is located on chromosome 13q12.3. It consists of 27 exons, of which exon 11 is remarkably large (4.9 kb). The open reading frame is 10,254 basepairs, encoding a protein of 3,418 aminoacids that has no significant similarity to any known protein. Exon 11 encodes a structural motif consisting of eight 'BRC' repeats, through which BRCA2 controls the function of RAD51, a recombinase enzyme, in pathways for DNA repair by homologous recombination.

Gene expression
A wide range of human tissues express *BRCA2* mRNA, in a pattern very similar to that of *BRCA1*, but the highest levels were observed in breast and thymus, with slightly lower levels in lung, ovary, and spleen {2891}. In normal cells, BRCA2 is a nuclear protein, preferentially expressed during the late-G1/early-S phase of the cell cycle {258,480,3012}. In mice, *Brca1* and *Brca2* are coordinately upregulated during ductal proliferation, morphogenesis and differentiation of breast epithelial cells occurring at puberty, pregnancy and lactation {1582,1769,

2323}. Both proteins co-exist with RAD51 in subnuclear foci during S phase, which redistribute following DNA damage {450,2193}.

Exon 12 of the messenger is alternatively spliced, and there is some suggestion that this splice variant is expressed at higher levels in about a third of sporadic breast tumour when compared to normal epithelial cells {266}. In sporadic breast tumours, *BRCA2* mRNA-expression was higher than that in normal surrounding tissues in 20% of the cases, and lower in 11% {267}. In agreement with this, no hypermethylation of the *BRCA2* promotor region has been detected in breast and ovarian cancer {541}.

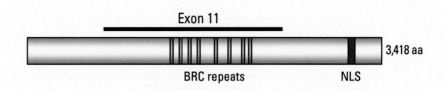

Fig. 8.09 Functional domains in *BRCA2*. There are 8 BRC repeats in the central region of the protein which interact with RAD51. NLS = nuclear localization signal. The proportion encoded by exon 11 is indicated.

Gene function

Loss, or mutational inactivation, of the single wild-type allele in heterozygous carriers of mutations in the *BRCA2* gene is a key step in tumourigenesis. The mechanism by which the encoded protein contributes to disease progression is not yet completely understood but is thought to be related, at least in part, to the proposed role of BRCA2 in the repair of damaged DNA.

BRCA2 encodes a very large (3,418 amino acids in humans) protein that is expressed during S phase of the cell cycle when it is present in the cell nucleus. Although the amino acid sequence of the BRCA2 protein presents few direct clues as to its normal cellular role, some functional domains have been defined. The C-terminal region of BRCA2 contains a functional nuclear localization sequence; many pathogenic truncating mutations in human *BRCA2* are proximal to this domain and would therefore be predicted to encode cytoplasmic proteins. The central part of the protein encoded by the large exon 11 contains eight copies of a novel sequence (the BRC repeat) that has been shown to be capable of binding RAD51 protein. RAD51 is a key protein involved in double-strand DNA break repair and homologous recombination and the interaction with BRCA2 was the first evidence implicating the protein in these processes. BRCA2-deficient cells and tumours characteristically accumulate aberrations in chromosome structure {3018}. These lesions include breaks involving one of the two sister chromatids, as well as tri-radial and quadri-radial chromosomes typical of Bloom syndrome and Fanconi anaemia. Thus, BRCA2 deficiency may be similar in its pathogenesis to other genetic diseases in which unstable chromosome structure is linked to cancer predisposition.

Chromatid-type breaks, tri-radial and quadri-radial chromosomes are thought to arise from defects in the repair of DNA double-strand breaks (DSBs) during the S phase of cell cycle. During S phase, DSB repair proceeds preferentially through mechanisms involving homologous recombination. These mechanisms enable error-free repair of broken DNA, taking advantage of the availability of the replicated sister chromatid as a substrate for recombination reactions. In BRCA2-deficient cells, DSB repair by homologous recombination is defective. However, alternative – but error-prone - mechanisms for DSB repair such as end-joining or strand-annealing are still present. The end result is that DSBs in BRCA2-deficient cells are mis-repaired, giving rise to mutations and chromosomal rearrangements including translocations or deletions. The resulting genetic instability is believed to potentiate the acquisition of mutations that transform a normal cell into a cancer cell. Thus, BRCA2 works as a tumour suppressor indirectly through its 'caretaker' role in protecting chromosomal stability.

BRCA2 is essential for homologous recombination because it controls the intra-cellular transport and activity of RAD51. In BRCA2-deficient cells, RAD51 fails to efficiently enter the nucleus. After exposure of BRCA2-deficient cells to DNA damaging agents, RAD51 fails to localize

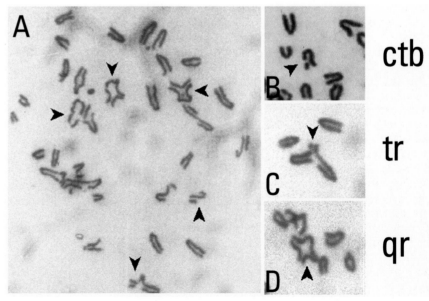

Fig. 8.10 Aberrations in chromosome structure reminiscent of Bloom syndrome and Fanconi anaemia accumulate during the division of BRCA2-deficient cells in culture. Enlargements of characteristic aberrations are shown in the panels on the right hand-side (ctb, chromatid break, tr, tri-radial and qr, quadri-radial). Reproduced from K.J. Patel et al. {2193}.

in typical nuclear foci that may represent sites for DNA damage processing. Moreover, BRCA2 controls the assembly of RAD51 into a nucleoprotein filament that coats DNA, a critical intermediate structure in recombination reactions.

Unexpected and potentially informative insight into the role of *BRCA1/2* genes in DNA repair in humans in vivo has come from recent studies on Fanconi anaemia (FA), a complex disorder characterized by congenital abnormalities, progressive bone marrow failure and cancer susceptibility. FA is a recessively inherited disorder which can result from mutation in at least 8 individual genes. It has recently been suggested that one of the previously unidentified FA genes, FANCD1, is in fact BRCA2 {1251}. The cellular consequences of homozygosity for *BRCA2* mutation, including spontaneous chromosome instability and hypersensitivity to DNA cross-linking agents, are rather similar to those observed in cells derived from FA patients. This is not the only link between FA and breast cancer susceptibility genes. Another FA gene product, FANCD2, can interact and co-localize with BRCA1 {958}. Thus it seems that the pathways disrupted in FA and breast cancer susceptibility are intimately connected. Only a small proportion of FA, which in itself is rare, is caused by *BRCA2* mutation but the importance of this finding is that it connects together two previously different bodies of work on DNA repair.

A current simplified model on how *BRCA2* and several other genes involved in breast cancer predisposition act coordinately to repair DNA damage is indicated in Fig. 8.08. ATM and CHEK2 protein kinases signal the presence of double-stranded DNA breaks and phosphorylate (red arrows) a number of downstream effector proteins, including BRCA1. This induces their migration to sites where DNA is repaired. BRCA2 carries the DNA-recombination enzyme RAD51 to the same sites, guided there by the DNA-binding structures formed between its C-terminal domain and Dss1 protein. A complex of Fanconi anaemia proteins – termed A, C, D2, E, F, and G – triggers the ubiquitination of the D2 protein alone and its colocalization with BRCA1.

Other roles for BRCA2 have been suggested in chromatin remodelling and gene transcription {1442}. Such functions – which remain very poorly charac-terized – may help to explain why cancer predisposition associated with *BRCA2* mutations should be specific to tissues such as the breast and ovary. However, notwithstanding these other potential functions, it seems likely that loss of BRCA2 function engenders genomic instability leading to oncogene activation and tumour suppressor loss that culminates in tumourigenic progression. A major challenge for future work will be to understand how this basic pathogenic mechanism plays out in the complex tissue environments of the breast, ovary or prostate, giving rise to site-specific epithelial malignancies.

Mutation spectrum
Germline mutations in *BRCA2* have been detected in 5-10% of clinic-based breast cancer families, and in similar frequencies of breast-ovarian cancer families {2657,3023}. Somatic mutations in sporadic breast and ovarian tumours are extremely rare. Mutations occur throughout the entire coding region, and hence the mutation spectrum did not provide immediate clues to functional gene domains. The majority of the mutations are predicted to lead to a prematurely truncated protein when translated. In conjunction with the observed loss of the wildtype allele in tumours arising in mutation carriers {560}, this indicates the importance of gene inactivation for tumourigenesis to occur. Despite the strong variability in mutations detected in families, founder effects have led to some mutations being very prevalent in certain populations of defined geographical or ethnic background. Examples are the 999del5 mutation, which is present in approximately 0.6% of all Icelandic individuals {2920}, and the 6174delT mutation found in an equal proportion of Ashkenazi Jews {2083}. As a result, mutation spectra may vary according to ethnic background of the sampled population {2824}. In recent years, an increasing number of missense changes are being detected in *BRCA2* of which the clinical significance is uncertain in the absence of a functional assay. These already comprise up to 50% of all known sequence changes in *BRCA2*. Although many of them are expected to be rare neutral polymorphisms, some might be associated with elevated levels of breast cancer risk. An example is the arginine for histidine substitution at codon 372 {1167}.

Many known deleterious *BRCA1* and *BRCA2* mutations affect splicing, and these typically lie near intron/exon boundaries. However, there are also potential internal exonic mutations that disrupt functional exonic splicing enhancer (ESE) sequences, resulting in exon skipping. A T2722R mutation segregated with affected individuals in a family with breast cancer and disrupted 3 potential ESE sites {816}. The mutation caused deleterious protein truncation and suggested a potentially useful method for determining the clinical significance of a subset of the many unclassified variants of *BRCA1* and *BRCA2*. As more functional and structural information on the BRCA1 and BRCA2 proteins accumulates, our understanding of genetic variation in these genes will improve. The Breast Cancer Information Core (BIC) maintains a website providing a central repository for information regarding mutations and polymorphisms (http://research.nhgri.nih.gov/bic/).

Genotype-phenotype correlations
Evidence is accumulating that the risks conferred by pathogenic *BRCA2* mutations are dependent on the position of the mutation in the gene, genetic variation in other genes, and environmental or lifestyle factors.

BRCA2 mutation position
Truncating mutations in families with the highest risk of ovarian cancer relative to breast cancer are clustered in a region of approximately 3.3 kb in exon 11 {972}. This region of *BRCA2*, bounded by nucleotides 3035 and 6629, was dubbed the 'ovarian cancer cluster region,' or OCCR. Notably, this region coincides with the BRC repeats that are critical for the functional interaction with the RAD51 protein. A much larger study of 164 families confirmed that OCCR mutations are associated with a lower risk of breast cancer and with a higher risk of ovarian cancer {2913}. The extent of risk modification is too moderate, however, to be used in genetic counseling.

Genetic risk-modifiers
A length-variation of the polyglutamine repeats in the estrogen receptor co-activator NCOA3 influences breast cancer risk in carriers of *BRCA1* and *BRCA2* {2345}. Although it should be noted that most of the carriers in these studies are *BRCA1* carriers, and there was insuffi-

cient power to determine the effect in *BRCA2* carriers alone. Similarly, the variant progesterone receptor allele named PROGINS was associated with an odds ratio of 2.4 for ovarian cancer among 214 *BRCA1/2* carriers with no past exposure to oral contraceptives, compared to women without ovarian cancer and with no PROGINS allele {2487}. A C/G polymorphism in the 5' untranslated region of *RAD51* was found to modify

both breast and ovarian cancer risk in carriers of *BRCA2* {1644,3053}. These results support the hypothesis that genetic variation in the genes constituting endocrine signalling and DNA repair pathways may modify *BRCA2*-associated cancer risk.

Hormonal risk modifiers
As in the BRCA1 syndrome, the breast cancer risk of BRCA2 carriers is influ-

enced by hormonal factors, including oral contraceptives and pregnancy (see page 56).

Prognosis and prevention
Life expectancy and preventive strategies are similar to those discussed for BRCA1 carriers (see page 56).

Li-Fraumeni syndrome

P. Hainaut
R. Eeles
H. Ohgaki
M. Olivier

Definition
Li-Fraumeni syndrome (LFS) is an inherited neoplastic disease with autosomal dominant trait. It is characterized by multiple primary neoplasms in children and young adults, with a predominance of soft tissue sarcomas, osteosarcomas, breast cancer, and an increased incidence of brain tumours, leukaemia and adrenocortical carcinoma. The majority of Li-Fraumeni cases is caused by a *TP53* germline mutation.

MIM Nos. {1835}
Li-Fraumeni syndrome	151623
TP53 mutations (germline and sporadic)	191170
CHEK2 mutations	604373

Synonym
Sarcoma family syndrome of Li and Fraumeni.

Incidence
From 1990 to 1998, 143 families with a *TP53* germline mutations were report-

ed {2086}. The IARC Database {www.iarc.fr/p53/germline.html} currently contains 223 families {2104a}.

Diagnostic criteria
The criteria used to identify an affected individual in a Li-Fraumeni family are: (i) occurrence of sarcoma before the age of 45 and (ii) at least one first degree relative with any tumour before age 45 and (iii) a second (or first) degree relative with cancer before age 45 or a sarcoma at any age {273,957,1650}.

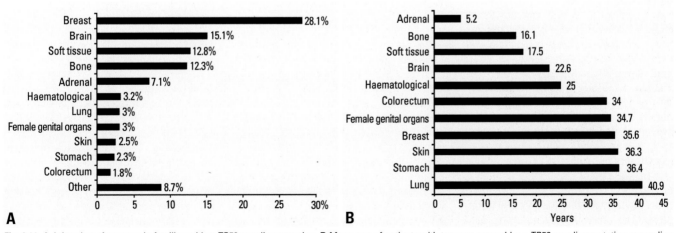

Fig. 8.11 A A fraction of tumours in families with a *TP53* germline mutation. **B** Mean age of patients with tumours caused by a *TP53* germline mutation, according to organ site.

Breast tumours

Frequency

Breast cancers are the most frequent neoplasms developed in families with a *TP53* germline mutation. Thirty-seven % of these families are defined as Li-Fraumeni syndrome and 30% as Li-Fraumeni-like syndrome. In the 219 families with a *TP53* germline mutation reported in 1990–2001 (IARC *TP53* database: www.iarc.fr/p53), a total of 562 tumours developed in individuals with a confirmed *TP53* germline mutation. Of these, 158 (28%) were breast tumours. Eighty-three (38%) families with a *TP53* mutation had at least one family member with a breast tumour. Among the families in which at least one case of breast cancer developed, the mean number of breast tumours per family was 1.9.

Age and sex distribution

Breast cancers associated with a *TP53* germline mutation develop earlier than their sporadic counterparts, with a mean age of 35+10 years (range 14-67 years old). The mean age of women with Li-Fraumeni-like syndrome (LFL) is approximately 8 years higher {2104a} However, breast cancers associated with *TP53* germline mutations never developed in young children, suggesting that hormonal stimulation of the mammary glands constitutes an important co-factor.

Sporadic breast tumours occur approximately 100 times more frequently in females than in males {1475}, and none occurred in males among the 158 reported breast cancer with *TP53* germline mutations.

Pathology

Of the 158 breast tumours recorded, the majority (146 cases, 92%) have not been classified histologically, but recorded as just breast cancers. Histologically classified cases included carcinoma in situ (4 cases), adenocarcinoma (1 case), Paget disease (2 cases), malignant phyllodes tumour (2 cases), comedocarcinoma (1 case), spindle cell sarcoma (1 case), and stromal sarcoma (1 case).

Prognosis and prognostic factors

The breast cancers that occur in LFS are of younger onset and so may have a poorer prognosis due to this early age at diagnosis. In mice, there is relative radioresistance in *p53* mutants, however, radioresistance due to germline

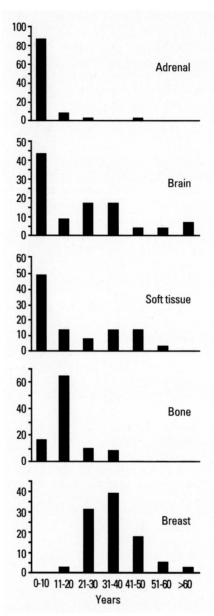

Fig. 8.12 Age distribution of patients with tumours caused by a *TP53* germline mutation.

mutation has not been convincingly shown in man.

Other tumours

Frequency

Following breast cancer, brain tumours and sarcomas (osteosarcomas and soft tissue sarcomas) are the next most frequent manifestations. The sporadic counterparts of these tumours also show somatic *TP53* mutations, suggesting that in these neoplasms, *TP53* mutations are capable of initiating the process of malignant transformation {1475,2087}.

Age distribution

In general, tumours associated with a *TP53* germline mutation develop earlier than their sporadic counterparts, but there are marked organ-specific differences. As with sporadic brain tumours, the age of patients with nervous system neoplasms associated with *TP53* germline mutations shows a bimodal distribution. The first peak of incidence (representing medulloblastomas and related primitive neuroectodermal tumours) is in children, and the second (mainly astrocytic brain tumours) in the third and fourth decades of life {2087}. Adrenocortical carcinomas associated with a *TP53* germline mutation develop almost exclusively in children, in contrast to sporadic adrenocortical carcinomas, which have a broad age distribution with a peak beyond age 40 {1475}.

Genetics – *TP53*

Chromosomal location

The *TP53* gene encompasses 20 kilobases on chromosome 17p13.1. *TP53* belongs to a family of growth suppressors that also comprises two other members, *TP73* and *TP63*. Whereas the two latter genes are mostly involved in the regulation of differentiation and development, *TP53* plays specialized functions as a tumour suppressor {1643}.

Gene structure

The gene contains 11 exons, the first one non-coding. The first intron is particularly large (10 kilobases). The coding sequence is concentrated over 1.3 kilobases. *TP53* is ubiquitously expressed, mostly as a single mRNA species (although rare alternatively spliced variants have been reported). The promoter does not contain a classical TATA box but shows binding elements for several common transcription factors, including c-Jun and NF-kappaB {1107}.

Gene expression

The p53 protein is constitutively expressed in most cell types but, in normal circumstances, does not accumulate to significant level due to rapid degradation by the proteasome machinery. In response to various types of cellular stress, the p53 protein undergoes a number of post-translational modifications that release p53 from the negative control of MDM2, a protein that binds to p53 and mediates its degradation.

These modifications result in the intranuclear accumulation of p53 and in its activation as a transcription factors. Two major signaling pathways can trigger *TP53* activation. The first, and best characterized, is the pathway of response to DNA damage, including large kinases of the phosphoinositol-3 kinase family such as *ATM* (ataxia telangiectasia mutated) and the cell-cycle regulatory kinase *CHEK2*. Both of these kinases phosphorylate p53 in the extreme N-terminus (serines 15, 20 and 37), within the region that binds to MDM2. The second is activated in response to the constitutive stimulation of growth-promoting signaling cascades. The central regulator in this pathway is p14ARF, the alternative product of the locus encoding the cyclin-kinase inhibitor *p16/CDKN2a*. p14ARF expression is activated by E2F transcription factors, and binds to MDM2, thus neutralizing its capacity to induce p53 degradation. This pathway may be part of a normal feedback control loop in which p53 is activated as a cell-cycle brake in cells exposed to hyperproliferative stimuli {2267}.

Gene function
After accumulation, the p53 protein acts as a transcriptional regulator for a panel of genes that differ according to the nature of the stimulus, its intensity and the cell type considered. Broadly speaking, the genes controlled by p53 fall into three main categories, including cell-cycle regulatory genes (*WAF1, GADD45, 14-3-3S, CYCLING*), pro-apoptotic genes (*FAS/APO1/CD95, KILLER/DR5, AIF1, PUMA, BAX*) and genes involved in DNA repair (*O⁶MGMT, MLH2*). The p53 protein also binds to compoments of the transcription, replication and repair machineries and may exert additional controls on DNA stability through the modulation of these mechanisms. Collectively, the p53 target genes mediate two type of cellular responses: cell-cycle arrest, followed by DNA repair in cells exposed to light forms of genotoxic stress, and apoptosis, in cells exposed to levels of damage that cannot be efficiently repaired. Both responses contribute to the transient or permanent suppression of cells that contain damaged, potentially oncogenic DNA. In the mouse, inactivation of *Tp53* by homologous recombination does not prevent normal growth but results in a strong pre-

disposition to early, multiple cancers, illustrating the crucial role of this gene as a tumour suppressor {714}.

Mutation spectrum
The *TP53* gene is frequently mutated in most forms of sporadic cancers, with prevalences that range from a few percents in cervical cancers and in malignant melanomas to over 50% in invasive carcinomas of the aero-digestive tract. Over 75% of the mutations are single base substitutions (missense or nonsense), clustering in exons 5 to 8 that encode the DNA-binding domain of the protein. Codons 175, 245, 248, 273 and 282 are major mutation hotspots in almost all types of cancers. Together, these codons contain over 25% of all known *TP53* mutations. Other codons are mutation hotspots in only specific tumour types, such as codon 249 in hepatocellular carcinoma and codon 157 in bronchial cancer. Mutation patterns can differ significantly between between different types cancers or between geographic areas for the same cancer type (as for example hepatocellular carcinoma). These observations have led to the concept that mutation patterns may reveal clues on the cellular or environmental mechanisms that have caused the mutations {1107}. In sporadic breast cancers, *TP53* is mutated in about 25% of the cases. However, several studies have reported accumulation of the p53 protein without mutation in up to 30-40% of inva-

sive ductal carcinoma in situ. The mutation pattern is similar to that of many other cancers and does not provide information on possible mutagenic events. There is limited evidence that the mutation prevalence is higher in *BRCA1* mutation carriers.
Germline *TP53* mutations have been identified in 223 families. Of these families, 83 match the strict LFS criteria, 67 correspond to the extended, LFL definition, 37 have a family history of cancer that does not fit within LFS or LFL definitions and 36 have germline mutations without documented familial history of cancer (IARC *TP53* mutation database, www.iarc.fr/p53). The codon distribution of germline *TP53* mutations show the same mutational hotspots as somatic mutations {1475}. The distribution of inherited mutations that predisposes to breast cancer are scattered along exons 5 to 8 with relative "hotspots" at codons 245, 248 and 273, which are also commonly mutated in somatic breast cancer. In contrast, a total of 16 breast cancers have been detected in 5 families with a germline mutation at codon 133, a position which is not a common mutation hotspot in somatic breast cancer. It remains to be established whether this mutant has particular functional properties that predispose to breast cancer.

Genotype-phenotype correlations
Brain tumours appear to be associated with missense TP53 mutations in the

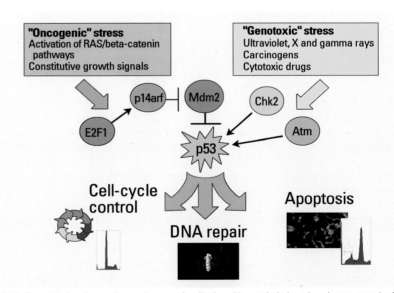

Fig. 8.13 The p53 signaling pathway. In normal cells the p53 protein is kept in a latent state by MDM2. Oncogenic and genotoxic stresses release p53 from the negative control of MDM2, resulting in p53 accumulation and activation. Active p53 acts as transcription factor for genes involved cell cycle control, DNA repair and apoptosis, thus exerting a broad range of antiproliferative effects.

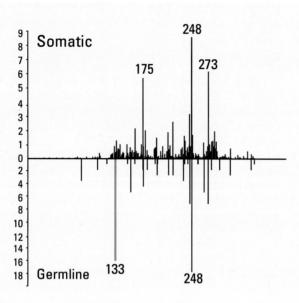

Fig. 8.14 Codon distribution of somatic (top) or germline (bottom) *TP53* mutations associated with breast cancers. Hotspot mutations are indicated. Mutation at codon 133 has been reported in 5 Li-Fraumeni families with breast cancers, but is not a frequent site for somatic mutation in breast cancer in the general population. Compiled from: IARC *TP53* database, www.iarc.fr/p53.

DNA-binding loop that contacts the minor groove, while early onset brain tumours were associated with mutations likely to result in absence of protein or loss of function {2104a}. Adrenocortical carcinomas were associated with missense mutations in the loops opposing the protein-DNA contact surface {2104a}.

Genetics – *CHEK2*
Chromosomal location
CHEK2 is on chromosome 22q12.1.

Gene structure
CHEK2 has 14 exons and there are several homologous loci, which encompass exons 10-14 of the gene, scattered throughout the genome. These gene fragment copies can present problems when analysing *CHEK2* for germline mutations in genomic DNA, and it is important to ensure that the correct copy is being amplified {2742}. This problem can be overcome by amplifying exons 10-14 by the use of a long range PCR using primers located in the non-duplicated region of the gene {2741}. The individual exons can then be subsequently amplified using the product of the long range PCR as a template.

Gene expression
CHEK2 is expressed in nonproliferating and terminally differentiated cells. It is homogenously expressed in renewing cell populations such as epidermis, esophagus, rectum, bladder, stomach, intestine and colon, and heterogenously in conditionally renewing tissues such as lung, breast kidney, salivary, thyroid, parathyroid, adrenal glands, pancreas, prostate, epididymis, sweat glands, endometruim, stromal mesenchymal cells, blood vessels, lymphoid tissues, smooth and cardiac muscle tissues and preipheral nerves. It is absent or cytoplasmic in static tissues such as muscle and brain. CHEK2 remains expressed and can be activated in all phases of the cell cycle in response to DNA damage {1714}.

Gene function
Human *CHEK2* is a homolog of the yeast G2-checkpoint kinases *CDS1* and *RAD53* {1791}. In response to DNA damage, CHEK2 propagates the checkpoint signal along several pathways, which eventually causes cell-cycle arrest in G1, S and G2/M phases {449,820}; activation of DNA repair {1609}, and in apoptotic cell death {1315}. Four of the downstream checkpoint effectors that are established as substrates of CHEK2 in vivo include p53, BRCA1 and Cdc25A and Cdc25C.

Mutation spectrum
Recently, heterozygous germline muta-

tions in *CHEK2* have been identified in three of a subset of individuals with the dominantly inherited Li-Fraumeni syndrome which do not harbour *TP53* mutations {209}. However, one of these was found to be in a pseudogene copy of the *CHEK2* gene. Another one appeared to be neutral polymorphism in the Finnish population. The third was a protein-truncating mutation, 1100delC in exon 10, which abolishes the kinase function of CHEK2. The possibility that this gene is only contributing to the breast cancer cases within LFS families rather than LFS *per se* has been raised {2740}.

The frequency of 1100delC has been estimated in healthy control populations, and was found to vary between 0.3% and 1.7% {1840,2084,2984}. This would also suggest that the 1100delC is a polymorphism, rather than a disease-causing mutation. Yet among unselected patients with breast cancer, its prevalence was found to be approximately 1.5-fold higher than in controls. Significantly elevated frequencies were found among patients with a positive family history and among patients with bilateral breast cancer {2984}. The strongest enrichment of 1100delC carriers (approximately 5-fold) was found among familial breast cancer patients in whom the presence of *BRCA1* or *BRCA2* mutations were excluded {1840,2984}. However, in families with the 1100delC mutation, it appears to cosegregate poorly with breast cancer. The results suggest that *CHEK2*1100delC* is a low risk breast cancer susceptibility allele which may make a significant contribution to familial clustering of breast cancer, including families with smaller numbers of affected cases. As it is enriched among multiple-case families, but unable to explain all breast cancer in families with at least one carrier case, it may interact with other, as yet unknown breast cancer susceptibility alleles.

Search for additional LFS genes
The paucity of large LFS kindreds makes classical linkage methodology difficult. A candidate approach is therefore being used. Candidate genes are those involved in cell cycle pathways, those commonly mutated in multiple tumour types and the breast cancer genes, as this site is commonly affected in LFS kindreds. Using these approaches, the genes *P16* and *PTEN* {379} have been analysed and no germline mutations found.

Cowden syndrome

C. Eng

Definition

Cowden syndrome (CS) is an autosomal dominant disorder caused by germline mutaions of the *PTEN* gene. It is characterized by multiple hamartomas involving organs derived from all three germ cell layers and a high risk of breast, uterine and non-medullary thyroid cancer. The classic hamartoma is the trichilemmoma and is pathognomonic for CS.

MIM No.   158350 {1835}

Synonyms

Cowden disease, multiple hamartoma syndrome.

Incidence

The single most comprehensive clinical epidemiologic study before the CS susceptibility gene was identified estimated the prevalence to be 1:1 000 000 {1990,2776}. Once the gene was identified {1654}, a molecular-based estimate of prevalence in the same population was 1:300 000 {1989}. Because of the difficulty in recognizing this syndrome, prevalence figures are likely underestimated.

Diagnostic criteria

Because of the variable and broad expression of CS and the lack of uniform diagnostic criteria prior to 1996, the International Cowden Consortium {1990} compiled operational diagnostic criteria for CS, based on the published literature and their own clinical experience {785}. These criteria have been recently revised in light of new data, and have been adopted by the US-based National Comprehensive Cancer Network Practice Guidelines {786,1299}. Trichilemommas and papillomatous papules are particularly important to recognize. CS usually presents by the late 20's. It has variable expression and, probably, an age-related penetrance although the exact penetrance is unknown. By the third decade, 99% of affected individuals would have developed the mucocutaneous stigmata although any of the features could be present already. Because the clinical literature on CS consists mostly of reports of the most florid and unusual families or case reports by subspecialists interested in their respective organ systems, the spectrum of component signs is unknown.

Despite this, the most commonly reported manifestations are mucocutaneous lesions, thyroid abnormalities, fibrocystic disease and carcinoma of the breast, gastrointestinal hamartomas, multiple, early-onset uterine leiomyoma, macrocephaly (specifically, megencephaly) and mental retardation {1133, 1693,1748,2776}. Recent data have suggested that endometrial carcinoma should be a component cancer of CS {657,786,1772}. What its frequency is in mutation carriers is as yet unknown.

Table 8.07
International Cowden Syndrome Consortium Operational Criteria for the Diagnosis of Cowden Syndrome (Ver. 2000)*.

Pathognomonic criteria	Mucocutaneous lesions:
	    Trichilemmomas, facial
	    Acral keratoses
	    Papillomatous papules
	    Mucosal lesions

Major criteria	Breast carcinoma Thyroid carcinoma (non-medullary), esp. follicular thyroid carcinoma Macrocephaly (Megalencephaly) (say, >97%ile) Lhermitte-Duclos disease (LDD) Endometrial carcinoma
Minor criteria	Other thyroid lesions (e.g. adenoma or multinodular goiter) Mental retardation (say, IQ < 75) GI hamartomas Fibrocystic disease of the breast Lipomas Fibromas GU tumours (e.g. renal cell carcinoma, uterine fibroids) or malformation

Operational diagnosis in an individual	1. Mucocutanous lesions alone if:
	    a) there are 6 or more facial papules, of which 3 or more must be trichilemmoma, or
	    b) cutaneous facial papules and oral mucosal papillomatosis, or
	    c) oral mucosal papillomatosis and acral keratoses, or
	    d) palmoplantar keratoses, 6 or more
	2. Two major criteria but one must include macrocephaly or LDD
	3. One major and 3 minor criteria
	4. Four minor criteria

Operational diagnosis in a family where one individual is diagnostic for Cowden	1. The pathognomonic criterion/ia 2. Any one major criterion with or without minor criteria 3. Two minor criteria

*Operational diagnostic criteria are reviewed and revised on a continuous basis as new clinical and genetic information becomes available. The 1995 version and 2000 version have been accepted by the US-based National Comprehensive Cancer Network High Risk/Genetics Panel.

Breast tumours

Age distribution and penetrance

Invasive carcinomas of the breast have been diagnosed as early as the age of 14 years and as late as in the 60's {1693}. However, the majority of CS-related breast cancers occur after the age of 30-35 years {786,788}. A single population-based clinical study, without the benefit of genetic analysis, suggested that benign breast disease can occur in two-thirds of affected women while CS females have a 25-50% lifetime risk of developing invasive breast cancer {786,2776}. Male breast cancer can occur in CS as well but the frequency is unknown {817,1771}.

Clinical features

It is believed that the clinical presentation of breast cancer in CS is no different from that of the general population. However, no formal data is currently available.

Pathology

Like other inherited cancer syndromes, multifocality and bilateral involvement is the rule. With regard to the individual cancers, even of the breast and thyroid, as of mid 1997, there has yet to be a systematic study published. There exists, however, one study which has attempted to look at benign and malignant breast pathology in CS patients. Although these are preliminary studies, without true matched controls, it is, to date, the only study that examines breast pathology in a series of CS cases. Breast histopathology from 59 cases belonging to 19 CS women was systematically analysed {2578}. Thirty-five specimens had some form of malignant pathology. Of these, 31 (90%) had ductal adenocarcinoma, one tubular carcinoma and one lobular carcinoma-in-situ. Sixteen of the 31 had both invasive and in situ (DCIS) components of ductal carcinoma while 12 had DCIS only and two only invasive adenocarcinoma. Interestingly, it was noted that 19 of these carcinomas appeared to have arisen in the midst of densely fibrotic hamartomatous tissue. Benign breast disease is more common than malignant, with the former believed to occur in 75% of affected females. Fibrocystic disease of the breast, breast hamartomas, and fibroadenomas are commonly seen.

Uterine tumours

Age distribution and penetrance

Since endometrial carcinomas have only recently been suggested to be a minor component of CS {786}, it is unknown what the true frequency is among mutation carriers or what the age distribution is. Anecdotal cases suggest that the frequency could be 6-10% in affected women.

Benign tumours of the uterus are common in CS. Uterine leiomyomas are believed to occur in almost half of affected women {1693}. They are usually multi-focal and occur at a young age, even in the 20's. Other benign uterine pathologies such as polyps and hyperplasias have been found in CS patients but are of unknown frequency.

Clinical features

There have been no systematic studies of uterine tumours in CS. Clinical observation and anecdotal reports suggest that the leiomyomas can become quite symptomatic, presenting with bleeding and pain. It is unclear if the clinical presentation of the endometrial carcinomas is different from that of sporadic cases.

Pathology

There have been no systematic studies of uterine tumours in CS although it is believed that the histopathology is no different from that of typical sporadic cases.

Prognosis and prognostic factors

Whether the prognosis differs from sporadic cases is unknown.

Thyroid tumours

Age of distribution and penetrance

Apart from breast cancer, the other major component cancer in CS is non-medullary thyroid cancer. Nonmedullary thyroid carcinomas occur at a frequency of 3-10% of affected individuals, regardless of sex, in non-systematic clinical series {1693,2776}. It is unclear, however, whether the age of onset is earlier than that of sporadic cases.

Benign thyroid disease occurs in approximately 70% of affected individuals. Component features include multinodular goitre and follicular adenomas. These benign tumours can occur at any age and can even manifest in teenagers.

Clinical features

Many of the benign tumours in CS individuals remain asymptomatic. However, the most common presenting sign or symptom would be a neck mass. Like many inherited syndromes, CS thyroid lesions can be multifocal and bilobar.

Pathology

No systematic studies have been performed to examine the thyroid in CS. However, clinical observations and clinical reports suggest that the histology of the nonmedullary thyroid carcinoma is predominantly of the follicular type {786, 2776}.

Other tumours

Dysplastic gangliocytoma of the cerebellum (Lhermitte-Duclos disease) is the major manifestation in the central nervous system. Peripheral lesions include verrucous skin changes, cobblestone-like papules, fibromas of the oral mucosa, multiple facial trichilemmomas and hamartomatous polyps of the colon.

Genetics

Chromosomal location and mode of transmission

CS is an autosomal dominant disorder, with age related penetrance and variable expression {787}. The CS susceptibility gene, PTEN, resides on 10q23.3 {1651, 1654,1990}.

Gene structure

PTEN/MMAC1/TEP1 is comprised of 9 exons spanning 120-150 kb of genomic distance {1649,1651,1654,2777}. It is believed that intron 1 occupies much of this (approximately 100 kb). PTEN encodes a transcript of 1.2 kb.

Gene expression

PTEN is expressed almost ubiquitously in the adult human. In normal human embryonic and foetal development, PTEN protein is expressed ubiquitously as well, although levels might change throughout development {1008}. PTEN is very highly expressed in the developing central nervous system as well as neural crest and its derivatives, e.g. enteric ganglia {1008}.

Gene function

PTEN encodes a dual specificity lipid and protein phosphatase [reviewed in {3043}]. It is the major 3-phosphatase acting in the phosphoinositol-3-kinase (PI3K)/Akt apoptotic pathway {1730, 2774}. To date, virtually all naturally occurring missense mutations tested abrogate both lipid and protein phosphatase activity, and one mutant, G129E, affects only lipid phosphatase activity [reviewed in {3043}]. Overexpression of PTEN results, for the most part, in phosphatase-dependent cell cycle arrest at G1 and/or apoptosis, depending on cell type [reviewed in {3043}]. There is also growing evidence that PTEN can mediate growth arrest independent of the PI3K/Akt pathway and perhaps independent of the lipid phosphatase activity {3096-3098} [reviewed in {3042}].

Murine models null for Pten result in early embryonic death {688,2268,2817}. Hemizygous knock-out of Pten result in various neoplasias, and the spectra are different depending on the particular model. While the neoplasias are reminiscent of the component tumours found in the human syndrome, none of the three models are similar to CS.

Mutation spectrum

As with most other tumour suppressor genes, the mutations found in *PTEN* are scattered throughout all 9 exons. They comprise loss-of-function mutations including missense, nonsense, frameshift and splice site mutations {309, 1771}. Approximately 30-40% of germline *PTEN* mutations are found in exon 5, although exon 5 represents 20% of the coding sequence. Further, approximately 65% of all mutations can

be found in one of exons 5, 7 or 8 {309, 1771}.

Although *PTEN* is the major susceptibility gene for CS, one CS family, without *PTEN* mutations, was found to have a germline mutation in *BMPR1A*, which is one of the susceptibility genes for juvenile polyposis syndrome {1250,3262}. Whether *BMPR1A* is a minor CS susceptiblity gene or whether this family with CS features actually has occult juvenile polyposis is as yet unknown.

Genotype-phenotype correlations

Approximately 70-80% of CS cases, as strictly defined by the Consortium criteria, have a germline *PTEN* mutation {1654,1771}. If the diagnostic criteria are relaxed, then mutation frequencies drop to 10-50% {1723,1991,2959}. A formal study which ascertained 64 unrelated CS-like cases revealed a mutation frequency of 2% if the criteria are not met, even if the diagnosis is made short of one criterion {1772}.

A single research centre study involving 37 unrelated CS families, ascertained according to the strict diagnostic criteria of the Consortium, revealed a mutation frequency of 80% {1771}. Exploratory genotype-phenotype analyses revealed that the presence of a germline mutation was associated with a familial risk of developing malignant breast disease {1771}. Further, missense mutations and/or mutations 5' of the phosphatase core motif seem to be associated with a surrogate for disease severity (multiorgan involvement). One other small study comprising 13 families, with 8

PTEN mutation positive, could not find any genotype-phenotype associations {1989}. However, it should be noted that this small sample size is not suitable for statistical analyses and no conclusions should be drawn.

Previously thought to be clinically distinct, Bannayan-Riley-Ruvalcaba syndrome (BRR, MIM 153480), which is characterized by macrocephaly, lipomatosis, haemangiomatosis and speckled penis, is likely allelic to CS {1773}. Approximately 60% of BRR families and isolated cases combined carry a germline *PTEN* mutation {1774}. Interestingly, there were 11 cases classified as true CS-BRR overlap families in this cohort, and 10 of the 11 had a PTEN mutation. The overlapping mutation spectrum, the existence of true overlap families and the genotype-phenotype associations which suggest that the presence of germline *PTEN* mutation is associated with cancer strongly suggest that CS and BRR are allelic and are along a single spectrum at the molecular level. The aggregate term of PTEN hamartoma tumour syndrome (PHTS) has been suggested {1774}.

Recently, the clinical spectrum of PHTS has expanded to include subsets of Proteus syndrome and Proteus-like (non-CS, non-BRR) syndromes {3260}. Germline *PTEN* mutations in one case of macrocephaly and autism and hydrocephaly associated with VATER association have been reported {625,2341}.

Hereditary non-polyposis colon cancer (HNPCC)

H.F.A. Vasen
H. Moreau
P. Peltomaki
R. Fodde

Definition

Hereditary nonpolyposis colorectal cancer (HNPCC) is an autosomal dominant disorder characterized by the development of colorectal cancer, endometrial cancer and other cancers due to inherited mutations in one of the DNA mismatch repair (MMR) genes {1725}.

MIM Nos. {1835}

Familial nonpolyposis colon
cancer, type 1   120435
Familial nonpolyposis colon
cancer, type 2   120436

Synonyms

Lynch syndrome, hereditary colorectal endometrial cancer syndrome {3007}, hereditary defective mismatch repair syndrome {595}.

Incidence

Approximately 2-5% of all cases of colorectal cancer are due to HNPCC {12}. The estimated frequency of carriers of a DNA mismatch repair gene mutation in the general population is one in 1000.

Diagnostic criteria

The International Collaborative Group on HNPCC (ICG-HNPCC) proposed a set of diagnostic criteria (Revised Amsterdam Criteria) to provide uniformity in clinical studies {3010}. These criteria identify families that are very likely to represent HNPCC. Other widely used criteria are the Bethesda Criteria that can be used to identify families suspected of HNPCC that need testing for microsatellite instability {2398}.

Endometrial tumours

Predisposed individuals from HNPCC families have a high risk (30-80%) of developing colorectal cancer. The most frequent extracolonic cancer is endometrial cancer. The lifetime risk of developing this cancer is 30-60% by age 70 {14,731,3009,3071}. HNPCC-associated endometrial cancer is diagnosed approx. 10 years earlier than in the general pop-

ulation. The mean age at diagnosis is 50 years. Patients with colorectal cancer associated with HNPCC have a better prognosis than patients with common sporadic colorectal cancer {2526,3070}. In contrast, a recent study showed that the survival of endometrial cancer associated with HNPCC does not differ significantly from endometrial cancer in the general population {305}.

Pathology of endometrial tumours

In patients from families with proven germline mutations in the MMR genes, *MLH1*, *MSH2*, *MSH6*, or from (suspected) HNPCC families, the majority of endometrial tumours were reported to be of the endometrioid type with diverse grading and staging {650,2174}. Certain histopathologic features such as mucinous differentiation, solid-cribriform growth pattern, high grade and possible necrosis might suggest that a tumour is due to a mismatch repair defect {1481, 2174,2206}.

Loss of MLH1 protein expression occurs in endometrial cancer associated with HNPCC {235,650,1276, 1768,2174,2264} but also in 15-30 % of sporadic cancers with somatic inactivation of MLH1 {2518,2772}.

Abrogation of MSH2 and/or MSH6 protein expression, especially at a young age seems to be a more specific indicator for HNPCC {235, 650, 2174,2264}. Already in the hyperplastic precursor lesions such loss of expression can be encountered {235, 650}.

Other cancers

Many other cancers have been reported in HNPCC {13,14,3009,3010}. The frequency of specific cancers depends on the prevalence of the cancer in the background population {2178}. Cancer of the stomach for example is frequently observed in families from Finland and Japan, both countries with a high prevalence of stomach cancer in population. The ages at diagnosis of most cancers reported are earlier than their sporadic counterparts.

Table 8.08
Revised Amsterdam Criteria.

There should be at least three relatives with colorectal cancer (CRC) or with an HNPCC-associated cancer: cancer of the endometrium, small bowel, ureter or renal pelvis.

- one relative should be a first degree relative of the other two,

- at least two successive generations should be affected,

- at least one tumour should be diagnosed before age 50,

- familial adenomatous polyposis should be excluded in the CRC case if any,

- tumours should be verified by histopathological examination.

Table 8.09
Bethesda Criteria.

1. Individuals with two HNPCC-related cancers, including synchronous and metachronous colorectal cancers or associated extracolonic cancers (endometrial, ovarian, gastric, hepatobiliary, small bowel cancer or transitional cell carcinoma of the renal pelvis or ureter)

2. Individuals with colorectal cancer and a first degree relative with colorectal cancer and/or HNPCC-related extracolonic cancer and/or colorectal adenoma; one of the cancers diagnosed at age <45 y, and the adenoma diagnosed at age <40 y

3. Individuals with colorectal cancer or endometrial cancer diagnosed at age <45 y

4. Individuals with right-sided colorectal cancer with an undifferentiated pattern on histopathology diagnosed at age <45 y

5. Individuals with signet-ring-cell-type colorectal cancer diagnosed at age <45 y

6. Individuals with adenomas diagnosed at age <40

Genetics of *MLH1, MSH2, MSH6*

Chromosomal location and structure

HNPCC is associated with germline mutations in five genes with verified or putative DNA mismatch repair function, viz. *MSH2* (MutS homologue 2), *MLH1* (MutL homologue 1), *PMS2* (Postmeiotic segregation 2), *MSH6* (MutS homologue 6), and possibly *MLH3* (MutL homologue 3). Structural characteristics of these genes are given in Table 8.11. Endometrial cancer appears to be part of the syndrome in families with mutations in any one of these genes, but is particularly associated with *MSH2* and *MSH6* germline mutations {236,3011,3114}.

Gene product

HNPCC genes show ubiquitous, nuclear expression in adult human tissues, and the expression is particularly prominent in the epithelium of the digestive tract as well as in testis and ovary {860,1602, 3132}. These genes are also expressed in normal endometrium, and loss of protein expression is an early change in endometrial tumorigenesis. Studies of *MSH2* or *MLH1* mutation carriers have shown that these proteins may be lost already in atypical hyperplasia (precursor lesion of endometrial cancer) or even in endometrial hyperplasia without atypia in several months before the diagnosis of endometrial cancer, suggesting that immunohistochemical analysis of MSH2 and MLH1 proteins may be useful for pre-screening purposes in HNPCC patients {235,1277}.

Gene function

The protein products of HNPCC genes are key players in the correction of mis-

Table 8.10
Extracolonic cancer in 144 HNPCC families known at the Dutch HNPCC Registry.

Cancer site	Number	Mean age (yrs)	Range (yrs)
Endometrium	87	49	24-78
Stomach	26	51	23-82
Ureter/pyelum	24	55	37-72
Small bowel	22	51	25-69
Ovarian cancer	28	48	19-75
Brain	18	42	2-78

Table 8.11
Characteristics of HNPCC-associated human DNA mismatch repair genes.

Gene	Chromosomal location	Length of cDNA (kb)	Number of exons	Genomic size (kb)	References
MSH2	2p21	2.8	16	73	{1495,1680 2213,2563}
MLH1	3p21-p23	2.3	19	58-100	{353,1121,1494 1666,1679,2167}
PMS2	7p22	2.6	15	16	{2008,2010}
MSH6	2p21	4.2	10	20	{30,2009. 2163,2563}
MLH3	14q24.3	4.3	12	37	{1674}

matches that arise during DNA replication {1496}. Two different MutS-related heterodimeric complexes are responsible for mismatch recognition: MSH2-MSH3 and MSH2-MSH6. While the presence of MSH2 in the complex is mandatory, MSH3 can replace MSH6 in the correction of insertion-deletion mismatches, but not single-base mispairs. Following mismatch binding, a heterodimeric complex of MutL-related proteins, MLH1-PMS2 or MLH1-MLH3, is recruited, and this larger complex, together with numerous other proteins, accomplishes mismatch repair. The observed functional redundancy in the DNA mismatch repair protein family may help explain why mutations in *MSH2* and *MLH1* are prevalent in HNPCC families, while those in *MSH6, PMS2* and *MLH3* are less frequent (and *MSH3* mutations completely absent), although alternative hypotheses (e.g. based on the differential participation of the DNA mismatch repair proteins in apoptosis signaling {863}) have also been proposed.

It is not known why some female HNPCC patients develop endometrial cancer, while others develop colon cancer. Comparison of these two tumour types originating from identical germline mutation carriers suggests the existence of some important tissue-specific differences that may indicate different pathogenetic mechanisms. For example, acquired loss of *MSH2* and *MSH6* appears to characterize endometrial, but not colon carcinomas developing in patients with inherited mutations of *MLH1* {2589}. Moreover, the general MSI patterns and target genes for MSI seem dif-

ferent in endometrial and colorectal cancers from HNPCC patients {1527}. Early inactivation of *PTEN* characterizes most endometrial cancers from HNPCC patients {3261} and tumorigenesis mediated by PTEN inactivation is accelerated by mismatch repair deficiency {3052}. Apart from biosynthetic errors, the DNA mismatch repair proteins also recognize and eliminate various types of endogenous and exogenous DNA damage, and differential exposure to such agents or variable capacity to correct lesions induced by them may also play a role in the organ-specific cancer susceptibility in HNPCC {655}.

Gene mutations

The International Collaborative Group on HNPCC maintains a database for HNPCC-associated mutations and polymorphisms (http://www.nfdht.nl). To date (May 2002), there are 155 different *MSH2* mutations (comprising 39% of all mutations) and 200 (50%) *MLH1* mutations reported to the database, together with 30 (8%), 5 (1%) and 10 (3%) mutations in *MSH6, PMS2*, and *MLH3*, respectively. Most *MSH2* and *MLH1* mutations are truncating {2214}. However, 30-40% of *MLH1* and *MSH6* mutations are of the missense type (leading only to an amino acid substitution), which constitutes a diagnostic problem concerning their pathogenicity. Besides commonly used theoretical predictions (evolutionary conservation status of the amino acid, conservativeness of the amino acid change, occurrence of the variant in the normal population, co-segregation with disease phenotype) functional tests may be necessary in the evaluation of the pathogenicity of missense changes.

Microsatellite instability

Microsatellite instability (MSI) is the hallmark of tumours that arise in carriers of *MLH1*, *MSH2*, of *MSH6* mutations. Overall, MSI is detected in approximately 15% of all colorectal cancers. It is measured as alterations in the length of simple repetitive genomic sequences, usually dinucleotide repeats, or mononucleotide runs. As these repeats have a tendency to form mismatches during DNA replication, a mismatch repair defect is expected to increase their mutation frequency. Because the definition of instability applied has been variable, in 1998 an international working group recommended the use of five markers to assess MSI {306}. Tumours are characterized as having high-frequency MSI (MSI-H) if two or more of the five markers show instability (i.e. have insertion/deletion mutations), or as having low-frequency MSI (MSI-L) if only one of the five markers shows instability. The distinction between microsatellite stable (MSS) and low frequency MSI (MSI-L) can only be accomplished if a greater number of markers is utilized. MSI analysis, in conjunction with immunohistochemistry, can greatly improve the efficacy of the molecular screening for HNPCC {650,2516}.

In one study, all 12 endometrial carcinomas from carriers of *MLH1* and *MSH2* germline mutations demonstrated an MSI-high phenotype involving all types of repeat markers, while this was found in only 4 out of 11 (36%) endometrial carcinomas from *MSH6* mutation carriers {650}. In another study, MSI-patterns in endometrial cancers differed from those in colorectal cancers, even though the patients had identical predisposing mutations in the MMR genes *MLH1* or *MSH2* {1527}. In endometrial cancers, the pattern was more heterogeneous and involved a lower proportion of unstable markers per tumour and shorter allelic shifts for BAT markers. These results might point to gene-specific and/or organ-specific differences that may be important determinants of the HNPCC tumour spectrum.

Mutation spectrum

Hereditary non polyposis colorectal cancer (HNPCC) is caused by germline mutations in one of 5 DNA mismatch repair genes (MMR): *MSH2* {864}, *MLH1* {353}, *PMS1* {2010}, *PMS2* {2010}, and *MSH6* (formerly GTBP) {53,1884}. Other genes like *EXO1* {3161}, *MLH3* {1674,3162} and *TGFbRII* {1705} have been reported to possibly cause HNPCC-like syndromes, although no definitive evidence has been delivered yet, both in terms of pathogenicity and/or cosegregation with the disease of the alleged germline mutations in affected families.

To date, more than 300 different predisposing mutations have been identified, most in *MSH2* and *MLH1* and in families complying with the clinical Amsterdam criteria (AMS+) {2214}. Many HNPCC families, however, do not fully comply with these criteria, and in most of these cases the disease-causing mutations are yet unknown. Mutations in *MSH6* have been found in atypical HNPCC families (see below).

In general, MMR mutations are scattered along the coding sequence of *MSH2* and *MLH1* and predict either the truncation of the corresponding protein products, or a subtler amino acid substitutions. These mutations appear evenly distributed throughout the coding regions of the main MMR genes, with some clustering in *MSH2* exon 12 {2214} and *MLH1* exon 16 {3115}. While most of the *MSH2* mutations consist of frameshift or nonsense changes, *MLH1* is mainly affected by frameshift or missense alterations. Most of the mutations found to date are unique, with a few common recurring ones {2214}. Genomic deletions have also been found at both loci {442,2070, 3116}. *MSH2* deletions appear to be a very frequent cause of HNPCC, contributing for up to a quarter of the families selected by Amsterdam criteria {3116}. *MLH1* deletions are less frequent than in *MSH2* {1793,2070}. Southern analysis and/or other PCR-based methods to detect larger rearrangements at the genomic level {443} should be routinely employed when approaching the mutation analyses of these major mismatch repair genes.

Genotype-phenotype correlations

The combination of clinical (number and type of tumours, age of onset, clinical course of the disease, etc.) and genetic (different mismatch repair genes, truncating and missense mutations) hetero-geneity in HNPCC represents an ideal opportunity to attempt the establishment of genotype-phenotype correlations. Unfortunately, and notwithstanding the large number of mutations and clinical data collected to date, no clear-cut correlations have been observed between specific MMR gene mutations and their clinical outcome. For example, the identification of identical mutations both in HNPCC and in Muir-Torre or Turcot syndrome does not support the existence of consistent genotype-phenotype correlations {179,1115,1494}.

The most reliable correlation found to date is the association between clear-cut pathogenic mutations at *MSH2*, *MLH1* and *MSH6*, and the resulting spectrum of colorectal and extracolonic tumours. HNPCC kindreds due to *MSH2* or *MLH1* germline mutations are characterized by high penetrance and early onset of colorectal and endometrial cancer. The diagnostic criteria, Amsterdam I and II, established by the International Collaborative Group on HNPCC {3008, 3010} well serve the purpose of selecting families with a high likelihood to carry *MSH2* and *MLH1* mutations {3117}. In addition to the fulfillment of the above criteria, other factors represent valid predictors of the presence of germline *MSH2* and *MLH1* mutations in HNPCC families. These include 1. young age at diagnosis of colorectal cancer, and 2. the occurrence of at least one patient with an extra-colonic cancer, such as those of the endometrium, small intestine, brain, and stomach, within an AMS+ HNPCC kindred. The frequency of mutations identified in these families increased to about 70% {3117}. Moreover, the occurrence of at least one patient with multiple synchronous or metachronous colorectal cancers, and the combined occurrence of colorectal cancer with endometrial cancer in one patient are very good predictors of *MSH2* or *MLH1* mutations {3117}.

The first reports on *MSH6* germline mutations already indicated that the clinical phenotype differed from the "classical" HNPCC caused by *MSH2* and *MLH1* mutations {53,1884}. More recently, *MSH6* germline mutations have been demonstrated in a considerable number of the atypical HNPCC families, i.e. not complying with the Amsterdam criteria (ACI and II) {1497,3039,3114,3160}. In general, the penetrance of colorectal cancer seemed to be reduced while endometrial cancer seems to represent a more important clinical manifestation among female *MSH6* mutation carriers. Also, the mean age of onset of colorectal and endometrial cancer appeared to be delayed in families with *MSH6* germline mutations {3011,3039,3114}. Notably,

MSI analysis of tumours from *MSH6* mutation carriers suggests a reduced penetrance of the MSI-H phenotype and preferential instability at mononucleotide repeats {650,1497,3114,3160}.

An additional *MSH6*-associated clinical phenotype is the papillary transitional cell carcinoma of the ureter and renal

pelvis, observed in approx. 10% of the carriers from an extended *MSH6* kindred {3039}. Notably, the lifetime cumulative risk of this tumour type in *MLH1* or *MSH2* mutation carriers is only 2.6% {2673}.

Ataxia telangiectasia syndrome

A. Broeks
L.J. van't Veer
A.L. Borresen-Dale
J. Hall

Definition

Ataxia telangiectasia syndrome (A-T) is a rare, progressive neurological disorder that manifests at the toddler stage. The disease is characterized by cerebellar degeneration (ataxia), dilated blood vessels in the eyes and skin (telangiectasia), immunodeficiency, chromosomal instability, increased sensitivity to ionizing radiation and a predisposition to cancer, in particular leukaemias and lymphomas. Germline mutations in the *ATM* gene (ataxia telangiectasia mutated), homozygous or compound heterozygous, are the cause of this autosomal recessive disorder. Heterozygous carriers are phenotypically unaffected but exhibit an increased risk to develop breast cancer and often display a variety of age related disorders which may result in reduced life expectancy {2808}.

MIM No.   208900 {1835}

Synonyms

Louis-Bar Syndrome, A-T complementation group A (ATA), group C (ATC), group D (ATD) and group E (ATE). The different complementation groups are all linked to the *ATM* gene.

Incidence

The rare A-T disease occurs in both genders and world wide among all races. The disease has an estimated incidence of one per 40,000 to one per 300,000 live births.

Approximately 0.2-1% of the general population has been estimated to be heterozygous carriers of a type of germline mutation in the *ATM* gene that in homozygous state causes the A-T syndrome.

Tumours in A-T patients

Individuals with A-T have a 50 to 150 fold excess risk of cancer, with approximately 70% being lymphomas and T cell leukaemias. In younger patients, an acute lymphoblastic leukaemia is most often of T-cell origin, although the pre-B common ALL of childhood has also been seen in A-T patients. When leukaemia develops in older A-T patients it is usually an aggressive T-cell leukaemia (T-PLL, T cell prolymphocytic leukaemia). Lymphomas are usually B cell types. A wide range of solid tumours makes up the remainder of the tumours seen in A-T patients and includes cancers of the breast, stomach, ovary and melanoma. The presence of missense mutations in A-T patients has been associated with a milder clinical phenotype and altered cancer predisposition. In two British A-T families a T>G tranversion at base pair 7271 was found to be associated with a milder clinical phenotype, lower radiosensitivity but an increased risk of breast cancer. This increased risk was observed in both the homozygote and heterozygotes carriers of this modification (RR 12.7 p=0.0025) {2775}. This sequence alteration has subsequently

been found in multiple-case breast cancer families. The expression and activity analyses of the ATM protein in heterozygous cell lines carrying this sequence change indicated that this mutation was dominant negative {462}.

Breast cancer in *ATM* heterozygotes

Heterozygous carriers of *ATM* mutations have a higher mortality rate and an earlier age at death from cancer and ischemic heart disease than non-carriers {2808}. A-T heterozygotes have been reported to have a 3 to 8 fold increased risk of breast cancer. The association between *ATM* heterozygosity and breast cancer risk was initially found among blood relatives of A-T patients {2820}, and in almost every study of A-T relatives since an increased breast cancer risk has been detected {318,741,981,1291, 1334,2105,2257,2819}. Paradoxically, in the years following the cloning of the *ATM* gene {2546}, several studies investigating large breast cancer cohorts failed to find an increased incidence of *ATM* mutations of the type found in A-T patients, and a controversy arose regarding the role of *ATM* in breast cancer susceptibility {194,281,884}. However, a number of recent studies, analysing the frequency of all type of *ATM* mutations, did confirm previous findings of an elevated breast cancer risk in *ATM* mutation carriers {129,351, 462,2592,2775}.

Age distribution and penetrance

Most of the studies finding an increased risk of breast cancer in A-T relatives point to an early onset of the disease. The penetrance has been difficult to estimate since most of the studies are small, and different mutations may have different effects. In several studies of A-T relatives, the elevated risk is restricted to obligate carriers (mothers), and is not increased in other relatives according to their probability of being a mutation carrier. This may point to an interaction with environmental and/or other genetic factors contributing to the elevated breast cancer risk.

Clinical and pathological features

No typical clinical or pathological features are so far known for *ATM* heterozygous breast cancer patients, other than early age at onset (before age 50) and frequent bilateral occurrence {351}.

Response to therapy and prognosis

ATM heterozygotes with breast cancer do not seem to exhibit acute radiation sensitivity as A-T patients do, and excessive toxicity has not been observed after radiotherapy {115,2331,3088}. It has however been speculated whether *ATM* heterozygous breast cancer patients have an increased risk of developing a second breast cancer after radiation treatment, and large multi-center studies are ongoing to answer this question.

There are only few studies evaluating the prognosis of A-T carriers with breast cancer, pointing to a long-term survival. This may be due to their tumours being more susceptible to cell killing by ionizing radiation than tumour cells in non-carriers {2809}.

ATM expression in breast cancer

Normal breast tissue shows a distinct pattern of ATM expression, the protein being found in the nucleus of the ductal epithelial cells and to a lesser extent in the surrounding myoepithelial cells. Decreased ATM expression is often observed in breast carcinomas {102, 1384} and *ATM* mRNA levels have also been found to be lower in invasive breast carcinomas than in normal tissues or benign lesions {3041}.

Significant loss of heterozygosity in sporadic breast tumours across chromosome 11q22-23 where the *ATM* gene is located has been reported {1118,1439, 1553,1754,2375}.

Table 8.12

Proposed *ATM* genotype / phenotype relationships {971}.

Genotype	Phenotype
ATM^wt/wt	Normal
ATM^trun/trun	Ataxia telangiectasia, High cancer risk
ATM^trun/mis	Ataxia telangiectasia, Variant A-T?, High cancer risk?
ATM^mis/mis	Ataxia telangiectasia? Variant A-T?, High cancer risk?
ATM^trun/wt	A-T relatives, Elevated breast cancer risk, Increased age related disorders?
ATM^mis/wt	Few A-T relatives, Moderate breast cancer risk? Increased age related disorders?

Genetics

Chromosomal location

The *ATM* gene is located on human chromosome 11q22-23.

Gene structure

The *ATM* gene has 66 exons scanning 150 kilobase of genomic DNA and is expressed in a wide range of tissues as an approximately 12-kilobase messenger RNA encoding a 350 kD serine/threonine protein kinase. The initiation codon falls within exon 4. The last exon is 3.8kb and contains the stop codon and a 3'-untranslated region of about 3600 nucleotides {2983}.

Gene expression

The major 13 kb *ATM* transcript is observed in every tissue tested to date. Northern blots and RT-PCR products from various tissues failed to disclose any evidence of alternative forms within the coding region. However the first four exons, which fall within the 5'-untranslated region (UTR), undergo extensive alternative splicing. Differential polyadenylation results in 3'UTRs of varying lengths. These structural features suggest that *ATM* expression might be subject to complex post-transcriptional regulation {2547}.

Gene function

The ATM protein plays a central role in sensing and signalling the presence of DNA double-strand breaks (DSBs) formed in cells as a result of normal DNA metabolism (e.g. meiotic or V(D)J recombination) or damage caused by external agents. The kinase domain in the carboxy-terminal region of the protein contains the signature motifs of phos-phatidylinositol 3-kinases. ATM's kinase activity is itself enhanced in response to DNA double-strand breaks resulting in a phosphorylation cascade activating many proteins each of which in turn affects a specific signalling pathway. These substrates include the protein products of a number of well characterized tumour-suppressor genes including *TP53*, *BRCA1* and *CHEK2* which play important roles in triggering cell cycle arrest, DNA repair or apoptosis (reviewed in Shiloh et al. {2660}). Additional DSB-induced responses that are ATM dependent include the activation of transcription factors such as AP-1, p73 and NFKB, and deacetylation of chromatin proteins (reviewed in Barzilai et al. {189}).

Mutation spectrum in A-T patients

Since the *ATM* gene was cloned {2546} more than 300 different A-T disease-causing mutations have been reported. The profile of these has revealed that most are unique and uniformly distributed along the length of the gene, no mutational hotspots have been detected. The majority of A-T patients are compound heterozygotes having two different *ATM* mutations and patients homozygous for the same *ATM* mutation are rare. The predominate type of mutation found in the *ATM* gene in A-T patients results in a truncated and unstable ATM protein. Some A-T patients have a milder phenotype (variant A-T) that may be related to the presence of missense mutations or mutations producing an ATM protein retaining some normal function {1825,2592}.

Genotype-phenotype correlations

Gatti et al. {971}, in distinguishing between truncating mutations where no

ATM protein is detected and missense substitutions where mutant protein of variable stability is observed, have suggested that this mutant protein could produce a dominant negative effect in heterozygotes, resulting in an altered phenotype and an increased breast cancer susceptibility. The expected phenotypes that might arise from having two types of A-T carriers in the general population are shown in Table 8.12.

The genotype $ATM^{trun/trun}$ with two truncating mutations causes the classical A-T disorder. The genotype $ATM^{mis/mis}$ with two missense mutations is also found in some children with the classical form of the disease, in particular when these are located within the ATM kinase domain (for instance Belzen et al. {2987}, Angele et al. {101}) but may also be associated with a variant A-T phenotype with some neurological features and cancer susceptibility. Two types of ATM heterozygotes exist and the phenotypes differ, i.e. those with truncating mutations that make no protein and those with missense mutations that make reduced amount or partly defective protein {115,462,971, 1825,2331,2592,2775,2809,3088}, and these two groups may have different breast cancer risks. If this proposed model is correct it necessitates a re-analyses of the epidemiological data stratifying for the two types of heterozygotes. The literature to date suggests that germline ATM missense mutations are more frequent than the 0.2-1% frequency of A-T causing mutations and hence contribute to a larger fraction of breast cancer patients {351,462,2592}.

Contributors

Dr Vera M. ABELER**
Department of Pathology
The Norwegian Radium Hospital
Montebello
0310 Oslo
NORWAY
Tel. +47 22 93 40 00
Fax. +47 22 93 54 26
v.m.abeler@labmed.uio.no

Dr Jorge ALBORES-SAAVEDRA
Department of Pathology
LSU Health Sciences Center
1501 Kings Highway
Shreveport, LA 71130
U.S.A
Tel. +1 318 675 7732
Fax. +1 318 675 7662
jalbor@lsuhsc.edu

Dr Isabel ALVARADO-CABRERO
Vicente Suárez 42-201
Colonia Condesa
CP 06140
MEXICO, DF
Tel. +52-56-27-69-00
Fax. +52 55-74-23-22
isa98@prodigy.net.mx

Dr Erik Søgaard ANDERSEN
Department of Obstetrics and
Gynaecology, Aalborg Hospital
Hobrovej
DK-9000 Aalborg
DENMARK
Tel. +45 9932 1218
Fax. +45 9932 1240
u19040@aas.nja.dk

Dr Alan ASHWORTH
The Breakthrough Breast Cancer Centre
The Institute of Cancer Research
237 Fulham Road
London SW3 6JB
UNITED KINGDOM
Tel. +44 207 153 5333
Fax. +44 207 153 5340
alan.ashworth@icr.ac.uk

Dr Jean-Pierre BELLOCQ*
Service d'Anatomie Pathologique
Hôpitaux Universitaires de Strasbourg
Avenue Molière
67098 Strasbourg
FRANCE
Tel. +33 3 88 12 70 53
Fax. +33 3 88 12 70 52
jean-pierre.bellocq@chru-strasbourg.fr

Dr Christine BERGERON**
Laboratoire Pasteur-Cerba
95066 Cergy Pontoise
Cedex 9
FRANCE
Tel. +33 1 34 40 21 17
Fax. +33 1 34 40 20 29
bergeron@pasteur-cerba.com

Dr Ross S. BERKOWITZ
Brigham and Women's Hospital
Harvard Medical School,
75 Francis St.
Boston, MA 02115
U.S.A
Tel. +1 617 732 8843
Fax. +1 617 738 5124
rberkowitz@partners.org

Dr Werner BÖCKER*
Gerhard Domagk Institute of Pathology
University of Münster
Domagkstrasse 17
D-48129 Münster
GERMANY
Tel. +49 251 835 54 40/1
Fax. +49 251 835 54 60
werner.boecker@uni-muenster.de

Dr Anne-Lise BØRRESEN-DALE
Department of Genetics
Institute for Cancer Research
The Norwegian Radium Hospital
0310 Oslo
NORWAY
Tel. +47 22 93 44 19
Fax. +47 22 93 44 40
alb@radium.uio.no

Dr Annegien BROEKS
Department of Molecular Pathology
Netherlands Cancer Institute
Plesmanlaan 121
1066 CX Amsterdam
THE NETHERLANDS
Tel. +31 20 5122754
Fax. +31 20 5122759
a.broeks@nki.nl

Dr C. Hilary BUCKLEY
Department of Gynecologic Pathology
St Mary's Hospital
Manchester M13 0JH
UNITED KINGDOM
Tel. +44 161 445 7132
Fax. +44 161 276 6348
chb@chbpath.fsnet.co.uk

Dr Gianni BUSSOLATI*
Istituto di Anatomia e Istologia Patologica
University of Turin
Via Santena 7
10126 Torino
ITALY
Tel. +39 011 670 65 05
Fax. +39 011 663 52 67
gianni.bussolati@unito.it

Dr Rosmarie CADUFF
Department of Pathology
University Hospital USZ
Schmelzbergstr. 12
8091 Zürich
SWITZERLAND
Tel. +41 1 255 25 05
Fax. +41 1 255 44 16
rosmarie.caduff@pty.usz.ch

Dr Maria-Luisa CARCANGIU
Department of Pathology
National Cancer Institute
Via G. Venezian 1
20133 Milano
ITALY
Tel. +39 02 239 02264
Fax. +39 02 239 02756
carcangiu@istitutotumori.mi.it

Dr Silvestro CARINELLI
Department of Pathology
Istituti Clinici di Perfezionamento
Via della Commenda 12
20122 Milano
ITALY
Tel. +39 02 5799 2415
Fax. +39 02 5799 2860
silvestro.carinelli@icp.mi.it

Dr Annie N. CHEUNG
Department of Pathology
Queen Mary Hospital
The University of Hong Kong
Hong Kong
CHINA
Tel. +852 2855 4876
Fax. +852 2872 5197
anycheun@hkucc.hku.hk

Dr Anne-Marie CLETON-JANSEN
Department of Pathology
Leiden University Medical Centre
P.O. Box 9600, L1-Q
2300 RC Leiden
THE NETHERLANDS
Tel. +31 71 5266515
Fax. +31 71 5248158
a.m.cleton-jansen@lumc.nl

Dr Cees J. CORNELISSE
Department of Pathology
Leiden University Medical Center
Albinusdreef 2 P.O. Box 9600
2300 RC Leiden
THE NETHERLANDS
Tel. +31 71 526 6624
Fax. +31 71 524 8158
c.j.cornelisse@lumc.nl

Dr Christopher P. CRUM
Department of Pathology
Brigham and Women's Hospital
75 Francis Street
Boston MA 02115
U.S.A
Tel. +1 617 732 75 30
Fax. +1 617 264 51 25
ccrum@partners.org

Dr Bruno CUTULI
Département de Radiothérapie
Polyclinique de Courlancy
38 rue de Courlancy
51100 Reims
FRANCE
Tel. +33 3 26 84 02 84
Fax. +33 3 26 84 70 20
b.cutuli@wanadoo.fr

Dr Peter DEVILEE*
Departments of Human and Clinical
Genetics and Pathology
Leiden University Medical Center
2333 AL Leiden
THE NETHERLANDS
Tel. +31 71 527 6117
Fax. +31 71 527 6075
p.devilee@lumc.nl

Dr Mojgan DEVOUASSOUX-SHISHEBORAN**
Service d'Anatomie et Cytologie
Hôpital de la Croix Rousse
103, Grande rue de la Croix Rousse
69317 Lyon
FRANCE
Tel. +33 4 72 07 18 78
Fax. +33 4 72 07 18 79
devouass@lsgrisn1.univ-lyon1.fr

Dr Manfred DIETEL**
Institute of Pathology
Charité University Hospital
Schumanstrasse 20/21
10117 Berlin
GERMANY
Tel. +49 30 4505 36001
Fax. +49 30 4505 36900
manfred.dietel@charite.de

Dr Stephen DOBBS
Department of Gynaecological Oncology
Belfast City Hospital
Lisburn Road
Belfast BT9 7AB
UNITED KINGDOM
Tel. +44 28 90 26 38 94
Fax. +44 28 90 26 39 53
stephen.dobbs@bch.n-i.nhs.uk

Dr Maria DRIJKONINGEN*
Department of Pathology
University Hospital St. Rafael
Catholic University Leuven
3000 Leuven
BELGIUM
Tel. +32 16 33 66 41
Fax. +3216336548
ria.drijkoningen@uz.kuleuven.ac.be

Dr Douglas EASTON
Cancer Research UK
Genetic Epidemiology Unit
University of Cambridge
Cambridge CB1 8RN
UNITED KINGDOM
Tel. +44 122 374 0160
Fax. +44 122 374 0159
douglas@srl.cam.ac.uk

* One asterisk indicates participation in the
Editorial and Consensus Conference on the
WHO classification of Tumours of the
Breast during January 12-16 in Lyon,
France. **Two asterisks indicate participa-
tion in the conference on the WHO classifi-
cation of Tumours of Female Genital
Organs during March 16-20, 2002.

Dr Rosalind EELES
Translational Cancer Genetics
Institute of Cancer Research and Royal
Marsden NHS Trust
Sutton, Surrey SM2 5PT
UNITED KINGDOM
Tel. +44 208 661 3642
Fax. +44 208 770 1489
rosalind.eeles@icr.ac.uk

Dr Ian O. ELLIS*
Department of Histopathology
University of Nottingham
City Hospital, Hucknall Road
Nottingham NG5 1PB
UNITED KINGDOM
Tel. +44 115 969 11 69 Ext. 46875
Fax. +44 115 962 77 68
Ian.ellis@nottingham.ac.uk

Dr Charis ENG
Division of Human Genetics
Department of Internal Medicine
The Ohio State University
Columbus, OH 43210
U.S.A.
Tel. +1 614 292 2347
Fax. +1 614 688 3582
eng.25@osu.edu

Dr Vincenzo EUSEBI*
M. Malphighi Department of Pathology
Ospedale Bellaria, University of Bologna
Via Altura 3
40139 Bologna
ITALY
Tel. +39 051 622 57 50/55 23
Fax. +39 051 622 57 59
vincenzo.eusebi@ausl.bologna.it

Dr Mathias FEHR
Department of Obstetrics and Gynecology
University Hospital
Frauenklinikstr. 10
8091 Zürich
SWITZERLAND
Tel. +41 1 255 57 07
Fax. +41 1 255 44 33
matias.fehr@usz.ch

Dr Rosemary A. FISHER
Department of Cancer Medicine
Imperial College London
Charing Cross Campus
London W6 8RF
UNITED KINGDOM
Tel. +44 20 8846 1413
Fax. +44 20 8748 5665
r.fisher@imperial.ac.uk

Dr Riccardo FODDE
Josephine Nefkens Institue
Erasmus University Medical Center
P.O. Box 1738
3000 DR Rotterdam
THE NETHERLANDS
Tel. +31 10 408 78 96
Fax. +31 10 408 84 50
t.wechgelaar@erasmusmc.nl

Dr Silvia FRANCESCHI
Unit of Field and Intervention Studies
International Agency for Research on
Cancer (IARC)
69008 Lyon
FRANCE
Tel. +33 4 72 73 84 02
Fax. +33 4 72 73 83 45
franceschi@iarc.fr

Dr Shingo FUJII
Department of Gynecology and Obstetrics
Kyoto University Graduate School of
Medicine
Sakyoku, Kyoto 606-8507
JAPAN
Tel. +81 75 751 3267
Fax. +81 75 751 3247
sfu@kuhp.kyoto-u.ac.jp

Dr David R. GENEST**
Dept. of Pathology
Brigham and Women's Hospital
75 Francis Street
Boston, MA 02115
U.S.A
Tel. +1 617 732 7542
Fax. +1 617 630 1145
dgenest@partners.org

Dr Deborah J. GERSELL
Department of Pathology
St. John's Mercy Medical Center
615 South New Ballas Road
St Louis, MO 63141
U.S.A
Tel. +1 314 569 6120
Fax. +1 314 995 4414
gersdj@stlo.smhs.com

Dr Blake GILKS
Department of Pathology and Laboratory
Medicine, Vancouver General Hospital
University of British Columbia
Vancouver V5M 1Z9
CANADA
Tel. +1 604 875 5555
Fax. +1 604 875 4797
bgilks@vanhosp.bc.ca

Dr David E. GOLDGAR
Unit of Genetic Epidemiology
International Agency for Research on
Cancer (IARC)
69008 Lyon
FRANCE
Tel. +33 4 7273 83 18
Fax. +33 4 7273 83 42
goldgar@iarc.fr

Dr Annekathryn GOODMAN
Gillette Center for Women's Cancer
Massachusetts General Hospital
100 Blossom St
Boston, MA 02114
U.S.A
Tel. +1 617 726 5997
Fax. +1 617 523 1247
agoodman@partners.org

Dr Pierre HAINAUT
Unit of Molecular Carcinogenesis
International Agency for Research on
Cancer (IARC)
69008 Lyon
FRANCE
Tel. +33 4 72 73 85 32
Fax. +33 4 72 73 83 22
hainaut@iarc.fr

Dr Janet HALL
DNA Repair Group
International Agency for Research on
Cancer (IARC)
69008 Lyon
FRANCE
Tel. +33 4 72 73 85 96
Fax. +33 4 72 73 83 22
hall@iarc.fr

Dr Urs HALLER
Departement of Obstetrics and Gynecology
University Hospital
Frauenklinikstr. 10
8091 Zürich
SWITZERLAND
Tel. +41 1 255 5200
Fax. +41 1 255 4433
urs.haller@usz.ch

Dr Antonius G.J.M. HANSELAAR**
Office of the Managing Director
Dutch Cancer Society
P.O. Box 75508
1070 AM Amsterdam
THE NETHERLANDS
Tel. +31 20 57 00 510
Fax. +31 20 67 50 302
directie@kankerbestrijding.nl

Dr Steffen HAUPTMANN
Institute of Pathology
Martin-Luther-University Halle-Wittenberg
Magdeburger Str. 14
06112 Halle (Saale)
GERMANY
Tel. +49-345-557-1880
Fax. +49-345-557-1295
steffen.hauptmann@medizin.uni-halle.de

Dr Michael R. HENDRICKSON**
Lab. of Surgical Pathology, H 2110
Stanford University Medical Center
300 Pasteur Drive
Stanford CA 94305-5243
U.S.A
Tel. +1 650 498 64 60
Fax. +1 650 725 69 02
michael.hendrickson@stanford.edu

Dr Sylvia H. HEYWANG-KöBRUNNER
Center for Breast Diagnosis and
Intervention
Technical University Munich
Klinikum Rechts der Isar
81675 Munich
GERMANY
Tel. +49 89 4140-0
Fax. +49-89-4140-4831

Dr Heinz HöFLER*
Institute of Pathology
Technical University Munich
Ismaninger Strasse 22
81675 Munich
GERMANY
Tel. +49 89 41 40 41 60
Fax. +49 89 41 40 48 65
hoefler@lrz.tu-muenchen.de

Dr Roland HOLLAND*
National Breast Cancer Screening Centre
Nÿmegen University Hospital
Geert Grooteplein 18, Postbus 9101
6500 HB Nÿmegen
THE NETHERLANDS
Tel. +31 24 361 6706
Fax. +31 24 354 0527
r.holland@lrcb.umcn.nl

Dr Jocelyne JACQUEMIER
Department of Pathology
Institut Paoli Calmettes
232, Boulevard Sainte Marguerite
13009 Marseille
FRANCE
Tel. +33 4 91 22 34 57
Fax. +33 4 91 22 35 73
jacquemierj@marseille.fnclcc.fr

Dr Rudolf KAAKS*
Hormones and Cancer Group
International Agency for Research on
Cancer (IARC)
69008 Lyon
FRANCE
Tel. +33 4 72 73 85 53
Fax. +33 4 72 73 83 61
kaaks@iarc.fr

Dr Apollon I. KARSELADZE**
Division of Human Tumour Pathology
Russian Oncological Center
Kashirskoye shosse, 24
115 478 Moscow
RUSSIA
Tel. +7 095 324 96 44
Fax. +7 095 323 57 10
karsela@aha.ru

Dr Richard L. KEMPSON**
Department of Pathology
Stanford University Medical Center
300 Pasteur Drive, Room L235
Stanford, CA 94305-5324
U.S.A
Tel. + 1 650 498 6460
Fax. +1 650 725 6902
rkempson@stanford.edu

Dr Takako KIYOKAWA
Department of Pathology
Jikei University School of Medecine
3-25-8-Nishishinbashi Minato-ku
Tokyo 105-8461
JAPAN
Tel. +81 3 3433 1111 ex5372
Fax. +81 3 5470 9380
takakok@jikei.ac.jp

Dr Paul KLEIHUES* **
International Agency for Research on
Cancer (IARC)
150, cours Albert Thomas
69008 Lyon
FRANCE
Tel. +33 4 72 73 81 77
Fax. +33 4 72 73 85 64
kleihues@iarc.fr

Dr Ikuo KONISHI
Department of Obstetrics and Gynecology
Shinshu University School of Medicine
Asahi
Matsumoto 390-8621
JAPAN
Tel. +81 263 37 2716
Fax. +81 263 34 0944
konishi@hsp.md.shinshu-u.ac.jp

Dr Rahel KUBIK-HUCH
Institute of Radiology
Cantonal Hospital
5404 Baden
SWITZERLAND
Tel. +41 56 486 38 03
Fax. +41 56 483 38 09
rahel.kubik@ksb.ch

Dr Robert J. KURMAN**
Departements of Pathology and
Gynecology & Obstetrics
The Johns Hopkins Hospital
Baltimore, MD 21231-2410
U.S.A.
Tel. +1 410 955 0471/2804
Fax. +1 410 614 1287
rkurman@jhmi.edu

Dr Carlo LA VECCHIA
Laboratory of Epidemiology
Istituto "Mario Negri"
Via Eritrea 62
I-20157 Milano
ITALY
Tel. +390 02 390 14527
Fax. +39 02 332 00231
lavecchia@marionegri.it

Dr Sunil R. LAKHANI*
The Breakthrough Toby Robins Breast
Cancer Research Centre
Chester Beatty Labs
London SW3 6JB
UNITED KINGDOM
Tel. +44 20 7153 5525
Fax. +44 20 7153 5533
sunil.lakhani@icr.ac.uk

Dr Janez LAMOVEC
Department of Pathology
Institute of Oncology
Zaloska 2
1105 Ljubljana
SLOVENIA
Tel. +386 1 4322 099
Fax. +386 1 4314 180
jlamovec@onko-i.si

Dr Salvatore LANZAFAME
Anatomia Patologica
Policlinoco Università di Catania
Via S. Sofia, 87
95123 Catania
ITALY
Tel. +39 095 310 241?
Fax. +39 095 256022
lanzafas@unict.it

Dr Sigurd LAX**
Department of Pathology
General Hospital Graz West
Goestinger Strasse 22
8020 Graz
AUSTRIA
Tel. +43 316 5466 4650
Fax. +43 316 5466 74652
sigurd.lax@uni-graz.at

Dr Kenneth R. LEE
Department of Pathology
Brigham and Women's Hospital
75 Francis Street
Boston MA 02115
U.S.A
Tel. +1 617 278 0736
Fax. +1 617 739 6192
krlee@partners.org

Dr Fabio LEVI
Unité d'Epidémiologie du Cancer
Institut Universitaire de Médecine
Sociale et Préventive, CHUV-Falaises 1
1011 Lausanne
SWITZERLAND
Tel. +41 213 147 311
Fax. +41 213 230 303
fabio.levi@hospvd.ch

Dr Gaëtan MacGROGAN*
Département de Pathologie
Institut Bergonié
229, Cours de l'Argonne
33076 Bordeaux cedex
FRANCE
Tel. +33 5 56 33 33 23
Fax. +33 5 56 33 0438
macgrogan@bergonie.org

Dr Gaetano MAGRO
Dipartimento G.F. INGRASSIA
Anatomia Patologica
Università di Catania
95123 Catania
ITALY
Tel. +39 952 56025
Fax. +39 95256023
gaetano.magro@tiscali.it

Dr Kien T. MAI
Laboratory Medicine, Room 113
1053 Carling Ave.
Ottawa, Ontario K1Y 4E9
CANADA
Tel. +1 613 761 43 44
Fax. +1613 761 48 46
ktmai@ottawahospital.an.ca

Dr W. Glenn McCLUGGAGE**
Department of Pathology
Royal Group of Hospitals Trust
Grosvenor Road
Belfast BT12 6BL
UNITED KINGDOM
Tel. +44 28 9063 2563
Fax. +44 28 9023 3643
glenn.mccluggage@bll.n-i.nhs.uk

Dr Hanne MEIJERS-HEIJBOER
Department of Clinical Genetics
Erasmus Medical Center Rotterdam
Westzeedijk 112
3016 AH Rotterdam
THE NETHERLANDS
Tel. +31 10 4636919
Fax. +31 10 4367133
h.meijers@erasmusmc.nl

Dr Rosemary R. MILLIS*
Hedley Atkins / Cancer Research UK
Breast Pathology Laboratory
Guy's Hospital
London SE1 9RT
UNITED KINGDOM
Tel. +44 207 955 4539
Fax. +44 207 955 8746
rosemary@millisr.fsnet.co.uk

Dr Farid MOINFAR*
Department of Pathology
University of Graz
Auenbruggerplatz 25
8036 Graz
AUSTRIA
Tel. +43 316 380 4453
Fax. +43 316 385 3432
farid.moinfar@uni-graz.at

Dr Samuel C. MOK
Department of Obstetrics, Gynecology &
Reproductive Biology
Brigham and Women's Hospital
Boston, MA 02115
U.S.A
Tel. +1 617 278 0196
Fax. +1 617 975 0818
scmok@rics.bwh.harvard.edu

Dr Alvaro N. MONTEIRO
Dept. of Cell and Developmental Biology
Weill Medical College, Cornell University
1300 York Avenue
New York, NY 10021
U.S.A
Tel. +1 212 734 0567 / ext 225
Fax. +1 212 472 9471
monteia@rockefeller.edu

Dr Eoghan E. MOONEY**
Department of Pathology and Laboratory
Medicine
National Maternity Hospital
Dublin 2
IRELAND
Tel. +353 1 63 735 31
Fax. +353 1 67 65 048
emooney@nmh.ie

Dr Philippe MORICE
Département de Chirurgie
Institut Gustave Roussy
39 rue Camille Desmoulins
94805 Villejuif
FRANCE
Tel. +33 1 42 11 54 41
Fax. +33 1 42 11 52 13
morice@igr.fr

Dr Hans MORREAU
Department of Pathology
Leiden University Medical Centre
PO Box 9600
2300 RC Leiden
THE NETHERLANDS
Tel. +33 71 52 66 625
Fax. +33 71 52 48 158
j.morreau@lumc.nl

Dr Kiyoshi MUKAI
First Department of Pathology
Tokyo Medical University
Shinjuku 6-1-1, Shinjuku-ku
160-8402 Tokyo
JAPAN
Tel. +81 3 3351 6141
Fax. +81 3 3352 6335
kmukai@tokyo-med.ac.jp

Dr Mary MURNAGHAN
Royal Jubilee Maternity Hospital
Royal Hospitals Trust
Grosvenor Road
Belfast BT12 6AA
UNITED KINGDOM
Tel. +44 28 90 632150
Fax. +44 28 90 235256
mmurnaghan@lineone.net

Dr George L. MUTTER**
Department of Pathology
Brigham and Women's Hospital
Harvard Medical School
Boston, MA 02115
U.S.A
Tel. +1 617 732 6096
Fax. +1 617 738 6996
gmutter@rics.bwh.harvard.edu

Dr Steven NAROD
The Center for Research in Women's
Health, University of Toronto
790 Bay Street, 7th floor
Toronto, Ontario M5G 1N8
CANADA
Tel. +1 416 351 37 32
Fax. +1 416 351 37 67
steven.narod@swchsc.on.ca

Dr Jahn M. NESLAND**
Department of Pathology, University Clinic
The Norwegian Radium Hospital
Montebello
0310 Oslo
NORWAY
Tel. +47 22 93 5620
Fax. +47 22 730 164
j.m.nesland@labmed.uio.no

Dr Edward S. NEWLANDS
Medical Oncology
Charing Cross Hospital
Imperial College School of Medicine
London W6 8RF
UNITED KINGDOM
Tel. +44 208 8461419
Fax. +44 208 7485665
enewlands@imperial.ac.uk

Dr Bernt B. NIELSEN
Institute of Pathology
Randers Hospital
Skovlyvej 1
8900 Randers
DENMARK
Tel. +45 8910 2351
Fax. +45 8642 7602
bbn@rc.aaa.dk

Dr Francisco F. NOGALES**
Department of Pathology
Granada University Faculty of Medicine
Avenida de Madrid, 11
18071 Granada
SPAIN
Tel. +34 9 58 243 508
Fax. +34 9 58 243 510
fnogales@ugr.es

Dr Hiroko OHGAKI* **
Unit of Molecular Pathology
International Agency for Research on
Cancer (IARC)
69008 Lyon
FRANCE
Tel. +33 4 72 73 85 34
Fax. +33 4 72 73 85 64
ohgaki@iarc.fr

Dr Magali OLIVIER
Unit of Molecular Carcinogenesis
International Agency for Research on
Cancer (IARC)
69008 Lyon
FRANCE
Tel. +33 4 72 73 86 69
Fax. +33 4 72 73 83 22
molivier@iarc.fr

Dr Andrew G. ÖSTÖR**** (Deceased)
Department of Pathology, Obstetrics and
Gynaecology
The University of Melbourne
48 Anderson Rd
3123 Hawthorn East, Vic.
AUSTRALIA
Tel. +61 3 9822 1145
Fax. +61 3 9882 0933

Dr Jorma PAAVONEN
Department of Obstetrics and Gynecology
University of Helsinki
Haartmaninkatu 2
00290 Helsinki
FINLAND
Tel. +358 9 4717 2807
Fax. +358 9 4717 4902
jorma.paavonen@helsinki.fi

Dr Paivi PELTOMAKI
Biomedicum Helsinki Department of
Medical Genetics, University of Helsinki
Haartmaninkatu 8, P. O. Box 63
00014 Helsinki
FINLAND
Tel. +358 9 19125092
Fax. +358 9 19125105
paivi.peltomaki@helsinki.fi

Dr Johannes L. PETERSE*
Department of Pathology
Netherlands Cancer Institute
Plesmanlaan 121
1066 CX Amsterdam
THE NETHERLANDS
Tel. +31 20 512 27 50
Fax +31 20 512 2759
j.peterse@nki.nl

Dr Jurgen J.M. PIEK
Department of Obstetrics and Gynaecology
VU University Medical Center
P.O. Box 7057
1007 MB Amsterdam
THE NETHERLANDS
Tel. +31 20 444 2828
Fax. +31 20 444 4811
jurgen.piek@vumc.nl

Dr Paola PISANI
Unit of Descriptive Epidemiology
International Agency for Research on
Cancer (IARC)
69008 Lyon
FRANCE
Tel. +33 4 72 73 85 22
Fax. +33 4 72 73 86 96
pisani@iarc.fr

Dr Steven PIVER
Department of Gynecology and Oncology
Sisters of Charity Hospital
2157 Main Street
New York, NY 14214
U.S.A.
Tel. +1 716-862 1000
Fax. +1 716-862 1899
mpiver@wnychs.org

Dr Jaime PRAT**
Department of Pathology
Hospital de la Sta Creu i Sant Pau
Autonomous University of Barcelona
08025 Barcelona
SPAIN
Tel. +34 93 291 90 23
Fax. +34 93 291 93 44
jprat@hsp.santpau.es

Dr Klaus PRECHTEL*
Pathologie Starnberg
Höhenweg 18a
82229 Seefeld
GERMANY
Tel. +49 8152 7740
Fax. +49 8152 7740
k.prechtel@t-online.de

Dr Dieter PRECHTEL
Gemeinschaftspraxis Pathologie
Am Fuchsengraben 3
82319 Starnberg
GERMANY
Tel. +49 8151/3612-0
Fax. +49 8151/78420
d.prechel@pathologie-starnberg.de

Dr Usha RAJU
Department of Pathology
Henry Ford Hospital
2799 WG Blvd
Detroit MI 48202
U.S.A
Tel. +1 313 916 1917
Fax. +1 313 916 9113
uraju1@hfhs.org

Dr Juan ROSAI*
Department of Pathology
National Cancer Institute
Via Venezian 1
20133 Milan
ITALY
Tel. +39 02 2390 2876
Fax. +39 02 2390 2877
juan.rosai@istitutotumori.mi.it

Dr Lawrence M. ROTH
Department of Pathology
Indiana University School of Medicine
550 North University Blvd., Room 3465
Indianapolis, Indiana 46202-5280
U.S.A.
Tel. +1 317 274 5784
Fax. +1 317 274 5346
lroth@iupui.edu

Dr Peter RUSSELL
Department of Anatomical Pathology
Royal Prince Alfred Hospital
Camperdown, NSW 2050
AUSTRALIA
Tel. +61 4 1822 2567
Fax. +61 2 9515 8405
peter.russell@email.cs.nsw.gov.au

Dr Joanne K.L. RUTGERS
Department of Pathology
Long Beach Memorial Medical Center
2801 Atlantic Ave.
Long Beach, CA 90801-1428
U.S.A
Tel. +1 562 933 0726
Fax. +1 562 933 0719
jrutgers@memorialcare.org

Dr Rengaswamy SANKARANARAYANAN
Unit of Descriptive Epidemiology
International Agency for Research on
Cancer (IARC)
69008 Lyon
FRANCE
Tel. +33 4 72 73 85 99
Fax. +33 4 72 73 85 18
sankar@iarc.fr

Dr Anna SAPINO
Department of Biomedical Sciences and
Oncology, University of Torino
Via Santena 7
10126 Torino
ITALY
Tel. +39-011-6706510
Fax. +390116635267
anna.sapino@unito.it

Dr Annie J. SASCO*
Unit of Epidemiology for Cancer Prevention
International Agency for Research on
Cancer (IARC)
69008 Lyon
FRANCE
Tel. +33 4 72 73 84 12
Fax. +33 4 72 73 83 42
sasco@iarc.fr

Dr Xavier SASTRE-GARAU*
Service de Pathologie
Institut Curie
26 rue d'Ulm
75248 Paris
FRANCE
Tel. +33 1 44 32 42 54 / 50
Fax. +33 1 44 32 40 72
xavier.sastre@curie.net

Dr Stuart J. SCHNITT*
Department of Pathology
Beth Israel Deaconess Medical Center
330 Brookline Avenue
Boston, MA 02215
U.S.A
Tel. +1 617 667 43 44
Fax. +1 617 975 56 20
sschnitt@bidmc.harvard.edu

Dr John O. SCHORGE
Gynecologic Oncology
Univ. of Texas Southwestern Medical Center
5323 Harry Hines Blvd, Room J7.124
Dallas TX 75390-9032
U.S.A
Tel. +1 214 648 3026
Fax. +1 214 648 8404
john.schorge@utsouthwestern.edu

Dr Peter E. SCHWARTZ**
Department of Obstetrics and Gynecology
Yale University School of Medicine
333 Cedar Street - FMB 316
New Haven, CT 06520-8063
U.S.A
Tel. +1 203 785 4014
Fax. +1 203 785 4135
peter.schwartz@yale.edu

Dr Robert E. SCULLY**
Department of Pathology
Massachusetts General Hospital
55 Fruit Street, Warren 242
Boston, MA 02114-2696
U.S.A
Tel. +1 617 724 14 59
Fax. +1 617 726 59 15
emelchionno@partners.org

Dr Hideto SENZAKI
Department of Pathology
Kansai Medical University
10-15 Fumizonocho, Moriguchi,
Osaka 570-8506
JAPAN
Tel. +81-6-6993-9432
Fax. +81-6-6992-5023
senzaki@takii.kmu.ac.jp

Dr Elvio G. SILVA
Dept. of Pathology
M.D. Anderson Cancer Center
1515 Holcombe Blvd.
Houston TX 77030
U.S.A
Tel. +1 713 792 31 54
Fax. +1 713 792 55 29
esilva@mdanderson.org

Dr Steven G. SILVERBERG**
Department of Pathology
University of Maryland Medical System
22 South Greene Street
Baltimore MD 21201
U.S.A
Tel. +1 410 328 50 72
Fax. +1 410 328 00 81
sboes001@umaryland.edu

Dr Jorge SOARES
Departamento de Patologia Morfológica
Instituto Português de Oncologia
Rua Professor Lima Basto
1099-023 Lisboa
PORTUGAL
Tel. +351 21 7229825
Fax. +351 21 7229825
jsoares.anpat@fcm.unl.pt

Dr Leslie H. SOBIN* **
Department of Hepatic and
Gastrointestinal Pathology
Armed Forces Institute of Pathology
Washington, DC 20306
U.S.A.
Tel. +1 202 782 2880
Fax. +1 202 782 9020
sobin@afip.osd.mil

Ms Nayanta SODHA MSc
Cancer Genetics Laboratory
Institute of Cancer Research
Cotswold Road
Sutton, Surrey SM2 5NG
UNITED KINGDOM
Tel. +44 208 643 8901
Fax. +44 208 770 1489
nayanta@icr.ac.uk

Dr Mike R. STRATTON
Cancer Genome Project
The Wellcome Trust Sanger Institute
Hinxton
Cambridge CB10 1SA
UNITED KINGDOM
Tel. +44 1223 494757
Fax. +44 1223 494969
mrs@sanger.ac.uk

Dr Csilla SZABO
Unit of Genetic Epidemiology
International Agency for Research on
Cancer (IARC)
69008 Lyon
FRANCE
Tel. +33 4 72 73 86 58
Fax. +33 4 72 73 83 42
szabo@iarc.fr

Dr László TABÁR
Mammography Department
Central Hospital
79182 Falun
SWEDEN
Tel. +46 23 49 2507
Fax. +46 23 49 0592
laszlo@mammographic.org

Dr Aleksander TALERMAN
Department of Pathology
Thomas Jefferson University
132 South 10th Street
Room 285Q / Main Building
Philadelphia, PA 19107-5244
U.S.A
Tel. +1 215 955 2433
Fax. +1 215 923 1969

Dr Colette TARANGER-CHARPIN
Service d'Anatomie et Cytologie
Pathologique, Hôpital Nord
Boulevard Dramard
13916 Marseille
FRANCE
Tel. +33 4 91 69 88 64
Fax. +33 4 91 69 89 53
colette.charpin@ap-hm.fr

Dr Fattaneh A. TAVASSOLI* **
Department of Pathology
Yale University School of Medicine
310 Cedar Street, Room # LH 222
New Haven, CT 06520
U.S.A
Tel. +1 203 785 5439
Fax. +1 203 785 7146
fattaneh.tavassoli@yale.edu

Dr Manuel TEIXEIRA
Department of Genetics
Portuguese Oncology Institute
Rua Dr. Antonio Bernardino Almeida
4200-072 Porto
PORTUGAL
Tel. +351 22 550 20 11/50 78
Fax. +351 22 502 64 89
mteixeir@ipoporto.min-saude.pt

Dr Massimo TOMMASINO
Unit of Infection and Cancer
International Agency for Research on
Cancer (IARC)
69008 Lyon
FRANCE
Tel. +33 4 72 73 81 91
Fax. +33 4 72 73 84 42
tommasino@iarc.fr

Dr Airo TSUBURA
Second Department of Pathology
Kansai Medical University
10-15 Fumizono, Moriguchi,
Osaka 570-8506
JAPAN
Tel. +81 6 6993 9431
Fax. +81 6 6992 5023
tsubura@takii.kmu.ac.jp

Dr Paul J. VAN DIEST
Department of Pathology
Universitair Medisch Centrum Ultrecht
Heidelberglaan 100
3508 GA Utrecht
THE NETHERLANDS
Tel. +31 30 250 6565
Fax. +31 30 254 4990
pj.vandiest@vumc.nl

Dr Laura J. VAN'T VEER
Department of Molecular Pathology
Netherlands Cancer Institute
Plesmanlaan 121
1066 CX Amsterdam
THE NETHERLANDS
Tel. +31 20 5122754
Fax. +31 20 5122759
lveer@nki.nl

Dr Russell S. VANG
Department of Gynecologic and Breast
Pathology, Building 54, Room 1072
Armed Forces Institute of Pathology
Washington, D.C. 20306-6000
U.S.A.
Tel. +1 202-782-1609
Fax. +1 202-782-3939
vangr@afip.osd.mil

Dr Hans F.A. VASEN
Netherlands Foundation for the Detection
of Hereditary Tumours
Poortgebouw Zuid, Rijnsburgerweg 10
2333 AA Leiden
THE NETHERLANDS
Tel. +31 71 5262687
Fax. +31 71 5212137
nfdht@xs4all.nl

Dr A.R. VENKITARAMAN
MRC Cancer Cell Unit
Dept. of Oncology, Hills Road
University of Cambridge
Cambridge CB2 2XZ
UNITED KINGDOM
Tel. +44 122 333 6901
Fax. +44 122 376 3374
arv22@cam.ac.uk

Dr René H.M. VERHEIJEN
Division of Gynaecologycal Oncology
VU University Medical Center
P.O. Box 7057
1007 MB Amsterdam
THE NETHERLANDS
Tel. +31 20 444 4851
Fax. +31 20 444 3333
r.verheijen@vumc.nl

Dr William R. WELCH
Department of Pathology
Brigham and Women's Hospital
75 Francis Street
Boston MA 02115
U.S.A
Tel. +1 617 732 4745
Fax. +1 617 734 8490
wrwelch@bics.bwh.harvard.edu

Dr Michael WELLS**
Academic Unit of Pathology
Medical School
Beech Hill Road
Sheffield S10 2RX
UNITED KINGDOM
Tel. +44 114 271 2397/2683
Fax. +44 114 226 1464
m.wells@sheffield.ac.uk

Dr Edward J. WILKINSON
Department of Pathology
University of Florida College of Medicine
1600 S.W. Archer Rd.
Gainesville, FL 32610-0275
U.S.A
Tel. +1 352 265 0238
Fax. +1 352 265 0437
wilkinso@pathology.ufl.edu

Dr Andrew WOTHERSPOON
Department of Histopathology
Royal Marsden Trust
Fulham Road
London SW3 6JJ
UNITED KINGDOM
Tel. +44 207 352 73 48
Fax. +44 207 352 73 48
andrew.wotherspoon@rmh.nthames.nhs.uk

Source of charts and photographs

01.01	IARC, Lyon
01.02	Dr. P. Pisani
01.03	Dr. A. Sasco
01.04	IARC, Lyon
01.05	Dr. R. Kaaks
01.06	Dr. R. Kaaks/ Dr. A. Sasco
01.07	Dr. I.O. Ellis
01.08A-01.10C	Dr. L. Tabár
01.11	Dr. R. Caduff
01.12A,B	Dr. S.J. Schnitt
01.12C	Dr. I.O. Ellis
01.13	Dr. J. Jacquemier
01.14A,B	Dr. F.A. Tavassoli
01.15-01.16A	Dr. J.L. Peterse
01.16B	Dr. S.J. Schnitt
01.17A,B	Dr. F.A. Tavassoli
01.18	Dr. X. Sastre-Garau
01.19A,B	Dr. L. Tabár
01.20-01.21C	Dr. X. Sastre-Garau
01.22A,B	Dr. F.A. Tavassoli
01.23	Dr. L. Tabár
01.24A-01.25	Dr. F.A. Tavassoli
01.26	Dr. L. Tabár
01.27	Dr. I.O. Ellis
01.28	Dr. X. Sastre-Garau
01.29A-C	Dr. L. Tabár
01.30	Dr. R. Caduff
01.31A-01.32D	Dr. F.A. Tavassoli
01.33A	Dr. S.J. Schnitt
01.33B-01.34	Dr. G. Bussolati
01.35A-C	Dr. L. Tabár
01.36A,B	Dr. F.A. Tavassoli
01.37-01.38C	Dr. J.L. Peterse
01.39-01.41	Dr. V. Eusebi
01.42-01.43	Dr. F.A. Tavassoli
01.44A	Dr. Okcu Institut für Pathologie, Karl-Franzens-Universität, Graz, Austria
01.44B-01.47	Dr. F.A. Tavassoli
01.48	Dr. U. Raju
01.49A	Dr. R. Caduff
01.49B-01.51B	Dr. F.A. Tavassoli
01.52-01.55	Dr. V. Eusebi
01.56	Dr. F.A. Tavassoli

01.57-01.61	Dr. V. Eusebi
01.62A-01.64	Dr. F.A. Tavassoli
01.65-01.068	Dr. P. Devilee
01.69	Dr. A.L. Borresen-Dale
01.70	Dr. F.A. Tavassoli
01.71	Dr. S.J. Schnitt
01.72	Dr. F.A. Tavassoli
01.73	Dr. L.J. van't Veer
01.74A-01.75C	Dr. F.A. Tavassoli
01.76	Dr. W. Boecker
01.77A-01.80B	Dr. F.A. Tavassoli
01.80C,D	Dr. W. Boecker
01.81-01.82	Dr. F.A. Tavassoli
01.83	Dr. R. Heywang-Koebrunner
01.84	Dr. W. Boecker
01.85A,B	Dr. F.A. Tavassoli
01.86A-D	Dr. R. Heywang-Koebrunner
01.87A,B	Dr. L. Tabár
01.88A,B	Dr. W. Boecker
01.89A-01.90B	Dr. F.A. Tavassoli
01.90C-D	Dr. W. Boecker
01.90E-01.91	Dr. F.A. Tavassoli
01.92-01.93	Dr. L. Tabár
01.94A	Dr. W. Boecker
01.94B-01.97C	Dr. F.A. Tavassoli
01.98-01.99B	Dr. G. MacGrogan
01.100-01.101C	Dr. U. Raju
01.102A,B	Dr. G. MacGrogan
01.103A-C	Dr. W. Boecker
01.103D	Dr. G. MacGrogan
01.104	Dr. U. Raju
01.105A-C	Dr. L. Tabár
01.106A	Dr. M. Drijkoningen
01.106B-D	Dr. G. MacGrogan
01.107	Dr. M. Drijkoningen
01.108-01.109A	Dr. B.B. Nielsen
01.109B	Dr. S.J. Schnitt
01.109C	Dr. M. Drijkoningen
01.110A,B	Dr. W. Boecker
01.111	Dr. B.B. Nielsen
01.112	Dr. F.A. Tavassoli
01.113	Dr. B.B. Nielsen
01.114-01.117	Dr. F.A. Tavassoli
01.118	Dr. W. Boecker
01.119	Dr. A.G.J.M. Hanselaar
01.120	Dr. M. Drijkoningen
01.121A-01.122B	Dr. G. Bussolati
01.123	Dr. F.A. Tavassoli
01.124	Dr. G. Bussolati
01.125A,B	Dr. F.A. Tavassoli
01.126A,B	Dr. B.B. Nielsen
01.127A-01.131B	Dr. F.A. Tavassoli

01.132	Dr. J.L. Peterse
01.133-01.136	Dr. F.A. Tavassoli
01.137A-01.139	Dr. J.P. Bellocq
01.140A-C	Dr. V. Eusebi
01.141-01.142	Dr. J.L. Peterse
01.143-01.145B	Dr. F.A. Tavassoli
01.146A-01.152C	Dr. J.P. Bellocq
01.153A,B	Dr. F.A. Tavassoli
01.154	Dr. J.P. Bellocq
01.155-01.157B	Dr. V. Eusebi
01.158A-C	Dr. K.T. Mai
01.159A-01.160	Dr. J. Lamovec
01.161	Dr. E.S. Jaffe NIH, National Cancer Institute, Bethesda MD, U.S.A
01.162	Dr. J. Lamovec
01.163	Dr. J. Jacquemier
01.164-01.166	Dr. K. Prechtel
01.167	Dr. F.A. Tavassoli

2.

02.01	IARC
02.02	Dr. R.A. Kubik-Huch
02.03A	Dr. J. Prat
02.03B	Dr. L. Roth
02.04A	Dr. F.A. Tavassoli
02.04B	Dr. S. Lax
02.05	Dr. J. Prat
02.06A.B	Dr. M. Dietel
02.07A	Dr. F.A. Tavassoli
02.07B	Dr. S. Lax
02.08	Dr. J. Prat
02.09A	Dr. F.A. Tavassoli
02.09B	Dr. M. Dietel
02.10A,B	Dr. J. Prat
02.11	Dr. M. Dietel
02.12	Dr. A.I. Karseladze
02.13	Dr. M. Dietel
02.14	Dr. R.H. Young Dept. Pathology Massachusetts General Hospital Boston, U.S.A
02.15	Dr. K. Lee
02.16A	Dr. J. Prat
02.16B	Dr. K. Lee
02.17	Dr. R.H. Young
02.18-02.19	Dr. K. Lee
02.20	Dr. J. Prat
02.21A	Dr. K. Lee
02.21B	Dr. J. Prat

02.22-02.24B	Dr. K. Lee
02.25	Dr. R.H. Young
02.26	Dr. K. Lee
02.27	Dr. J. Prat
02.28A,B	Dr. S. Lax
02.29A,B	Dr. J. Prat
02.30A	Dr. S. Lax
02.30B-02.31A	Dr. J. Prat
02.31B	Dr. L. Roth
02.32-02.34	Dr. J. Prat
02.35	Dr. C.H. Buckley
02.36	Dr. F.A. Tavassoli
02.37A	Dr. S. Lax
02.37B	Dr. J. Prat
02.38	Dr. S. Lax
02.39A	Dr. A.I. Karseladze
02.39B	Dr. L. Roth
02.40	Dr. A.I. Karseladze
02.41	Dr. J. Prat
02.42	Dr. R. Vang
02.43	Dr. V. Abeler
02.44A,B	Dr. J. Prat
02.45	Dr. R.A. Kubik-Huch
02.46	Dr. R. Vang
02.47	Dr. J. Prat
02.48A,B	Dr. D.J. Gersell
02.49	Dr. J. Prat
02.50-02.53A	Dr. D.J. Gersell
02.53B	Dr. J. Prat
02.53C	Dr. D.J. Gersell
02.54A,B	Dr. E.G. Silva
02.55	Dr. R.A. Kubik-Huch
02.56A-02.63B	Dr. F.A. Tavassoli
02.64A-02.65	Dr. D.J. Gersell
02.66	Dr. F.A. Tavassoli
02.67A-02.69	Dr. D.J. Gersell
02.70	Dr. F.A. Tavassoli
02.71	Dr. L. Roth
02.72A-02.73	Dr. F.A. Tavassoli
02.74-02.75A	Dr. E. Mooney
02.75B	Dr. F.A. Tavassoli
02.75C-02.78	Dr. E. Mooney
02.79A-02.80	Dr. F.A. Tavassoli
02.81	Dr. E. Mooney
02.82	Dr. F.A. Tavassoli
02.83-02.84A	Dr. L. Roth
02.84B	Dr. S. Lax
02.85	Dr. E. Mooney
02.86	Dr. L. Roth
02.87A,B	Dr. P.E. Schwartz
02.88A-02.97	Dr. F. Nogales
02.98A,B	Dr. F.A. Tavassoli
02.99	Dr. R.A. Kubik-Huch

02.100	Dr. A. Ostor
02.101	Dr. F.A. Tavassoli
02.102A,B	Dr. M. Devouassoux-Shisheboran
02.103	Dr. S. Lax
02.104-02.106	Dr. M. Devouassoux-Shisheboran
02.107-02.109B	Dr. F.A. Tavassoli
02.110-02.113	Dr. A. Talerman
02.114-02.116B	Dr. F. Nogales
02.117-02.118B	Dr. L. Roth
02.119A,B	Dr. H. Senzaki/ Dr. A. Tsubura
02.120-02.121	Dr. L. Roth
02.122A,B	Dr. M. Devouassoux-Shisheboran
02.123-02.126	Dr. L. Roth
02.127	Dr. F.A. Tavassoli
02.128A-02.129B	Dr. R. Vang
02.130A-02.131A	Dr. J. Prat
02.131B	Dr. L. Roth
02.131C-02.134	Dr. J. Prat
02.135	Dr. L. Roth
02.136-02.137C	Dr. J. Prat
02.138A	Dr. L. Roth
02.138B	Dr. F. Nogales
02.139A,B	Dr. L. Roth
02.140A-C	Dr. F.A. Tavassoli
02.141	Dr. M.R. Hendrickson
02.142A	Dr. F.A. Tavassoli
02.142B	Dr. L. Roth
02.143A-02.144	Dr. M.R. Hendrickson
02.145	Dr. F.A. Tavassoli

3.

03.01	Dr. R. Caduff
03.02A-03.04C	Dr. I. Alvarado-Cabrero
03.05A-03.06	Dr. L. Roth
03.07	Dr. A. Cheung
03.08	Dr. L. Roth
03.09	Dr. A. Cheung
03.10	Dr. L. Roth
03.11A,B	Dr. F.A. Tavassoli
03.12-03.13	Dr. L. Roth
03.14A	Dr. M. Devouassoux-Shisheboran
03.14B	Dr. L. Roth
03.15A,B	Dr. F.A. Tavassoli
03.16	Dr. R. Vang
03.17A,B	Dr. L. Roth

4.

04.01	IARC
04.02A,B	Dr. F.A. Tavassoli
04.03-04.04	Dr. S.G. Silverberg
04.05	Dr. S. Lax
04.06	Dr. F.A. Tavassoli
04.07	Dr. S.G. Silverberg
04.08	Dr. F. Nogales
04.09-04.12	Dr. S.G. Silverberg
04.13	Dr. F.A. Tavassoli
04.14	Dr. S.G. Silverberg
04.15A	Dr. M. Márquez Hospital Clinic Barcelona, Spain
04.15B	Dr. F. Nogales
04.16A	Dr. E. Mendoza Hospital Virgen del Rocio, Sevilla, Spain
04.16B-04.18A	Dr. F. Nogales
04.18B	Dr. F.A. Tavassoli
04.19-04.21	Dr. F. Nogales
04.22	Dr. S. Lax
04.23-04.24	Dr. G.L. Mutter
04.25A-C	Dr. M.R. Hendrickson
04.26A	Dr. S.G. Silverberg
04.26B-04.28B	Dr. M.R. Hendrickson
04.28C,D	Dr. F.A. Tavassoli
04.29	Dr. S.G. Silverberg
04.30A	Dr. M.R. Hendrickson
04.30B-C	Dr. S.G. Silverberg
04.30D-04.32B	Dr. M.R. Hendrickson
04.32C	Dr. S.G. Silverberg
04.33	Dr. R.A. Kubik-Huch
04.34	Dr. M.R. Hendrickson
04.35-04.36	Dr. S.G. Silverberg
04.37-04.38C	Dr. M.R. Hendrickson
04.39	Dr. S.G. Silverberg
04.40A-C	Dr. R. Vang
04.41	Dr. W.G. McCluggage
04.42-04.43B	Dr. F.A. Tavassoli
04.43C,D	Dr. R. Vang
04.44A	Dr. L. Roth
04.44B-04.45	Dr. R. Vang
04.46A,B	Dr. D. Genest
04.47A	Dr. A. Ostor
04.47B	Dr. L. Roth
04.48A	Dr. D. Genest
04.48B	Dr. M. Wells
04.49A	Dr. A. Ostor
04.49B	Dr. D. Genest
04.50A	Dr. A. Ostor

04.50B	Dr. D. Genest
04.51	Dr. R.A. Kubik-Huch
04.52-04.55	Dr. D. Genest
04.56A-04.57B	Dr. F. Nogales
04.58A,B	Dr. F.A. Tavassoli
04.59A-04.60	Dr. V. Abeler

5.

05.01-05.02	IARC, Lyon
05.03	Dr. M. Tommasino
05.04	Dr. N. Muñoz, IARC, Lyon
05.05	Dr. S. Franceschi
05.06	Dr. R.A. Kubik-Huch
05.07	Dr. E.J. Wilkinson
05.08-05.09	Dr. A.G. Hanselaar
05.10	Dr. A. Ostor
05.11-05.12	Dr. C.P. Crum
05.13	Dr. M. Wells
05.14A,B	Dr. C.P. Crum
05.15A	Dr. S. Lax
05.15B-05.19	Dr. A.G.J.M. Hanselaar
05.20A,B	Dr. A. Ostor
05.20C	Dr. A.G.J.M. Hanselaar
05.21	Dr. L. Roth
05.22A,B	Dr. A. Ostor
05.23A-C	Dr. R. Vang
05.24-05.27	Dr. A. Ostor
05.28	Dr. M. Wells
05.29-05.30	Dr. A. Ostor
05.31-05.32A	Dr. J. Nesland
05.32B	Dr. C.P. Crum
05.33-05.34	Dr. M. Wells
05.35A,B	Dr. T.P. Rollason Dept. Histopathology, Birmingham Women's Hospital, Birmingham, UK
05.36A-05.41	Dr. M.L. Carcangiu
05.42	Dr. R.A. Kubik-Huch
05.43-05.44	Dr. F.A. Tavassoli
05.45-05.48B	Dr. B. Gilks

6.

06.01A,B	Dr. E. Andersen
06.02-06.09	Dr. J. Paavonen/ Dr. C. Bergeron
06.10	Dr. F.A. Tavassoli
06.11A	Dr. R.L. Kempson
06.11B	Dr. L. Roth
06.12A-06.15	Dr. A.G.J.M. Hanselaar

06.16	Dr. A. Ostor
06.17A-06.19	Dr. R.L. Kempson
06.20	Dr. L. Roth
06.21A,B	Dr. R. Vang
06.22	Dr. F.A. Tavassoli
06.23A-06.25	Dr. R. Vang

7.

07.01-07.02	Dr. E.J. Wilkinson
07.03A	Dr. F.A. Tavassoli
07.03B-07.09A	Dr. E.J. Wilkinson
07.09B	Dr. L. Roth
07.09C	Dr. R.L. Kempson
07.10A,B	Dr. E.J. Wilkinson
07.11	Dr. L. Roth
07.12A,B	Dr. E.J. Wilkinson
07.12C	Dr. F.A. Tavassoli
07.13A-07.14	Dr. E.J. Wilkinson
07.15	Dr. R.L. Kempson
07.16A-07.17C	Dr. L. Roth
07.18A-07.19	Dr. R.L. Kempson
07.20A-07.22	Dr. E.J. Wilkinson
07.23A,B	Dr. M. Wells

8.

08.01-08.02	Dr. D. Easton
08.03-08.05	Dr. J. Piek
08.06	Dr. P. Devilee
08.07	Dr. S. Narod
08.08	Dr. A.R. Venkitaraman {4116}
08.09	Dr. P. Devilee
08.10	Dr. A.R. Venkitaraman
08.11A-08.12	Dr. H. Ohgaki
08.13-08.14	Dr. P. Hainaut

References

1. Anon. (1982). The World Health Organization Histological Typing of Breast Tumors-Second Edition. The World Health Organization. *Am J Clin Pathol* 78: 806-816.

2. Anon. (1987). The reduction in risk of ovarian cancer associated with oral-contraceptive use. The Cancer and Steroid Hormone Study of the Centers for Disease Control and the National Institute of Child Health and Human Development. *N Engl J Med* 316: 650-655.

3. Anon. (1990). Surgical-procedure terminology for the vulva and vagina. Report of an International Society for the Study of Vulvar Disease Task Force. *J Reprod Med* 35: 1033-1034.

4. Anon. (1992). Systemic treatment of early breast cancer by hormonal, cytotoxic, or immune therapy. 133 randomised trials involving 31,000 recurrences and 24,000 deaths among 75,000 women. Early Breast Cancer Trialists' Collaborative Group. *Lancet* 339: 1-15.

5. Anon. (1996). Clinical practice guidelines for the use of tumor markers in breast and colorectal cancer. Adopted on May 17, 1996 by the American Society of Clinical Oncology. *J Clin Oncol* 14: 2843-2877.

6. Anon. (1997). Consensus conference on the classification of ductal carcinoma in situ. *Hum Pathol* 28: 1221-1225.

7. Anon. (1997). Consensus Conference on the classification of ductal carcinoma in situ. The Consensus Conference Committee. *Cancer* 80: 1798-1802.

8. Anon. (1997). Pathology of familial breast cancer: differences between breast cancers in carriers of BRCA1 or BRCA2 mutations and sporadic cases. Breast Cancer Linkage Consortium. *Lancet* 349: 1505-1510.

9. Anon. (1998). 1997 update of recommendations for the use of tumor markers in breast and colorectal cancer. Adopted on November 7, 1997 by the American Society of Clinical Oncology. *J Clin Oncol* 16: 793-795.

10. Anon. (1998). Tamoxifen for early breast cancer: an overview of the randomised trials. Early Breast Cancer Trialists' Collaborative Group. *Lancet* 351: 1451-1467.

11. Anon. (1999). Cancer risks in BRCA2 mutation carriers. The Breast Cancer Linkage Consortium. *J Natl Cancer Inst* 91: 1310-1316.

12. Aaltonen LA, Salovaara R, Kristo P, Canzian F, Hemminki A, Peltomaki P, Chadwick RB, Kaariainen H, Eskelinen M, Jarvinen H, Mecklin JP, de la CA (1998). Incidence of hereditary nonpolyposis colorectal cancer and the feasibility of molecular screening for the disease. *N Engl J Med* 338: 1481-1487.

13. Aarnio M, Mecklin JP, Aaltonen LA, Nystrom-Lahti M, Jarvinen HJ (1995). Lifetime risk of different cancers in hereditary non-polyposis colorectal cancer (HNPCC) syndrome. *Int J Cancer* 64: 430-433.

14. Aarnio M, Sankila R, Pukkala E, Salovaara R, Aaltonen LA, de la CA, Peltomaki P, Mecklin JP, Jarvinen HJ (1999). Cancer risk in mutation carriers of DNA-mismatch-repair genes. *Int J Cancer* 81: 214-218.

15. Aaro CA, Jacobson LJ, Soule EH (1963). Endocervical polyps. *Obstet Gynecol* 21: 659-665.

16. Aas T, Borresen AL, Geisler S, Smith-Sorensen B, Johnsen H, Varhaug JE, Akslen LA, Lonning PE (1996). Specific P53 mutations are associated with de novo resistance to doxorubicin in breast cancer patients. *Nat Med* 2: 811-814.

17. Abati AD, Kimmel M, Rosen PP (1990). Apocrine mammary carcinoma. A clinicopathologic study of 72 cases. *Am J Clin Pathol* 94: 371-377.

18. Abbondanzo SL, Seidman JD, Lefkowitz M, Tavassoli FA, Krishnan J (1996). Primary diffuse large B-cell lymphoma of the breast. A clinicopathologic study of 31 cases. *Pathol Res Pract* 192: 37-43.

19. Abbott TM, Hermann WJJr., Scully RE (1984). Ovarian fetiform teratoma (homunculus) in a 9-year-old girl. *Int J Gynecol Pathol* 2: 392-402.

20. Abdul-Karim FW, Bazi TM, Sorensen K, Nasr MF (1987). Sarcoma of the uterine cervix: clinicopathologic findings in three cases. *Gynecol Oncol* 26: 103-111.

21. Abeler V, Nesland JM (1989). Alveolar soft-part sarcoma in the uterine cervix. *Arch Pathol Lab Med* 113: 1179-1183.

22. Abeler VM, Holm R, Nesland JM, Kjorstad KE (1994). Small cell carcinoma of the cervix. A clinicopathologic study of 26 patients. *Cancer* 73: 672-677.

23. Abeler VM, Kjorstad KE, Nesland JM (1991). Undifferentiated carcinoma of the endometrium. A histopathologic and clinical study of 31 cases. *Cancer* 68: 98-105.

24. Abeler VM, Vergote IB, Kjorstad KE, Trope CG (1996). Clear cell carcinoma of the endometrium. Prognosis and metastatic pattern. *Cancer* 78: 1740-1747.

25. Abell MR, Ramirez JA (1973). Sarcomas and carcinosarcomas of the uterine cervix. *Cancer* 31: 1176-1192.

26. Abeln EC, Smit VT, Wessels JW, de Leeuw WJ, Cornelisse CJ, Fleuren GJ (1997). Molecular genetic evidence for the conversion hypothesis of the origin of malignant mixed mullerian tumours. *J Pathol* 183: 424-431.

27. Abner AL, Collins L, Peiro G, Recht A, Come S, Shulman LN, Silver B, Nixon A, Harris JR, Schnitt SJ, Connolly JL (1998). Correlation of tumor size and axillary lymph node involvement with prognosis in patients with T1 breast carcinoma. *Cancer* 83: 2502-2508.

28. Aboumrad MH, Horn RC, Fine G (1963). Lipid-secreting mammary carcinoma. *Cancer* 16: 521-525.

29. Abrams J, Talcott J, Corson JM (1989). Pulmonary metastases in patients with low-grade endometrial stromal sarcoma. Clinicopathologic findings with immunohistochemical characterization. *Am J Surg Pathol* 13: 133-140.

30. Acharya S, Wilson T, Gradia S, Kane MF, Guerrette S, Marsischky GT, Kolodner R, Fishel R (1996). hMSH2 forms specific mispair-binding complexes with hMSH3 and hMSH6. *Proc Natl Acad Sci USA* 93: 13629-13634.

31. Ackerman AB, Mihara I (1985). Dysplasia, dysplastic melanocytes, dysplastic nevi, the dysplastic nevus syndrome, and the relation between dysplastic nevi and malignant melanomas. *Hum Pathol* 16: 87-91.

32. Ackerman LV, Katzenstein AL (1977). The concept of minimal breast cancer and the pathologist's role in the diagnosis of "early carcinoma". *Cancer* 39: 2755-2763.

33. Acosta-Sison H (1970). Chorioadenoma destruens. A report of 41 case. *Am J Obstet Gynecol* 80: 176.

34. Acs G, Lawton TJ, Rebbeck TR, LiVolsi VA, Zhang PJ (2001). Differential expression of E-cadherin in lobular and ductal neoplasms of the breast and its biologic and diagnostic implications. *Am J Clin Pathol* 115: 85-98.

35. Adami HO, Bergstrom R, Hansen J (1985). Age at first primary as a determinant of the incidence of bilateral breast cancer. Cumulative and relative risks in a population-based case-control study. *Cancer* 55: 643-647.

36. Adami HO, Signorello LB, Trichopoulos D (1998). Towards an understanding of breast cancer etiology. *Semin Cancer Biol* 8: 255-262.

37. Adami HO, Sparen P, Bergstrom R, Holmberg L, Krusemo UB, Ponten J (1989). Increasing survival trend after cancer diagnosis in Sweden: 1960-1984. *J Natl Cancer Inst* 81: 1640-1647.

38. Adashi EY, Rosenshein NB, Parmley TH, Woodruff JD (1980). Histogenesis of the broad ligament adrenal rest. *Int J Gynaecol Obstet* 18: 102-104.

39. Adeniji KA, Adelusola KA, Odesanmi WO, Fadiran OA (1997). Histopathological analysis of carcinoma of the male breast in Ile-Ife, Nigeria. *East Afr Med J* 74: 455-457.

40. Adeyinka A, Mertens F, Idvall I, Bondeson L, Ingvar C, Heim S, Mitelman F, Pandis N (1998). Cytogenetic findings in invasive breast carcinomas with prognostically favourable histology: a less complex karyotypic pattern? *Int J Cancer* 79: 361-364.

41. Adnane J, Gaudray P, Dionne CA, Crumley G, Jaye M, Schlessinger J, Jeanteur P, Birnbaum D, Theillet C (1991). BEK and FLG, two receptors to members of the FGF family, are amplified in subsets of human breast cancers. *Oncogene* 6: 659-663.

42. Agathanggelou A, Honorio S, Macartney DP, Martinez A, Dallol A, Rader J, Fullwood P, Chauhan A, Walker R, Shaw JA, Hosoe S, Lerman MI, Minna JD, Maher ER, Latif F (2001). Methylation associated inactivation of RASSF1A from region 3p21.3 in lung, breast and ovarian tumours. *Oncogene* 20: 1509-1518.

43. Agnarsson BA, Jonasson JG, Bjornsdottir IB, Barkardottir RB, Egilsson V, Sigurdsson H (1998). Inherited BRCA2 mutation associated with high grade breast cancer. *Breast Cancer Res Treat* 47: 121-127.

44. Agoff SN, Grieco VS, Garcia R, Gown AM (2001). Immunohistochemical distinction of endometrial stromal sarcoma and cellular leiomyoma. *Appl Immunohistochem Mol Morphol* 9: 164-169.

45. Aguirre P, Scully RE, Wolfe HJ, DeLellis RA (1986). Argyrophil cells in Brenner tumors: histochemical and immunohistochemical analysis. *Int J Gynecol Pathol* 5: 223-234.

46. Aguirre P, Thor AD, Scully RE (1989). Ovarian small cell carcinoma. Histogenetic considerations based on immunohistochemical and other findings. *Am J Clin Pathol* 92: 140-149.

47. Ahern JK, Allen NH (1978). Cervical hemangioma: a case report and review of the literature. *J Reprod Med* 21: 228-231.

48. Ahmed AA, Swan RW, Owen A, Kraus FT, Patrick F (1997). Uterus-like mass arising in the broad ligament: a metaplasia or mullerian duct anomaly? *Int J Gynecol Pathol* 16: 279-281.

49. Aho M, Vesterinen E, Meyer B, Purola E, Paavonen J (1991). Natural history of vaginal intraepithelial neoplasia. *Cancer* 68: 195-197.

50. Aida H, Takakuwa K, Nagata H, Tsuneki I, Takano M, Tsuji S, Takahashi T, Sonoda T, Hatae M, Takahashi K, Hasegawa K, Mizunuma H, Toyoda N, Kamata H, Torii Y, Saito N, Tanaka K, Yakushiji M, Araki T, Tanaka K (1998). Clinical features of ovarian cancer in Japanese women with germline mutations of BRCA1. *Clin Cancer Res* 4: 235-240.

51. AJCC (2002). *AJCC Cancer Staging Manual.* Sixth ed. Springer Verlag: New York.

52. Akhtar M, Robinson C, Ashraf Ali M, Godwin JT (1983). Secretory carcinoma of the breast in adults. *Cancer* 51: 2245-2254.

53. Akiyama Y, Sato H, Yamada T, Nagasaki H, Tsuchiya A, Abe R, Yuasa Y (1997). Germ-line mutation of the hMSH6/GTBP gene in an atypical hereditary nonpolyposis colorectal cancer kindred. *Cancer Res* 57: 3920-3923.

54. Al Jafari MS, Panton HM, Gradwell E (1985). Phaeochromocytoma of the broad ligament. Case report. *Br J Obstet Gynaecol* 92: 649-651.

55. Al Kurdi M, Monaghan JM (1981). Thirty-two years experience in management of primary tumours of the vagina. *Br J Obstet Gynaecol* 88: 1145-1150.

56. Al Nafussi AI, Al Yusif R (1998). Papillary squamotransitional cell carcinoma of the uterine cervix: an advanced stage disease despite superficial location: report of two cases and review of the literature. *Eur J Gynaecol Oncol* 19: 455-457.

57. Al Nafussi AI, Hughes DE (1994). Histological features of CIN3 and their value in predicting invasive microinvasive squamous carcinoma. *J Clin Pathol* 47: 799-804.

58. Alamowitch B, Mausset V, Ruiz A, Tissier F, Fourmestraux J, Bouillot JL, Bethoux JP (1999). [Non-secreting pheochromocytoma of the broad ligament revealed by appendicular peritonitis]. *Presse Med* 28: 225-228.

59. Albain KS, Allred DC, Clark GM (1994). Breast cancer outcome and predictors of outcome: are there age differentials? *J Natl Cancer Inst Monogr* 35-42.

60. Albertson DG, Ylstra B, Segraves R, Collins C, Dairkee SH, Kowbel D, Kuo WL, Gray JW, Pinkel D (2000). Quantitative mapping of amplicon structure by array CGH identifies CYP24 as a candidate oncogene. *Nat Genet* 25: 144-146.

61. Albonico G, Querzoli P, Ferretti S, Rinaldi R, Nenci I (1996). Biological heterogeneity of breast carcinoma in situ. *Ann N Y Acad Sci* 784: 458-461.

62. Albonico G, Querzoli P, Ferretti S, Rinaldi R, Nenci I (1998). Biological profile of in situ breast cancer investigated by immunohistochemical technique. *Cancer Detect Prev* 22: 313-318.

63. Albores-Saavedra J, Gersell D, Gilks CB, Henson DE, Lindberg G, Santiago H, Scully RE, Silva E, Sobin LH, Tavassoli FJ, Travis WD, Woodruff JM (1997). Terminology of endocrine tumors of the uterine cervix: results of a workshop sponsored by the College of American Pathologists and the National Cancer Institute. *Arch Pathol Lab Med* 121: 34-39.

64. Albores-Saavedra J, Gilcrease M (1999). Glomus tumor of the uterine cervix. *Int J Gynecol Pathol* 18: 69-72.

65. Albores-Saavedra J, Manivel C, Mora A, Vuitch F, Milchgrub S, Gould E (1992). The solid variant of adenoid cystic carcinoma of the cervix. *Int J Gynecol Pathol* 11: 2-10.

66. Albores-Saavedra J, Young RH (1995). Transitional cell neoplasms (carcinomas and inverted papillomas) of the uterine cervix. A report of five cases. *Am J Surg Pathol* 19: 1138-1145.

67. Alderson MR, Hamlin I, Staunton MD (1971). The relative significance of prognostic factors in breast carcinoma. *Br J Cancer* 25: 646-656.

68. Alfsen GC, Kristensen GB, Skovlund E, Pettersen EO, Abeler VM (2001). Histologic subtype has minor importance for overall survival in patients with adenocarcinoma of the uterine cervix: a population-based study of prognostic factors in 505 patients with nonsquamous cell carcinomas of the cervix. *Cancer* 92: 2471-2483.

69. Alizadeh AA, Ross DT, Perou CM, van de Rijn M (2001). Towards a novel classification of human malignancies based on gene expression patterns. *J Pathol* 195: 41-52.

70. Allaire AD, Majmudar B (1993). Dracunculosis of the broad ligament. A case of a "parasitic leiomyoma". *Am J Surg Pathol* 17: 937-940.

71. Allred DC, Elledge RM (1999). Caution concerning micrometastatic breast carcinoma in sentinel lymph nodes. *Cancer* 86: 905-907.

72. Allred DC, Mohsin SK, Fuqua SA (2001). Histological and biological evolution of human premalignant breast disease. *Endocr Relat Cancer* 8: 47-61.

73. Altaras MM, Jaffe R, Corduba M, Holtzinger M, Bahary C (1990). Primary paraovarian cystadenocarcinoma: clinical and management aspects and literature review. *Gynecol Oncol* 38: 268-272.

74. Alvarado-Cabrero I, Navani SS, Young RH, Scully RE (1997). Tumors of the fimbriated end of the fallopian tube: a clinicopathologic analysis of 20 cases, including nine carcinomas. *Int J Gynecol Pathol* 16: 189-196.

75. Alvarado-Cabrero I, Young RH, Vamvakas EC, Scully RE (1999). Carcinoma of the fallopian tube: a clinicopathological study of 105 cases with observations on staging and prognostic factors. *Gynecol Oncol* 72: 367-379.

76. Alvarez-Fernandez E, Salinero-Paniagua E (1981). Vascular tumors of the mammary gland. A histochemical and ultrastructural study. *Virchows Arch A Pathol Anat Histol* 394: 31-47.

77. Amant F, Moerman P, Davel GH, De Vos R, Vergote I, Lindeque BG, de Jonge E (2001). Uterine carcinosarcoma with melanocytic differentiation. *Int J Gynecol Pathol* 20: 186-190.

78. Ambros RA, Kurman RJ (1992). Combined assessment of vascular and myometrial invasion as a model to predict prognosis in stage I endometrioid adenocarcinoma of the uterine corpus. *Cancer* 69: 1424-1431.

79. Ambros RA, Sherman ME, Zahn CM, Bitterman P, Kurman RJ (1995). Endometrial intraepithelial carcinoma: a distinctive lesion specifically associated with tumors displaying serous differentiation. *Hum Pathol* 26: 1260-1267.

80. American Joint Committee on Cancer (1997). *AJCC Cancer Staging Manual.* 5th ed. Lippincott-Raven: Philadelphia.

81. Amr SS, Elmallah KO (1995). Agressive angiomyxoma of the vagina. *Int J Gynaecol Obstet* 42: 207-210.

82. Anan K, Mitsuyama S, Tamae K, Nishihara K, Iwashita T, Abe Y, Ihara T, Nakahara S, Katsumoto F, Toyoshima S (2001). Pathological features of mucinous carcinoma of the breast are favourable for breast-conserving therapy. *Eur J Surg Oncol* 27: 459-463.

83. Anand S, Penrhyn-Lowe S, Venkitaraman AR (2003). AURORA-A amplification overrides the mitotic spindle assembly checkpoint, inducing resistance to Taxol. *Cancer Cell* 3: 51-62.

84. Anastassiades OT, Bouropoulou V, Kontogeorgos G, Tsakraklides EV (1979). Duct elastosis in infiltrating carcinoma of the breast. *Pathol Res Pract* 165: 411-421.

85. Anbazhagan R, Fujii H, Gabrielson E (1999). Microsatellite instability is uncommon in breast cancer. *Clin Cancer Res* 5: 839-844.

86. Andersen JA (1974). Lobular carcinoma in situ of the breast with ductal involvement. Frequency and possible influence on prognosis. *Acta Pathol Microbiol Scand [A]* 82: 655-662. **87.** Andersen JA (1974). Lobular carcinoma in situ. A histologic study of 52 cases. *Acta Pathol Microbiol Scand [A]* 82: 735-741.

88. Andersen JA (1974). Lobular carcinoma in situ. A long-term follow-up in 52 cases. *Acta Pathol Microbiol Scand [A]* 82: 519-533.

89. Andersen JA, Vendelboe ML (1981). Cytoplasmic mucous globules in lobular carcinoma in situ. Diagnosis and prognosis. *Am J Surg Pathol* 5: 251-255.

90. Anderson B, Turner DA, Benda J (1987). Ovarian sarcoma. *Gynecol Oncol* 26: 183-192.

91. Anderson BO, Petrek JA, Byrd DR, Senie RT, Borgen PI (1996). Pregnancy influences breast cancer stage at diagnosis in women 30 years of age and younger. *Ann Surg Oncol* 3: 204-211.

92. Anderson C, Ricci A Jr., Pedersen CA, Cartun RW (1991). Immunocytochemical analysis of estrogen and progesterone receptors in benign stromal lesions of the breast. Evidence for hormonal etiology in pseudoangiomatous hyperplasia of mammary stroma. *Am J Surg Pathol* 15: 145-149. **92a.** Anderson DE (1971). Some characteristics of familial breast cancer. *Cancer* 28: 1500-1504.

93. Anderson DE (1974). Genetic study of breast cancer: identification of a high risk group. *Cancer* 34: 1090-1097.

94. Anderson DE, Badzioch MD (1992). Breast cancer risks in relatives of male breast cancer patients. *J Natl Cancer Inst* 84: 1114-1117.

95. Anderson DE, Badzioch MD (1993). Familial effects of prostate and other cancers on lifetime breast cancer risk. *Breast Cancer Res Treat* 28: 107-113.

96. Anderson MC, Rees DA (1975). Gynandroblastoma of the ovary. *Br J Obstet Gynaecol* 82: 68-73.

97. Anderson TJ, Lamb J, Donnan P, Alexander FE, Huggins A, Muir BB, Kirkpatrick AE, Chetty U, Hepburn W, Smith A, Prescott RJ, Forrest P. (1991). Comparative pathology of breast cancer in a randomised trial of screening. *Br J Cancer* 64: 108-113.

98. Andrac-Meyer L, Solere K, Sappa P, Garcia S, Charpin C (2000). [Infiltrating syringoadenoma of the nipple: a new case]. *Ann Pathol* 20: 142-144.

99. Andrassy RJ, Wiener ES, Raney RB, Hays DM, Arndt CA, Lobe TE, Lawrence W, Anderson JR, Qualman SJ, Crist WM (1999). Progress in the surgical management of vaginal rhabdomyosarcoma: a 25-year review from the Intergroup Rhabdomyosarcoma Study Group. *J Pediatr Surg* 34: 731-734.

100. Andreasson B, Bock JE, Strom KV, Visfeldt J (1983). Verrucous carcinoma of the vulval region. *Acta Obstet Gynecol Scand* 62: 183-186.

101. Angele S, Lauge A, Fernet M, Moullan N, Beauvais P, Couturier J, Stoppa-Lyonnet D, Hall J (2003). Phenotypic cellular characterization of an ataxia telangiectasia patient carrying a causal homozygous missense mutation. *Hum Mutat* 21: 169-170.

102. Angele S, Treilleux I, Taniere P, Martel-Planche G, Vuillaume M, Bailly C, Bremond A, Montesano R, Hall J (2000). Abnormal expression of the ATM and TP53 genes in sporadic breast carcinomas. *Clin Cancer Res* 6: 3536-3544.

103. Ansah-Boateng Y, Wells M, Poole DR (1985). Coexistent immature teratoma of the uterus and endometrial adenocarcinoma complicated by gliomatosis peritonei. *Gynecol Oncol* 21: 106-110.

104. Anteby EY, Ron M, Revel A, Shimonovitz S, Ariel I, Hurwitz A (1994). Germ cell tumors of the ovary arising after dermoid cyst resection: a long-term follow-up study. *Obstet Gynecol* 83: 605-608.

105. Anthony PP, James PD (1975). Adenoid cystic carcinoma of the breast: prevalence, diagnostic criteria, and histogenesis. *J Clin Pathol* 28: 647-655.

106. Antoniou A, Pharoah PD, Narod S, Risch HA, Eyfjord JE, Hopper JL, Loman N, Olsson H, Johannsson O, Borg A, Pasini B, Radice P, Manoukian S, Eccles DM, Tang N, Olah E, Anton-Culver H, Warner E, Lubinski J, Gronwald J, Gorski B, Tulinius H, Thorlacius S, Eerola H, Nevanlinna H, Syrjakoski K, Kallioniemi OP, Thompson D, Evans C, Peto J, Lalloo F, Evans DG, Easton DF (2003). Average risks of breast and ovarian cancer associated with BRCA1 or BRCA2 mutations detected in case series unselected for family history: a combined analysis of 22 studies. *Am J Hum Genet* 72: 1117-1130.

107. Antoniou AC, Pharoah PD, McMullan G, Day NE, Ponder BA, Easton D (2001). Evidence for further breast cancer susceptibility genes in addition to BRCA1 and BRCA2 in a population-based study. *Genet Epidemiol* 21: 1-18.

108. Anttila T, Saikku P, Koskela P, Bloigu A, Dillner J, Ikaheimo I, Jellum E, Lehtinen M, Lenner P, Hakulinen T, Narvanen A, Pukkala E, Thoresen S, Youngman L, Paavonen J (2001). Serotypes of Chlamydia trachomatis and risk for development of cervical squamous cell carcinoma. *JAMA* 285: 47-51.

109. Anzick SL, Kononen J, Walker RL, Azorsa DO, Tanner MM, Guan XY, Sauter G, Kallioniemi OP, Trent JM, Meltzer PS (1997). AIB1, a steroid receptor coactivator amplified in breast and ovarian cancer. *Science* 277: 965-968.

110. Aoyama C, Peters J, Senadheera S, Liu P, Shimada H (1998). Uterine cervical dysplasia and cancer: identification of c-myc status by quantitative polymerase chain reaction. *Diagn Mol Pathol* 7: 324-330.

111. Aoyama T, Mizuno T, Andoh K, Takagi T, Mizuno T, Eimoto T (1996). alpha-Fetoprotein-producing (hepatoid) carcinoma of the fallopian tube. *Gynecol Oncol* 63: 261-266.

112. Aozasa K, Ito H, Kohro T, Ha K, Nakamura M, Okada A (1981). Chorio-carcinoma in infant and mother. *Acta Pathol Jpn* 31: 317-322.

113. Aozasa K, Ohsawa M, Saeki K, Horiuchi K, Kawano K, Taguchi T (1992). Malignant lymphoma of the breast. Immunologic type and association with lymphocytic mastopathy. *Am J Clin Pathol* 97: 699-704.

114. Aozasa K, Saeki K, Ohsawa M, Horiuchi K, Mishima K, Tsujimoto M (1993). Malignant lymphoma of the uterus. Report of seven cases with immunohistochemical study. *Cancer* 72: 1959-1964.

115. Appleby JM, Barber JB, Levine E, Varley JM, Taylor AM, Stankovic T, Heighway J, Warren C, Scott D (1997). Absence of mutations in the ATM gene in breast cancer patients with severe responses to radiotherapy. *Br J Cancer* 76: 1546-1549.

116. Arbabi L, Warhol MJ (1982). Pleomorphic liposarcoma following radiotherapy for breast carcinoma. *Cancer* 49: 878-880.

117. Arber DA, Simpson JF, Weiss LM, Rappaport H (1994). Non-Hodgkin's lymphoma involving the breast. *Am J Surg Pathol* 18: 288-295.

118. Arias-Stella J Jr., Rosen PP (1988). Hemangiopericytoma of the breast. *Mod Pathol* 1: 98-103.

119. Ariel IM, Kempner R (1989). The prognosis of patients who become pregnant after mastectomy for breast cancer. *Int Surg* 74: 185-187.

120. Ariyoshi K, Kawauchi S, Kaku T, Nakano H, Tsuneyoshi M (2000). Prognostic factors in ovarian carcinosarcoma: a clinicopathological and immunohistochemical analysis of 23 cases. *Histopathology* 37: 427-436.

121. Armes JE, Egan AJ, Southey MC, Dite GS, McCredie MR, Giles GG, Hopper JL, Venter DJ (1998). The histologic phenotypes of breast carcinoma occurring before age 40 years in women with and without BRCA1 or BRCA2 germline mutations: a population-based study. *Cancer* 83: 2335-2345.

122. Aron DC, Marks WM, Alper PR, Karam JH (1980). Pheochromocytoma of the broad ligament. Localization by computerized tomography and ultrasonography. *Arch Intern Med* 140: 550-552.

123. Arora DS, Haldane S (1996). Carcinosarcoma arising in a dermoid cyst of the ovary. *J Clin Pathol* 49: 519-521.

124. Arroyo JG, Harris W, Laden SA (1998). Recurrent mixed germ cell-sex cord-stromal tumor of the ovary in an adult. *Int J Gynecol Pathol* 17: 281-283.

125. Asgeirsson KS, Jonasson JG, Tryggvadottir L, Olafsdottir K, Sigurgeirsdottir JR, Ingvarsson S, Ogmundsdottir HM (2000). Altered expression of E-cadherin in breast cancer: patterns, mechanisms and clinical significance. *Eur J Cancer* 36: 1098-1106.

126. Ashikari R, Huvos AG, Urban JA, Robbins GF (1973). Infiltrating lobular carcinoma of the breast. *Cancer* 31: 110-116.

127. Aslani M, Ahn GH, Scully RE (1988). Serous papillary cystadenoma of borderline malignancy of broad ligament. A report of 25 cases. *Int J Gynecol Pathol* 7: 131-138.

127a. Aslani M, Scully RE (1989). Primary carcinoma of the broad ligament. Report of four cases and review of the literature. *Cancer* 64: 1540-1545.

128. Athale UH, Shurtleff SA, Jenkins JJ, Poquette CA, Tan M, Downing JR, Pappo AS (2001). Use of reverse transcriptase polymerase chain reaction for diagnosis and staging of alveolar rhabdomyosarcoma, Ewing sarcoma family of tumors, and desmoplastic small round cell tumor. *Am J Pediatr Hematol Oncol* 23: 99-104.

129. Athma P, Rappaport R, Swift M (1996). Molecular genotyping shows that ataxia-telangiectasia heterozygotes are predisposed to breast cancer. *Cancer Genet Cytogenet* 92: 130-134.

130. Atkins K, Bell S, Kempson R, Hendrickson M (2001). Epithelioid smooth muscle tumors of the uterus. *Modern Pathol* 14: 132A.

131. Atkins K, Bell S, Kempson R, Hendrickson M (2001). Myxoid smooth muscle tumors of the uterus. *Modern Pathol* 14: 132A.

132. Atlas I, Gajewski W, Falkenberry S, Granai CO, Steinhoff MM (1998). Absence of estrogen and progesterone receptors in glassy cell carcinoma of the cervix. *Obstet Gynecol* 91: 136-138.

133. Atri M, Nazarnia S, Aldis AE, Reinhold C, Bret PM, Kintzen G (1994). Transvaginal US appearance of endometrial abnormalities. *Radiographics* 14: 483-492.

134. Aubele M, Mattis A, Zitzelsberger H, Walch A, Kremer M, Welzl G, Hofler H, Werner M (2000). Extensive ductal carcinoma In situ with small foci of invasive ductal carcinoma: evidence of genetic resemblance by CGH. *Int J Cancer* 85: 82-86.

135. Aubele M, Werner M (1999). Heterogeneity in breast cancer and the problem of relevance of findings. *Anal Cell Pathol* 19: 53-58.

136. Aubele MM, Cummings MC, Mattis AE, Zitzelsberger HF, Walch AK, Kremer M, Hofler H, Werner M (2000). Accumulation of chromosomal imbalances from intraductal proliferative lesions to adjacent in situ and invasive ductal breast cancer. *Diagn Mol Pathol* 9: 14-19.

137. Aure JC, Høeg K, Kolstad P (1971). Clinical and histologic studies of ovarian carcinoma. Long-term follow-up of 990 cases. *Obstet Gynecol* 37: 1-9.

138. Austin RM, Dupree WB (1986). Liposarcoma of the breast: a clinicopathologic study of 20 cases. *Hum Pathol* 17: 906-913.

139. Austin RM, Norris HJ (1987). Malignant Brenner tumor and transitional cell carcinoma of the ovary: a comparison. *Int J Gynecol Pathol* 6: 29-39.

140. Avinoach I, Zirkin HJ, Glezerman M (1989). Proliferating trichilemmal tumor of the vulva. Case report and review of the literature. *Int J Gynecol Pathol* 8: 163-168.

141. Axe S, Parmley T, Woodruff JD, Hlopak B (1986). Adenomas in minor vestibular glands. *Obstet Gynecol* 68: 16-18.

142. Axe SR, Klein VR, Woodruff JD (1985). Choriocarcinoma of the ovary. *Obstet Gynecol* 66: 111-114.

143. Axiotis CA, Lippes HA, Merino MJ, deLanerolle NC, Stewart AF, Kinder B (1987). Corticotroph cell pituitary adenoma within an ovarian teratoma. A new cause of Cushing's syndrome. *Am J Surg Pathol* 11: 218-224.

144. Aziz S, Kuperstein G, Rosen B, Cole D, Nedelcu R, McLaughlin J, Narod SA (2001). A genetic epidemiological study of carcinoma of the fallopian tube. *Gynecol Oncol* 80: 341-345.

145. Azoury RS, Woodruff JD (1971). Primary ovarian sarcomas. Report of 43 cases from the Emil Novak Ovarian Tumor Registry. *Obstet Gynecol* 37: 920-941.

146. Azuma C, Saji F, Tokugawa Y, Kimura T, Nobunaga T, Takemura M, Kameda T, Tanizawa O (1991). Application of gene amplification by polymerase chain reaction to genetic analysis of molar mitochondrial DNA: the detection of anuclear empty ovum as the cause of complete mole. *Gynecol Oncol* 40: 29-33.

147. Azzopardi AG (1979). *Problems in Breast Pathology. Classification of Primary Breast Carcinoma.* AG Azzopardi (Ed.) WB Saunders: Philadelphia.

148. Azzopardi JG (1979). Papilloma and papillary carcinoma. In: *Problems in Breast Pathology.* JG Azzopardi (Ed.) WB Saunders: London, pp. 150-166.

149. Azzopardi JG, Ahmed A, Millis RR (1979). *Problems in Breast Pathology.* AG Azzopardi (Ed.) WB Saunders: London/Philadelphia.

150. Azzopardi JG, Eusebi V (1977). Melanocyte colonization and pigmentation of breast carcinoma. *Histopathology* 1: 21-30.

151. Azzopardi JG, Salm R (1984). Ductal adenoma of the breast: a lesion which can mimic carcinoma. *J Pathol* 144: 15-23.

152. Azzopardi JG, Smith, OD (1959). Salivary gland tumours and their mucins. *J Pathol Bacteriol* 77: 131-140.

153. Baak JP, Nauta JJ, Wisse-Brekelmans EC, Bezemer PD (1988). Architectural and nuclear morphometrical features together are more important prognosticators in endometrial hyperplasias than nuclear morphometrical features alone. *J Pathol* 154: 335-341.

154. Baak JP, Orbo A, van Diest PJ, Jiwa M, de Bruin P, Broeckaert M, Snijders W, Boodt PJ, Fons G, Burger C, Verheijen RH, Houben PW, The HS, Kenemans P (2001). Prospective multicenter evaluation of the morphometric D-score for prediction of the outcome of endometrial hyperplasias. *Am J Surg Pathol* 25: 930-935.

155. Babin EA, Davis JR, Hatch KD, Hallum AV III (2000). Wilms' tumor of the cervix: a case report and review of the literature. *Gynecol Oncol* 76: 107-111.

156. Bacus SS, Zelnick CR, Chin DM, Yarden Y, Kaminsky DB, Bennington J, Wen D, Marcus JN, Page DL (1994). Medullary carcinoma is associated with expression of intercellular adhesion molecule-1. Implication to its morphology and its clinical behavior. *Am J Pathol* 145: 1337-1348.

157. Badve S, Sloane JP (1995). Pseudoangiomatous hyperplasia of male breast. *Histopathology* 26: 463-466.

158. Baekelandt M, Jorunn NA, Kristensen GB, Trope CG, Abeler VM (2000). Carcinoma of the fallopian tube. *Cancer* 89: 2076-2084.

159. Baer R, Ludwig T (2002). The BRCA1/BARD1 heterodimer, a tumor suppressor complex with ubiquitin E3 ligase activity. *Curr Opin Genet Dev* 12: 86-91.

160. Baergen RN, Warren CD, Isacson C, Ellenson LH (2001). Early uterine serous carcinoma: clonal origin of extrauterine disease. *Int J Gynecol Pathol* 20: 214-219.

161. Bagshawe KD, Dent J, Webb J (1986). Hydatidiform mole in England and Wales 1973-83. *Lancet* 2: 673-677.

162. Bagshawe KD, Rawlins G, Pike MC, Lawler SD (1971). ABO blood-groups in trophoblastic neoplasia. *Lancet* 1: 553-556.

163. Bague S, Rodriguez IM, Prat J (2002). Sarcoma-like mural nodules in mucinous cystic tumors of the ovary revisited: a clinicopathologic analysis of 10 additional cases. *Am J Surg Pathol* 26: 1467-1476.

164. Bailey MJ, Royce C, Sloane JP, Ford HT, Powles TJ, Gazet JC (1980). Bilateral carcinoma of the breast. *Br J Surg* 67: 514-516.

165. Baker BA, Frickey L, Yu IT, Hawkins EP, Cushing B, Perlman EJ (1998). DNA content of ovarian immature teratomas and malignant germ cell tumors. *Gynecol Oncol* 71: 14-18.

166. Baker PM, Oliva E, Young RH, Talerman A, Scully RE (2001). Ovarian mucinous carcinoids including some with a carcinomatous component: a report of 17 cases. *Am J Surg Pathol* 25: 557-568.

167. Baker RJ, Hildebrandt RH, Rouse RV, Hendrickson MR, Longacre TA (1999). Inhibin and CD99 (MIC2) expression in uterine stromal neoplasms with sex-cord-like elements. *Hum Pathol* 30: 671-679.

168. Bakri Y, Berkowitz RS, Goldstein DP, Subhi J, Senoussi M, von Sinner W, Jabbar FA (1994). Brain metastases of gestational trophoblastic tumor. *J Reprod Med* 39: 179-184.

169. Balasa RW, Adcock LL, Prem KA, Dehner LP (1977). The Brenner tumor: a clinicopathologic review. *Obstet Gynecol* 50: 120-128.

170. Balat O, Balat A, Verschraegen C, Tornos C, Edwards CL (1996). Sarcoma botryoides of the uterine endocervix: long-term results of conservative surgery. *Eur J Gynaecol Oncol* 17: 335-337.

171. Ball HG, Berman ML (1982). Management of primary vaginal carcinoma. *Gynecol Oncol* 14: 154-163.

172. Ballance WA, Ro JY, el Naggar AK, Grignon DJ, Ayala AG, Romsdahl MG (1990). Pleomorphic adenoma (benign mixed tumor) of the breast. An immunohistochemical, flow cytometric, and ultrastructural study and review of the literature. *Am J Clin Pathol* 93: 795-801.

173. Ballerini P, Recchione C, Cavalleri A, Moneta R, Saccozzi R, Secreto G (1990). Hormones in male breast cancer. *Tumori* 76: 26-28.

174. Balzi D, Buiatti E, Geddes M, Khlat M, Masuyer E, Parkin DM (1993). Summary of the results by site. In: *Cancer in Italian Migrant Populations*, IARC Scientific Publication No 123, International Agency for Research on Cancer: Lyon, pp. 193-292.

175. Bandera CA, Muto MG, Schorge JO, Berkowitz RS, Rubin SC, Mok SC (1998). BRCA1 gene mutations in women with papillary serous carcinoma of the peritoneum. *Obstet Gynecol* 92: 596-600.

176. Bandera CA, Muto MG, Welch WR, Berkowitz RS, Mok SC (1998). Genetic imbalance on chromosome 17 in papillary serous carcinoma of the peritoneum. *Oncogene* 16: 3455-3459.

177. Banik S, Bishop PW, Ormerod LP, O'Brien TE (1986). Sarcoidosis of the breast. *J Clin Pathol* 39: 446-448.

178. Bannatyne P, Russell P (1981). Early adenocarcinoma of the fallopian tubes. A case for multifocal tumorigenesis. *Diagn Gynecol Obstet* 3: 49-60.

179. Bapat B, Xia L, Madlensky L, Mitri A, Tonin P, Narod SA, Gallinger S (1996). The genetic basis of Muir-Torre syndrome includes the hMLH1 locus. *Am J Hum Genet* 59: 736-739.

180. Bapat K, Brustein S (1989). Uterine sarcoma with liposarcomatous differentiation: report of a case and review of the literature. *Int J Gynaecol Obstet* 28: 71-75.

181. Barlund M, Monni O, Kononen J, Cornelison R, Torhorst J, Sauter G, Kallioniemi OLLI, Kallioniemi A (2000). Multiple genes at 17q23 undergo amplification and overexpression in breast cancer. *Cancer Res* 60: 5340-5344.

182. Baron JA (1984). Smoking and estrogen-related disease. *Am J Epidemiol* 119: 9-22.

183. Barrett TL, Smith KJ, Hodge JJ, Butler R, Hall FW, Skelton HG (1997). Immunohistochemical nuclear staining for p53, PCNA, and Ki-67 in different histologic variants of basal cell carcinoma. *J Am Acad Dermatol* 37: 430-437.

184. Barry TS, Schnitt SJ, Ellis I, Eusebi V, Gown AM (1999). Absence of myoepithelium in microglandular adenosis of the breast confirmed with new myoepithelial markers. *Lab Invest* 79: 16A.

185. Barter JF, Smith EB, Szpak CA, Hinshaw W, Clarke-Pearson DL, Creasman WT (1985). Leiomyosarcoma of the uterus: clinicopathologic study of 21 cases. *Gynecol Oncol* 21: 220-227.

186. Barth RJ Jr. (1999). Histologic features predict local recurrence after breast conserving therapy of phyllodes tumors. *Breast Cancer Res Treat* 57: 291-295.

186a. Barth A, Craig PH, Silverstein MJ (1997). Predictors of axillary lymph node metastases in patients with T1 breast carcinoma. *Cancer* 79: 1918-1922.

187. Bartnik J, Powell WS, Moriber-Katz S, Amenta PS (1989). Metaplastic papillary tumor of the fallopian tube. Case report, immunohistochemical features, and review of the literature. *Arch Pathol Lab Med* 113: 545-547.

188. Barwick KW, LiVolsi VA (1979). Heterologous mixed mullerian tumor confined to an endometrial polyp. *Obstet Gynecol* 53: 512-514.

189. Barzilai A, Rotman G, Shiloh Y (2002). ATM deficiency and oxidative stress: a new dimension of defective response to DNA damage. *DNA Repair (Amst)* 1: 3-25.

190. Baschinsky DY, Niemann TH, Eaton LA, Frankel WL (1999). Malignant mixed Mullerian tumor with rhabdoid features: a report of two cases and a review of the literature. *Gynecol Oncol* 73: 145-150.

191. Bassler R, Katzer B (1992). Histopathology of myoepithelial (basocellular) hyperplasias in adenosis and epitheliosis of the breast demonstrated by the reactivity of cytokeratins and S100 protein. An analysis of heterogenic cell proliferations in 90 cases of benign and malignant breast diseases. *Virchows Arch A Pathol Anat Histopathol* 421: 435-442.

192. Bauer RD, McCoy CP, Roberts DK, Fritz G (1984). Malignant melanoma metastatic to the endometrium. *Obstet Gynecol* 63: 264-268.

193. Bayo S, Bosch FX, de Sanjose S, Munoz N, Combita AL, Coursaget P, Diaz M, Dolo A, van den Brule AJ, Meijer CJ (2002). Risk factors of invasive cervical cancer in Mali. *Int J Epidemiol* 31: 202-209.

194. Bebb DG, Yu Z, Chen J, Telatar M, Gelmon K, Phillips N, Gatti RA, Glickman BW (1999). Absence of mutations in the ATM gene in forty-seven cases of sporadic breast cancer. *Br J Cancer* 80: 1979-1981.

195. Becker JL, Papenhausen PR, Widen RH (1997). Cytogenetic, morphologic and oncogene analysis of a cell line derived from a heterologous mixed mullerian tumor of the ovary. *In Vitro Cell Dev Biol Anim* 33: 325-331.

196. Beckmann MW, Niederacher D, Schnurch HG, Gusterson BA, Bender HG (1997). Multistep carcinogenesis of breast cancer and tumour heterogeneity. *J Mol Med* 75: 429-439. **197.** Beerman H, Smit VT, Kluin PM, Bonsing BA, Hermans J, Cornelisse CJ (1991). Flow cytometric analysis of DNA stemline heterogeneity in primary and metastatic breast cancer. *Cytometry* 12: 147-154.

198. Begin LR, Clement PB, Kirk ME, Jothy S, McCaughey WT, Ferenczy A (1985). Aggressive angiomyxoma of pelvic soft parts: a clinicopathologic study of nine cases. *Hum Pathol* 16: 621-628.

199. Beilby JO, Parkinson C (1975). Features of prognostic significance in solid ovarian teratoma. *Cancer* 36: 2147-2154.

200. Bell DA (1991). Mucinous adenofibromas of the ovary. A report of 10 cases. *Am J Surg Pathol* 15: 227-232.

201. Bell DA, Scully RE (1985). Atypical and borderline endometrioid adenofibromas of the ovary. A report of 27 cases. *Am J Surg Pathol* 9: 205-214.

202. Bell DA, Scully RE (1985). Benign and borderline clear cell adenofibromas of the ovary. *Cancer* 56: 2922-2931.

203. Bell DA, Scully RE (1990). Ovarian serous borderline tumors with stromal microinvasion: a report of 21 cases. *Hum Pathol* 21: 397-403.

204. Bell DA, Scully RE (1990). Serous borderline tumors of the peritoneum. *Am J Surg Pathol* 14: 230-239.

205. Bell DA, Scully RE (1994). Early de novo ovarian carcinoma. A study of fourteen cases. *Cancer* 73: 1859-1864.

206. Bell DA, Shimm DS, Gang DL (1985). Wilms' tumor of the endocervix. *Arch Pathol Lab Med* 109: 371-373.

207. Bell DA, Weinstock MA, Scully RE (1988). Peritoneal implants of ovarian serous borderline tumors. Histologic features and prognosis. *Cancer* 62: 2212-2222.

208. Bell DA, Woodruff JM, Scully RE (1984). Ependymoma of the broad ligament. A report of two cases. *Am J Surg Pathol* 8: 203-209.

209. Bell DW, Varley JM, Szydlo TE, Kang DH, Wahrer DC, Shannon KE, Lubratovich M, Verselis SJ, Isselbacher KJ, Fraumeni JF, Birch JM, Li FP, Garber JE, Haber DA (1999). Heterozygous germ line hCHK2 mutations in Li-Fraumeni syndrome. *Science* 286: 2528-2531.

210. Bell KA, Smith Sehdev AE, Kurman RJ (2001). Refined diagnostic criteria for implants associated with ovarian atypical proliferative serous tumors (borderline) and micropapillary serous carcinomas. *Am J Surg Pathol* 25: 419-432.

211. Bell SW, Kempson RL, Hendrickson MR (1994). Problematic uterine smooth muscle neoplasms. A clinicopathologic study of 213 cases. *Am J Surg Pathol* 18: 535-558.

212. Ben David M, Dekel A, Gal R, Dicker D, Feldberg D, Goldman JA (1988). Prolapsed cervical leiomyosarcoma. *Obstet Gynecol Surv* 43: 642-644.

213. Ben David Y, Chetrit A, Hirsh-Yechezkel G, Friedman E, Beck BD, Beller U, Ben Baruch G, Fishman A, Levavi H, Lubin F, Menczer J, Piura B, Struewing JP, Modan B (2002). Effect of BRCA mutations on the length of survival in epithelial ovarian tumors. *J Clin Oncol* 20: 463-466.

214. Ben Ezra J, Sheibani K (1987). Antigenic phenotype of the lymphocytic component of medullary carcinoma of the breast. *Cancer* 59: 2037-2041.

215. Benatar B, Wright C, Freinkel AL, Cooper K (1998). Primary extrarenal Wilms' tumor of the uterus presenting as a cervical polyp. *Int J Gynecol Pathol* 17: 277-280.

216. Benda JA, Platz CE, Anderson B (1986). Malignant melanoma of the vulva: a clinical-pathologic review of 16 cases. *Int J Gynecol Pathol* 5: 202-216.

217. Benedet JL, Bender H, Jones H III, Ngan HY, Pecorelli S (2000). FIGO staging classifications and clinical practice guidelines in the management of gynecologic cancers. FIGO Committee on Gynecologic Oncology. *Int J Gynaecol Obstet* 70: 209-262.

218. Benedet JL, Ehlen TG (2001). *Vulvar Cancer* In: *Prognostic Factors in Cancer.* MK Gospodarowicz, DE Henson, RV Hutter, B O'Sullivan, LH Oblin, CH Wittekink (Eds.) 2nd ed. Willey- Liss: New York, pp. 489-500.

219. Benedet JL, Miller DM, Ehlen TG, Bertrand MA (1997). Basal cell carcinoma of the vulva: clinical features and treatment results in 28 patients. *Obstet Gynecol* 90: 765-768.

220. Benedet JL, Murphy KJ, Fairey RN, Boyes DA (1983). Primary invasive carcinoma of the vagina. *Obstet Gynecol* 62: 715-719.

221. Benedetti-Panici P, Maneschi F, D'Andrea G, Cutillo G, Rabitti C, Congiu M, Coronetta F, Capelli A (2000). Early cervical carcinoma: the natural history of lymph node involvement redefined on the basis of thorough parametrectomy and giant section study. *Cancer* 88: 2267-2274.

222. Bennett HGJ, Ehrlich MM (1941). Myoma of the vagina. *Am J Obstet Gynecol* 42: 314-320.

223. Bentz JS, Yassa N, Clayton F (1998). Pleomorphic lobular carcinoma of the breast: clinicopathologic features of 12 cases. *Mod Pathol* 11: 814-822.

224. Beral V (2002). Breast cancer and breastfeeding: collaborative reanalysis of individual data from 47 epidemiological studies in 30 countries, including 50302 women with breast cancer and 96973 women without the disease. *Lancet* 360: 187-195.

225. Beral V, Banks E, Reeves G, Appleby P (1999). Use of HRT and the subsequent risk of cancer. *J Epidemiol Biostat* 4: 191-210.

226. Beral V, Hermon C, Munoz N, Devesa SS (1994). Cervical cancer. *Cancer surv* 19-20: 265-285.

227. Beral V, Reeves G (1993). Childbearing, oral contraceptive use, and breast cancer. *Lancet* 341: 1102.

228. Berchuck A, Boyd J (1995). Molecular basis of endometrial cancer. *Cancer* 76: 2034-2040.

229. Berchuck A, Heron KA, Carney ME, Lancaster JM, Fraser EG, Vinson VL, Deffenbaugh AM, Miron A, Marks JR, Futreal PA, Frank TS (1998). Frequency of germline and somatic BRCA1 mutations in ovarian cancer. *Clin Cancer Res* 4: 2433-2437.

230. Berchuck A, Kohler MF, Marks JR, Wiseman R, Boyd J, Bast RC Jr. (1994). The p53 tumor suppressor gene frequently is altered in gynecologic cancers. *Am J Obstet Gynecol* 170: 246-252.

231. Berchuck A, Rubin SC, Hoskins WJ, Saigo PE, Pierce VK, Lewis JL Jr. (1988). Treatment of uterine leiomyosarcoma. *Obstet Gynecol* 71: 845-850.

232. Berchuck A, Rubin SC, Hoskins WJ, Saigo PE, Pierce VK, Lewis JL Jr. (1990). Treatment of endometrial stromal tumors. *Gynecol Oncol* 36: 60-65.

233. Berean K, Tron VA, Churg A, Clement PB (1986). Mammary fibroadenoma with multinucleated stromal giant cells. *Am J Surg Pathol* 10: 823-827.

234. Berek J, Adashi PA, Hillart PA (1996). *Novak's Gynaecology.* XII ed. Williams & Wilkins: Baltimore, Maryland.

235. Berends MJ, Hollema H, Wu Y, Van der Sluis T, Mensink RG, ten Hoor KA, Sijmons RH, de Vries EG, Pras E, Mourits MJ, Hofstra RM, Buys CH, Kleibeuker JH, Der Zee AG (2001). MLH1 and MSH2 protein expression as a pre-screening marker in hereditary and non-hereditary endometrial hyperplasia and cancer. *Int J Cancer* 92: 398-403.

236. Berends MJ, Wu Y, Sijmons RH, Mensink RG, Van Der Sluis T, Hordijk-Hos JM, de Vries EG, Hollema H, Karrenbeld A, Buys CH, van der Zee AG, Hofstra RM, Kleibeuker JH (2002). Molecular and clinical characteristics of MSH6 variants: an analysis of 25 index carriers of a germline variant. *Am J Hum Genet* 70: 26-37.

237. Berezowski K, Stastny JF, Kornstein MJ (1996). Cytokeratins 7 and 20 and carcinoembryonic antigen in ovarian and colonic carcinoma. *Mod Pathol* 9: 426-429.

238. Bergeron C, Ferenczy A, Richart RM, Guralnick M (1990). Micropapillomatosis labialis appears unrelated to human papillomavirus. *Obstet Gynecol* 76: 281-286.

239. Bergeron C, Ferenczy A, Shah KV, Naghashfar Z (1987). Multicentric human papillomavirus infections of the female genital tract: correlation of viral types with abnormal mitotic figures, colposcopic presentation, and location. *Obstet Gynecol* 69: 736-742.

240. Bergeron C, Nogales FF, Masseroli M, Abeler V, Duvillard P, Muller-Holzner E, Pickartz H, Wells M (1999). A multicentric European study testing the reproducibility of the WHO classification of endometrial hyperplasia with a proposal of a simplified working classification for biopsy and curettage specimens. *Am J Surg Pathol* 23: 1102-1108.

241. Bergh J, Norberg T, Sjogren S, Lindgren A, Holmberg L (1995). Complete sequencing of the p53 gene provides prognostic information in breast cancer patients, particularly in relation to adjuvant systemic therapy and radiotherapy. *Nat Med* 1: 1029-1034.

241a. Bergstrom A, Pisani P, Tenet V, Wolk A, Adami HO (2001). Overweight as an avoidable cause of cancer in Europe. *Int J Cancer* 91: 421-430.

242. Berkey CS, Frazier AL, Gardner JD, Colditz GA (1999). Adolescence and breast carcinoma risk. *Cancer* 85: 2400-2409.

243. Berkowitz RS, Bernstein MR, Laborde O, Goldstein DP (1994). Subsequent pregnancy experience in patients with gestational trophoblastic disease. New England Trophoblastic Disease Center, 1965-1992. *J Reprod Med* 39: 228-232.

244. Berkowitz RS, Cramer DW, Bernstein MR, Cassells S, Driscoll SG, Goldstein DP (1985). Risk factors for complete molar pregnancy from a case-control study. *Am J Obstet Gynecol* 152: 1016-1020.
245. Berkowitz RS, Ehrmann RL, Knapp RC (1978). Endometrial stromal sarcoma arising from vaginal endometriosis. *Obstet Gynecol* 51: 34s-37s.
246. Berliant II (1970). [Neurofibroma of the broad ligament of the uterus]. *Akush Ginekol* (Mosk) 46: 70-71.
247. Berman ML, Soper JT, Creasman WT, Olt GT, Disaia PJ (1989). Conservative surgical management of superficially invasive stage I vulvar carcinoma. *Gynecol Oncol* 35: 352-357.
248. Bermudez A, Vighi S, Garcia A, Sardi J (2001). Neuroendocrine cervical carcinoma: a diagnostic and therapeutic challenge. *Gynecol Oncol* 82: 32-39.
249. Berns EM, Foekens JA, Vossen R, Look MP, Devilee P, Henzen-Logmans SC, van Staveren IL, van Putten WL, Inganas M, Meijer-van Gelder ME, Cornelisse C, Claassen CJ, Portengen H, Bakker B, Klijn JG (2000). Complete sequencing of TP53 predicts poor response to systemic therapy of advanced breast cancer. *Cancer Res* 60: 2155-2162.
250. Berns EM, Klijn JG, van Putten WL, van Staveren IL, Portengen H, Foekens JA (1992). c-myc amplification is a better prognostic factor than HER2/neu amplification in primary breast cancer. *Cancer Res* 52: 1107-1113.
251. Berns EM, van Staveren IL, Look MP, Smid M, Klijn JG, Foekens JA (1998). Mutations in residues of TP53 that directly contact DNA predict poor outcome in human primary breast cancer. *Br J Cancer* 77: 1130-1136.
252. Bernstein JL, Thompson WD, Risch N, Holford TR (1992). Risk factors predicting the incidence of second primary breast cancer among women diagnosed with a first primary breast cancer. *Am J Epidemiol* 136: 925-936.
253. Bernstein JL, Thompson WD, Risch N, Holford TR (1992). The genetic epidemiology of second primary breast cancer. *Am J Epidemiol* 136: 937-948.
254. Bernstein L, Deapen D, Ross RK (1993). The descriptive epidemiology of malignant cystosarcoma phyllodes tumors of the breast. *Cancer* 71: 3020-3024.
255. Bernstein L, Ross RK (1993). Endogenous hormones and breast cancer risk. *Epidemiol Rev* 15: 48-65.
256. Berrino F, Capocaccia R, Esteve J, Gatta G, Hakulinen T, Micheli A, Sant M, Verdecchia A (1999). *Survival of Cancer patients in Europe: The EUROCARE-2 Study.* IARC Scientific Publication No 151. International Agency for Research on Cancer: Lyon.
257. Bertucci F, Nasser V, Granjeaud S, Eisinger F, Adelaide J, Tagett R, Loriod B, Giaconia A, Benziane A, Devilard E, Jacquemier J, Viens P, Nguyen C, Birnbaum D, Houlgatte R (2002). Gene expression profiles of poor-prognosis primary breast cancer correlate with survival. *Hum Mol Genet* 11: 863-872.
258. Bertwistle D, Swift S, Marston NJ, Jackson LE, Crossland S, Crompton MR, Marshall CJ, Ashworth A (1997). Nuclear location and cell cycle regulation of the BRCA2 protein. *Cancer Res 57*: 5485-5488.
259. Berx G, Becker KF, Hofler H, van Roy F (1998). Mutations of the human E-cadherin (CDH1) gene. *Hum Mutat* 12: 226-237.
260. Berx G, Cleton-Jansen AM, Nollet F, de Leeuw WJ, van de Vijvert M, Cornelisse C, van Roy F (1995). E-cadherin is a tumour/invasion suppressor gene mutated in human lobular breast cancers. *EMBO J* 14: 6107-6115.
261. Berx G, Cleton-Jansen AM, Strumane K, de Leeuw WJ, Nollet F, van Roy F, Cornelisse C (1996). E-cadherin is inactivated in a majority of invasive human lobular breast cancers by truncation mutations throughout its extracellular domain. *Oncogene* 13: 1919-1925.
262. Bethwaite PB, Holloway LJ, Yeong ML, Thornton A (1993). Effect of tumour associated tissue eosinophilia on survival of women with stage IB carcinoma of the uterine cervix. *J Clin Pathol* 46: 1016-1020.
263. Bethwaite PB, Koreth J, Herrington CS, McGee JO (1995). Loss of heterozygosity occurs at the D11S29 locus on chromosome 11q23 in invasive cervical carcinoma. *Br J Cancer* 71: 814-818.
264. Biankin SA, O'Toole VE, Fung C, Russell P (2000). Bizarre leimyoma of the vagina: Report of a case. *Int J Gynecol Pathol* 19: 186-187.
265. Bieche I, Lidereau R (1995). Genetic alterations in breast cancer. *Genes Chromosomes Cancer* 14: 227-251.
266. Bieche I, Lidereau R (1999). Increased level of exon 12 alternatively spliced BRCA2 transcripts in tumor breast tissue compared with normal tissue. *Cancer Res* 59: 2546-2550.
267. Bieche I, Nogues C, Lidereau R (1999). Overexpression of BRCA2 gene in sporadic breast tumours. *Oncogene* 18: 5232-5238.
268. Bienenstock J, Befus AD (1980). Mucosal immunology. *Immunology* 41: 249-270.
269. Biernat W, Jablkowski W (2000). Syringomatous adenoma of the nipple. Pol *J Pathol* 51: 201-202.
270. Bijker N, Peterse JL, Duchateau L, Robanus-Maandag EC, Bosch CA, Duval C, Pilotti S, Van de Vijver MJ (2001). Histological type and marker expression of the primary tumour compared with its local recurrence after breast-conserving therapy for ductal carcinoma in situ. *Br J Cancer* 84: 539-544.
271. Bijker N, Rutgers EJ, Peterse JL, Fentiman IS, Julien JP, Duchateau L, van Dongen JA (2001). Variations in diagnostic and therapeutic procedures in a multicentre, randomized clinical trial (EORTC 10853) investigating breast-conserving treatment for DCIS. *Eur J Surg Oncol* 27: 135-140.
272. Bingham C, Roberts D, Hamilton TC (2001). The role of molecular biology in understanding ovarian cancer initiation and progression. *Int J Gynecol Cancer* 11 Suppl 1: 7-11.
273. Birch JM, Hartley AL, Blair V, Kelsey AM, Harris M, Teare MD, Jones PH (1990). Cancer in the families of children with soft tissue sarcoma. *Cancer* 66: 2239-2248.
274. Birkeland SA, Storm HH, Lamm LU, Barlow L, Blohme I, Forsberg B, Eklund B, Fjeldborg O, Friedberg M, Frodin L, Glattre E, Halvorsen S, Holm NV, Jakobsen A, Jorgensen HE, Ladefoged J, Lindholm T, Lundgren G, Pukkala E. (1995). Cancer risk after renal transplantation in the Nordic countries, 1964-1986. *Int J Cancer* 60: 183-189.
275. Bisceglia M, Attino V, D'Addetta C, Murgo R, Fletcher CD (1996). [Early stage Stewart-Treves syndrome: report of 2 cases and review of the literature]. *Pathologica* 88: 483-490.
276. Bisceglia M, Fusilli S, Zaffarano L, Fiorentino F, Tardio B (1995). [Inflammatory pseudotumor of the breast. Report of a case and review of the literature]. *Pathologica* 87: 59-64.
277. Biscotti CV, Hart WR (1989). Juvenile granulosa cell tumors of the ovary. Arch *Pathol Lab Med* 113: 40-46.
278. Biscotti CV, Hart WR (1992). Peritoneal serous micropapillomatosis of low malignant potential (serous borderline tumors of the peritoneum). A clinicopathologic study of 17 cases. *Am J Surg Pathol* 16: 467-475.
279. Biscotti CV, Hart WR (1998). Apoptotic bodies: a consistent morphologic feature of endocervical adenocarcinoma in situ. *Am J Surg Pathol* 22: 434-439.
280. Bishara M, Scapa E (1997). [Stromal uterine sarcoma arising from intestinal endometriosis after abdominal hysterectomy and salpingo-oophorectomy]. *Harefuah* 133: 353-355.
281. Bishop DT, Hopper J (1997). AT-tributable risks? *Nat Genet* 15: 226.
282. Bitterman P, Chun B, Kurman RJ (1990). The significance of epithelial differentiation in mixed mesodermal tumors of the uterus. A clinicopathologic and immunohistochemical study. *Am J Surg Pathol* 14: 317-328.
283. Bjorkholm E, Silfversward C (1980). Theca-cell tumors. Clinical features and prognosis. *Acta Radiol Oncol* 19: 241-244.
284. Bjorkholm E, Silfversward C (1981). Prognostic factors in granulosa-cell tumors. *Gynecol Oncol* 11: 261-274.
285. Black CL, Morris DM, Goldman LI, McDonald JC (1983). The significance of lymph node involvement in patients with medullary carcinoma of the breast. *Surg Gynecol Obstet* 157: 497-499.
286. Black MM, Barclay TH, Hankey BF (1975). Prognosis in breast cancer utilizing histologic characteristics of the primary tumor. *Cancer* 36: 2048-2055.
287. Blaker H, Graf M, Rieker RJ, Otto HF (1999). Comparison of losses of heterozygosity and replication errors in primary colorectal carcinomas and corresponding liver metastases. *J Pathol* 188: 258-262.
288. Blamey RW (1998). *Clinical aspects of malignant breast lesions In: Systemic Pathology,* CW Elston, IO Ellis (Eds.). 3rd ed. Churchill Livingstone: Edinburgh, pp. 501-513.
289. Bloch T, Roth LM, Stehman FB, Hull MT, Schwenk GR Jr. (1988). Osteosarcoma of the uterine cervix associated with hyperplastic and atypical mesonephric rests. *Cancer* 62: 1594-1600.
290. Block E (1947). Squamous cell carcinoma of the fallopian tube. *Acta Radiol* 28: 49-68.
291. Blom R, Guerrieri C, Stal O, Malmstrom H, Simonsen E (1998). Leiomyosarcoma of the uterus: A clinicopathologic, DNA flow cytometric, p53, and mdm-2 analysis of 49 cases. *Gynecol Oncol* 68: 54-61.
292. Blom R, Malmstrom H, Guerrieri C (1999). Endometrial stromal sarcoma of the uterus: a clinicopathologic, DNA flow cytometric, p53, and mdm-2 analysis of 17 cases. *Int J Gynecol Cancer* 9: 98-104.
293. Bloom HJ, Richardson WW (1957). Histological grading and prognosis in breast cancer. *Br J Cancer* 11: 359-377.
294. Bloom HJ, Richardson WW, Field JR (1970). Host resistance and survival in carcinoma of breast: a study of 104 cases of medullary carcinoma in a series of 1,411 cases of breast cancer followed for 20 years. *Br Med J* 3: 181-188.
295. Boardman CH, Webb MJ, Jefferies JA (2000). Low-grade endometrial stromal sarcoma of the ectocervix after therapy for breast cancer. *Gynecol Oncol* 79: 120-123.
296. Bobrow LG, Richards MA, Happerfield LC, Diss TC, Isaacson PG, Lammie GA, Millis RR (1993). Breast lymphomas: a clinicopathologic review. *Hum Pathol* 24: 274-278.
297. Bochar DA, Wang L, Beniya H, Kinev A, Xue Y, Lane WS, Wang W, Kashanchi F, Shiekhattar R (2000). BRCA1 is associated with a human SWI/SNF-related complex: linking chromatin remodeling to breast cancer. *Cell* 102: 257-265.
298. Bodian CA, Perzin KH, Lattes R (1996). Lobular neoplasia. Long term risk of breast cancer and relation to other factors. *Cancer* 78: 1024-1034.
299. Bodian CA, Perzin KH, Lattes R, Hoffmann P, Abernathy TG (1993). Prognostic significance of benign proliferative breast disease. *Cancer* 71: 3896-3907.
300. Bodner K, Bodner-Adler B, Obermair A, Windbichler G, Petru E, Mayerhofer S, Czerwenka K, Leodolter S, Kainz C, Mayerhofer K (2001). Prognostic parameters in endometrial stromal sarcoma: a clinicopathologic study in 31 patients. *Gynecol Oncol* 81: 160-165.
301. Boecker W, Buerger H, Schmitz K, Ellis IA, van Diest PJ, Sinn H-P, Geradts J, Diallo R, Poremba C, Herbst H (2001). Ductal epithelial proliferations of the breast: a biological continuum? Comparative genomic hybridization an high-molecular-weight cytokeratin expression patterns. *J Pathol* 195: 415-421.
302. Bohm J, Roder-Weber M, Hofler H, Kolben M (1991). Bilateral stromal Leydig cell tumour of the ovary. Case report and literature review. *Pathol Res Pract* 187: 348-352.
303. Boice JD Jr., Engholm G, Kleinerman RA, Blettner M, Stovall M, Lisco H, Moloney WC, Austin DF, Bosch A, Cookfair DL, Krementz ET, Latourettte HB, Merrill JA, Peters LJ, Schultz MD, Strom HH, Bjorkholm E, Pettersson F, Bell CMJ, Coleman MP, Fraser P, Neal FE, Prior P, Choi NW, Hislop TG, Koch M, Kreiger N, Robb D, Robson D, Thomson DH, Lochmuller H, Vonfournier D, Frischkorn R, Kjorstad KE, Rimpela A, Pejovic MH, Kirn VP, Stankusova H, Berrino F, Sigurdsson K, Hutchinson GB, Macmahon B (1988). Radiation dose and second cancer risk in patients treated for cancer of the cervix. *Radiat Res* 116: 3-55.
304. Boice JD Jr., Preston D, Davis FG, Monson RR (1991). Frequent chest X-ray fluoroscopy and breast cancer incidence among tuberculosis patients in Massachusetts. *Radiat Res* 125: 214-222.
305. Boks D.E., Trujillo A.P., Voogd AC, Morreau H, Kenter GG, Vasen HF (2002). Survival analysis of endometrial carcinoma asociated with hereditary nonpolyposis colorectal cancer. *Int J Cancer* 102: 198-200.
306. Boland CR, Thibodeau SN, Hamilton SR, Sidransky D, Eshleman JR, Burt RW, Meltzer SJ, Rodriguez-Bigas MA, Fodde R, Ranzani GN, Srivastava S (1998). A National Cancer Institute Workshop on Microsatellite Instability for cancer detection and familial predisposition: development of international criteria for the determination of microsatellite instability in colorectal cancer. *Cancer Res* 58: 5248-5257.

307. Bolis GB, Maccio T (2000). Clear cell adenocarcinoma of the vulva arising in endometriosis. A case report. *Eur J Gynaecol Oncol* 21: 416-417.
308. Bonfiglio TA, Patten SF Jr., Woodworth FE (1976). Fibroxanthosarcoma of the uterine cervix: cytopathologic and histopathologic manifestations. *Acta Cytol* 20: 501-504.
309. Bonneau D, Longy M (2000). Mutations of the human PTEN gene. *Hum Mutat* 16: 109-122.
310. Bonnet M, Guinebretiere JM, Kremmer E, Grunewald V, Benhamou E, Contesso G, Joab I (1999). Detection of Epstein-Barr virus in invasive breast cancers. *J Natl Cancer Inst* 91: 1376-1381.
311. Bonnier P, Romain S, Dilhuydy JM, Bonichon F, Julien JP, Charpin C, Lejeune C, Martin PM, Piana L (1997). Influence of pregnancy on the outcome of breast cancer: a case-control study. Societe Francaise de Senologie et de Pathologie Mammaire Study Group. *Int J Cancer* 72: 720-727.
312. Bonnier P, Romain S, Giacalone PL, Laffargue F, Martin PM, Piana L (1995). Clinical and biologic prognostic factors in breast cancer diagnosed during postmenopausal hormone replacement therapy. *Obstet Gynecol* 85: 11-17.
313. Bonsing BA, Corver WE, Fleuren GJ, Cleton-Jansen AM, Devilee P, Cornelisse CJ (2000). Allelotype analysis of flow-sorted breast cancer cells demonstrates genetically related diploid and aneuploid subpopulations in primary tumors and lymph node metastases. *Genes Chromosomes Cancer* 28: 173-183.
314. Borazjani G, Prem KA, Okagaki T, Twiggs LB, Adcock LL (1990). Primary malignant melanoma of the vagina: a clinicopathological analysis of 10 cases. *Gynecol Oncol* 37: 264-267.
315. Borgen PI, Senie RT, McKinnon WM, Rosen PP (1997). Carcinoma of the male breast: analysis of prognosis compared with matched female patients. *Ann Surg Oncol* 4: 385-388.
316. Bork P, Hofmann K, Bucher P, Neuwald AF, Altschul SF, Koonin EV (1997). A superfamily of conserved domains in DNA damage-responsive cell cycle checkpoint proteins. *FASEB J* 11: 68-76.
317. Borresen AL, Andersen TI, Eyfjord JE, Cornelis RS, Thorlacius S, Borg A, Johansson U, Theillet C, Scherneck S, Hartman S, Cornelisse CJ, Hovig E, Devilee P (1995). TP53 mutations and breast cancer prognosis: particularly poor survival rates for cases with mutations in the zinc-binding domains. *Genes Chromosomes Cancer* 14: 71-75.
318. Borresen AL, Andersen TI, Tretli S, Heiberg A, Moller P (1990). Breast cancer and other cancers in Norwegian families with ataxia-telangiectasia. *Genes Chromosomes Cancer* 2: 339-340.
319. Borst MJ, Ingold JA (1993). Metastatic patterns of invasive lobular versus invasive ductal carcinoma of the breast. *Surgery* 114: 637-641.
320. Bosch FX, Lorincz A, Munoz N, Meijer CJ, Shah KV (2002). The causal relation between human papillomavirus and cervical cancer. *J Clin Pathol* 55: 244-265.
321. Bose S, Derosa CM, Ozzello L (1999). Immunostaining of type IV collagen and smooth muscle actin as an aid in the diagnosis of breast lesions. *Breast J* 5: 194-201.
322. Bostwick DG, Tazelaar HD, Ballon SC, Hendrickson MR, Kempson RL (1986). Ovarian epithelial tumors of borderline malignancy. A clinical and pathologic study of 109 cases. *Cancer* 58: 2052-2065.
323. Botta G, Fessia L, Ghiringhello B (1982). Juvenile milk protein secreting carcinoma. *Virchows Arch A Pathol Anat Histol* 395: 145-152.
324. Bottles K, Lacey CG, Goldberg J, Lanner-Cusin K, Hom J, Miller TR (1984). Merkel cell carcinoma of the vulva. *Obstet Gynecol* 63: 61S-65S.
325. Boulat J, Mathoulin MP, Vacheret H, Andrac L, Habib MC, Pellissier JF, Piana L, Charpin C (1994). [Granular cell tumors of the breast]. *Ann Pathol* 14: 93-100.
326. Boussen H, Kochbati L, Besbes M, Dhiab T, Makhlouf R, Jerbi G, Gamoudi A, Benna F, Rahal K, Maalej M, Ben Ayed F (2000). [Male secondary breast cancer after treatment for Hodgkin's disease. Case report and review of the literature]. *Cancer Radiother* 4: 465-468.
327. Bouvet M, Ollila DW, Hunt KK, Babiera GV, Spitz FR, Giuliano AE, Strom EA, Ames FC, Ross MI, Singletary SE (1997). Role of conservation therapy for invasive lobular carcinoma of the breast. *Ann Surg Oncol* 4: 650-654.
328. Bower JF, Erickson ER (1967). Bilateral ovarian fibromas in a 5-year-old. *Am J Obstet Gynecol* 99: 880-882.
329. Boyd J, Sonoda Y, Federici MG, Bogomolniy F, Rhei E, Maresco DL, Saigo PE, Almadrones LA, Barakat RR, Brown CL, Chi DS, Curtin JP, Poynor EA, Hoskins WJ (2000). Clinicopathologic features of BRCA-linked and sporadic ovarian cancer. *JAMA* 283: 2260-2265.
330. Boyd J, Takahashi H, Waggoner SE, Jones LA, Hajek RA, Wharton JT, Liu FS, Fujino T, Barrett JC, McLachlan JA (1996). Molecular genetic analysis of clear cell adenocarcinomas of the vagina and cervix associated and unassociated with diethylstilbestrol exposure in utero. *Cancer* 77: 507-513.
331. Boyer CV, Navin JJ (1965). Extraskeletal osteogenic sarcoma. A late complication of radiation therapy. *Cancer* 18: 628-633.
332. Brainard JA, Hart WR (1998). Adenoid basal epitheliomas of the uterine cervix: a reevaluation of distinctive cervical basaloid lesions currently classified as adenoid basal carcinoma and adenoid basal hyperplasia. *Am J Surg Pathol* 22: 965-975.
333. Brand E, Berek JS, Nieberg RK, Hacker NF (1987). Rhabdomyosarcoma of the uterine cervix. Sarcoma botryoides. *Cancer* 60: 1552-1560.
334. Brandfass RJ, Everts-Suarez EA (1955). Lipomatous tumors of the uterus: a review of the world's literature with a case report of true lipoma. *Am J Obstet Gynecol* 70: 359-367.
335. Branton PA, Tavassoli FA (1993). Spindle cell epithelioma, the so-called mixed tumor of the vagina. A clinicopathologic, immunohistochemical, and ultrastructural analysis of 28 cases. *Am J Surg Pathol* 17: 509-515.
336. Bratthauer GL, Lininger RA, Man YG, Tavassoli FA (2002). Androgen and estrogen receptor mRNA status in apocrine carcinomas. *Diagn Mol Pathol* 11: 113-118.
337. Bratthauer GL, Moinfar F, Stamatakos MD, Mezzetti TP, Shekitka KM, Man Y-G, Tavassoli FA (2002). Combined E-cadherin and high molecular weight cytokeratin immunoprofile differentiates lobular, ductal and hybrid mammary intraepithelial neoplasia. *Hum Pathol* 33: 620-627.
338. Bratthauer GL, Tavassoli FA (2002). Lobular neoplasia: previously unexplored aspects assessed in 775 cases and their clinical implications. *Virchows Arch* 440: 134-138.
339. Braun S, Pantel K, Muller P, Janni W, Hepp F, Kentenich CR, Gastroph S, Wischnik A, Dimpfl T, Kindermann G, Riethmuller G, Schlimok G (2000). Cytokeratin-positive cells in the bone marrow and survival of patients with stage I, II, or III breast cancer. *N Engl J Med* 342: 525-533.
340. Breen JL, Neubecker RD (1962). Tumors of the round ligament. A review of the literature and a report of 25 cases. *Obstet Gynecol* 19: 771-780.
341. Brescia RJ, Dubin N, Demopoulos RI (1989). Endometrioid and clear cell carcinoma of the ovary. Factors affecting survival. *Int J Gynecol Pathol* 8: 132-138.
342. Bret AJ, Grepinet J (1967). [Endometrial polyps of the intramural portion of the Fallopian tube. Their relation to sterility and endometriosis]. *Sem Hop* 43: 183-192.
343. Brewer JI, Mazur MT (1981). Gestational choriocarcinoma. Its origin in the placenta during seemingly normal pregnancy. *Am J Surg Pathol* 5: 267-277.
344. Briest S, Horn LC, Haupt R, Schneider JP, Schneider U, Hockel M (1999). Metastasizing signet ring cell carcinoma of the stomach-mimicking bilateral inflammatory breast cancer. *Gynecol Oncol* 74: 491-494.
345. Brinck U, Jakob C, Bau O, Fuzesi L (2000). Papillary squamous cell carcinoma of the uterine cervix: report of three cases and a review of its classification. *Int J Gynecol Pathol* 19: 231-235.
346. Brinkmann U (1998). CAS, the human homologue of the yeast chromosome-segregation gene CSE1, in proliferation, apoptosis, and cancer. *Am J Hum Genet* 62: 509-513.
346 a. Brinton LA, Hoover R, Fraumeni JF Jr. (1982). Interaction of familial and hormonal risk factors for breast cancer. *J Natl Cancer Inst* 69: 817-822.
347. Brinton LA, Nasca PC, Mallin K, Schairer C, Rosenthal J, Rothenberg R, Yordan E Jr., Richart RM (1990). Case-control study of in situ and invasive carcinoma of the vagina. *Gynecol Oncol* 38: 49-54.
348. Brisigotti M, Moreno A, Murcia C, Matias-Guiu X, Prat J (1989). Verrucous carcinoma of the vulva. A clinicopathologic and immunohistochemical study of five cases. *Int J Gynecol Pathol* 8: 1-7.
349. Brocca PP (1866). *Traité des Tumeurs.*
350. Broders AC (2002). Squamous cell epithelioma of the skin. A study of 256 cases. *Ann Surg* 73: 141-160.
351. Broeks A, Urbanus JH, Floore AN, Dahler EC, Klijn JG, Rutgers EJ, Devilee P, Russell NS, van Leeuwen FE, van't Veer LJ (2000). ATM-heterozygous germline mutations contribute to breast cancer-susceptibility. *Am J Hum Genet* 66: 494-500.
352. Brogi E, Harris NL (1999). Lymphomas of the breast: pathology and clinical behavior. *Semin Oncol* 26: 357-364.
353. Bronner CE, Baker SM, Morrison PT, Warren G, Smith LG, Lescoe MK, Kane M, Earabino C, Lipford J, Lindblom A, Tannergard P, Bollag AG, Godwin AR, Ward DC, Nordenskjold M, Fishel R, Kolodner R, Liskay RM. (1994). Mutation in the DNA mismatch repair gene homologue hMLH1 is associated with hereditary non-polyposis colon cancer. *Nature* 368: 258-261.
354. Brooks JJ, LiVolsi VA (1987). Liposarcoma presenting on the vulva. *Am J Obstet Gynecol* 156: 73-75.
355. Brown H, Vlastos G, Newman LA, Benderly M, Singletary E, Sahin A (2000). Histopathological features of bilateral and unilateral breast carcinoma: a comparative study. *Mod Pathol* 13: 18A.
356. Brown MA, Xu CF, Nicolai H, Griffiths B, Chambers JA, Black D, Solomon E (1996). The 5' end of the BRCA1 gene lies within a duplicated region of human chromosome 17q21. *Oncogene* 12: 2507-2513.
357. Brown RS, Marley JL, Cassoni AM (1998). Pseudo-Meigs' syndrome due to broad ligament leiomyoma: a mimic of metastatic ovarian carcinoma. *Clin Oncol* (R Coll Radiol) 10: 198-201.
358. Brown VL, Proby CM, Barnes DM, Kelsell DP (2002). Lack of mutations within ST7 gene in tumour-derived cell lines and primary epithelial tumours. *Br J Cancer* 87: 208-211.
359. Brustein S, Filippa DA, Kimmel M, Lieberman PH, Rosen PP (1987). Malignant lymphoma of the breast. A study of 53 patients. *Ann Surg* 205: 144-150.
360. Bryson SC, Colgan TJ, Vernon CP (1986). Invasive squamous cell carcinoma of the vulva: Delineation of high-risk group requiring adjuvant radiotherapy. *J Reprod Med* 31: 976-978.
361. Buchwalter CL, Jenison EL, Fromm M, Mehta VT, Hart WR (1997). Pure embryonal rhabdomyosarcoma of the fallopian tube. *Gynecol Oncol* 67: 95-101.
362. Buckley CH (2000). Tumours of the cervix - tumours of the female genital tract. In: *Diagnostic Histopathology of Tumours,* CDM Fletcher (Ed.) Churchill Livingstone: London. pp. 685-705.
363. Buckley JD (1984). The epidemiology of molar pregnancy and choriocarcinoma. *Clin Obstet Gynecol* 27: 153-159.
364. Buckshee K, Dhond AJ, Mittal S, Bose S (1990). Pseudo-Meigs' syndrome secondary to broad ligament leiomyoma: a case report. *Asia Oceania J Obstet Gynaecol* 16: 201-205.
365. Buerger H, Mommers EC, Littmann R, Simon R, Diallo R, Poremba C, Dockhorn-Dworniczak B, van Diest PJ, Boecker W (2001). Ductal invasive G2 and G3 carcinomas of the breast are the end stages of at least two different lines of genetic evolution. *J Pathol* 194: 165-170.
366. Buerger H, Otterbach F, Simon R, Poremba C, Diallo R, Decker T, Riethdorf L, Brinkschmidt C, Dockhorn-Dworniczak B, Boecker W (1999). Comparative genomic hybridization of ductal carcinoma in situ of the breast-evidence of multiple genetic pathways. *J Pathol* 187: 396-402.
367. Bullón A, Arseneau J, Prat J, Young RH, Scully RE (1981). Tubular Krukenberg tumor. A problem in histopathologic diagnosis. *Am J Surg Pathol* 5: 225-232.
368. Bundred NJ (2001). Prognostic and predictive factors in breast cancer. *Cancer Treat Rev* 27: 137-142.

369. Bur ME, Zimarowski MJ, Schnitt SJ, Baker S, Lew R (1992). Estrogen receptor immunohistochemistry in carcinoma in situ of the breast. *Cancer* 69: 1174-1181.

370. Burghardt E, Baltzer J, Tulusan AH, Haas J (1992). Results of surgical treatment of 1028 cervical cancers studied with volumetry. *Cancer* 70: 648-655.

371. Burghardt E, Östör AG, Fox H (1997). The new FIGO definition of cervical cancer stage IA: a critique. *Gynecol Oncol* 65: 1-5.

372. Burghardt E, Pickel H, Girardi F (1998). *Colposcopy-Cervical Pathology Textbook and Atlas*. 3rd ed. Thieme: New York.

373. Burke TW, Eifel PJ, McGuire P, et al. (2000). Vulva. In: *Principles and Practice of Gynecologic Oncology*. WJ Hoskins, CA Perez, RC Young (Eds.). 3rd ed. pp. 775-810.Williams & Wilkins: Philadelphia,

374. Burke TW, Stringer CA, Gershenson DM, Edwards CL, Morris M, Wharton JT (1990). Radical wide excision and selective inguinal node dissection for squamous cell carcinoma of the vulva. *Gynecol Oncol* 38: 328-332.

375. Burki N, Buser M, Emmons LR, Gencik A, Haner M, Torhorst JK, Weber W, Muller H (1990). Malignancies in families of women with medullary, tubular and invasive ductal breast cancer. *Eur J Cancer* 26: 295-303.

376. Burks RT, Sherman ME, Kurman RJ (1996). Micropapillary serous carcinoma of the ovary. A distinctive low-grade carcinoma related to serous borderline tumors. *Am J Surg Pathol* 20: 1319-1330.

377. Burns B, Curry RH, Bell ME (1979). Morphologic features of prognostic significance in uterine smooth muscle tumors: a review of eighty-four cases. *Am J Obstet Gynecol* 135: 109-114.

378. Burrell HC, Sibbering DM, Wilson AR (1995). Case report: fibromatosis of the breast in a male patient. *Br J Radiol* 68: 1128-1129.

379. Burt EC, McGown G, Thorncroft M, James LA, Birch JM, Varley JM (1999). Exclusion of the genes CDKN2 and PTEN as causative gene defects in Li-Fraumeni syndrome. *Br J Cancer* 80: 9-10.

380. Burt RL, Prichard RW, Kim BS (1976). Fibroepithelial polyp of the vagina. A report of five cases. *Obstet Gynecol* 47: 52S-54S.

381. Busby JG (1952). Neurofibromatosis of the cervix. *Am J Obstet Gynecol* 63: 674-675.

382. Bussolati G, Gugliotta P, Sapino A, Eusebi V, Lloyd RV (1985). Chromogranin-reactive endocrine cells in argyrophilic carcinomas ("carcinoids") and normal tissue of the breast. *Am J Pathol* 120: 186-192.

383. Butnor KJ, Sporn TA, Hammar SP, Roggli VL (2001). Well-differentiated papillary mesothelioma. *Am J Surg Pathol* 25: 1304-1309.

384. Byrne P, Vella EJ, Rollason T, Frampton J (1989). Ovarian fibromatosis with minor sex cord elements. Case report. *Br J Obstet Gynaecol* 96: 245-248.

385. Byskov AG, Skakkebaek NE, Stafanger G, Peters H (1977). Influence of ovarian surface epithelium and rete ovarii on follicle formation. *J Anat* 123: 77-86.

386. Calabresi E, De Giuli G, Becciolini A, Giannotti P, Lombardi G, Serio M (1976). Plasma estrogens and androgens in male breast cancer. *J Steroid Biochem* 7: 605-609.

387. Calle EE, Murphy TK, Rodriguez C, Thun MJ, Heath CWJ (1998). Occupation and breast cancer mortality in a prospective cohort of US women. *Am J Epidemiol* 148: 191-197.

388. Calle EE, Rodriguez C, Walker-Thurmond K, Thun MJ (2003). Overweight, obesity, and mortality from cancer in a prospectively studied cohort of U.S. adults. *N Engl J Med* 348: 1625-1638.

389. Calonje E, Guerin D, McCormick D, Fletcher CD (1999). Superficial angiomyxoma: clinicopathologic analysis of a series of distinctive but poorly recognized cutaneous tumors with tendency for recurrence. *Am J Surg Pathol* 23: 910-917.

390. Cameron CT, Adair FE (1965). The clinical features and diagnosis of the common breast tumours. *Med J Aust* 2: 651-654.

391. Campello TR, Fittipaldi H, O'Valle F, Carvia RE, Nogales FF (1998). Extrauterine (tubal) placental site nodule. *Histopathology* 32: 562-565.

392. Cancellieri A, Eusebi V, Mambelli V, Ricotti G, Gardini G, Pasquinelli G (1991). Well-differentiated angiosarcoma of the skin following radiotherapy. Report of two cases. *Pathol Res Pract* 187: 301-306.

393. Cangiarella J, Symmans WF, Cohen JM, Goldenberg A, Shapiro RL, Waisman J (1998). Malignant melanoma metastatic to the breast: a report of seven cases diagnosed by fine-needle aspiration cytology. *Cancer* 84: 160-162.

394. Cannistra SA (1993). Cancer of the ovary. *N Engl J Med* 329: 1550-1559.

395. Canola T, Kirkis EJ, Meckes PF, Pitts SB (1994). Interdisciplinary group approach to occupational safety and health administration standard: reductions in cost and duplication of effort. *Am J Infect Control* 22: 182-187.

396. Cantuaria G, Angioli R, Nahmias J, Estape R, Penalver M (1999). Primary malignant melanoma of the uterine cervix: case report and review of the literature. *Gynecol Oncol* 75: 170-174.

397. Capella C, Usellini L, Papotti M, Macri L, Finzi G, Eusebi V, Bussolati G (1990). Ultrastructural features of neuroendocrine differentiated carcinomas of the breast. *Ultrastruct Pathol* 14: 321-334.

398. Cappello F, Barbato F, Tomasino RM (2000). Mature teratoma of the uterine corpus with thyroid differentiation. *Pathol Int* 50: 546-548.

399. Carapeto R, Nogales FF Jr., Matilla A (1978). Ectopic pregnancy coexisting with a primary carcinoma of the Fallopian tube: a case report. *Int J Gynaecol Obstet* 16: 263-264.

400. Carcangiu ML, Chambers JT (1995). Early pathologic stage clear cell carcinoma and uterine papillary serous carcinoma of the endometrium: comparison of clinicopathologic features and survival. *Int J Gynecol Pathol* 14: 30-38.

401. Cardenosa G, Eklund GW (1991). Benign papillary neoplasms of the breast: mammographic findings. *Radiology* 181: 751-755.

402. Carinelli SG, Giudici MN, Brioschi D, Cefis F (1990). Alveolar soft part sarcoma of the vagina. *Tumori* 76: 77-80.

403. Carlson JA, Ambros R, Malfetano J, Ross J, Grabowski R, Lamb P, Figge H, Mihm MC Jr. (1998). Vulvar lichen sclerosus and squamous cell carcinoma: a cohort, case control, and investigational study with historical perspective; implications for chronic inflammation and sclerosis in the development of neoplasia. *Hum Pathol* 29: 932-948.

404. Carlson JA Jr., Wheeler JE (1993). Primary ovarian melanoma arising in a dermoid stage IIIc: long-term disease-free survival with aggressive surgery and platinum therapy. *Gynecol Oncol* 48: 397-401.

405. Carlson JW, McGlennen RC, Gomez R, Longbella C, Carter J, Carson LF (1996). Sebaceous carcinoma of the vulva: a case report and review of the literature. *Gynecol Oncol* 60: 489-491.

406. Carlson RW, Favret AM (1999). Multidisciplinary management of locally advanced breast cancer. *Breast J* 5: 303-307.

407. Carney JA, Young WF Jr. (1992). Primary pigmented nodular adrenocortical disease and its associated conditions. *Endocrinologist* 2: 6-21.

408. Carpenter R, Gibbs N, Matthews J, Cooke T (1987). Importance of cellular DNA content in pre-malignant breast disease and pre-invasive carcinoma of the female breast. *Br J Surg* 74: 905-906.

409. Carstens PH, Greenberg RA, Francis D, Lyon H (1985). Tubular carcinoma of the breast. A long term follow-up. *Histopathology* 9: 271-280.

410. Carstens PH, Huvos AG, Foote FW Jr., Ashikari R (1972). Tubular carcinoma of the breast: a clinicopathologic study of 35 cases. *Am J Clin Pathol* 58: 231-238.

411. Carter BA, Page DL, Schuyler P, Parl FF, Simpson JF, Jensen RA, Dupont WD (2001). No elevation in long-term breast carcinoma risk for women with fibroadenomas that contain atypical hyperplasia. *Cancer* 92: 30-36.

412. Carter CL, Corle DK, Micozzi MS, Schatzkin A, Taylor PR (1988). A prospective study of the development of breast cancer in 16,692 women with benign breast disease. *Am J Epidemiol* 128: 467-477.

412a. Carter CL, Jones DY, Schatzkin A, Brinton LA (1989). A prospective study of reproductive, familial and socioeconomic risk factors for breast cancer using NHANES I data. *Public Health Rep* 104: 45-50.

413. Carter D, Orr SL, Merino MJ (1983). Intracystic papillary carcinoma of the breast. After mastectomy, radiotherapy or excisional biopsy alone. *Cancer* 52: 14-19.

414. Carter D, Pipkin RD, Shepard RH, Elkins RC, Abbey H (1978). Relationship of necrosis and tumor border to lymph node metastases and 10-year survival in carcinoma of the breast. *Am J Surg Pathol* 2: 39-46.

415. Carter J, Elliott P (1990). Syringoma-an unusual cause of pruritus vulvae. *Aust NZ J Obstet Gynaecol* 30: 382-383.

416. Carter J, Elliott P, Russell P (1992). Bilateral fibroepithelial polypi of labium minus with atypical stromal cells. *Pathology* 24: 37-39.

417. Cartier R, Cartier I (1993). Practical Colposcopy. 3rd ed. Laboratoire Cartier: Paris.

418. Casagrande JT, Hanisch R, Pike MC, Ross RK, Brown JB, Henderson BE (1988). A case-control study of male breast cancer. *Cancer Res* 48: 1326-1330.

419. Cashell AW, Cohen ML (1991). Masculinizing sclerosing stromal tumor of the ovary during pregnancy. *Gynecol Oncol* 43: 281-285.

420. Casper GR, Östör AG, Quinn MA (1997). A clinicopathologic study of glandular dysplasia of the cervix. *Gynecol Oncol* 64: 166-170.

421. Cass I, Baldwin RL, Fasylova E, Fields AL, Klinger HP, Runowicz CD, Karlan BY (2001). Allelotype of papillary serous peritoneal carcinomas. *Gynecol Oncol* 82: 69-76.

422. Cass I, Baldwin RL, Varkey T, Moslehi R, Narod SA, Karlan BY (2003). Improved survival in women with BRCA-associated ovarian carcinoma. *Cancer* 97: 2187-2195.

423. Castellsague X, Bosch FX, Munoz N, Meijer CJ, Shah KV, de Sanjose S, Eluf-Neto J, Ngelangel CA, Chichareon S, Smith JS, Herrero R, Moreno V, Franceschi S (2002). Male circumcision, penile human papillomavirus infection, and cervical cancer in female partners. *N Engl J Med* 346: 1105-1112.

424. Castrillon DH, Lee KR, Nucci MR (2002). Distinction between endometrial and endocervical adenocarcinoma: an immunohistochemical study. *Int J Gynecol Pathol* 21: 4-10.

425. Castrillon DH, Sun D, Weremowicz S, Fisher RA, Crum CP, Genest DR (2001). Discrimination of complete hydatidiform mole from its mimics by immunohistochemistry of the paternally imprinted gene product p57KIP2. *Am J Surg Pathol* 25: 1225-1230.

426. Catteau A, Harris WH, Xu CF, Solomon E (1999). Methylation of the BRCA1 promoter region in sporadic breast and ovarian cancer: correlation with disease characteristics. *Oncogene* 18: 1957-1965.

427. Cavalli LR, Rogatto SR, Rainho CA, dos Santos MJ, Cavalli IJ, Grimaldi DM (1995). Cytogenetic report of a male breast cancer. *Cancer Genet Cytogenet* 81: 66-71.

428. Cecalupo AJ, Frankel LS, Sullivan MP (1982). Pelvic and ovarian extramedullary leukemic relapse in young girls: a report of four cases and review of the literature. *Cancer* 50: 587-593.

429. Cerhan JR, Kushi LH, Olson JE, Rich SS, Zheng W, Folsom AR, Sellers TA (2000). Twinship and risk of postmenopausal breast cancer. *J Natl Cancer Inst* 92: 261-265.

430. Chachlani N, Yue CT, Gerardo LT (1997). Granular cell tumor of the breast in a male. A case report. Acta Cytol 41: 1807-1810.

431. Chafe W, Richards A, Morgan L, Wilkinson E (1988). Unrecognized invasive carcinoma in vulvar intraepithelial neoplasia (VIN). *Gynecol Oncol* 31: 154-165.

432. Chalvardjian A, Derzko C (1982). Gynandroblastoma: its ultrastructure. *Cancer* 50: 710-721.

433. Chalvardjian A, Scully RE (1973). Sclerosing stromal tumors of the ovary. *Cancer* 31: 664-670.

434. Chandraratnam E, Leong AS (1983). Papillary serous cystadenoma of borderline malignancy arising in a parovarian paramesonephric cyst. Light microscopic and ultrastructural observations. *Histopathology* 7: 601-611.

435. Chang-Claude J, Eby N, Kiechle M, Bastert G, Becher H (2000). Breastfeeding and breast cancer risk by age 50 among women in Germany. *Cancer Causes Control* 11: 687-695.

436. Chang J, Sharpe JC, A'Hern RP, Fisher C, Blake P, Shepherd J, Gore ME (1995). Carcinosarcoma of the ovary: incidence, prognosis, treatment and survival of patients. *Ann Oncol* 6: 755-758.
437. Chang KL, Crabtree GS, Lim-Tan SK, Kempson RL, Hendrickson MR (1990). Primary uterine endometrial stromal neoplasms. A clinicopathologic study of 117 cases. *Am J Surg Pathol* 14: 415-438.
438. Chang KL, Crabtree GS, Lim-Tan SK, Kempson RL, Hendrickson MR (1993). Primary extrauterine endometrial stromal neoplasms: a clinicopathologic study of 20 cases and a review of the literature. *Int J Gynecol Pathol* 12: 282-296.
439. Chang YC, Hricak H, Thurnher S, Lacey CG (1988). Vagina: evaluation with MR imaging. Part II. Neoplasms. *Radiology* 169: 175-179.
440. Chano T, Kontani K, Teramoto K, Okabe H, Ikegawa S (2002). Truncating mutations of RB1CC1 in human breast cancer. *Nat Genet* 31: 285-288.
441. Chappuis PO, Rosenblatt J, Foulkes WD (1999). The influence of familial and hereditary factors on the prognosis of breast cancer. *Ann Oncol* 10: 1163-1170.
442. Charbonnier F, Olschwang S, Wang Q, Boisson C, Martin C, Buisine MP, Puisieux A, Frebourg T (2002). MSH2 in contrast to MLH1 and MSH6 is frequently inactivated by exonic and promoter rearrangements in hereditary nonpolyposis colorectal cancer. *Cancer Res* 62: 848-853.
443. Charbonnier F, Raux G, Wang Q, Drouot N, Cordier F, Limacher JM, Saurin JC, Puisieux A, Olschwang S, Frebourg T (2000). Detection of exon deletions and duplications of the mismatch repair genes in hereditary nonpolyposis colorectal cancer families using multiplex polymerase chain reaction of short fluorescent fragments. *Cancer Res* 60: 2760-2763.
444. Charpin C, Bonnier P, Garcia S, Andrac L, Crebassa B, Dorel M, Lavaut MN, Allasia C (1999). E-cadherin and beta-catenin expression in breast medullary carcinomas. *Int J Oncol* 15: 285-292.
445. Charpin C, Bonnier P, Khouzami A, Vacheret H, Andrac L, Lavaut MN, Allasia C, Piana L (1992). Inflammatory breast carcinoma: an immunohistochemical study using monoclonal anti-pHER-2/neu, pS2, cathepsin, ER and PR. *Anticancer Res* 12: 591-597.
446. Charpin C, Mathoulin MP, Andrac L, Barberis J, Boulat J, Sarradour B, Bonnier P, Piana L (1994). Reappraisal of breast hamartomas. A morphological study of 41 cases. *Pathol Res Pract* 190: 362-371.
447. Chatterjee A, Pulido HA, Koul S, Beleno N, Perilla A, Posso H, Manusukhani M, Murty VV (2001). Mapping the sites of putative tumor suppressor genes at 6p25 and 6p21.3 in cervical carcinoma: occurrence of allelic deletions in precancerous lesions. *Cancer Res* 61: 2119-2123.
448. Chaudary MA, Millis RR, Hoskins EO, Halder M, Bulbrook RD, Cuzick J, Hayward JL (1984). Bilateral primary breast cancer: a prospective study of disease incidence. *Br J Surg* 71: 711-714.
449. Chehab NH, Malikzay A, Appel M, Halazonetis TD (2000). Chk2/hCds1 functions as a DNA damage checkpoint in G(1) by stabilizing p53. *Genes Dev* 14: 278-288.
450. Chen J, Silver DP, Walpita D, Cantor SB, Gazdar AF, Tomlinson G, Couch FJ, Weber BL, Ashley T, Livingston DM, Scully R (1998). Stable interaction between the products of the BRCA1 and BRCA2 tumor suppressor genes in mitotic and meiotic cells. *Mol Cell* 2: 317-328.
451. Chen KT (1981). Bilateral papillary adenofibroma of the fallopian tube. *Am J Clin Pathol* 75: 229-231.
452. Chen KT (1984). Bilateral malignant Brenner tumor of the ovary. *J Surg Oncol* 26: 194-197.
453. Chen KT (1986). Female genital tract tumors in Peutz-Jeghers syndrome. *Hum Pathol* 17: 858-861.
454. Chen KT (1990). Pleomorphic adenoma of the breast. *Am J Clin Pathol* 93: 792-794.
455. Chen KT (2000). Composite Large-Cell Neuroendocrine Carcinoma and Surface Epithelial-Stromal Neoplasm of the Ovary. *Int J Surg Pathol* 8: 169-174.
456. Chen KT, Hafez GR, Gilbert EF (1980). Myxoid variant of epithelioid smooth muscle tumor. *Am J Clin Pathol* 74: 350-353.
457. Chen KT, Kirkegaard DD, Bocian JJ (1980). Angiosarcoma of the breast. *Cancer* 46: 368-371.
458. Chen KT, Kuo TT, Hoffmann KD (1981). Leiomyosarcoma of the breast: a case of long survival and late hepatic metastasis. *Cancer* 47: 1883-1886.
459. Chen KT, Vergon JM (1981). Carcinomesenchymoma of the uterus. *Am J Clin Pathol* 75: 746-748.
460. Chen T, Sahin A, Aldaz CM (1996). Deletion map of chromosome 16q in ductal carcinoma in situ of the breast: refining a putative tumor suppressor gene region. *Cancer Res* 56: 5605-5609. **461.** Chen YY, Schnitt SJ (1998). Prognostic factors for patients with breast cancers 1cm and smaller. *Breast Cancer Res Treat* 51: 209-225.
462. Chenevix-Trench G, Spurdle AB, Gatei M, Kelly H, Marsh A, Chen X, Donn K, Cummings M, Nyholt D, Jenkins MA, Scott C, Pupo GM, Dork T, Bendix R, Kirk J, Tucker K, McCredie MR, Hopper JL, Sambrook J, Mann GJ, Khanna KK (2002). Dominant negative ATM mutations in breast cancer families. *J Natl Cancer Inst* 94: 205-215.
463. Cheng J, Saku T, Okabe H, Furthmayr H (1992). Basement membranes in adenoid cystic carcinoma. An immunohistochemical study. *Cancer* 69: 2631-2640.
464. Cheng PC, Gosewehr JA, Kim TM, Velicescu M, Wan M, Zheng J, Felix JC, Cofer KF, Luo P, Biela BH, Godorov G, Dubeau L (1996). Potential role of the inactivated X chromosome in ovarian epithelial tumor development. *J Natl Cancer Inst* 88: 510-518.
465. Cheng WF, Lin HH, Chen CK, Chang DY, Huang SC (1995). Leiomyosarcoma of the broad ligament: a case report and literature review. *Gynecol Oncol* 56: 85-89.
466. Chestnut DH, Szpak CA, Fortier KJ, Hammond CB (1988). Uterine hemangioma associated with infertility. *South Med J* 81: 926-928.
467. Chetty R, Govender D (1997). Inflammatory pseudotumor of the breast. *Pathology* 29: 270-271.
468. Chetty R, Kalan MR (1992). Malignant granular cell tumor of the breast. *J Surg Oncol* 49: 135-137.
469. Cheung AN, Shen DH, Khoo US, Wong LC, Ngan HY (1998). p21WAF1/CIP1 expression in gestational trophoblastic disease: correlation with clinicopathological parameters, and Ki67 and p53 gene expression. *J Clin Pathol* 51: 159-162.
470. Cheung AN, So KF, Ngan HY, Wong LC (1994). Primary squamous cell carcinoma of fallopian tube. *Int J Gynecol Pathol* 13: 92-95.
471. Cheung AN, Srivastava G, Chung LP, Ngan HY, Man TK, Liu YT, Chen WZ, Collins RJ, Wong LC, Ma HK (1994). Expression of the p53 gene in trophoblastic cells in hydatidiform moles and normal human placentas. *J Reprod Med* 39: 223-227.
472. Cheung AN, Young RH, Scully RE (1994). Pseudocarcinomatous hyperplasia of the fallopian tube associated with salpingitis. A report of 14 cases. *Am J Surg Pathol* 18: 1125-1130.
473. Chevallier B, Asselain B, Kunlin A, Veyret C, Bastit P, Graic Y (1987). Inflammatory breast cancer. Determination of prognostic factors by univariate and multivariate analysis. *Cancer* 60: 897-902.
474. Chhieng C, Cranor M, Lesser ME, Rosen PP (1998). Metaplastic carcinoma of the breast with osteocartilaginous heterologous elements. *Am J Surg Pathol* 22: 188-194.
475. Chiarle R, Godio L, Fusi D, Soldati T, Palestro G (1997). Pure alveolar rhabdomyosarcoma of the corpus uteri: description of a case with increased serum level of CA-125. *Gynecol Oncol* 66: 320-323.
476. Chiba N, Parvin JD (2001). Redistribution of BRCA1 among four different protein complexes following replication blockage. *J Biol Chem* 276: 38549-38554.
477. Chico A, Garcia JL, Matias-Guiu X, Webb SM, Rodriguez J, Prat J, Calaf J (1995). A gonadotrophin dependent stromal luteoma: a rare cause of post-menopausal virilization. *Clin Endocrinol (Oxf)* 43: 645-649.
478. Cho D, Woodruff JD (1988). Trichoepithelioma of the vulva. A report of two cases. *J Reprod Med* 33: 317-319.
479. Cho SB, Park CM, Park SW, Kim SH, Kim KA, Cha SH, Chung IJ, Kim YW, Yoon YK, Kim JS (2001). Malignant mixed mullerian tumor of the ovary: imaging findings. *Eur Radiol* 11: 1147-1150.
480. Chodosh LA (1998). Expression of BRCA1 and BRCA2 in normal and neoplastic cells. *J Mammary Gland Biol Neoplasia* 3: 389-402.
481. Choi-Hong SR, Genest DR, Crum CP, Berkowitz R, Goldstein DP, Schofield DE (1995). Twin pregnancies with complete hydatidiform mole and coexisting fetus: use of fluorescent in situ hybridization to evaluate placental X- and Y-chromosomal content. *Hum Pathol* 26: 1175-1180.
482. Choi YL, Kim HS, Ahn G (2000). Immunoexpression of inhibin alpha subunit, inhibin/activin betaA subunit and CD99 in ovarian tumors. *Arch Pathol Lab Med* 124: 563-569.
483. Chorlton I, Norris HJ, King FM (1974). Malignant reticuloendothelial disease involving the ovary as a primary manifestation: a series of 19 lymphomas and 1 granulocytic sarcoma. *Cancer* 34: 397-407.
484. Christman JE, Ballon SC (1990). Ovarian fibrosarcoma associated with Maffucci's syndrome. *Gynecol Oncol* 37: 290-291.
485. Chu KC, Tarone RE, Kessler LG, Ries LA, Hankey BF, Miller BA, Edwards BK (1996). Recent trends in U.S. breast cancer incidence, survival, and mortality rates. *J Natl Cancer Inst* 88: 1571-1579.
486. Chu PG, Arber DA, Weiss LM, Chang KL (2001). Utility of CD10 in distinguishing between endometrial stromal sarcoma and uterine smooth muscle tumors: an immunohistochemical comparison of 34 cases. *Mod Pathol* 14: 465-471.
487. Chua CL, Thomas A, Ng BK (1988). Cystosarcoma phyllodes--Asian variations. *Aust N Z J Surg* 58: 301-305.
488. Chuang SS, Lin CN, Li CY, Wu CH (2001). Uterine leiomyoma with massive lymphocytic infiltration simulating malignant lymphoma. A case report with immunohistochemical study showing that the infiltrating lymphocytes are cytotoxic T cells. *Pathol Res Pract* 197: 135-138.
489. Chuaqui R, Silva M, Emmert-Buck M (2001). Allelic deletion mapping on chromosome 6q and X chromosome inactivation clonality patterns in cervical intraepithelial neoplasia and invasive carcinoma. *Gynecol Oncol* 80: 364-371.
490. Chuaqui RF, Sanz-Ortega J, Vocke C, Linehan WM, Sanz-Esponera J, Zhuang Z, Emmert-Buck MR, Merino MJ (1995). Loss of heterozygosity on the short arm of chromosome 8 in male breast carcinomas. *Cancer Res* 55: 4995-4998.
491. Chumas JC, Scully RE (1991). Sebaceous tumors arising in ovarian dermoid cysts. *Int J Gynecol Pathol* 10: 356-363.
492. Chung AF, Casey MJ, Flannery JT, Woodruff JM, Lewis JL Jr. (1980). Malignant melanoma of the vagina--report of 19 cases. *Obstet Gynecol* 55: 720-727.
493. Churg A, Colby TV, Cagle P, Corson J, Gibbs AR, Gilks B, Grimes M, Hammar S, Roggli V, Travis WD (2000). The separation of benign and malignant mesothelial proliferations. *Am J Surg Pathol* 24: 1183-1200.
494. Ciano PS, Antonioli DA, Critchlow J, Burke L, Goldman H (1987). Villous adenoma presenting as a vaginal polyp in a rectovaginal tract. *Hum Pathol* 18: 863-866.
495. Cina SJ, Richardson MS, Austin RM, Kurman RJ (1997). Immunohistochemical staining for Ki-67 antigen, carcinoembryonic antigen, and p53 in the differential diagnosis of glandular lesions of the cervix. *Mod Pathol* 10: 176-180.
496. Cinel L, Taner D, Nabaei SM, Dogan M (2000). Aggressive angiomyxoma of the vagina. Report of a distinctive type gynecologic soft tissue neoplasm. *Acta Obstet Gynecol Scand* 79: 232-233.
497. Cirisano FD Jr., Robboy SJ, Dodge RK, Bentley RC, Krigman HR, Synan IS, Soper JT, Clarke-Pearson DL (2000). The outcome of stage I-II clinically and surgically staged papillary serous and clear cell endometrial cancers when compared with endometrioid carcinoma. *Gynecol Oncol* 77: 55-65.
498. Clark WH Jr., Hood AF, Tucker MA, Jampel RM (1998). Atypical melanocytic nevi of the genital type with a discussion of reciprocal parenchymal-stromal interactions in the biology of neoplasia. *Hum Pathol* 29: S1-24.
499. Claus EB, Risch N, Thompson WD (1994). Autosomal dominant inheritance of early-onset breast cancer. Implications for risk prediction. *Cancer* 73: 643-651.
500. Claus EB, Risch N, Thompson WD, Carter D (1993). Relationship between breast histopathology and family history of breast cancer. *Cancer* 71: 147-153.

501. Claus EB, Risch NJ, Thompson WD (1990). Age at onset as an indicator of familial risk of breast cancer. *Am J Epidemiol* 131: 961-972.
502. Clayton F (1986). Pure mucinous carcinomas of breast: morphologic features and prognostic correlates. *Hum Pathol* 17: 34-38.
503. Clayton F, Bodian CA, Banogon P, Goetz H, Kancherla P, Lazarovic B. (1992). Reproducibility of diagnosis in noninvasive breast disease. *Lab Invest* 66: 12A.
504. Clement PB (1988). Postoperative spindle-cell nodule of the endometrium. *Arch Pathol Lab Med* 112: 566-568.
505. Clement PB (1993). Tumor-like lesions of the ovary associated with pregnancy. *Int J Gynecol Pathol* 12: 108-115.
506. Clement PB (1994). Diseases of the peritoneum (including endometriosis). In: *Blaustein's Pathology of the Female Genital Tract*, RJ Kurman (Ed.) 4th ed. Springer-Verlag: New York. pp. 647-703.
507. Clement PB, Azzopardi JG (1983). Microglandular adenosis of the breast--a lesion simulating tubular carcinoma. *Histopathology* 7: 169-180.
508. Clement PB, Dimmick JE (1979). Endodermal variant of mature cystic teratoma of the ovary: report of a case. *Cancer* 43: 383-385.
509. Clement PB, Oliva E, Young RH (1996). Mullerian adenosarcoma of the uterine corpus associated with tamoxifen therapy: a report of six cases and a review of tamoxifen-associated endometrial lesions. *Int J Gynecol Pathol* 15: 222-229.
510. Clement PB, Scully RE (1974). Mullerian adenosarcoma of the uterus. A clinicopathologic analysis of ten cases of a distinctive type of mullerian mixed tumor. *Cancer* 34: 1138-1149.
511. Clement PB, Scully RE (1976). Uterine tumors resembling ovarian sex-cord tumors. A clinicopathologic analysis of fourteen cases. *Am J Clin Pathol* 66: 512-525.
512. Clement PB, Scully RE (1978). Extrauterine mesodermal (mullerian) adenosarcoma: a clinicopathologic analysis of five cases. *Am J Clin Pathol* 69: 276-283.
513. Clement PB, Scully RE (1980). Large solitary luteinized follicle cyst of pregnancy and puerperium: A clinicopathological analysis of eight cases. *Am J Surg Pathol* 4: 431-438.
514. Clement PB, Scully RE (1990). Mullerian adenofibroma of the uterus with invasion of myometrium and pelvic veins. *Int J Gynecol Pathol* 9: 363-371.
515. Clement PB, Scully RE (1990). Mullerian adenosarcoma of the uterus: a clinicopathologic analysis of 100 cases with a review of the literature. *Hum Pathol* 21: 363-381.
516. Clement PB, Scully RE (1992). Endometrial stromal sarcomas of the uterus with extensive endometrioid glandular differentiation: a report of three cases that caused problems in differential diagnosis. *Int J Gynecol Pathol* 11: 163-173.
517. Clement PB, Young RH (1987). Atypical polypoid adenomyoma of the uterus associated with Turner's syndrome. A report of three cases, including a review of "estrogen-associated" endometrial neoplasms and neoplasms associated with Turner's syndrome. *Int J Gynecol Pathol* 6: 104-113.
518. Clement PB, Young RH (1987). Diffuse leiomyomatosis of the uterus: a report of four cases. *Int J Gynecol Pathol* 6: 322-330.
518 a. Clement PB, Young RH (1999). Florid cystic endosalpingiosis with tumor-like manifestations: a report of four cases including the first reported cases of transmural endosalpingiosis of the uterus. *Am J Surg Pathol* 23: 166-175.
519. Clement PB, Young RH, Azzopardi JG (1987). Collagenous spherulosis of the breast. *Am J Surg Pathol* 11: 411-417.
520. Clement PB, Young RH, Hanna W, Scully RE (1994). Sclerosing peritonitis associated with luteinized thecomas of the ovary. A clinicopathological analysis of six cases. *Am J Surg Pathol* 18: 1-13.
521. Clement PB, Young RH, Keh P, Östör AG, Scully RE (1995). Malignant mesonephric neoplasms of the uterine cervix. A report of eight cases, including four with a malignant spindle cell component. *Am J Surg Pathol* 19: 1158-1171.
522. Clement PB, Young RH, Scully RE (1987). Endometrioid-like variant of ovarian yolk sac tumor. A clinicopathological analysis of eight cases. *Am J Surg Pathol* 11: 767-778.
523. Clement PB, Young RH, Scully RE (1988). Intravenous leiomyomatosis of the uterus. A clinicopathological analysis of 16 cases with unusual histologic features. *Am J Surg Pathol* 12: 932-945.
524. Clement PB, Young RH, Scully RE (1988). Ovarian granulosa cell proliferations of pregnancy: a report of nine cases. *Hum Pathol* 19: 657-662.
525. Clement PB, Young RH, Scully RE (1992). Diffuse, perinodular, and other patterns of hydropic degeneration within and adjacent to uterine leiomyomas. Problems in differential diagnosis. *Am J Surg Pathol* 16: 26-32.
526. Clement PB, Young RH, Scully RE (1996). Malignant mesotheliomas presenting as ovarian masses. A report of nine cases, including two primary ovarian mesotheliomas. *Am J Surg Pathol* 20: 1067-1080.
527. Clement PB, Zubovits JT, Young RH, Scully RE (1998). Malignant mullerian mixed tumors of the uterine cervix: a report of nine cases of a neoplasm with morphology often different from its counterpart in the corpus. *Int J Gynecol Pathol* 17: 211-222.
528. Clifford GM, Smith JS, Plummer M, Munoz N, Franceschi S (2003). Human papillomavirus types in invasive cervical cancer worldwide: a meta-analysis. *Br J Cancer* 88: 63-73.
529. Cobleigh MA, Vogel CL, Tripathy D, Robert NJ, Scholl S, Fehrenbacher L, Wolter JM, Paton V, Shak S, Lieberman G, Slamon DJ (1999). Multinational study of the efficacy and safety of humanized anti-HER2 monoclonal antibody in women who have HER2-overexpressing metastatic breast cancer that has progressed after chemotherapy for metastatic disease. *J Clin Oncol* 17: 2639-2648.
530. Cohen C, Guarner J, DeRose PB (1993). Mammary Paget's disease and associated carcinoma. An immunohistochemical study. *Arch Pathol Lab Med* 117: 291-294.
531. Cohen I, Altaras MM, Shapira J, Tepper R, Rosen DJ, Cordoba M, Zalel Y, Figer A, Yigael D, Beyth Y (1996). Time-dependent effect of tamoxifen therapy on endometrial pathology in asymptomatic postmenopausal breast cancer patients. *Int J Gynecol Pathol* 15: 152-157.
532. Cohen MA, Morris EA, Rosen PP, Dershaw DD, Liberman L, Abramson AF (1996). Pseudoangiomatous stromal hyperplasia: mammographic, sonographic, and clinical patterns. *Radiology* 198: 117-120.
533. Cohen MB, Mulchahey KM, Molnar JJ (1986). Ovarian endodermal sinus tumor with intestinal differentiation. *Cancer* 57: 1580-1583.
534. Cohen PL, Brooks JJ (1991). Lymphomas of the breast. A clinicopathologic and immunohistochemical study of primary and secondary cases. *Cancer* 67: 1359-1369.
535. Cohen PR, Kohn SR, Kurzrock R (1991). Association of sebaceous gland tumors and internal malignancy: the Muir-Torre syndrome. *Am J Med* 90: 606-613.
536. Cohn-Cedermark G, Rutqvist LE, Rosendahl I, Silfversward C (1991). Prognostic factors in cystosarcoma phyllodes. A clinicopathologic study of 77 patients. *Cancer* 68: 2017-2022.
537. Cokelaere K, Michielsen P, De Vos R, Sciot R (2001). Primary mesenteric malignant mixed mesodermal (mullerian) tumor with neuroendocrine differentiation. *Mod Pathol* 14: 515-520.
538. Colgan TJ (1998). Vulvar intraepithelial neoplasia: a synopsis of recent developments. *J Lower Genital Tract Disease* 2: 31-36.
539. Collaborative Group on Hormonal Factors in Breast Cancer (1996). Breast cancer and hormonal contraceptives: collaborative reanalysis of individual data on 53 297 women with breast cancer and 100 239 women without breast cancer from 54 epidemiological studies. *Lancet* 347: 1713-1727.
540. Collaborative Group on Hormonal Factors in Breast Cancer (1997). Breast cancer and hormone replacement therapy: collaborative reanalysis of data from 51 epidemiological studies of 52,705 women with breast cancer and 108,411 women without breast cancer. *Lancet* 350: 1047-1059.
541. Collins N, Wooster R, Stratton MR (1997). Absence of methylation of CpG dinucleotides within the promoter of the breast cancer susceptibility gene BRCA2 in normal tissues and in breast and ovarian cancers. *Br J Cancer* 76: 1150-1156.
542. Collins RJ, Cheung A, Ngan HY, Wong LC, Chan SY, Ma HK (1991). Primary mixed neuroendocrine and mucinous carcinoma of the ovary. *Arch Gynecol Obstet* 248: 139-143.
543. Colombat M, Sevestre H, Gontier MF (2001). Epithelioid leiomyosarcoma of the uterine cervix. Report of a case. *Ann Pathol* 21: 48-50.
544. Colome MI, Ro JY, Ayala AG, El-Nagger A, Siddiqui RT, Ordonez NG (1996). Adenoid cystic carcinoma of the breast metastatic tio the kidney. *J Pathol Bacteriol* 4: 69-78.
545. Colpaert C, Vermeulen P, Jeuris W, van Beest P, Goovaerts G, Weyler J, Van Dam P, Dirix L, Van Marck E (2001). Early distant relapse in "node-negative" breast cancer patients is not predicted by occult axillary lymph node metastases, but by the features of the primary tumour. *J Pathol* 193: 442-449.
546. Comerci JT Jr., Licciardi F, Bergh PA, Gregori C, Breen JL (1994). Mature cystic teratoma: a clinicopathologic evaluation of 517 cases and review of the literature. *Obstet Gynecol* 84: 22-28.
547. Conant EF, Dillon RL, Palazzo J, Ehrlich SM, Feig SA (1994). Imaging findings in mucin-containing carcinomas of the breast: correlation with pathologic features. *AJR Am J Roentgenol* 163: 821-824.
548. Connolly DC, Katabuchi H, Cliby WA, Cho KR (2000). Somatic mutations in the STK11/LKB1 gene are uncommon in rare gynecological tumor types associated with Peutz-Jegher's syndrome. *Am J Pathol* 156: 339-345.
549. Conran RM, Hitchcock CL, Popek EJ, Norris HJ, Griffin JL, Geissel A, McCarthy WF (1993). Diagnostic considerations in molar gestations. *Hum Pathol* 24: 41-48.
550. Contesso G, Mouriesse H, Friedman S, Genin J, Sarrazin D, Rouesse J (1987). The importance of histologic grade in long-term prognosis of breast cancer: a study of 1,010 patients, uniformly treated at the Institut Gustave-Roussy. *J Clin Oncol* 5: 1378-1386.
551. Cook DL, Weaver DL (1995). Comparison of DNA content, S-phase fraction, and survival between medullary and ductal carcinoma of the breast. *Am J Clin Pathol* 104: 17-22.
552. Cooper HS, Patchefsky AS, Krall RA (1978). Tubular carcinoma of the breast. *Cancer* 42: 2334-2342.
553. Copas P, Dyer M, Hall DJ, Diddle AW (1981). Granular cell myoblastoma of the uterine cervix. *Diagn Gynecol Obstet* 3: 251-254.
554. Copeland LJ, Cleary K, Sneige N, Edwards CL (1985). Neuroendocrine (Merkel cell) carcinoma of the vulva: a case report and review of the literature. *Gynecol Oncol* 22: 367-378.
555. Copeland LJ, Gershenson DM, Saul PB, Sneige N, Stringer CA, Edwards CL (1985). Sarcoma botryoides of the female genital tract. *Obstet Gynecol* 66: 262-266.
556. Copeland LJ, Sneige N, Gershenson DM, Saul PB, Stringer CA, Seski JC (1986). Adenoid cystic carcinoma of Bartholin gland. *Obstet Gynecol* 67: 115-120.
557. Copeland LJ, Sneige N, Ordonez NG, Hancock KC, Gershenson DM, Saul PB, Kavanagh JJ (1985). Endodermal sinus tumor of the vagina and cervix. *Cancer* 55: 2558-2565.
558. Copeland LJ, Sneige N, Stringer CA, Gershenson DM, Saul PB, Kavanagh JJ (1985). Alveolar rhabdomyosarcoma of the female genitalia. *Cancer* 56: 849-855.
559. Cornelis RS, Devilee P, van Vliet M, Kuipers-Dijkshoorn N, Kersenmaeker A, Bardoel A, Khan PM, Cornelisse CJ (1993). Allele loss patterns on chromosome 17q in 109 breast carcinomas indicate at least two distinct target regions. *Oncogene* 8: 781-785.
560. Cornelis RS, Neuhausen SL, Johansson O, Arason A, Kelsell D, Ponder BA, Tonin P, Hamann U, Lindblom A, Lalle P, Longy M, Olah E, Scherneck S, Bignon YJ, Sobol H, Changclaude J, Larsson C, Spurr N, Borg A, Barkardottir RB, Narod S, Devilee P. (1995). High allele loss rates at 17q12-q21 in breast and ovarian tumors from BRCAl-linked families. The Breast Cancer Linkage Consortium. *Genes Chromosomes Cancer* 13: 203-210.
561. Costa A (1974). [A little known variant of pure adenoma of the breast: pure apocrine cell adenoma (with a classification of breast adenomas)]. *Arch De Vecchi Anat Patol* 60: 393-401.

562. Costa MJ, Ames PF, Walls J, Roth LM (1997). Inhibin immunohistochemistry applied to ovarian neoplasms: a novel, effective, diagnostic tool. *Hum Pathol* 28: 1247-1254.

563. Costa MJ, DeRose PB, Roth LM, Brescia RJ, Zaloudek CJ, Cohen C (1994). Immunohistochemical phenotype of ovarian granulosa cell tumors: absence of epithelial membrane antigen has diagnostic value. *Hum Pathol* 25: 60-66.

564. Costa MJ, Hansen C, Dickerman A, Scudder SA (1998). Clinicopathologic significance of transitional cell carcinoma pattern in nonlocalized ovarian epithelial tumors (stages 2-4). *Am J Clin Pathol* 109: 173-180.

565. Costa MJ, McIlnay KR, Trelford J (1995). Cervical carcinoma with glandular differentiation: histological evaluation predicts disease recurrence in clinical stage I or II patients. *Hum Pathol* 26: 829-837.

566. Costa MJ, Silverberg SG (1989). Oncocytic carcinoma of the male breast. *Arch Pathol Lab Med* 113: 1396-1399.

567. Costa MJ, Thomas W, Majmudar B, Hewan-Lowe K (1992). Ovarian myxoma: ultrastructural and immunohistochemical findings. *Ultrastruct Pathol* 16: 429-438.

568. Coukos G, Makrigiannakis A, Chung J, Randall TC, Rubin SC, Benjamin I (1999). Complete hydatidiform mole. A disease with a changing profile. *J Reprod Med* 44: 698-704.

569. Coyne J.D. (2001). Apocrine ductal carcinoma in-situ with an unusual morphological presentation. *Histopathology* 38: 277-280.

570. Cozen W, Bernstein L, Wang F, Press MF, Mack TM (1999). The risk of angiosarcoma following primary breast cancer. *Br J Cancer* 81: 532-536.

571. Craig JR, Hart WR (1979). Extragenital adenomatoid tumor: Evidence for the mesothelial theory of origin. *Cancer* 43: 1678-1681.

572. Cramer SF, Roth LM, Ulbright TM, Mazur MT, Nunez CA, Gersell DJ, Mills SE, Kraus FT (1987). Evaluation of the reproducibility of the World Health Organization classification of common ovarian cancers. With emphasis on methodology. *Arch Pathol Lab Med* 111: 819-829.

573. Crawford D, Nimmo M, Clement PB, Thomson T, Benedet JL, Miller D, Gilks CB (1999). Prognostic factors in Paget's disease of the vulva: a study of 21 cases. *Int J Gynecol Pathol* 18: 351-359.

574. Creasman W, Ondicino F, Maisonneuve P, Benefet J, Shepherd J (1998). Carcinoma of the corpus uteri: Annual report on the results of treatment in gynaecological cancer. *J Epidemiol Biostat* 3: 46-47.

575. Creasman WT (1993). Prognostic significance of hormone receptors in endometrial cancer. *Cancer* 71: 1467-1470.

576. Creasman WT, Odicino F, Maisonneuve P, Beller U, Benedet JL, Heintz AP, Ngan HY, Sideri M, Pecorelli S (2001). Carcinoma of the corpus uteri. *J Epidemiol Biostat* 6: 47-86.

577. Creasman WT, Phillips JL, Menck HR (1998). The National Cancer Data Base report on cancer of the vagina. *Cancer* 83: 1033-1040.

578. Crichlow RW, Galt SW (1990). Male breast cancer. *Surg Clin North Am* 70: 1165-1177.

579. Crissman JD, Visscher DW, Kubus J (1990). Image cytophotometric DNA analysis of atypical hyperplasias and intraductal carcinomas of the breast. *Arch Pathol Lab Med* 114: 1249-1253.

580. Crook T, Brooks LA, Crossland S, Osin P, Barker KT, Waller J, Philp E, Smith PD, Yulug I, Peto J, Parker G, Allday MJ, Crompton MR, Gusterson BA (1998). p53 mutation with frequent novel condons but not a mutator phenotype in B. *Oncogene* 17: 1681-1689.

581. Crook T, Crossland S, Crompton MR, Osin P, Gusterson BA (1997). p53 mutations in BRCA1-associated familial breast cancer. *Lancet* 350: 638-639.

582. Crowe J, Hakes T, Rosen PP, Rosen PP, Kinne DW, Robbins GF. (1985). Changing trends in the management of inflammatory breast cancer: a clinical-pathological review of 69 patients. *Am J Clin Oncol* 8: 21.

583. Crozier MA, Copeland LJ, Silva EG, Gershenson DM, Stringer CA (1989). Clear cell carcinoma of the ovary: a study of 59 cases. *Gynecol Oncol* 35: 199-203.

584. Crum CP (1992). Carcinoma of the vulva: epidemiology and pathogenesis. *Obstet Gynecol* 79: 448-454.

585. Crum CP, Fu YS, Levine RU, Richart RM, Townsend DE, Fenoglio CM (1982). Intraepithelial squamous lesions of the vulva: biologic and histologic criteria for the distinction of condylomas from vulvar intraepithelial neoplasia. *Am J Obstet Gynecol* 144: 77-83.

586. Crum CP, Ikenberg H, Richart RM, Gissman L (1984). Human papillomavirus type 16 and early cervical neoplasia. *N Engl J Med* 310: 880-883.

587. Crum CP, Mitao M, Levine RU, Silverstein S (1985). Cervical papillomaviruses segregate within morphologically distinct precancerous lesions. *J Virol* 54: 675-681.

588. Crum CP, Rogers BH, Andersen W (1980). Osteosarcoma of the uterus: case report and review of the literature. *Gynecol Oncol* 9: 256-268.

589. Cuatrecasas M, Erill N, Musulen E, Costa I, Matias-Guiu X, Prat J (1998). K-ras mutations in nonmucinous ovarian epithelial tumors: a molecular analysis and clinicopathologic study of 144 patients. *Cancer* 82: 1088-1095.

590. Cuatrecasas M, Matias-Guiu X, Prat J (1996). Synchronous mucinous tumors of the appendix and the ovary associated with pseudomyxoma peritonei. A clinicopathologic study of six cases with comparative analysis of c-Ki-ras mutations. *Am J Surg Pathol* 20: 739-746.

591. Cuatrecasas M, Villanueva A, Matias-Guiu X, Prat J (1997). K-ras mutations in mucinous ovarian tumors: a clinicopathologic and molecular study of 95 cases. *Cancer* 79: 1581-1586.

592. Cui J, Antoniou AC, Dite GS, Southey MC, Venter DJ, Easton DF, Giles GG, McCredie MR, Hopper JL (2001). After BRCA1 and BRCA2-what next? Multifactorial segregation analyses of three-generation, population-based Australian families affected by female breast cancer. *Am J Hum Genet* 68: 420-431.

592a. Cui S, Lespinasse P, Cracchiolo B, Sama J, Kreitzer MS, Heller DS (2001). Large cell neuroendocrine carcinoma of the cervix associated with adenocarcinoma in situ: evidence of a common origin. *Int J Gynecol Pathol* 20: 311-312.

593. Cummings MC, Aubele M, Mattis A, Purdie D, Hutzler P, Hofler H, Werner M (2000). Increasing chromosome 1 copy number parallels histological progression in breast carcinogenesis. *Br J Cancer* 82: 1204-1210.

594. Cunha TM, Felix A, Cabral I (2001). Preoperative assessment of deep myometrial and cervical invasion in endometrial carcinoma: comparison of magnetic resonance imaging and gross visual inspection. *Int J Gynecol Cancer* 11: 130-136.

595. Cunningham JM, Kim CY, Christensen ER, Tester DJ, Parc Y, Burgart LJ, Halling KC, McDonnell SK, Schaid DJ, Walsh VC, Kubly V, Nelson H, Michels VV, Thibodeau SN (2001). The frequency of hereditary defective mismatch repair in a prospective series of unselected colorectal carcinomas. *Am J Hum Genet* 69: 780-790.

596. Cuny M, Kramar A, Courjal F, Johannsdottir V, Iacopetta B, Fontaine H, Grenier J, Culine S, Theillet C (2000). Relating genotype and phenotype in breast cancer: an analysis of the prognostic significance of amplification at eight different genes or loci and of p53 mutations. *Cancer Res* 60: 1077-1083.

597. Curry JL, Olejnik JL, Wojcik EM (2001). Cellular angiofibroma of the vulva with DNA ploidy analysis. *Int J Gynecol Pathol* 20: 200-203.

598. Curtin JP, Rubin SC, Hoskins WJ, Hakes TB, Lewis JL Jr. (1989). Second-look laparotomy in endodermal sinus tumor: a report of two patients with normal levels of alpha-fetoprotein and residual tumor at reexploration. *Obstet Gynecol* 73: 893-895.

599. Curtin JP, Saigo P, Slucher B, Venkatraman ES, Mychalczak B, Hoskins WJ (1995). Soft-tissue sarcoma of the vagina and vulva: a clinicopathologic study. *Obstet Gynecol* 86: 269-272.

600. Cushing B, Giller R, Ablin A, Cohen L, Cullen J, Hawkins E, Heifetz SA, Krailo M, Lauer SJ, Marina N, Rao PV, Rescorla F, Vinocur CD, Weetman RM, Castleberry RP (1999). Surgical resection alone is effective treatment for ovarian immature teratoma in children and adolescents: a report of the pediatric oncology group and the children's cancer group. *Am J Obstet Gynecol* 181: 353-358.

601. Cutuli B, Borel C, Dhermain F, Magrini SM, Wasserman TH, Bogart JA, Provencio M, de Lafontan B, de la RA, Cellai E, Graic Y, Kerbrat P, Alzieu C, Teissier E, Dilhuydy JM, Mignotte H, Velten M (2001). Breast cancer occurred after treatment for Hodgkin's disease: analysis of 133 cases. *Radiother Oncol* 59: 247-255.

602. Cutuli B, Dilhuydy JM, de Lafontan B, Berlie J, Lacroze M, Lesaunier F, Graic Y, Tortochaux J, Resbeut M, Lesimple T, Gamelin E, Campana F, Reme-Saumon M, Moncho-Bernier V, Cuilliere JC, Marchal C, De Gislain G, N'Guyen TD, Teissier E, Velten M (1997). Ductal carcinoma in situ of the male breast. Analysis of 31 cases. *Eur J Cancer* 33: 35-38.

603. Czernobilsky B (1967). Intracystic carcinoma of the female breast. *Surg Gynecol Obstet* 124: 93-98.

604. Czernobilsky B, Gillespie JJ, Roth LM (1982). Adenosarcoma of the ovary. A light- and electron-microscopic study with review of the literature. *Diagn Gynecol Obstet* 4: 25-36.

604a. Czernobilsky B, Lancet M (1972). Broad ligament adenocarcinoma of Mullerian origin. *Obstet Gynecol* 40: 238-242.

605. Czernobilsky B, Moll R, Levy R, Franke WW (1985). Co-expression of cytokeratin and vimentin filaments in mesothelial, granulosa and rete ovarii cells of the human ovary. *Eur J Cell Biol* 37: 175-190.

606. d'Ablaing G III, Klatt EC, DiRocco G, Hibbard LT (1983). Broad ligament serous tumor of low malignant potential. *Int J Gynecol Pathol* 2: 93-99.

607. D'Avanzo B, La Vecchia C (1995). Risk factors for male breast cancer. *Br J Cancer* 71: 1359-1362.

608. D'Orsi CJ, Feldhaus L, Sonnenfeld M (1983). Unusual lesions of the breast. *Radiol Clin North Am* 21: 67-80.

609. Dal Cin P, Timmerman D, Van den Berghe H, Wanschura S, Kazmierczak B, Vergote I, Deprest J, Neven P, Moerman P, Bullerdiek J, Van den Berghe H (1998). Genomic changes in endometrial polyps associated with tamoxifen show no evidence for its action as an external carcinogen. *Cancer Res* 58: 2278-2281.

610. Dalal P, Shousha S (1995). Keratin 19 in paraffin sections of medullary carcinoma and other benign and malignant breast lesions. *Mod Pathol* 8: 413-416.

611. Daling JR, Sherman KJ, Hislop TG, Maden C, Mandelson MT, Beckmann AM, Weiss NS (1992). Cigarette smoking and the risk of anogenital cancer. *Am J Epidemiol* 135: 180-189.

612. Dalton LW, Page DL, Dupont WD (1994). Histologic grading of breast carcinoma. A reproducibility study. *Cancer* 73: 2765-2770.

613. Daly MB (1992). Ovarian Cancer. *Hematology/oncology clinics of North America. The epidemiology of ovarian cancer*. WB Saunders: Philadelphia.

614. Damajanov I, Drobnjak P, Grizelj V, Longhino N (1975). Sclerosing stromal tumor of the ovary: A hormonal and ultrastructural analysis. *Obstet Gynecol* 45: 675-679.

615. Damiani S, Dina R, Eusebi V (1999). Eosinophilic and granular cell tumors of the breast. *Semin Diagn Pathol* 16: 117-125.

616. Damiani S, Eusebi V, Losi L, D'Adda T, Rosai J (1998). Oncocytic carcinoma (malignant oncocytoma) of the breast. *Am J Surg Pathol* 22: 221-230.

617. Damiani S, Koerner FC, Dickersin GR, Cook MG, Eusebi V (1992). Granular cell tumour of the breast. *Virchows Arch A Pathol Anat Histopathol* 420: 219-226.

618. Damiani S, Panarelli M (1996). Mammary adenohibernoma. *Histopathology* 28: 554-555.

619. Damiani S, Pasquinelli G, Lamovec J, Peterse JL, Eusebi V (2000). Acinic cell carcinoma of the breast: an immunohistochemical and ultrastructural study. *Virchows Arch* 437: 74-81.

620. Damjanov I, Amenta PS, Zarghami F (1984). Transformation of an AFP-positive yolk sac carcinoma into an AFP-negative neoplasm. Evidence for in vivo cloning of the human parietal yolk sac carcinoma. *Cancer* 53: 1902-1907.

621. Dammann R, Li C, Yoon JH, Chin PL, Bates S, Pfeifer GP (2000). Epigenetic inactivation of a RAS association domain family protein from the lung tumour suppressor locus 3p21.3. *Nat Genet* 25: 315-319.

622. Dammann R, Yang G, Pfeifer GP (2001). Hypermethylation of the cpG island of Ras association domain family 1A (RASSF1A), a putative tumor suppressor gene from the 3p21.3 locus, occurs in a large percentage of human breast cancers. *Cancer Res* 61: 3105-3109.

623. Daroca PJ Jr. (1987). Medullary carcinoma of the breast with granulomatous stroma. *Hum Pathol* 18: 761-763.
624. Daroca PJ Jr., Reed RJ, Love GL, Kraus SD (1985). Myoid hamartomas of the breast. *Hum Pathol* 16: 212-219.
625. Dasouki M, Ishmael H, Eng C (2001). Macrocephaly, macrosomia and autistic behavior due to a de novo PTEN germline mutation. *Am J Hum Genet* 69S: 280.
626. Davies JD, Mera SL (1987). Elastosis in breast carcinoma: II. Association of protease inhibitors with immature elastic fibres. *J Pathol* 153: 317-324.
627. Davis BW, Gelber R, Goldhirsch A, Hartmann WH, Hollaway L, Russell I, Rudenstam CM (1985). Prognostic significance of peritumoral vessel invasion in clinical trials of adjuvant therapy for breast cancer with axillary lymph node metastasis. *Hum Pathol* 16: 1212-1218.
628. Davis DL, Bradlow HL, Wolff M, Woodruff T, Hoel DG, Anton-Culver H (1993). Medical hypothesis: xenoestrogens as preventable causes of breast cancer. *Environ Health Perspect* 101: 372-377.
629. Davis GD, Patton WS (1983). Capillary hemangioma of the cervix and vagina: management with carbon dioxide laser. *Obstet Gynecol* 62: 95s-96s.
630. Davis GL (1996). Malignant melanoma arising in mature ovarian cystic teratoma (dermoid cyst). Report of two cases and literature analysis. *Int J Gynecol Pathol* 15: 356-362.
631. Davis KP, Hartmann LK, Keeney GL, Shapiro H (1996). Primary ovarian carcinoid tumors. *Gynecol Oncol* 61: 259-265.
632. Davis S, Mirick DK, Stevens RG (2001). Night shift work, light at night, and risk of breast cancer. *J Natl Cancer Inst* 93: 1557-1562.
633. Davos I, Abell MR (1976). Sarcomas of the vagina. *Obstet Gynecol* 47: 342-350.
634. Daw E (1971). Primary carcinoma of the vagina. *J Obstet Gynaecol Br Commonw* 78: 853-856.
635. Dawson PJ, Ferguson DJ, Karrison T (1982). The pathological findings of breast cancer in patients surviving 25 years after radical mastectomy. *Cancer* 50: 2131-2138.
636. Dawson PJ, Schroer KR, Wolman SR (1996). ras and p53 genes in male breast cancer. *Mod Pathol* 9: 367-370.
637. Daya D (1994). Malignant female adnexal tumor of probable wolffian origin with review of the literature. *Arch Pathol Lab Med* 118: 310-312.
638. Daya D, Lukka H, Clement PB (1992). Primitive neuroectodermal tumors of the uterus: a report of four cases. *Hum Pathol* 23: 1120-1129.
639. Daya D, Nazerali L, Frank GL (1992). Metastatic ovarian carcinoma of large intestinal origin simulating primary ovarian carcinoma. A clinicopathologic study of 25 cases. *Am J Clin Pathol* 97: 751-758.
640. Daya D, Sabet L (1991). The use of cytokeratin as a sensitive and reliable marker for trophoblastic tissue. *Am J Clin Pathol* 95: 137-141.
641. Daya D, Young RH, Scully RE (1992). Endometrioid carcinoma of the fallopian tube resembling an adnexal tumor of probable wolffian origin: a report of six cases. *Int J Gynecol Pathol* 11: 122-130.
642. Daya DA, Scully RE (1988). Sarcoma botryoides of the uterine cervix in young women: a clinicopathological study of 13 cases. *Gynecol Oncol* 29: 290-304.
643. de Cremoux P, Salomon AV, Liva S, Dendale R, Bouchind'homme B, Martin E, Sastre-Garau X, Magdelenat H, Fourquet A, Soussi T (1999). p53 mutation as a genetic trait of typical medullary breast carcinoma. *J Natl Cancer Inst* 91: 641-643.
644. de Deus JM, Focchi J, Stavale JN, de Lima GR (1995). Histologic and biomolecular aspects of papillomatosis of the vulvar vestibule in relation to human papillomavirus. *Obstet Gynecol* 86: 758-763.
645. de Fusco PA, Gaffey TA, Malkasian GD Jr., Long HJ, Cha SS (1989). Endometrial stromal sarcoma: review of Mayo Clinic experience, 1945-1980. *Gynecol Oncol* 35: 8-14.
646. de Hullu JA, Doting E, Piers DA, Hollema H, Aalders JG, Koops HS, Boonstra H, van der Zee AG (1998). Sentinel lymph node identification with technetium-99m-labeled nanocolloid in squamous cell cancer of the vulva. *J Nucl Med* 39: 1381-1385.
647. de la Fuente AA (1982). Benign mixed Mullerian tumour--adenofibroma of the fallopian tube. *Histopathology* 6: 661-666.
648. de la Rochefordiere A, Asselain B, Scholl S, Campana F, Ucla L, Vilcoq JR, Durand JC, Pouillart P, Fourquet A (1994). Simultaneous bilateral breast carcinomas: a retrospective review of 149 cases. *Int J Radiat Oncol Biol Phys* 30: 35-41.
649. de Leeuw WJ, Berx G, Vos CB, Peterse JL, Van de Vijver MJ, Litvinov S, van Roy F, Cornelisse CJ, Cleton-Jansen AM (1997). Simultaneous loss of E-cadherin and catenins in invasive lobular breast cancer and lobular carcinoma in situ. *J Pathol* 183: 404-411.
650. de Leeuw WJ, Dierssen J, Vasen HF, Wijnen JT, Kenter GG, Meijers-Heijboer H, Brocker-Vriends A, Stormorken A, Moller P, Menko F, Cornelisse CJ, Morreau H (2000). Prediction of a mismatch repair gene defect by microsatellite instability and immunohistochemical analysis in endometrial tumours from HNPCC patients. *J Pathol* 192: 328-335.
651. de Nictolis M, Curatola A, Tommasoni S, Magiera G (1994). High-grade endometrial stromal sarcoma: clinicopathologic and immunohistochemical study of a case. *Pathologica* 86: 217-221.
652. de Nictolis M, Montironi R, Tommasoni S, Carinelli S, Ojeda B, Matias-Guiu X, Prat J (1992). Serous borderline tumors of the ovary. A clinicopathologic, immunohistochemical, and quantitative study of 44 cases. *Cancer* 70: 152-160.
653. de Nictolis M, Montironi R, Tommasoni S, Valli M, Pisani E, Fabris G, Prat J (1994). Benign, borderline, and well-differentiated malignant intestinal mucinous tumors of the ovary: a clinicopathologic, histochemical, immunohistochemical, and nuclear quantitative study of 57 cases. *Int J Gynecol Pathol* 13: 10-21.
654. de Rosa G, Boscaino A, Terracciano LM, Giordano G (1992). Giant adenomatoid tumors of the uterus. *Int J Gynecol Pathol* 11: 156-160.
655. de Wind N, Dekker M, van Rossum A, van der Valk M, te Riele H (1998). Mouse models for hereditary nonpolyposis colorectal cancer. *Cancer Res* 58: 248-255.
656. de Mascarel I, MacGrogan G, Mathoulin-Pelissier S, Soubeyran I, Picot V, Coindre JM (2002). Breast ductal carcinoma in situ with microinvasion: a definition supported by a long-term study of 1248 serially sectioned ductal carcinomas. *Cancer* 94: 2134-2142.
657. de Vivo I, Gertig DM, Nagase S, Hankinson SE, O'Brien R, Speizer FE, Parsons R, Hunter DJ (2000). Novel germline mutations in the PTEN tumour suppressor gene found in women with multiple cancers. *J Med Genet* 37: 336-341.
658. Deavers MT, Gershenson DM, Tortolero-Luna G, Malpica A, Lu KH, Silva EG (2002). Micropapillary and cribriform patterns in ovarian serous tumors of low malignant potential: a study of 99 advanced stage cases. *Am J Surg Pathol* 26: 1129-1141.
659. de Hoop TA, Mira J, Thomas MA (1997). Endosalpingiosis and chronic pelvic pain. *J Reprod Med* 42: 613-616.
660. Dekel A, van Iddekinge B, Isaacson C, Dicker D, Feldberg D, Goldman J (1986). Primary choriocarcinoma of the fallopian tube. Report of a case with survival and postoperative delivery. Review of the literature. *Obstet Gynecol Surv* 41: 142-148.
661. Del Giudice ME, Fantus IG, Ezzat S, McKeown-Eyssen G, Page D, Goodwin PJ (1998). Insulin and related factors in premenopausal breast cancer risk. *Breast Cancer Res Treat* 47: 111-120.
662. Delaloye JF, Ruzicka J, de Grandi P (1993). An ovarian tumor of probable Wolffian origin. *Acta Obstet Gynecol Scand* 72: 314-316.
663. Delgado G, Bundy B, Zaino R, Sevin BU, Creasman WT, Major F (1990). Prospective surgical-pathological study of disease-free interval in patients with stage IB squamous cell carcinoma of the cervix: a Gynecologic Oncology Group study. *Gynecol Oncol* 38: 352-357.
664. Deligdisch L, Hirschmann S, Altchek A (1997). Pathologic changes in gonadotropin releasing hormone agonist analogue treated uterine leiomyomata. *Fertil Steril* 67: 837-841.
665. Deligdisch L, Kalir T, Cohen CJ, de Latour M, Le Bouedec G, Penault-Llorca F (2000). Endometrial histopathology in 700 patients treated with tamoxifen for breast cancer. *Gynecol Oncol* 78: 181-186.
666. Dellas A, Schultheiss E, Holzgreve W, Oberholzer M, Torhorst J, Gudat F (1997). Investigation of the Bcl-2 and C-myc expression in relationship to the Ki-67 labelling index in cervical intraepithelial neoplasia. *Int J Gynecol Pathol* 16: 212-218.
667. de Matos P, Tyler D, Seigler HF (1998). Mucosal melanoma of the female genitalia: a clinicopathologic study of forty-three cases at Duke University Medical Center. *Surgery* 124: 38-48.
668. de May RM, Kay S (1984). Granular cell tumor of the breast. *Pathol Annu 19 Pt* 2: 121-148.
669. Demers PA, Thomas DB, Rosenblatt KA, Jimenez LM, McTiernan A, Stalsberg H, Stemhagen A, Thompson WD, Curnen MG, Satariano W, Austin DF, Isacson P, Greenberg RS, Key C, Kolonel LN, West DW. (1991). Occupational exposure to electromagnetic fields and breast cancer in men. *Am J Epidemiol* 134: 340-347.
670. Demopoulos RI, Sitelman A, Flotte T, Bigelow B (1980). Ultrastructural study of a female adnexal tumor of probable wolffian origin. *Cancer* 46: 2273-2280.
671. Deng G, Lu Y, Zlotnikov G, Thor AD, Smith HS (1996). Loss of heterozygosity in normal tissue adjacent to breast carcinomas. *Science* 274: 2057-2059.
672. Denley H, Pinder SE, Tan PH, Sim CS, Brown R, Barker T, Gearty J, Elston CW, Ellis IO (2000). Metaplastic carcinoma of the breast arising within complex sclerosing lesion: a report of five cases. *Histopathology* 36: 203-209.
673. Denton AS, Bond SJ, Matthews S, Bentzen SM, Maher EJ (2000). National audit of the management and outcome of carcinoma of the cervix treated with radiotherapy in 1993. *Clin Oncol (R Coll Radiol)* 12: 347-353.
674. Department of Health (1998). Report on health and social subjects No. 48. Nutritional aspects of the development of cancer. The Stationery Office: Norwich.
675. DePasquale SE, McGuinness TB, Mangan CE, Husson M, Woodland MB (1996). Adenoid cystic carcinoma of Bartholin's gland: a review of the literature and report of a patient. *Gynecol Oncol* 61: 122-125.
676. DePriest PD, Banks ER, Powell DE, van Nagell JR Jr., Gallion HH, Puls LE, Hunter JE, Kryscio RJ, Royalty MB (1992). Endometrioid carcinoma of the ovary and endometriosis: the association in postmenopausal women. *Gynecol Oncol* 47: 71-75.
677. Devaney K, Snyder R, Norris HJ, Tavassoli FA (1993). Proliferative and histologically malignant struma ovarii: a clinicopathologic study of 54 cases. *Int J Gynecol Pathol* 12: 333-343.
678. Devaney K, Tavassoli FA (1991). Immunohistochemistry as a diagnostic aid in the interpretation of unusual mesenchymal tumors of the uterus. *Mod Pathol* 4: 225-231.
679. Devilee P, Cleton-Jansen A, Cornelisse CJ (2001). Ever since Knudson. *Trends Genet* 17: 569-573.
680. Devilee P, Cornelisse CJ (1994). Somatic genetic changes in human breast cancer. *Biochim Biophys Acta* 1198: 113-130.
681. Devouassoux-Shisheboran M, Schammel MD, Man YG, Tavassoli FA (2000). Fibromatosis of the breast: age-correlated morphofunctional features of 33 cases. *Arch Pathol Lab Med* 124: 276-280.
682. Devouassoux-Shisheboran M, Silver SA, Tavassoli FA (1999). Wolffian adnexal tumor, so-called female adnexal tumor of probable Wolffian origin (FATWO): immunohistochemical evidence in support of a Wolffian origin. *Hum Pathol* 30: 856-863.
683. Devouassoux-Shisheboran M, Vortmeyer AO, Silver SA, Zhuang Z, Tavassoli FA (2000). Teratomatous genotype detected in malignancies of a non-germ cell phenotype. *Lab Invest* 80: 81-86.
684. Dgani R, Shoham Z, Czernobilsky B, Singer D, Shani A, Lancet M (1989). Endolymphatic stromal myosis (endometrial low-grade stromal sarcoma) presenting with hematuria: a diagnostic challenge. *Gynecol Oncol* 35: 263-266.
685. Dhaliwal LK, Das I, Gopalan S (1992). Recurrent leiomyoma of the vagina. *Int J Gynaecol Obstet* 37: 281-283.
686. Dharkar DD, Kraft JR, Gangadharam D (1981). Uterine lipomas. *Arch Pathol Lab Med* 105: 43-45.
687. Di Bonito L, Patriarca S, Falconieri G (1992). Aggressive "breast-like" adenocarcinoma of vulva. *Pathol Res Pract* 188: 211-214.
688. Di Cristofano A, Pesce B, Cordon-Cardo C, Pandolfi PP (1998). Pten is essential for embryonic development and tumour suppression. *Nat Genet* 19: 348-355.

689. Di Domenico A, Stangl F, Bennington J (1982). Leiomyosarcoma of the broad ligament. *Gynecol Oncol* 13: 412-415. 690. Di Sant'Agnese PA, Knowles DM (1980). Extracardiac rhabdomyoma: a clinicopathologic study and review of the literature. *Cancer* 46: 780-789.
691. Diab SG, Clark GM, Osborne CK, Libby A, Allred DC, Elledge RM (1999). Tumor characteristics and clinical outcome of tubular and mucinous breast carcinomas. *J Clin Oncol* 17: 1442-1448.
692. Diaz NM, McDivitt RW, Wick MR (1991). Microglandular adenosis of the breast. An immunohistochemical comparison with tubular carcinoma. *Arch Pathol Lab Med* 115: 578-582.
693. Diaz NM, Palmer JO, McDivitt RW (1991). Carcinoma arising within fibroadenomas of the breast. A clinicopathologic study of 105 patients. *Am J Clin Pathol* 95: 614-622.
694. Dickersin GR, Maluf HM, Koerner FC (1997). Solid papillary carcinoma of breast: an ultrastructural study. *Ultrastruct Pathol* 21: 153-161.
695. Dickersin GR, Scully RE (1993). An update on the electron microscopy of small cell carcinoma of the ovary with hypercalcemia. *Ultrastruct Pathol* 17: 411-422.
696. Dickersin GR, Scully RE (1998). Ovarian small cell tumors: an electron microscopic review. *Ultrastruct Pathol* 22: 199-226.
697. Dickersin GR, Young RH, Scully RE (1995). Signet-ring stromal and related tumors of the ovary. *Ultrastruct Pathol* 19: 401-419.
698. Dickson JM, Mansel RE (2000). *ABC of Breast Diseases. Symptoms, Assessment and Guidelines for Referral.* 2nd ed. BMJ Books: London, pp. 1-5.
699. DiCostanzo D, Rosen PP, Gareen I, Franklin S, Lesser M (1990). Prognosis in infiltrating lobular carcinoma. An analysis of "classical" and variant tumors. *Am J Surg Pathol* 14: 12-23.
700. Dietl J, Horny HP, Ruck P, Kaiserling E (1993). Dysgerminoma of the ovary. An immunohistochemical study of tumor-infiltrating lymphoreticular cells and tumor cells. *Cancer* 71: 2562-2568.
701. Dietrich CU, Pandis N, Teixeira MR, Bardi G, Gerdes AM, Andersen JA, Heim S (1995). Chromosome abnormalities in benign hyperproliferative disorders of epithelial and stromal breast tissue. *Int J Cancer* 60: 49-53.
702. Dina R, Eusebi V (1997). Clear cell tumors of the breast. *Semin Diagn Pathol* 14: 175-182.
703. Dinh TV, Slavin RE, Bhagavan BS, Hannigan EV, Tiamson EM, Yandell RB (1989). Mixed mullerian tumors of the uterus: a clinicopathologic study. *Obstet Gynecol* 74: 388-392.
704. Dixon AR, Ellis IO, Elston CW, Blamey RW (1991). A comparison of the clinical metastatic patterns of invasive lobular and ductal carcinomas of the breast. *Br J Cancer* 63: 634-635.
705. Dixon JM, Anderson TJ, Page DL, Lee D, Duffy SW (1982). Infiltrating lobular carcinoma of the breast. *Histopathology* 6: 149-161.
706. Dixon JM, Lumsden AB, Krajewski A, Elton RA, Anderson TJ (1987). Primary lymphoma of the breast. *Br J Surg* 74: 214-216.
707. Dixon JM, Sainsbury JRC (1998). *Handbook of Diseases of the Breast.* 2nd ed. Churchill Livingstone: Edinburgh.
708. Dobbs SP, Shaw PA, Brown LJ, Ireland D (1998). Borderline malignant change in recurrent mullerian papilloma of the vagina. *J Clin Pathol* 51: 875-877.
709. Dockerty MB, Masson JC (1944). Ovarian fibromas: a clinical and pathological study of two hundred-and eighty-three cases. *Am J Obstet Gynecol* 47: 741-752.
710. Dodge JA, Eltabbakh GH, Mount SL, Walker RP, Morgan A (2001). Clinical features and risk of recurrence among patients with vaginal intraepithelial neoplasia. *Gynecol Oncol* 83: 363-369.
711. Domagala W, Harezga B, Szadowska A, Markiewski M, Weber K, Osborn M (1993). Nuclear p53 protein accumulates preferentially in medullary and high-grade ductal but rarely in lobular breast carcinomas. *Am J Pathol* 142: 669-674.
712. Done SJ, Eskandarian S, Bull S, Redston M, Andrulis IL (2001). p53 missense mutations in microdissected high-grade ductal carcinoma in situ of the breast. *J Natl Cancer Inst* 93: 700-704.
713. Donegan WL, Redlich PN, Lang PJ, Gall MT (1998). Carcinoma of the breast in males: a multiinstitutional survey. *Cancer* 83: 498-509.
714. Donehower LA, Harvey M, Slagle BL, McArthur MJ, Montgomery CA Jr., Butel JS, Bradley A (1992). Mice deficient for p53 are developmentally normal but susceptible to spontaneous tumours. *Nature* 356: 215-221.
715. Dong C, Hemminki K (2001). Modification of cancer risks in offspring by sibling and parental cancers from 2,112,616 nuclear families. *Int J Cancer* 92: 144-150.
715 a. Dong HJ, Li JG, Zeng JH, Huang SZ (1986). Papillary adenocarcinoma of the broad ligament. Report of a case and review of literature. *Chin Med J (Engl)* 99: 431-432.
716. Donkers B, Kazzaz BA, Meijering JH (1972). Rhabdomyosarcoma of the corpus uteri. Report of two cases with review of the literature. *Am J Obstet Gynecol* 114: 1025-1030.
717. Donnell RM, Rosen PP, Lieberman PH, Kaufman RJ, Kay S, Braun DW Jr., Kinne DW (1981). Angiosarcoma and other vascular tumors of the breast. *Am J Surg Pathol* 5: 629-642.
718. Dougherty CM, Cunningham C, Mickal A (1978). Choriocarcinoma with metastasis in a postmenopausal woman. *Am J Obstet Gynecol* 132: 700-701.
719. Douglas-Jones AG, Pace DP (1997). Pathology of R4 spiculated lesions in the breast screening programme. *Histopathology* 30: 214-220.
720. Downey GO, Okagaki T, Ostrow RS, Clark BA, Twiggs LB, Faras AJ (1988). Condylomatous carcinoma of the vulva with special reference to human papillomavirus DNA. *Obstet Gynecol* 72: 68-73.
721. Drew PA, al Abbadi MA, Orlando CA, Hendricks JB, Kubilis PS, Wilkinson EJ (1996). Prognostic factors in carcinoma of the vulva: a clinicopathologic and DNA flow cytometric study. *Int J Gynecol Pathol* 15: 235-241.
722. Driscoll SG (1963). Choriocarcinoma. An "incidental finding" within a term placenta. *Obstet Gynecol* 21: 96-101.
723. Droufakou S, Deshmane V, Roylance R, Hanby A, Tomlinson I, Hart IR (2001). Multiple ways of silencing E-cadherin gene expression in lobular carcinoma of the breast. *Int J Cancer* 92: 404-408.
724. Droulias CA, Sewell CW, McSweeney MB, Powell RW (1976). Inflammatory carcinoma of the breast: A correlation of clinical, radiologic and pathogic findings. *Ann Surg* 184: 217-222.
725. du Toit RS, Locker AP, Ellis IO, Elston CW, Nicholson RI, Blamey RW (1989). Invasive lobular carcinomas of the breast--the prognosis of histopathological subtypes. *Br J Cancer* 60: 605-609.
726. Dubeau L (1999). The cell of origin of ovarian epithelial tumors and the ovarian surface epithelium dogma: does the emperor have no clothes? *Gynecol Oncol* 72: 437-442.
727. Duggan MA, Hugh J, Nation JG, Robertson DI, Stuart GC (1989). Ependymoma of the uterosacral ligament. *Cancer* 64: 2565-2571.
728. Dumont-Herskowitz RA, Safaii HS, Senior B (1978). Ovarian fibromata in four successive generations. *J Pediatr* 93: 621-624.
729. Dunaif A, Hoffman AR, Scully RE, Flier JS, Longcope C, Levy LJ, Crowley WF Jr. (1985). Clinical, biochemical, and ovarian morphologic features in women with acanthosis nigricans and masculinization. *Obstet Gynecol* 66: 545-552.
730. Dungar CF, Wilkinson EJ (1995). Vaginal columnar cell metaplasia. An acquired adenosis associated with topical 5-fluorouracil therapy. *J Reprod Med* 40: 361-366.
731. Dunlop MG, Farrington SM, Carothers AD, Wyllie AH, Sharp L, Burn J, Liu B, Kinzler KW, Vogelstein B (1997). Cancer risk associated with germline DNA mismatch repair gene mutations. *Hum Mol Genet* 6: 105-110.
732. Dupont WD, Page DL (1985). Risk factors for breast cancer in women with proliferative breast disease. *N Engl J Med* 312: 146-151.
733. Dupont WD, Page DL (1987). Breast cancer risk associated with proliferative disease, age at first birth, and a family history of breast cancer. *Am J Epidemiol* 125: 769-779.
734. Dupont WD, Page DL, Parl FF, Vnencak-Jones CL, Plummer WD Jr., Rados MS, Schuyler PA (1994). Long-term risk of breast cancer in women with fibroadenoma. *N Engl J Med* 331: 10-15.
735. Dupont WD, Parl FF, Hartmann WH, Brinton LA, Winfield AC, Worrell JA, Schuyler PA, Plummer WD (1993). Breast cancer risk associated with proliferative breast disease and atypical hyperplasia. *Cancer* 71: 1258-1265.
736. Durkop H, Foss HD, Eitelbach F, Anagnostopoulos I, Latza U, Pileri S, Stein H (2000). Expression of the CD30 antigen in non-lymphoid tissues and cells. *J Pathol* 190: 613-618.
737. Durst M, Gissmann L, Ikenberg H, zur Hausen H (1983). A papillomavirus DNA from a cervical carcinoma and its prevalence in cancer biopsy samples from different geographic regions. *Proc Natl Acad Sci USA* 80: 3812-3815.
738. Duska LR, Flynn C, Goodman A (1998). Masculinizing sclerosing stromal cell tumor in pregnancy: report of a case and review of the literature. *Eur J Gynaecol Oncol* 19: 441-443.
739. Duun S (1994). Bilateral virilizing hilus (Leydig) cell tumors of the ovary. Acta *Obstet Gynecol Scand* 73: 76-77.
740. Duvall E, Survis JA (1983). Borderline tumour of the broad ligament. Case report. *Br J Obstet Gynaecol* 90: 372-375.
741. Easton DF (1994). Cancer risks in A-T heterozygotes. Int J Radiat Biol 66: S177-S182.
742. Easton DF, Ford D, Bishop DT (1995). Breast and ovarian cancer incidence in BRCA1-mutation carriers. Breast Cancer Linkage Consortium. *Am J Hum Genet* 56: 265-271.
743. Easton DF, Matthews FE, Ford D, Swerdlow AJ, Peto J (1996). Cancer mortality in relatives of women with ovarian cancer: the OPCS Study. Office of Population Censuses and Surveys. *Int J Cancer* 65: 284-294.
744. Easton DF, Steele L, Fields P, Ormiston W, Averill D, Daly PA, McManus R, Neuhausen SL, Ford D, Wooster R, Cannon-Albright LA, Stratton MR, Goldgar DE (1997). Cancer risks in two large breast cancer families linked to BRCA2 on chromosome 13q12-13. *Am J Hum Genet* 61: 120-128.
745. Ebrahim S, Daponte A, Smith TH, Tiltman A, Guidozzi F (2001). Primary mucinous adenocarcinoma of the vagina. *Gynecol Oncol* 80: 89-92.
746. Eckstein RP, Paradinas FJ, Bagshawe KD (1982). Placental site trophoblastic tumour (trophoblastic pseudotumour): a study of four cases requiring hysterectomy including one fatal case. *Histopathology* 6: 211-226. 747. Eckstein RP, Russell P, Friedlander ML, Tattersall MH, Bradfield A (1985). Metastasizing placental site trophoblastic tumor: a case study. *Hum Pathol* 16: 632-636.
748. Eddy GL, Marks RD Jr., Miller MC III, Underwood PB Jr. (1991). Primary invasive vaginal carcinoma. *Am J Obstet Gynecol* 165: 292-296.
749. Eeles RA (1999). Screening for hereditary cancer and genetic testing, epitomized by breast cancer. *Eur J Cancer* 35: 1954-1962.
750. Egan AJ, Russell P (1996). Transitional (urothelial) cell metaplasia of the fallopian tube mucosa: morphological assessment of three cases. *Int J Gynecol Pathol* 15: 72-76.
751. Egan RL (1976). Bilateral breast carcinomas: Role of mammography. *Cancer* 38: 931-938.
752. Eggers JW, Chesney TM (1984). Squamous cell carcinoma of the breast: a clinicopathologic analysis of eight cases and review of the literature. *Hum Pathol* 15: 526-531.
753. Ehrlich CE, Roth LM (1971). The Brenner tumor. A clinicopathologic study of 57 cases. *Cancer* 27: 332-342.
754. Eichhorn JH, Bell DA, Young RH, Scully RE (1999). Ovarian serous borderline tumors with micropapillary and cribriform patterns: a study of 40 cases and comparison with 44 cases without these patterns. *Am J Surg Pathol* 23: 397-409.
755. Eichhorn JH, Bell DA, Young RH, Swymer CM, Flotte TJ, Preffer RI, Scully RE (1992). DNA content and proliferative activity in ovarian small cell carcinomas of the hypercalcemic type. Implications for diagnosis, prognosis, and histogenesis. *Am J Clin Pathol* 98: 579-586.
756. Eichhorn JH, Lawrence WD, Young RH, Scully RE (1996). Ovarian neuroendocrine carcinomas of non-small-cell type associated with surface epithelial adenocarcinomas. A study of five cases and review of the literature. *Int J Gynecol Pathol* 15: 303-314.

757. Eichhorn JH, Scully RE (1991). Ovarian myxoma: clinicopathologic and immunocytologic analysis of five cases and a review of the literature. *Int J Gynecol Pathol* 10: 156-169.

758. Eichhorn JH, Scully RE (1995). "Adenoid cystic" and basaloid carcinomas of the ovary: evidence for a surface epithelial lineage. A report of 12 cases. *Mod Pathol* 8: 731-740.

759. Eichhorn JH, Scully RE (1996). Endometrioid ciliated-cell tumors of the ovary: a report of five cases. *Int J Gynecol Pathol* 15: 248-256.

760. Eichhorn JH, Young RH, Clement PB, Scully RE (2002). Mesodermal (mullerian) adenosarcoma of the ovary: a clinicopathologic analysis of 40 cases and a review of the literature. *Am J Surg Pathol* 26: 1243-1258.

761. Eichhorn JH, Young RH, Scully RE (1992). Primary ovarian small cell carcinoma of pulmonary type. A clinicopathologic, immunohistologic, and flow cytometric analysis of 11 cases. *Am J Surg Pathol* 16: 926-938.

762. Eifel P, Hendrickson M, Ross J, Ballon S, Martinez A, Kempson R (1982). Simultaneous presentation of carcinoma involving the ovary and the uterine corpus. *Cancer* 50: 163-170.

763. Eisen A, Rebbeck TR, Lynch HT, Lerman C, Ghadirian P, Dube MP (2000). Reduction in Breast Cancer Risk following Bilateral Prophylactic Oophorectomy in BRCA1 and BRCA2 Mutation Carriers. *Am J Hum Genet* 67: 58.

764. Eisinger F, Jacquemier J, Charpin C, Stoppa-Lyonnet D, Bressac-de Paillerets B, Peyrat JP, Longy M, Guinebretiere JM, Sauvan R, Noguchi T, Birnbaum D, Sobol H (1998). Mutations at BRCA1: the medullary breast carcinoma revisited. *Cancer Res* 58: 1588-1592.

765. Eisinger F, Jacquemier J, Guinebretiere JM, Birnbaum D, Sobol H (1997). p53 involvement in BRCA1-associated breast cancer. *Lancet* 350: 1101.

766. Eisinger F, Jacquemier J, Nogues C, Birnbaum D, Sobol H (1999). Steroid receptors in hereditary breast carcinomas associated with BRCA1 or BRCA2 mutations or unknown susceptibility genes. *Cancer* 85: 2291-2295.

767. Eisner RF, Nieberg RK, Berek JS (1989). Synchronous primary neoplasms of the female reproductive tract. *Gynecol Oncol* 33: 335-339.

768. Elliott P, Coppleson M, Russell P, Liouros P, Carter J, MacLeod C, Jones M (2000). Early invasive (FIGO stage IA) carcinoma of the cervix: a clinico-pathologic study of 476 cases. *Int J Gynecol Cancer* 10: 42-52.

769. Ellis DL, Teitelbaum SL (1974). Inflammatory carcinoma of the breast. A pathologic definition. *Cancer* 33: 1045-1047.

770. Ellis IO, Elston CW, Goulding H, et al. (1998). Miscellaneous benign lesions. In: *The Breast*. CW Elston and IO Ellis (Ed.) 1st ed. Churchill Livingstone: Edinburgh, p. 224.

771. Ellis IO, Galea M, Broughton N, Locker A, Blamey RW, Elston CW (1992). Pathological prognostic factors in breast cancer. II. Histological type. Relationship with survival in a large study with long-term follow-up. *Histopathology* 20: 479-489.

772. Ellis IO, Galea MH, Locker A, Roebuck EJ, Elston CW, Blamey RW, Wilson ARM (1993). Early experience in breast cancer screening: Emphasis on development of protocols for triple assessment. *Breast* 2: 148-153.

773. Elsheikh A, Keramopoulos A, Lazaris D, Ambela C, Louvrou N, Michalas S (2000). Breast tumors during adolescence. *Eur J Gynaecol Oncol* 21: 408-410.

774. Elston C.W, Ellis I.O. (1998). Classification of malignant breast disease. In: *The Breast*. Systemic Pathology. CW Elston and IO Ellis (Eds.) 3rd ed. Churchill Livingstone: Edinburgh, pp. 239-247.

775. Elston C.W, Ellis I.O. (1998). Fibroadenoma and related conditions. In: *The Breast*. CW Elston and IO Ellis (Ed.) Churchill Livingstone: Edinburgh.

775a. Elston CW, Bagshawe KD (1972). The diagnosis of trophoblastic tumours from uterine curettings. *J Clin Pathol* 25: 111-118.

776. Elston CW, Bagshawe KD (1972). The value of histological grading in the management of hydatidiform mole. *J Obstet Gynaecol Br Commonw* 79: 717-724.

777. Elston CW, Ellis IO (1991). Pathological prognostic factors in breast cancer. I. The value of histological grade in breast cancer: experience from a large study with long-term follow-up. *Histopathology* 19: 403-410.

778. Elston CW, Ellis IO (1998). Metastases within the breast. In: *The Breast*. CW Elston and IO Ellis (Eds.) Churchill Livingstone: Edinburgh.

779. Elston CW, Ellis IO (1998). Systemic pathology 3E. In: *The Breast*. CW Elston and IO Ellis (Eds.) Churchill Livingstone: Edinburgh.

780. Elston CW, Sloane JP, Amendoeira I, Apostolikas N, Bellocq JP, Bianchi S, Boecker W, Bussolati G, Coleman D, Connolly CE, Dervan P, Drijkoningen M, Eusebi V, Faverly D, Holland R, Jacquemier J, Lacerda M, Martinez-Penuela J, De Miguel C, Mossi S, Munt C, Peterse JL, Rank F, Reiner A, Sylvan M, Wells CA, Zafrani B (2000). Causes of inconsistency in diagnosing and classifying intraductal proliferations of the breast. European Commission Working Group on Breast Screening Pathology. *Eur J Cancer* 36: 1769-1772.

781. Emerich J, Senkus E, Konefka T (1996). Alveolar rhabdomyosarcoma of the uterine cervix. *Gynecol Oncol* 63: 398-403.

782. Emery JD, Kennedy AW, Tubbs RR, Castellani WJ, Hussein MA (1999). Plasmacytoma of the ovary: a case report and literature review. *Gynecol Oncol* 73: 151-154.

783. Emmert-Buck MR, Chuaqui R, Zhuang Z, Nogales F, Liotta LA, Merino MJ (1997). Molecular analysis of synchronous uterine and ovarian endometrioid tumors. *Int J Gynecol Pathol* 16: 143-148.

784. Emoto M, Iwasaki H, Kawarabayashi T, Egami D, Yoshitake H, Kikuchi M, Shirakawa K (1994). Primary osteosarcoma of the uterus: report of a case with immunohistochemical analysis. *Gynecol Oncol* 54: 385-388.

785. Eng C (1997). Cowden syndrome. *J Genet Counsel* 6: 181-191.

786. Eng C (2000). Will the real Cowden syndrome please stand up: revised diagnostic criteria. *J Med Genet* 37: 828-830.

787. Eng C, Parsons R (1998). Cowden syndrome. In: *The Genetic Basis of Human Cancer*. B Vogelstein, K Kinzler (Eds.) New York: McGraw-Hill, pp. 519-526.

788. Eng C, Parsons R (2001). Cowden syndrome. In: *Metabolic and Molecular Bases of Inherited Disease*. C Scriver, AL Beaudet, WS Sly, D Valle (Eds.) 8th ed. McGraw-Hill: New York , pp. 979-988.

789. Enomoto T, Haba T, Fujita M, Hamada T, Yoshino K, Nakashima R, Wada H, Kurachi H, Wakasa K, Sakurai M, Murata Y, Shroyer KR (1997). Clonal analysis of high-grade squamous intra-epithelial lesions of the uterine cervix. *Int J Cancer* 73: 339-344.

790. Enzinger FM, Shiraki M (1967). Musculo-aponeurotic fibromatosis of the shoulder girdle (extra-abdominal desmoid). Analysis of thirty cases followed up for ten or more years. *Cancer* 20: 1131-1140.

791. Erdreich LS, Asal NR, Hoge AF (1980). Morphologic types of breast cancer: age, bilaterality, and family history. *South Med J* 73: 28-32.

792. Eriksson ET, Schimmelpenning H, Aspenblad U, Zetterberg A, Auer GU (1994). Immunohistochemical expression of the mutant p53 protein and nuclear DNA content during the transition from benign to malignant breast disease. *Hum Pathol* 25: 1228-1233.

793. Erlandson RA, Rosen PP (1982). Infiltrating myoepithelioma of the breast. *Am J Surg Pathol* 6: 785-793.

794. Ernster VL, Barclay J, Kerlikowske K, Wilkie H, Ballard-Barbash R (2000). Mortality among women with ductal carcinoma in situ of the breast in the population-based surveillance, epidemiology and end results program. *Arch Intern Med* 160: 953-958.

795. Escalonilla P, Grilli R, Canamero M, Soriano ML, Farina MC, Manzarbeitia F, Sainz R, Matsukura T, Requena L (1999). Sebaceous carcinoma of the vulva. *Am J Dermatopathol* 21: 468-472.

796. Esche C, Kruse R, Lamberti C, Friedl W, Propping P, Lehmann P, Ruzicka T (1997). Muir-Torre syndrome: clinical features and molecular genetic analysis. *Br J Dermatol* 136: 913-917.

797. Essary LR, Kaarami M, Page DL, Wick MR (1999). Immunohistology of variant adenosis & pseudoinvasive epithelial proliferations of the breast: helpful or not? *Lab Invest* 79.

798. Esteban JM, Allen WM, Schaerf RH (1999). Benign metastasizing leiomyoma of the uterus: histologic and immunohistochemical characterization of primary and metastatic lesions. *Arch Pathol Lab Med* 123: 960-962.

799. Esteller M, Levine R, Baylin SB, Ellenson LH, Herman JG (1998). MLH1 promoter hypermethylation is associated with the microsatellite instability phenotype in sporadic endometrial carcinomas. *Oncogene* 17: 2413-2417.

800. Etzell JE, Devries S, Chew K, Florendo C, Molinaro A, Ljung BM, Waldman FM (2001). Loss of chromosome 16q in lobular carcinoma in situ. *Hum Pathol* 32: 292-296.

801. Eusebi V, Azzopardi JG (1980). Lobular endocrine neoplasia in fibroadenoma of the breast. *Histopathology* 4: 413-428.

802. Eusebi V, Betts CM, Haagensen DE, Gugliotta P, Bussolati G, Azzopardi JG (1984). Apocrine differentiation in lobular carcinoma of the breast. *Hum Pathol* 15: 134-140.

803. Eusebi V, Casadei GP, Bussolati G, Azzopardi JG (1986). Adenomyoepithelioma of the breast with a distinctive type of apocrine adenosis. *Histopathology* 11: 305-315.

804. Eusebi V, Damiani S, Losi L, Millis RR (1997). Apocrine differentiation in breast epithelium. *Advances Anat Pathol* 4: 139-155.

805. Eusebi V, Damiani S, Losi L, Millis RR (1997). Apocrine differentiation in breast epithelium. *Advances in Anatomic Pathology* 4: 139-155.

806. Eusebi V, Foschini MP, Bussolati G, Rosen PP (1995). Myoblastomatoid (histiocytoid) carcinoma of the breast. A type of apocrine carcinoma. *Am J Surg Pathol* 19: 553-562.

807. Eusebi V, Lamovec J, Cattani MG, Fedeli F, Millis RR (1986). Acantholytic variant of squamous-cell carcinoma of the breast. *Am J Surg Pathol* 10: 855-861.

808. Eusebi V, Magalhaes F, Azzopardi AG (1992). Pleomorphic lobular carcinoma of the breast: an aggressive tumour showing apocrine differentiation. *Hum Pathol* 23: 655-662.

809. Eusebi V, Millis RR, Cattani MG, Bussolati G, Azzopardi JG (1986). Apocrine carcinoma of the breast. A morphologic and immunocytochemical study. *Am J Pathol* 123: 532-541.

810. Evans AJ, Pinder SE, Ellis IO, Wilson AR (2001). Screen detected ductal carcinoma in situ (DCIS): overdiagnosis or an obligate precursor of invasive disease? *J Med Screen* 8: 149-151. **811.** Evans HL (1982). Endometrial stromal sarcoma and poorly differentiated endometrial sarcoma. *Cancer* 50: 2170-2182.

812. Evans HL, Chawla SP, Simpson C, Finn KP (1988). Smooth muscle neoplasms of the uterus other than ordinary leiomyoma. A study of 46 cases, with emphasis on diagnostic criteria and prognostic factors. *Cancer* 62: 2239-2247.

813. Evans MJ, Langlois NE, Kitchener HC, Miller ID (1995). Is there an association between long-term tamoxifen treatment and the development of carcinosarcoma (malignant mixed Mullerian tumor) of the uterus? *Int J Gynecol Cancer* 5: 310-313.

814. Ewertz M, Holmberg L, Karjalainen S, Tretli S, Adami HO (1989). Incidence of male breast cancer in Scandinavia, 1943-1982. *Int J Cancer* 43: 27-31.

815. Ewertz M, Holmberg L, Tretli S, Pedersen BV, Kristensen A (2001). Risk factors for male breast cancer - a case-control study from Scandinavia. *Acta Oncol* 40: 467-471.

816. Fackenthal JD, Cartegni L, Krainer AR, Olopade OI (2002). BRCA2 T2722R is a deleterious allele that causes exon skipping. *Am J Hum Genet* 71: 625-631.

817. Fackenthal JD, Marsh DJ, Richardson AL, Cummings SA, Eng C, Robinson BG, Olopade OI (2001). Male breast cancer in Cowden syndrome patients with germline PTEN mutations. *J Med Genet* 38: 159-164.

818. Fagundes H, Perez CA, Grigsby PW, Lockett MA (1992). Distant metastases after irradiation alone in carcinoma of the uterine cervix. *Int J Radiat Oncol Biol Phys* 24: 197-204.

819. Fairfield KM, Hankinson SE, Rosner BA, Hunter DJ, Colditz GA, Willett WC (2001). Risk of ovarian carcinoma and consumption of vitamins A, C, and E and specific carotenoids: a prospective analysis. *Cancer* 92: 2318-2326.

820. Falck J, Petrini JH, Williams BR, Lukas J, Bartek J (2002). The DNA damage-dependent intra-S phase checkpoint is regulated by parallel pathways. *Nat Genet* 30: 290-294.
821. Falconieri G, Della LD, Zanconati F, Bittesini L (1997). Leiomyosarcoma of the female breast: report of two new cases and a review of the literature. *Am J Clin Pathol* 108: 19-25.
822. Falkenberry SS, Steinhoff MM, Gordinier M, Rappoport S, Gajewski W, Granai CO (1996). Synchronous endometrioid tumors of the ovary and endometrium. A clinicopathologic study of 22 cases. *J Reprod Med* 41: 713-718.
823. Fan LD, Zang HY, Zhang XS (1996). Ovarian epidermoid cyst: report of eight cases. *Int J Gynecol Pathol* 15: 69-71.
824. Fanburg-Smith JC, Meis-Kindblom JM, Fante R, Kindblom LG (1998). Malignant granular cell tumor of soft tissue: diagnostic criteria and clinicopathologic correlation. *Am J Surg Pathol* 22: 779-794.
825. Fanning J, Lambert HC, Hale TM, Morris PC, Schuerch C (1999). Paget's disease of the vulva: prevalence of associated vulvar adenocarcinoma, invasive Paget's disease, and recurrence after surgical excision. *Am J Obstet Gynecol* 180: 24-27.
826. Faquin WC, Fitzgerald JT, Lin MC, Boynton KA, Muto MG, Mutter GL (2000). Sporadic microsatellite instability is specific to neoplastic and preneoplastic endometrial tissues. *Am J Clin Pathol* 113: 576-582.
827. Farshid G, Moinfar F, Meredith DJ, Peiterse S, Tavassoli FA (2001). Spindle cell ductal carcinoma in situ. An unusual variant of ductal intra-epithelial neoplasia that simulates ductal hyperplasia or a myoepithelial proliferation. *Virchows Arch* 439: 70-77.
828. Fastenberg NA, Martin RG, Buzdar AU, Hortobagyi GN, Montague ED, Blumenschein GR, Jessup JM (1985). Management of inflammatory carcinoma of the breast. A combined modality approach. *Am J Clin Oncol* 8: 134-141.
829. Fathalla MF (1967). The occurrence of granulosa and theca tumours in clinically normal ovaries. A study of 25 cases. *J Obstet Gynaecol Br Commonw* 74: 278-282.
830. Faul C, Kounelis S, Karasek K, Papadaki H, Greeenberger J, Jones MW (1996). Small cell carcinoma of the uterine cervix: Overespression of p53, Bcl2, and CD 44. *Int J Gynecol Cancer* 6: 369-375.
831. Faverly DR, Burgers L, Bult P, Holland R (1994). Three dimensional imaging of mammary ductal carcinoma in situ: clinical implications. *Semin Diagn Pathol* 11: 193-198.
832. Fawcett FJ, Kimbell NK (1971). Phaeochromocytoma of the ovary. *J Obstet Gynaecol Br Commonw* 78: 458-459.
833. Feakins RM, Lowe DG (1997). Basal cell carcinoma of the vulva: a clinicopathologic study of 45 cases. *Int J Gynecol Pathol* 16: 319-324.
834. Fechner RE (1972). Infiltrating lobular carcinoma without lobular carcinoma in situ. *Cancer* 29: 1539-1545.
835. Fechner RE (1975). Histologic variants of infiltrating lobular carcinoma of the breast. *Hum Pathol* 6: 373-378.
836. Fechner RE, Mills SE (1990). Breast Pathology Benign Proliferations, Atypias In Situ Carcinomas. ASCP Press - American Society of Clinical Pathologist: Chicago.
837. Feczko JD, Jentz DL, Roth LM (1996). Adenoid cystic ovarian carcinoma compared with other adenoid cystic carcinomas of the female genital tract. *Mod Pathol* 9: 413-417.
838. Feeley KM, Wells M (2001). Precursor lesions of ovarian epithelial malignancy. *Histopathology* 38: 87-95.
839. Fein DA, Fowble BL, Hanlon AL, Hooks MA, Hoffman JP, Sigurdson ER, Jardines LA, Eisenberg BL (1997). Identification of women with T1-T2 breast cancer at low risk of positive axillary nodes. *J Surg Oncol* 65: 34-39.
840. Feinmesser M, Sulkes A, Morgenstern S, Sulkes J, Stern S, Okon E (2000). HLA-DR and beta 2 microglobulin expression in medullary and atypical medullary carcinoma of the breast: histopathologically similar but biologically distinct entities. *J Clin Pathol* 53: 286-291.
841. Feldman LD, Hortobagyi GN, Buzdar AU, Ames FC, Blumenschein GR (1986). Pathological assessment of response to induction chemotherapy in breast cancer. *Cancer Res* 46: 2578-2581.
842. Feltmate CM, Genest DR, Wise L, Bernstein MR, Goldstein DP, Berkowitz RS (2001). Placental site trophoblastic tumor: a 17-year experience at the New England Trophoblastic Disease Center. *Gynecol Oncol* 82: 415-419.
843. Fenoglio C, Lattes R (1974). Sclerosing papillary proliferations in the female breast. A benign lesion often mistaken for carcinoma. *Cancer* 33: 691-700.
844. Fentiman IS, Millis RR, Smith P, Ellul JP, Lampejo O (1997). Mucoid breast carcinomas: histology and prognosis. *Br J Cancer* 75: 1061-1065.
845. Ferguson AW, Katabuchi H, Ronnett BM, Cho KR (2001). Glial implants in gliomatosis peritonei arise from normal tissue, not from the associated teratoma. *Am J Pathol* 159: 51-55.
846. Ferlay J, Bray F, Pisani P, Parkin DM (2001). *Globocan 2000*. Cancer Incidence, Mortality and Prevalence Worlwide. IARCPress: Lyon.
847. Fernandez FA, Val-Bernal F, Garijo-Ayensa F (1989). Mixed lipomas of the uterus and the broad ligament. *Appl Pathol* 7: 70-71.
848. Feroze M, Aravindan KP, Thomas M (1997). Mullerian adenosarcoma of the uterine cervix. *Indian J Cancer* 34: 68-72.
849. Ferry JA, Scully RE (1988). "Adenoid cystic" carcinoma and adenoid basal carcinoma of the uterine cervix. A study of 28 cases. *Am J Surg Pathol* 12: 134-144.
850. Ferry JA, Scully RE (1990). Mesonephric remnants, hyperplasia, and neoplasia in the uterine cervix. A study of 49 cases. *Am J Surg Pathol* 14: 1100-1111.
851. Ferry JA, Young RH (1991). Malignant lymphoma, pseudolymphoma, and hematopoietic disorders of the female genital tract. *Pathol Annu 26 Pt* 1: 227-263.
852. Ferry JA, Young RH, Engel G, Scully RE (1994). Oxyphilic Sertoli cell tumor of the ovary: a report of three cases, two in patients with the Peutz-Jeghers syndrome. *Int J Gynecol Pathol* 13: 259-266.
853. Fetsch JF, Laskin WB, Lefkowitz M, Kindblom LG, Meis-Kindblom JM (1996). Aggressive angiomyxoma: a clinicopathologic study of 29 female patients. *Cancer* 78: 79-90.
854. Fetsch JF, Laskin WB, Tavassoli FA (1997). Superficial angiomyxoma (cutaneous myxoma): a clinicopathologic study of 17 cases arising in the genital region. *Int J Gynecol Pathol* 16: 325-334.
855. Feyrter F, Hartmann G (1963). Uber die carcinoide Wuchsform des Carcinoma mammae, insbesondere das Carcinoma solidum (gelatinosum) mamma. *Fradf Z Pathol* 73: 24-30.
856. Fiche M, Avet-Loiseau H, Maugard CM, Sagan C, Heymann MF, Leblanc M, Classe JM, Fumoleau P, Dravet F, Mahe M, Dutrillaux B (2000). Gene amplifications detected by fluorescence in situ hybridization in pure intraductal breast carcinomas: relation to morphology, cell proliferation and expression of breast cancer-related genes. *Int J Cancer* 89: 403-410.
857. Fina F, Romain S, Ouafik L, Palmari J, Ben Ayed F, Benharkat S, Bonnier P, Spyratos F, Foekens JA, Rose C, Buisson M, Gerard H, Reymond MO, Seigneurin JM, Martin PM (2001). Frequency and genome load of Epstein-Barr virus in 509 breast cancers from different geographical areas. *Br J Cancer* 84: 783-790.
858. Fingerland A (1938). Ganglioneuroma of the cervix uteri. *J Pathol Bacteriol* 47: 631-634.
859. Fink D, Kubik-Huch RA, Wildermuth S (2001). Juvenile granulosa cell tumor. *Abdom Imaging* 26: 550-552.
860. Fink D, Nebel S, Aebi S, Zheng H, Kim HK, Christen RD, Howell SB (1997). Expression of the DNA mismatch repair proteins hMLH1 and hPMS2 in normal human tissues. *Br J Cancer* 76: 890-893.
861. Finkler NJ, Berkowitz RS, Driscoll SG, Goldstein DP, Bernstein MR (1988). Clinical experience with placental site trophoblastic tumors at the New England Trophoblastic Disease Center. *Obstet Gynecol* 71: 854-857.
862. Finn WF, Javert CT (1949). Primary and metastatic cancer of the fallopian tube. *Cancer* 2: 803-814.
863. Fishel R (2001). The selection for mismatch repair defects in hereditary nonpolyposis colorectal cancer: revising the mutator hypothesis. *Cancer Res* 61: 7369-7374.
864. Fishel R, Lescoe MK, Rao MR, Copeland NG, Jenkins NA, Garber J, Kane M, Kolodner R (1993). The human mutator gene homolog MSH2 and its association with hereditary nonpolyposis colon cancer. *Cell* 75: 1027-1038.
865. Fisher B, Costantino JP, Wickerham DL, Redmond CK, Kavanah M, Cronin WM, Vogel V, Robidoux A, Dimitrov N, Atkins J, Daly M, Wieand S, Tan-Chiu E, Ford L, Wolmark N (1998). Tamoxifen for prevention of breast cancer: report of the National Surgical Adjuvant Breast and Bowel Project P-1 Study. *J Natl Cancer Inst* 90: 1371-1388.
866. Fisher B, Dignam J, Wolmark N, Wickerham DL, Fisher ER, Mamounas E, Smith R, Begovic M, Dimitrov NV, Margolese RG, Kardinal CG, Kavanah MT, Fehrenbacher L, Oishi RH (1999). Tamoxifen in treatment of intraductal breast cancer: National Surgical Adjuvant Breast and Bowel Project B-24 randomised controlled trial. *Lancet* 353: 1993-2000.
867. Fisher CJ, Hanby AM, Robinson L, Millis RR (1992). Mammary hamartoma--a review of 35 cases. *Histopathology* 20: 99-106.
868. Fisher ER, Anderson S, Redmond C, Fisher B (1993). Pathologic findings from the National Surgical Adjuvant Breast Project protocol B-06. 10-year pathologic and clinical prognostic discriminants. *Cancer* 71: 2507-2514.
869. Fisher ER, Costantino J, Fisher B, Palekar AS, Paik SM, Suarez CM, Wolmark N (1996). Pathologic findings from the National Surgical Adjuvant Breast Project (NSABP) Protocol B-17. Five-year observations concerning lobular carcinoma in situ. *Cancer* 78: 1403-1416.
870. Fisher ER, Costantino J, Fisher B, Palekar AS, Redmond C, Mamounas E (1995). Pathologic findings from the National Surgical Adjuvant Breast Project (NSABP) Protocol B-17. Intraductal carcinoma (ductal carcinoma in situ). The National Surgical Adjuvant Breast and Bowel Project Collaborating Investigators. *Cancer* 75: 1310-1319.
871. Fisher ER, Costantino J, Fisher B, Redmond C (1993). Pathologic findings from the National Surgical Adjuvant Breast Project (Protocol 4). Discriminants for 15-year survival. National Surgical Adjuvant Breast and Bowel Project Investigators. *Cancer* 71: 2141-2150.
872. Fisher ER, Fisher B, Sass R, Wickerham L (1984). Pathologic findings from the National Surgical Adjuvant Breast Project (Protocol No. 4). XI. Bilateral breast cancer. *Cancer* 54: 3002-3011.
873. Fisher ER, Gregorio R, Kim WS, Redmond C (1977). Lipid in invasive cancer of the breast. *Am J Clin Pathol* 68: 558-561.
874. Fisher ER, Gregorio RM, Fisher B, Redmond C, Vellios F, Sommers SC (1975). The pathology of invasive breast cancer. A syllabus derived from findings of the National Surgical Adjuvant Breast Project (protocol no. 4). *Cancer* 36: 1-85.
875. Fisher ER, Gregorio RM, Redmond C, Fisher B (1977). Tubulolobular invasive breast cancer: a variant of lobular invasive cancer. *Hum Pathol* 8: 679-683.
876. Fisher ER, Kenny JP, Sass R, Dimitrov NV, Siderits RH, Fisher B (1990). Medullary cancer of the breast revisited. *Breast Cancer Res Treat* 16: 215-229.
877. Fisher ER, Palekar AS, Gregorio RM, Redmond C, Fisher B (1978). Pathological findings from the National Surgical Adjuvant Breast Project (Protocol No 4) IV. Significance of tumour necrosis. *Hum Pathol* 9: 523-530.
878. Fisher ER, Palekar AS, Gregorio RM, Paulson JD (1983). Mucoepidermoid and squamous cell carcinomas of breast with reference to squamous metaplasia and giant cell tumors. *Am J Surg Pathol* 7: 15-27.
879. Fisher ER, Palekar AS, Redmond C, Barton B, Fisher B (1980). Pathologic findings from the National Surgical Adjuvant Breast Project (protocol no. 4). VI. Invasive papillary cancer. *Am J Clin Pathol* 73: 313-322.
880. Fisher ER, Tavares J, Bulatao IS, Sass R, Fisher B (1985). Glycogen-rich, clear cell breast cancer: with comments concerning other clear cell variants. *Hum Pathol* 16: 1085-1090.
881. Fisher PE, Estabrook A, Cohen MB (1990). Fine needle aspiration biopsy of intramammary neurilemoma. *Acta Cytol* 34: 35-37.

882. Fisher RA, Lawler SD, Ormerod MG, Imrie PR, Povey S (1987). Flow cytometry used to distinguish between complete and partial hydatidiform moles. *Placenta* 8: 249-256.

883. Fishman DA, Schwartz PE (1994). Current approaches to diagnosis and treatment of ovarian germ cell malignancies. *Curr Opin Obstet Gynecol* 6: 98-104.

884. FitzGerald MG, Bean JM, Hegde SR, Unsal H, MacDonald DJ, Harkin DP, Finkelstein DM, Isselbacher KJ, Haber DA (1997). Heterozygous ATM mutations do not contribute to early onset of breast cancer. *Nat Genet* 15: 307-310.

885. Fitzgibbons PL, Henson DE, Hutter RV (1998). Benign breast changes and the risk for subsequent breast cancer: an update of the 1985 consensus statement. Cancer Committee of the College of American Pathologists. *Arch Pathol Lab Med* 122: 1053-1055.

886. Fitzgibbons PL, Page DL, Weaver D, Thor AD, Allred DC, Clark GM, Ruby SG, O'Malley F, Simpson JF, Connolly JL, Hayes DF, Edge SB, Lichter A, Schnitt SJ (2000). Prognostic factors in breast cancer. College of American Pathologists Consensus Statement 1999. *Arch Pathol Lab Med* 124: 966-978.

887. Flagiello D, Gerbault-Seureau M, Sastre-Garau X, Padoy E, Vielh P, Dutrillaux B (1998). Highly recurrent der(1;16)(q10;p10) and other 16q arm alterations in lobular breast cancer. *Genes Chromosomes Cancer* 23: 300-306.

888. Flanagan CW, Parker JR, Mannel RS, Min KW, Kida M (1997). Primary endodermal sinus tumor of the vulva: a case report and review of the literature. *Gynecol Oncol* 66: 515-518.

889. Flemming P, Wellmann A, Maschek H, Lang H, Georgii A (1995). Monoclonal antibodies against inhibin represent key markers of adult granulosa cell tumors of the ovary even in their metastases. A report of three cases with late metastasis, being previously misinterpreted as hemangiopericytoma. *Am J Surg Pathol* 19: 927-933.

890. Fletcher CD, Tsang WY, Fisher C, Lee KC, Chan JK (1992). Angiomyofibroblastoma of the vulva. A benign neoplasm distinct from aggressive angiomyxoma. *Am J Surg Pathol* 16: 373-382.

891. Fletcher JA, Pinkus JL, Lage JM, Morton CC, Pinkus GS (1992). Clonal 6p21 rearrangement is restricted to the mesenchymal component of an endometrial polyp. *Genes Chromosomes Cancer* 5: 260-263.

892. Flint A, Gikas PW, Roberts JA (1985). Alveolar soft part sarcoma of the uterine cervix. *Gynecol Oncol* 22: 263-267.

893. Flint A, Oberman HA (1984). Infarction and squamous metaplasia of intraductal papilloma: a benign breast lesion that may simulate carcinoma. *Hum Pathol* 15: 764-767.

894. Fogt F, Vortmeyer AO, Ahn G, De Girolami U, Hunt RB, Daly T, Loda M (1994). Neural cyst of the ovary with central nervous system microvasculature. *Histopathology* 24: 477-480.

895. Foote FW, Stewart FW (1946). A histologic classification of carcinoma of the breast. *Surgery* 19: 74-99.

896. Ford D, Easton DF, Bishop DT, Narod SA, Goldgar DE (1994). Risks of cancer in BRCA1-mutation carriers. Breast Cancer Linkage Consortium. *Lancet* 343: 692-695.

897. Ford D, Easton DF, Peto J (1995). Estimates of the gene frequency of BRCA1 and its contribution to breast and ovarian cancer incidence. *Am J Hum Genet* 57: 1457-1462.

898. Ford D, Easton DF, Stratton M, Narod S, Goldgar D, Devilee P, Bishop DT, Weber B, Lenoir G, Chang-Claude J, Sobol H, Teare MD, Struewing J, Arason A, Scherneck S, Peto J, Rebbeck TR, Tonin P, Neuhausen S, Barkardottir R, Eyfjord J, Lynch H, Ponder BA, Gayther SA, Zelada-Hedman M, Birch JM, Lindblom A, Stoppa-Lyonnet D, Bignon Y, Borg A, Hamann U, Haites N, Scott RJ, Maugard CM, Vasen H (1998). Genetic heterogeneity and penetrance analysis of the BRCA1 and BRCA2 genes in breast cancer families. The Breast Cancer Linkage Consortium. *Am J Hum Genet* 62: 676-689.

899. Ford D, Easton DF, Stratton M, Narod S, Goldgar D, Devilee P, Bishop DT, Weber B, Lenoir G, Chang-Claude J, Sobol H, Teare MD, Struewing J, Arason A, Scherneck S, Peto J, Rebbeck TR, Tonin P, Neuhausen S, Barkardottir R, Eyfjord J, Lynch H, Ponder BA, Gayther SA, Zelada-Hedman M (1998). Genetic heterogeneity and penetrance analysis of the BRCA1 and BRCA2 genes in breast cancer families. The Breast Cancer Linkage Consortium. *Am J Hum Genet* 62: 676-689.

900. Foschini MP, Eusebi V (1998). Carcinomas of the breast showing myoepithelial cell differentiation. A review of the literature. *Virchows Arch* 432: 303-310.

901. Foschini MP, Eusebi V, Tison V (1989). Alveolar soft part sarcoma of the cervix uteri. A case report. *Pathol Res Pract* 184: 354-358.

902. Foschini MP, Marucci G, Eusebi V (2002). Low-grade mucoepidermoid carcinoma of salivary glands: characteristic immunohistochemical profile and evidence of striated duct differentiation. *Virchows Arch* 440: 536-542.

903. Foschini MP, Pizzicannella G, Peterse JL, Eusebi V (1995). Adenomyoepithelioma of the breast associated with low-grade adenosquamous and sarcomatoid carcinomas. *Virchows Arch* 427: 243-250.

904. Foulkes WD, Wong N, Brunet JS, Narod SA (1998). BRCA mutations and survival in breast cancer. *J Clin Oncol* 16: 3206-3208.

905. Fox H, Agrawal K, Langley FA (1972). The Brenner tumour of the ovary. A clinicopathological study of 54 cases. *J Obstet Gynaecol Br Commonw* 79: 661-665.

906. Fox H, Agrawal K, Langley FA (1975). A clinicopathologic study of 92 cases of granulosa cell tumor of the ovary with special reference to the factors influencing prognosis. *Cancer* 35: 231-241.

907. Fox H, Laurini RN (1988). Intraplacental choriocarcinoma: a report of two cases. *J Clin Pathol* 41: 1085-1088.

908. Fox H, Sen DK (1967). A Krukenberg tumour of the uterine cervix. *J Obstet Gynaecol Br Commonw* 74: 449-450.

909. Fox H, Wells M, Harris M, McWilliam LJ, Anderson GS (1988). Enteric tumours of the lower female genital tract: a report of three cases. *Histopathology* 12: 167-176.

910. Frable WJ, Kay S (1968). Carcinoma of the breast. Histologic and clinical features of apocrine tumors. *Cancer* 21: 756-763.

911. Fracchia AA, Robinson D, Legaspi A, Greenall MJ, Kinne DW, Groshen S (1985). Survival in bilateral breast cancer. *Cancer* 55: 1414-1421.

912. Fraga M, Prieto O, Garcia-Caballero T, Beiras A, Forteza J (1994). Myxoid leiomyosarcoma of the uterine cervix. *Histopathology* 25: 381-384.

913. Franceschi S, Dal Maso L, Arniani S, Crosignani P, Vercelli M, Simonato L, Falcini F, Zanetti R, Barchielli A, Serraino D, Rezza G (1998). Risk of cancer other than Kaposi's sarcoma and non-Hodgkin's lymphoma in persons with AIDS in Italy. Cancer and AIDS Registry Linkage Study. *Br J Cancer* 78: 966-970.

914. Franquemont DW, Frierson HF Jr., Mills SE (1991). An immunohistochemical study of normal endometrial stroma and endometrial stromal neoplasms. Evidence for smooth muscle differentiation. *Am J Surg Pathol* 15: 861-870.

915. Fraser JL, Raza S, Chorny K, Connolly JL, Schnitt SJ (1998). Columnar alteration with prominent apical snouts and secretions: a spectrum of changes frequently present in breast biopsies performed for microcalcifications. *Am J Surg Pathol* 22: 1521-1527.

916. Frei KA, Kinkel K (2001). Staging endometrial cancer: role of magnetic resonance imaging. *J Magn Reson Imaging* 13: 850-855.

917. Friedman HD, Mazur MT (1991). Primary ovarian leiomyosarcoma. An immunohistochemical and ultrastructural study. *Arch Pathol Lab Med* 115: 941-945.

918. Friedman LS, Gayther SA, Kurosaki T, Gordon D, Noble B, Casey G, Ponder BA, Anton-Culver H (1997). Mutation analysis of BRCA1 and BRCA2 in a male breast cancer population. *Am J Hum Genet* 60: 313-319.

919. Friedrich EG Jr., Wilkinson EJ, Fu YS (1980). Carcinoma in situ of the vulva: a continuing challenge. *Am J Obstet Gynecol* 136: 830-843.

920. Frisch M, Biggar RJ, Goedert JJ (2000). Human papillomavirus-associated cancers in patients with human immunodeficiency virus infection and acquired immunodeficiency syndrome. *J Natl Cancer Inst* 92: 1500-1510.

921. Fritz A, Percy C, Jack A, Shanmugaratnam K, Sobin LH, Parkin DM, Whelan S (2000). *International Classification of Diseases for Oncology (ICD-O)*. 3rd ed. World Health Organization: Geneva.

922. Frixen UH, Behrens J, Sachs M, Eberle G, Voss B, Warda A, Lochner D, Birchmeier W (1991). E-cadherin-mediated cell-cell adhesion prevents invasiveness of human carcinoma cells. *J Cell Biol* 113: 173-185.

923. Fujii H, Matsumoto T, Yoshida M, Furugen Y, Takagaki T, Iwabuchi K, Nakata Y, Takagi Y, Moriya T, Ohtsuji N, Ohtsuji M, Hirose S, Shirai T (2002). Genetics of synchronous uterine and ovarian endometrioid carcinoma: combined analyses of loss of heterozygosity, PTEN mutation, and microsatellite instability. *Hum Pathol* 33: 421-428.

924. Fujii H, Szumel R, Marsh C, Zhou W, Gabrielson E (1996). Genetic progression, histological grade, and allelic loss in ductal carcinoma in situ of the breast. *Cancer Res* 56: 5260-5265.

925. Fujii H, Yoshida M, Gong ZX, Matsumoto T, Hamano Y, Fukunaga M, Hruban RH, Gabrielson E, Shirai T (2000). Frequent genetic heterogeneity in the clonal evolution of gynecological carcinosarcoma and its influence on phenotypic diversity. *Cancer Res* 60: 114-120.

926. Fujita M, Enomoto T, Wada H, Inoue M, Okudaira Y, Shroyer KR (1996). Application of clonal analysis. Differential diagnosis for synchronous primary ovarian and endometrial cancers and metastatic cancer. *Am J Clin Pathol* 105: 350-359.

927. Fujiwaki R, Yoshida M, Iida K, Ohnishi Y, Ryuko K, Miyazaki K (1998). Epithelioid leiomyosarcoma of the uterine cervix. *Acta Obstet Gynecol Scand* 77: 246-248.

928. Fukunaga M (2001). Pseudoangiomatous hyperplasia of mammary stroma: a case of pure type after removal of fibroadenoma. *APMIS* 109: 113-116.

929. Fukunaga M, Ishihara A, Ushigome S (1998). Extrauterine low-grade endometrial stromal sarcoma: report of three cases. *Pathol Int* 48: 297-302.

930. Fukunaga M, Miyazawa Y, Ushigome S (1997). Endometrial low-grade stromal sarcoma with ovarian sex cord-like differentiation: report of two cases with an immunohistochemical and flow cytometric study. *Pathol Int* 47: 412-415.

931. Fukunaga M, Nomura K, Endo Y, Ushigome S, Aizawa S (1996). Carcino-sarcoma of the uterus with extensive neuroectodermal differentiation. *Histopathology* 29: 565-570.

932. Fukunaga M, Nomura K, Ishikawa E, Ushigome S (1997). Ovarian atypical endometriosis: its close association with malignant epithelial tumours. *Histopathology* 30: 249-255.

933. Fukunaga M, Ushigome S (1993). Malignant trophoblastic tumors: immunohistochemical and flow cytometric comparison of choriocarcinoma and placental site trophoblastic tumors. *Hum Pathol* 24: 1098-1106.

934. Fukunaga M, Ushigome S (1997). Myofibroblastoma of the breast with diverse differentiations. *Arch Pathol Lab Med* 121: 599-603.

935. Fukunaga M, Ushigome S, Fukunaga M, Sugishita M (1993). Application of flow cytometry in diagnosis of hydatidiform moles. *Mod Pathol* 6: 353-359.

936. Fukushima M, Twiggs LB, Okagaki T (1986). Mixed intestinal adenocarcinoma-argentaffin carcinoma of the vagina. *Gynecol Oncol* 23: 387-394.

937. Fulop V, Mok SC, Genest DR, Gati I, Doszpod J, Berkowitz RS (1998). p53, p21, Rb and mdm2 oncoproteins. Expression in normal placenta, partial and complete mole, and choriocarcinoma. *J Reprod Med* 43: 119-127.

938. Fulop V, Mok SC, Genest DR, Szigetvari I, Cseh I, Berkowitz RS (1998). c-myc, c-erbB-2, c-fms and bcl-2 oncoproteins. Expression in normal placenta, partial and complete mole, and choriocarcinoma. *J Reprod Med* 43: 101-110.

939. Funk KC, Heiken JP (1989). Papillary cystadenoma of the broad ligament in a patient with von Hippel-Lindau disease. *AJR Am J Roentgenol* 153: 527-528.

940. Furuya M, Shimizu M, Nishihara H, Ito T, Sakuragi N, Ishikura H, Yoshiki T (2001). Clear cell variant of malignant melanoma of the uterine cervix: a case report and review of the literature. *Gynecol Oncol* 80: 409-412.

941. Gabbay-Moore M, Ovadia Y, Neri A (1982). Accessory ovaries with bilateral dermoid cysts. *Eur J Obstet Gynecol Reprod Biol* 14: 171-173.

942. Gaber LW, Redline RW, Mostoufi-Zadeh M, Driscoll SG (1986). Invasive partial mole. *Am J Clin Pathol* 85: 722-724.

943. Gad A, Azzopardi JG (1975). Lobular carcinoma of the breast: a special variant of mucin-secreting carcinoma. *J Clin Pathol* 28: 711-716.
944. Gad S, Caux-Moncoutier V, Pages-Berhouet S, Gauthier-Villars M, Coupier I, Pujol P, Frenay M, Gilbert B, Maugard C, Bignon YJ, Chevrier A, Rossi A, Fricker JP, Nguyen TD, Demange L, Aurias A, Bensimon A, Stoppa-Lyonnet D (2002). Significant contribution of large BRCA1 gene rearrangements in 120 French breast and ovarian cancer families. *Oncogene* 21: 6841-6847.
945. Gadaleanu V, Craciun C (1987). Malignant oncocytoma of the breast. *Zentralbl Allg Pathol* 133: 279-283.
946. Gadducci A, Ferdeghini M, Prontera C, Moretti L, Mariani G, Bianchi R, Fioretti P (1992). The concomitant determination of different tumor markers in patients with epithelial ovarian cancer and benign ovarian masses: relevance for differential diagnosis. *Gynecol Oncol* 44: 147-154.
947. Gadducci A, Landoni F, Sartori E, Zola P, Maggino T, Lissoni A, Bazzurini L, Arisio R, Romagnolo C, Cristofani R (1996). Uterine leiomyosarcoma: analysis of treatment failures and survival. *Gynecol Oncol* 62: 25-32.
948. Gaertner EM, Farley JH, Taylor RR, Silver SA (1999). Collision of uterine rhabdoid tumor and endometrioid adenocarcinoma: a case report and review of the literature. *Int J Gynecol Pathol* 18: 396-401.
949. Gaffey MJ, Mills SE, Boyd JC (1994). Aggressive papillary tumor of middle ear/temporal bone and adnexal papillary cystadenoma. Manifestations of von Hippel-Lindau disease. *Am J Surg Pathol* 18: 1254-1260.
950. Gaffey MJ, Mills SE, Frierson HF Jr., Zarbo RJ, Boyd JC, Simpson JF, Weiss LM (1995). Medullary carcinoma of the breast: interobserver variability in histopathologic diagnosis. *Mod Pathol* 8: 31-38.
951. Gagnon Y, Tetu B (1989). Ovarian metastases of breast carcinoma. A clinicopathologic study of 59 cases. *Cancer* 64: 892-898.
952. Gal R, Dekel A, Ben David M, Goldman JA, Kessler E (1988). Granular cell myoblastoma of the cervix. Case report. *Br J Obstet Gynaecol* 95: 720-722.
953. Galant C, Mazy S, Berliere M, Mazy G, Wallon J, Marbaix E (1997). Two schwannomas presenting as lumps in the same breast. *Diagn Cytopathol* 16: 281-284.
954. Galea MH, Blamey RW, Elston CE, Ellis IO (1992). The Nottingham Prognostic Index in primary breast cancer. *Breast Cancer Res Treat* 22: 207-219.
955. Gamallo C, Palacios J, Moreno G, Calvo dM, Suarez A, Armas A (1999). beta-catenin expression pattern in stage I and II ovarian carcinomas : relationship with beta-catenin gene mutations, clinicopathological features, and clinical outcome. *Am J Pathol* 155: 527-536.
956. Gamallo C, Palacios J, Suarez A, Pizarro A, Navarro P, Quintanilla M, Cano A (1993). Correlation of E-cadherin expression with differentiation grade and histological type in breast carcinoma. *Am J Pathol* 142: 987-993.
957. Garber JE, Goldstein AM, Kantor AF, Dreyfus MG, Fraumeni JF Jr., Li FP (1991). Follow-up study of twenty-four families with Li-Fraumeni syndrome. *Cancer Res* 51: 6094-6097.
958. Garcia-Higuera I, Taniguchi T, Ganesan S, Meyn MS, Timmers C, Hejna J, Grompe M, D'Andrea AD (2001). Interaction of the Fanconi anemia proteins and BRCA1 in a common pathway. *Mol Cell* 7: 249-262.
959. Garcia A, Bussaglia E, Machin P, Matias-Guiu X, Prat J (2000). Loss of heterozygosity on chromosome 17q in epithelial ovarian tumors: association with carcinomas with serous differentiation. *Int J Gynecol Pathol* 19: 152-157.
960. Garcia R, Troyas RG, Bercero EA (1995). Mullerian adenosarcoma of the cervix: differential diagnosis, histogenesis and review of the literature. *Pathol Int* 45: 890-894.
961. Gardella C, Chumas JC, Pearl ML (1996). Ovarian lipoma of teratomatous origin. *Obstet Gynecol* 87: 874-875.
962. Gardner GH, Greene RR, Peckham BM (1948). Normal and cystic structures of the broad ligament. *Am J Obstet Gynecol* 55: 917-939.
963. Garg PP, Kerlikowske K, Subak L, Grady D (1998). Hormone replacement therapy and the risk of epithelial ovarian carcinoma: a meta-analysis. *Obstet Gynecol* 92: 472-479.
964. Garrett AP, Lee KR, Colitti CR, Muto MG, Berkowitz RS, Mok SC (2001). k-ras mutation may be an early event in mucinous ovarian tumorigenesis. *Int J Gynecol Pathol* 20: 244-251.
965. Garrett AP, Ng SW, Muto MG, Welch WR, Bell DA, Berkowitz RS, Mok SC (2000). ras gene activation and infrequent mutation in papillary serous carcinoma of the peritoneum. *Gynecol Oncol* 77: 105-111.
966. Garzetti GG, Ciavattini A, Goteri G, Stramazzoti D, Fabris G, Mannello B, Romanini C (1996). Proliferating cell nuclear antigen (PCNA) immunoreactivity in stage I endometrial cancer: A new prognostic factor. *Int J Gynecol Cancer* 6: 186-192.
967. Garzetti GG, Ciavattini A, Goteri G, Menzo S, de Nictolis M, Clementi M, Brugia M, Romanini C (1994). Vaginal micropapillary lesions are not related to human papillomavirus infection: in situ hybridization and polymerase chain reaction detection techniques. *Gynecol Obstet Invest* 38: 134-139.
968. Gatalica Z, Norris BA, Kovatich AJ (2000). Immunohistochemical localization of prostate-specific antigen in ductal epithelium of male breast. Potential diagnostic pitfall in patients with gynecomastia. *Appl Immunohistochem Molecul Morphol* 8: 158-161.
969. Gatchell FG, Dockerty MB, Clagett OT (1958). Intracystic carcinoma of the breast. *Surg Gynecol Obstet* 106: 347.
970. Gatta G, Lasota MB, Verdecchia A (1998). Survival of European women with gynaecological tumours, during the period 1978-1989. *Eur J Cancer* 34: 2218-2225.
971. Gatti RA, Tward A, Concannon P (1999). Cancer risk in ATM heterozygotes: a model of phenotypic and mechanistic differences between missense and truncating mutations. *Mol Genet Metab* 68: 419-423.
972. Gayther SA, Mangion J, Russell P, Seal S, Barfoot R, Ponder BA, Stratton MR, Easton D (1997). Variation of risks of breast and ovarian cancer associated with different germline mutations of the BRCA2 gene. *Nat Genet* 15: 103-105.
973. Gayther SA, Russell P, Harrington P, Antoniou AC, Easton DF, Ponder BA (1999). The contribution of germline BRCA1 and BRCA2 mutations to familial ovarian cancer: no evidence for other ovarian cancer-susceptibility genes. *Am J Hum Genet* 65: 1021-1029.
974. Gayther SA, Warren W, Mazoyer S, Russell PA, Harrington PA, Chiano M, Seal S, Hamoudi R, van Rensburg EJ, Dunning AM, Love R, Evans G, Easton D, Clayton D, Stratton MR, Ponder BAJ (1995). Germline mutations of the BRCA1 gene in breast and ovarian cancer families provide evidence for a genotype-phenotype correlation. *Nat Genet* 11: 428-433.
975. Gehrig PA, Groben PA, Fowler WC Jr., Walton LA, Van Le L (2001). Noninvasive papillary serous carcinoma of the endometrium. *Obstet Gynecol* 97: 153-157.
976. Geisler S, Lonning PE, Aas T, Johnsen H, Fluge O, Haugen DF, Lillehaug JR, Akslen LA, Borresen-Dale AL (2001). Influence of TP53 gene alterations and c-erbB-2 expression on the response to treatment with doxorubicin in locally advanced breast cancer. *Cancer Res* 61: 2505-2512.
977. Genest DR (2001). Partial hydatidiform mole: clinicopathological features, differential diagnosis, ploidy and molecular studies, and gold standards for diagnosis. *Int J Gynecol Pathol* 20: 315-322.
978. Genest DR, Laborde O, Berkowitz RS, Goldstein DP, Bernstein MR, Lage J (1991). A clinicopathologic study of 153 cases of complete hydatidiform mole (1980-1990): histologic grade lacks prognostic significance. *Obstet Gynecol* 78: 402-409.
979. Geng L, Connolly DC, Isacson C, Ronnett BM, Cho KR (1999). Atypical immature metaplasia (AIM) of the cervix: is it related to high-grade squamous intraepithelial lesion (HSIL)? *Hum Pathol* 30: 345-351.
980. Gentile G, Formelli G, Pelusi G, Flamigni C (1997). Is vestibular micropapillomatosis associated with human papillomavirus infection? *Eur J Gynaecol Oncol* 18: 523-525.
981. Geoffroy-Perez B, Janin N, Ossian K, Lauge A, Croquette MF, Griscelli C, Debre M, Bressac-de-Paillerets B, Aurias A, Stoppa-Lyonnet D, Andrieu N (2001). Cancer risk in heterozygotes for ataxia-telangiectasia. *Int J Cancer* 93: 288-293.
982. Georgiannos SN, Chin Aleong J, Goode AW, Sheaff M (2001). Secondary Neoplasms of the Breast: A survey of the 20th Century. *Cancer* 92: 2259-2266.
983. Geraads A, Tary P, Cloup N (1991). [Demons-Meigs syndrome caused by ovarian goiter]. *Rev Pneumol Clin* 47: 194-196.
984. Gerald WL, Miller HK, Battifora H, Miettinen M, Silva EG, Rosai J (1991). Intra-abdominal desmoplastic small round-cell tumor. Report of 19 cases of a distinctive type of high-grade polyphenotypic malignancy affecting young individuals. *Am J Surg Pathol* 15: 499-513.
985. Gernow A, Ahrentsen OD (1989). Adenoid cystic carcinoma of the endometrium. *Histopathology* 15: 197-198.
986. Gersell DJ, Fulling KH (1989). Localized neurofibromatosis of the female genitourinary tract. *Am J Surg Pathol* 13: 873-878.
987. Gersell DJ, Katzenstein AL (1981). Spindle cell carcinoma of the breast. A clinocopathologic and ultrastructural study. *Hum Pathol* 12: 550-561.
988. Gersell DJ, King TC (1988). Papillary cystadenoma of the mesosalpinx in von Hippel-Lindau disease. *Am J Surg Pathol* 12: 145-149.
989. Gershenson DM, del Junco G, Silva EG, Copeland LJ, Wharton JT, Rutledge FN (1986). Immature teratoma of the ovary. *Obstet Gynecol* 68: 624-629.
990. Ghadially FN (1985). *Diagnostic Electron Microscopy of Tumors.* Butterworth & Company: London.
991. Ghazali S (1973). Embryonic rhabdomyosarcoma of the urogenital tract. *Br J Surg* 60: 124-128.
992. Giannacopoulos K, Giannacopoulou C, Matalliotakis I, Neonaki M, Papanicolaou N, Koumantakis E (1998). Pseudo-Meigs' syndrome caused by paraovarian fibroma. *Eur J Gynaecol Oncol* 19: 389-390.
993. Giannotti FO, Miiji LN, Vainchenker M, Gordan AN (2001). Breast cancer with choriocarcinomatous and neuroendocrine features. *Sao Paulo Med J* 119: 154-155.
994. Giardini R, Piccolo C, Rilke F (1992). Primary non-Hodgkin's lymphomas of the female breast. *Cancer* 69: 725-735.
995. Gibbons D, Leitch M, Coscia J, Lindberg G, Molberg K, Ashfaq R, Saboorian MH (2000). Fine Needle Aspiration Cytology and Histologic Findings of Granular Cell Tumor of the Breast: Review of 19 Cases with Clinical/Radiologic Correlation. *Breast J* 6: 27-30.
996. Gil-Moreno A, Garcia-Jimenez A, Gonzalez-Bosquet J, Esteller M, Castellvi-Vives J, Martinez Palones JM, Xercavins J (1997). Merkel cell carcinoma of the vulva. *Gynecol Oncol* 64: 526-532.
997. Gilbey S, Moore DH, Look KY, Sutton GP (1997). Vulvar keratoacanthoma. *Obstet Gynecol* 89: 848-850.
998. Gilchrist KW, Gould VE, Hirschl S, Imbriglia JE, Patchefsky AS, Penner DW, Pickren J, Schwartz IS, Wheeler JE, Barnes JM, Mansour EG (1982). Interobserver variation in the identification of breast carcinoma in intramammary lymphatics. *Hum Pathol* 13: 170-172.
999. Gilchrist KW, Gray R, Fowble B, Tormey DC, Taylor SG (1993). Tumor necrosis is a prognostic predictor for early recurrence and death in lymph node-positive breast cancer: a 10-year follow-up study of 728 Eastern Cooperative Oncology Group patients. *J Clin Oncol* 11: 1929-1935.
1000. Gilks CB, Alkushi A, Yue JJ, Lanvin D, Ehlen TG, Miller DM (2003). Advanced-stage serous borderline tumors of the ovary: a clinicopathological study of 49 cases. *Int J Gynecol Pathol* 22: 29-36.
1001. Gilks CB, Bell DA, Scully RE (1990). Serous psammocarcinoma of the ovary and peritoneum. *Int J Gynecol Pathol* 9: 110-121.
1002. Gilks CB, Clement PB, Hart WR, Young RH (2000). Uterine adenomyomas excluding atypical polypoid adenomyomas and adenomyomas of endocervical type: a clinicopathologic study of 30 cases of an underemphasized lesion that may cause diagnostic problems with brief consideration of adenomyomas of other female genital tract sites. *Int J Gynecol Pathol* 19: 195-205.
1003. Gilks CB, Clement PB, Wood WS (1989). Trichoblastic fibroma. A clinicopathologic study of three cases. *Am J Dermatopathol* 11: 397-402.

1004. Gilks CB, Young RH, Aguirre P, DeLellis RA, Scully RE (1989). Adenoma malignum (minimal deviation adenocarcinoma) of the uterine cervix. A clinicopathological and immunohistochemical analysis of 26 cases. *Am J Surg Pathol* 13: 717-729.
1005. Gilks CB, Young RH, Clement PB, Hart WR, Scully RE (1996). Adenomyomas of the uterine cervix of of endocervical type: a report of ten cases of a benign cervical tumor that may be confused with adenoma malignum. *Mod Pathol* 9: 220-224.
1006. Gilks CB, Young RH, Gersell DJ, Clement PB (1997). Large cell neuroendocrine carcinoma of the uterine cervix: a clinicopathologic study of 12 cases. *Am J Surg Pathol* 21: 905-914.
1007. Gillett CE, Lee AH, Millis RR, Barnes DM (1998). Cyclin D1 and associated proteins in mammary ductal carcinoma in situ and atypical ductal hyperplasia. *J Pathol* 184: 396-400.
1008. Gimm O, Attie-Bitach T, Lees JA, Vekemans M, Eng C (2000). Expression of the PTEN tumour suppressor protein during human development. *Hum Mol Genet* 9: 1633-1639.
1009. Ginolhac SM, Gad S, Corbex M, Bressac-de-Paillerets B, Chompret A, Bignon YJ, Peyrat JP, Fournier J, Lasset C, Giraud S, Muller D, Fricker JP, Hardouin A, Berthet P, Maugard C, Nogues C, Lidereau R, Longy M, Olschwang S, Toulas C, Guimbaud R, Yannoukakos D, Szabo C, Durocher F, Moisan AM, Simard J, Mazoyer S, Lynch HT, Goldgar D, Stoppa-Lyonnet D, Lenoir GM, Sinilnikova OM (2003). BRCA1 wild-type allele modifies risk of ovarian cancer in carriers of BRCA1 germ-line mutations. *Cancer Epidemiol Biomarkers Prev* 12: 90-95.
1010. Giri DD, Dundas SA, Nottingham JF, Underwood JC (1989). Oestrogen receptors in benign epithelial lesions and intraduct carcinomas of the breast: an immunohistological study. *Histopathology* 15: 575-584.
1011. Giroud F, Haroske G, Reith A, Bocking A (1998). 1997 ESACP consensus report on diagnostic DNA image cytometry. Part II: Specific recommendations for quality assurance. European Society for Analytical Cellular Pathology. *Anal Cell Pathol* 17: 201-208.
1012. Gisser SD (1986). Obstructing fallopian tube papilloma. *Int J Gynecol Pathol* 5: 179-182.
1013. Gissmann L, deVilliers EM, zur Hausen H (1982). Analysis of human genital warts (condylomata acuminata) and other genital tumors for human papillomavirus type 6 DNA. *Int J Cancer* 29: 143-146.
1014. Gissmann L, Wolnik L, Ikenberg H, Koldovsky U, Schnurch HG, zur Hausen H (1983). Human papillomavirus types 6 and 11 DNA sequences in genital and laryngeal papillomas and in some cervical cancers. *Proc Natl Acad Sci USA* 80: 560-563.
1015. Glaser SL, Ambinder RF, DiGiuseppe JA, Horn-Ross PL, Hsu JL (1998). Absence of Epstein-Barr virus EBER-1 transcripts in an epidemiologically diverse group of breast cancers. *Int J Cancer* 75: 555-558.
1016. Glaubitz LC, Bowen JH, Cox EB, McCarty KS Jr. (1984). Elastosis in human breast cancer. Correlation with sex steroid receptors and comparison with clinical outcome. *Arch Pathol Lab Med* 108: 27-30.
1017. Gleeson NC, Ruffolo EH, Hoffman MS, Cavanagh D (1994). Basal cell carcinoma of the vulva with groin node metastasis. *Gynecol Oncol* 53: 366-368.
1018. Gloor E, Dialdas J, Hurlimann J, Ribolzi J, Barrelet L (1983). Placental site trophoblastic tumor (trophoblastic pseudotumor) of the uterus with metastases and fatal outcome. Clinical and autopsy observations of a case. *Am J Surg Pathol* 7: 483-486.
1019. Gloor E, Hurlimann J (1981). Trophoblastic pseudotumor of the uterus: clinicopathologic report with immunohistochemical and ultrastructural studies. *Am J Surg Pathol* 5: 5-13.
1020. Glorieux I, Chabbert V, Rubie H, Baunin C, Gaspard MH, Guitard J, Duga I, Suc A, Puget C, Robert A (1998). [Autoimmune hemolytic anemia associated with a mature ovarian teratoma]. Arch Pediatr 5: 41-44.
1021. Glusac EJ, Hendrickson MS, Smoller BR (1994). Apocrine cystadenoma of the vulva. *J Am Acad Dermatol* 31: 498-499.
1022. Gobbi H, Simpson JF, Borowsky A, Jensen RA, Page DL (1999). Metaplastic breast tumors with a dominant fibromatosis-like phenotype have a high risk of local recurrence. *Cancer* 85: 2170-2182.
1023. Gocht A, Bosmuller HC, Bassler R, Tavassoli FA, Moinfar F, Katenkamp D, Schirrmacher K, Luders P, Saeger W (1999). Breast tumors with myofibroblastic differentiation: clinico-pathological observations in myofibroblastoma and myofibrosarcoma. *Pathol Res Pract* 195: 1-10.
1024. Goff BA, Mandel L, Muntz HG, Melancon CH (2000). Ovarian carcinoma diagnosis. *Cancer* 89: 2068-2075.
1025. Goffin J, Chappuis PO, Wong N, Foulkes WD (2001). Re: Magnetic resonance imaging and mammography in women with a hereditary risk of breast cancer. *J Natl Cancer Inst* 93: 1754-1755.
1026. Golbang P, Khan A, Scurry J, MacIsaac I, Planner R (1997). Cervical sarcoma botryoides and ovarian Sertoli-Leydig cell tumor. *Gynecol Oncol* 67: 102-106.
1027. Goldblum J, Hart WR (1995). Localized and diffuse mesotheliomas of the genital tract and peritoneum in women. A clinicopathologic study of nineteen true mesothelial neoplasms, other than adenomatoid tumors, multicystic mesotheliomas, and localized fibrous tumors. *Am J Surg Pathol* 19: 1124-1137.
1028. Goldblum JR, Hart WR (1998). Perianal Paget's disease: a histologic and immunohistochemical study of 11 cases with and without associated rectal adenocarcinoma. *Am J Surg Pathol* 22: 170-179.
1029. Goldgar DE, Easton DF, Cannon-Albright LA, Skolnick MH (1994). Systematic population-based assessment of cancer risk in first-degree relatives of cancer probands. *J Natl Cancer Inst* 86: 1600-1608.
1030. Goldhirsch A, Glick JH, Gelber RD, Coates AS, Senn HJ (2001). Meeting highlights: International Consensus Panel on the Treatment of Primary Breast Cancer. Seventh International Conference on Adjuvant Therapy of Primary Breast Cancer. *J Clin Oncol* 19: 3817-3827.
1031. Goldhirsch A, Glick JH, Gelber RD, Senn HJ (1998). Meeting highlights: International consensus panel on the treatment of primary breast cancer. *J Natl Cancer Inst* 90: 1601-1608.
1032. Goldstein NS, Ahmad E, Hussain M, Hankin RC, Perez-Reyes N (1998). Endocervical glandular atypia: does a preneoplastic lesion of adenocarcinoma in situ exist? *Am J Clin Pathol* 110: 200-209.
1033. Goldstein NS, Bassi D, Watts JC, Layfield LJ, Yaziji H, Gown AM (2001). E-cadherin reactivity of 95 noninvasive ductal and lobular lesions of the breast. Implications for the interpretation of problematic lesions. *Am J Clin Pathol* 115: 534-542.
1034. Goldstein NS, O'Malley BA (1997). Cancerization of small ectatic ducts of the breast by ductal carcinoma in situ cells with apocrine snouts: a lesion associated with tubular carcinoma. *Am J Clin Pathol* 107: 561-566.
1035. Gollamudi SV, Gelman RS, Peiro G, Schneider LJ, Schnitt SJ, Recht A, Silver BJ, Harris JR, Connolly JL (1997). Breast-conserving therapy for stage I-II synchronous bilateral breast carcinoma. *Cancer* 79: 1362-1369.
1036. Gollard R, Kosty M, Bordin G, Wax A, Lacey C (1995). Two unusual presentations of mullerian adenosarcoma: case reports, literature review, and treatment considerations. *Gynecol Oncol* 59: 412-422.
1037. Gong G, Devries S, Chew KL, Cha I, Ljung BM, Waldman FM (2001). Genetic changes in paired atypical and usual ductal hyperplasia of the breast by comparative genomic hybridization. *Clin Cancer Res* 7: 2410-2414.
1038. Gonzalez-Crussi F, Crawford SE, Sun CC (1990). Intraabdominal desmoplastic small-cell tumors with divergent differentiation. Observations on three cases of childhood. *Am J Surg Pathol* 14: 633-642.
1039. Gonzalez-Moreno S, Yan H, Alcorn KW, Sugarbaker PH (2002). Malignant transformation of "benign" cystic mesothelioma of the peritoneum. *J Surg Oncol* 79: 243-251.
1040. Goodman ZD, Taxy JB (1981). Fibroadenomas of the breast with prominent smooth muscle. *Am J Surg Pathol* 5: 99-101.
1041. Gordon AN, Montag TW (1990). Sarcoma botryoides of the cervix: excision followed by adjuvant chemotherapy for preservation of reproductive function. *Gynecol Oncol* 36: 119-124.
1042. Gorlin RJ (1987). Nevoid basal-cell carcinoma syndrome. *Medicine (Baltimore)* 66: 98-113.
1043. Gorski GK, McMorrow LE, Blumstein L, Faasse D, Donaldson MH (1992). Trisomy 14 in two cases of granulosa cell tumor of the ovary. *Cancer Genet Cytogenet* 60: 202-205.
1044. Gotlieb WH, Friedman E, Bar-Sade RB, Kruglikova A, Hirsh-Yechezkel G, Modan B, Inbar M, Davidson B, Kopolovic J, Novikov I, Ben Baruch G (1998). Rates of Jewish ancestral mutations in BRCA1 and BRCA2 in borderline ovarian tumors. *J Natl Cancer Inst* 90: 995-1000.
1045. Gotoh T, Kikuchi Y, Takano M, Kita T, Ogata S, Aida S (2001). Epithelioid leiomyosarcoma of the uterine cervix. *Gynecol Oncol* 82: 400-405.
1046. Gottlieb C, Raju U, Greenwald KA (1990). Myoepithelial cells in the differential diagnosis of complex benign and malignant breast lesions: an immunohistochemical study. *Mod Pathol* 3: 135-140.
1047. Gould S (1967). Neurilemmoma within the broad ligament. A case report. *J S C Med Assoc* 63: 6-8.
1048. Govender NS, Goldstein DP (1977). Metastatic tubal mole and coexisting intrauterine pregnancy. *Obstet Gynecol* 49: 67-69.
1049. Govoni E, Pileri S, Bazzocchi F, Severi B, Martinelli G (1981). Postmastectomy angiosarcoma: ultrastructural study of a case. *Tumori* 67: 79-86.
1051. Goyert G, Budev H, Wright C, Jones A, Deppe G (1987). Vaginal mullerian stromal sarcoma. A case report. *J Reprod Med* 32: 129-130.
1052. Gradishar WJ (1996). Inflammatory breast cancer: the evolution of multimodality treatment strategies. *Semin Surg Oncol* 12: 352-363.
1053. Graham MD, Yelland A, Peacock J, Beck N, Ford H, Gazet JC (1993). Bilateral carcinoma of the breast. *Eur J Surg Oncol* 19: 259-264.
1054. Granter SR, Nucci MR, Fletcher CD (1997). Aggressive angiomyxoma: reappraisal of its relationship to angiomyofibroblastoma in a series of 16 cases. *Histopathology* 30: 3-10.
1055. Gras E, Catasus L, Arguelles R, Moreno-Bueno G, Palacios J, Gamallo C, Matias-Guiu X, Prat J (2001). Microsatellite instability, MLH-1 promoter hypermethylation, and frameshift mutations at coding mononucleotide repeat microsatellites in ovarian tumors. *Cancer* 92: 2829-2836.
1056. Gray GF Jr., Glick AD, Kurtin PJ, Jones HW III (1986). Alveolar soft part sarcoma of the uterus. *Hum Pathol* 17: 297-300.
1057. Grayson W, Cooper K (2002). A reappraisal of "Basaloid Carcinoma" of the cervix, and the differential diagnosis of basaloid cervical neoplasms. *Adv Anat Pathol* 9: 290-300.
1058. Grayson W, Fourie J, Tiltman AJ (1998). Xanthomatous leiomyosarcoma of the uterine cervix. *Int J Gynecol Pathol* 17: 89-90.
1059. Grayson W, Taylor LF, Cooper K (1999). Adenoid cystic and adenoid basal carcinoma of the uterine cervix: comparative morphologic, mucin, and immunohistochemical profile of two rare neoplasms of putative 'reserve cell' origin. *Am J Surg Pathol* 23: 448-458.
1060. Grayson W, Taylor LF, Cooper K (2001). Carcinosarcoma of the uterine cervix: a report of eight cases with immunohistochemical analysis and evaluation of human papillomavirus status. *Am J Surg Pathol* 25: 338-347.
1061. Green DM (1990). Mucoid carcinoma of the breast with choriocarcinoma in its metastases. *Histopathology* 16: 504-506.
1062. Green I, McCormick B, Cranor M, Rosen PP (1997). A comparative study of pure tubular and tubulolobular carcinoma of the breast. *Am J Surg Pathol* 21: 653-657.
1063. Green JA, Kirwan JM, Tierney JF, Symonds P, Fresco L, Collingwood M, Williams CJ (2001). Survival and recurrence after concomitant chemotherapy and radiotherapy for cancer of the uterine cervix: a systematic review and meta-analysis. *Lancet* 358: 781-786.
1064. Green LK, Kott ML (1989). Histopathologic findings in ectopic tubal pregnancy. *Int J Gynecol Pathol* 8: 255-262.
1065. Greene JB, McCue SA (1978). Chorioadenoma destruens. *Ann N Y Acad Sci* 80: 143.
1066. Greenlee RT, Hill-Harmon MB, Murray T, Thun M (2001). Cancer statistics, 2001. *CA Cancer J Clin* 51: 15-36.

1067. Grimes MM (1992). Cystosarcoma phyllodes of the breast: histologic features, flow cytometric analysis, and clinical correlations. *Mod Pathol* 5: 232-239.
1068. Grody WW, Nieberg RK, Bhuta S (1985). Ependymoma-like tumor of the mesovarium. *Arch Pathol Lab Med* 109: 291-293.
1069. Gronroos M, Meurman L, Kahra K (1983). Proliferating glia and other heterotopic tissues in the uterus: fetal homografts? *Obstet Gynecol* 61: 261-266.
1070. Gross GE, Barrasso R (1997). Human Pamilloma Virus Infection - A Clinical Atlas. Berlin.
1071. Gruber SB, Thompson WD (1996). A population-based study of endometrial cancer and familial risk in younger women. Cancer and Steroid Hormone Study Group. *Cancer Epidemiol Biomarkers Prev* 5: 411-417.
1072. Gruvberger S, Ringner M, Chen Y, Panavally S, Saal LH, Borg A, Ferno M, Peterson C, Meltzer PS (2001). Estrogen receptor status in breast cancer is associated with remarkably distinct gene expression patterns. *Cancer Res* 61: 5979-5984.
1073. Gudmundsson J, Barkardottir RB, Eiriksdottir G, Baldursson T, Arason A, Egilsson V, Ingvarsson S (1995). Loss of heterozygosity at chromosome 11 in breast cancer: association of prognostic factors with genetic alterations. *Br J Cancer* 72: 696-701.
1074. Guerin M, Gabillot M, Mathieu MC, Travagli JP, Spielmann M, Andrieu N, Riou G (1989). Structure and expression of c-erbB-2 and EGF receptor genes in inflammatory and non-inflammatory breast cancer: prognostic significance. *Int J Cancer* 43: 201-208.
1075. Guerrieri C, Franlund B, Boeryd B (1995). Expression of cytokeratin 7 in simultaneous mucinous tumors of the ovary and appendix. *Mod Pathol* 8: 573-576.
1076. Guerrieri C, Hogberg T, Wingren S, Fristedt S, Simonsen E, Boeryd B (1994). Mucinous borderline and malignant tumors of the ovary. A clinicopathologic and DNA ploidy study of 92 cases. *Cancer* 74: 2329-2340.
1077. Guerrieri C, Jarlsfelt I (1993). Ependymoma of the ovary. A case report with immunohistochemical, ultrastructural, and DNA cytometric findings, as well as histogenetic considerations. *Am J Surg Pathol* 17: 623-632.
1078. Guillou L, Wadden C, Coindre JM, Krausz T, Fletcher CD (1997). "Proximal-type" epithelioid sarcoma, a distinctive aggressive neoplasm showing rhabdoid features. Clinicopathologic, immunohistochemical, and ultrastructural study of a series. *Am J Surg Pathol* 21: 130-146.
1079. Guinee VF, Olsson H, Moller T, Hess KR, Taylor SH, Fahey T, Gladikov JV, van den Blink JW, Bonichon F, Dische S, Yates JW, Cleaton FJ (1994). Effect of pregnancy on prognosis for young women with breast cancer. *Lancet* 343: 1587-1589.
1080. Guinet C, Ghossain MA, Buy JN, Malbec L, Hugol D, Truc JB, Vadrot D (1995). Mature cystic teratomas of the ovary: CT and MR findings. *Eur J Radiol* 20: 137-143.
1081. Gultekin SH, Cody HS III, Hoda SA (1996). Schwannoma of the breast. *South Med J* 89: 238-239.
1082. Gump FE (1990). Lobular carcinoma in situ. Pathology and treatment. *Surg Clin North Am* 70: 873-883.
1083. Gump FE, Sternschein MJ, Wolff M (1981). Fibromatosis of the breast. *Surg Gynecol Obstet* 153: 57-60.
1084. Gunn RA, Gallager HS (1980). Vulvar Paget's disease: a topographic study. *Cancer* 46: 590-594.
1085. Gunther K, Merkelbach-Bruse S, Amo-Takyi BK, Handt S, Schroder W, Tietze L (2001). Differences in genetic alterations between primary lobular and ductal breast cancers detected by comparative genomic hybridization. *J Pathol* 193: 40-47.
1086. Guo Z, Thunberg U, Sallstrom J, Wilander E, Ponten J (1998). Clonality analysis of cervical cancer on microdissected archival materials by PCR-based X-chromosome inactivation approach. *Int J Oncol* 12: 1327-1332.
1087. Gupta D, Balsara G (1999). Extrauterine malignancies. Role of Pap smears in diagnosis and management. *Acta Cytol* 43: 806-813.
1088. Gupta JW, Saito K, Saito A, Fu YS, Shah KV (1989). Human papillomaviruses and the pathogenesis of cervical neoplasia. A study by in situ hybridization. *Cancer* 64: 2104-2110.
1089. Gupta RK (1996). Aspiration cytodiagnosis of a rare carcinoma of breast with bizarre malignant giant cells. *Diagn Cytopathol* 15: 66-69.
1090. Gupta SK, Douglas-Jones AG, Jasani B, Morgan JM, Pignatelli M, Mansel RE (1997). E-cadherin (E-cad) expression in duct carcinoma in situ (DCIS) of the breast. *Virchows Arch* 430: 23-28.
1091. Gustafson ML, Lee MM, Scully RE, Moncure AC, Hirakawa T, Goodman A, Muntz HG, Donahoe PK, MacLaughlin DT, Fuller AF Jr. (1992). Mullerian inhibiting substance as a marker for ovarian sex-cord tumor. *N Engl J Med* 326: 466-471.
1092. Gustafsson A, Tartter PI, Brower ST, Lesnick G (1994). Prognosis of patients with bilateral carcinoma of the breast. *J Am Coll Surg* 178: 111-116.
1093. Gwavava NJ, Traub AI (1980). A neurilemmoma of the cervix. *Br J Obstet Gynaecol* 87: 444-446.
1094. Ha HK, Baek SY, Kim SH, Kim HH, Chung EC, Yeon KM (1995). Krukenberg's tumor of the ovary: MR imaging features. *AJR Am J Roentgenol* 164: 1435-1439.
1095. Haagensen CD (1971). Inflammatory Carcinoma. In: *Diseases of the Breast.* CD Haagensen (Ed.) 2nd ed. WB Sauders: Philadelphia, pp. 576-584.
1096. Haagensen CD (1986). *Diseases of the Breast.* 3rd ed. WB Saunders: Philadelphia.
1097. Haagensen CD (1986). Multiple intraductal papilloma. In: *Diseases of the Breast.* 3rd ed. WB Saunders: Philadelphia, pp. 176-191.
1098. Haagensen CD (1986). Solitary intraductal papilloma. In: *Diseases of the Breast.* 3rd ed. WB Saunders: Philadelphia, pp. 136-175.
1099. Haagensen CD, Lane N, Lattes R (1972). Neoplastic proliferation of the epithelium of the mammary lobules: adenosis, lobular neoplasia, and small cell carcinoma. *Surg Clin North Am* 52: 497-524.
1100. Haagensen CD, Lane N, Lattes R, Bodian C (1978). Lobular neoplasia (so-called lobular carcinoma in situ) of the breast. *Cancer* 42: 737-769.
1101. Haberal A, Turgut F, Ozbey B, Kucukali T, Sapmaz M (1995). Granular cell myoblastoma of the cervix in a 14 year old girl. *Cent Afr J Med* 41: 298-300.
1102. Hachi H, Othmany A, Douayri A, Bouchikhi C, Tijami F, Laalou L, Chami M, Boughtab A, Jalil A, Benjelloun S, Ahyoud F, Kettani F, Souadka A (2002). [Association of ovarian juvenile granulosa cell tumor with Maffucci's syndrome]. *Gynecol Obstet Fertil* 30: 692-695.
1103. Hachisuga T, Sugimori H, Kaku T, Matsukuma K, Tsukamoto N, Nakano H (1990). Glassy cell carcinoma of the endometrium. *Gynecol Oncol* 36: 134-138.
1104. Hacker NF (2000). Uterine cancer. In: *Practical Gynecologic Oncology.* 3rd ed. Lippincott, William & Wilkins: Philadelphia, pp. 407-455.
1105. Hacker NF, Berek JS, Lagasse LD, Nieberg RK, Leuchter RS (1984). Individualization of treatment for stage I squamous cell vulvar carcinoma. *Obstet Gynecol* 63: 155-162.
1106. Haefner HK, Tate JE, McLachlin CM, Crum CP (1995). Vulvar intraepithelial neoplasia: age, morphological phenotype, papillomavirus DNA, and coexisting invasive carcinoma. *Hum Pathol* 26: 147-154.
1107. Hainaut P, Hollstein M (2000). p53 and human cancer: the first ten thousand mutations. *Adv Cancer Res* 77: 81-137.
1108. Hakem R, de la Pompa JL, Elia A, Potter J, Mak TW (1997). Partial rescue of Brca1 (5-6) early embryonic lethality by p53 or p21 null mutation. *Nat Genet* 16: 298-302.
1109. Hall JM, Lee MK, Newman B, Morrow JE, Anderson LA, Huey B, King MC (1990). Linkage of early-onset familial breast cancer to chromosome 17q21. *Science* 250: 1684-1689.
1110. Hallgrimsson J, Scully RE (1972). Borderline and malignant Brenner tumours of the ovary. A report of 15 cases. *Acta Pathol Microbiol Scand [A]* 233: 56-66.
1111. Hamby LS, McGrath PC, Cibull ML, Schwartz RW (1991). Gastric carcinoma metastatic to the breast. *J Surg Oncol* 48: 117-121.
1112. Hameed K, Burslem MR (1970). A melanotic ovarian neoplasm resembling the "retinal anlage" tumor. *Cancer* 25: 564-567.
1113. Hamele-Bena D, Cranor ML, Sciotto C, Erlandson R, Rosen PP (1996). Uncommon presentation of mammary myofibroblastoma. *Mod Pathol* 9: 786-790.
1114. Hamilton S, Aaltonen L (2000). *WHO Classification of Tumours. Pathology and Genetics of Tumours of the Digestive System.* IARC Press: Lyon.
1115. Hamilton SR, Liu B, Parsons RE, Papadopoulos N, Jen J, Powell SM, Krush AJ, Berk T, Cohen Z, Tetu B, Burger PC, Wood PA, Taqi F, Booker SV, Petersen GM, Offerhaus GJA, Tersmette AC, Giardiello FM, Volgelstein B, Kinzler KW. (1995). The molecular basis of Turcot's syndrome. *N Engl J Med* 332: 839-847.
1116. Hamm B, Kubik-Huch RA, Fleige B (1999). MR imaging and CT of the female pelvis: radiologic-pathologic correlation. *Eur Radiol* 9: 3-15.
1117. Hampl M, Hampl JA, Reiss G, Schackert G, Saeger HD, Schackert HK (1999). Loss of heterozygosity accumulation in primary breast carcinomas and additionally in corresponding distant metastases is associated with poor outcome. *Clin Cancer Res* 5: 1417-1425.
1118. Hampton GM, Mannermaa A, Winquist R, Alavaikko M, Blanco G, Taskinen PJ, Kiviniemi H, Newsham I, Cavenee WK, Evans GA (1994). Loss of heterozygosity in sporadic human breast carcinoma: a common region between 11q22 and 11q23.3. *Cancer Res* 54: 4586-4589.
1119. Hampton GM, Penny LA, Baergen RN, Larson A, Brewer C, Liao S, Busby-Earle RM, Williams AW, Steel CM, Bird CC, Stanbridge EJ, Evans GA. (1994). Loss of heterozygosity in cervical carcinoma: subchromosomal localization of a putative tumor-suppressor gene to chromosome 11q22-q24. *Proc Natl Acad Sci USA* 91: 6953-6957.
1120. Hampton HL, Huffman HT, Meeks GR (1992). Extraovarian Brenner tumor. *Obstet Gynecol* 79: 844-846.
1121. Han HJ, Maruyama M, Baba S, Park JG, Nakamura Y (1995). Genomic structure of human mismatch repair gene, hMLH1, and its mutation analysis in patients with hereditary non-polyposis colorectal cancer (HNPCC). *Hum Mol Genet* 4: 237-242.
1122. Han HS, Park IA, Kim SH, Lee HP (1998). The clear cell variant of epithelioid intravenous leiomyomatosis of the uterus: report of a case. *Pathol Int* 48: 892-896.
1123. Hancock BW, Welch EM, Gillespie AM, Newlands ES (2000). A retrospective comparison of current and proposed staging and scoring systems for persistent gestational trophoblastic disease. *Int J Gynecol Cancer* 10: 318-322.
1124. Hanjani P, Petersen RO, Bonnell SA (1980). Malignant mixed Mullerian tumor of the fallopian tube. Report of a case and review of literature. *Gynecol Oncol* 9: 381-393.
1125. Hankins GR, De Souza AT, Bentley RC, Patel MR, Marks JR, Iglehart JD, Jirtle RL (1996). M6P/IGF2 receptor: a candidate breast tumor suppressor gene. *Oncogene* 12: 2003-2009.
1126. Hankinson SE, Hunter DJ, Colditz GA, Willett WC, Stampfer MJ, Rosner B, Hennekens CH, Speizer FE (1993). Tubal ligation, hysterectomy, and risk of ovarian cancer. A prospective study. *JAMA* 270: 2813-2818.
1127. Hankinson SE, Willett WC, Colditz GA, Hunter DJ, Michaud DS, Deroo B, Rosner B, Speizer FE, Pollak M (1998). Circulating concentrations of insulin-like growth factor-I and risk of breast cancer. *Lancet* 351: 1393-1396.
1128. Hankinson SE, Willett WC, Manson JE, Colditz GA, Hunter DJ, Spiegelman D, Barbieri RL, Speizer FE (1998). Plasma sex steroid hormone levels and risk of breast cancer in postmenopausal women. *J Natl Cancer Inst* 90: 1292-1299.
1129. Hanna NN, O'Donnell K, Wolfe GR (1996). Alveolar soft part sarcoma metastatic to the breast. *J Surg Oncol* 61: 159-162.
1130. Hanna W, Kahn HJ (1985). Ultrastructural and immunohistochemical characteristics of mucoepidermoid carcinoma of the breast. *Hum Pathol* 16: 941-946.
1131. Hanselaar A, van Loosbroek M, Schuurbiers O, Helmerhorst T, Bulten J, Bernhelm J (1997). Clear cell adenocarcinoma of the vagina and cervix. An update of the central Netherlands registry showing twin age incidence peaks. *Cancer* 79: 2229-2236.

1132. Hanselaar AG, Boss EA, Massuger LF, Bernheim JL (1999). Cytologic examination to detect clear cell adenocarcinoma of the vagina or cervix. *Gynecol Oncol* 75: 338-344.

1133. Hanssen AM, Fryns JP (1995). Cowden syndrome. *J Med Genet* 32: 117-119.

1134. Harada Y, Katagiri T, Ito I, Akiyama F, Sakamoto G, Kasumi F, Nakamura Y, Emi M (1994). Genetic studies of 457 breast cancers. Clinicopathologic parameters compared with genetic alterations. *Cancer* 74: 2281-2286.

1135. Hardesty LA, Sumkin JH, Hakim C, Johns C, Nath M (2001). The ability of helical CT to preoperatively stage endometrial carcinoma. *Am J Roentgenol* 176: 603-606.

1136. Hardesty LA, Sumkin JH, Nath ME, Edwards RP, Price FV, Chang TS, Johns CM, Kelley JL (2000). Use of preoperative MR imaging in the management of endometrial carcinoma: cost analysis. *Radiology* 215: 45-49.

1137. Hardisson D, Simon RS, Burgos E (2001). Primary osteosarcoma of the uterine corpus: report of a case with immunohistochemical and ultrastructural study. *Gynecol Oncol* 82: 181-186.

1138. Harkin DP, Bean JM, Miklos D, Song YH, Truong VB, Englert C, Christians FC, Ellisen LW, Maheswaran S, Oliner JD, Haber DA (1999). Induction of GADD45 and JNK/SAPK-dependent apoptosis following inducible expression of BRCA1. *Cell* 97: 575-586.

1139. Harlow BL, Weiss NS, Lofton S (1986). The epidemiology of sarcomas of the uterus. *J Natl Cancer Inst* 76: 399-402.

1140. Harnden P, Kennedy W, Andrew AC, Southgate J (1999). Immunophenotype of transitional metaplasia of the uterine cervix. *Int J Gynecol Pathol* 18: 125-129.

1141. Haroske G, Giroud F, Reith A, Bocking A (1998). 1997 ESACP consensus report on diagnostic DNA image cytometry. Part I: basic considerations and recommendations for preparation, measurement and interpretation. European Society for Analytical Cellular Pathology. *Anal Cell Pathol* 17: 189-200.

1142. Harris M, Howell A, Chrissohou M, Swindell RI, Hudson M, Sellwood RA (1984). A comparison of the metastatic pattern of infiltrating lobular carcinoma and infiltrating duct carcinoma of the breast. *Br J Cancer* 50: 23-30.

1143. Harris M, Wells S, Vasudev KS (1978). Primary signet ring cell carcinoma of the breast. *Histopathology* 2: 171-176.

1144. Harris NL, Jaffe ES, Diebold J, Flandrin G, Muller-Hermelink HK, Vardiman J, Lister TA, Bloomfield CD (2000). The World Health Organization classification of hematological malignancies report of the Clinical Advisory Committee Meeting, Airlie House, Virginia, November 1997. *Mod Pathol* 13: 193-207.

1145. Harris NL, Scully RE (1984). Malignant lymphoma and granulocytic sarcoma of the uterus and vagina. A clinicopathologic analysis of 27 cases. *Cancer* 53: 2530-2545.

1146. Harrison M, Magee HM, O'Loughlin J, Gorey TF, Dervan PA (1995). Chromosome 1 aneusomy, identified by interphase cytogenetics, in mammographically detected ductal carcinoma in situ of the breast. *J Pathol* 175: 303-309.

1147. Hart WR (1977). Ovarian epithelial tumors of borderline malignancy (carcinomas of low malignant potential). *Hum Pathol* 8: 541-549.

1148. Hart WR, Billman JK Jr. (1978). A reassessment of uterine neoplasms originally diagnosed as leiomyosarcomas. *Cancer* 41: 1902-1910.

1149. Hart WR, Craig JR (1978). Rhabdomyosarcomas of the uterus. *Am J Clin Pathol* 70: 217-223.

1150. Hart WR, Norris HJ (1973). Borderline and malignant mucinous tumors of the ovary. Histologic criteria and clinical behavior. *Cancer* 31: 1031-1045.

1151. Hartge P, Struewing JP, Wacholder S, Brody LC, Tucker MA (1999). The prevalence of common BRCA1 and BRCA2 mutations among Ashkenazi Jews. *Am J Hum Genet* 64: 963-970.

1152. Hartveit E (1990). Attenuated cells in breast stroma: the missing lymphatic system of the breast. *Histopathology* 16: 533-543.

1153. Hasebe T, Mukai K, Tsuda H, Ochiai A (2000). New prognostic histological parameter of invasive ductal carcinoma of the breast: clinicopathological significance of fibrotic focus. *Pathol Int* 50: 263-272.

1154. Hashiguchi J, Ito M, Kishikawa M, Sekine I, Kase Y (1994). Intravascular leiomyomatosis with uterine lipoleiomyoma. *Gynecol Oncol* 52: 94-98.

1155. Haskel S, Chen SS, Spiegel G (1989). Vaginal endometrioid adenocarcinoma arising in vaginal endometriosis: a case report and literature review. *Gynecol Oncol* 34: 232-236.

1156. Hastrup N, Sehested M (1985). High-grade mucoepidermoid carcinoma of the breast. *Histopathology* 9: 887-892.

1157. Haswani P, Arseneau J, Ferenczy A (1998). Primary signet cell carcinoma of the uterine cervix: a clinicopathologic study of two cases with review of the literature. *Int J Gynecol Cancer* 8: 374-379.

1158. Hata JI, Ueyama Y, Tamaoki N, Akatsuka A, Yoshimura S, Shimuzu K, Morikawa Y, Furukawa T (1980). Human yolk sac tumor serially transplanted in nude mice: its morphologic and functional properties. *Cancer* 46: 2446-2455.

1159. Hauptmann S, Dietel M (2001). Serous tumors of low malignant potential of the ovary-molecular pathology: part 2. *Virchows Arch* 438: 539-551.

1160. Hausen H. (2000). Papillomaviruses causing cancer: evasion from host-cell control in early events in carcinogenesis. *J Natl Cancer Inst* 92: 690-698.

1161. Hawkins RE, Schofield JB, Fisher C, Wiltshaw E, McKinna JA (1992). The clinical and histologic criteria that predict metastases from cystosarcoma phyllodes. *Cancer* 69: 141-147.

1162. Hayashi K, Bracken MB, Freeman DH Jr., Hellenbrand K (1982). Hydatidiform mole in the United States (1970-1977): a statistical and theoretical analysis. *Am J Epidemiol* 115: 67-77.

1163. Hayes MC, Scully RE (1987). Ovarian steroid cell tumors (not otherwise specified). A clinicopathological analysis of 63 cases. *Am J Surg Pathol* 11: 835-845.

1164. Hayes MC, Scully RE (1987). Stromal luteoma of the ovary: a clinicopathological analysis of 25 cases. *Int J Gynecol Pathol* 6: 313-321.

1165. Hayes MM, Seidman JD, Ashton MA (1995). Glycogen-rich clear cell carcinoma of the breast. A clinicopathologic study of 21 cases. *Am J Surg Pathol* 19: 904-911.

1166. Hays DM, Donaldson SS, Shimada H, Crist WM, Newton WA Jr., Andrassy RJ, Wiener E, Green J, Triche T, Maurer HM (1997). Primary and metastatic rhabdomyosarcoma in the breast: neoplasms of adolescent females, a report from the Intergroup Rhabdomyosarcoma Study. *Med Pediatr Oncol* 29: 181-189.

1167. Healey CS, Dunning AM, Teare MD, Chase D, Parker L, Burn J, Chang-Claude J, Mannermaa A, Kataja V, Huntsman DG, Pharoah PD, Luben RN, Easton DF, Ponder BA (2000). A common variant in BRCA2 is associated with both breast cancer risk and prenatal viability. *Nat Genet* 26: 362-364.

1168. Healey EA, Cook EF, Orav EJ, Schnitt SJ, Connolly JL, Harris JR (1993). Contralateral breast cancer: clinical characteristics and impact on prognosis. *J Clin Oncol* 11: 1545-1552.

1169. Heatley MK (2000). Adenomatous hyperplasia of the rete ovarii. *Histopathology* 36: 383-384.

1170. Heatley MK (2001). Polyp of the fallopian tube. *Pathology* 33: 538-539.

1171. Hedenfalk I, Duggan D, Chen Y, Radmacher M, Bittner M, Simon R, Meltzer P, Gusterson B, Esteller M, Kallioniemi OP, Wilfond B, Borg A, Trent J (2001). Gene-expression profiles in hereditary breast cancer. *N Engl J Med* 344: 539-548.

1172. Heffelfinger SC, Yassin R, Miller MA, Lower EE (2000). Cyclin D1, retinoblastoma, p53, and Her2/neu protein expression in preinvasive breast pathologies: correlation with vascularity. *Pathobiology* 68: 129-136.

1173. Hefler LA, Rosen AC, Graf AH, Lahousen M, Klein M, Leodolter S, Reinthaller A, Kainz C, Tempfer CB (2000). The clinical value of serum concentrations of cancer antigen 125 in patients with primary fallopian tube carcinoma: a multicenter study. *Cancer* 89: 1555-1560.

1174. Heifetz SA, Cushing B, Giller R, Shuster JJ, Stolar CJ, Vinocur CD, Hawkins EP (1998). Immature teratomas in children: pathologic considerations: a report from the combined Pediatric Oncology Group/Children's Cancer Group. *Am J Surg Pathol* 22: 1115-1124.

1175. Heim S, Teixeira MR, Dietrich CU, Pandis N (1997). Cytogenetic polyclonality in tumors of the breast. *Cancer Genet Cytogenet* 95: 16-19.

1176. Heimann R, Lan F, McBride R, Hellman S (2000). Separating favorable from unfavorable prognostic markers in breast cancer: the role of E-cadherin. *Cancer Res* 60: 298-304.

1177. Heintz AP, Schaberg A, Engelsman E, van Hall EV (1985). Placental-site trophoblastic tumor: diagnosis, treatment, and biological behavior. *Int J Gynecol Pathol* 4: 75-82.

1178. Helland A, Karlsen F, Due EU, Holm R, Kristensen G, Borresen-Dale A (1998). Mutations in the TP53 gene and protein expression of p53, MDM 2 and p21/WAF-1 in primary cervical carcinomas with no or low human papillomavirus load. *Br J Cancer* 78: 69-72.

1179. Heller DS, Keohane M, Bessim S, Jagirdar J, Deligdisch L (1989). Pituitary-containing benign cystic teratoma arising from the uterosacral ligament. *Arch Pathol Lab Med* 113: 802-804.

1180. Heller DS, Rubinstein N, Dikman S, Deligdisch L, Moss R (1991). Adenomatous polyp of the fallopian tube. A case report. *J Reprod Med* 36: 82-84.

1181. Hellman S, Harris JR (1987). The appropriate breast cancer paradigm. *Cancer Res* 47: 339-342.

1181 a. Hellstrom AC, Hue J, Silfversward C, Auer G (1994). DNA-ploidy and mutant p53 overexpression in primary fallopian tube cancer. *Int J Gynecol Cancer* 4: 408-413.

1182. Hellstrom AC, Tegerstedt G, Silfversward C, Pettersson F (1999). Malignant mixed mullerian tumors of the ovary: histopathologic and clinical review of 36 cases. *Int J Gynecol Cancer* 9: 312-316.

1183. Helzlsouer KJ, Alberg AJ, Bush TL, Longcope C, Gordon GB, Comstock GW (1994). A prospective study of endogenous hormones and breast cancer. *Cancer Detect Prev* 18: 79-85.

1184. Hemminki K, Dong C, Vaittinen P (1999). Familial risks in cervical cancer: is there a hereditary component? *Int J Cancer* 82: 775-781.

1185. Hemminki K, Vaittinen P (1999). Male breast cancer: risk to daughters. *Lancet* 353: 1186-1187.

1186. Hendrickson M, Ross J, Eifel P, Martinez A, Kempson R (1982). Uterine papillary serous carcinoma: a highly malignant form of endometrial adenocarcinoma. *Am J Surg Pathol* 6: 93-108.

1187. Hendrickson MR, Kempson RL (1983). Ciliated carcinoma--a variant of endometrial adenocarcinoma: a report of 10 cases. *Int J Gynecol Pathol* 2: 1-12.

1188. Hendrickson MR, Scheithauer BW (1986). Primitive neuroectodermal tumor of the endometrium: report of two cases, one with electron microscopic observations. *Int J Gynecol Pathol* 5: 249-259.

1189. Hennig Y, Caselitz J, Bartnitzke S, Bullerdiek J (1997). A third case of a low-grade endometrial stromal sarcoma with a t(7;17)(p14 approximately 21;q11.2 approximately 21). *Cancer Genet Cytogenet* 98: 84-86.

1190. Henson DE, Ries L, Freedman LS, Carriaga M (1991). Relationship among outcome, stage of disease, and histologic grade for 22,616 cases of breast cancer. The basis for a prognostic index. *Cancer* 68: 2142-2149.

1191. Herbold DR, Axelrod JH, Bobowski SJ, Freel JH (1988). Glassy cell carcinoma of the fallopian tube. A case report. *Int J Gynecol Pathol* 7: 384-390.

1192. Herbold DR, Fu YS, Silbert SW (1983). Leiomyosarcoma of the broad ligament. A case report and literature review with follow-up. *Am J Surg Pathol* 7: 285-292.

1193. Herbst AL, Green TH Jr., Ulfelder H (1970). Primary carcinoma of the vagina. An analysis of 68 cases. *Am J Obstet Gynecol* 106: 210-218.

1194. Herbst AL, Ulfelder H, Poskanzer DC (1971). Adenocarcinoma of the vagina. Association of maternal stilbestrol therapy with tumor appearance in young women. *N Engl J Med* 284: 878-881.

1195. Hermanek P, Hutter RV, Sobin LH, Wittekind C (1999). International Union Against Cancer. Classification of isolated tumor cells and micrometastasis. *Cancer* 86: 2668-2673.

1196. Hernandez-Boussard TR-TPMRHP (2001). IARC p53 mutation database: a relational database to compile and analyze p53 mutations in human tumors and cell lines (R5 version). WHO/IARC http://www.iarc.fr/P53.

1197. Herod JJ, Shafi MI, Rollason TP, Jordan JA, Luesley DM (1996). Vulvar intraepithelial neoplasia with superficially invasive carcinoma of the vulva. *Br J Obstet Gynaecol* 103: 453-456.

1198. Herrera LJ, Lugo-Vicente H (1998). Primary embryonal rhabdomyosarcoma of the breast in an adolescent female: a case report. *J Pediatr Surg* 33: 1582-1584.

1199. Herrero R, Munoz N (1999). Human papillomavirus and cancer. *Cancer surv* 33: 75-98.

1200. Herrington CS, Tarin D, Buley I, Athanasou N (1994). Osteosarcomatous differentiation in carcinoma of the breast: a case of 'metaplastic' carcinoma with osteoclasts and osteoclast-like giant cells. *Histopathology* 24: 282-285.

1201. Herrington CS, Wells M (2002). Premalignant and malignant squamous lesions of the cervix. In: *Haines and Taylor Obstetrical and Gynaecological Pathology*. H Fox, M Wells (Eds.) Fifth ed. Churchill Livingstone: Edinburgh, pp. 297-338.

1202. Hertel BF, Zaloudek C, Kempson RL (1976). Breast adenomas. *Cancer* 37: 2891-2905.

1203. Hertig AT, Mansell H (1956). Tumours of the female sex organs. Part I Hydatidiform mole and choriocarcinoma. In: Atlas of Tumour Pathology, AFIP (Ed.) AFIP: Washington,DC.

1204. Hessler C, Schnyder P, Ozzello L (1978). Hamartoma of the breast: diagnostic observation of 16 cases. *Radiology* 126: 95-98.

1205. Hetzel DJ, Wilson TO, Keeney GL, Roche PC, Cha SS, Podratz KC (1992). HER-2/neu expression: a major prognostic factor in endometrial cancer. *Gynecol Oncol* 47: 179-185.

1206. Heywang-Kobrunner SH, Dershaw DD, Schreer I (2000). *Diagnostic Breast Imaging*. 2nd ed. Thieme: New York.

1207. Hibberd AD, Horwood LJ, Wells JE (1983). Long term prognosis of women with breast cancer in New Zealand: study of survival to 30 years. *Br Med J (Clin Res Ed)* 286: 1777-1779.

1208. Hidalgo A, Schewe C, Petersen S, Salcedo M, Gariglio P, Schluns K, Dietel M, Petersen I (2000). Human papilloma virus status and chromosomal imbalances in primary cervical carcinomas and tumour cell lines. *Eur J Cancer* 36: 542-548.

1209. Hierro I, Blanes A, Matilla A, Munoz S, Vicioso L, Nogales FF (2000). Merkel cell (neuroendocrine) carcinoma of the vulva. A case report with immunohistochemical and ultrastructural findings and review of the literature. *Pathol Res Pract* 196: 503-509.

1210. Hill A, Yagmur Y, Tran KN, Bolton JS, Robson M, Borgen PI (1999). Localized male breast carcinoma and family history. An analysis of 142 patients. *Cancer* 86: 821-825.

1211. Hill RP, Miller FN (1954). With case report of carcinomatous transformation in an adenoma. *Cancer* 7: 318-324.

1212. Hinkula M, Pukkala E, Kyyronen P, Kauppila A (2002). Grand multiparity and incidence of endometrial cancer: a population-based study in Finland. *Int J Cancer* 98: 912-915.

1213. Hiort O, Naber SP, Lehners A, Muletta-Feurer S, Sinnecker GH, Zollner A, Komminoth P (1996). The role of androgen receptor gene mutations in male breast carcinoma. *J Clin Endocrinol Metab* 81: 3404-3407.

1214. Hirakawa T, Tsuneyoshi M, Enjoji M (1989). Squamous cell carcinoma arising in mature cystic teratoma of the ovary. Clinicopathologic and topographic analysis. *Am J Surg Pathol* 13: 397-405.

1215. Hirakawa T, Tsuneyoshi M, Enjoji M, Shigyo R (1988). Ovarian sarcoma with histologic features of telangiectatic osteosarcoma of the bone. *Am J Surg Pathol* 12: 567-572.

1216. Hirano A, Emi M, Tsuneizumi M, Utada Y, Yoshimoto M, Kasumi F, Akiyama F, Sakamoto G, Haga S, Kajiwara T, Nakamura Y (2001). Allelic losses of loci at 3p25.1, 8p22, 13q12, 17p13.3, and 22q13 correlate with postoperative recurrence in breast cancer. *Clin Cancer Res* 7: 876-882.

1217. Hirohashi S (1998). Inactivation of the E-cadherin-mediated cell adhesion system in human cancers. *Am J Pathol* 153: 333-339.

1218. Hiroi H, Yasugi T, Matsumoto K, Fujii T, Watanabe T, Yoshikawa H, Taketani Y (2001). Mucinous adenocarcinoma arising in a neovagina using the sigmoid colon thirty years after operation: a case report. *J Surg Oncol* 77: 61-64.

1219. Hislop TG, Elwood JM, Coldman AJ, Spinelli JJ, Worth AJ, Ellison LG (1984). Second primary cancers of the breast: incidence and risk factors. *Br J Cancer* 49: 79-85.

1220. Hitchcock CL, Norris HJ (1992). Flow cytometric analysis of endometrial stromal sarcoma. *Am J Clin Pathol* 97: 267-271.

1221. Hittmair AP, Lininger RA, Tavassoli FA (1998). Ductal carcinoma in situ (DCIS) in the male breast: a morphologic study of 84 cases of pure DCIS and 30 cases of DCIS associated with invasive carcinoma--a preliminary report. *Cancer* 83: 2139-2149.

1222. Ho YB, Robertson DI, Clement PB, Mincey EK (1982). Sclerosing stromal tumor of the ovary. *Obstet Gynecol* 60: 252-256.

1223. Hock YL, Mohamid W (1995). Myxoid neurofibroma of the male breast: fine needle aspiration cytodiagnosis. *Cytopathology* 6: 44-47.

1224. Hocking GR, Hayman JA, Östör AG (1996). Adenocarcinoma in situ of the uterine cervix progressing to invasive adenocarcinoma. *Aust N Z J Obstet Gynaecol* 36: 218-220.

1225. Hoda SA, Cranor ML, Rosen PP (1992). Hemangiomas of the breast with atypical histological features. Further analysis of histological subtypes confirming their benign character. *Am J Surg Pathol* 16: 553-560.

1226. Hoda SA, Prasad ML, Moore A, Hoda RS, Giri D (1999). Microinvasive carcinoma of the breast: can it be diagnosed reliably and is it clinically significant? *Histopathology* 35: 468-470.

1227. Hodak E, Jones RE, Ackerman AB (1993). Solitary keratoacanthoma is a squamous-cell carcinoma: three examples with metastases. *Am J Dermatopathol* 15: 332-342.

1228. Hoerl HD, Hart WR (1998). Primary ovarian mucinous cystadenocarcinomas: a clinicopathologic study of 49 cases with long-term follow-up. *Am J Surg Pathol* 22: 1449-1462.

1229. Hogervorst FB, Nederlof PM, Gille JJ, McElgunn CJ, Grippeling M, Pruntel R, Regnerus R, van Welsem T, van Spaendonk R, Menko FH, Kluijt I, Dommering C, Verhoef S, Schouten JP, van't Veer LJ, Pals G (2003). Large genomic deletions and duplications in the BRCA1 gene identified by a novel quantitative method. *Cancer Res* 63: 1449-1453.

1230. Holland R, Faverly D (1997). Whole organ studies. In: *Ductal Carcinoma in Situ of the Breast*. MJ Silverstein (Ed.) Williams & Wilkins: Baltimore. pp. 233-240.

1230a. Holland R, Faverly D (1997). The local distribution of ductal carcinoma in situ of the breast. In: *Ductal Carcinoma in Situ of the Breast*. MJ Silverstein (Ed.) Williams & Wilkins: Baltimore. pp. 233-240.

1231. Holland R, Hendriks JH (1994). Microcalcifications associated with ductal carcinoma in situ: mammographic-pathologic correlation. *Semin Diagn Pathol* 11: 181-192.

1232. Hollingsworth HC, Steinberg SM, Silverberg SG, Merino MJ (1996). Advanced stage transitional cell carcinoma of the ovary. *Hum Pathol* 27: 1267-1272.

1233. Holmberg L, Adami HO, Ekbom A, Bergstrom R, Sandstrom A, Lindgren A (1988). Prognosis in bilateral breast cancer. Effects of time interval between first and second primary tumours. *Br J Cancer* 58: 191-194.

1234. Holway AH, Rieger-Christ KM, Miner WR, Cain JW, Dugan JM, Pezza JA, Silverman ML, Shapter A, McLellan R, Summerhayes IC (2000). Somatic mutation of PTEN in vulvar cancer. *Clin Cancer Res* 6: 3228-3235.

1235. Homesley HD, Bundy BN, Sedlis A, Yordan E, Berek JS, Jahshan A, Mortel R (1993). Prognostic factors for groin node metastasis in squamous cell carcinoma of the vulva (a Gynecologic Oncology Group study). *Gynecol Oncol* 49: 279-283.

1236. Honore LH, Nickerson KG (1976). Papillary serous cystadenoma arising in a paramesonephric cyst of the parovarium. *Am J Obstet Gynecol* 125: 870-871.

1237. Hopkins M, Nunez C, Murphy JR, Wentz WB (1985). Malignant placental site trophoblastic tumor. *Obstet Gynecol* 66: 95S-100S.

1238. Hopper JL, Carlin JB (1992). Familial aggregation of a disease consequent upon correlation between relatives in a risk factor measured on a continuous scale. *Am J Epidemiol* 136: 1138-1147.

1239. Horie Y, Ikawa S, Kadowaki K, Minagawa Y, Kigawa J, Terakawa N (1995). Lipoadenofibroma of the uterine corpus. Report of a new variant of adenofibroma (benign mullerian mixed tumor). *Arch Pathol Lab Med* 119: 274-276.

1240. Horn LC, Einenkel J, Baier D (2000). Endometrial metastasis from breast cancer in a patient receiving tamoxifen therapy. *Gynecol Obstet Invest* 50: 136-138.

1241. Horn PL, Thompson WD (1988). Risk of contralateral breast cancer. Associations with histologic, clinical, and therapeutic factors. *Cancer* 62: 412-424.

1242. Horn T, Jao W, Keh PC (1983). Benign cystic teratoma of the fallopian tube. *Arch Pathol Lab Med* 107: 48.

1243. Horne CH, Reid IN, Milne GD (1976). Prognostic significance of inappropriate production of pregnancy proteins by breast cancers. *Lancet* 2: 279-282.

1244. Horsfall DJ, Tilley WD, Orell SR, Marshall VR, Cant EL (1986). Relationship between ploidy and steroid hormone receptors in primary invasive breast cancer. *Br J Cancer* 53: 23-28.

1245. Houghton CR, Iversen T (1982). Squamous cell carcinoma of the vagina: a clinical study of the location of the tumor. *Gynecol Oncol* 13: 365-372.

1246. Houlston RS, McCarter E, Parbhoo S, Scurr JH, Slack J (1992). Family history and risk of breast cancer. *J Med Genet* 29: 154-157.

1247. Houvras Y, Benezra M, Zhang H, Manfredi JJ, Weber BL, Licht JD (2000). BRCA1 physically and functionally interacts with ATF1. *J Biol Chem* 275: 36230-36237.

1248. Howarth CB, Caces JN, Pratt CB (1980). Breast metastases in children with rhabdomyosarcoma. *Cancer* 46: 2520-2524.

1249. Howat AJ, Armour A, Ellis IO (2000). Microinvasive lobular carcinoma of the breast. *Histopathology* 37: 477-478.

1250. Howe JR, Bair JL, Sayed MG, Anderson ME, Mitros FA, Petersen GM, Velculescu VE, Traverso G, Vogelstein B (2001). Germline mutations of the gene encoding bone morphogenetic protein receptor 1A in juvenile polyposis. *Nat Genet* 28: 184-187.

1251. Howlett NG, Taniguchi T, Olson S, Cox B, Waisfisz Q, Die-Smulders C, Persky N, Grompe M, Joenje H, Pals G, Ikeda H, Fox EA, D'Andrea AD (2002). Biallelic inactivation of BRCA2 in Fanconi anemia. *Science* 297: 606-609.

1252. Hrynchak M, Horsman D, Salski C, Berean K, Benedet JL (1994). Complex karyotypic alterations in an endometrial stromal sarcoma. *Cancer Genet Cytogenet* 77: 45-49.

1253. Hsing AW, McLaughlin JK, Cocco P, Co Chien HT, Fraumeni JFJr. (1998). Risk factors for male breast cancer (United States). *Cancer Causes Control* 9: 269-275.

1254. Hsu SM, Raine L, Nayak RN (1981). Medullary carcinoma of breast: an immunohistochemical study of its lymphoid stroma. *Cancer* 48: 1368-1376.

1255. Hsueh S, Chang TC (1996). Malignant rhabdoid tumor of the uterine corpus. *Gynecol Oncol* 61: 142-146.

1256. Hu CY, Taymor ML, Hertig AT (1950). Primary carcinoma of the fallopian tube. *Am J Obstet Gynecol* 59: 58-60.

1257. Huang E, Cheng SH, Dressman H, Pittman J, Tsou MH, Horng CF, Bild A, Iversen ES, Liao M, Chen CM, West M, Nevins JR, Huang AT (2003). Gene expression predictors of breast cancer outcomes. *Lancet* 361: 1590-1596.

1258. Huang KT, Chen CA, Cheng WF, Wu CC, Jou HJ, Hsieh CY, Lin GJ, Hsieh FJ (1996). Sonographic characteristics of adenofibroma of the endometrium following tamoxifen therapy for breast cancer: two case reports. *Ultrasound Obstet Gynecol* 7: 363-366.

1259. Huang LW, Garrett AP, Schorge JO, Muto MG, Bell DA, Welch WR, Berkowitz RS, Mok SC (2000). Distinct allelic loss patterns in papillary serous carcinoma of the peritoneum. *Am J Clin Pathol* 114: 93-99.

1260. Huettner PC, Gersell DJ (1994). Placental site nodule: a clinicopathologic study of 38 cases. *Int J Gynecol Pathol* 13: 191-198.

1261. Hugh JC, Jackson FI, Hanson J, Poppema S (1990). Primary breast lymphoma. An immunohistologic study of 20 new cases. *Cancer* 66: 2602-2611.

1262. Hughesdon PE (1982). Ovarian tumours of Wolffian or allied nature: their place in ovarian oncology. *J Clin Pathol* 35: 526-535.

1263. Hugues FC, Gourlot C, Le Jeunne C (2000). [Drug-induced gynecomastia]. *Ann Med Interne (Paris)* 151: 10-17.

1264. Hull MT, Warfel KA (1986). Glycogen-rich clear cell carcinomas of the breast. A clinicopathologic and ultrastructural study. *Am J Surg Pathol* 10: 553-559.

1265. Hull MT, Warfel KA (1987). Mucinous breast carcinomas with abundant intracytoplasmic mucin and neuroendocrine features: light microscopic, immunohistochemical, and ultrastructural study. *Ultrastruct Pathol* 11: 29-38.

1266. Humeniuk V, Forrest AP, Hawkins RA, Prescott R (1983). Elastosis and primary breast cancer. *Cancer* 52: 1448-1452.

1267. Hunt CR, Hale RJ, Armstrong C, Rajkumar T, Gullick WJ, Buckley CH (1995). c-erbB-3 proto-oncogene expression in uterine cervical carcinoma. *Int J Gynecol Cancer* 5: 282-285.

1268. Hunt SJ, Santa Cruz DJ, Barr RJ (1990). Cellular angiolipoma. *Am J Surg Pathol* 14: 75-81.

1269. Hunter CE Jr., Sawyers JL (1980). Intracystic papillary carcinoma of the breast. *South Med J* 73: 1484-1486.

1270. Huntington RW Jr., Bullock WK (1970). Yolk sac tumors of extragonadal origin. *Cancer* 25: 1368-1376.

1271. Huntsman DG, Clement PB, Gilks CB, Scully RE (1994). Small-cell carcinoma of the endometrium. A clinicopathological study of sixteen cases. *Am J Surg Pathol* 18: 364-375.

1272. Husseinzadeh N, Recinto C (1999). Frequency of invasive cancer in surgically excised vulvar lesions with intraepithelial neoplasia (VIN 3). *Gynecol Oncol* 73: 119-120.

1273. Huvos AG, Lucas JC Jr., Foote FW Jr. (1973). Metaplastic breast carcinoma. Rare form of mammary cancer. *N Y State J Med* 73: 1078-1082.

1274. Iacocca MV, Maia DM (2001). Bilateral infiltrating lobular carcinoma of the breast with osteoclast-like giant cells. *Breast J* 7: 60-65.

1275. Ibrahim RE, Sciotto CG, Weidner N (1989). Pseudoangiomatous hyperplasia of mammary stroma. Some observations regarding its clinicopathologic spectrum. *Cancer* 63: 1154-1160.

1275a. Ichihara S, Aoyama H (1994). Intraductal carcinoma of the breast arising in sclerosing adenosis. *Pathol Int* 44: 722-726.

1276. Ichikawa Y, Lemon SJ, Wang S, Franklin B, Watson P, Knezetic JA, Bewtra C, Lynch HT (1999). Microsatellite instability and expression of MLH1 and MSH2 in normal and malignant endometrial and ovarian epithelium in hereditary nonpolyposis colorectal cancer family members. *Cancer Genet Cytogenet* 112: 2-8.

1277. Ichikawa Y, Tsunoda H, Takano K, Oki A, Yoshikawa H (2002). Microsatellite instability and immunohistochemical analysis of MLH1 and MSH2 in normal endometrium, endometrial hyperplasia and endometrial cancer from a hereditary nonpolyposis colorectal cancer patient. *Jpn J Clin Oncol* 32: 110-112.

1278. Ichinohasama R, Teshima S, Kishi K, Mukai K, Tsunematsu R, Ishii-Ohba H, Shimosato Y (1989). Leydig cell tumor of the ovary associated with endometrial carcinoma and containing 17 beta-hydroxysteroid dehydrogenase. *Int J Gynecol Pathol* 8: 64-71.

1279. Iczkowski KA, Han AC, Edelson MI, Rosenblum NG (2000). Primary, localized vulvar B-cell lymphoma expressing CD44 variant 6 but not cadherins. A case report. *J Reprod Med* 45: 853-856.

1280. Idvall I, Andersson C, Fallenius G, Ingvar C, Ringberg A, Strand C, Akerman M, Ferno M (2001). Histopathological and cell biological factors of ductal carcinoma in situ before and after the introduction of mammographic screening. *Acta Oncol* 40: 653-659.

1280a. Ihara N, Togashi K, Todo G, Nakai A, Kojima N, Ishigaki T, Suginami N, Kinoshita M, Shintaku M (1999). Sclerosing stromal tumor of the ovary: MRI. *J Comput Assist Tomogr* 23: 555-557.

1281. Ihekwaba FN (1994). Breast cancer in men in black Africa: a report of 73 cases. *J R Coll Surg Edinb* 39: 344-347.

1282. Imachi M, Tsukamoto N, Amagase H, Shigematsu T, Amada S, Nakano H (1993). Metastatic adenocarcinoma to the uterine cervix from gastric cancer. A clinicopathologic analysis of 16 cases. *Cancer* 71: 3472-3477.

1283. Imachi M, Tsukamoto N, Shigematsu T, Nakano H (1992). Cytologic diagnosis of primary adenocarcinoma of Bartholin's gland. A case report. *Acta Cytol* 36: 167-170.

1284. Imachi M, Tsukamoto N, Shigematsu T, Watanabe T, Uehira K, Amada S, Umezu T, Nakano H (1992). Malignant mixed Mullerian tumor of the fallopian tube: report of two cases and review of literature. *Gynecol Oncol* 47: 114-124.

1285. Imachi M, Tsukamoto N, Shimamoto T, Hirakawa T, Uehira K, Nakano H (1991). Clear cell carcinoma of the ovary: a clinicopathological analysis of 34 cases. *Int J Gynecol Cancer* 1: 113-119.

1286. Imai H, Kitamura H, Nananura T, Watanabe M, Koyama T, Kitamura H (1999). Mullerian carcinofibroma of the uterus. A case report. *Acta Cytol* 43: 667-674.

1287. Inaji H, Koyama H (1991). [Tumor markers. Personal experience--screening of breast cancer by determining CEA in nipple discharge]. *Gan To Kagaku Ryoho* 18: 313-317.

1288. Innes KE, Byers TE (1999). Preeclampsia and breast cancer risk. *Epidemiology* 10: 722-732.

1289. Inoue H, Kikuchi Y, Hori T, Nabuchi K, Kobayashi M, Nagata I (1995). An ovarian tumor of probable Wolffian origin with hormonal function. *Gynecol Oncol* 59: 304-308.

1290. Inoue T, Nabeshima K, Shimao Y, Akiyama Y, Ohtsuka T, Koono M (2001). Tubal ectopic pregnancy associated with an adenomatoid tumor. *Pathol Int* 51: 211-214.

1291. Inskip HM, Kinlen LJ, Taylor AM, Woods CG, Arlett CF (1999). Risk of breast cancer and other cancers in heterozygotes for ataxia-telangiectasia. *Br J Cancer* 79: 1304-1307.

1292. International Agency for Research on Cancer (2002). IARC Handbooks of Cancer Prevention Vol. 6: *Weight Control and Physical Activity*. IARC Press: Lyon.

1293. International Agency for Research on Cancer (1995). IARC Monographs on the Evaluation of the Carcinogenic Risks to Humans. Volume 64: *Human papillomaviruses*. IARC Press: Lyon.

1294. International Agency for Research on Cancer (1999). Hormonal contraceptives, progestogens only. In: IARC Monographs on the Evaluation of Carcinogenic Risks to Humans Vol. 72 *Hormonal Contraception and Post-Menopausal Hormonal Therapy*. IARC Press: Lyon , pp. 339-397.

1295. International Agency for Research on Cancer (1999). IARC Monograph on the Evaluation of Carcinogenic Risk to Humans. Volume 72: *Hormonal contraception and post menopausal Hormonal Therapy*. IARC Press: Lyon.

1296. International Agency for Research on Cancer (1999). Oral contraceptives, combined. In: IARC Monographs on the Evaluation of Carcinogenic Risks to Humans Vol. 72 *Hormonal Contraception and Post-Menopausal Hormonal Therapy*. IARC Press: Lyon, pp. 49-338.

1297. International Agency for Research on Cancer (1999). Post-menopausal oestrogen-progestogen therapy. In: IARC Monographs on the Evaluation of Carcinogenic Risks to Humans Vol. 72 *Hormonal Contraception and Post-Menopausal Hormonal Therapy*. IARC Press: Lyon, pp. 531-628.

1298. International Agency for Research on Cancer (1999). Post-menopausal oestrogen therapy. In: IARC Monographs on the Evaluation of Carcinogenic Risks to Humans Vol. 72 *Hormonal Contraception and Post-Menopausal Hormonal Therapy*. IARC Press: Lyon, pp. 399-530.

1299. International Cowden's Syndrome Consortium, Operational Criteria for the Diagnosis of CS, Daly M (1999). NCCN practice guidelines: Genetics/familial high-risk cancer screening. *Oncology* 13: 161-186.

1300. International Federation of Gynecology and Obstretrics (1995). Modifications in the Staging for Stage I Vulvar and Stage I Cervical Cancer. Reports of the FIGO Committee on Gynaecologic Oncology. *Int J Gynaecol Obstet* 50: 215-216.

1301. Iqbal M, Davies MP, Shoker BS, Jarvis C, Sibson DR, Sloane JP (2001). Subgroups of non-atypical hyperplasia of breast defined by proliferation of oestrogen receptor-positive cells. *J Pathol* 193: 333-338.

1302. Iraniha S, Shen V, Kruppe CN, Downey EC (1999). Uterine cervical extrarenal Wilms tumor managed without hysterectomy. *J Pediatr Hematol Oncol* 21: 548-550.

1303. Isaac MA, Vijayalakshmi S, Madhu CS, Bosincu L, Nogales FF (2000). Pure cystic nephroblastoma of the ovary with a review of extrarenal Wilms' tumors. *Hum Pathol* 31: 761-764.

1304. Isaacs C, Stearns V, Hayes DF (2001). New prognostic factors for breast cancer recurrence. *Semin Oncol* 28: 53-67.

1305. Isaacson PG, Spencer J (1987). Malignant lymphoma of mucosa-associated lymphoid tissue. *Histopathology* 11: 445-462.

1306. Ishikura H, Kojo T, Ichimura H, Yoshiki T (1998). Desmoplastic malignant melanoma of the uterine cervix: a rare primary malignancy in the uterus mimicking a sarcoma. *Histopathology* 33: 93-94.

1307. Ishikura H, Scully RE (1987). Hepatoid carcinoma of the ovary. A newly described tumor. *Cancer* 60: 2775-2784.

1308. Ismail SM, Walker SM (1990). Bilateral virilizing sclerosing stromal tumours of the ovary in a pregnant woman with Gorlin's syndrome: implications for pathogenesis of ovarian stromal neoplasms. *Histopathology* 17: 159-163.

1309. Ito K, Watanabe K, Nasim S, Sasano H, Sato S, Yajima A, Silverberg SG, Garrett CT (1994). Prognostic significance of p53 overexpression in endometrial cancer. *Cancer Res* 54: 4667-4670.

1310. Ito T, Saga S, Nagayoshi S, Imai M, Aoyama A, Yokoi T, Hoshino M (1986). Class distribution of immunoglobulin-containing plasma cells in the stroma of medullary carcinoma of breast. *Breast Cancer Res Treat* 7: 97-103.

1311. Itoh T, Mochizuki M, Kumazaki S, Ishihara T, Fukayama M (1997). Cystic pulmonary metastases of endometrial stromal sarcoma of the uterus, mimicking lymphangiomyomatosis: a case report with immunohistochemistry of HMB45. *Pathol Int* 47: 725-729.

1312. Iversen T, Tretli S (1998). Intraepithelial and invasive squamous cell neoplasia of the vulva: trends in incidence, recurrence, and survival rate in Norway. *Obstet Gynecol* 91: 969-972.

1313. Iversen UM (1996). Two cases of benign vaginal rhabdomyoma. Case reports. *APMIS* 104: 575-578.

1314. Iwasaka T, Yokoyama M, Ohuchida M, Matsuo N, Hara K, Fukuyama K, Hachisuga T, Fukuda K, Sugimori H (1992). Detection of human papillomavirus genome and analysis of expression of c-myc and Ha-ras oncogenes in invasive cervical carcinomas. *Gynecol Oncol* 46: 298-303.

1315. Jack MT, Woo RA, Hirao A, Cheung A, Mak TW, Lee PW (2002). Chk2 is dispensable for p53-mediated G1 arrest but is required for a latent p53-mediated apoptotic response. *Proc Natl Acad Sci USA* . 99:9825-9829.

1316. Jackson-York GL, Ramzy I (1992). Synchronous papillary mucinous adenocarcinoma of the endocervix and fallopian tubes. *Int J Gynecol Pathol* 11: 63-67.

1317. Jacobs AJ, Newland JR, Green RK (1982). Pure choriocarcinoma of the ovary. *Obstet Gynecol Surv* 37: 603-609.

1318. Jacobs DM, Sandles LG, Leboit PE (1986). Sebaceous carcinoma arising from Bowen's disease of the vulva. *Arch Dermatol* 122: 1191-1193.

1319. Jacobs PA, Szulman AE, Funkhouser J, Matsuura JS, Wilson CC (1982). Human triploidy: relationship between parental origin of the additional haploid complement and development of partial hydatidiform mole. *Ann Hum Genet* 46: 223-231.

1320. Jacobs TW, Byrne C, Colditz G, Connolly JL, Schnitt SJ (1999). Radial scars in benign breast-biopsy specimens and the risk of breast cancer. *N Engl J Med* 340: 430-436.

1321. Jacobsen GK, Braendstrup O, Talerman A (1991). Bilateral mixed germ cell sex-cord stroma tumour in a young adult woman. Case report. *APMIS Suppl* 23: 132-137.

1321a. Jacobsen O (1946). *Heredity and Breast Cancer*. London.

1322. Jacoby AF, Fuller AF Jr., Thor AD, Muntz HG (1993). Primary leiomyosarcoma of the fallopian tube. *Gynecol Oncol* 51: 404-407.

1323. Jacques SM, Qureshi F, Ramirez NC, Malviya VK, Lawrence WD (1997). Tumors of the uterine isthmus: clinicopathologic features and immunohistochemical characterization of p53 expression and hormone receptors. *Int J Gynecol Pathol* 16: 38-44.

1324. Jaffe R, Altaras M, Bernheim J, Ben Aderet N (1985). Endocervical stromal sarcoma--a case report. *Gynecol Oncol* 22: 105-108.

1325. Jafri NH, Niemann TH, Nicklin JL, Copeland LJ (1998). A carcinoid tumor of the broad ligament. *Obstet Gynecol* 92: 708.

1326. Jain AN, Chin K, Borresen-Dale AL, Erikstein BK, Eynstein LP, Kaaresen R, Gray JW (2001). Quantitative analysis of chromosomal CGH in human breast tumors associates copy number abnormalities with p53 status and patient survival. *Proc Natl Acad Sci USA* 98: 7952-7957.

1327. Jain S, Fisher C, Smith P, Millis RR, Rubens RD (1993). Patterns of metastatic breast cancer in relation to histological type. *Eur J Cancer* 29A: 2155-2157.

1328. Jakubowska A, Narod SA, Goldgar DE, Mierzejewski M, Masojc B, Nej K, Huzarska J, Byrski T, Gorski B, Lubinski J (2003). Breast Cancer Risk Reduction Associated with the RAD51 Polymorphism among Carriers of the BRCA1 5382insC Mutation in Poland. *Cancer Epidemiol Biomarkers Prev* 12: 457-459.

1329. Jamal AA (2001). Pattern of breast diseases in a teaching hospital in Jeddah, Saudi Arabia. *Saudi Med J* 22: 110-113.

1330. Jamal S, Mushtaq S, Malik IA, Khan AH, Mamoon N (1994). Malignant tumours of the male breast - a review of 50 cases. *J Pak Med Assoc* 44: 275-277.

1331. James BA, Cranor MI, Rosen PP (1993). Carcinoma of the breast arising in microglandular adenosis. *Am J Clin Pathol* 100: 507-513.

1332. James K, Bridger J, Anthony PP (1988). Breast tumour of pregnancy ('lactating' adenoma). *J Pathol* 156: 37-44.

1333. James LA, Mitchell EL, Menasce L, Varley JM (1997). Comparative genomic hybridisation of ductal carcinoma in situ of the breast: identification of regions of DNA amplification and deletion in common with invasive breast carcinoma. *Oncogene* 14: 1059-1065.

1334. Janin N, Andrieu N, Ossian K, Lauge A, Croquette MF, Griscelli C, Debre M, Bressac-de-Paillerets B, Aurias A, Stoppa-Lyonnet D (1999). Breast cancer risk in ataxia telangiectasia (AT) heterozygotes: haplotype study in French AT families. *Br J Cancer* 80: 1042-1045.

1335. Janvoski NA, Paramanandhan TL (1973). Ovarian Tumors. Tumors and tumor-like conditions of the ovaries, fallopian tubes and ligaments of the uterus. Major problems in obstetrics and gynecology. WB Sauders: Philadelphia.

1336. Japaze H, Van Dinh T, Woodruff JD (1982). Verrucous carcinoma of the vulva: study of 24 cases. *Obstet Gynecol* 60: 462-466.

1337. Jauniaux E, Nicolaides KH, Hustin J (1997). Perinatal features associated with placental mesenchymal dysplasia. *Placenta* 18: 701-706.

1338. Jee KJ, Kim YT, Kim KR, Kim HS, Yan A, Knuutila S (2001). Loss in 3p and 4p and gain of 3q are concomitant aberrations in squamous cell carcinoma of the vulva. *Mod Pathol* 14: 377-381.

1339. Jensen ML, Kiaer H, Andersen J, Jensen V, Melsen F (1997). Prognostic comparison of three classifications for medullary carcinomas of the breast. *Histopathology* 30: 523-532.

1340. Jensen ML, Kiaer H, Melsen F (1996). Medullary breast carcinoma vs. poorly differentiated ductal carcinoma: an immunohistochemical study with keratin 19 and oestrogen receptor staining. *Histopathology* 29: 241-245.

1341. Jensen ML, Nielsen MN (1989). Broad ligament mucinous and serous cystadenomas of borderline malignancy. *Acta Obstet Gynecol Scand* 68: 663-667.

1342. Jensen ML, Nielsen MN (1990). Broad ligament mucinous cystadenoma of borderline malignancy. *Histopathology* 16: 89-91.

1343. Jensen PA, Dockerty MB, Symmonds RE, Wilson RB (1966). Endometrioid sarcoma ("stromal endometriosis"). Report of 15 cases including 5 with metastases. *Am J Obstet Gynecol* 95: 79-90.

1344. Jensen RD, Norris HJ, Fraumeni JF Jr. (1974). Familial arrhenoblastoma and thyroid adenoma. *Cancer* 33: 218-223.

1345. Jensen V, Jensen ML, Kiaer H, Andersen J, Melsen F (1997). MIB-1 expression in breast carcinomas with medullary features. An immunohistological study including correlations with p53 and bcl-2. *Virchows Arch* 431: 125-130.

1346. Jeon HJ, Akagi T, Hoshida Y, Hayashi K, Yoshino T, Tanaka T, Ito J, Kamei T, Kawabata K (1992). Primary non-Hodgkin malignant lymphoma of the breast. An immunohistochemical study of seven patients and literature review of 152 patients with breast lymphoma in Japan. *Cancer* 70: 2451-2459.

1347. Jernstrom H (2001). Breast-feeding and the Risk of Breast Cancer in BRCA1 and BRCA2 Carriers. *Am J Hum Genet* 69: 9.

1348. Jernstrom H, Lerman C, Ghadirian P, Lynch HT, Weber B, Garber J, Daly M, Olopade OI, Foulkes WD, Warner E, Brunet JS, Narod SA (1999). Pregnancy and risk of early breast cancer in carriers of BRCA1 and BRCA2. *Lancet* 354: 1846-1850.

1349. Jhala DN, Atkinson BF, Balsara GR, Hernandez E, Jhala NC (2001). Role of DNA ploidy analysis in endometrial adenocarcinoma. *Ann Diagn Pathol* 5: 267-273.

1350. Jiao YF, Nakamura S, Oikawa T, Sugai T, Uesugi N (2001). Sebaceous gland metaplasia in intraductal papilloma of the breast. *Virchows Arch* 438: 505-508.

1351. Johannsson O, Loman N, Borg A, Olsson H (1998). Pregnancy-associated breast cancer in BRCA1 and BRCA2 germline mutation carriers. *Lancet* 352: 1359-1360.

1352. Johannsson OT, Idvall I, Anderson C, Borg A, Barkardottir RB, Egilsson V, Olsson H (1997). Tumour biological features of BRCA1-induced breast and ovarian cancer. *Eur J Cancer* 33: 362-371.

1353. Johannsson OT, Ranstam J, Borg A, Olsson H (1998). Survival of BRCA1 breast and ovarian cancer patients: a population-based study from southern Sweden. *J Clin Oncol* 16: 397-404.

1354. Johnson AD, Hebert AA, Esterly NB (1986). Nevoid basal cell carcinoma syndrome: bilateral ovarian fibromas in a 3 1/2-year-old girl. *J Am Acad Dermatol* 14: 371-374.

1355. Johnson TL, Kumar NB, White CD, Morley GW (1986). Prognostic features of vulvar melanoma: a clinicopathologic analysis. *Int J Gynecol Pathol* 5: 110-118.

1356. Jones D.B. (1955). Florid papillomatosis of the nipple ducts. *Cancer* 8: 315-319.

1357. Jones C, Damiani S, Wells D, Chaggar R, Lakhani SR, Eusebi V (2001). Molecular cytogenetic comparison of apocrine hyperplasia and apocrine carcinoma of the breast. *Am J Pathol* 158: 207-214.

1358. Jones C, Merrett S, Thomas VA, Barker TH, Lakhani SR (2003). Comparative genomic hybridization analysis of bilateral hyperplasia of usual type of the breast. *J Pathol* 199: 152-156.

1359. Jones HW, III (1999). The importance of grading in endometrial cancer. *Gynecol Oncol* 74: 1-2.

1360. Jones HW, III, Droegemueller W, Makowski EL (1971). A primary melanocarcinoma of the cervix. *Am J Obstet Gynecol* 111: 959-963.

1361. Jones MA, Mann EW, Caldwell CL, Tarraza HM, Dickersin GR, Young RH (1990). Small cell neuroendocrine carcinoma of Bartholin's gland. *Am J Clin Pathol* 94: 439-442.

1362. Jones MA, Young RH, Scully RE (1991). Diffuse laminar endocervical glandular hyperplasia. A benign lesion often confused with adenoma malignum (minimal deviation adenocarcinoma). *Am J Surg Pathol* 15: 1123-1129.

1363. Jones MW, Kounelis S, Papadaki H, Bakker A, Swalsky PA, Woods J, Finkelstein SD (2000). Well-differentiated villoglandular adenocarcinoma of the uterine cervix: oncogene/tumor suppressor gene alterations and human papillomavirus genotyping. *Int J Gynecol Pathol* 19: 110-117.

1364. Jones MW, Norris HJ (1995). Clinicopathologic study of 28 uterine leiomyosarcomas with metastasis. *Int J Gynecol Pathol* 14: 243-249.

1365. Jones MW, Norris HJ, Snyder RC (1989). Infiltrating syringomatous adenoma of the nipple. A clinical and pathological study of 11 cases. *Am J Surg Pathol* 13: 197-201.

1366. Jones MW, Silverberg SG, Kurman RJ (1993). Well-differentiated villoglandular adenocarcinoma of the uterine cervix: a clinicopathological study of 24 cases. *Int J Gynecol Pathol* 12: 1-7.

1367. Jones MW, Tavassoli FA (1995). Coexistence of nipple duct adenoma and breast carcinoma: a clinicopathologic study of five cases and review of the literature. *Mod Pathol* 8: 633-636.

1368. Jones PA, Laird PW (1999). Cancer epigenetics comes of age. *Nat Genet* 21: 163-167.

1369. Jones RW, Rowan DM (1994). Vulvar intraepithelial neoplasia III: a clinical study of the outcome in 113 cases with relation to the later development of invasive vulvar carcinoma. *Obstet Gynecol* 84: 741-745.

1370. Jordan LB, Abdul-Kader M, al Nafussi A (2001). Uterine serous papillary carcinoma: histopathologic changes within the female genital tract. *Int J Gynecol Cancer* 11: 283-289.

1371. Joseph RE, Enghardt MH, Doering DL, Brown BF, Shaffer DW, Raval HB (1992). Small cell neuroendocrine carcinoma of the vagina. *Cancer* 70: 784-789.

1372. Joshi MG, Lee AK, Pedersen CA, Schnitt S, Camus MG, Hughes KS (1996). The role of immunocytochemical markers in the differential diagnosis of proliferative and neoplastic lesions of the breast. *Mod Pathol* 9: 57-62.

1373. Jozefczyk MA, Rosen PP (1985). Vascular tumors of the breast. II. Perilobular hemangiomas and hemangiomas. *Am J Surg Pathol* 9: 491-503.

1374. Julien M, Trojani M, Coindre JM (1994). [Myofibroblastoma of the breast. Report of 8 cases]. *Ann Pathol* 14: 143-147.

1375. Junge J, Horn T, Bock J (1989). Primary malignant Schwannoma of the uterine cervix. Case report. *Br J Obstet Gynaecol* 96: 111-116.

1376. Kaaks R (1996). Nutrition, hormones, and breast cancer: is insulin the missing link? *Cancer Causes Control* 7: 605-625.

1377. Kaaks R, Lundin E, Manjer J, Rinaldi S, Biessy C, Soderberg S, Lenner P, Janzon L, Riboli E, Berglund G, Hallmans G (2002). Prospective study of IGF-I, IGF-binding proteins and breast cancer risk, in northern and southern Sweden. *Cancer Causes Control* 13: 307-316.

1378. Kachel G, Bornkamm GW, Hermanek P, Kaduk B, Schricker KT (1980). [Burkitt lymphoma of African type in Europe (author's transl)]. *Dtsch Med Wochenschr* 105: 413-417.

1379. Kader HA, Jackson J, Mates D, Andersen S, Hayes M, Olivotto IA (2001). Tubular carcinoma of the breast: a population-based study of nodal metastases at presentation and of patterns of relapse. *Breast J* 7: 8-13.

1380. Kaern J, Trope CG, Kristensen GB, Abeler VM, Pettersen EO (1993). DNA ploidy; the most important prognostic factor in patients with borderline tumors of the ovary. *Int J Gynecol Cancer* 3: 349-358.

1381. Kahanpaa KV, Wahlstrom T, Grohn P, Heinonen E, Nieminen U, Widholm O (1986). Sarcomas of the uterus: a clinicopathologic study of 119 patients. *Obstet Gynecol* 67: 417-424.

1382. Kahner S, Ferenczy A, Richart RM (1975). Homologous mixed Mullerian tumors (carcinosarcomal) confined to endometrial polyps. *Am J Obstet Gynecol* 121: 278-279.

1383. Kainu T, Juo SH, Desper R, Schaffer AA, Gillanders E, Rozenblum E, Freas-Lutz D, Weaver D, Stephan D, Bailey-Wilson J, Kallioniemi OP, Tirkkonen M, Syrjakoski K, Kuukasjarvi T, Koivisto P, Karhu R, Holli K, Arason A, Johannesdottir G, Bergthorsson JT, Johannsdottir H, Egilsson V, Barkardottir RB, Johannsson O, Haraldsson K, Sandberg T, Holmberg E, Gronberg H, Olsson H, Borg A, Vehmanen P, Eerola H, Heikkila P, Pyrhonen S, Nevanlinna H (2000). Somatic deletions in hereditary breast cancers implicate 13q21 as a putative novel breast cancer susceptibility locus. *Proc Natl Acad Sci USA* 97: 9603-9608.

1384. Kairouz R, Clarke RA, Marr PJ, Watters D, Lavin MF, Kearsley JH, Lee CS (1999). ATM protein synthesis patterns in sporadic breast cancer. *Mol Pathol* 52: 252-256.

1385. Kajii T, Ohama K (1977). Androgenetic origin of hydatidiform mole. *Nature* 268: 633-634.

1386. Kajiwara M, Toyoshima S, Yao T, Tanaka M, Tsuneyoshi M (1999). Apoptosis and cell proliferation in medullary carcinoma of the breast: a comparative study between medullary and non-medullary carcinoma using the TUNEL method and immunohistochemistry. *J Surg Oncol* 70: 209-216.

1387. Kaku T, Kamura T, Shigematsu T, Sakai K, Nakanami N, Uehira K, Amada S, Kobayashi H, Saito T, Nakano H (1997). Adenocarcinoma of the uterine cervix with predominantly villogladular papillary growth pattern. *Gynecol Oncol* 64: 147-152.
1388. Kaku T, Silverberg SG, Major FJ, Miller A, Fetter B, Brady MF (1992). Adenosarcoma of the uterus: a Gynecologic Oncology Group clinicopathologic study of 31 cases. *Int J Gynecol Pathol* 11: 75-88.
1389. Kallenberg GA, Pesce CM, Norman B, Ratner RE, Silvergerg SG (1990). Ectopic hyperprolactinemia resulting from an ovarian teratoma. *JAMA* 263: 2472-2474.
1390. Kalstone CE, Jaffe RB, Abell MR (1969). Massive edema of the ovary simulating fibroma. *Obstet Gynecol* 34: 564-571.
1391. Kaminski PF, Norris HJ (1983). Minimal deviation carcinoma (adenoma malignum) of the cervix. *Int J Gynecol Pathol* 2: 141-152.
1392. Kaminski PF, Norris HJ (1984). Coexistence of ovarian neoplasms and endocervical adenocarcinoma. *Obstet Gynecol* 64: 553-556.
1393. Kamoi S, Iskander M, Akin MR, Silverberg SG (1998). Immunohistochemical distinction between endometrial and endocervical adenocarcinomas: Site of origin versus pathway of differentiation. *Mod Pathol* 11: 106 A.
1394. Kanai Y, Oda T, Tsuda H, Ochiai A, Hirohashi S (1994). Point mutation of the E-cadherin gene in invasive lobular carcinoma of the breast. *Jpn J Cancer Res* 85: 1035-1039.
1395. Kang Y, Siegel PM, Shu W, Drobnjak M, Kakonen SM, Cordon-Cardo C, Guise TA, Massague J (2003). A multigenic program mediating breast cancer metastasis to bone. *Cancer Cell* 3: 537-549.
1396. Kao GF, Norris HJ (1978). Benign and low grade variants of mixed mesodermal tumor (adenosarcoma) of the ovary and adnexal region. *Cancer* 42: 1314-1324.
1397. Kapadia SB, Norris HJ (1993). Rhabdomyoma of the vagina. *Mod Pathol* 6: 75A.
1398. Kaplan EJ, Caputo TA, Shen PU, Sassoon RI, Soslow RA (1998). Familial papillary serous carcinoma of the cervix, peritoneum, and ovary: a report of the first case. *Gynecol Oncol* 70: 289-294.
1399. Karayiannakis AJ, Bastounis EA, Chatzigianni EB, Makri GG, Alexiou D, Karamanakos P (1996). Immunohistochemical detection of oestrogen receptors in ductal carcinoma in situ of the breast. *Eur J Surg Oncol* 22: 578-582.
1400. Kariminejad MH, Scully RE (1973). Female adnexal tumor of probable Wolffian origin. A distinctive pathologic entity. *Cancer* 31: 671-677.
1401. Karl SR, Ballentine TVN, Hershey RZ (1985). Juvenile secretory carcinoma of the breast. *J Ped Surg* 20: 368-371.
1402. Karlan BY, Baldwin RL, Lopez-Luevanos E, Raffel LJ, Barbuto D, Narod S, Platt LD (1999). Peritoneal serous papillary carcinoma, a phenotypic variant of familial ovarian cancer: implications for ovarian cancer screening. *Am J Obstet Gynecol* 180: 917-928.
1403. Karseladze AI (2001). On the site of origin of epithelial tumors of the ovary. *Eur J Gynaecol Oncol* 22: 110-115.
1404. Karseladze AI, Zakharova TI, Navarro S, Llombart-Bosch A (2000). Malignant fibrous histiocytoma of the uterus. *Eur J Gynaecol Oncol* 21: 588-590.
1405. Kasamatsu T, Shiromizu K, Takahashi M, Kikuchi A, Uehara T (1998). Leiomyosarcoma of the uterine cervix. *Gynecol Oncol* 69: 169-171.
1406. Kasami M, Olson SJ, Simpson JF, Page DL (1998). Maintenance of polarity and a dual cell population in adenoid cystic carcinoma of the breast: an immunohistochemical study. *Histopathology* 32: 232-238.
1407. Kaspersen P, Buhl L, Moller BR (1988). Fallopian tube papilloma in a patient with primary sterility. Acta Obstet Gynecol Scand 67: 93-94.
1408. Katabuchi H, Tashiro H, Cho KR, Kurman RJ, Hedrick EL (1998). Micropapillary serous carcinoma of the ovary: an immunohistochemical and mutational analysis of p53. *Int J Gynecol Pathol* 17: 54-60.
1409. Katsube Y, Berg JW, Silverberg SG (1982). Epidemiologic pathology of ovarian tumors: a histopathologic review of primary ovarian neoplasms diagnosed in the Denver Standard Metropolitan Statistical Area, 1 July-31 December 1969 and 1 July-31 December 1979. *Int J Gynecol Pathol* 1: 3-16.
1409 a. Katsube Y, Iwaoki Y, Silverberg SG, Fujiwara A (1988). Sclerosing stromal tumor of the ovary associated with endometrial adenocarcinoma: a case report. *Gynecol Oncol* 29: 392-398.
1410. Katsube Y, Mukai K, Silverberg SG (1982). Cystic mesothelioma of the peritoneum: a report of five cases and review of the literature. *Cancer* 50: 1615-1622.
1411. Katz L, Merino MJ, Sakamoto H, Schwartz PE (1987). Endometrial stromal sarcoma: a clinicopathologic study of 11 cases with determination of estrogen and progestin receptor levels in three tumors. *Gynecol Oncol* 26: 87-97.
1412. Katzenstein AL, Mazur MT, Morgan TE, Kao MS (1978). Proliferative serous tumors of the ovary. Histologic features and prognosis. *Am J Surg Pathol* 2: 339-355.
1413. Kauff ND, Satagopan JM, Robson ME, Scheuer L, Hensley M, Hudis CA, Ellis NA, Boyd J, Borgen PI, Barakat RR, Norton L, Castiel M, Nafa K, Offit K (2002). Risk-reducing salpingo-oophorectomy in women with a BRCA1 or BRCA2 mutation. *N Engl J Med* 346: 1609-1615.
1414. Kaufman MW, Marti JR, Gallager HS, Hoehn JL (1984). Carcinoma of the breast with pseudosarcomatous metaplasia. *Cancer* 53: 1908-1917.
1415. Kaufman SL, Stout AP (1960). Hemangiopericytoma in children. *Cancer* 13: 695-710.
1416. Kawai K, Horiguchi H, Sekido N, Akaza H, Koiso K (1996). Leiomyosarcoma of the ovarian vein: an unusual cause of severe abdominal and flank pain. *Int J Urol* 3: 234-236.
1417. Kawamoto S, Urban BA, Fishman EK (1999). CT of epithelial ovarian tumors. Radiographics 19 Spec No: S85-102.
1418. Kawauchi S, Fukuda T, Miyamoto S, Yoshioka J, Shirahama S, Saito T, Tsukamoto N (1998). Peripheral primitive neuroectodermal tumor of the ovary confirmed by CD99 immunostaining, karyotypic analysis, and RT-PCR for EWS/FLI-1 chimeric mRNA. *Am J Surg Pathol* 22: 1417-1422.
1419. Kawauchi S, Tsuji T, Kaku T, Kamura T, Nakano H, Tsuneyoshi M (1998). Sclerosing stromal tumor of the ovary: a clinicopathologic, immunohistochemical, ultrastructural, and cytogenetic analysis with special reference to its vasculature. *Am J Surg Pathol* 22: 83-92.
1420. Kay S, Schneider V (1985). Reactive spindle cell nodule of the endocervix simulating uterine sarcoma. *Int J Gynecol Pathol* 4: 255-257.
1421. Kayaalp E, Heller DS, Majmudar B (2000). Serous tumor of low malignant potential of the fallopian tube. *Int J Gynecol Pathol* 19: 398-400.
1422. Keating JT, Cviko A, Riethdorf S, Riethdorf L, Quade BJ, Sun D, Duensing S, Sheets EE, Munger K, Crum CP (2001). Ki-67, cyclin E, and p16INK4 are complimentary surrogate biomarkers for human papilloma virus-related cervical neoplasia. *Am J Surg Pathol* 25: 884-891.
1423. Keatings L, Sinclair J, Wright C, Corbett IP, Watchorn C, Hennessy C, Angus B, Lennard T, Horne CH (1990). c-erbB-2 oncoprotein expression in mammary and extramammary Paget's disease. *Histopathology* 17: 243-247.
1424. Keel SB, Clement PB, Prat J, Young RH (1998). Malignant schwannoma of the uterine cervix: a study of three cases. *Int J Gynecol Pathol* 17: 223-230.
1424a. Keelan PA, Myers JL, Wold LE, Katzmann JA, Gibney DJ (1992). Phyllodes tumor: clinicopathologic review of 60 patients and flow cytometric analysis in 30 patients. *Hum Pathol* 23: 1048-1054.
1425. Keeney GL, Thrasher TV (1988). Metaplastic papillary tumor of the fallopian tube: a case report with ultrastructure. *Int J Gynecol Pathol* 7: 86-92.
1426. Keep D, Zaragoza MV, Hassold T, Redline RW (1996). Very early complete hydatidiform mole. *Hum Pathol* 27: 708-713.
1427. Keitoku M, Konishi I, Nanbu K, Yamamoto S, Mandai M, Kataoka N, Oishi T, Mori T (1997). Extraovarian sex cord-stromal tumor: case report and review of the literature. *Int J Gynecol Pathol* 16: 180-185.
1428. Kelley JL, III, Burke TW, Tornos C, Morris M, Gershenson DM, Silva EG, Wharton JT (1992). Minimally invasive vulvar carcinoma: an indication for conservative surgical therapy. *Gynecol Oncol* 44: 240-244.
1429. Kelly RR, Scully RE (1961). Cancer developing in dermoid cysts of the ovary. A report of 8 cases, including a carcinoid and a leiomyosarcoma. *Cancer* 14: 989-1000.
1430. Kelsey JL, Gammon MD, John EM (1993). Reproductive factors and breast cancer. *Epidemiol Rev* 15: 36-47.
1431. Kempson RL, Fletcher CDM, Evans HL, Hendrikson MR, Sibley RK (2001). *Tumours of the Soft Tissues.* AFIP: Washington, DC.
1432. Kempson RL, Hendrickson MR (2000). Smooth muscle, endometrial stromal, and mixed Mullerian tumors of the uterus. *Mod Pathol* 13: 328-342.
1433. Kendall BS, Ronnett BM, Isacson C, Cho KR, Hedrick L, Diener-West M, Kurman RJ (1998). Reproducibility of the diagnosis of endometrial hyperplasia, atypical hyperplasia, and well-differentiated carcinoma. *Am J Surg Pathol* 22: 1012-1019.
1434. Kennebeck CH, Alagoz T (1998). Signet ring breast carcinoma metastases limited to the endometrium and cervix. *Gynecol Oncol* 71: 461-464.
1435. Kennedy AW, Biscotti CV, Hart WR, Webster KD (1989). Ovarian clear cell adenocarcinoma. *Gynecol Oncol* 32: 342-349.
1436. Kennedy AW, Markman M, Webster KD, Kulp B, Peterson G, Rybicki LA, Belinson JL (1998). Experience with platinum-paclitaxel chemotherapy in the initial management of papillary serous carcinoma of the peritoneum. *Gynecol Oncol* 71: 288-290.
1437. Kennedy MM, Baigrie CF, Manek S (1999). Tamoxifen and the endometrium: review of 102 cases and comparison with HRT-related and non-HRT-related endometrial pathology. *Int J Gynecol Pathol* 18: 130-137.
1438. Kenny-Moynihan MB, Hagen J, Richman B, McIntosh DG, Bridge JA (1996). Loss of an X chromosome in aggressive angiomyxoma of female soft parts: a case report. *Cancer Genet Cytogenet* 89: 61-64.
1439. Kerangueven F, Eisinger F, Noguchi T, Allione F, Wargniez V, Eng C, Padberg G, Theillet C, Jacquemier J, Longy M, Sobol H, Birnbaum D (1997). Loss of heterozygosity in human breast carcinomas in the ataxia telangiectasia, Cowden disease and BRCA1 gene regions. *Oncogene* 14: 339-347.
1439a. Kerlikowske K, Barclay J, Grady D, Sickles EA, Ernster V (1997). Comparison of risk factors for ductal carcinoma in situ and invasive breast cancer. *J Natl Cancer Inst* 89: 76-82.
1440. Kermarec J, Plouvier S, Duplay H, Daniel R (1973). [Myoepithelial cell breast tumor. Ultrastructural study]. *Arch Anat Pathol (Paris)* 21: 225-231.
1441. Kerner H, Sabo E, Friedman M, Beck D, Samare O, Lichtig C (1995). An immunohistochemical study of estrogen and progesterone receptors in adenocarcinoma of the endometrium and in the adjacent mucosa. *Int J Gynecol Cancer* 5: 275-281.
1442. Kerr P, Ashworth A (2001). New complexities for BRCA1 and BRCA2. *Curr Biol* 11: R668-R676.
1443. Kerrigan SA, Turnnir RT, Clement PB, Young RH, Churg A (2002). Diffuse malignant epithelial mesotheliomas of the peritoneum in women: a clinicopathologic study of 25 patients. *Cancer* 94: 378-385.
1444. Kersemaekers AM, Hermans J, Fleuren GJ, Van de Vijver MJ (1998). Loss of heterozygosity for defined regions on chromosomes 3, 11 and 17 in carcinomas of the uterine cervix. *Br J Cancer* 77: 192-200.
1445. Kersemaekers AM, Van de Vijver MJ, Kenter GG, Fleuren GJ (1999). Genetic alterations during the progression of squamous cell carcinomas of the uterine cervix. *Genes Chromosomes Cancer* 26: 346-354.
1446. Key TJ (1999). Serum oestradiol and breast cancer risk. *Endocr Relat Cancer* 6: 175-180.
1447. Key TJ, Pike MC (1988). The role of oestrogens and progestagens in the epidemiology and prevention of breast cancer. *Eur J Cancer Clin Oncol* 24: 29-43.
1448. Khalifa MA, Hansen CH, Moore JL Jr., Rusnock EJ, Lage JM (1996). Endometrial stromal sarcoma with focal smooth muscle differentiation: recurrence after 17 years: a follow-up report with discussion of the nomenclature. *Int J Gynecol Pathol* 15: 171-176.

1449. Khalifa MA, Mannel RS, Haraway SD, Walker J, Min KW (1994). Expression of EGFR, HER-2/neu, P53, and PCNA in endometrioid, serous papillary, and clear cell endometrial adenocarcinomas. *Gynecol Oncol* 53: 84-92.
1450. Khan MS, Dodson AR, Heatley MK (1999). Ki-67, oestrogen receptor, and progesterone receptor proteins in the human rete ovarii and in endometriosis. *J Clin Pathol* 52: 517-520.
1451. Khoor A, Fleming MV, Purcell CA, Seidman JD, Ashton AH, Weaver DL (1995). Mature teratoma of the uterine cervix with pulmonary differentiation. *Arch Pathol Lab Med* 119: 848-850.
1452. Khoury S, Odeh M, Ophir E, Cohen H, Oettinger M (1997). Uterine metastasis from gastric cancer. *Acta Obstet Gynecol Scand* 76: 803.
1453. Khunamornpong S, Russell P, Dalrymple JC (1999). Proliferating (LMP) mucinous tumours of the ovaries with microinvasion: morphological assessment of 13 cases. *Int J Gynecol Pathol* 18: 238-246.
1454. Kiaer H, Nielsen B, Paulsen S, Sorensen IM, Dyreborg U, Blichert-Toft M (1984). Adenomyoepithelial adenosis and low-grade malignant adenomyoepithelioma of the breast. *Virchows Arch A Pathol Anat Histopathol* 405: 55-67.
1455. Kiaer W, Holm-Jensen S (1972). Metastases to the uterus. Five cases diagnosed on the basis of curettings. *Acta Pathol Microbiol Scand [A]* 80: 835-840.
1456. Kido A, Togashi K, Konishi I, Kataoka ML, Koyama T, Ueda H, Fujii S, Konishi J (1999). Dermoid cysts of the ovary with malignant transformation: MR appearance. *AJR Am J Roentgenol* 172: 445-449.
1457. Kiechle-Schwarz M, Kommoss F, Schmidt J, Lukovic L, Walz L, Bauknecht T, Pfleiderer A (1992). Cytogenetic analysis of an adenoid cystic carcinoma of the Bartholin's gland. A rare, semimalignant tumor of the female genitourinary tract. *Cancer Genet Cytogenet* 61: 26-30.
1458. Kikkawa F, Kawai M, Tamakoshi K, Suganuma N, Nakashima N, Furuhashi Y, Kuzuya K, Hattori S, Arii Y, Tomoda Y (1996). Mucinous carcinoma of the ovary. Clinicopathologic analysis. *Oncology* 53: 303-307.
1459. Kim KR, Scully RE (1990). Peritoneal keratin granulomas with carcinomas of endometrium and ovary and atypical polypoid adenomyoma of endometrium. A clinicopathological analysis of 22 cases. *Am J Surg Pathol* 14: 925-932.
1460. Kim SH, Kim WH, Park KJ, Lee JK, Kim JS (1996). CT and MR findings of Krukenberg tumors: comparison with primary ovarian tumors. *J Comput Assist Tomogr* 20: 393-398.
1461. Kim YT, Thomas NF, Kessis TD, Wilkinson EJ, Hedrick L, Cho KR (1996). p53 mutations and clonality in vulvar carcinomas and squamous hyperplasias: evidence suggesting that squamous hyperplasias do not serve as direct precursors of human papillomavirus-negative vulvar carcinomas. *Hum Pathol* 27: 389-395.
1462. Kindblom LG, Stenman G, Angervall L (1991). Morphological and cytogenetic studies of angiosarcoma in Stewart-Treves syndrome. *Virchows Arch A Pathol Anat Histopathol* 419: 439-445.
1463. King BF, Enders AC (1993). *The Human Yolk Sac and Yolk Sac* Tumours. Springer: Berlin.
1464. King MC, Wieand S, Hale K, Lee M, Walsh T, Owens K, Tait J, Ford L, Dunn BK, Costantino J, Wickerham L, Wolmark N, Fisher B (2001). Tamoxifen and breast cancer incidence among women with inherited mutations in BRCA1 and BRCA2: National Surgical Adjuvant Breast and Bowel Project (NSABP-P1) Breast Cancer Prevention Trial. *JAMA* 286: 2251-2256.
1465. King ME, Dickersin GR, Scully RE (1982). Myxoid leiomyosarcoma of the uterus. A report of six cases. *Am J Surg Pathol* 6: 589-598.
1466. King ME, Micha JP, Allen SL, Mouradian JA, Chaganti RS (1985). Immature teratoma of the ovary with predominant malignant retinal anlage component. A parthenogenically derived tumor. *Am J Surg Pathol* 9: 221-231.
1467. Kinne DW, Petrek JA, Osborne MP, Fracchia AA, DePalo AA, Rosen PP (1989). Breast carcinoma in situ. *Arch Surg* 124: 33-36.
1468. Kinzler K, Vogelstein B (1998). *The Genetic Basis of Human Cancer.* McGraw Hill: Toronto.
1469. Kirchhoff M, Rose H, Petersen BL, Maahr J, Gerdes T, Lundsteen C, Bryndorf T, Kryger-Baggesen N, Christensen L, Engelholm SA, Philip J (1999). Comparative genomic hybridization reveals a recurrent pattern of chromosomal aberrations in severe dysplasia/carcinoma in situ of the cervix and in advanced-stage cervical carcinoma. *Genes Chromosomes Cancer* 24: 144-150.
1470. Kister SJ, Sommers SC, Haagensen CD, Cooley E (1966). Reevaluation of blood vessel invasion and lymphocytic infiltrates ni breast carcinoma. *Cancer* 19: 1213-1216.
1471. Kitchen PR, Smith TH, Henderson MA, Goldhirsch A, Castiglione-Gertsch M, Coates AS, Gusterson B, Brown RW, Gelber RD, Collins JP (2001). Tubular carcinoma of the breast: prognosis and response to adjuvant systemic therapy. *Aust N Z J Surg* 71: 27-31.
1472. Klauber-DeMore N, Tan LK, Liberman L, Kaptain S, Fey J, Borgen P, Heerdt A, Montgomery L, Paglia M, Petrek JA, Cody HS, Van Zee KJ (2000). Sentinel lymph node biopsy: is it indicated in patients with high-risk ductal carcinoma-in-situ and ductal carcinoma-in-situ with microinvasion? *Ann Surg Oncol* 7: 636-642.
1473. Kleer CG, Giordano TJ, Braun T, Oberman HA (2001). Pathologic, immunohistochemical, and molecular features of benign and malignant phyllodes tumors of the breast. *Mod Pathol* 14: 185-190.
1474. Kleihues P, Cavenee WK (2000). *WHO Classification of Tumours. Pathology and Genetics of Tumours of the Nervous System.* IARC Press: Lyon, France.
1475. Kleihues P, Schauble B, zur Hausen A, Esteve J, Ohgaki H (1997). Tumors associated with p53 germline mutations: a synopsis of 91 families. *Am J Pathol* 150: 1-13.
1476. Kleinman GM, Young RH, Scully RE (1993). Primary neuroectodermal tumors of the ovary. A report of 25 cases. *Am J Surg Pathol* 17: 764-778.
1477. Klemi PJ, Gronroos M (1979). Endometrioid carcinoma of the ovary. A clinicopathologic, histochemical, and electron microscopic study. *Obstet Gynecol* 53: 572-579.
1478. Kliewer EV, Smith KR (1995). Breast cancer mortality among immigrants in Australia and Canada. *J Natl Cancer Inst* 87: 1154-1161.
1479. Kline RC, Wharton JT, Atkinson EN, Burke TW, Gershenson DM, Edwards CL (1990). Endometrioid carcinoma of the ovary: retrospective review of 145 cases. *Gynecol Oncol* 39: 337-346.
1480. Ko SF, Wan YL, Ng SH, Lee TY, Lin JW, Chen WJ, Kung FT, Tsai CC (1999). Adult ovarian granulosa cell tumors: spectrum of sonographic and CT findings with pathologic correlation. *AJR Am J Roentgenol* 172: 1227-1233.
1481. Kobayashi K, Sagae S, Kudo R, Saito H, Koi S, Nakamura Y (1995). Microsatellite instability in endometrial carcinomas: frequent replication errors in tumors of early onset and/or of poorly differentiated type. *Genes Chromosomes Cancer* 14: 128-132.
1481a. Kobayashi Y, Yamazaki K, Shinohara M, Iwahashi K, Suzuki A, Fujii T, Sasaki H, Shiraishi S (1996). Undifferentiated carcinoma of the broad ligament in a 28-year-old woman--a case report and results of immunohistochemical and electron-microscopic studies. *Gynecol Oncol* 63: 382-387.
1482. Kocova L, Skalova A, Fakan F, Rousarova M (1998). Phyllodes tumour of the breast: immunohistochemical study of 37 tumours using MIB1 antibody. *Pathol Res Pract* 194: 97-104.
1483. Koenig C, Dadmanesh F, Bratthauer GL, Tavassoli FA (2000). Carcinoma arising in microglandular adenosis: an immunohistochemical analysis of 20 intraepithelial and invasive neoplasms. *Int J Surg Pathol* 8: 303-315.
1485. Koenig C, Demopoulos RI, Vamvakas EC, Mittal KR, Feiner HD, Espiritu EC (1993). Flow cytometric DNA ploidy and quantitative histopathology in partial moles. *Int J Gynecol Pathol* 12: 235-240.
1486. Koenig C, Tavassoli FA (1998). Mucinous cystadenocarcinoma of the breast. *Am J Surg Pathol* 22: 698-703.
1487. Koenig C, Tavassoli FA (1998). Nodular hyperplasia, adenoma, and adenomyoma of Bartholin's gland. *Int J Gynecol Pathol* 17: 289-294.
1488. Koenig C, Turnicky RP, Kankam CF, Tavassoli FA (1997). Papillary squamotransitional cell carcinoma of the cervix: a report of 32 cases. *Am J Surg Pathol* 21: 915-921.
1489. Kofinas AD, Suarez J, Calame RJ, Chipeco Z (1984). Chondrosarcoma of the uterus. *Gynecol Oncol* 19: 231-237.
1490. Kokal WA, Hill LR, Porudominsky D, Beatty JD, Kemeny MM, Riihimaki DU, Terz JJ (1985). Inflammatory breast carcinoma: a distinct entity? *J Surg Oncol* 30: 152-155.
1491. Kollias J, Ellis IO, Elston CW, Blamey RW (1999). Clinical and histological predictors of contralateral breast cancer. *Eur J Surg Oncol* 25: 584-589.
1492. Kollias J, Ellis IO, Elston CW, Blamey RW (2001). Prognostic significance of synchronous and metachronous bilateral breast cancer. *World J Surg* 25: 1117-1124.
1493. Kollias J, Elston CW, Ellis IO, Robertson JF, Blamey RW (1997). Early-onset breast cancer--histopathological and prognostic considerations. *Br J Cancer* 75: 1318-1323.
1494. Kolodner RD, Hall NR, Lipford J, Kane MF, Morrison PT, Finan PJ, Burn J, Chapman P, Earabino C, Merchant E, Bishop DT. (1995). Structure of the human MLH1 locus and analysis of a large hereditary nonpolyposis colorectal carcinoma kindred for mlh1 mutations. *Cancer Res* 55: 242-248.
1495. Kolodner RD, Hall NR, Lipford J, Kane MF, Rao MR, Morrison P, Wirth L, Finan PJ, Burn J, Chapman P (1994). Structure of the human MSH2 locus and analysis of two Muir-Torre kindreds for msh2 mutations. *Genomics* 24: 516-526.
1496. Kolodner RD, Marsischky GT (1999). Eukaryotic DNA mismatch repair. *Curr Opin Genet Dev* 9: 89-96.
1497. Kolodner RD, Tytell JD, Schmeits JL, Kane MF, Gupta RD, Weger J, Wahlberg S, Fox EA, Peel D, Ziogas A, Garber JE, Syngal S, Anton-Culver H, Li FP (1999). Germ-line msh6 mutations in colorectal cancer families. *Cancer Res* 59: 5068-5074.
1498. Komaki K, Sakamoto G, Sugano H, Morimoto T, Monden Y (1988). Mucinous carcinoma of the breast in Japan. A prognostic analysis based on morphologic features. *Cancer* 61: 989-996.
1499. Kommoss F, Oliva E, Bhan AK, Young RH, Scully RE (1998). Inhibin expression in ovarian tumors and tumor-like lesions: an immunohistochemical study. *Mod Pathol* 11: 656-664.
1500. Kommoss F, Schmidt M, Merz E, Knapstein PG, Young RH, Scully RE (1999). Ovarian endometrioid-like yolk sac tumor treated by surgery alone, with recurrence at 12 years. *Gynecol Oncol* 72: 421-424.
1501. Kondi-Paphitis A, Deligeorgi-Politi H, Liapis A, Plemenou-Frangou M (1998). Human papilloma virus in verrucus carcinoma of the vulva: an immunopathological study of three cases. *Eur J Gynaecol Oncol* 19: 319-320.
1502. Koonings PP, Campbell K, Mishell DR Jr., Grimes DA (1989). Relative frequency of primary ovarian neoplasms: a 10-year review. *Obstet Gynecol* 74: 921-926.
1503. Koontz JI, Soreng AL, Nucci M, Kuo FC, Pauwels P, Van den Berghe H, Cin PD, Fletcher JA, Sklar J (2001). Frequent fusion of the JAZF1 and JJAZ1 genes in endometrial stromal tumors. *Proc Natl Acad Sci USA* 98: 6348-6353.
1504. Kopolovic J, Weiss DB, Dolberg L, Brezinsky A, Ne'eman Z, Anteby SO (1987). Alveolar soft-part sarcoma of the female genital tract. Case report with ultrastructural findings. *Arch Gynecol* 240: 125-129.
1505. Korn WT, Schatzki SC, DiSciullo AJ, Scully RE (1990). Papillary cystadenoma of the broad ligament in von Hippel-Lindau disease. *Am J Obstet Gynecol* 163: 596-598.
1506. Kosary CL (1994). FIGO stage, histology, histologic grade, age and race as prognostic factors in determining survival for cancers of the female gynecological system: an analysis of 1973-87 SEER cases of cancers of the endometrium, cervix, ovary, vulva, and vagina. *Semin Surg Oncol* 10: 31-46.
1507. Koss LG, Brannan CD, Ashikari R (1970). Histologic and ultrastructural features of adenoid cystic carcinoma of the breast. *Cancer* 26: 1271-1279.
1508. Koss LG, Durfee GR (1956). Unusual patterns of squamous epithelium of the uterine cervix and pathological study of kaoilocytotic atypia. *Ann N Y Acad Sci* 63: 1245-1261.
1509. Koss LG, ShapiroR.H., Brunschwig A (1965). Endometrial stromal sarcoma. *Surg Gynecol Obstet* 121: 531-537.
1510. Kotlan B, Gruel N, Zafrani B, Furedi G, Foldi J, Petranyi G, Fridman W, Teillaud J (1999). Immunoglobulin variable regions usage by B-lymphocytes infiltrating a human breast medullary carcinoma. *Immunology Letters* 65: 143-151.

1511. Kotylo PK, Michael H, Davis TE, Sutton GP, Mark PR, Roth LM (1992). Flow cytometric DNA analysis of placental-site trophoblastic tumors. *Int J Gynecol Pathol* 11: 245-252.

1512. Kounelis S, Kapranos N, Kouri E, Coppola D, Papadaki H, Jones MW (2000). Immunohistochemical profile of endometrial adenocarcinoma: a study of 61 cases and review of the literature. *Mod Pathol* 13: 379-388.

1513. Koutsky LA, Holmes KK, Critchlow CW, Stevens CE, Paavonen J, Beckmann AM, DeRouen TA, Galloway DA, Vernon D, Kiviat NB (1992). A cohort study of the risk of cervical intraepithelial neoplasia grade 2 or 3 in relation to papillomavirus infection. *N Engl J Med* 327: 1272-1278.

1514. Kouvidou C, Karayianni M, Liapi-Avgeri G, Toufexi H, Karaiossifidi H (2000). Old ectopic pregnancy remnants with morphological features of placental site nodule occurring in fallopian tube and broad ligament. *Pathol Res Pract* 196: 329-332.

1515. Kovi J, Duong HD, Leffall LS Jr. (1981). High-grade mucoepidermoid carcinoma of the breast. *Arch Pathol Lab Med* 105: 612-614.

1516. Koyama M, Kurotaki H, Yagihashi N, Aizawa S, Sugai M, Kamata Y, Oyama T, Yagihashi S (1997). Immunohistochemical assessment of proliferative activity in mammary adenomyoepithelioma. *Histopathology* 31: 134-139.

1517. Kraemer BB, Silva EG, Sneige N (1984). Fibrosarcoma of ovary. A new component in the nevoid basal-cell carcinoma syndrome. *Am J Surg Pathol* 8: 231-236.

1518. Kraggerud SM, Szymanska J, Abeler VM, Kaern J, Eknaes M, Heim S, Teixeira MR, Trope CG, Peltomaki P, Lothe RA (2000). DNA copy number changes in malignant ovarian germ cell tumors. *Cancer Res* 60: 3025-3030.

1519. Krausz T, Jenkins D, Grontoft O, Pollock DJ, Azzopardi JG (1989). Secretory carcinoma of the breast in adults: emphasis on late recurrence and metastasis. *Histopathology* 14: 25-36.

1520. Krieger N, Hiatt RA (1992). Risk of breast cancer after benign breast diseases. Variation by histologic type, degree of atypia, age at biopsy, and length of follow-up. *Am J Epidemiol* 135: 619-631.

1521. Krishnamurthy S, Jungbluth AA, Busam KJ, Rosai J (1998). Uterine tumors resembling ovarian sex-cord tumors have an immunophenotype consistent with true sex-cord differentiation. *Am J Surg Pathol* 22: 1078-1082.

1521 a. Krivak TC, McBroom JW, Sundborg MJ, Crothers B, Parker MF (2001). Large cell neuroendocrine cervical carcinoma: a report of two cases and review of the literature. *Gynecol Oncol* 82: 187-191.

1522. Kubik-Huch RA, Dorffler W, von Schulthess GK, Marincek B, Kochli OR, Seifert B, Haller U, Steinert HC (2000). Value of (18F)-FDG positron emission tomography, computed tomography, and magnetic resonance imaging in diagnosing primary and recurrent ovarian carcinoma. *Eur Radiol* 10: 761-767.

1523. Kucera E, Speiser P, Gnant M, Szabo L, Samonigg H, Hausmaninger H, Mittlbock M, Fridrik M, Seifert M, Kubista E, Reiner A, Zeillinger R, Jakesz R (1999). Prognostic significance of mutations in the p53 gene, particularly in the zinc-binding domains, in lymph node- and steroid receptor positive breast cancer patients. Austrian Breast Cancer Study Group. *Eur J Cancer* 35: 398-405.

1524. Kucera H, Langer M, Smekal G, Weghaupt K (1985). Radiotherapy of primary carcinoma of the vagina: management and results of different therapy schemes. *Gynecol Oncol* 21: 87-93.

1525. Kuijper A, Mommers EC, van der Wall E, van Diest PJ (2001). Histopathology of fibroadenoma of the breast. *Am J Clin Pathol* 115: 736-742.

1526. Kuiper GG, Enmark E, Pelto-Huikko M, Nilsson S, Gustafsson JA (1996). Cloning of a novel receptor expressed in rat prostate and ovary. *Proc Natl Acad Sci USA* 93: 5925-5930.

1527. Kuismanen SA, Moisio AL, Schweizer P, Truninger K, Salovaara R, Arola J, Butzow R, Jiricny J, Nystrom-Lahti M, Peltomaki P (2002). Endometrial and colorectal tumors from patients with hereditary nonpolyposis colon cancer display different patterns of microsatellite instability. *Am J Pathol* 160: 1953-1958.

1528. Kulski JK, Demeter T, Rakoczy P, Sterrett GF, Pixley EC (1989). Human papillomavirus coinfections of the vulva and uterine cervix. *J Med Virol* 27: 244-251.

1529. Kumar A, Schneider V (1983). Metastases to the uterus from extrapelvic primary tumors. *Int J Gynecol Pathol* 2: 134-140.

1530. Kumar L, Pokharel YH, Dawar R, Thulkar S (1999). Cervical cancer metastatic to the breast: a case report and review of the literature. *Clin Oncol (R Coll Radiol)* 11: 414-416.

1531. Kumar NB, Hart WR (1982). Metastases to the uterine corpus from extragenital cancers. A clinicopathologic study of 63 cases. *Cancer* 50: 2163-2169.

1532. Kupets R, Covens A (2001). Is the International Federation of Gynecology and Obstetrics staging system for cervical carcinoma able to predict survival in patients with cervical carcinoma?: an assessment of clinimetric properties. *Cancer* 92: 796-804.

1533. Kupryjanczyk J, Kujawa M (1992). Signet-ring cells in squamous cell carcinoma of the cervix and in non-neoplastic ectocervical epithelium. *Int J Gynecol Cancer* 2: 152-156.

1534. Kurian K, al Nafussi A (1999). Relation of cervical glandular intraepithelial neoplasia to microinvasive and invasive adenocarcinoma of the uterine cervix: a study of 121 cases. *J Clin Pathol* 52: 112-117.

1535. Kurman RJ, Kaminski PF, Norris HJ (1985). The behavior of endometrial hyperplasia. A long-term study of "untreated" hyperplasia in 170 patients. *Cancer* 56: 403-412.

1536. Kurman RJ, Norris HJ (1976). Embryonal carcinoma of the ovary: a clinicopathologic entity distinct from endodermal sinus tumor resembling embryonal carcinoma of the adult testis. *Cancer* 38: 2420-2433.

1537. Kurman RJ, Norris HJ (1976). Endodermal sinus tumor of the ovary: a clinical and pathologic analysis of 71 cases. *Cancer* 38: 2404-2419.

1538. Kurman RJ, Norris HJ (1976). Mesenchymal tumors of the uterus. VI. Epithelioid smooth muscle tumors including leiomyoblastoma and clear-cell leiomyoma: a clinical and pathologic analysis of 26 cases. *Cancer* 37: 1853-1865.

1539. Kurman RJ, Norris HJ, Wilkinson E (1992). Tumours of the cervix, vagina, and vulva. In: *Atlas of Tumour Pathology*, AFIP, ed., AFIP: Washington,DC .

1540. Kurman RJ, Scully RE, Norris HJ (1976). Trophoblastic pseudotumor of the uterus: an exaggerated form of "syncytial endometritis" simulating a malignant tumor. *Cancer* 38: 1214-1226.

1541. Kurman RJ, Toki T, Schiffman MH (1993). Basaloid and warty carcinomas of the vulva. Distinctive types of squamous cell carcinoma frequently associated with human papillomaviruses. *Am J Surg Pathol* 17: 133-145.

1542. Kurman RJ, Trimble CL (1993). The behavior of serous tumors of low malignant potential: are they ever malignant? *Int J Gynecol Pathol* 12: 120-127.

1543. Kurman RJ, Young RH, Norris HJ, Main CS, Lawrence WD, Scully RE (1984). Immunocytochemical localization of placental lactogen and chorionic gonadotropin in the normal placenta and trophoblastic tumors, with emphasis on intermediate trophoblast and the placental site trophoblastic tumor. *Int J Gynecol Pathol* 3: 101-121. **1544.** Kuroda N, Hirano K, Inui Y, Yamasaki Y, Toi M, Nakayama H, Hiroi M, Enzan H (2001). Compound melanocytic nevus arising in a mature cystic teratoma of the ovary. *Pathol Int* 51: 902-904.

1545. Kurose K, Hoshaw-Woodard S, Adeyinka A, Lemeshow S, Watson PH, Eng C (2001). Genetic model of multi-step breast carcinogenesis involving the epithelium and stroma: clues to tumour-microenvironment interactions. *Hum Mol Genet* 10: 1907-1913.

1546. Kurosumi M, Ishida T, Kurebayashi J, Kawai T, Joshita T, Honjo T, Izuo M (1988). Lipid-secreting mammary carcinoma: a light and electon microscopic investigation. *J Clin Electron Microscopy* 21: 147-156.

1547. Kushner BH, LaQuaglia MP, Wollner N, Meyers PA, Lindsley KL, Ghavimi F, Merchant TE, Boulad F, Cheung NK, Bonilla MA, Crouch G, Kelleher JF Jr., Steinherz PG, Gerald WL (1996). Desmoplastic small round-cell tumor: prolonged progression-free survival with aggressive multimodality therapy. *J Clin Oncol* 14: 1526-1531.

1548. Kuukasjarvi T, Tanner M, Pennanen S, Karhu R, Kallioniemi OP, Isola J (1997). Genetic changes in intraductal breast cancer detected by comparative genomic hybridization. *Am J Pathol* 150: 1465-1471.

1549. Kuwabara H, Uda H (1997). Clear cell mammary malignant myoepithelioma with abundant glycogens. *J Clin Pathol* 50: 700-702.

1550. Kwiatkowska E, Teresiak M, Lamperska KM, Karczewska A, Breborowicz D, Stawicka M, Godlewski D, Krzyzosiak WJ, Mackiewicz A (2001). BRCA2 germline mutations in male breast cancer patients in the Polish population. *Hum Mutat* 17: 73.

1551. La Vecchia C, Levi F, Lucchini F (1992). Descriptive epidemiology of male breast cancer in Europe. *Int J Cancer* 51: 62-66.

1551 a. La Vecchia C, Parazzini F, Franceschi S, Decarli A (1985). Risk factors for benign breast disease and their relation with breast cancer risk. Pooled information from epidemiologic studies. *Tumori* 71: 167-178.

1552. Laake K, Launonen V, Niederacher D, Gudlaugsdottir S, Seitz S, Rio P, Champeme MH, Bieche I, Birnbaum D, White G, Sztan M, Sever N, Plummer S, Osorio A, Broeks A, Huusko P, Spurr N, Borg A, Cleton-Jansen AM, van't Veer L, Benitez J, Casey G, Peterlin B, Olah E, Varley J, Bignon YJ, Scherneck S, Sigurdardottir V, Lidereau R, Eyfjord J, Beckmann MW, Winqvist R, Skovlund E, Borresen-Dale AL. (1999). Loss of heterozygosity at 11q23.1 and survival in breast cancer: results of a large European study. Breast Cancer Somatic Genetics Consortium. *Genes Chromosomes Cancer* 25: 212-221.

1553. Laake K, Odegard A, Andersen TI, Bukholm IK, Karesen R, Nesland JM, Ottestad L, Shiloh Y, Borresen-Dale AL (1997). Loss of heterozygosity at 11q23.1 in breast carcinomas: indication for involvement of a gene distal and close to ATM. *Genes Chromosomes Cancer* 18: 175-180.

1554. Labonte S, Tetu B, Boucher D, Larue H (2001). Transitional cell carcinoma of the endometrium associated with a benign ovarian Brenner tumor: a case report. *Hum Pathol* 32: 230-232.

1555. Lack EE, Goldstein DP (1984). Primary ovarian tumours in childhood and adolescence. *Current Probl Obstet Gynecol* 7: 9-36.

1556. Lacson AG, Gillis DA, Shawwa A (1988). Malignant mixed germ-cell-sex cord-stromal tumors of the ovary associated with isosexual precocious puberty. *Cancer* 61: 2122-2133.

1557. Lage JM (1991). Placentomegaly with massive hydrops of placental stem villi, diploid DNA content, and fetal omphaloceles: possible association with Beckwith-Wiedemann syndrome. *Hum Pathol* 22: 591-597.

1558. Lage JM, Berkowitz RS, Rice LW, Goldstein DP, Bernstein MR, Weinberg DS (1991). Flow cytometric analysis of DNA content in partial hydatidiform moles with persistent gestational trophoblastic tumor. *Obstet Gynecol* 77: 111-115.

1559. Lage JM, Driscoll SG, Yavner DL, Olivier AP, Mark SD, Weinberg DS (1988). Hydatidiform moles. Application of flow cytometry in diagnosis. *Am J Clin Pathol* 89: 596-600.

1560. Lage JM, Mark SD, Roberts DJ, Goldstein DP, Bernstein MR, Berkowitz RS (1992). A flow cytometric study of 137 fresh hydropic placentas: correlation between types of hydatidiform moles and nuclear DNA ploidy. *Obstet Gynecol* 79: 403-410.

1561. Lage JM, Popek EJ (1993). The role of DNA flow cytometry in evaluation of partial and complete hydatidiform moles and hydropic abortions. *Semin Diagn Pathol* 10: 267-274.

1562. Lage JM, Roberts DJ (1993). Choriocarcinoma in a term placenta: pathologic diagnosis of tumor in an asymptomatic patient with metastatic disease. *Int J Gynecol Pathol* 12: 80-85.

1563. Lage JM, Weinberg DS, Yavner DL, Bieber FR (1989). The biology of tetraploid hydatidiform moles: histopathology, cytogenetics, and flow cytometry. *Hum Pathol* 20: 419-425.

1564. Lagios MD (1977). Multicentricity of breast carcinoma demonstrated by routine correlated serial subgross and radiographic examination. *Cancer* 40: 1726-1734.
1565. Lagios MD, Margolin FR, Westdahl PR, Rose MR (1989). Mammographically detected duct carcinoma in situ. Frequency of local recurrence following tylectomy and prognostic effect of nuclear grade on local recurrence. *Cancer* 63: 618-624.
1566. Lagios MD, Rose MR, Margolin FR (1980). Tubular carcinoma of the breast: association with multicentricity, bilaterality, and family history of mammary carcinoma. *Am J Clin Pathol* 73: 25-30.
1567. Lakhani SR (1999). The transition from hyperplasia to invasive carcinoma of the breast. *J Pathol* 187: 272-278.
1568. Lakhani SR, Chaggar R, Davies S, Jones C, Collins N, Odel C, Stratton MR, O'Hare MJ (1999). Genetic alterations in 'normal' luminal and myoepithelial cells of the breast. *J Pathol* 189: 496-503.
1569. Lakhani SR, Collins N, Sloane JP, Stratton MR (1995). Loss of heterozygosity in lobular carcinoma in situ of the breast. *Jounal of Clinical Pathology:Molecular Pathology* 48: M74-M78.
1570. Lakhani SR, Collins N, Stratton MR, Sloane JP (1995). Atypical ductal hyperplasia of the breast: clonal proliferation with loss of heterozygosity on chromosomes 16q and 17p. *J Clin Pathol* 48: 611-615.
1571. Lakhani SR, Gusterson BA, Jacquemier J, Sloane JP, Anderson TJ, Van de Vijver MJ, Venter D, Freeman A, Antoniou A, McGuffog L, Smyth E, Steel CM, Haites N, Scott RJ, Goldgar D, Neuhausen S, Daly PA, Ormiston W, McManus R, Scherneck S, Ponder BA, Futreal PA, Peto J, Stoppa-Lyonnet D, Bignon YJ, Stratton MR (2000). The pathology of familial breast cancer: histological features of cancers in families not attributable to mutations in BRCA1 or BRCA2. *Clin Cancer Res* 6: 782-789.
1572. Lakhani SR, Jacquemier J, Sloane JP, Gusterson BA, Anderson TJ, Van de Vijver MJ, Farid LM, Venter D, Antoniou A, Storfer-Isser A, Smyth E, Steel CM, Haites N, Scott RJ, Goldgar D, Neuhausen S, Daly PA, Ormiston W, McManus R, Scherneck S, Ponder BA, Ford D, Peto J, Stoppa-Lyonnet D, Bignon YJ, Struewing JP, Spurr NK, Bishop DT, Klijn JGM, Devilee P, Cornelisse CJ, Lasset C, Lenoir G, Barkardottir RB, Egilsson V, Hamann U, Chang-claude J, Sobol H, Weber B, Stratton MR, Easton DF. (1998). Multifactorial analysis of differences between sporadic breast cancers and cancers involving BRCA1 and BRCA2 mutations. *J Natl Cancer Inst* 90: 1138-1145.
1573. Lakhani SR, O'Hare MJ, Monaghan P, Winehouse J, Gazet JC, Sloane JP (1995). Malignant myoepithelioma (myoepithelial carcinoma) of the breast: a detailed cytokeratin study. *J Clin Pathol* 48: 164-167.
1574. Lakhani SR, Van de Vijver MJ, Jacquemier J, Anderson TJ, Osin PP, McGuffog L, Easton DF (2002). The pathology of familial breast cancer: predictive value of immunohistochemical markers estrogen receptor, progesterone receptor, HER-2, and p53 in patients with mutations in BRCA1 and BRCA2. *J Clin Oncol* 20: 2310-2318.
1575. Lam RM, Geittmann P (1988). Sclerosing stromal tumor of the ovary. A light, electron microscopic and enzyme histochemical study. *Int J Gynecol Pathol* 7: 280-290.
1576. Lambot MA, Eddafali B, Simon P, Fayt I, Noel JC (2001). Metastasis from apocrine carcinoma of the breast to an endometrial polyp. *Virchows Arch* 438: 517-518.
1577. Lammie GA, Millis RR (1989). Ductal adenoma of the breast--a review of fifteen cases. *Hum Pathol* 20: 903-908.
1578. Lamovec J, Bracko M (1991). Metastatic pattern of infiltrating lobular carcinoma of the breast: an autopsy study. *J Surg Oncol* 48: 28-33.
1579. Lamovec J, Bracko M (1994). Secretory carcinoma of the breast: light microscopical, immunohistochemical and flow cytometric study. *Mod Pathol* 7: 475-479.
1580. Lamovec J, Jancar J (1987). Primary malignant lymphoma of the breast. Lymphoma of the mucosa-associated lymphoid tissue. *Cancer* 60: 3033-3041.
1581. Lamovec J, Us-Krasovec M, Zidar A, Kljun A (1989). Adenoid cystic carcinoma of the breast: a histologic, cytologic, and immunohistochemical study. *Semin Diagn Pathol* 6: 153-164.
1582. Lane TF, Deng C, Elson A, Lyu MS, Kozak CA, Leder P (1995). Expression of Brca1 is associated with terminal differentiation of ectodermally and mesodermally derived tissues in mice. *Genes Dev* 9: 2712-2722.
1583. Laricchia R, Wierdis T, Loiudice L, Trisolini A, Riezzo A (1977). [Vulvar neoplasms (myeloblastoma) as the first manifestation of acute myeloblastic leukemia]. *Minerva Ginecol* 29: 957-961.
1584. Larson AA, Liao SY, Stanbridge EJ, Cavenee WK, Hampton GM (1997). Genetic alterations accumulate during cervical tumorigenesis and indicate a common origin for multifocal lesions. *Cancer Res* 57: 4171-4176.
1585. Larson B, Silfversward C, Nilsson B, Pettersson F (1990). Prognostic factors in uterine leiomyosarcoma. A clinical and histopathological study of 143 cases. The Radiumhemmet series 1936-1981. *Acta Oncol* 29: 185-191.
1586. Larson PS, de las MA, Cupples LA, Huang K, Rosenberg CL (1998). Genetically abnormal clones in histologically normal breast tissue. *Am J Pathol* 152: 1591-1598.
1587. Lash RH, Hart WR (1987). Intestinal adenocarcinomas metastatic to the ovaries. A clinicopathologic evaluation of 22 cases. *Am J Surg Pathol* 11: 114-121.
1588. Lathrop JC (1967). Malignant pelvic lymphomas. *Obstet Gynecol* 30: 137-145.
1589. Lathrop JC, Lauchlan S, Nayak R, Ambler M (1988). Clinical characteristics of placental site trophoblastic tumor (PSTT). *Gynecol Oncol* 31: 32-42.
1590. Lauchlan SC (1981). Tubal (serous) carcinoma of the endometrium. *Arch Pathol Lab Med* 105: 615-618.
1591. Laufer MR, Heerema AE, Parsons KE, Barbieri RL (1998). Endosalpingiosis: clinical presentation and follow-up. *Gynecol Obstet Invest* 46: 195-198.
1592. Lauria R, Perrone F, Carlomagno C, De Laurentiis M, Morabito A, Gallo C, Varriale E, Pettinato G, Panico L, Petrella G, Bianco AR, Deplacido S. (1995). The prognostic value of lymphatic and blood vessel invasion in operable breast cancer. *Cancer* 76: 1772-1778.
1593. Lawler SD, Fisher RA, Dent J (1991). A prospective genetic study of complete and partial hydatidiform moles. *Am J Obstet Gynecol* 164: 1270-1277.
1594. Lax SF, Kendall B, Tashiro H, Slebos RJ, Hedrick L (2000). The frequency of p53, K-ras mutations, and microsatellite instability differs in uterine endometrioid and serous carcinoma: evidence of distinct molecular genetic pathways. *Cancer* 88: 814-824.
1595. Lax SF, Pizer ES, Ronnett BM, Kurman RJ (1998). Clear cell carcinoma of the endometrium is characterized by a distinctive profile of p53, Ki-67, estrogen, and progesterone receptor expression. *Hum Pathol* 29: 551-558.
1596. Layfield LJ, Hart J, Neuwirth H, Bohman R, Trumbull WE, Giuliano AE (1989). Relation between DNA ploidy and the clinical behavior of phyllodes tumors. *Cancer* 64: 1486-1489.
1597. Lazure T, Alsamad IA, Meuric S, Orbach D, Fabre M (2001). [Primary uterine and vulvar Ewing's sarcoma/peripheral neuroectodermal tumors in children: two unusual locations]. *Ann Pathol* 21: 263-266.
1598. Le Bouedec G, de Latour M, Levrel O, Dauplat J (1997). [Krukenberg tumors of breast origin. 10 cases]. *Presse Med* 26: 454-457.
1599. Le Gal M, Ollivier L, Asselain B, Meunier M, Laurent M, Vielh P, Neuenschwander S (1992). Mammographic features of 455 invasive lobular carcinomas. *Radiology* 185: 705-708.
1600. Le Gal Y (1961). Adenoma of the Breast. *Am Surg* 27: 14-22.
1601. Le Doussal V, Tubiana-Hulin M, Friedman S, Hacene K, Spyratos F, Brunet M (1989). Prognostic value of histologic grade nuclear components of Scarff-Bloom-Richardson (SBR). An improved score modification based on a multivariate analysis of 1262 invasive ductal breast carcinomas. *Cancer* 64: 1914-1921.
1602. Leach FS, Polyak K, Burrell M, Johnson KA, Hill D, Dunlop MG, Wyllie AH, Peltomaki P, de la CA, Hamilton SR, Kinzler KW, Vogelstein B (1996). Expression of the human mismatch repair gene hMSH2 in normal and neoplastic tissues. *Cancer Res* 56: 235-240.
1603. Leake J, Woolas RP, Daniel J, Oram DH, Brown CL (1994). Immunocytochemical and serological expression of CA 125: a clinicopathological study of 40 malignant ovarian epithelial tumours. *Histopathology* 24: 57-64.
1604. Leal C, Costa I, Fonseca D, Lopes P, Bento MJ, Lopes C (1998). Intracystic (encysted) papillary carcinoma of the breast: a clinical, pathological, and immunohistochemical study. *Hum Pathol* 29: 1097-1104.
1605. Leal C, Henrique R, Monteiro P, Lopes C, Bento MJ, De Sousa CP, Lopes P, Olson S, Silva MD, Page DL (2001). Apocrine ductal carcinoma in situ of the breast: histologic classification and expression of biologic markers. *Hum Pathol* 32: 487-493.
1606. Lee A.K.C., Loda M, Mackarem G, Bosari S., DeLellis R.A., Heatley G.J., Hughes K. (1997). Lymph node negative invasive breast carcinoma 1 centimeter or less in size: clinicopathological features and outcome. *Cancer* 79: 761-771.
1607. Lee BJ, Tannenbaum E (1924). Inflammatory carcinoma of the breast: a report of twenty-eight cases from the breast clinic of the Memorial Hospital. *Surg Gynecol Obstet* 39: 580-595.
1608. Lee JF, Yang YC, Lee YN, Wang KL, Lin YN (1991). Leiomyosarcoma of the broad ligament--report of two cases. *Zhonghua Yi Xue Za Zhi (Taipei)* 48: 59-65.
1609. Lee JS, Collins KM, Brown AL, Lee CH, Chung JH (2000). hCds1-mediated phosphorylation of BRCA1 regulates the DNA damage response. *Nature* 404: 201-204.
1610. Lee JY, Dong SM, Kim HS, Kim SY, Na EY, Shin MS, Lee SH, Park WS, Kim KM, Lee YS, Jang JJ, Yoo NJ (1998). A distinct region of chromosome 19p13.3 associated with the sporadic form of adenoma malignum of the uterine cervix. *Cancer Res* 58: 1140-1143.
1611. Lee KR, Flynn CE (2000). Early invasive adenocarcinoma of the cervix. *Cancer* 89: 1048-1055.
1612. Lee KR, Minter LJ, Crum CP (1997). Koilocytotic atypia in Papanicolaou smears. Reproducibility and biopsy correlations. *Cancer* 81: 10-15.
1613. Lee KR, Scully RE (2000). Mucinous tumors of the ovary: a clinicopathologic study of 196 borderline tumors (of intestinal type) and carcinomas, including an evaluation of 11 cases with 'pseudomyxoma peritonei'. *Am J Surg Pathol* 24: 1447-1464.
1614. Lee KR, Young RH (2003). The distinction between primary and metastatic mucinous carcinomas of the ovary: gross and histologic findings in 50 cases. *Am J Surg Pathol* 27: 281-292.
1615. Lee WL, Wang PH (2001). Torsion of benign serous cystadenoma of the fallopian tube: a challenge in differential diagnosis of abdominal pain in women during their childbearing years--a case report. *Kaohsiung J Med Sci* 17: 270-273.
1616. Lee YS (1995). p53 expression in gestational trophoblastic disease. *Int J Gynecol Pathol* 14: 119-124.
1617. Leeper K, Garcia R, Swisher E, Goff B, Greer B, Paley P (2002). Pathologic findings in prophylactic oophorectomy specimens in high-risk women. *Gynecol Oncol* 87: 52-56.
1618. Lefkowitz M, Lefkowitz W, Wargotz ES (1994). Intraductal (intracystic) papillary carcinoma of the breast and its variants: a clinicopathological study of 77 cases. *Hum Pathol* 25: 802-809.
1619. Lehman MB, Hart WR (2001). Simple and complex hyperplastic papillary proliferations of the endometrium: a clinicopathologic study of nine cases of apparently localized papillary lesions with fibrovascular stromal cores and epithelial metaplasia. *Am J Surg Pathol* 25: 1347-1354.
1620. Leiberman J, Chaim W, Cohen A, Czernobilsky B (1975). Primary carcinoma of stomach with uterine metastasis. *Br J Obstet Gynaecol* 82: 917-921.
1621. Leibowitch M, Neill S, Pelisse M, Moyal-Baracco M (1990). The epithelial changes associated with squamous cell carcinoma of the vulva: a review of the clinical, histological and viral findings in 78 women. *Br J Obstet Gynaecol* 97: 1135-1139.
1622. Leibsohn S, d'Ablaing G, Mishell DR Jr., Schlaerth JB (1990). Leiomyosarcoma in a series of hysterectomies performed for presumed uterine leiomyomas. *Am J Obstet Gynecol* 162: 968-974.
1623. Leitner SP, Swern AS, Weinberger D, Duncan LJ, Hutter RV (1995). Predictors of recurrence for patients with small (one centimeter or less) localized breast cancer (T1a,b N0 M0). *Cancer* 76: 2266-2274.

1624. Lele SB, Piver MS, Barlow JJ, Tsukada Y (1978). Squamous cell carcinoma arising in ovarian endometriosis. *Gynecol Oncol* 6: 290-293.

1625. Lemoine NR, Hall PA (1986). Epithelial tumors metastatic to the uterine cervix. A study of 33 cases and review of the literature. *Cancer* 57: 2002-2005.

1626. Lenehan PM, Meffe F, Lickrish GM (1986). Vaginal intraepithelial neoplasia: biologic aspects and management. *Obstet Gynecol* 68: 333-337.

1627. Lenfant-Pejovic MH, Mlika-Cabanne N, Bouchardy C, Auquier A (1990). Risk factors for male breast cancer: a Franco-Swiss case-control study. *Int J Cancer* 45: 661-665.

1628. Leoncini L (1980). [Brenner tumor of the broad ligament]. *Arch De Vecchi Anat Patol* 64: 97-102.

1629. Leong AS, Williams JA (1985). Mucoepidermoid carcinoma of the breast: high grade variant. *Pathology* 17: 516-521.

1630. Leppien G (1987). Non-uterine gynecological sarcomas. *Arch Gynecol Obstet* 241: 25-32.

1631. Lerner LB, Andrews SJ, Gonzalez JL, Heaney JA, Currie JL (1999). Vulvar metastases secondary to transitional cell carcinoma of the bladder. A case report. *J Reprod Med* 44: 729-732.

1632. Lesser ML, Rosen PP, Kinne DW (1982). Multicentricity and bilaterality in invasive breast carcinoma. *Surgery* 91: 234-240.

1633. Lesueur GC, Brown RW, Bhathal PS (1983). Incidence of perilobular hemangioma in the female breast. *Arch Pathol Lab Med* 107: 308-310.

1634. Leuchter RS, Hacker NF, Voet RL, Berek JS, Townsend DE, Lagasse LD (1982). Primary carcinoma of the Bartholin gland: a report of 14 cases and review of the literature. *Obstet Gynecol* 60: 361-368.

1635. Leung WY, Schwartz PE, Ng HT, Yang-Feng TL (1990). Trisomy 12 in benign fibroma and granulosa cell tumor of the ovary. *Gynecol Oncol* 38: 28-31.

1636. Levi F, La Vecchia C, Gulie C, Negri E (1993). Dietary factors and breast cancer risk in Vaud, Switzerland. *Nutr Cancer* 19: 327-335.

1637. Levi F, Lucchini F, Negri E, Boyle P, La Vecchia C (1999). Cancer mortality in Europe, 1990-1994, and an overview of trends from 1955 to 1994. *Eur J Cancer* 35: 1477-1516.

1638. Levi F, Lucchini F, Negri E, Franceschi S, La Vecchia C (2000). Cervical cancer mortality in young women in Europe: patterns and trends. *Eur J Cancer* 36: 2266-2271.

1639. Levi F, Pasche C, Lucchini F, La Vecchia C (2001). Dietary intake of selected micronutrients and breast-cancer risk. *Int J Cancer* 91: 260-263.

1640. Levi F, Randimbison L, Te VC, La Vecchia C (1994). Incidence of breast cancer in women with fibroadenoma. *Int J Cancer* 57: 681-683.

1641. Levine PH, Steinhorn SC, Ries LG, Aron JL (1985). Inflammatory breast cancer: the experience of the surveillance, epidemiology, and end results (SEER) program. *J Natl Cancer Inst* 74: 291-297.

1642. Levine RL, Cargile CB, Blazes MS, van Rees B, Kurman RJ, Ellenson LH (1998). PTEN mutations and microsatellite instability in complex atypical hyperplasia, a precursor lesion to uterine endometrioid carcinoma. *Cancer Res* 58: 3254-3258.

1643. Levrero M, De Laurenzi V, Costanzo A, Gong J, Wang JY, Melino G (2000). The p53/p63/p73 family of transcription factors: overlapping and distinct functions. *J Cell Sci* 113: 1661-1670.

1644. Levy-Lahad E, Lahad A, Eisenberg S, Dagan E, Paperna T, Kasinetz L, Catane R, Kaufman B, Beller U, Renbaum P, Gershoni-Baruch R (2001). A single nucleotide polymorphism in the RAD51 gene modifies cancer risk in BRCA2 but not BRCA1 carriers. *Proc Natl Acad Sci USA* 98: 3232-3236.

1645. Lew WY (1993). Spindle cell lipoma of the breast: a case report and literature review. *Diagn Cytopathol* 9: 434-437.

1646. Lewis TL (1971). Colloid (mucus secreting) carcinoma of the cervix. *J Obstet Gynaecol Br Commonw* 78: 1128-1132.

1647. Li CI, Anderson BO, Porter P, Holt SK, Daling JR, Moe RE (2000). Changing incidence rate of invasive lobular breast carcinoma among older women. *Cancer* 88: 2561-2569.

1648. Li CI, Weiss NS, Stanford JL, Daling JR (2000). Hormone replacement therapy in relation to risk of lobular and ductal breast carcinoma in middle-aged women. *Cancer* 88: 2570-2577.

1649. Li DM, Sun H (1997). TEP1, encoded by a candidate tumor suppressor locus, is a novel protein tyrosine phosphatase regulated by transforming growth factor beta. *Cancer Res* 57: 2124-2129.

1650. Li FP, Fraumeni JF Jr., Mulvihill JJ, Blattner WA, Dreyfus MG, Tucker MA, Miller RW (1988). A cancer family syndrome in twenty-four kindreds. *Cancer Res* 48: 5358-5362.

1651. Li J, Yen C, Liaw D, Podsypanina K, Bose S, Wang SI, Puc J, Miliaresis C, Rodgers L, McCombie R, Bigner SH, Giovanella BC, Ittmann M, Tycko B, Hibshoosh H, Wigler MH, Parsons R (1997). PTEN, a putative protein tyrosine phosphatase gene mutated in human brain, breast, and prostate cancer. *Science* 275: 1943-1947.

1652. Li S, Zimmerman RL, LiVolsi VA (1999). Mixed malignant germ cell tumor of the fallopian tube. *Int J Gynecol Pathol* 18: 183-185.

1653. Liang SB, Sonobe H, Taguchi T, Takeuchi T, Furihata M, Yuri K, Ohtsuki Y (2001). Tetrasomy 12 in ovarian tumors of thecoma-fibroma group: A fluorescence in situ hybridization analysis using paraffin sections. *Pathol Int* 51: 37-42.

1654. Liaw D, Marsh DJ, Li J, Dahia PL, Wang SI, Zheng Z, Bose S, Call KM, Tsou HC, Peacocke M, Eng C, Parsons R (1997). Germline mutations of the PTEN gene in Cowden disease, an inherited breast and thyroid cancer syndrome. *Nat Genet* 16: 64-67.

1655. Liberman L (2000). Pathologic analysis of sentinel lymph nodes in breast carcinoma. *Cancer* 88: 971-977.

1656. Liberman L, Dershaw DD, Kaufman RJ, Rosen PP (1992). Angiosarcoma of the breast. *Radiology* 183: 649-654.

1657. Liberman L, Giess CS, Dershaw DD, Louie DC, Deutch BM (1994). Non-Hodgkin lymphoma of the breast: imaging characteristics and correlation with histopathologic findings. *Radiology* 192: 157-160.

1658. Lichtenstein P, Holm NV, Verkasalo PK, Iliadou A, Kaprio J, Koskenvuo M, Pukkala E, Skytthe A, Hemminki K (2000). Environmental and heritable factors in the causation of cancer--analyses of cohorts of twins from Sweden, Denmark, and Finland. *N Engl J Med* 343: 78-85.

1659. Lie AK, Skarsvag S, Skomedal H, Haugen OA, Holm R (1999). Expression of p53, MDM2, and p21 proteins in high-grade cervical intraepithelial neoplasia and relationship to human papillomavirus infection. *Int J Gynecol Pathol* 18: 5-11.

1660. Lifschitz-Mercer B, Walt H, Kushnir I, Jacob N, Diener PA, Moll R, Czernobilsky B (1995). Differentiation potential of ovarian dysgerminoma: an immunohistochemical study of 15 cases. *Hum Pathol* 26: 62-66.

1661. Lillemoe TJ, Perrone T, Norris HJ, Dehner LP (1991). Myogenous phenotype of epithelial-like areas in endometrial stromal sarcomas. *Arch Pathol Lab Med* 115: 215-219.

1662. Lim CL, Walker MJ, Mehta RR, Das Gupta TK (1986). Estrogen and antiestrogen binding sites in desmoid tumors. *Eur J Cancer Clin Oncol* 22: 583-587.

1663. Lin MC, Mutter GL, Trivijisilp P, Boynton KA, Sun D, Crum CP (1998). Patterns of allelic loss (LOH) in vulvar squamous carcinomas and adjacent non-invasive epithelia. *Am J Pathol* 152: 1313-1318.

1664. Lin WM, Forgacs E, Warshal DP, Yeh IT, Martin JS, Ashfaq R, Muller CY (1998). Loss of heterozygosity and mutational analysis of the PTEN/MMAC1 gene in synchronous endometrial and ovarian carcinomas. *Clin Cancer Res* 4: 2577-2583.

1665. Lin Y, Govindan R, Hess JL (1997). Malignant hematopoietic breast tumors. *Am J Clin Pathol* 107: 177-186.

1666. Lindblom A, Tannergard P, Werelius B, Nordenskjold M (1993). Genetic mapping of a second locus predisposing to hereditary non-polyposis colon cancer. *Nat Genet* 5: 279-282.

1667. Linder D, Power J (1970). Further evidence for post-meiotic origin of teratomas in the human female. *Ann Hum Genet* 34: 21-30.

1668. Linell F, Ljungberg O, Andersson I (1980). Breast carcinoma. Aspects of early stages, progression and related problems. *Acta Pathol Microbiol Scand Suppl* 1-233.

1669. Lininger RA, Ashfaq R, Albores-Saavedra J, Tavassoli FA (1997). Transitional cell carcinoma of the endometrium and endometrial carcinoma with transitional cell differentiation. *Cancer* 79: 1933-1943.

1670. Lininger RA, Fujii H, Man YG, Gabrielson E, Tavassoli FA (1998). Comparison of loss heterozygosity in primary and recurrent ductal carcinoma in situ of the breast. *Mod Pathol* 11: 1151-1159.

1671. Lininger RA, Park WS, Man YG, Pham T, MacGrogan G, Zhuang Z, Tavassoli FA (1998). LOH at 16p13 is a novel chromosomal alteration detected in benign and malignant microdissected papillary neoplasms of the breast. *Hum Pathol* 29: 1113-1118.

1672. Lininger RA, Wistuba I, Gazdar A, Koenig C, Tavassoli FA, Albores-Saavedra J (1998). Human papillomavirus type 16 is detected in transitional cell carcinomas and squamotransitional cell carcinomas of the cervix and endometrium. *Cancer* 83: 521-527.

1673. Lininger RA, Zhuang Z, Man Y, Park WS, Emmert-Buck M, Tavassoli FA (1999). Loss of heterozygosity is detected at chromosomes 1p35-36 (NB), 3p25 (VHL), 16p13 (TSC2/PKD1), and 17p13 (TP53) in microdissected apocrine carcinomas of the breast. *Mod Pathol* 12: 1083-1089.

1674. Lipkin SM, Wang V, Jacoby R, Banerjee-Basu S, Baxevanis AD, Lynch HT, Elliott RM, Collins FS (2000). MLH3: a DNA mismatch repair gene associated with mammalian microsatellite instability. *Nat Genet* 24: 27-35.

1675. Lipper S, Wilson C, Copeland KC (1981). Pseudogynecomastia due to neurofibromatosis: a light microscopic and ultrastructural study. *Hum Pathol* 12: 755-759.

1676. Lipworth L, Hsieh CC, Wide L, Ekbom A, Yu SZ, Yu GP, Xu B, Hellerstein S, Carlstrom K, Trichopoulos D, Adami HO (1999). Maternal pregnancy hormone levels in an area with a high incidence (Boston, USA) and in an area with a low incidence (Shanghai, China) of breast cancer. *Br J Cancer* 79: 7-12.

1677. Lissoni A, Cormio G, Perego P, Gabriele A, Cantu MG, Bratina G (1997). Conservative management of endometrial stromal sarcoma en young women. *Int J Gynecol Cancer* 7: 364-367.

1678. Little MP, Boice JDJ (1999). Comparison of breast cancer incidence in the Massachusetts tuberculosis fluoroscopy cohort and in the Japanese atomic bomb survivors. *Radiat Res* 151: 218-224.

1679. Liu B, Nicolaides NC, Markowitz S, Willson JK, Parsons RE, Jen J, Papadopolous N, Peltomaki P, de la Chapelle A, Hamilton SR, Kinzler KW, Vogelstein B (1995). Mismatch repair gene defects in sporadic colorectal cancers with microsatellite instability. *Nat Genet* 9: 48-55.

1680. Liu B, Parsons RE, Hamilton SR, Petersen GM, Lynch HT, Watson P, Markowitz S, Willson JK, Green J, de la Chapelle A, Kinzler KW, Vogelstein B (1994). hMSH2 mutations in hereditary nonpolyposis colorectal cancer kindreds. *Cancer Res* 54: 4590-4594.

1681. Liu FS, Kohler MF, Marks JR, Bast RC Jr., Boyd J, Berchuck A (1994). Mutation and overexpression of the p53 tumor suppressor gene frequently occurs in uterine and ovarian sarcomas. *Obstet Gynecol* 83: 118-124.

1682. Liu MM (1988). Fibromyoma of the vagina. *Eur J Obstet Gynecol Reprod Biol* 29: 321-328.

1683. Liu WM, Chen CJ, Kan YY, Chao KC, Yuan CC, Ng HT (1989). Simultaneous endometrioid carcinoma of the uterine corpus and ovary. *Zhonghua Yi Xue Za Zhi (Taipei)* 44: 38-44.

1684. LiVolsi VA, Kelsey JL, Fischer DB, Holford TR, Mostow ED, Goldenberg IS (1982). Effect of age at first childbirth on risk of developing specific histologic subtype of breast cancer. *Cancer* 49: 1937-1940.

1685. Lloreta J, Prat J (1992). Endometrial stromal nodule with smooth and skeletal muscle components simulating stromal sarcoma. *Int J Gynecol Pathol* 11: 293-298.

1686. Lobaccaro JM, Lumbroso S, Belon C, Galtier-Dereure F, Bringer J, Lesimple T, Namer M, Cutuli BF, Pujol H, Sultan C (1993). Androgen receptor gene mutation in male breast cancer. *Hum Mol Genet* 2: 1799-1802.

1687. Loman N, Johannsson O, Kristoffersson U, Olsson H, Borg A (2001). Family history of breast and ovarian cancers and BRCA1 and BRCA2 mutations in a population-based series of early-onset breast cancer. *J Natl Cancer Inst* 93: 1215-1223.

1688. London SJ, Connolly JL, Schnitt SJ, Colditz GA (1992). A prospective study of benign breast disease and the risk of breast cancer. *JAMA* 267: 941-944.

1689. Longacre TA, Chung MH, Jensen DN, Hendrickson MR (1995). Proposed criteria for the diagnosis of well-differentiated endometrial carcinoma. A diagnostic test for myoinvasion. *Am J Surg Pathol* 19: 371-406.

1690. Longacre TA, Chung MH, Rouse RV, Hendrickson MR (1996). Atypical polypoid adenomyofibromas (atypical polypoid adenomyomas) of the uterus. A clinicopathologic study of 55 cases. *Am J Surg Pathol* 20: 1-20.

1691. Longnecker MP (1994). Alcoholic beverage consumption in relation to risk of breast cancer: meta-analysis and review. *Cancer Causes Control* 5: 73-82.

1692. Longway SR, Lind HM, Haghighi P (1986). Extraskeletal Ewing's sarcoma arising in the broad ligament. *Arch Pathol Lab Med* 110: 1058-1061.

1693. Longy M, Lacombe D (1996). Cowden disease. Report of a family and review. *Ann Genet* 39: 35-42.

1694. Look KY, Roth LM, Sutton GP (1993). Vulvar melanoma reconsidered. *Cancer* 72: 143-146.

1695. Loose JH, Patchefsky AS, Hollander IJ, Lavin LS, Cooper HS, Katz SM (1992). Adenomyoepithelioma of the breast. A spectrum of biologic behavior. *Am J Surg Pathol* 16: 868-876.

1695a. Lopes JM, Seruca R, Hall AP, Branco P, Castedo SM (1990). Cytogenetic study of a sclerosing stromal tumor of the ovary. *Cancer Genet Cytogenet* 49: 103-106.

1696. Lopez-Rios F, Miguel PS, Bellas C, Ballestin C, Hernandez L (2000). Lymphoepithelioma-like carcinoma of the uterine cervix: a case report studied by in situ hybridization and polymerase chain reaction for Epstein-Barr virus. *Arch Pathol Lab Med* 124: 746-747.

1697. Lorenz G (1978). [Adenomatoid tumor of the ovary and vagina (author's transl)]. *Zentralbl Gynakol* 100: 1412-1416.

1698. Lorigan PC, Grierson AJ, Goepel JR, Coleman RE, Goyns MH (1996). Gestational choriocarcinoma of the ovary diagnosed by analysis of tumour DNA. *Cancer Lett* 104: 27-30.

1699. Lorincz AT, Reid R, Jenson AB, Greenberg MD, Lancaster W, Kurman RJ (1992). Human papillomavirus infection of the cervix: relative risk associations of 15 common anogenital types. *Obstet Gynecol* 79: 328-337.

1700. Losi L., Lorenzini R., Eusebi V, Bussolati G (1995). Apocrine differentiation in invasive carcinoma of the breast. *Appl Immunohistochem* 3: 91-98.

1701. Lotocki RJ, Krepart GV, Paraskevas M, Vadas G, Heywood M, Fung FK (1992). Glassy cell carcinoma of the cervix: a bimodal treatment strategy. *Gynecol Oncol* 44: 254-259.

1702. Loverro G, Cormio G, Renzulli G, Lepera A, Ricco R, Selvaggi L (1997). Serous papillary cystadenoma of borderline malignancy of the broad ligament. *Eur J Obstet Gynecol Reprod Biol* 74: 211-213.

1703. Loy TS, Calaluce RD, Keeney GL (1996). Cytokeratin immunostaining in differentiating primary ovarian carcinoma from metastatic colonic adenocarcinoma. *Mod Pathol* 9: 1040-1044.

1704. Lu KH, Cramer DW, Muto MG, Li EY, Niloff J, Mok SC (1999). A population-based study of BRCA1 and BRCA2 mutations in Jewish women with epithelial ovarian cancer. *Obstet Gynecol* 93: 34-37.

1705. Lu SL, Kawabata M, Imamura T, Akiyama Y, Nomizu T, Miyazono K, Yuasa Y (1998). HNPCC associated with germline mutation in the TGF-beta type II receptor gene. *Nat Genet* 19: 17-18.

1706. Lu X, Nikaido T, Toki T, Zhai YL, Kita N, Konishi I, Fujii S (2000). Loss of heterozygosity among tumor suppressor genes in invasive and in situ carcinoma of the uterine cervix. *Int J Gynecol Cancer* 10: 452-458.

1707. Lu YJ, Osin P, Lakhani SR, Di Palma S, Gusterson BA, Shipley JM (1998). Comparative genomic hybridization analysis of lobular carcinoma in situ and atypical lobular hyperplasia and potential roles for gains and losses of genetic material in breast neoplasia. *Cancer Res* 58: 4721-4727.

1708. Lucas FV, Perez-Mesa C (1978). Inflammatory carcinoma of the breast. *Cancer* 41: 1595-1605.

1709. Luchtrath H, Moll R (1989). Mucoepidermoid mammary carcinoma. Immunohistochemical and biochemical analyses of intermediate filaments. *Virchows Arch A Pathol Anat Histopathol* 416: 105-113.

1710. Ludwig T, Chapman DL, Papaioannou VE, Efstratiadis A (1997). Targeted mutations of breast cancer susceptibility gene homologs in mice: lethal phenotypes of Brca1, Brca2, Brca1/Brca2, Brca1/p53, and Brca2/p53 nullizygous embryos. *Genes Dev* 11: 1226-1241.

1711. Luevano-Flores E, Sotelo J, Tena-Suck M (1985). Glial polyp (glioma) of the uterine cervix, report of a case with demonstration of glial fibrillary acidic protein. *Gynecol Oncol* 21: 385-390.

1712. Luft F, Gebert J, Schneider A, Melsheimer P, von Knebel DM (1999). Frequent allelic imbalance of tumor suppressor gene loci in cervical dysplasia. *Int J Gynecol Pathol* 18: 374-380.

1713. Lui M, Dahlstrom JE, Bell S, James DT (2001). Apocrine adenoma of the breast: diagnosis on large core needle biopsy. *Pathology* 33: 149-152.

1714. Lukas C, Bartkova J, Latella L, Falck J, Mailand N, Schroeder T, Sehested M, Lukas J, Bartek J (2001). DNA damage-activated kinase Chk2 is independent of proliferation or differentiation yet correlates with tissue biology. *Cancer Res* 61: 4990-4993.

1715. Luna-More S, Gonzalez B, Acedo C, Rodrigo I, Luna C (1994). Invasive micropapillary carcinoma of the breast. A new special type of invasive mammary carcinoma. *Pathol Res Pract* 190: 668-674.

1716. Lund B, Thomsen HK, Olsen J (1991). Reproducibility of histopathological evaluation in epithelial ovarian carcinoma. Clinical implications. *APMIS* 99: 353-358.

1717. Lurain JR, Brewer JI, Torok EE, Halpern B (1982). Gestational trophoblastic disease: treatment results at the Brewer Trophoblastic Disease Center. *Obstet Gynecol* 60: 354-360.

1718. Luton JP, Clerc J, Paoli V, Bonnin A, Dumez Y, Vacher-Lavenu MC (1991). [Bilateral Leydig cell tumor of the ovary in a woman with congenital adrenal hyperplasia. The first reported case]. *Presse Med* 20: 109-112.

1719. Luttges JE, Lubke M (1994). Recurrent benign Mullerian papilloma of the vagina. Immunohistological findings and histogenesis. *Arch Gynecol Obstet* 255: 157-160.

1720. Luxman D, Jossiphov J, Cohen JR, Wolf Y, David MP (1997). Uterine metastasis from vulvar malignant melanoma. A case report. *J Reprod Med* 42: 244-246.

1721. Luzzi V, Holtschlag V, Watson MA (2001). Expression profiling of ductal carcinoma in situ by laser capture microdissection and high-density oligonucleotide arrays. *Am J Pathol* 158: 2005-2010.

1722. Lyday RO (1952). Fibroma of the ovary with abdominal implants. *Am J Surg* 84: 737-738.

1723. Lynch ED, Ostermeyer EA, Lee MK, Arena JF, Ji H, Dann J, Swisshelm K, Suchard D, MacLeod PM, Kvinnsland S, Gjertsen BT, Heimdal K, Lubs H, Moller P, King MC (1997). Inherited mutations in PTEN that are associated with breast cancer, cowden disease, and juvenile polyposis. *Am J Hum Genet* 61: 1254-1260.

1724. Lynch HT, Albano WA, Heieck JJ, Mulcahy GM, Lynch JF, Layton MA, Danes BS (1984). Genetics, biomarkers, and control of breast cancer: a review. *Cancer Genet Cytogenet* 13: 43-92.

1725. Lynch HT, de la Chapelle A (1999). Genetic susceptibility to non-polyposis colorectal cancer. *J Med Genet* 36: 801-818.

1726. Mabuchi K, Bross DS, Kessler II (1985). Risk factors for male breast cancer. *J Natl Cancer Inst* 74: 371-375.

1727. MacLachlan TK, Somasundaram K, Sgagias M, Shifman Y, Muschel RJ, Cowan KH, El Deiry WS (2000). BRCA1 effects on the cell cycle and the DNA damage response are linked to altered gene expression. *J Biol Chem* 275: 2777-2785.

1728. MacSweeney JE, King DM (1994). Computed tomography, diagnosis, staging and follow-up of pure granulosa cell tumour of the ovary. *Clin Radiol* 49: 241-245.

1729. Madison T, Schottenfeld D, Baker V (1998). Cancer of the corpus uteri in white and black women in Michigan, 1985-1994: an analysis of trends in incidence and mortality and their relation to histologic subtype and stage. *Cancer* 83: 1546-1554.

1730. Maehama T, Dixon JE (1998). The tumor suppressor, PTEN/MMAC1, dephosphorylates the lipid second messenger, phosphatidylinositol 3,4,5-trisphosphate. *J Biol Chem* 273: 13375-13378.

1731. Magi-Galluzi C, O'Connor JT, Neffen F, Sun D, Quade BJ, Crum CP, Nucci MR (2001). Are mucinous cystadenomas of the ovary derived from germ cells ? *Mod Pathol* 14: 140 A.

1732. Magrina JF, Gonzalez-Bosquet J, Weaver AL, Gaffey TA, Leslie KO, Webb MJ, Podratz KC (2000). Squamous cell carcinoma of the vulva stage IA: long-term results. *Gynecol Oncol* 76: 24-27.

1733. Magro G, Bisceglia M, Michal M (2000). Expression of steroid hormone receptors, their regulated proteins, and bcl-2 protein in myofibroblastoma of the breast. *Histopathology* 36: 515-521.

1734. Magro G, Fraggetta F, Torrisi A, Emmanuele C, Lanzafame S (1999). Myofibroblastoma of the breast with hemangiopericytoma-like pattern and pleomorphic lipoma-like areas. Report of a case with diagnostic and histogenetic considerations. *Pathol Res Pract* 195: 257-262.

1735. Magro G, Michal M, Bisceglia M (2001). Benign spindle cell tumors of the mammary stroma: diagnostic criteria, classification, and histogenesis. *Pathol Res Pract* 197: 453-466.

1736. Magro G, Michal M, Vasquez E, Bisceglia M (2000). Lipomatous myofibroblastoma: a potential diagnostic pitfall in the spectrum of the spindle cell lesions of the breast. *Virchows Arch* 437: 540-544.

1737. Mahmoud-Ahmed AS, Suh JH, Barnett GH, Webster KD, Kennedy AW (2001). Tumor distribution and survival in six patients with brain metastases from cervical carcinoma. *Gynecol Oncol* 81: 196-200.

1738. Mai KT, Yazdi HM, Bertrand MA, LeSaux N, Cathcart LL (1996). Bilateral primary ovarian squamous cell carcinoma associated with human papilloma virus infection and vulvar and cervical intraepithelial neoplasia. A case report with review of the literature. *Am J Surg Pathol* 20: 767-772.

1739. Maier RC, Norris HJ (1980). Coexistence of cervical intraepithelial neoplasia with primary adenocarcinoma of the endocervix. *Obstet Gynecol* 56: 361-364.

1740. Maier WP, Rosemond GP, Goldman LI, Kaplan GF, Tyson RR (1977). A ten year study of medullary carcinoma of the breast. *Surg Gynecol Obstet* 144: 695-698.

1741. Maiorano E, Ricco R, Virgintino D, et al. (1994). Infiltrating myoepithelioma of the breast. *Appl Immunohistochem* 2: 130-136.

1742. Maitra A, Wistuba II, Gibbons D, Gazdar AF, Albores-Saavedra J (1999). Allelic losses at chromosome 3p are seen in human papilloma virus 16 associated transitional cell carcinoma of the cervix. *Gynecol Oncol* 74: 361-368.

1743. Maitra A, Wistuba II, Washington C, Virmani AK, Ashfaq R, Milchgrub S, Gazdar AF, Minna JD (2001). High-resolution chromosome 3p allelotyping of breast carcinomas and precursor lesions demonstrates frequent loss of heterozygosity and a discontinuous pattern of allele loss. *Am J Pathol* 159: 119-130.

1744. Majmudar B, Ross RJ, Gorelkin L (1979). Benign blue nevus of the uterine cervix. *Am J Obstet Gynecol* 134: 600-601.

1745. Major FJ, Blessing JA, Silverberg SG, Morrow CP, Creasman WT, Currie JL, Yordan E, Brady MF (1993). Prognostic factors in early-stage uterine sarcoma. A Gynecologic Oncology Group study. *Cancer* 71: 1702-1709.

1746. Malik SN, Wilkinson EJ (1999). Pseudo-Paget's disease of the vulva: a case report. *J Lower Genital Tract Disease* 3: 201-203.

1747. Malinak LR, Miller GV, Armstrong JT (1966). Primary squamous cell carcinoma of the Fallopian tube. *Am J Obstet Gynecol* 95: 1167-1168.

1748. Mallory SB (1995). Cowden syndrome (multiple hamartoma syndrome). *Dermatol Clin* 13: 27-31.

1749. Malmstrom H, Janson H, Simonsen E, Stenson S, Stendahl U (1990). Prognostic factors in invasive squamous cell carcinoma of the vulva treated with surgery and irradiation. *Acta Oncol* 29: 915-919.

1750. Maluf FC, Sabbatini P, Schwartz L, Xia J, Aghajanian C (2001). Endometrial stromal sarcoma: objective response to letrozole. *Gynecol Oncol* 82: 384-388.

1751. Maluf HM, Koerner FC (1994). Carcinomas of the breast with endocrine differentiation: a review. *Virchows Arch* 425: 449-457.

1752. Maluf HM, Koerner FC (1995). Solid papillary carcinoma of the breast. A form of intraductal carcinoma with endocrine differentiation frequently associated with mucinous carcinoma. *Am J Surg Pathol* 19: 1237-1244.

1753. Mambo NC, Burke JS, Butler JJ (1977). Primary malignant lymphomas of the breast. *Cancer* 39: 2033-2040.

1754. Man S, Ellis IO, Sibbering M, Blamey RW, Brook JD (1996). High levels of allele loss at the FHIT and ATM genes in non-comedo ductal carcinoma in situ and grade I tubular invasive breast cancers. *Cancer Res* 56: 5484-5489.

1755. Mandai M, Konishi I, Kuroda H, Komatsu T, Yamamoto S, Nanbu K, Matsushita K, Fukumoto M, Yamabe H, Mori T (1998). Heterogeneous distribution of K-ras-mutated epithelia in mucinous ovarian tumors with special reference to histopathology. *Hum Pathol* 29: 34-40.

1756. Manegold E, Tietze L, Gunther K, Fleischer A, Amo-Takyi BK, Schroder W, Handt S (2001). Trisomy 8 as sole karyotypic aberration in an ovarian metastasizing Sertoli-Leydig cell tumor. *Hum Pathol* 32: 559-562.

1757. Manhoff DT, Schiffman R, Haupt HM (1995). Adenoid cystic carcinoma of the uterine cervix with malignant stroma. An unusual variant of carcinosarcoma? *Am J Surg Pathol* 19: 229-233.

1758. Manini C, Pietribiasi F, Sapino A, Donadio S (1998). [Serous cystadenocarcinoma of the ovary with simultaneous breast metastases. Description of a case]. *Pathologica* 90: 152-155.

1759. Manivel JC, Niehans G, Wick MR, Dehner LP (1987). Intermediate trophoblast in germ cell neoplasms. *Am J Surg Pathol* 11: 693-701.

1760. Manjer J, Malina J, Berglund G, Bondeson L, Garne JP, Janzon L (2001). Increased incidence of small and well-differentiated breast tumours in post-menopausal women following hormone-replacement therapy. *Int J Cancer* 92: 919-922.

1761. Mannion C, Park WS, Man YG, Zhuang Z, Albores-Saavedra J, Tavassoli FA (1998). Endocrine tumors of the cervix: morphologic assessment, expression of human papillomavirus, and evaluation for loss of heterozygosity on 1p, 3p, 11q, and 17p. *Cancer* 83: 1391-1400.

1762. Manson CM, Hirsch PJ, Coyne JD (1995). Post-operative spindle cell nodule of the vulva. *Histopathology* 26: 571-574.

1763. Mansour EG, Ravdin PM, Dressler L (1994). Prognostic factors in early breast carcinoma. *Cancer* 74: 381-400.

1764. Marchal C, Weber B, de Lafontan B, Resbeut M, Mignotte H, du Chatelard PP, Cutuli B, Reme-Saumon M, Broussier-Leroux A, Chaplain G, Lesaunier F, Dilhuydy JM, Lagrange JL (1999). Nine breast angiosarcomas after conservative treatment for breast carcinoma: a survey from French comprehensive Cancer Centers. *Int J Radiat Oncol Biol Phys* 44: 113-119.

1765. Marchese MJ, Liskow AS, Crum CP, McCaffrey RM, Frick HC (1984). Uterine sarcomas: a clinicopathologic study, 1965-1981. *Gynecol Oncol* 18: 299-312.

1766. Marchetti A, Buttitta F, Pellegrini S, Campani D, Diella F, Cecchetti D, Callahan R, Bistocchi M (1993). p53 mutations and histological type of invasive breast carcinoma. *Cancer Res* 53: 4665-4669.

1767. Marcus JN, Watson P, Page DL, Narod SA, Lenoir GM, Tonin P, Linder-Stephenson L, Salerno G, Conway TA, Lynch HT (1996). Hereditary breast cancer: pathobiology, prognosis, and BRCA1 and BRCA2 gene linkage. *Cancer* 77: 697-709.

1768. Marcus VA, Madlensky L, Gryfe R, Kim H, So K, Millar A, Temple LK, Hsieh E, Hiruki T, Narod S, Bapat BV, Gallinger S, Redston M (1999). Immunohistochemistry for hMLH1 and hMSH2: a practical test for DNA mismatch repair-deficient tumors. *Am J Surg Pathol* 23: 1248-1255.

1769. Marquis ST, Rajan JV, Wynshaw-Boris A, Xu J, Yin GY, Abel KJ, Weber BL, Chodosh LA (1995). The developmental pattern of Brca1 expression implies a role in differentiation of the breast and other tissues. *Nat Genet* 11: 17-26.

1770. Marsden DE, Friedlander M, Hacker NF (2000). Current management of epithelial ovarian carcinoma: a review. *Semin Surg Oncol* 19: 11-19.

1771. Marsh DJ, Coulon V, Lunetta KL, Rocca-Serra P, Dahia PL, Zheng Z, Liaw D, Caron S, Duboue B, Lin AY, Richardson AL, Bonnetblanc JM, Bressieux JM, Cabarrot-Moreau A, Chompret A, Demange L, Eeles RA, Yahanda AM, Fearon ER, Fricker JP, Gorlin RJ, Hodgson SV, Huson S, Lacombe D, Leprat F, Odent S, Toulouse C, Olopade OI, Sobol H, Tishler S, Woods CG, Robinson BG, Weber HC, Parsons R, Peacocke M, Longy M, Eng C (1998). Mutation spectrum and genotype-phenotype analyses in Cowden disease and Bannayan-Zonana syndrome, two hamartoma syndromes with germline PTEN mutation. *Hum Mol Genet* 7: 507-515.

1772. Marsh DJ, Dahia PL, Caron S, Kum JB, Frayling IM, Tomlinson IP, Hughes KS, Eeles RA, Hodgson SV, Murday VA, Houlston R, Eng C (1998). Germline PTEN mutations in Cowden syndrome-like families. *J Med Genet* 35: 881-885.

1773. Marsh DJ, Dahia PL, Zheng Z, Liaw D, Parsons R, Gorlin RJ, Eng C (1997). Germline mutations in PTEN are present in Bannayan-Zonana syndrome. *Nat Genet* 16: 333-334.

1774. Marsh DJ, Kum JB, Lunetta KL, Bennett MJ, Gorlin RJ, Ahmed SF, Bodurtha J, Crowe C, Curtis MA, Dasouki M, Dunn T, Feit H, Geraghty MT, Graham JM Jr., Hodgson SV, Hunter A, Korf BR, Manchester D, Miesfeldt S, Murday VA, Nathanson KL, Parisi M, Pober B, Romano C, Tolmie JL, Trembath R, Winter RM, Zackai EH, Zori RT, Weng LP, Dahia PLM, Eng C (1999). PTEN mutation spectrum and genotype-phenotype correlations in Bannayan-Riley-Ruvalcaba syndrome suggest a single entity with Cowden syndrome. *Hum Mol Genet* 8: 1461-1472.

1774a. Marsh WL, Jr., Lucas JG, Olsen J (1989). Chondrolipoma of the breast. *Arch Pathol Lab Med* 113: 369-371

1775. Marshall LM, Hunter DJ, Connolly JL, Schnitt SJ, Byrne C, London SJ, Colditz GA (1997). Risk of breast cancer associated with atypical hyperplasia of lobular and ductal types. *Cancer Epidemiol Biomarkers Prev* 6: 297-301.

1776. Marshall RJ, Braye SG, Jones DB (1986). Leiomyosarcoma of the uterus with giant cells resembling osteoclasts. *Int J Gynecol Pathol* 5: 260-268.

1777. Martin-Hirsch PL, Paraskevaidis E, Kitchener H (2001). *Surgery for cervical intraepithelial neoplasia* (Cochrane Review). The Cochrane Library.

1778. Martinelli G, Govoni E, Pileri S, Grigioni FW, Doglioni C, Pelusi G (1983). Sclerosing stromal tumor of the ovary. A hormonal, histochemical and ultrastructural study. *Virchows Arch A Pathol Anat Histopathol* 402: 155-161.

1779. Martinez A, Walker RA, Shaw JA, Dearing SJ, Maher ER, Latif F (2001). Chromosome 3p allele loss in early invasive breast cancer: detailed mapping and association with clinicopathological features. *Mol Pathol* 54: 300-306.

1780. Martinez V, Azzopardi JG (1979). Invasive lobular carcinoma of the breast: incidence and variants. *Histopathology* 3: 467-488.

1781. Martino A, Zamparelli M, Santinelli A, Cobellis G, Rossi L, Amici G (2001). Unusual clinical presentation of a rare case of phyllodes tumor of the breast in an adolescent girl. *J Pediatr Surg* 36: 941-943.

1782. Mascarello JT, Cajulis TR, Billman GF, Spruce WE (1993). Ovarian germ cell tumor evolving to myelodysplasia. *Genes Chromosomes Cancer* 7: 227-230.

1783. Massarelli G, Bosincu L, Costanzi G, Onida GA (1999). Uterine Wilms' tumor. *Int J Gynecol Pathol* 18: 402-403.

1784. Matanoski GM, Breysse PN, Elliott EA (1991). Electromagnetic field exposure and male breast cancer. *Lancet* 337: 737.

1785. Mathoulin-Portier MP, Penault-Llorca F, Labit-Bouvier C, Charafe E, Martin F, Hassoun J, Jacquemier J (1998). Malignant mullerian mixed tumor of the uterine cervix with adenoid cystic component. *Int J Gynecol Pathol* 17: 91-92.

1786. Matias-Guiu X, Bussaglia E, Catasus L, Lagarda H, Gras E, Machin P, Prat J (2000). Correspondence re: W.M. Lin et al., loss of heterozygosity and mutational analysis of the PTEN/MMAC1 gene in synchronous endometrial and ovarian carcinomas. Clin. Cancer Res., 4: 2577-2583, 1998. *Clin Cancer Res* 6: 1598-1600.

1787. Matias-Guiu X, Catasus L, Bussaglia E, Lagarda H, Garcia A, Pons C, Munoz J, Arguelles R, Machin P, Prat J (2001). Molecular pathology of endometrial hyperplasia and carcinoma. *Hum Pathol* 32: 569-577.

1788. Matias-Guiu X, Lagarda H, Catasus LI, Bussaglia E, Gallardo A, Gras E, Prat J (2002). Clonality analysis in synchronous or metachronous tumors of the female genital tract. *Int J Gynecol Pathol* 21: 205-211.

1789. Matias-Guiu X, Pons C, Prat J (1998). Mullerian inhibiting substance, alpha-inhibin, and CD99 expression in sex cord-stromal tumors and endometrioid ovarian carcinomas resembling sex cord-stromal tumors. *Hum Pathol* 29: 840-845.

1790. Matias-Guiu X, Prat J (1990). Ovarian tumors with functioning stroma. An immunohistochemical study of 100 cases with human chorionic gonadotropin monoclonal and polyclonal antibodies. *Cancer* 65: 2001-2005.

1791. Matsuoka S, Huang M, Elledge SJ (1998). Linkage of ATM to cell cycle regulation by the Chk2 protein kinase. *Science* 282: 1893-1897.

1792. Mattia AR, Ferry JA, Harris NL (1993). Breast lymphoma. A B-cell spectrum including the low grade B-cell lymphoma of mucosa associated lymphoid tissue. *Am J Surg Pathol* 17: 574-587.

1793. Mauillon JL, Michel P, Limacher JM, Latouche JB, Dechelotte P, Charbonnier F, Martin C, Moreau V, Metayer J, Paillot B, Frebourg T (1996). Identification of novel germline hMLH1 mutations including a 22 kb Alu-mediated deletion in patients with familial colorectal cancer. *Cancer Res* 56: 5728-5733.

1794. Mauz-Korholz C, Harms D, Calaminus G, Gobel U (2000). Primary chemotherapy and conservative surgery for vaginal yolk-sac tumour. Maligne Keimzelltumoren Study Group. *Lancet* 355: 625.

1795. Mawhinney RR, Powell MC, Worthington BS, Symonds EM (1988). Magnetic resonance imaging of benign ovarian masses. *Br J Radiol* 61: 179-186.

1796. Mayall F, Rutty K, Campbell F, Goddard H (1994). p53 immunostaining suggests that uterine carcinosarcomas are monoclonal. *Histopathology* 24: 211-214.

1797. Mayerhofer K, Obermair A, Windbichler G, Petru E, Kaider A, Hefler L, Czerwenka K, Leodolter S, Kainz C (1999). Leiomyosarcoma of the uterus: a clinico-pathologic multicenter study of 71 cases. *Gynecol Oncol* 74: 196-201.

1798. Maymon E, Piura B, Mazor M, Bashiri A, Silberstein T, Yanai-Inbar I (1998). Primary hepatoid carcinoma of ovary in pregnancy. *Am J Obstet Gynecol* 179: 820-822.

1799. Mayorga M, Garcia-Valtuille A, Fernandez I, et al. (1997). Adenocarcinoma of the uterine cervix with massive signet-ring cell differentiation. *Int J Surg Pathol* 5: 95-100.

1800. Mazoujian G, Pinkus GS, Davis S, Haagensen DE Jr. (1983). Immunohistochemistry of a gross cystic disease fluid protein (GCDFP-15) of the breast. A marker of apocrine epithelium and breast carcinomas with apocrine features. *Am J Pathol* 110: 105-112.

1801. Mazur MT (1981). Atypical polypoid adenomyomas of the endometrium. *Am J Surg Pathol* 5: 473-482.

1801a. Mazur MT (1989). Metastatic gestational choriocarcinoma. Unusual pathologic variant following therapy. *Cancer* 63: 1370-1377.

1802. Mazur MT, Hsueh S, Gersell DJ (1984). Metastases to the female genital tract. Analysis of 325 cases. *Cancer* 53: 1978-1984.

1802a. Mazur MT, Lurain JR, Brewer JI (1982). Fatal gestational choriocarcinoma. Clinicopathologic study of patients treated at a trophoblastic disease center. *Cancer* 50: 1833-1846.

1803. Mazzella FM, Sieber SC, Braza F (1995). Ductal carcinoma of male breast with prominent lipid-rich component. *Pathology* 27: 280-283.

1804. McAdam JA, Stewart F, Reid R (1998). Vaginal epithelioid angiosarcoma. *J Clin Pathol* 51: 928-930.

1805. McBride CM, Hortobagyi GN (1985). Primary inflammatory carcinoma of the female breast: staging and treatment possibilities. *Surgery* 98: 792-798.

1806. McCarthy JH, Aga R (1988). A fallopian tube lesion of borderline malignancy associated with pseudo-myxoma peritonei. *Histopathology* 13: 223-225.

1807. McCluggage G, McBride H, Maxwell P, Bharucha H (1997). Immunohistochemical detection of p53 and bcl-2 proteins in neoplastic and non-neoplastic endocervical glandular lesions. *Int J Gynecol Pathol* 16: 22-27.

1808. McCluggage WG (1999). Uterine tumours resembling ovarian sex cord tumours: immunohistochemical evidence for true sex cord differentiation. *Histopathology* 34: 375-376.

1809. McCluggage WG (2002). Malignant biphasic uterine tumours: carcinosarcomas or metaplastic carcinomas (Review article). *J Clin Pathol* 55: 321-325.

1810. McCluggage WG (2002). Uterine carcinosarcomas (malignant mixed Mullerian tumors) are metaplastic carcinomas. *Int J Gynecol Cancer* 12: 687-690.

1811. McCluggage WG, Abdulkader M, Price JH, Kelehan P, Hamilton S, Beattie J, al Nafussi A (2000). Uterine carcinosarcomas in patients receiving tamoxifen. A report of 19 cases. *Int J Gynecol Cancer* 10: 280-284.

1812. McCluggage WG, Cromie AJ, Bryson C, Traub AI (2001). Uterine endometrial stromal sarcoma with smooth muscle and glandular differentiation. *J Clin Pathol* 54: 481-483.

1813. McCluggage WG, Date A, Bharucha H, Toner PG (1996). Endometrial stromal sarcoma with sex cord-like areas and focal rhabdoid differentiation. *Histopathology* 29: 369-374.

1814. McCluggage WG, Lioe TF, McClelland HR, Lamki H (2002). Rhabdomyosarcoma of the uterus: report of two cases including one of the spindle cell variant. *Int J Gynecol Cancer* 12: 128-132.

1815. McCluggage WG, Maxwell P (2001). Immunohistochemical staining for calretinin is useful in the diagnosis of ovarian sex cord-stromal tumours. *Histopathology* 38: 403-408.

1816. McCluggage WG, Maxwell P, Sloan JM (1997). Immunohistochemical staining of ovarian granulosa cell tumors with monoclonal antibody against inhibin. *Hum Pathol* 28: 1034-1038.

1817. McCluggage WG, Nirmala V, Radhakumari K (1999). Intramural mullerian papilloma of the vagina. *Int J Gynecol Pathol* 18: 94-95.

1818. McCluggage WG, Perenyei M, Irwin ST (2002). Recurrent cellular angiofibroma of the vulva. *J Clin Pathol* 55: 477-479.

1819. McCluggage WG, Sloan JM, Boyle DD, Toner PG (1998). Malignant fibrothecomatous tumour of the ovary: diagnostic value of anti-inhibin immunostaining. *J Clin Pathol* 51: 868-871.

1820. McCluggage WG, Sloan JM, Murnaghan M, White R (1996). Gynandroblastoma of ovary with juvenile granulosa cell component and heterologous intestinal type glands. *Histopathology* 29: 253-257.

1821. McCluggage WG, Sumathi VP, Maxwell P (2001). CD10 is a sensitive and diagnostically useful immunohistochemical marker of normal endometrial stroma and of endometrial stromal neoplasms. *Histopathology* 39: 273-278.

1822. McCluggage WG, Sumathi VP, McBride HA, Patterson A (2002). A panel of immunohistochemical stains, including carcinoembryonic antigen, vimentin, and estrogen receptor, aids in the distinction between primary endometrial and endocervical adenocarcinomas. *Int J Gynecol Pathol* 21: 11-15.

1823. McCluskey LL, Dubeau L (1997). Biology of ovarian cancer. *Curr Opin Oncol* 9: 465-470.

1824. McConnell DT, Miller ID, Parkin DE, Murray GI (1997). p53 protein expression in a population-based series of primary vulval squamous cell carcinoma and immediate adjacent field change. *Gynecol Oncol* 67: 248-254.

1825. McConville CM, Stankovic T, Byrd PJ, McGuire GM, Yao QY, Lennox GG, Taylor MR (1996). Mutations associated with variant phenotypes in ataxia-telangiectasia. *Am J Hum Genet* 59: 320-330.

1826. McCready DR, Hortobagyi GN, Kau SW, Smith TL, Buzdar AU, Balch CM (1989). The prognostic significance of lymph node metastases after preoperative chemotherapy for locally advanced breast cancer. *Arch Surg* 124: 21-25.

1827. McCulloch GL, Evans AJ, Yeoman L, Wilson AR, Pinder SE, Ellis IO, Elston CW (1997). Radiological features of papillary carcinoma of the breast. *Clin Radiol* 52: 865-868.

1828. McCullough K, Froats ER, Falk HC (1946). Epidermoid carcinoma arising in an endometrial cyst of the ovary. *Arch Pathol Lab Med* 41: 335-337.

1829. McDivitt RW, Boyce W, Gersell D (1982). Tubular carcinoma of the breast. Clinical and pathological observations concerning 135 cases. *Am J Surg Pathol* 6: 401-411.

1830. McDivitt RW, Stevens JA, Lee NC, Wingo PA, Rubin GL, Gersell D (1992). Histologic types of benign breast disease and the risk for breast cancer. The Cancer and Steroid Hormone Study Group. *Cancer* 69: 1408-1414.

1831. McDivitt RW, Stewart FW (1966). Breast carcinoma in children. *JAMA* 195: 388-390.

1832. McDivitt RW, Stewart FW, Berg JW (1968). *Atlas of Tumour Pathology*. 2nd series ed. Washington.

1833. McGuire WL, Clark GM (1992). Prognostic factors and treatment decisions in axillary node-negative breast cancer. *N Engl J Med* 326: 1756-1761.

1834. McKittrick JE, Doane WA, Failing RM (1969). Intracystic papillary carcinoma of the breast. *Am Surg* 35: 195-202.

1835. McKusick VA (1998). *Mendelian Inheritance in Man. Catalogs of Human Genes and Genetic Disorders*. 12th ed. John Hopkins University Press: Baltimore.

1836. McLachlan SA, Erlichman C, Liu FF, Miller N, Pintilie M (1996). Male breast cancer: an 11 year review of 66 patients. *Breast Cancer Res Treat* 40: 225-230.

1837. McLachlin CM, Kozakewich H, Craighill M, O'Connell B, Crum CP (1994). Histologic correlates of vulvar human papillomavirus infection in children and young adults. *Am J Surg Pathol* 18: 728-735.

1838. Meier-Ruge W (1992). Epidemiology of congenital innervation defects of the distal colon. *Virchows Arch A Pathol Anat Histopathol* 420: 171-177.

1839. Meigs JV (1954). Fibroma of the ovary with ascites and hydrothorax. Meigs' syndrome. *Am J Obstet Gynecol* 67: 962-987.

1840. Meijers-Heijboer H, van den Ouweland A, Klijn J, Wasielewski M, de Snoo A, Oldenburg R, Hollestelle A, Houben M, Crepin E, Veghel-Plandsoen M, Elstrodt F, van Duijn C, Bartels C, Meijers C, Schutte M, McGuffog L, Thompson D, Easton D, Sodha N, Seal S, Barfoot R, Mangion J, Chang-Claude J, Eccles D, Eeles R, Evans DG, Houlston R, Murday V, Narod S, Peretz T, Peto J, Phelan C, Zhang HX, Szabo C, Devilee P, Goldgar D, Futreal PA, Nathanson KL, Weber B, Rahman N, Stratton MR (2002). Low-penetrance susceptibility to breast cancer due to CHEK2(*)1100delC in noncarriers of BRCA1 or BRCA2 mutations. *Nat Genet* 31: 55-59.

1841. Meisels A, Fortin R (1976). Condylomatous lesions of the cervix and vagina. I. Cytologic patterns. *Acta Cytol* 20: 505-509.

1842. Melhem MF, Tobon H (1987). Mucinous adenocarcinoma of the endometrium: a clinico-pathological review of 18 cases. *Int J Gynecol Pathol* 6: 347-355.

1843. Melnick S, Cole P, Anderson D, Herbst A (1987). Rates and risks of diethylstilbestrol-related clear-cell adenocarcinoma of the vagina and cervix. An update. *N Engl J Med* 316: 514-516.

1844. Mendez LE, Joy S, Angioli R, Estape R, Penalver M (1999). Primary uterine angiosarcoma. *Gynecol Oncol* 75: 272-276.

1845. Mentzel T (2001). Myofibroblastic sarcomas: a brief review of sarcomas showing a myofibroblastic line of differentiation and discussion of the differential diagnosis. *Current Diagn Pathol* 7: 17-24.

1846. Merajver SD, Pham TM, Caduff RF, Chen M, Poy EL, Cooney KA, Weber BL, Collins FS, Johnston C, Frank TS (1995). Somatic mutations in the BRCA1 gene in sporadic ovarian tumours. *Nat Genet* 9: 439-443.

1846 a. Merina MJ, Llombart-Bosch A, Menteagudo C (1990). Malignant changes associated with sclerosing adenosis: a morphologic and immunohistocheical analysis of seven cases. *Mod Pathol* 7.

1847. Merino MJ, Carter D, Berman M (1983). Angiosarcoma of the breast. *Am J Surg Pathol* 7: 53-60.

1848. Merino MJ, Edmonds P, LiVolsi V (1985). Appendiceal carcinoma metastatic to the ovaries and mimicking primary ovarian tumors. *Int J Gynecol Pathol* 4: 110-120.

1849. Merino MJ, LiVolsi VA (1981). Signet ring carcinoma of the female breast: a clinicopathologic analysis of 24 cases. *Cancer* 48: 1830-1837.

1850. Merino MJ, LiVolsi VA, Schwartz PE, Rudnicki J (1982). Adenoid basal cell carcinoma of the vulva. *Int J Gynecol Pathol* 1: 299-306.

1850 a. Merrill JA (1959). Carcinoma of the broad ligament. *Obstet Gynecol* 13: 472-476.

1851. Meyer AC, Dokerty MB, Harrington SW (1948). Inflammatory carcinoma of the breast. A correlation of clinical radiologic and pathological findings. *Surg Gynecol Obstet* 87: 417-424.

1852. Meyer JE, Lester SC, DiPrio PJ, Ferraro FA, Frenna TH, Denison CM (1995). Occult calcified fibroadenomas. *Breast disease* 8: 29-38.

1853. Meyer JS (1986). Cell kinetics of histologic variants of in situ breast carcinoma. *Breast Cancer Res Treat* 7: 171-180.

1854. Michael H, Ulbright TM, Brodhecker CA (1989). The pluripotential nature of the mesenchyme-like component of yolk sac tumor. *Arch Pathol Lab Med* 113: 1115-1119.

1855. Michaels BM, Nunn CR, Roses DF (1994). Lobular carcinoma of the male breast. *Surgery* 115: 402-405.

1856. Micheletti L, Preti M, Bogliatto F, Chieppa P (2000). [Vestibular papillomatosis]. *Minerva Ginecol* 52: 87-91.

1857. Michels KB, Trichopoulos D, Robins JM, Rosner BA, Manson JE, Hunter DJ, Colditz GA, Hankinson SE, Speizer FE, Willett WC (1996). Birthweight as a risk factor for breast cancer. *Lancet* 348: 1542-1546.

1858. Middleton LP, Palacios DM, Bryant BR, Krebs P, Otis CN, Merino MJ (2000). Pleomorphic lobular carcinoma: morphology, immunohistochemistry, and molecular analysis. *Am J Surg Pathol* 24: 1650-1656.

1859. Middleton LP, Palacios DM, Bryant BR, Krebs P, Otis CN, Merino MJ (2000). Pleomorphic lobular carcinoma: morphology, immunohistochemistry, and molecular analysis. *Am J Surg Pathol* 24: 1650-1656.

1860. Mies C (1993). Recurrent secretory carcinoma in residual mammary tissue after mastectomy. *Am J Surg Pathol* 17: 715-721.

1861. Mies C, Rosen PP (1987). Juvenile fibroadenoma with atypical epithelial hyperplasia. *Am J Surg Pathol* 11: 184-190.

1862. Miettinen M, Lehto VP, Virtanen I (1983). Postmastectomy angiosarcoma (Stewart-Treves syndrome). Light-microscopic, immunohistological, and ultrastructural characteristics of two cases. *Am J Surg Pathol* 7: 329-339.

1863. Mikami M, Ezawa S, Sakaiya N, Komuro Y, Tei C, Fukuchi T, Mukai M (2000). Response of glassy-cell carcinoma of the cervix to cisplatin, epirubicin, and mitomycin C. *Lancet* 355: 1159-1160.

1864. Miki Y, Swensen J, Shattuck-Eidens D, Futreal PA, Harshman K, Tavtigian S, Liu Q, Cochran C, Bennett LM, Ding W, Bell R, Rosenthal J, Hussey C, Tran T, McClure M, Frye C, Hattier T, Phelps R, Haugenstrano A, Katcher H, Dayananth P, Ward J, Tonin P, Narod S, Bristow PK, Norris FH, Helvering L, Morrison P, Rostek P, Lai M, Barrett JC, Lewis C, Neuhasen S, Cannonalbright L, Goldgar D, Wiseman R, Kamb A, Skolnick MH. (1994). A strong candidate for the breast and ovarian cancer susceptibility gene BRCA1. *Science* 266: 66-71.

1865. Milanezi MF, Saggioro FP, Zanati SG, Bazan R, Schmitt FC (1998). Pseudoangiomatous hyperplasia of mammary stroma associated with gynaecomastia. *J Clin Pathol* 51: 204-206.

1866. Milde-Langosch K, Albrecht K, Joram S, Schlechte H, Giessing M, Loning T (1995). Presence and persistence of HPV infection and p53 mutation in cancer of the cervix uteri and the vulva. *Int J Cancer* 63: 639-645.

1867. Miles PA, Kiley KC, Mena H (1985). Giant fibrosarcoma of the ovary. *Int J Gynecol Pathol* 4: 83-87.

1868. Miles PA, Norris HJ (1972). Proliferative and malignant Brenner tumors of the ovary. *Cancer* 30: 174-186.

1869. Miliauskas JR, Leong AS (1992). Small cell (neuroendocrine) carcinoma of the vagina. *Histopathology* 21: 371-374.

1870. Miller B, Flax S, Dockter M, Photopulos G (1994). Nucleolar organizer regions in adenocarcinoma of the uterine cervix. *Cancer* 74: 3142-3145.
1871. Miller BE, Barron BA, Dockter ME, Delmore JE, Silva EG, Gershenson DM (2001). Parameters of differentiation and proliferation in adult granulosa cell tumors of the ovary. *Cancer Detect Prev* 25: 48-54.
1872. Miller ES, Fairley JA, Neuburg M (1997). Vulvar basal cell carcinoma. *Dermatol Surg* 23: 207-209.
1873. Miller KN, McClure SP (1992). Papillary adenofibroma of the uterus. Report of a case involved by adenocarcinoma and review of the literature. *Am J Clin Pathol* 97: 806-809.
1874. Miller WR, Telford J, Dixon JM, Shivas AA (1985). Androgen metabolism and apocrine differentiation in human breast cancer. *Breast Cancer Res Treat* 5: 67-73.
1875. Minato H, Shimizu M, Hirokawa M, Fujiwara K, Kohno I, Manabe T (1998). Adenocarcinoma in situ of the fallopian tube. A case report. *Acta Cytol* 42: 1455-1457.
1876. Miremadi A, Pinder SE, Lee A, Bell JA, Paish EC, Wencyk P, Elston CW, Nicholson RI, Blamey RW, Robertson JF, Ellis IO (2002). Neuroendocrine differentiation and prognosis in breast adenocarcinoma. *Histopathology* 40: 215-222.
1877. Mirhashemi R, Kratz A, Weir MM, Molpus KL, Goodman AK (1998). Vaginal small cell carcinoma mimicking a Bartholin's gland abscess: a case report. *Gynecol Oncol* 68: 297-300.
1878. Mitao M, Nagai N, Levine RU, Silverstein SJ, Crum CP (1986). Human papillomavirus type 16 infection: a morphological spectrum with evidence for late gene expression. *Int J Gynecol Pathol* 5: 287-296.
1879. Mitelman F, Johansson B, Mertens F (2001). Mitelman Database of Chromosome Aberrations in Cancer. on-line http://cgap.nci.nih.gov/Chromosomes/Mitelman.
1880. Mitnick JS, Vazquez MF, Harris MN, Schechter S, Roses DF (1990). Invasive papillary carcinoma of the breast: mammographic appearance. *Radiology* 177: 803-806.
1881. Mittal K, Mesia A, Demopoulos RI (1999). MIB-1 expression is useful in distinguishing dysplasia from atrophy in elderly women. *Int J Gynecol Pathol* 18: 122-124.
1882. Mittal KR, Peng XC, Wallach RC, Demopoulos RI (1995). Coexistent atypical polypoid adenomyoma and endometrial adenocarcinoma. *Hum Pathol* 26: 574-576.
1883. Mittendorf R (1995). Teratogen update: carcinogenesis and teratogenesis associated with exposure to diethylstilbestrol (DES) in utero. *Teratology* 51: 435-445.
1884. Miyaki M, Konishi M, Tanaka K, Kikuchi-Yanoshita R, Muraoka M, Yasuno M, Igari T, Koike M, Chiba M, Mori T (1997). Germline mutation of MSH6 as the cause of hereditary nonpolyposis colorectal cancer. *Nat Genet* 17: 271-272.
1885. Miyoshi Y, Iwao K, Egawa C, Noguchi S (2001). Association of centrosomal kinase STK15/BTAK mRNA expression with chromosomal instability in human breast cancers. *Int J Cancer* 92: 370-373.
1886. Modan B, Hartge P, Hirsh-Yechezkel G, Chetrit A, Lubin F, Beller U, Ben Baruch G, Fishman A, Menczer J, Ebbers SM, Tucker MA, Wacholder S, Struewing JP, Friedman E, Piura B (2001). Parity, oral contraceptives, and the risk of ovarian cancer among carriers and noncarriers of a BRCA1 or BRCA2 mutation. *N Engl J Med* 345: 235-240.
1887. Moffat CJ, Pinder SE, Dixon AR, Elston CW, Blamey RW, Ellis IO (1995). Phyllodes tumours of the breast: a clinicopathological review of thirty-two cases. *Histopathology* 27: 205-218.
1888. Moffatt EJ, Kerns BJ, Madden JM, Layfield LJ (1997). Prognostic factors for fibromatoses: a correlation of proliferation index, estrogen receptor, p53, retinoblastoma, and src gene products and clinical features with outcome. *J Surg Oncol* 65: 117-122.
1889. Moinfar F, Man YG, Arnould L, Bratthauer GL, Ratschek M, Tavassoli FA (2000). Concurrent and independent genetic alterations in the stromal and epithelial cells of mammary carcinoma: implications for tumorigenesis. *Cancer Res* 60: 2562-2566.
1890. Moinfar F, Man YG, Lininger RA, Bodian C, Tavassoli FA (1999). Use of keratin 35betaE12 as an adjunct in the diagnosis of mammary intraepithelial neoplasia-ductal type--benign and malignant intraductal proliferations. *Am J Surg Pathol* 23: 1048-1058.
1891. Mok SC, Bell DA, Knapp RC, Fishbaugh PM, Welch WR, Muto MG, Berkowitz RS, Tsao SW (1993). Mutation of K-ras protooncogene in human ovarian epithelial tumors of borderline malignancy. *Cancer Res* 53: 1489-1492.
1892. Moll R, Mitze M, Frixen UH, Birchmeier W (1993). Differential loss of E-cadherin expression in infiltrating ductal and lobular breast carcinomas. *Am J Pathol* 143: 1731-1742.
1893. Moll UM, Chumas JC, Mann WJ, Patsner B (1990). Primary signet ring cell carcinoma of the uterine cervix. *N Y State J Med* 90: 559-560.
1894. Molyneux AJ, Deen S, Sundaresan V (1992). Primitive neuroectodermal tumour of the uterus. *Histopathology* 21: 584-585.
1895. Monk BJ, Nieberg R, Berek JS (1993). Primary leiomyosarcoma of the ovary in a perimenarchal female. *Gynecol Oncol* 48: 389-393.
1896. Monni O, Barlund M, Mousses S, Kononen J, Sauter G, Heiskanen M, Paavola P, Avela K, Chen Y, Bittner ML, Kallioniemi A (2001). Comprehensive copy number and gene expression profiling of the 17q23 amplicon in human breast cancer. *Proc Natl Acad Sci USA* 98: 5711-5716.
1897. Montag AG, Jenison EL, Griffiths CT, Welch WR, Lavin PT, Knapp RC (1989). Ovarian clear cell carcinoma. A clinicopathologic analysis of 44 cases. *Int J Gynecol Pathol* 8: 85-96.
1898. Montag TW, d'Ablaing G, Schlaerth JB, Gaddis O Jr., Morrow CP (1986). Embryonal rhabdomyosarcoma of the uterine corpus and cervix. *Gynecol Oncol* 25: 171-194.
1899. Monteiro AN (2000). BRCA1: exploring the links to transcription. *Trends Biochem Sci* 25: 469-474.
1900. Monterroso V, Jaffe ES, Merino MJ, Medeiros LJ (1993). Malignant lymphomas involving the ovary. A clinicopathologic analysis of 39 cases. *Am J Surg Pathol* 17: 154-170.
1901. Montes M, Roberts D, Berkowitz RS, Genest DR (1996). Prevalence and significance of implantation site trophoblastic atypia in hydatidiform moles and spontaneous abortions. *Am J Clin Pathol* 105: 411-416.
1902. Mooney EE, Man YG, Bratthauer GL, Tavassoli FA (1999). Evidence that Leydig cells in Sertoli-Leydig cell tumors have a reactive rather than a neoplastic profile. *Cancer* 86: 2312-2319.
1903. Mooney EE, Nogales FF, Bergeron C, Tavassoli FA (2002). Retiform Sertoli-Leydig cell Tumours: Clinical, Morphological, and Immunohistochemical Findings. *Histopathology* 41: 110-117.
1904. Mooney EE, Nogales FF, Tavassoli FA (1999). Hepatocytic differentiation in retiform Sertoli-Leydig cell tumors: distinguishing a heterologous element from Leydig cells. *Hum Pathol* 30: 611-617.
1905. Mooney EE, Tavassoli FA (1999). Papillary transitional cell carcinoma of the breast: a report of five cases with distinction from eccrine acrospiroma. *Mod Pathol* 12: 287-294.
1906. Moore DH, Michael H, Furlin JJ, Von Stein A (1998). Adenoid basal carcinoma of the vagina. *Int J Gynecol Cancer* 8: 261-263.
1907. Moore MP, Ihde JK, Crowe JP Jr., Hakes TP, Kinne DW (1991). Inflammatory breast cancer. *Arch Surg* 126: 304-306.
1908. Moore OS, Foote FW (1949). The relatively favorable prognosis of medullary carcinoma of the breast. *Cancer* 2: 635-642.
1909. Moreno-Bueno G, Gamallo C, Perez-Gallego L, de Mora JC, Suarez A, Palacios J (2001). beta-Catenin expression pattern, beta-catenin gene mutations, and microsatellite instability in endometrioid ovarian carcinomas and synchronous endometrial carcinomas. *Diagn Mol Pathol* 10: 116-122.
1910. Moreno-Rodriguez M, Perez-Sicilia M, Delinois R (1999). Lipoma of the endocervix. *Histopathology* 35: 483-484.
1911. Moreno V, Bosch FX, Munoz N, Meijer CJ, Shah KV, Walboomers JM, Herrero R, Franceschi S, International Agency for Research on Cancer. Multicentric Cervical Cancer Study Group (2002). Effect of oral contraceptives on risk of cervical cancer in women with papillomavirus infection: the IARC multicentric case-control study. *Lancet* 30: 1085-1092.
1912. Morgan LS, Joslyn P, Chafe W, Ferguson K (1988). A report on 18 cases of primary malignant melanoma of the vulva. *Colposcopy and Gynecologic Laser Surgery 4 (3) and Laser Surg* 4: 161-170.
1913. Morgan MB, Pitha JV (1998). Myofibroblastoma of the breast revisited: an etiologic association with androgens? *Hum Pathol* 29: 347-351.
1914. Morice P, Haie-Meder C, Pautier P, Lhomme C, Castaigne D (2001). Ovarian metastasis on transposed ovary in patients treated for squamous cell carcinoma of the uterine cervix: report of two cases and surgical implications. *Gynecol Oncol* 83: 605-607.
1915. Morikawa K, Hatabu H, Togashi K, Kataoka ML, Mori T, Konishi J (1997). Granulosa cell tumor of the ovary: MR findings. *J Comput Assist Tomogr* 21: 1001-1004.
1916. Morimitsu Y, Tanaka H, Iwanaga S, Kojiro M (1993). Alveolar soft part sarcoma of the uterine cervix. *Acta Pathol Jpn* 43: 204-208.
1917. Morimoto T, Komaki K, Yamakawa T, Tanaka T, Oomine Y, Konishi Y, Mori T, Monden Y (1990). Cancer of the male breast. *J Surg Oncol* 44: 180-184.
1918. Morimura Y, Honda T, Hoshi K, Yamada J, Nemoto K, Sato A (1995). A case of uterine cervical adenoid cystic carcinoma: immunohistochemical study for basement membrane material. *Obstet Gynecol* 85: 903-905.
1919. Moross T, Lang AP, Mahoney L (1983). Tubular adenoma of breast. *Arch Pathol Lab Med* 107: 84-86.
1920. Morrison JG, Gray GF Jr., Dao AH, Adkins RB Jr. (1987). Granular cell tumors. *Am Surg* 53: 156-160.
1921. Morrow M, Berger D, Thelmo W (1988). Diffuse cystic angiomatosis of the breast. *Cancer* 62: 2392-2396.
1922. Moscovic EA, Azar HA (1967). Multiple granular cell tumors ("myoblastomas"). Case report with electron microscopic observations and review of the literature. *Cancer* 20: 2032-2047.
1923. Mosher R, Genest DR (1997). Primary intraplacental chorioacarcinoma: clinical and pathological features of seven case (1967-1996) and discussion of the differential diagnosis. *J Surg Pathol* 2: 83-97.
1924. Mosher R, Goldstein DP, Berkowitz R, Bernstein M, Genest DR (1998). Complete hydatidiform mole. Comparison of clinicopathologic features, current and past. *J Reprod Med* 43: 21-27.
1925. Mosselman S, Polman J, Dijkema R (1996). ER beta: identification and characterization of a novel human estrogen receptor. *FEBS Lett* 392: 49-53.
1926. Mossler JA, Barton TK, Brinkhous AD, McCarty KS, Moylan JA, McCarty KS Jr. (1980). Apocrine differentiation in human mammary carcinoma. *Cancer* 46: 2463-2471.
1927. Mostoufizadeh M, Scully RE (1980). Malignant tumors arising in endometriosis. *Clin Obstet Gynecol* 23: 951-963.
1928. Motoyama T, Watanabe H (1996). Extremely well differentiated squamous cell carcinoma of the breast. Report of a case with a comparative study of an epidermal cyst. *Acta Cytol* 40: 729-733.
1929. Mount PM, Norris HJ (1982). *Overial Tumouren.* Springer: Berlin.
1930. Moyal-Barracco M, Leibowitch M, Orth G (1990). Vestibular papillae of the vulva. Lack of evidence for human papillomavirus etiology. *Arch Dermatol* 126: 1594-1598.
1931. Moynahan ME, Chiu JW, Koller BH, Jasin M (1999). Brca1 controls homology-directed DNA repair. *Mol Cell* 4: 511-518.
1932. Mrad K, Driss M, Maalej M, Romdhane KB (2000). Bilateral cystosarcoma phyllodes of the breast: a case report of malignant form with contralateral benign form. *Ann Diagn Pathol* 4: 370-372.
1933. Mrad K, Morice P, Fabre A, Pautier P, Lhomme C, Duvillard P, Sabourin JC (2000). Krukenberg tumor: a clinico-pathological study of 15 cases. *Ann Pathol* 20: 202-206.
1934. Muc RS, Grayson W, Grobbelaar JJ (2001). Adult extrarenal Wilms tumor occurring in the uterus. *Arch Pathol Lab Med* 125: 1081-1083.
1935. Mudhar HS, Smith JH, Tidy J (2001). Primary vaginal adenocarcinoma of intestinal type arising from an adenoma: case report and review of the literature. *Int J Gynecol Pathol* 20: 204-209.
1936. Mueller CB, Ames F (1978). Bilateral carcinoma of the breast: frequency and mortality. *Can J Surg* 21: 459-465.

1937. Mukai M, Torikata C, Iri H (1990). Alveolar soft part sarcoma: an electron microscopic study especially of uncrystallized granules using a tannic acid-containing fixative. *Ultrastruct Pathol* 14: 41-50.
1938. Muller CY, O'Boyle JD, Fong KM, Wistuba II, Biesterveld E, Ahmadian M, Miller DS, Gazdar AF, Minna JD (1998). Abnormalities of fragile histidine triad genomic and complementary DNAs in cervical cancer: association with human papillomavirus type. *J Natl Cancer Inst* 90: 433-439.
1939. Mulvany NJ, Nirenberg A, Östör AG (1996). Non-primary cervical adenocarcinomas. *Pathology* 28: 293-297.
1940. Mulvany NJ, Slavin JL, Östör AG, Fortune DW (1994). Intravenous leiomyomatosis of the uterus: a clinicopathologic study of 22 cases. *Int J Gynecol Pathol* 13: 1-9.
1941. Munkarah A, Malone JM Jr., Budev HD, Evans TN (1994). Mucinous adenocarcinoma arising in a neovagina. *Gynecol Oncol* 52: 272-275.
1942. Munn KE, Walker RA, Varley JM (1995). Frequent alterations of chromosome 1 in ductal carcinoma in situ of the breast. *Oncogene* 10: 1653-1657.
1943. Munoz N, Franceschi S, Bosetti C, Moreno V, Herrero R, Shah KV, Smith J, Meijer CJ, for the IARC Multi-centre Cervical Cancer Study Group (2001). The role of parity and HPV in cervical cancer: The IARC multi-centric cas-control study. *Lancet*.
1944. Munoz N, Franceschi S, Bosetti C, Moreno V, Herrero R, Smith JS, Shah KV, Meijer CJ, Bosch FX (2002). Role of parity and human papillomavirus in cervical cancer: the IARC multicentric case-control study. *Lancet* 359: 1093-1101.
1945. Murad TM, Contesso G, Mouriesse H (1981). Papillary tumors of large lactiferous ducts. *Cancer* 48: 122-133.
1946. Murao T, Nakai M, Hamada E (1986). [Intravascular papillary endothelial hyperplasia of the breast--report of a case with scanning electron microscopic observations]. *Gan No Rinsho* 32: 1471-1474.
1947. Murase E, Siegelman ES, Outwater EK, Perez-Jaffe LA, Tureck RW (1999). Uterine leiomyomas: histopathologic features, MR imaging findings, differential diagnosis, and treatment. *Radiographics* 19: 1179-1197.
1948. Murayama Y, Yamamoto Y, Shimojima N, Takahara T, Kikuchi K, Iida S, Kondo Y (1999). T1 Breast Cancer Associated with Von Recklinghausen's Neurofibromatosis. *Breast Cancer* 6: 227-230.
1949. Murphy DS, Hoare SF, Going JJ, Mallon EE, George WD, Kaye SB, Brown R, Black DM, Keith WN (1995). Characterization of extensive genetic alterations in ductal carcinoma in situ by fluorescence in situ hybridization and molecular analysis. *J Natl Cancer Inst* 87: 1694-1704.
1950. Murphy GF, Elder DE (1991). *Non-melanocytic Tumors of the Skin. Atlas of Tumor Pathology,* 3rd series, Fascicle 1 AFIP: Washington,D.C.
1951. Musgrave MA, Aronson KJ, Narod S, Hanna W, Miller AB, McCready DR (1998). Breast cancer and organochlorines: a marker for susceptibility? *Surg Oncol* 7: 1-4.
1952. Mussurakis S, Carleton PJ, Turnbull LW (1997). MR imaging of primary non-Hodgkin's breast lymphoma. A case report. *Acta Radiol* 38: 104-107.
1953. Muto MG, Lage JM, Berkowitz RS, Goldstein DP, Bernstein MR (1991). Gestational trophoblastic disease of the fallopian tube. *J Reprod Med* 36: 57-60.
1954. Muto MG, Welch WR, Mok SC, Bandera CA, Fishbaugh PM, Tsao SW, Lau CC, Goodman HM, Knapp RC, Berkowitz RS (1995). Evidence for a multifocal origin of papillary serous carcinoma of the peritoneum. *Cancer Res* 55: 490-492.
1955. Mutter GL (2000). Endometrial intraepithelial neoplasia (EIN): will it bring order to chaos? The Endometrial Collaborative Group. *Gynecol Oncol* 76: 287-290.
1956. Mutter GL (2000). Histopathology of genetically defined endometrial precancers. *Int J Gynecol Pathol* 19: 301-309.
1957. Mutter GL (2001). Pten, a protean tumor suppressor. *Am J Pathol* 158: 1895-1898.
1958. Mutter GL, Baak JP, Crum CP, Richart RM, Ferenczy A, Faquin WC (2000). Endometrial precancer diagnosis by histopathology, clonal analysis, and computerized morphometry. *J Pathol* 190: 462-469.
1959. Mutter GL, Ince TA, Baak JP, Kust GA, Zhou XP, Eng C (2001). Molecular identification of latent precancers in histologically normal endometrium. *Cancer Res* 61: 4311-4314.
1960. Myles JL, Hart WR (1985). Apoplectic leiomyomas of the uterus. A clinicopathologic study of five distinctive hemorrhagic leiomyomas associated with oral contraceptive usage. *Am J Surg Pathol* 9: 798-805.
1961. Naganawa S, Endo T, Aoyama H, Ichihara S (1996). MR Imaging of the Primary Breast Lymphoma: A Case Report. *Breast Cancer* 3: 209-213.
1962. Nagasaki K, Maass N, Manabe T, Hanzawa H, Tsukada T, Kikuchi K, Yamaguchi K (1999). Identification of a novel gene, DAM1, amplified at chromosome 1p13.3-21 region in human breast cancer cell lines. *Cancer Lett* 140: 219-226.
1963. Nagle RB, Bocker W, Davis JR, Heid HW, Kaufmann M, Lucas DO, Jarasch ED (1986). Characterization of breast carcinomas by two monoclonal antibodies distinguishing myoepithelial from luminal epithelial cells. *J Histochem Cytochem* 34: 869-881.
1964. Nakagawa S, Yoshikawa H, Kimura M, Kawana K, Matsumoto K, Onda T, Kino N, Yamada M, Yasugi T, Taketani Y (1999). A possible involvement of aberrant expression of the FHIT gene in the carcinogenesis of squamous cell carcinoma of the uterine cervix. *Br J Cancer* 79: 589-594.
1965. Nakamura Y, Nakashima T, Nakashima H, Hashimoto T (1981). Bilateral cystic nephroblastomas and botryoid sarcoma involving vagina and urinary bladder in a child with microcephaly, arhinencephaly, and bilateral cataracts. *Cancer* 48: 1012-1015.
1966. Nakanishi T, Wakai K, Ishikawa H, Nawa A, Suzuki Y, Nakamura S, Kuzuya K (2001). A comparison of ovarian metastasis between squamous cell carcinoma and adenocarcinoma of the uterine cervix. *Gynecol Oncol* 82: 504-509.
1967. Nakano T, Oka K, Ishikawa A, Morita S (1997). Correlation of cervical carcinoma c-erb B-2 oncogene with cell proliferation parameters in patients treated with radiation therapy for cervical carcinoma. *Cancer* 79: 513-520.
1968. Nakashima N, Fukatsu T, Nagasaka T, Sobue M, Takeuchi J (1987). The frequency and histology of hepatic tissue in germ cell tumors. *Am J Surg Pathol* 11: 682-692.
1969. Nakashima N, Murakami S, Fukatsu T, Nagasaka T, Fukata S, Ohiwa N, Nara Y, Sobue M, Takeuchi J (1988). Characteristics of "embryoid body" in human gonadal germ cell tumors. *Hum Pathol* 19: 1144-1154.
1970. Nakashima N, Nagasaka T, Fukata S, Oiwa N, Nara Y, Fukatsu T, Takeuchi J (1990). Study of ovarian tumors treated at Nagoya University Hospital, 1965-1988. *Gynecol Oncol* 37: 103-111.
1971. Nakashima N, Young RH, Scully RE (1984). Androgenic granulosa cell tumors of the ovary. A clinicopathologic analysis of 17 cases and review of the literature. *Arch Pathol Lab Med* 108: 786-791.
1972. Nanbu K, Konishi I, Yamamoto S, Koshiyama M, Mandai M, Komatsu T, Li W, Tokushige M, Higuchi K, Mori T (1995). Minimal deviation adenocarcinoma of endometrioid type may arise in the isthmus: clinicopathological and immunohistochemical study of two cases. *Gynecol Oncol* 58: 136-141.
1973. Naresh KN, Ahuja VK, Rao CR, Mukherjee G, Bhargava MK (1991). Squamous cell carcinoma arising in endometriosis of the ovary. *J Clin Pathol* 44: 958-959.
1974. Narod S, Tonin P, Lynch H, Watson P, Feunteun J, Lenoir G (1994). Histology of BRCA1-associated ovarian tumours. *Lancet* 343: 236.
1975. Narod SA (2002). Modifiers of risk of hereditary breast and ovarian cancer. *Nat Rev Cancer* 2: 113-123.
1976. Narod SA, Brunet JS, Ghadirian P, Robson M, Heimdal K, Neuhausen SL, Stoppa-Lyonnet D, Lerman C, Pasini B, de los Rios P, Weber B, Lynch H (2000). Tamoxifen and risk of contralateral breast cancer in BRCA1 and BRCA2 mutation carriers: a case-control study. Hereditary Breast Cancer Clinical Study Group. *Lancet* 356: 1876-1881.
1977. Narod SA, Dube MP, Klijn J, Lubinski J, Lynch HT, Ghadirian P, Provencher D, Heimdal K, Moller P, Robson M, Offit K, Isaacs C, Weber B, Friedman E, Gershoni-Baruch R, Rennert G, Pasini B, Wagner T, Daly M, Garber JE, Neuhausen SL, Ainsworth P, Olsson H, Evans G, Osborne M, Couch F, Foulkes WD, Warner E, Kim-Sing C, Olopade O, Tung N, Saal HM, Weitzel J, Merajver S, Gauthier-Villars M, Jernstrom H, Sun P, Brunet JS (2002). Oral contraceptives and the risk of breast cancer in BRCA1 and BRCA2 mutations carriers. *J Natl Cancer Inst* 94: 1773-1779.
1978. Narod SA, Goldgar D, Cannon-Albright L, Weber B, Moslehi R, Ives E, Lenoir G, Lynch H (1995). Risk modifiers in carriers of BRCA1 mutations. *Int J Cancer* 64: 394-398.
1979. Narod SA, Risch H, Moslehi R, Dorum A, Neuhausen S, Olsson H, Provencher D, Radice P, Evans G, Bishop S, Brunet JS, Ponder BA (1998). Oral contraceptives and the risk of hereditary ovarian cancer. Hereditary Ovarian Cancer Clinical Study Group. *N Engl J Med* 339: 424-428.
1980. Narod SA, Sun P, Ghadirian P, Lynch H, Isaacs C, Garber J, Weber B, Karlan B, Fishman D, Rosen B, Tung N, Neuhausen SL (2001). Tubal ligation and risk of ovarian cancer in carriers of BRCA1 or BRCA2 mutations: a case-control study. *Lancet* 357: 1467-1470.
1981. Nascimento AG, Karas M, Rosen PP, Caron AG (1979). Leiomyoma of the nipple. *Am J Surg Pathol* 3: 151-154.
1982. Nassar H, Wallis T, Andea A, Dey J, Adsay V, Visscher D (2001). Clinicopathologic analysis of invasive micropapillary differentiation in breast carcinoma. *Mod Pathol* 14: 836-841.
1983. Nasu M, Inoue J, Matsui M, Minoura S, Matsubara O (2000). Ovarian leiomyosarcoma: an autopsy case report. *Pathol Int* 50: 162-165.
1984. National Co-ordinating Group for Breast Screening Pathology (1995). Pathology Reporting. In: *Breast Screening Pathology, Breast Screening Pathology,* 2nd ed. ed. NHSBSP Publications.
1985. Navani SS, Alvarado-Cabrero I, Young RH, Scully RE (1996). Endometrioid carcinoma of the fallopian tube: a clinicopathologic analysis of 26 cases. *Gynecol Oncol* 63: 371-378.
1986. Naves AE, Monti JA, Chichoni E (1980). Basal cell-like carcinoma in the upper third of the vagina. *Am J Obstet Gynecol* 137: 136-137.
1987. Nayar R, Siriaunkgul S, Robbins KM, McGowan L, Ginzan S, Silverberg SG (1996). Microinvasion in low malignant potential tumors of the ovary. *Hum Pathol* 27: 521-527.
1988. Nayar R, Zhuang Z, Merino MJ, Silverberg SG (1997). Loss of heterozygosity on chromosome 11q13 in lobular lesions of the breast using tissue microdissection and polymerase chain reaction. *Hum Pathol* 28: 277-282.
1989. Nelen MR, Kremer H, Konings IB, Schoute F, van Essen AJ, Koch R, Woods CG, Fryns JP, Hamel B, Hoefsloot LH, Peeters EA, Padberg GW (1999). Novel PTEN mutations in patients with Cowden disease: absence of clear genotype-phenotype correlations. *Eur J Hum Genet* 7: 267-273.
1990. Nelen MR, Padberg GW, Peeters EA, Lin AY, van den Helm B, Frants RR, Coulon V, Goldstein AM, van Reen MM, Easton DF, Eeles RA, Hodgsen S, Mulvihill JJ, Murday VA, Tucker MA, Mariman EC, Starink TM, Ponder BA, Ropers HH, Kremer H, Longy M, Eng C (1996). Localization of the gene for Cowden disease to chromosome 10q22-23. *Nat Genet* 13: 114-116.
1991. Nelen MR, van Staveren WC, Peeters EA, Hassel MB, Gorlin RJ, Hamm H, Lindboe CF, Fryns JP, Sijmons RH, Woods DG, Mariman EC, Padberg GW, Kremer H (1997). Germline mutations in the PTEN/MMAC1 gene in patients with Cowden disease. *Hum Mol Genet* 6: 1383-1387.
1992. Nelson CL, Sellers TA, Rich SS, Potter JD, McGovern PG, Kushi LH (1993). Familial clustering of colon, breast, uterine, and ovarian cancers as assessed by family history. *Genet Epidemiol* 10: 235-244.
1993. Nemoto T, Castillo N, Tsukada Y, Koul A, Eckhert KH Jr., Bauer RL (1998). Lobular carcinoma in situ with microinvasion. *J Surg Oncol* 67: 41-46.
1994. Nesland JM, Holm R, Johannessen JV (1985). Ultrastructural and immunohistochemical features of lobular carcinoma of the breast. *J Pathol* 145: 39-52.

1995. Nesland JM, Lunde S, Holm R, Johannessen JV (1987). Electron microscopy and immunostaining of the normal breast and its benign lesions. A search for neuroendocrine cells. *Histol Histopathol* 2: 73-77.
1996. Neubecker RD, Breen JL (1962). Gynandroblastoma. A report of five cases with a discussion of the histogenesis ans classification of ovarian tumours. *Am J Clin Pathol* 38: 60-69.
1997. Neuhausen SL, Godwin AK, Gershoni-Baruch R, Schubert E, Garber J, Stoppa-Lyonnet D, Olah E, Csokay B, Serova O, Lalloo F, Osorio A, Stratton M, Offit K, Boyd J, Caligo MA, Scott RJ, Schofield A, Teugels E, Schwab M, Cannon-Albright L, Bishop T, Easton D, Benitez J, King MC, Ponder BAJ, Weber B, Devilee P, Borg A, Narod SA, Goldgar D. (1998). Haplotype and phenotype analysis of nine recurrent BRCA2 mutations in 111 families: results of an international study. *Am J Hum Genet* 62: 1381-1388.
1998. Nevin J, Laing D, Kaye P, McCulloch T, Barnard R, Silcocks P, Blackett T, Paterson M, Sharp F, Cruse P (1999). The significance of Erb-b2 immunostaining in cervical cancer. *Gynecol Oncol* 73: 354-358.
1999. Newcomer JR (1998). Ampullary tubal hydatidiform mole treated with linear salpingotomy. A case report. *J Reprod Med* 43: 913-915.
2000. Newman PL, Fletcher CD (1991). Smooth muscle tumours of the external genitalia: clinicopathological analysis of a series. *Histopathology* 18: 523-529.
2001. Newman W (1966). Lobular carcinoma of the female breast. Report of 73 cases. *Ann Surg* 164: 305-314.
2002. Newton WA Jr., Gehan EA, Webber BL, Marsden HB, van Unnik AJ, Hamoudi AB, Tsokos MG, Shimada H, Harms D, Schmidt D, Ninfo V, Cavazzana AO, Gonzalezcrussi F, Parham DM, Reiman HM, Asmar L, Beltangady MS, Sachs NE, Triche TJ, Maurer HM. (1995). Classification of rhabdomyosarcomas and related sarcomas. Pathologic aspects and proposal for a new classification--an Intergroup Rhabdomyosarcoma Study. *Cancer* 76: 1073-1085.
2003. Ng WK (2001). Fine needle aspiration cytology of invasive cribriform carcinoma of the breast with osteoclastlike giant cells: a case report. *Acta Cytol* 45: 593-598.
2004. Ngan HY, Liu SS, Yu H, Liu KL, Cheung AN (1999). Proto-oncogenes and p53 protein expression in normal cervical stratified squamous epithelium and cervical intra-epithelial neoplasia. *Eur J Cancer* 35: 1546-1550.
2005. Nguyen NP, Sallah S, Karlsson U, Vos P, Ludin A, Semer D, Tait D, Salehpour M, Jendrasiak G, Robiou C (2001). Prognosis for papillary serous carcinoma of the endometrium after surgical staging. Int J *Gynecol Cancer* 11: 305-311.
2006. Ngwalle KE, Hirakawa T, Tsuneyoshi M, Enjoji M (1990). Osteosarcoma arising in a benign dermoid cyst of the ovary. *Gynecol Oncol* 37: 143-147.
2007. Nichols GE, Mills SE, Ulbright TM, Czernobilsky B, Roth LM (1991). Spindle cell mural nodules in cystic ovarian mucinous tumors. A clinicopathologic and immunohistochemical study of five cases. *Am J Surg Pathol* 15: 1055-1062.
2008. Nicolaides NC, Carter KC, Shell BK, Papadopoulos N, Vogelstein B, Kinzler KW (1995). Genomic organization of the human PMS2 gene family. *Genomics* 30: 195-206.
2009. Nicolaides NC, Palombo F, Kinzler KW, Vogelstein B, Jiricny J (1996). Molecular cloning of the N-terminus of GTBP. *Genomics* 31: 395-397.
2010. Nicolaides NC, Papadopoulos N, Liu B, Wei YF, Carter KC, Ruben SM, Rosen CA, Haseltine WA, Fleischmann RD, Fraser CM, Adams MD, Venter JC, Dunlop MG, Hamilton SR, Petersen GM, de la Chapelle A, Vogelstein B, Kinzler KW. (1994). Mutations of two PMS homologues in hereditary nonpolyposis colon cancer. *Nature* 371: 75-80.
2011. Niehans GA, Manivel JC, Copland GT, Scheithauer BW, Wick MR (1988). Immunohistochemistry of germ cell and trophoblastic neoplasms. *Cancer* 62: 1113-1123.
2012. Nielsen AL, Nyholm HC, Engel P (1994). Expression of MIB-1 (paraffin ki-67) and AgNOR morphology in endometrial adenocarcinomas of endometrioid type. *Int J Gynecol Pathol* 13: 37-44.
2013. Nielsen BB (1981). Oncocytic breast papilloma. *Virchows Arch A Pathol Anat* 393: 345-351.
2014. Nielsen BB (1984). Leiomyosarcoma of the breast with late dissemination. *Virchows Arch A Pathol Anat Histopathol* 403: 241-245.
2015. Nielsen BB (1987). Adenosis tumour of the breast--a clinicopathological investigation of 27 cases. *Histopathology* 11: 1259-1275.
2016. Nielsen BB, Holm-Nielsen P, Kiaer HR (1993). Microglandular adenosis of the breast concomitant with secretory carcinoma. *Pathol Res Pract* 189: 769.
2017. Nielsen GP, Oliva E, Young RH, Rosenberg AE, Dickersin GR, Scully RE (1995). Alveolar soft-part sarcoma of the female genital tract: a report of nine cases and review of the literature. *Int J Gynecol Pathol* 14: 283-292.
2018. Nielsen GP, Oliva E, Young RH, Rosenberg AE, Prat J, Scully RE (1998). Primary ovarian rhabdomyosarcoma: a report of 13 cases. *Int J Gynecol Pathol* 17: 113-119.
2019. Nielsen GP, Rosenberg AE, Young RH, Dickersin GR, Clement PB, Scully RE (1996). Angiomyofibroblastoma of the vulva and vagina. *Mod Pathol* 9: 284-291.
2020. Nielsen GP, Young RH (2001). Mesenchymal tumors and tumor-like lesions of the female genital tract: a selective review with emphasis on recently described entities. *Int J Gynecol Pathol* 20: 105-127.
2021. Nielsen GP, Young RH, Prat J, Scully RE (1997). Primary angiosarcoma of the ovary: a report of seven cases and review of the literature. *Int J Gynecol Pathol* 16: 378-382.
2022. Nielsen M, Andersen JA, Henriksen FW, Kristensen PB, Lorentzen M, Ravn V, Schiodt T, Thorborg JV, Ornvold K (1981). Metastases to the breast from extramammary carcinomas. *Acta Pathol Microbiol Scand [A]* 89: 251-256.
2023. Nielsen VT, Andreasen C (1987). Phyllodes tumour of the male breast. *Histopathology* 11: 761-762.
2024. Nirmul D, Pegoraro RJ, Jialal I, Naidoo C, Joubert SM (1983). The sex hormone profile of male patients with breast cancer. *Br J Cancer* 48: 423-427.
2024 a. Nishikawa Y, Kaseki S, Tomoda Y, Ishizuka T, Asai Y, Suzuki T, Ushijima H (1985). Histopathologic classification of uterine choriocarcinoma. *Cancer* 55: 1044-1051.
2025. Nishimori H, Sasaki M, Hirata K, Zembutsu H, Yasoshima T, Fukui R, Kobayashi K (2000). Tubular adenoma of the breast in a 73-year-old woman. *Breast Cancer* 7: 169-172.
2026. Nishioka T, West CM, Gupta N, Wilks DP, Hendry JH, Davidson SE, Hunter RD (1999). Prognostic significance of c-erbB-2 protein expression in carcinoma of the cervix treated with radiotherapy. *J Cancer Res Clin Oncol* 125: 96-100.
2027. Nishizaki T, Chew K, Chu L, Isola J, Kallioniemi A, Weidner N, Waldman FM (1997). Genetic alterations in lobular breast cancer by comparative genomic hybridization. *Int J Cancer* 74: 513-517.
2028. Nishizaki T, Devries S, Chew K, Goodson WH, III, Ljung BM, Thor A, Waldman FM (1997). Genetic alterations in primary breast cancers and their metastases: direct comparison using modified comparative genomic hybridization. *Genes Chromosomes Cancer* 19: 267-272.
2029. Nixon AJ, Neuberg D, Hayes DF, Gelman R, Connolly JL, Schnitt S, Abner A, Recht A, Vicini F, Harris JR (1994). Relationship of patient age to pathologic features of the tumor and prognosis for patients with stage I or II breast cancer. *J Clin Oncol* 12: 888-894.
2030. Nixon AJ, Schnitt SJ, Gelman R, Gage I, Bornstein B, Hetelekidis S, Recht A, Silver B, Harris JR, Connolly JL (1996). Relationship of tumor grade to other pathologic features and to treatment outcome of patients with early stage breast carcinoma treated with breast-conserving therapy. *Cancer* 78: 1426-1431.
2031. Nobukawa B, Fujii H, Hirai S, Kumasaka T, Shimizu H, Matsumoto T, Suda K, Futagawa S (1999). Breast carcinoma diverging to aberrant melanocytic differentiation: a case report with histopathologic and loss of heterozygosity analyses. *Am J Surg Pathol* 23: 1280-1287.
2032. Nogales-Fernandez F, Silverberg SG, Bloustein PA, Martinez-Hernandez A, Pierce GB (1977). Yolk sac carcinoma (endodermal sinus tumor): ultrastructure and histogenesis of gonadal and extragonadal tumors in comparison with normal human yolk sac. *Cancer* 39: 1462-1474.
2033. Nogales-Ortiz F, Puerta J, Nogales FF Jr. (1978). The normal menstrual cycle. Chronology and mechanism of endometrial desquamation. *Obstet Gynecol* 51: 259-264.
2034. Nogales FF, Isaac MA (2002). Functioning uterine sex cord tumour. *Histopathology* 41: 277-279.
2035. Nogales FF (1993). Embryologic clues to human yolk sac tumors: a review. *Int J Gynecol Pathol* 12: 101-107.
2036. Nogales FF (1995). Mesonephric (Wolffian) Tumours of the Female Genital Tract : is Mesonephric Histogenesis a Mirage and a Trap ? *Current Diagn Pathol* 2: 94-100.
2037. Nogales FF, Ayala A, Ruiz-Avila I, Sirvent JJ (1991). Myxoid leiomyosarcoma of the ovary: analysis of three cases. *Hum Pathol* 22: 1268-1273.
2038. Nogales FF, Beltran E, Pavcovich M (1993). Pathology of ovarian yolk sac tumours. In: The Human Yolk Sac and Yolk Sac Tumours, FF Nogales (ed.), Springer-Verlag: Berlin , pp. 228-244.
2039. Nogales FF, Bergeron C, Carvia RE, Alvaro T, Fulwood HR (1996). Ovarian endometrioid tumors with yolk sac tumor component, an unusual form of ovarian neoplasm. Analysis of six cases. *Am J Surg Pathol* 20: 1056-1066.
2040. Nogales FF, Carvia RE, Donne C, Campello TR, Vidal M, Martin A (1997). Adenomas of the rete ovarii. *Hum Pathol* 28: 1428-1433.
2041. Nogales FF, Isaac MA, Hardisson D, Bosincu L, Palacios J, Ordi J, Mendoza E, Manzarbeitia F, Olivera H, O'Valle F, Krasevic M, Marquez M (2002). Adenomatoid tumors of the uterus: an analysis of 60 cases. *Int J Gynecol Pathol* 21: 34-40.
2042. Nogales FF, Ruiz A, I, Concha A, del Moral E (1993). Immature endodermal teratoma of the ovary: embryologic correlations and immunohistochemistry. *Hum Pathol* 24: 364-370.
2043. Nogales FF Jr., Matilla A, Nogales Ortiz F, Galera-Davidson H (1978). Yolk sac tumors with pure and mixed polyvesicular vitelline patterns. *Hum Pathol* 9: 553-566.
2044. Nogueira M, Andre S, Mendonca E (1998). Metaplastic carcinomas of the breast--fine needle aspiration (FNA) cytology findings. *Cytopathology* 9: 291-300.
2045. Nola M, Babic D, Ilic J, Marusic M, Uzarevic B, Petrovecki M, Sabioncello A, Kovac D, Jukic S (1996). Prognostic parameters for survival of patients with malignant mesenchymal tumors of the uterus. *Cancer* 78: 2543-2550.
2046. Noller KL (1993). Role of colposcopy in the examination of diethylstilbestrol-exposed women. *Obstet Gynecol Clin North Am* 20: 165-176.
2047. Nomura K, Aizawa S (2000). Noninvasive, microinvasive, and invasive mucinous carcinomas of the ovary: a clinicopathologic analysis of 40 cases. *Cancer* 89: 1541-1546.
2048. Nordal RN, Kjorstad KE, Stenwig AE, Trope CG (1993). Leiomyosarcoma (LMS) and endometrial stromal sarcoma (ESS) of the uterus. A survey of patients treated in the Norwegian Radium Hospital 1976-1985. *Int J Gynecol Cancer* 3: 110-115.
2049. Nordal RR, Kristensen GB, Kaern J, Stenwig AE, Pettersen EO, Trope CG (1995). The prognostic significance of stage, tumor size, cellular atypia and DNA ploidy in uterine leiomyosarcoma. *Acta Oncol* 34: 797-802.
2050. Norris HJ, Hilliard GD, Irey NS (1988). Hemorrhagic cellular leiomyomas ("apoplectic leiomyoma") of the uterus associated with pregnancy and oral contraceptives. *Int J Gynecol Pathol* 7: 212-224.
2051. Norris HJ, Parmley T (1975). Mesenchymal tumors of the uterus. V. Intravenous leiomyomatosis. A clinical and pathologic study of 14 cases. *Cancer* 36: 2164-2178.
2052. Norris HJ, Robinowitz M (1971). Ovarian adenocarcinoma of mesonephric type. *Cancer* 28: 1074-1081.
2053. Norris HJ, Taylor HB (1965). Prognosis of mucinous (gelatinous) carcinoma of the breast. *Cancer* 18: 879-885.
2054. Norris HJ, Taylor HB (1966). Mesenchymal tumors of the uterus. I. A clinical and pathological study of 53 endometrial stromal tumors. *Cancer* 19: 755-766.
2055. Norris HJ, Taylor HB (1966). Polyps of the vagina. A benign lesion resembling sarcoma botryoides. *Cancer* 19: 227-232.

2056. Norris HJ, Taylor HB (1967). Nodular theca-lutein hyperplasia of pregnancy (so-called "pregnancy luteoma"). A clinical and pathologic study of 15 cases. *Am J Clin Pathol* 47: 557-566.

2057. Norris HJ, Taylor HB (1967). Relationship of histologic features to behavior of cystosarcoma phyllodes. Analysis of ninety-four cases. *Cancer* 20: 2090-2099.

2058. Norris HJ, Taylor HB (1968). Prognosis of granulosa-theca tumors of the ovary. *Cancer* 21: 255-263.

2059. Norris HJ, Taylor HB (1969). Virilization associated with cystic granulosa tumors. *Obstet Gynecol* 34: 629-635.

2060. Norris HJ, Zirkin HJ, Benson WL (1976). Immature (malignant) teratoma of the ovary: a clinical and pathologic study of 58 cases. *Cancer* 37: 2359-2372.

2061. Nucci MR, Clement PB, Young RH (1999). Lobular endocervical glandular hyperplasia, not otherwise specified: a clinicopathologic analysis of thirteen cases of a distinctive pseudoneoplastic lesion and comparison with fourteen cases of adenoma malignum. *Am J Surg Pathol* 23: 886-891.

2062. Nucci MR, Fletcher CD (1998). Liposarcoma (atypical lipomatous tumors) of the vulva: a clinicopathologic study of six cases. *Int J Gynecol Pathol* 17: 17-23.

2063. Nucci MR, Granter SR, Fletcher CD (1997). Cellular angiofibroma: a benign neoplasm distinct from angiomyofibroblastoma and spindle cell lipoma. *Am J Surg Pathol* 21: 636-644.

2064. Nucci MR, Krausz T, Lifschitz-Mercer B, Chan JK, Fletcher CD (1998). Angiosarcoma of the ovary: clinicopathologic and immunohistochemical analysis of four cases with a broad morphologic spectrum. *Am J Surg Pathol* 22: 620-630.

2065. Nucci MR, O'Connell JT, Huettner PC, Cviko A, Sun D, Quade BJ (2001). h-Caldesmon expression effectively distinguishes endometrial stromal tumors from uterine smooth muscle tumors. *Am J Surg Pathol* 25: 455-463.

2066. Nucci MR, Prasad CJ, Crum CP, Mutter GL (1999). Mucinous endometrial epithelial proliferations: a morphologic spectrum of changes with diverse clinical significance. *Mod Pathol* 12: 1137-1142.

2067. Nucci MR, Young RH, Fletcher CD (2000). Cellular pseudosarcomatous fibroepithelial stromal polyps of the lower female genital tract: an underrecognized lesion often misdiagnosed as sarcoma. *Am J Surg Pathol* 24: 231-240.

2068. Nuovo J, Melnikow J, Willan AR, Chan BK (2000). Treatment outcomes for squamous intraepithelial lesions. *Int J Gynaecol Obstet* 68: 25-33.

2069. Nuovo MA, Nuovo GJ, Smith D, Lewis SH (1990). Benign mesenchymoma of the round ligament. A report of two cases with immunohistochemistry. *Am J Clin Pathol* 93: 421-424.

2070. Nystrom-Lahti M, Kristo P, Nicolaides NC, Chang SY, Aaltonen LA, Moisio AL, Jarvinen HJ, Mecklin JP, Kinzler KW, Vogelstein B, de la Chapelle A, Peltomaki P. (1995). Founding mutations and Alu-mediated recombination in hereditary colon cancer. *Nat Med* 1: 1203-1206.

2071. O'Connell P, Pekkel V, Fuqua SA, Osborne CK, Clark GM, Allred DC (1998). Analysis of loss of heterozygosity in 399 premalignant breast lesions at 15 genetic loci. *J Natl Cancer Inst* 90: 697-703.

2072. O'Connor DM, Norris HJ (1994). The influence of grade on the outcome of stage I ovarian immature (malignant) teratomas and the reproducibility of grading. *Int J Gynecol Pathol* 13: 283-289.

2073. O'Connor IF, Shembekar MV, Shousha S (1998). Breast carcinoma developing in patients on hormone replacement therapy: a histological and immunohistological study. *J Clin Pathol* 51: 935-938.

2074. O'Hara MF, Page DL (1985). Adenomas of the breast and ectopic breast under lactational influences. *Hum Pathol* 16: 707-712.

2075. Obata K, Morland SJ, Watson RH, Hitchcock A, Chenevix-Trench G, Thomas EJ, Campbell IG (1998). Frequent PTEN/MMAC mutations in endometrioid but not serous or mucinous epithelial ovarian tumors. *Cancer Res* 58: 2095-2097.

2076. Obata N, Sasaki A, Takeuchi S, Ishiguro Y (1987). Clinico-pathologic study on the early diagnosis of cervical adenocarcinoma. *Nippon Sanka Fujinka Gakkai Zasshi* 39: 771-776.

2077. Obata NH, Nakashima N, Kawai M, Kikkawa F, Mamba S, Tomoda Y (1995). Gonadoblastoma with dysgerminoma in one ovary and gonadoblastoma with dysgerminoma and yolk sac tumor in the contralateral ovary in a girl with 46XX karyotype. *Gynecol Oncol* 58: 124-128.

2077a. Ober WB, Edgcomb JH, Price EB Jr. (1971). The pathology of choriocarcinoma. *Ann N Y Acad Sci* 172: 299-426.

2078. Ober WB, Maier RC (1981). Gestational choriocarcinoma of the fallopian tube. *Diagn Gynecol Obstet* 3: 213-231.

2079. Oberman HA (1965). Cystosarcoma phyllodes. A clinicopathological study of hypercellular periductal stromal neoplasms of breast. *Cancer* 18: 697-710.

2080. Oberman HA (1980). Secretory carcinoma of the breast in adults. *Am J Surg Pathol* 4: 465-470.

2081. Oberman HA, Fidler WJ Jr. (1979). Tubular carcinoma of the breast. *Am J Surg Pathol* 3: 387-395.

2082. Ockner DM, Sayadi H, Swanson PE, Ritter JH, Wick MR (1997). Genital angiomyofibroblastoma. Comparison with aggressive angiomyxoma and other myxoid neoplasms of skin and soft tissue. *Am J Clin Pathol* 107: 36-44.

2083. Oddoux C, Struewing JP, Clayton CM, Neuhausen S, Brody LC, Kaback M, Haas B, Norton L, Borgen P, Jhanwar S, Goldgar D, Ostrer H, Offit K (1996). The carrier frequency of the BRCA2 6174delT mutation among Ashkenazi Jewish individuals is approximately 1%. *Nat Genet* 14: 188-190.

2084. Offit K, Pierce H, Kirchhoff T, Kolachana P, Rapaport B, Gregersen P, Johnson S, Yossepowitch O, Huang H, Satagopan J, Robson M, Scheuer L, Nafa K, Ellis N (2003). Frequency of CHEK2*1100delC in New York breast cancer cases and controls. *BMC Med Genet* 4: 1.

2085. Ogawa K, Johansson SL, Cohen SM (1999). Immunohistochemical analysis of uroplakins, urothelial specific proteins, in ovarian Brenner tumors, normal tissues, and benign and neoplastic lesions of the female genital tract. *Am J Pathol* 155: 1047-1050.

2086. Ohgaki H, Hernandez T, Kleihues P, Hainaut P (1999). p53 germline mutations and the molecular basis of Li-Fraumeni syndrome. In: *Molecular Biology in Cancer Medicine*, R Kurzrock, M Talpaz (eds.), 2nd ed. Martin Dunitz: London, pp. 477-492.

2087. Ohgaki H, Vital A, Kleihues P, Hainaut P (2000). Familial tumour syndromes involving the nervous system. Li-Fraumeni syndrome and TP53 germline mutations. In: *WHO Classification of Tumours. Pathology and Genetics of the Tumours of the Nervous System*, P Kleihues, WK Cavenee (eds.), 1st ed. IARC Press: Lyon, France, pp. 231-234.

2088. Ohnishi T, Watanabe S (2000). The use of cytokeratins 7 and 20 in the diagnosis of primary and secondary extramammary Paget's disease. *Br J Dermatol* 142: 243-247.

2089. Ohtake T, Abe R, Kimijima I, Fukushima T, Tsuchiya A, Hoshi K, Wakasa H (1995). Intraductal extension of primary invasive breast carcinoma treated by breast-conservative surgery. Computer graphic three-dimensional reconstruction of the mammary duct-lobular systems. *Cancer* 76: 32-45.

2090. Ohuchi N (1999). Breast-conserving surgery for invasive cancer: a principle based on segmental anatomy. *Tohoku J Exp Med* 188: 103-118.

2091. Ohuchi N, Abe R, Kasai M (1984). Possible cancerous change of intraductal papillomas of the breast. A 3-D reconstruction study of 25 cases. *Cancer* 54: 605-611.

2092. Ohuchi N, Abe R, Takahashi T, Tezuka F (1984). Origin and extension of intraductal papillomas of the breast: a three-dimensional reconstruction study. *Breast Cancer Res Treat* 4: 117-128.

2093. Ohuchi N, Furuta A, Mori S (1994). Management of ductal carcinoma in situ with nipple discharge. Intraductal spreading of carcinoma is an unfavorable pathologic factor for breast-conserving surgery. *Cancer* 74: 1294-1302.

2094. Oka H, Shiozaki H, Kobayashi K, Inoue M, Tahara H, Kobayashi T, Takatsuka Y, Matsuyoshi N, Hirano S, Takeichi M, Mori T (1993). Expression of E-cadherin cell adhesion molecules in human breast cancer and its relationship to metastasis. *Cancer Res* 53: 1696-1701.

2095. Okagaki T, Ishida T, Hilgers RD (1976). A malignant tumor of the vagina resembling synovial sarcoma: a light and electron microscopic study. *Cancer* 37: 2306-2320.

2096. Olah KS, Dunn JA, Gee H (1992). Leiomyosarcomas have a poorer prognosis than mixed mesodermal tumours when adjusting for known prognostic factors: the result of a retrospective study of 423 cases of uterine sarcoma. *Br J Obstet Gynaecol* 99: 590-594.

2097. Oliva E, Clement PB, Young RH (2000). Endometrial stromal tumors: an update on a group of tumors with a protean phenotype. *Adv Anat Pathol* 7: 257-281.

2098. Oliva E, Clement PB, Young RH, Scully RE (1998). Mixed endometrial stromal and smooth muscle tumors of the uterus: a clinicopathologic study of 15 cases. *Am J Surg Pathol* 22: 997-1005.

2099. Oliva E, Ferry JA, Young RH, Prat J, Srigley JR, Scully RE (1997). Granulocytic sarcoma of the female genital tract: a clinicopathologic study of 11 cases. *Am J Surg Pathol* 21: 1156-1165.

2100. Oliva E, Musulen E, Prat J, Young RH (1995). Transitional cell carinoma of the renal pelvis with symptomatic ovarian metastases. *Int J Surg Pathol* 2: 231-236.

2101. Oliva E, Young RH, Clement PB, Bhan AK, Scully RE (1995). Cellular benign mesenchymal tumors of the uterus. A comparative morphologic and immunohistochemical analysis of 33 highly cellular leiomyomas and six endometrial stromal nodules, two frequently confused tumors. *Am J Surg Pathol* 19: 757-768.

2102. Oliva E, Young RH, Clement PB, Scully RE (1999). Myxoid and fibrous endometrial stromal tumors of the uterus: a report of 10 cases. *Int J Gynecol Pathol* 18: 310-319.

2103. Olive DL, Lurain JR, Brewer JI (1984). Choriocarcinoma associated with term gestation. *Am J Obstet Gynecol* 148: 711-716.

2104. Olivier M, Eeles R, Hollstein M, Khan MA, Harris CC, Hainaut P (2002). The IARC TP53 database: new online mutation analysis and recommendations to users. *Hum Mutat* 19: 607-614.

2104a. Olivier M, Goldgar DE, Sodha N, Ohgaki H, Kleihues P, Hainaut P, Eeles RA (2003). Li-Fraumeni and related syndromes: correlation between tumour type, family structure and TP53 genotype. *Cancer Res* (in press).

2105. Olsen JH, Hahnemann JM, Borresen-Dale AL, Brondum-Nielsen K, Hammarstrom L, Kleinerman R, Kaariainen H, Lonnqvist T, Sankila R, Seersholm N, Tretli S, Yuen J, Boice JD Jr., Tucker M (2001). Cancer in patients with ataxia-telangiectasia and in their relatives in the nordic countries. *J Natl Cancer Inst* 93: 121-127.

2106. Olson SH, Mignone L, Nakraseive C, Caputo TA, Barakat RR, Harlap S (2001). Symptoms of ovarian cancer. *Obstet Gynecol* 98: 212-217.

2107. Olsson H, Alm P, Aspegren K, Gullberg B, Jonsson PE, Ranstam J (1990). Increased plasma prolactin levels in a group of men with breast cancer--a preliminary study. *Anticancer Res* 10: 59-62.

2108. Olszewski W, Darzynkiewicz Z, Rosen PP, Schwartz MK, Melamed MR (1981). Flow cytometry of breast carcinoma: I. Relation of DNA ploidy level to histology and estrogen receptor. *Cancer* 48: 980-984.

2109. Orbo A, Stalsberg H, Kunde D (1990). Topographic criteria in the diagnosis of tumor emboli in intramammary lymphatics. *Cancer* 66: 972-977.

2110. Ordi J, Nogales FF, Palacin A, Marquez M, Pahisa J, Vanrell JA, Cardesa A (2001). Mesonephric adenocarcinoma of the uterine corpus: CD10 expression as evidence of mesonephric differentiation. *Am J Surg Pathol* 25: 1540-1545.

2111. Ordi J, Schammel DP, Rasekh L, Tavassoli FA (1999). Sertoliform endometrioid carcinomas of the ovary: a clinicopathologic and immunohistochemical study of 13 cases. *Mod Pathol* 12: 933-940.

2112. Ordi J, Stamatakos MD, Tavassoli FA (1997). Pure pleomorphic rhabdomyosarcomas of the uterus. *Int J Gynecol Pathol* 16: 369-377.

2113. Ordonez NG (1998). Role of immunohistochemistry in distinguishing epithelial peritoneal mesotheliomas from peritoneal and ovarian serous carcinomas. *Am J Surg Pathol* 22: 1203-1214.

2114. Ordonez NG (1999). Granular cell tumor: a review and update. *Adv Anat Pathol* 6: 186-203.

2115. Ordonez NG (2000). Transitional cell carcinomas of the ovary and bladder are immunophenotypically different. *Histopathology* 36: 433-438.

2116. Ordonez NG, Mackay B (2000). Brenner tumor of the ovary: a comparative immunohistochemical and ultrastructural study with transitional cell carcinoma of the bladder. *Ultrastruct Pathol* 24: 157-167.
2117. Ordonez NG, Manning JT, Luna MA (1981). Mixed tumor of the vulva: a report of two cases probably arising in Bartholin's gland. *Cancer* 48: 181-186.
2118. Origoni M, Rossi M, Ferrari D, Lillo F, Ferrari AG (1999). Human papillomavirus with co-existing vulvar vestibulitis syndrome and vestibular papillomatosis. *Int J Gynaecol Obstet* 64: 259-263.
2119. Osborne BM, Robboy SJ (1983). Lymphomas or leukemia presenting as ovarian tumors. An analysis of 42 cases. *Cancer* 52: 1933-1943.
2120. Osborne CK (1998). Steroid hormone receptors in breast cancer management. *Breast Cancer Res Treat* 51: 227-238.
2121. Osin P, Crook T, Powles T, Peto J, Gusterson B (1998). Hormone status of in-situ cancer in BRCA1 and BRCA2 mutation carriers. *Lancet* 351: 1487.
2122. Osin P, Gusterson BA, Philp E, Waller J, Bartek J, Peto J, Crook T (1998). Predicted anti-oestrogen resistance in BRCA-associated familial breast cancers. *Eur J Cancer* 34: 1683-1686.
2123. Otis CN (1996). Uterine adenomatoid tumors: immunohistochemical characteristics with emphasis on Ber-EP4 immunoreactivity and distinction from adenocarcinoma. *Int J Gynecol Pathol* 15: 146-151.
2124. Otis CN, Powell JL, Barbuto D, Carcangiu ML (1992). Intermediate filamentous proteins in adult granulosa cell tumors. An immunohistochemical study of 25 cases. *Am J Surg Pathol* 16: 962-968.
2125. Ott G, Katzenberger T, Greiner A, Kalla J, Rosenwald A, Heinrich U, Ott MM, Muller-Hermelink HK (1997). The t(11;18)(q21;q21) chromosome translocation is a frequent and specific aberration in low-grade but not high-grade malignant non-Hodgkin's lymphomas of the mucosa-associated lymphoid tissue (MALT)- type. *Cancer Res* 57: 3944-3948.
2126. Otterbach F, Bankfalvi A, Bergner S, Decker T, Krech R, Boecker W (2000). Cytokeratin 5/6 immunohistochemistry assists the differential diagnosis of atypical proliferations of the breast. *Histopathology* 37: 232-240.
2127. Ottesen GL, Graversen HP, Blichert-Toft M, Christensen IJ, Andersen JA (2000). Carcinoma in situ of the female breast. 10 year follow-up results of a prospective nationwide study. *Breast Cancer Res Treat* 62: 197-210.
2128. Ottesen GL, Graversen HP, Blichert-Toft M, Zedeler K, Andersen JA (1993). Lobular carcinoma in situ of the female breast. Short-term results of a prospective nationwide study. The Danish Breast Cancer Cooperative Group. *Am J Surg Pathol* 17: 14-21.
2129. Ottman R, Pike MC, King MC, Casagrande JT, Henderson BE (1986). Familial breast cancer in a population-based series. *Am J Epidemiol* 123: 15-21.
2130. Ouchi T, Monteiro AN, August A, Aaronson SA, Hanafusa H (1998). BRCA1 regulates p53-dependent gene expression. *Proc Natl Acad Sci USA* 95: 2302-2306.
2131. Outwater EK, Marchetto B, Wagner BJ (2000). Virilizing tumors of the ovary: imaging features. *Ultrasound Obstet Gynecol* 15: 365-371.
2132. Outwater EK, Siegelman ES, Hunt JL (2001). Ovarian teratomas: tumor types and imaging characteristics. *Radiographics* 21: 475-490.
2133. Oyama T, Kashiwabara K, Yoshimoto K, Arnold A, Koerner F (1998). Frequent overexpression of the cyclin D1 oncogene in invasive lobular carcinoma of the breast. *Cancer Res* 58: 2876-2880.
2134. Ozguroglu M, Ersavasti G, Ilvan S, Hatemi G, Demir G, Demirelli FH (1999). Bilateral inflammatory breast metastases of epithelial ovarian cancer. *Am J Clin Oncol* 22: 408-410.
2135. Ozguroglu M, Ozaras R, Tahan V, Demirkesen C, Demir G, Dogusoy G, Buyukunal E, Serdengecti S, Berkarda B (1999). Anorectal melanoma metastatic to the breast. *J Clin Gastroenterol* 29: 197-199.
2136. Ozzello L, Gump FE (1985). The management of patients with carcinomas in fibroadenomatous tumors of the breast. *Surg Gynecol Obstet* 160: 99-104.
2137. Östör AG (1993). Natural history of cervical intraepithelial neoplasia: a critical review. *Int J Gynecol Pathol* 12: 186-192.
2138. Östör AG (1995). Pandora's box or Ariadne's thread? Definition and prognostic significance of microinvasion in the uterine cervix. Squamous lesions. *Pathol Annu* 30: 103-136.
2139. Östör AG (2000). Early invasive adenocarcinoma of the uterine cervix. *Int J Gynecol Pathol* 19: 29-38.
2140. Östör AG, Duncan A, Quinn M, Rome R (2000). Adenocarcinoma in situ of the uterine cervix: an experience with 100 cases. *Gynecol Oncol* 79: 207-210.
2141. Östör AG, Fortune DW, Riley CB (1988). Fibroepithelial polyps with atypical stromal cells (pseudosarcoma botryoides) of vulva and vagina. A report of 13 cases. *Int J Gynecol Pathol* 7: 351-360.
2142. Östör AG, Pagano R, Davoren RA, Fortune DW, Chanen W, Rome R (1984). Adenocarcinoma in situ of the cervix. *Int J Gynecol Pathol* 3: 179-190.
2143. Östör AG, Rome R, Quinn M (1997). Microinvasive adenocarcinoma of the cervix: a clinicopathologic study of 77 women. *Obstet Gynecol* 89: 88-93.
2144. Paavonen J (1985). Colposcopic findings associated with human papillomavirus infection of the vagina and the cervix. *Obstet Gynecol Surv* 40: 185-189.
2145. Padberg BC, Stegner HE, von Sengbusch S, Arps H, Schroder S (1992). DNA-cytophotometry and immunocytochemistry in ovarian tumours of borderline malignancy and related peritoneal lesions. *Virchows Arch A Pathol Anat Histopathol* 421: 497-503.
2146. Padmore RF, Lara JF, Ackerman DJ, Gales T, Sigurdson ER, Ehya H, Cooper HS, Patchefsky AS (1996). Primary combined malignant melanoma and ductal carcinoma of the breast. A report of two cases. *Cancer* 78: 2515-2525.
2147. Page DL, Anderson TJ, Sakamoto G (1987). *Infiltrating Carcinoma:Major Histoligical Types*. WB Saunders: London.
2148. Page DL, Dixon JM, Anderson T, Lee D, Stwewart H (1993). Invasive cribriform carcinoma of the breast. *Histopathology* 7: 525-536.
2149. Page DL, Dupont WD (1990). Anatomic markers of human premalignancy and risk of breast cancer. *Cancer* 66: 1326-1335.
2150. Page DL, Kidd TE Jr., Dupont WD, Simpson JF, Rogers LW (1991). Lobular neoplasia of the breast: higher risk for subsequent invasive cancer predicted by more extensive disease. *Hum Pathol* 22: 1232-1239.
2151. Page DL, Salhany KE, Jensen RA, Dupont WD (1996). Subsequent breast carcinoma risk after biopsy with atypia in a breast papilloma. *Cancer* 78: 258-266.
2152. Palacios J, Benito N, Pizarro A, Suarez A, Espada J, Cano A, Gamallo C (1995). Anomalous expression of P-Cadherin in breast carcinoma. Correlation with E-Cadherin expression and pathological features. *Am J Pathol* 146: 605-612.
2153. Palacios J, Gamallo C (1998). Mutations in the beta-catenin gene (CTNNB1) in endometrioid ovarian carcinomas. *Cancer Res* 58: 1344-1347.
2154. Palangie T, Mosseri V, Mihura J, Campana F, Beuzeboc P, Dorval T, Garcia-Giralt E, Jouve M, Scholl S, Asselain B, Pouillart P. (1994). Prognostic factors in inflammatory breast cancer and therapeutic implications. *Eur J Cancer* 30A: 921-927.
2155. Palazzo J, Hyslop T (1998). Hyperplastic ductal and lobular lesions and carcinoma in situ of the breast: Reproducibility of current diagnostic criteria among community and academic based pathologists. *Breast J* 4: 230-237.
2156. Palazzo JP, Gibas Z, Dunton CJ, Talerman A (1993). Cytogenetic study of botryoid rhabdomyosarcoma of the uterine cervix. *Virchows Arch A Pathol Anat Histopathol* 422: 87-91.
2157. Palli D, Galli M, Bianchi S, Bussolati G, Di Palma S, Eusebi V, Gambacorta M, Rosselli DT (1996). Reproducibility of histological diagnosis of breast lesions: results of a panel in Italy. *Eur J Cancer* 32A: 603-607.
2158. Palli D, Rosselli DT, Simoncini R, Bianchi S (1991). Benign breast disease and breast cancer: a case-control study in a cohort in Italy. *Int J Cancer* 47: 703-706.
2159. Pallis L, Wilking N, Cedermark B, Rutqvist LE, Skoog L (1992). Receptors for estrogen and progesterone in breast carcinoma in situ. *Anticancer Res* 12: 2113-2115.
2160. Palmer JP, Biback SM (1954). Primary cancer of the vagina. *Am J Obstet Gynecol* 67: 377-397.
2161. Palmer JR, Anderson D, Helmrich SP, Herbst AL (2000). Risk factors for diethylstilbestrol-associated clear cell adenocarcinoma. *Obstet Gynecol* 95: 814-820.
2162. Palmer PE, Bogojavlensky S, Bhan AK, Scully RE (1990). Prolactinoma in wall of ovarian dermoid cyst with hyperprolactinemia. *Obstet Gynecol* 75: 540-543.
2163. Palombo F, Gallinari P, Iaccarino I, Lettieri T, Hughes M, D'Arrigo A, Truong O, Hsuan JJ, Jiricny J (1995). GTBP, a 160-kilodalton protein essential for mismatch-binding activity in human cells. *Science* 268: 1912-1914.
2164. Pantoja E, Rodriguez-Ibanez I, Axtmayer RW, Noy MA, Pelegrina I (1975). Complications of dermoid tumors of the ovary. *Obstet Gynecol* 45: 89-94.
2165. Paoletti M, Pridjian G, Okagaki T, Talerman A (1987). A stromal Leydig cell tumor of the ovary occurring in a pregnant 15-year-old girl. Ultrastructural findings. *Cancer* 60: 2806-2810.
2166. Papadatos G, Rangan AM, Psarianos T, Ung O, Taylor R, Boyages J (2001). Probability of axillary node involvement in patients with tubular carcinoma of the breast. *Br J Surg* 88: 860-864.
2167. Papadopoulos N, Nicolaides NC, Wei YF, Ruben SM, Carter KC, Rosen CA, Haseltine WA, Fleischmann RD, Fraser CM, Adams MD, Venter JC, Hamilton SR, Petersen GM, Watson P, Lynch HT, Peltomaki T, Mecklin JP, de la Chapelle A, Kinzler KW, Vogelstein B. (1994). Mutation of a mutL homolog in hereditary colon cancer. *Science* 263: 1625-1629.
2168. Papchristou DN, Kinne DW, Ashikari R, Fortner JG (1979). Melanoma of the nipple and aerola. *Br J Surg (4)* 66: 287-288.
2169. Papotti M, Macri L, Bussolati G, Reubi JC (1989). Correlative study on neuro-endocrine differentiation and presence of somatostatin receptors in breast carcinomas. *Int J Cancer* 43: 365-369.
2170. Paradinas FJ, Browne P, Fisher RA, Foskett M, Bagshawe KD, Newlands E (1996). A clinical, histopathological and flow cytometric study of 149 complete moles, 146 partial moles and 107 non-molar hydropic abortions. *Histopathology* 28: 101-110.
2171. Paraskevas M, Scully RE (1989). Hilus cell tumor of the ovary. A clinicopathological analysis of 12 Reinke crystal-positive and nine crystal-negative cases. *Int J Gynecol Pathol* 8: 299-310.
2172. Parazzini F, Franceschi S, La Vecchia C, Fasoli M (1991). The epidemiology of ovarian cancer. *Gynecol Oncol* 43: 9-23.
2173. Parazzini F, La Vecchia C, Moroni S, Chatenoud L, Ricci E (1994). Family history and the risk of endometrial cancer. *Int J Cancer* 59: 460-462.
2174. Parc YR, Halling KC, Burgart LJ, McDonnell SK, Schaid DJ, Thibodeau SN, Halling AC (2000). Microsatellite instability and hMLH1/hMSH2 expression in young endometrial carcinoma patients: associations with family history and histopathology. *Int J Cancer* 86: 60-66.
2175. Parham DM, Hagen N, Brown RA (1992). Simplified method of grading primary carcinomas of the breast. *J Clin Pathol* 45: 517-520.
2176. Park CC, Mitsumori M, Nixon A, Recht A, Connolly J, Gelman R, Silver B, Hetelekidis S, Abner A, Harris JR, Schnitt SJ (2000). Outcome at 8 years after breast-conserving surgery and radiation therapy for invasive breast cancer: influence of margin status and systemic therapy on local recurrence. *J Clin Oncol* 18: 1668-1675.
2177. Park J, Sun D, Genest DR, Trivijitsilp P, Suh I, Crum CP (1998). Coexistence of low and high grade squamous intraepithelial lesions of the cervix: morphologic progression or multiple papillomaviruses? *Gynecol Oncol* 70: 386-391.
2178. Park JG, Park YJ, Wijnen JT, Vasen HF (1999). Gene-environment interaction in hereditary nonpolyposis colorectal cancer with implications for diagnosis and genetic testing. *Int J Cancer* 82: 516-519.
2179. Park JJ, Genest DR, Sun D, Crum CP (1999). Atypical immature metaplastic-like proliferations of the cervix: diagnostic reproducibility and viral (HPV) correlates. *Hum Pathol* 30: 1161-1165.

2180. Park JS, Jones RW, McLean MR, Currie JL, Woodruff JD, Shah KV, Kurman RJ (1991). Possible etiologic heterogeneity of vulvar intraepithelial neoplasia. A correlation of pathologic characteristics with human papillomavirus detection by in situ hybridization and polymerase chain reaction. *Cancer* 67: 1599-1607.
2181. Park SH, Kim I (1994). Histogenetic consideration of ovarian sex cord-stromal tumors analyzed by expression pattern of cytokeratins, vimentin, and laminin. Correlation studies with human gonads. *Pathol Res Pract* 190: 449-456.
2182. Park SK, Yoo KY, Lee SJ, Kim SU, Ahn SH, Noh DY, Choe KJ, Strickland PT, Hirvonen A, Kang D (2000). Alcohol consumption, glutathione S-transferase M1 and T1 genetic polymorphisms and breast cancer risk. *Pharmacogenetics* 10: 301-309.
2183. Park SY, Kim HS, Hong EK, Kim WH (2002). Expression of cytokeratins 7 and 20 in primary carcinomas of the stomach and colorectum and their value in the differential diagnosis of metastatic carcinomas to the ovary. *Hum Pathol* 33: 1078-1085.
2184. Park TW, Richart RM, Sun XW, Wright TC Jr. (1996). Association between human papillomavirus type and clonal status of cervical squamous intraepithelial lesions. *J Natl Cancer Inst* 88: 355-358.
2185. Parkash V, Carcangiu ML (1995). Transformation of ovarian dysgerminoma to yolk sac tumor: evidence for a histogenetic continuum. *Mod Pathol* 8: 881-887.
2186. Parker RG, Grimm P, Enstrom JE (1989). Contralateral breast cancers following treatment for initial breast cancers in women. *Am J Clin Oncol* 12: 213-216.
2187. Parker WH, Fu YS, Berek JS (1994). Uterine sarcoma in patients operated on for presumed leiomyoma and rapidly growing leiomyoma. *Obstet Gynecol* 83: 414-418.
2188. Parkin DM, Bray F, Ferlay J, Pisani P (2001). Estimating the world cancer burden: Globocan 2000. *Int J Cancer* 94: 153-156.
2189. Parkin DM, Whelan SL, Ferlay J, Raymond L, Young J (1997). *Cancer Incidence in Five Continents, Vol. VII* (IARC Scientific Publication N°143). International Agency for Research on Cancer: Lyon, France.
2190. Parl FF, Richardson LD (1983). The histologic and biologic spectrum of tubular carcinoma of the breast. *Hum Pathol* 14: 694-698.
2191. Patchefsky AS, Frauenhoffer CM, Krall RA, Cooper HS (1979). Low-grade mucoepidermoid carcinoma of the breast. *Arch Pathol Lab Med* 103: 196-198.
2192. Patchefsky AS, Shaber GS, Schwartz GF, Feig SA, Nerlinger RE (1977). The pathology of breast cancer detected by mass population screening. *Cancer* 40: 1659-1670.
2193. Patel KJ, Yu VP, Lee H, Corcoran A, Thistlethwaite FC, Evans MJ, Colledge WH, Friedman LS, Ponder BA, Venkitaraman AR (1998). Involvement of Brca2 in DNA repair. *Mol Cell* 1: 347-357.
2194. Paterakos M, Watkin WG, Edgerton SM, Moore DH, Thor AD (1999). Invasive micropapillary carcinoma of the breast: a prognostic study. *Hum Pathol* 30: 1459-1463.
2195. Patey DH, Scarff RW (1928). The position of histology in the prognosis of carcinoma of the breast. *Lancet* 1: 801-804.
2196. Patsner B (2001). Primary endodermal sinus tumor of the endometrium presenting as "recurrent" endometrial adenocarcinoma. *Gynecol Oncol* 80: 93-95.
2197. Pattillo RA, Sasaki S, Katayama KP, Roesler M, Mattingly RF (1981). Genesis of 46,XY hydatidiform mole. *Am J Obstet Gynecol* 141: 104-105.
2198. Paull TT, Cortez D, Bowers B, Elledge SJ, Gellert M (2001). From the Cover: Direct DNA binding by Brca1. *Proc Natl Acad Sci USA 98:* 6086-6091.
2199. Paulus DD (1990). Lymphoma of the breast. *Radiol Clin North Am* 28: 833-840.
2200. Pautier P, Genestie C, Rey A, Morice P, Roche B, Lhomme C, Haie-Meder C, Duvillard P (2000). Analysis of clinicopathologic prognostic factors for 157 uterine sarcomas and evaluation of a grading score validated for soft tissue sarcoma. *Cancer* 88: 1425-1431.
2201. Pedersen L, Holck S, Schiodt T, Zedeler K, Mouridsen HT (1994). Medullary carcinoma of the breast, prognostic importance of characteristic histopathological features evaluated in a multivariate Cox analysis. *Eur J Cancer 30A:* 1792-1797.
2202. Pedersen L, Larsen JK, Christensen IJ, Lykkesfeldt A, Holck S, Schiodt T (1994). DNA ploidy and S-phase fraction in medullary carcinoma of the breast--a flow cytometric analysis using archival material. *Breast Cancer Res Treat* 29: 297-306.
2203. Pedersen L, Zedeler K, Holck S, Schiodt T, Mouridsen HT (1991). Medullary carcinoma of the breast, proposal for a new simplified histopathological definition. Based on prognostic observations and observations on inter- and intraobserver variability of 11 histopathological characteristics in 131 breast carcinomas with medullary features. *Br J Cancer* 63: 591-595.
2204. Pedersen L, Zedeler K, Holck S, Schiodt T, Mouridsen HT (1995). Medullary carcinoma of the breast. Prevalence and prognostic importance of classical risk factors in breast cancer. *Eur J Cancer 31A*: 2289-2295.
2204a. Pedeutour F, Ligon AH, Morton CC (1999). [Genetics of uterine leiomyomata]. *Bull Cancer* 86: 920-928.
2205. Peiro G, Bornstein BA, Connolly JL, Gelman R, Hetelekidis S, Nixon AJ, Recht A, Silver B, Harris JR, Schnitt SJ (2000). The influence of infiltrating lobular carcinoma on the outcome of patients treated with breast-conserving surgery and radiation therapy. *Breast Cancer Res Treat* 59: 49-54.
2206. Peiro G, Diebold J, Lohse P, Ruebsamen H, Lohse P, Baretton GB, Lohrs U (2002). Microsatellite instability, loss of heterozygosity, and loss of hMLH1 and hMSH2 protein expression in endometrial carcinoma. *Hum Pathol* 33: 347-354.
2207. Pejovic T, Burki N, Odunsi K, Fiedler P, Achong N, Schwartz PE, Ward DC (1999). Well-differentiated mucinous carcinoma of the ovary and a coexisting Brenner tumor both exhibit amplification of 12q14-21 by comparative genomic hybridization. *Gynecol Oncol* 74: 134-137.
2208. Pejovic T, Heim S, Alm P, Iosif S, Himmelmann A, Skjaerris J, Mitelman F (1993). Isochromosome 1q as the sole karyotypic abnormality in a Sertoli cell tumor of the ovary. *Cancer Genet Cytogenet* 65: 79-80.
2209. Pejovic T, Heim S, Mandahl N, Elmfors B, Floderus UM, Furgyik S, Helm G, Willen H, Mitelman F (1990). Trisomy 12 is a consistent chromosomal aberration in benign ovarian tumors. *Genes Chromosomes Cancer* 2: 48-52.
2210. Pekin T, Eren F, Pekin O (2000). Leiomyosarcoma of the broad ligament: case report and literature review. *Eur J Gynaecol Oncol* 21: 318-319.
2211. Pelkey TJ, Frierson HF Jr., Mills SE, Stoler MH (1998). The diagnostic utility of inhibin staining in ovarian neoplasms. *Int J Gynecol Pathol* 17: 97-105.
2212. Pelosi G, Martignoni G, Bonetti F (1991). Intraductal carcinoma of mammary-type apocrine epithelium arising within a papillary hydradenoma of the vulva. Report of a case and review of the literature. *Arch Pathol Lab Med* 115: 1249-1254.
2213. Peltomaki P, Aaltonen LA, Sistonen P, Pylkkanen L, Mecklin JP, Jarvinen H, Green JS, Jass JR, Weber JL, Leach FS, Petersen GM, Hamilton SR, de la Chapelle A, Vogelstein B. (1993). Genetic mapping of a locus predisposing to human colorectal cancer. *Science* 260: 810-812.
2214. Peltomaki P, Vasen HF (1997). Mutations predisposing to hereditary nonpolyposis colorectal cancer: database and results of a collaborative study. The International Collaborative Group on Hereditary Nonpolyposis Colorectal Cancer. *Gastroenterology* 113: 1146-1158.
2214a. Penrose LS, Mackenzie JH, Karn MN (1948). A genetical study of human mammary cancer. *Ann Euegenics* 14: 234-266.
2215. Pensler JM, Silverman BL, Sanghavi J, Goolsby C, Speck G, Brizio-Molteni L, Molteni A (2000). Estrogen and progesterone receptors in gynecomastia. *Plast Reconstr Surg* 106: 1011-1013.
2216. Pereira H, Pinder SE, Sibbering DM, Galea MH, Elston CW, Blamey RW, Robertson JF, Ellis IO (1995). Pathological prognostic factors in breast cancer. IV: Should you be a typer or a grader? A comparative study of two histological prognostic features in operable breast carcinoma. *Histopathology* 27: 219-226.
2217. Perez CA, Arneson AN, Dehner LP, Galakatos A (1974). Radiation therapy in carcinoma of the vagina. *Obstet Gynecol* 44: 862-872.
2218. Perou CM, Sorlie T, Eisen MB, van de Rijn M, Jeffrey SS, Rees CA, Pollack JR, Ross DT, Johnsen H, Akslen LA, Fluge O, Pergamenschikov A, Williams C, Zhu SX, Lonning PE, Borresen-Dale AL, Brown PO, Botstein D (2000). Molecular portraits of human breast tumours. *Nature* 406: 747-752.
2219. Perrin L, Ward B (1995). Small cell carcinoma of the cervix. *Int J Gynecol Cancer* 5: 200-203.
2220. Persaud V, Anderson MF (1977). Endometrial stromal sarcoma of the broad ligament arising in an area of endometriosis in a paramesonephric cyst. Case report. *Br J Obstet Gynaecol* 84: 149-152.
2221. Persons DL, Hartmann LC, Herath JF, Keeney GL, Jenkins RB (1994). Fluorescence in situ hybridization analysis of trisomy 12 in ovarian tumors. *Am J Clin Pathol* 102: 775-779.
2222. Perzin KH, Lattes R (1972). Papillary adenoma of the nipple (florid papillomatosis, adenoma, adenomatosis). A clinicopathologic study. *Cancer* 29: 996-1009.
2223. Peters GN, Wolff M (1983). Adenoid cystic carcinoma of the breast. Report of 11 new cases: review of the literature and discussion of biological behavior. *Cancer* 52: 680-686.
2224. Peters GN, Wolff M, Haagensen CD (1981). Tubular carcinoma of the breast. Clinical pathologic correlations based on 100 cases. *Ann Surg* 193: 138-149.
2225. Peters WA, III, Andersen WA, Hopkins MP, Kumar NB, Morley GW (1988). Prognostic features of carcinoma of the fallopian tube. *Obstet Gynecol* 71: 757-762.
2226. Peters WA, III, Kumar NB, Andersen WA, Morley GW (1985). Primary sarcoma of the adult vagina: a clinicopathologic study. *Obstet Gynecol* 65: 699-704.
2227. Peters WA, III, Kumar NB, Morley GW (1985). Carcinoma of the vagina. Factors influencing treatment outcome. *Cancer* 55: 892-897.
2228. Peters WM, Wells M, Bryce FC (1984). Mullerian clear cell carcinofibroma of the uterine corpus. *Histopathology* 8: 1069-1078.
2229. Peterse JL (1993). Breast carcinoma with an unexpected inside out growth pattern, rotation of polarisation associated with angioinvasion. *Pathol Res Pract* 189: 780.
2230. Peto J, Collins N, Barfoot R, Seal S, Warren W, Rahman N, Easton DF, Evans C, Deacon J, Stratton MR (1999). Prevalence of BRCA1 and BRCA2 gene mutations in patients with early-onset breast cancer. *J Natl Cancer Inst* 91: 943-949.
2231. Petridou E, Giokas G, Kuper H, Mucci LA, Trichopoulos D (2000). Endocrine correlates of male breast cancer risk: a case-control study in Athens, Greece. *Br J Cancer* 83: 1234-1237.
2232. Petru E, Pickel H, Heydarfadai M, Lahousen M, Haas J, Schaider H, Tamussino K (1992). Nongenital cancers metastatic to the ovary. *Gynecol Oncol* 44: 83-86.
2233. Petterson F (1991). *Annual Report of the Treatment in Gynecological Cancer.* International Federation of Gynecology and Obstetrics: Stockholm.
2234. Pettinato G, Insabato L, De Chiara A, Manco A, Petrella G (1989). High-grade mucoepidermoid carcinoma of the breast. Fine needle aspiration cytology and clinicopathologic study of a case. *Acta Cytol* 33: 195-200.
2235. Pettinato G, Manivel JC, Insabato L, De Chiara A, Petrella G (1988). Plasma cell granuloma (inflammatory pseudotumor) of the breast. *Am J Clin Pathol* 90: 627-632.
2236. Pharoah PD, Antoniou A, Bobrow M, Zimmern RL, Easton DF, Ponder BA (2002). Polygenic susceptibility to breast cancer and implications for prevention. *Nat Genet* 31: 33-36.
2237. Pharoah PD, Day NE, Caldas C (1999). Somatic mutations in the p53 gene and prognosis in breast cancer: a meta-analysis. *Br J Cancer* 80: 1968-1973.
2238. Pharoah PD, Day NE, Duffy S, Easton DF, Ponder BA (1997). Family history and the risk of breast cancer: a systematic review and meta-analysis. *Int J Cancer* 71: 800-809.
2239. Pharoah PD, Easton DF, Stockton DL, Gayther S, Ponder BA (1999). Survival in familial, BRCA1-associated, and BRCA2-associated epithelial ovarian cancer. United Kingdom Coordinating Committee for Cancer Research (UKCCCR) Familial Ovarian Cancer Study Group. *Cancer Res* 59: 868-871.

2240. Phelan CM, Rebbeck TR, Weber BL, Devilee P, Ruttledge MH, Lynch HT, Lenoir GM, Stratton MR, Easton DF, Ponder BA, Cannon-Albright L, Larsson C, Goldgar DE, Narod SA (1996). Ovarian cancer risk in BRCA1 carriers is modified by the HRAS1 variable number of tandem repeat (VNTR) locus. *Nat Genet* 12: 309-311.

2241. Phillipson J, Ostrzega N (1994). Fine needle aspiration of invasive cribriform carcinoma with benign osteoclast-like giant cells of histiocytic origin. A case report. *Acta Cytol* 38: 479-482.

2242. Piana S, Nogales FF, Corrado S, Cardinale L, Gusolfino D, Rivasi F (1999). Pregnancy luteoma with granulosa cell proliferation: an unusual hyperplastic lesion arising in pregnancy and mimicking an ovarian neoplasia. *Pathol Res Pract* 195: 859-863.

2243. Picciocchi A, Masetti R, Terribile D, Ausili-Cefaro G, Antinori A, Marra A, Magistrelli P (1994). Inflammatory breast carcinoma: contribution of surgery as part of a combined modality approach. *Breast disease* 7: 143-149.

2244. Pickel H, Reich O, Tamussino K (1998). Bilateral atypical hyperplasia of the fallopian tube associated with tamoxifen: a report of two cases. *Int J Gynecol Pathol* 17: 284-285.

2245. Pickel H, Thalhammer M (1971). [Chondrosarcoma of the Fallopian tube]. *Geburtshilfe Frauenheilkd* 31: 1243-1248.

2246. Piek JM, van Diest PJ, Zweemer RP, Jansen JW, Poort-Keesom RJ, Menko FH, Gille JJ, Jongsma AP, Pals G, Kenemans P, Verheijen RH (2001). Dysplastic changes in prophylactically removed Fallopian tubes of women predisposed to developing ovarian cancer. *J Pathol* 195: 451-456.

2247. Piek JM, van Diest PJ, Zweemer RP, Kenemans P, Verheijen RH (2001). Tubal ligation and risk of ovarian cancer. *Lancet* 358: 844.

2248. Pierce GB (1974). Neoplasms, differentiations and mutations. *Am J Pathol* 77: 103-118.

2249. Pietruszka M, Barnes L (1978). Cystosarcoma phyllodes: a clinicopathologic analysis of 42 cases. *Cancer* 41: 1974-1983.

2250. Pike AM, Oberman HA (1985). Juvenile (cellular) adenofibromas. A clinicopathologic study. *Am J Surg Pathol* 9: 730-736.

2251. Pillai MR, Jayaprakash PG, Nair MK (1999). bcl-2 immunoreactivity but not p53 accumulation associated with tumour response to radiotherapy in cervical carcinoma. *J Cancer Res Clin Oncol* 125: 55-60.

2252. Pina L, Apesteguia L, Cojo R, Cojo F, Arias-Camison I, Rezola R, De Miguel C (1997). Myofibroblastoma of male breast: report of three cases and review of the literature. *Eur Radiol* 7: 931-934.

2253. Pinder SE, Ellis IO, Galea M, O'Rouke S, Blamey RW, Elston CW (1994). Pathological prognostic factors in breast cancer. III. Vascular invasion: relationship with recurrence and survival in a large study with long-term follow-up. *Histopathology* 24: 41-47.

2254. Pinder SE, Murray S, Ellis IO, Trihia H, Elston CW, Gelber RD, Goldhirsch A, Lindtner J, Cortes-Funes H, Simoncini E, Byrne MJ, Golouh R, Rudenstam CM, Castiglione-Gertsch M, Gusterson BA (1998). The importance of the histologic grade of invasive breast carcinoma and response to chemotherapy. *Cancer* 83: 1529-1539.

2255. Pins MR, Young RH, Daly WJ, Scully RE (1996). Primary squamous cell carcinoma of the ovary. Report of 37 cases. *Am J Surg Pathol* 20: 823-833.

2256. Pinto AP, Lin MC, Sheets EE, Muto MG, Sun D, Crum CP (2000). Allelic imbalance in lichen sclerosus, hyperplasia, and intraepithelial neoplasia of the vulva. *Gynecol Oncol* 77: 171-176.

2257. Pippard EC, Hall AJ, Barker DJ, Bridges BA (1988). Cancer in homozygotes and heterozygotes of ataxia-telangiectasia and xeroderma pigmentosum in Britain. *Cancer Res* 48: 2929-2932.

2258. Pitman MB, Young RH, Clement PB, Dickersin GR, Scully RE (1994). Endometrioid carcinoma of the ovary and endometrium, oxyphilic cell type: a report of nine cases. *Int J Gynecol Pathol* 13: 290-301.

2259. Pitts WC, Rojas VA, Gaffey MJ, Rouse RV, Esteban J, Frierson HF, Kempson RL, Weiss LM (1991). Carcinomas with metaplasia and sarcomas of the breast. *Am J Clin Pathol* 95: 623-632.

2260. Piura B, Rabinovich A, Dgani R (1999). Basal cell carcinoma of the vulva. *J Surg Oncol* 70: 172-176.

2261. Piura B, Rabinovich A, Dgani R (1999). Malignant melanoma of the vulva: report of six cases and review of the literature. *Eur J Gynaecol Oncol* 20: 182-186.

2262. Piver MS, Jishi MF, Tsukada Y, Nava G (1993). Primary peritoneal carcinoma after prophylactic oophorectomy in women with a family history of ovarian cancer. A report of the Gilda Radner Familial Ovarian Cancer Registry. *Cancer* 71: 2751-2755.

2263. Piver MS, Rutledge FN, Copeland L, Webster K, Blumenson L, Suh O (1984). Uterine endolymphatic stromal myosis: a collaborative study. *Obstet Gynecol* 64: 173-178.

2264. Planck M, Rambech E, Moslein G, Muller W, Olsson H, Nilbert M (2002). High frequency of microsatellite instability and loss of mismatch-repair protein expression in patients with double primary tumors of the endometrium and colorectum. *Cancer* 94: 2502-2510.

2265. Plentl AA, Frideman EA (1971). *Lymphatic System of the Female Genitali - The Morphological Basis of Oncologic Diagnosis and Therapy.* WB Saunders: Philadelphia.

2266. Plouffe L Jr., Tulandi T, Rosenberg A, Ferenczy A (1984). Non-Hodgkin's lymphoma in Bartholin's gland: case report and review of literature. *Am J Obstet Gynecol* 148: 608-609.

2267. Pluquet O, Hainaut P (2001). Genotoxic and non-genotoxic pathways of p53 induction. *Cancer Lett* 174: 1-15.

2268. Podsypanina K, Ellenson LH, Nemes A, Gu J, Tamura M, Yamada KM, Cordon-Cardo C, Catoretti G, Fisher PE, Parsons R (1999). Mutation of Pten/Mmac1 in mice causes neoplasia in multiple organ systems. *Proc Natl Acad Sci USA* 96: 1563-1568.

2269. Poen JC, Tran L, Juillard G, Selch MT, Giuliano A, Silverstein M, Fingerhut A, Lewinsky B, Parker RG (1992). Conservation therapy for invasive lobular carcinoma of the breast. *Cancer* 69: 2789-2795.

2270. Polger MR, Denison CM, Lester S, Meyer JE (1996). Pseudoangiomatous stromal hyperplasia: mammographic and sonographic appearances. *AJR Am J Roentgenol* 166: 349-352.

2271. Polk P, Parker KM, Biggs PJ (1996). Soft tissue oncocytoma. *Hum Pathol* 27: 206-208.

2272. Ponsky JL, Gliga L, Reynolds S (1984). Medullary carcinoma of the breast: an association with negative hormonal receptors. *J Surg Oncol* 25: 76-78.

2273. Pope TL Jr., Fechner RE, Wilhelm MC, Wanebo HJ, de Paredes ES (1988). Lobular carcinoma in situ of the breast: mammographic features. *Radiology* 168: 63-66.

2274. Porter PL, Garcia R, Moe R, Corwin DJ, Gown AM (1991). C-erbB-2 oncogene protein in in situ and invasive lobular breast neoplasia. *Cancer* 68: 331-334.

2275. Pothuri B, Leitao M, Barakat R, Akram M, Bogomolny F, Olvera N, Lin O, Soslow R, Robson ME, Offit K, Boyd J (2001). Genetic analysis of ovarian carcinoma histogenesis. *Gynecol Oncol* 80: 277.

2276. Potischman N, Hoover RN, Brinton LA, Siiteri P, Dorgan JF, Swanson CA, Berman ML, Mortel R, Twiggs LB, Barrett RJ, Wilbanks GD, Persky V, Lurain JR (1996). Case-control study of endogenous steroid hormones and endometrial cancer. *J Natl Cancer Inst* 88: 1127-1135.

2277. Potkul RK, Lancaster WD, Kurman RJ, Lewandowski G, Weck PK, Delgado G (1990). Vulvar condylomas and squamous vestibular micropapilloma. Differences in appearance and response to treatment. *J Reprod Med* 35: 1019-1022.

2278. Powell CM, Cranor ML, Rosen PP (1994). Multinucleated stromal giant cells in mammary fibroepithelial neoplasms. A study of 11 patients. *Arch Pathol Lab Med* 118: 912-916.

2279. Powell CM, Cranor ML, Rosen PP (1995). Pseudoangiomatous stromal hyperplasia (PASH). A mammary stromal tumor with myofibroblastic differentiation. *Am J Surg Pathol* 19: 270-277.

2280. Powers CN, Stastny JF, Frable WJ (1996). Adenoid basal carcinoma of the cervix: a potential pitfall in cervicovaginal cytology. *Diagn Cytopathol* 14: 172-177.

2281. Prasad CJ, Ray JA, Kessler S (1992). Primary small cell carcinoma of the vagina arising in a background of atypical adenosis. *Cancer* 70: 2484-2487.

2282. Prasad ML, Osborne MP, Giri DD, Hoda SA (2000). Microinvasive carcinoma (T1mic) of the breast: clinicopathologic profile of 21 cases. *Am J Surg Pathol* 24: 422-428.

2283. Prat J (2002). Clonality analysis in synchronous tumors of the female genital tract. *Hum Pathol* 33: 383-385.

2284. Prat J, Bhan AK, Dickersin GR, Robboy SJ, Scully RE (1982). Hepatoid yolk sac tumor of the ovary (endodermal sinus tumor with hepatoid differentiation): a light microscopic, ultrastructural and immunohistochemical study of seven cases. *Cancer* 50: 2355-2368.

2285. Prat J, de Nictolis M (2002). Serous borderline tumors of the ovary: a long-term follow-up study of 137 cases, including 18 with a micropapillary pattern and 20 with microinvasion. *Am J Surg Pathol* 26: 1111-1128.

2286. Prat J, Matias-Guiu X, Barreto J (1991). Simultaneous carcinoma involving the endometrium and the ovary. A clinicopathologic, immunohistochemical, and DNA flow cytometric study of 18 cases. *Cancer* 68: 2455-2459.

2287. Prat J, Matias-Guiu X, Scully RE (1989). Hepatic yolc sac differentiation in an ovarian polyembryoma. *Surgical Pathology* 2: 147-150.

2287a. Prat J, Rodriguez IM, Ota S, Matias-Guiu X (2003). Endometrioid, clear cell, and mixed carcinomas of the ovary with and without endometriosis: a comparative clinicopathological and molecular analysis of 113 cases. *Mod Pathol* 207A.

2288. Prat J, Scully RE (1979). Sarcomas in ovarian mucinous tumors: a report of two cases. *Cancer* 44: 1327-1331.

2289. Prat J, Scully RE (1981). Cellular fibromas and fibrosarcomas of the ovary: a comparative clinicopathologic analysis of seventeen cases. *Cancer* 47: 2663-2670.

2290. Prat J, Young RH, Scully RE (1982). Ovarian mucinous tumors with foci of anaplastic carcinoma. *Cancer* 50: 300-304.

2291. Prat J, Young RH, Scully RE (1982). Ovarian Sertoli-Leydig cell tumors with heterologous elements. II. Cartilage and skeletal muscle: a clinicopathologic analysis of twelve cases. *Cancer* 50: 2465-2475.

2292. Prayson RA, Goldblum JR, Hart WR (1997). Epithelioid smooth-muscle tumors of the uterus: a clinicopathologic study of 18 patients. *Am J Surg Pathol* 21: 383-391.

2293. Prayson RA, Hart WR (1992). Mitotically active leiomyomas of the uterus. *Am J Clin Pathol* 97: 14-20.

2294. Prayson RA, Hart WR, Petras RE (1994). Pseudomyxoma peritonei. A clinicopathologic study of 19 cases with emphasis on site of origin and nature of associated ovarian tumors. *Am J Surg Pathol* 18: 591-603.

2295. Prayson RA, Stoler MH, Hart WR (1995). Vulvar vestibulitis. A histopathologic study of 36 cases, including human papillomavirus in situ hybridization analysis. *Am J Surg Pathol* 19: 154-160.

2296. Prechtel D, Werenskiold AK, Prechtel K, Keller G, Hofler H (1998). Frequent loss of heterozygosity at chromosome 13q12-13 with BRCA2 markers in sporadic male breast cancer. *Diagn Mol Pathol* 7: 57-62.

2297. Prechtel K, Prechtel V (1997). [Breast carcinoma in the man. Current results from the viewpoint of clinic and pathology]. *Pathologe* 18: 45-52.

2298. Prempree T, Tang CK, Hatef A, Forster S (1983). Angiosarcoma of the vagina: a clinicopathologic report. A reappraisal of the radiation treatment of angiosarcomas of the female genital tract. *Cancer* 51: 618-622.

2299. Prendiville W, Cullimore J, Norman S (1989). Large loop excision of the transformation zone (LLETZ). A new method of management for women with cervical intraepithelial neoplasia. *Br J Obstet Gynaecol* 96: 1054-1060.

2300. Press MF, Scully RE (1985). Endometrial "sarcomas" complicating ovarian thecoma, polycystic ovarian disease and estrogen therapy. *Gynecol Oncol* 21: 135-154.

2301. Pride GL, Schultz AE, Chuprevich TW, Buchler DA (1979). Primary invasive squamous carcinoma of the vagina. *Obstet Gynecol* 53: 218-225.

2302. Pschera H, Wikstrom B (1991). Extraovarian Brenner tumor coexisting with serous cystadenoma. Case report. *Gynecol Obstet Invest* 31: 185-187.

2303. Puget N, Gad S, Perrin-Vidoz L, Sinilnikova OM, Stoppa-Lyonnet D, Lenoir GM, Mazoyer S (2002). Distinct BRCA1 rearrangements involving the BRCA1 pseudogene suggest the existence of a recombination hot spot. *Am J Hum Genet* 70: 858-865.

2304. Puls LE, Hamous J, Morrow MS, Schneyer A, MacLaughlin DT, Castracane VD (1994). Recurrent ovarian sex cord tumor with annular tubules: tumor marker and chemotherapy experience. *Gynecol Oncol* 54: 396-401.
2305. Purola E, Savia E (1977). Cytology of gynecologic condyloma acuminatum. *Acta Cytol* 21: 26-31.
2306. Pysher TJ, Hitch DC, Krous HF (1981). Bilateral juvenile granulosa cell tumors in a 4-month-old dysmorphic infant. A clinical, histologic, and ultrastructural study. *Am J Surg Pathol* 5: 789-794.
2307. Qiao S, Nagasaka T, Harada T, Nakashima N (1998). p53, Bax and Bcl-2 expression, and apoptosis in gestational trophoblast of complete hydatidiform mole. *Placenta* 19: 361-369.
2308. Qizilbash AH (1976). Cystosarcoma phyllodes with liposarcomatous stroma. *Am J Clin Pathol* 65: 321-327.
2309. Qizilbash AH, Patterson MC, Oliveira KF (1977). Adenoid cystic carcinoma of the breast. Light and electron microscopy and a brief review of the literature. *Arch Pathol Lab Med* 101: 302-306.
2310. Quaglia MP, Brennan MF (2000). The clinical approach to desmoplastic small round cell tumor. *Surg Oncol* 9: 77-81.
2311. Quigley JC, Hart WR (1981). Adenomatoid tumors of the uterus. *Am J Clin Pathol* 76: 627-635.
2312. Quincey C, Raitt N, Bell J, Ellis IO (1991). Intracytoplasmic lumina--a useful diagnostic feature of adenocarcinomas. *Histopathology* 19: 83-87.
2313. Quinn JM, McGee JO, Athanasou NA (1998). Human tumour-associated macrophages differentiate into osteoclastic bone-resorbing cells. *J Pathol* 184: 31-36.
2314. Quinn MA (1997). Adenocarcinoma of the cervix--are there arguments for a different treatment policy? *Curr Opin Obstet Gynecol* 9: 21-24.
2315. Quinn MA, Oster AO, Fortune D, Hudson B (1981). Sclerosing stromal tumour of the ovary case report with endocrine studies. *Br J Obstet Gynaecol* 88: 555-558.
2316. Raber G, Mempel V, Jackisch C, Hundeiker M, Heinecke A, Kurzl R, Glaubitz M, Rompel R, Schneider HP (1996). Malignant melanoma of the vulva. Report of 89 patients. *Cancer* 78: 2353-2358.
2317. Radford DM, Fair KL, Phillips NJ, Ritter JH, Steinbrueck T, Holt MS, Donis-Keller H (1995). Allelotyping of ductal carcinoma in situ of the breast: deletion of loci on 8p, 13q, 16q, 17p and 17q. *Cancer Res* 55: 3399-3405.
2318. Radhi JM (2000). Immunohistochemical analysis of pleomorphic lobular carcinoma: higher expression of p53 and chromogranin and lower expression of ER and PgR. *Histopathology* 36: 156-160.
2319. Radig K, Buhtz P, Roessner A (1998). Alveolar soft part sarcoma of the uterine corpus. Report of two cases and review of the literature. *Pathol Res Pract* 194: 59-63.
2320. Ragnarsson-Olding BK, Nilsson BR, Kanter-Lewensohn LR, Lagerlof B, Ringborg UK (1999). Malignant melanoma of the vulva in a nationwide, 25-year study of 219 Swedish females: predictors of survival. *Cancer* 86: 1285-1293.
2321. Rahilly MA, Williams AR, Krausz T, al Nafussi A (1995). Female adnexal tumour of probable Wolffian origin: a clinicopathological and immunohistochemical study of three cases. *Histopathology* 26: 69-74.
2322. Rajakariar R, Walker RA (1995). Pathological and biological features of mammographically detected invasive breast carcinomas. *Br J Cancer* 71: 150-154.
2323. Rajan JV, Marquis ST, Gardner HP, Chodosh LA (1997). Developmental expression of Brca2 colocalizes with Brca1 and is associated with proliferation and differentiation in multiple tissues. *Dev Biol* 184: 385-401.
2324. Rajkumar T, Franceschi S, Vaccarella S, Gajalakshmi V, Sharmila A, Snijders PJ, Munoz N, Meijer CJ, Herrero R (2003). Role of paan chewing and dietary habits in cervical carcinoma in Chennai, India. *Br J Cancer* 88: 1388-1393.
2325. Raju U, Shah V, Perveen N, Linden M (2001). Evaluation of Breast Core Needle Biopsies with CK 5/6, E-cadherin and Calponin. *Mod Pathol* 14: 34A.
2326. Raju U, Vertes D (1996). Breast papillomas with atypical ductal hyperplasia: a clinicopathologic study. *Hum Pathol* 27: 1231-1238.
2327. Raju UB, Lee MW, Zarbo RJ, Crissman JD (1989). Papillary neoplasia of the breast: immunohistochemically defined myoepithelial cells in the diagnosis of benign and malignant papillary breast neoplasms. *Mod Pathol* 2: 569-576.
2327 a. Ramachandra S, Machin L, Ashley S, Monaghan P, Gusterson BA (1990). Immunohistochemical distribution of c-erbB-2 in in situ breast carcinoma--a detailed morphological analysis. *J Pathol* 161: 7-14.
2328. Ramaswamy S, Ross KN, Lander ES, Golub TR (2003). A molecular signature of metastasis in primary solid tumors. *Nat Genet* 33: 49-54.
2329. Ramesh V, Iyengar B (1990). Proliferating trichilemmal cysts over the vulva. *Cutis* 45: 187-189.
2330. Ramos CV, Taylor HB (1974). Lipid-rich carcinoma of the breast. A clinicopathologic analysis of 13 examples. *Cancer* 33: 812-819.
2331. Ramsay J, Birrell G, Lavin M (1998). Testing for mutations of the ataxia telangiectasia gene in radiosensitive breast cancer patients. *Radiother Oncol* 47: 125-128.
2332. Ramzy I (1976). Signet-ring stromal tumor of ovary. Histochemical, light, and electron microscopic study. *Cancer* 38: 166-172.
2333. Randall ME, Kim JA, Mills SE, Hahn SS, Constable WC (1986). Uncommon variants of cervical carcinoma treated with radical irradiation. A clinicopathologic study of 66 cases. *Cancer* 57: 816-822.
2334. Rapin V, Contesso G, Mouriesse H, Bertin F, Lacombe MJ, Piekarski JD, Travagli JP, Gadenne C, Friedman S (1988). Medullary breast carcinoma. A reevaluation of 95 cases of breast cancer with inflammatory stroma. *Cancer* 61: 2503-2510.
2335. Rasbridge SA, Gillett CE, Millis RR (1993). Oestrogen and progesterone receptor expression in mammary fibromatosis. *J Clin Pathol* 46: 349-351.
2336. Rasbridge SA, Gillett CE, Sampson SA, Walsh FS, Millis RR (1993). Epithelial (E-) and placental (P-) cadherin cell adhesion molecule expression in breast carcinoma. *J Pathol* 169: 245-250.
2336 a. Rasbridge SA, Millis RR (1995). Carcinoma in situ involving sclerosing adenosis: a mimic of invasive breast carcinoma. *Histopathology* 27: 269-273.
2337. Rasbridge SA, Millis RR, Sampson SA, Walsh FS (1992). Epithelial cadherin expression in breast carcinomas. *J Pathol* 167: 149.
2338. Rasmussen BB, Rose C, Thorpe SM, Andersen KW, Hou-Jensen K (1985). Argyrophilic cells in 202 human mucinous breast carcinomas. Relation to histopathologic and clinical factors. *Am J Clin Pathol* 84: 737-740.
2339. Rastkar G, Okagaki T, Twiggs LB, Clark BA (1982). Early invasive and in situ warty carcinoma of the vulva: clinical, histologic, and electron microscopic study with particular reference to viral association. *Am J Obstet Gynecol* 143: 814-820.
2340. Rauscher FJ, III, Benjamin LE, Fredericks WJ, Morris JF (1994). Novel oncogenic mutations in the WT1 Wilms' tumor suppressor gene: a t(11;22) fuses the Ewing's sarcoma gene, EWS1, to WT1 in desmoplastic small round cell tumor. *Cold Spring Harb Symp Quant Biol* 59: 137-146.
2341. Reardon W, Zhou XP, Eng C (2001). A novel germline mutation of the PTEN gene in a patient with macrocephaly, ventricular dilatation, and features of VATER association. *J Med Genet* 38: 820-823.
2342. Rebbeck TR, Kantoff PW, Krithivas K, Neuhausen S, Blackwood MA, Godwin AK, Daly MB, Narod SA, Garber JE, Lynch HT, Weber BL, Brown M (1999). Modification of BRCA1-associated breast cancer risk by the polymorphic androgen-receptor CAG repeat. *Am J Hum Genet* 64: 1371-1377.
2343. Rebbeck TR, Levin AM, Eisen A, Snyder C, Watson P, Cannon-Albright L, Isaacs C, Olopade O, Garber JE, Godwin AK, Daly MB, Narod SA, Neuhausen SL, Lynch HT, Weber BL (1999). Breast cancer risk after bilateral prophylactic oophorectomy in BRCA1 mutation carriers. *J Natl Cancer Inst* 91: 1475-1479.
2344. Rebbeck TR, Lynch HT, Neuhausen SL, Narod SA, van't Veer L, Garber JE, Evans G, Isaacs C, Daly MB, Matloff E, Olopade OI, Weber BL (2002). Prophylactic oophorectomy in carriers of BRCA1 or BRCA2 mutations. *N Engl J Med* 346: 1616-1622.
2345. Rebbeck TR, Wang Y, Kantoff PW, Krithivas K, Neuhausen SL, Godwin AK, Daly MB, Narod SA, Brunet JS, Vesprini D, Garber JE, Lynch HT, Weber BL, Brown M (2001). Modification of BRCA1- and BRCA2-associated breast cancer risk by AIB1 genotype and reproductive history. *Cancer Res* 61: 5420-5424.
2346. Recht A, Rutgers EJ, Fentiman IS, Kurtz JM, Mansel RE, Sloane JP (1998). The fourth EORTC DCIS Consensus meeting (Chateau Marquette, Heemskerk, The Netherlands, 23-24 January 1998)--conference report. *Eur J Cancer* 34: 1664-1669.
2347. Reddy DB, Rao DB, Sarojini JS (1963). Extra-ovarian granulosa cell tumour. *J Indian Med Assoc* 41: 254-257.
2348. Redline RW, Hassold T, Zaragoza MV (1998). Prevalence of the partial molar phenotype in triploidy of maternal and paternal origin. *Hum Pathol* 29: 505-511.
2349. Reich O, Pickel H, Tamussino K, Winter R (2001). Microinvasive carcinoma of the cervix: site of first focus of invasion. *Obstet Gynecol* 97: 890-892.
2350. Reich O, Regauer S, Urdl W, Lahousen M, Winter R (2000). Expression of oestrogen and progesterone receptors in low-grade endometrial stromal sarcomas. *Br J Cancer* 82: 1030-1034.
2351. Reiner A, Reiner G, Spona J, Schemper M, Holzner JH (1988). Histopathologic characterization of human breast cancer in correlation with estrogen receptor status. A comparison of immunocytochemical and biochemical analysis. *Cancer* 61: 1149-1154.
2352. Reinfuss M, Stelmach A, Mitus J, Rys J, Duda K (1995). Typical medullary carcinoma of the breast: a clinical and pathological analysis of 52 cases. *J Surg Oncol* 60: 89-94.
2353. Reitamo JJ, Scheinin TM, Hayry P (1986). The desmoid syndrome. New aspects in the cause, pathogenesis and treatment of the desmoid tumor. *Am J Surg* 151: 230-237.
2354. Renno SI, Moreland WS, Pettenati MJ, Beaty MW, Keung YK (2002). Primary malignant lymphoma of uterine corpus: case report and review of the literature. *Ann Hematol* 81: 44-47.
2355. Report of an Advisory Group on Non-ionising Radiation (2001). Electromagnetic Fields and the Risk of Cancer. Doc NRBP, *Vol. 12(1)*: 3-179.
2356. Resnick M, Lester S, Tate JE, Sheets EE, Sparks C, Crum CP (1996). Viral and histopathologic correlates of MN and MIB-1 expression in cervical intraepithelial neoplasia. *Hum Pathol* 27: 234-239.
2357. Resta L, Maiorano E, Piscitelli D, Botticella MA (1994). Lipomatous tumors of the uterus. Clinico-pathological features of 10 cases with immunocytochemical study of histogenesis. *Pathol Res Pract* 190: 378-383.
2358. Revillion F, Bonneterre J, Peyrat J (1998). ERBB2 oncogene in human breast cancer and its clinical significance. *European Journal of Cancer* 34: 791-808.
2359. Reymundo C, Toro M, Morales C, Lopez-Beltran A, Nogales F, Nogales F Jr. (1993). Hyaline globules in uterine malignant mixed mullerian tumours. A diagnostic aid? *Pathol Res Pract* 189: 1063-1066.
2360. Rhatigan RM, Mojadidi Q (1973). Adenosquamous carcinomas of the vulva and vagina. *Am J Clin Pathol* 60: 208-217.
2361. Rhatigan RM, Nuss RC (1985). Keratoacanthoma of the vulva. *Gynecol Oncol* 21: 118-123.
2361 a. Rhemtula H, Grayson W, van Iddekinge B, Tiltman A (2001). Large-cell neuroendocrine carcinoma of the uterine cervix--a clinicopathological study of five cases. *S Afr Med J* 91: 525-528.
2362. Rhodes AR, Mihm MC Jr., Weinstock MA (1989). Dysplastic melanocytic nevi: a reproducible histologic definition emphasizing cellular morphology. *Mod Pathol* 2: 306-319.
2363. Ribeiro GG, Phillips HV, Skinner LG (1980). Serum oestradiol-17 beta, testosterone, luteinizing hormone and follicle-stimulating hormone in males with breast cancer. *Br J Cancer* 41: 474-477.
2364. Rice BF, Barclay DL, Sternberg WH (1969). Luteoma of pregnancy: steroidogenic and morphologic considerations. *Am J Obstet Gynecol* 104: 871-878.
2365. Rice LW, Berkowitz RS, Lage JM, Goldstein DP, Bernstein MR (1990). Persistent gestational trophoblastic tumor after partial hydatidiform mole. *Gynecol Oncol* 36: 358-362.
2366. Richard F, Pacyna-Gengelbach M, Schluns K, Fleige B, Winzer KJ, Szymas J, Dietel M, Petersen I, Schwendel A (2000). Patterns of chromosomal imbalances in invasive breast cancer. *Int J Cancer* 89: 305-310.

2367. Richardson WW (1956). Medullary carcinoma of the breast. A distinctive tumour type with a relatively good prognosis following radical mastectomy. *Br J Cancer* 10: 415-423.
2368. Richart RM (1973). Cervical intraepithelial neoplasia. *Pathol Annu* 8: 301-328.
2369. Ridley CM, Neill SM (1999). Non-infective cutaneous conditions of vulva in The Vulva. 2nd ed. Malden, MA Blackwell Science: Oxford.
2370. Ridolfi RL, Rosen PP, Port A, Kinne D, Mike V (1977). Medullary carcinoma of the breast: a clinicopathologic study with 10 year follow-up. *Cancer* 40: 1365-1385.
2371. Riedel I, Czernobilsky B, Lifschitz-Mercer B, Roth LM, Wu XR, Sun TT, Moll R (2001). Brenner tumors but not transitional cell carcinomas of the ovary show urothelial differentiation: immunohistochemical staining of urothelial markers, including cytokeratins and uroplakins. *Virchows Arch* 438: 181-191.
2372. Rigaud C, Theobald S, Noel P, Badreddine J, Barlier C, Delobelle A, Gentile A, Jacquemier J, Maisongrosse V, Peffault de Latour M, Trojani M, Zafrani B (1993). Medullary carcinoma of the breast. A multicenter study of its diagnostic consistency. *Arch Pathol Lab Med* 117: 1005-1008.
2373. Riman T, Dickman PW, Nilsson S, Correia N, Nordlinder H, Magnusson CM, Weiderpass E, Persson IR (2002). Hormone replacement therapy and the risk of invasive epithelial ovarian cancer in Swedish women. *J Natl Cancer Inst* 94: 497-504.
2374. Rimm DL, Sinard JH, Morrow JS (1995). Reduced alpha-catenin and E-cadherin expression in breast cancer. *Lab Invest* 72: 506-512.
2375. Rio PG, Pernin D, Bay JO, Albuisson E, Kwiatkowski F, de Latour M, Bernard-Gallon DJ, Bignon YJ (1998). Loss of heterozygosity of BRCA1, BRCA2 and ATM genes in sporadic invasive ductal breast carcinoma. *Int J Oncol* 13: 849-853.
2376. Riopel MA, Perlman EJ, Seidman JD, Kurman RJ, Sherman ME (1998). Inhibin and epithelial membrane antigen immunohistochemistry assist in the diagnosis of sex cord-stromal tumors and provide clues to the histogenesis of hypercalcemic small cell carcinomas. *Int J Gynecol Pathol* 17: 46-53.
2377. Riopel MA, Ronnett BM, Kurman RJ (1999). Evaluation of diagnostic criteria and behavior of ovarian intestinal-type mucinous tumors: atypical proliferative (borderline) tumors and intraepithelial, microinvasive, invasive, and metastatic carcinomas. *Am J Surg Pathol* 23: 617-635.
2378. Riopel MA, Spellerberg A, Griffin CA, Perlman EJ (1998). Genetic analysis of ovarian germ cell tumors by comparative genomic hybridization. *Cancer Res* 58: 3105-3110.
2379. Rishi M, Howard LN, Bratthauer GL, Tavassoli FA (1997). Use of monoclonal antibody against human inhibin as a marker for sex cord-stromal tumors of the ovary. *Am J Surg Pathol* 21: 583-589.
2380. Risinger JI, Berchuck A, Kohler MF, Boyd J (1994). Mutations of the E-cadherin gene in human gynecologic cancers. *Nat Genet* 7: 98-102.
2381. Ro JY, Silva EG, Gallager HS (1987). Adenoid cystic carcinoma of the breast. *Hum Pathol* 18: 1276-1281.
2382. Roa BB, Boyd AA, Volcik K, Richards CS (1996). Ashkenazi Jewish population frequencies for common mutations in BRCA1 and BRCA2. *Nat Genet* 14: 185-187.
2383. Robbins GF, Berg JW (1964). Bilateral primary breast cancers. A propective clinico-pathological study. *Cancer* 17: 1502-1527.
2384. Robbins GF, Shah J, Rosen P, Chu F, Taylor J (1974). Inflammatory carcinoma of the breast. *Surg Clin North Am* 54: 801-810.
2385. Robbins P, Pinder S, de Klerk N, Dawkins H, Harvey J, Sterrett G, Ellis I, Elston C (1995). Histological grading of breast carcinomas: a study of interobserver agreement. *Hum Pathol* 26: 873-879.
2386. Robboy SJ, Kaufman RH, Prat J, Welch WR, Gaffey T, Scully RE, Richart R, Fenoglio CM, Virata R, Tilley BC (1979). Pathologic findings in young women enrolled in the National Cooperative Diethylstilbestrol Adenosis (DESAD) project. *Obstet Gynecol* 53: 309-317.
2387. Robboy SJ, Krigman HR, Donohue J, Scully RE (1995). Prognostic indices in malignant struma ovarii: a clinicopathological analysis of 36 patients with 20-year follow up. *Mod Pathol* 8: 95A.
2388. Robboy SJ, Norris HJ, Scully RE (1975). Insular carcinoid primary in the ovary. A clinicopathologic analysis of 48 cases. *Cancer* 36: 404-418.
2389. Robboy SJ, Scully RE (1970). Ovarian teratoma with glial implants on the peritoneum. An analysis of 12 cases. *Hum Pathol* 1: 643-653.
2390. Robboy SJ, Scully RE (1980). Strumal carcinoid of the ovary: an analysis of 50 cases of a distinctive tumor composed of thyroid tissue and carcinoid. *Cancer* 46: 2019-2034.
2391. Robboy SJ, Scully RE, Norris HJ (1974). Carcinoid metastatic to the ovary. A clinocopathologic analysis of 35 cases. *Cancer* 33: 798-811.
2392. Robboy SJ, Scully RE, Norris HJ (1977). Primary trabecular carcinoid of the ovary. *Obstet Gynecol* 49: 202-207.
2393. Robertson AJ, Brown RA, Cree IA, MacGillivray JB, Slidders W, Beck JS (1981). Prognostic value of measurement of elastosis in breast carcinoma. *J Clin Pathol* 34: 738-743.
2394. Robles-Frias A, Severin CE, Robles-Frias MJ, Garrido JL (2001). Diffuse uterine leiomyomatosis with ovarian and parametrial involvement. *Obstet Gynecol* 97: 834-835.
2395. Robles SC, White F, Peruga A (1996). Trends in cervical cancer mortality in the Americas. *Bull Pan Am Health Organ* 30: 290-301.
2396. Roca AN, Guajardo M, Estrada WJ (1980). Glial polyp of the cervix and endometrium. Report of a case and review of the literature. *Am J Clin Pathol* 73: 718-720.
2397. Rodolakis A, Papaspyrou I, Sotiropoulou M, Markaki S, Michalas S (2001). Primary squamous cell carcinoma of the endometrium. A report of 3 cases. *Eur J Gynaecol Oncol* 22: 143-146.
2398. Rodriguez-Bigas MA, Boland CR, Hamilton SR, Henson DE, Jass JR, Khan PM, Lynch H, Perucho M, Smyrk T, Sobin L, Srivastava S (1997). A National Cancer Institute Workshop on Hereditary Nonpolyposis Colorectal Cancer Syndrome: meeting highlights and Bethesda guidelines. *J Natl Cancer Inst* 89: 1758-1762.
2399. Rodriguez C, Patel AV, Calle EE, Jacob EJ, Thun MJ (2001). Estrogen replacement therapy and ovarian cancer mortality in a large prospective study of US women. *JAMA* 285: 1460-1465.
2400. Rodriguez HA, Ackerman LV (1968). Cellular blue nevus. Clinicopathologic study of forty-five cases. *Cancer* 21: 393-405.
2401. Rodriguez IM, Prat J (2002). Mucinous tumors of the ovary: a clinicopathologic analysis of 75 borderline tumors (of intestinal type) and carcinomas. *Am J Surg Pathol* 26: 139-152.
2402. Rogers DA, Lobe TE, Rao BN, Fleming ID, Schropp KP, Pratt AS, Pappo AS (1994). Breast malignancy in children. *J Pediatr Surg* 29: 48-51.
2402a. Rojansky N, Ophir E, Sharony A, Spira H, Suprun H (1985). Broad ligament adenocarcinoma--its origin and clinical behavior. A literature review and report of a case. *Obstet Gynecol Surv* 40: 665-671.
2403. Rome RM, England PG (2000). Management of vaginal intraepithelial neoplasia: A series of 132 cases with long-term follow-up. *Int J Gynecol Cancer* 10: 382-390.
2404. Roncaroli F, Lamovec J, Zidar A, Eusebi V (1996). Acinic cell-like carcinoma of the breast. *Virchows Arch* 429: 69-74.
2405. Roncaroli F, Riccioni L, Cerati M, Capella C, Calbucci F, Trevisan C, Eusebi V (1997). Oncocytic meningioma. *Am J Surg Pathol* 21: 375-382.
2406. Ronnett BM, Kurman RJ, Shmookler BM, Sugarbaker PH, Young RH (1997). The morphologic spectrum of ovarian metastases of appendiceal adenocarcinomas: a clinicopathologic and immunohistochemical analysis of tumors often misinterpreted as primary ovarian tumors or metastatic tumors from other gastrointestinal sites. *Am J Surg Pathol* 21: 1144-1155.
2407. Ronnett BM, Kurman RJ, Zahn CM, Shmookler BM, Jablonski KA, Kass ME, Sugarbaker PH (1995). Pseudomyxoma peritonei in women: a clinicopathologic analysis of 30 cases with emphasis on site of origin, prognosis, and relationship to ovarian mucinous tumors of low malignant potential. *Hum Pathol* 26: 509-524.
2408. Ronnett BM, Shmookler BM, Diener-West M, Sugarbaker PH, Kurman RJ (1997). Immunohistochemical evidence supporting the appendiceal origin of pseudomyxoma peritonei in women. *Int J Gynecol Pathol* 16: 1-9.
2409. Ronnett BM, Zahn CM, Kurman RJ, Kass ME, Sugarbaker PH, Shmookler BM (1995). Disseminated peritoneal adenomucinosis and peritoneal mucinous carcinomatosis. A clinicopathologic analysis of 109 cases with emphasis on distinguishing pathologic features, site of origin, prognosis, and relationship to "pseudomyxoma peritonei". *Am J Surg Pathol* 19: 1390-1408.
2410. Rorat E, Wallach RC (1984). Mixed tumors of the vulva: clinical outcome and pathology. *Int J Gynecol Pathol* 3: 323-328.
2411. Rosai J (1991). Borderline epithelial lesions of the breast. *Am J Surg Pathol* 15: 209-221.
2412. Rose PG, Arafah B, Abdul-Karim FW (1998). Malignant struma ovarii: recurrence and response to treatment monitored by thyroglobulin levels. *Gynecol Oncol* 70: 425-427.
2413. Rosen PP (1983). Microglandular adenosis, a benign lesion simultating invasive mammary carcinoma. *Am J Surg Pathol* 7: 137-144.
2414. Rosen PP (1983). Syringomatous adenoma of the nipple. *Am J Surg Pathol* 7: 739-745.
2415. Rosen PP (1983). Tumor emboli in intramammary lymphatics in breast carcinoma: pathologic criteria for diagnosis and clinical significance. *Pathol Annu 18 Pt* 2:215-32.: 215-232.
2416. Rosen PP (1985). Vascular tumors of the breast. III. Angiomatosis. *Am J Surg Pathol* 9: 652-658.
2417. Rosen PP (1986). Mucocele-like tumors of the breast. *Am J Surg Pathol* 10: 464-469.
2418. Rosen PP (1987). Adenomyoepithelioma of the breast. *Hum Pathol* 18: 1232-1237.
2419. Rosen PP (1989). Adenoid cystic carcinoma of the breast. A morphologically heterogeneous neoplasm. *Pathol Annu 24 Pt* 2: 237-254.
2420. Rosen PP (1997). Benign papillary tumors. In: *Breast Pathology*, PP Rosen (ed.), 1st ed. Lippincott-Raven: Philadelphia , pp. 67-104.
2421. Rosen PP (1997). Carcinoma with metaplasia. In: *Rosen's Breast Pathology, PP Rosen* (ed.), Lippincott-Raven: Philadelphia, pp. 375-395.
2422. Rosen PP (1997). Glycogen-rich carcinoma. In: *Breast Pathology*, PP Rosen (ed.), Lipincott-Raven, ed., Philadelphia/New York .
2423. Rosen PP (1997). Mammary carcinoma with osteoclast-like giant cells. In: *Breast Pathology*, PP Rosen (ed.), Lippincott-Raven, ed., Philadelphia/New York .
2424. Rosen PP (1997). Metastases in the breast from non-mammary malignant neoplasms. In: *Breast Pathology*, PP Rosen (ed.), Lippincott-Raven, ed., Philadelphia/New York .
2425. Rosen PP (1997). *Rosen's Breast Pathology*. Lippincott-Raven: Philadelphia.
2426. Rosen PP (1997). *Rosen's Breast Pathology*. 2nd ed. Philadelphia.
2427. Rosen PP (2001). *Rosen's Breast Pathology*. Lippincott Williams and Wilkins: Philadelphia.
2428. Rosen PP, Braun DW Jr., Lyngholm B, Urban JA, Kinne DW (1981). Lobular carcinoma in situ of the breast: preliminary results of treatment by ipsilateral mastectomy and contralateral breast biopsy. *Cancer* 47: 813-819.
2429. Rosen PP, Caicco JA (1986). Florid papillomatosis of the nipple. A study of 51 patients, including nine with mammary carcinoma. *Am J Surg Pathol* 10: 87-101.
2430. Rosen PP, Cranor ML (1991). Secretory carcinoma of the breast. *Arch Pathol Lab Med* 115: 141-144.
2431. Rosen PP, Ernsberger D (1987). Low-grade adenosquamous carcinoma. A variant of metaplastic mammary carcinoma. *Am J Surg Pathol* 11: 351-358.
2432. Rosen PP, Ernsberger D (1989). Mammary fibromatosis. A benign spindle-cell tumor with significant risk for local recurrence. *Cancer* 63: 1363-1369.
2433. Rosen PP, Groshen S, Kinne DW, Norton L (1993). Factors influencing prognosis in node-negative breast carcinoma: analysis of 767 T1N0M0/T2N0M0 patients with long-term follow-up. *J Clin Oncol* 11: 2090-2100.

2434. Rosen PP, Groshen S, Saigo PE, Kinne DW, Hellman S (1989). Pathological prognostic factors in stage I (T1N0M0) and stage II (T1N1M0) breast carcinoma: a study of 644 patients with median follow-up of 18 years. *J Clin Oncol* 7: 1239-1251.

2435. Rosen PP, Jozefczyk MA, Boram LH (1985). Vascular tumors of the breast. IV. The venous hemangioma. *Am J Surg Pathol* 9: 659-665.

2436. Rosen PP, Kimmel M, Ernsberger D (1988). Mammary angiosarcoma. The prognostic significance of tumor differentiation. *Cancer* 62: 2145-2151.

2437. Rosen PP, Kinne DW, Lesser M, Hellman S (1986). Are prognostic factors for local control of breast cancer treated by primary radiotherapy significant for patients treated by mastectomy? *Cancer* 57: 1415-1420.

2438. Rosen PP, Kosloff C, Lieberman PH, Adair F, Braun DW Jr. (1978). Lobular carcinoma in situ of the breast. Detailed analysis of 99 patients with average follow-up of 24 years. *Am J Surg Pathol* 2: 225-251.

2439. Rosen PP, Lesser ML, Arroyo CD, Cranor M, Borgen P, Norton L (1995). Immunohistochemical detection of HER2/neu in patients with axillary lymph node negative breast carcinoma. A study of epidemiologic risk factors, histologic features, and prognosis. *Cancer* 75: 1320-1326.

2440. Rosen PP, Lesser ML, Arroyo CD, Cranor M, Borgen P, Norton L (1995). p53 in node-negative breast carcinoma: an immunohistochemical study of epidemiologic risk factors, histologic features, and prognosis. *J Clin Oncol* 13: 821-830.

2441. Rosen PP, Lesser ML, Senie RT, Kinne DW (1982). Epidemiology of breast carcinoma III: relationship of family history to tumor type. *Cancer* 50: 171-179.

2442. Rosen PP, Oberman HA (1993). *Atlas of Tumour Pathology*. Tumour of the Mammary Gland. Washington,D.C.

2443. Rosen PP, Ridolfi RL (1977). The perilobular hemangioma. A benign microscopic vascular lesion of the breast. *Am J Clin Pathol* 68: 21-23.

2444. Rosen PP, Saigo PE, Braun DW Jr., Weathers E, Kinne DW (1981). Prognosis in stage II (T1N1M0) breast cancer. *Ann Surg* 194: 576-584.

2445. Rosen PP, Saigo PE, Braun DW Jr., Weathers E, DePalo A (1981). Predictors of recurrence in stage I (T1N0M0) breast carcinoma. *Ann Surg* 193: 15-25.

2446. Rosen PP, Senie R, Schottenfeld D, Ashikari R (1979). Noninvasive breast carcinoma: frequency of unsuspected invasion and implications for treatment. *Ann Surg* 189: 377-382.

2447. Rosen PP, Wang T-Y (1980). Colloid carcinoma of the breast. Analysis of 64 patients with long term followup. *Am J Clin Pathol* 73: 304.

2448. Rosenberg CR, Pasternack BS, Shore RE, Koenig KL, Toniolo PG (1994). Premenopausal estradiol levels and the risk of breast cancer: a new method of controlling for day of the menstrual cycle. *Am J Epidemiol* 140: 518-525.

2449. Rosenblatt KA, Thomas DB, McTiernan A, Austin MA, Stalsberg H, Stemhagen A, Thompson WD, Curnen MG, Satariano W, Austin DF, et al. (1991). Breast cancer in men: aspects of familial aggregation. *J Natl Cancer Inst* 83: 849-854.

2450. Rosenblatt KA, Weiss NS, Schwartz SM (1989). Incidence of malignant fallopian tube tumors. *Gynecol Oncol* 35: 236-239.

2451. Rosenfeld WD, Rose E, Vermund SH, Schreiber K, Burk RD (1992). Follow-up evaluation of cervicovaginal human papillomavirus infection in adolescents. *J Pediatr* 121: 307-311.

2452. Roses DF, Bell DA, Flotte TJ, Taylor R, Ratech H, Dubin N (1982). Pathologic predictors of recurrence in stage 1 (TINOMO) breast cancer. *Am J Clin Pathol* 78: 817-820.

2453. Rosner D, Lane WW, Penetrante R (1991). Ductal carcinoma in situ with microinvasion. A curable entity using surgery alone without need for adjuvant therapy. *Cancer* 67: 1498-1503.

2454. Ross JC, Eifel PJ, Cox RS, Kempson RL, Hendrickson MR (1983). Primary mucinous adenocarcinoma of the endometrium. A clinicopathologic and histochemical study. *Am J Surg Pathol* 7: 715-729.

2455. Ross LD (1984). Hilus cell tumour of the ovary with an associated endometrial carcinoma, presenting with male pattern baldness and postmenopausal bleeding. Case report. *Br J Obstet Gynaecol* 91: 1266-1268.

2456. Ross MJ, Welch WR, Scully RE (1989). Multilocular peritoneal inclusion cysts (so-called cystic mesotheliomas). *Cancer* 64: 1336-1346.

2457. Rossi G, Bonacorsi G, Longo L, Artusi T, Rivasi F (2001). Primary high-grade mucosa-associated lymphoid tissue-type lymphoma of the cervix presenting as a common endocervical polyp. *Arch Pathol Lab Med* 125: 537-540.

2458. Rossing MA, Daling JR, Weiss NS, Moore DE, Self SG (1994). Ovarian tumors in a cohort of infertile women. *N Engl J Med* 331: 771-776.

2459. Roth LM, Anderson MC, Govan AD, Langley FA, Gowing NF, Woodcock AS (1981). Sertoli-Leydig cell tumors: a clinicopathologic study of 34 cases. *Cancer* 48: 187-197.

2460. Roth LM, Czernobilsky B (1985). Ovarian Brenner tumors. II. Malignant. *Cancer* 56: 592-601.

2461. Roth LM, Dallenbach-Hellweg G, Czernobilsky B (1985). Ovarian Brenner tumors. I. Metaplastic, proliferating, and of low malignant potential. *Cancer* 56: 582-591.

2462. Roth LM, Davis MM, Sutton GP (1996). Steroid cell tumor of the broad ligament arising in an accessory ovary. *Arch Pathol Lab Med* 120: 405-409.

2463. Roth LM, Deaton RL, Sternberg WH (1979). Massive ovarian edema. A clinicopathologic study of five cases including ultrastructural observations and review of the literature. *Am J Surg Pathol* 3: 11-21.

2464. Roth LM, Gersell DJ, Ulbright TM (1993). Ovarian Brenner tumors and transitional cell carcinoma: recent developments. *Int J Gynecol Pathol* 12: 128-133.

2465. Roth LM, Gersell DJ, Ulbright TM (1996). Transitional cell carcinoma and other transitional cell tumors of the ovary. *Anat Pathol* 1: 179-191.

2466. Roth LM, Liban E, Czernobilsky B (1982). Ovarian endometrioid tumors mimicking Sertoli and Sertoli-Leydig cell tumors: Sertoliform variant of endometrioid carcinoma. *Cancer* 50: 1322-1331.

2467. Roth LM, Look KY (2000). Inverted follicular keratosis of the vulvar skin: a lesion that can be confused with squamous cell carcinoma. *Int J Gynecol Pathol* 19: 369-373.

2468. Roth LM, Nicholas TR, Ehrlich CE (1979). Juvenile granulosa cell tumor: a clinicopathologic study of three cases with ultrastructural observations. *Cancer* 44: 2194-2205.

2469. Roth LM, Reed RJ (1999). Dissecting leiomyomas of the uterus other than cotyledonoid dissecting leiomyomas: a report of eight cases. *Am J Surg Pathol* 23: 1032-1039.

2470. Roth LM, Reed RJ, Sternberg WH (1996). Cotyledonoid dissecting leiomyoma of the uterus. The Sternberg tumor. *Am J Surg Pathol* 20: 1455-1461.

2471. Roth LM, Slayton RE, Brady LW, Blessing JA, Johnson G (1985). Retiform differentiation in ovarian Sertoli-Leydig cell tumors. A clinicopathologic study of six cases from a Gynecologic Oncology Group study. *Cancer* 55: 1093-1098.

2472. Roth LM, Sternberg WH (1973). Ovarian stromal tumors containing Leydig cells. II. Pure Leydig cell tumor, non-hilar type. *Cancer* 32: 952-960.

2473. Rothbard MJ, Markham EH (1974). Leiomyosarcoma of the cervix: report of a case. *Am J Obstet Gynecol* 120: 853-854.

2474. Royar J, Becher H, Chang-Claude J (2001). Low-dose oral contraceptives: protective effect on ovarian cancer risk. *Int J Cancer* 95: 370-374.

2475. Roylance R, Gorman P, Hanby A, Tomlinson I (2002). Allelic imbalance analysis of chromosome 16q shows that grade I and grade III invasive ductal breast cancers follow different genetic pathways. *J Pathol* 196: 32-36.

2476. Roylance R, Gorman P, Harris W, Liebmann R, Barnes D, Hanby A, Sheer D (1999). Comparative genomic hybridization of breast tumors stratified by histological grade reveals new insights into the biological progression of breast cancer. *Cancer Res* 59: 1433-1436.

2477. Rozan S, Vincent-Salomon A, Zafrani B, Validire P, de Cremoux P, Bernoux A, Nieruchalski M, Fourquet A, Clough K, Dieras V, Pouillart P, Sastre-Garau X (1998). No significant predictive value of c-erbB-2 or p53 expression regarding sensitivity to primary chemotherapy or radiotherapy in breast cancer. *Int J Cancer* 79: 27-33.

2478. Rubens JR, Lewandrowski KB, Kopans DB, Koerner FC, Hall DA, McCarthy KA (1990). Medullary carcinoma of the breast. Overdiagnosis of a prognostically favorable neoplasm. *Arch Surg* 125: 601-604.

2479. Rubin SC, Benjamin I, Behbakht K, Takahashi H, Morgan MA, LiVolsi VA, Berchuck A, Muto MG, Garber JE, Weber BL, Lynch HT, Boyd J (1996). Clinical and pathological features of ovarian cancer in women with germ-line mutations of BRCA1. *N Engl J Med* 335: 1413-1416.

2480. Rubin SC, Young J, Mikuta JJ (1985). Squamous carcinoma of the vagina: treatment, complications, and long-term followup. *Gynecol Oncol* 20: 346-353.

2481. Rubio IT, Korourian S, Brown H, Cowan C, Klimberg VS (1998). Carcinoid tumor metastatic to the breast. *Arch Surg* 133: 1117-1119.

2482. Rudan I, Rudan N, Skoric T, Sarcevic B (1996). Fibromatosis of male breast. *Acta Med Croatica* 50: 157-159.

2483. Rudas M, Neumayer R, Gnant MF, Mittelbock M, Jakesz R, Reiner A (1997). p53 protein expression, cell proliferation and steroid hormone receptors in ductal and lobular in situ carcinomas of the breast. *Eur J Cancer* 33: 39-44.

2484. Rudas M, Schmidinger M, Wenzel C, Okamoto I, Budinsky A, Fazeny B, Marosi C (2000). Karyotypic findings in two cases of male breast cancer. *Cancer Genet Cytogenet* 121: 190-193.

2485. Ruffolo EF, Koerner FC, Maluf HM (1997). Metaplastic carcinoma of the breast with melanocytic differentiation. *Mod Pathol* 10: 592-596.

2486. Ruggieri AM, Brody JM, Curhan RP (1996). Vaginal leiomyoma. A case report with imaging findings. *J Reprod Med* 41: 875-877.

2487. Runnebaum IB, Wang-Gohrke S, Vesprini D, Kreienberg R, Lynch H, Moslehi R, Ghadirian P, Weber B, Godwin AK, Risch H, Garber J, Lerman C, Olopade OI, Foulkes WD, Karlan B, Warner E, Rosen B, Rebbeck T, Tonin P, Dube MP, Kieback DG, Narod SA (2001). Progesterone receptor variant increases ovarian cancer risk in BRCA1 and BRCA2 mutation carriers who were never exposed to oral contraceptives. *Pharmacogenetics* 11: 635-638.

2488. Rush DS, Tan J, Baergen RN, Soslow RA (2001). h-Caldesmon, a novel smooth muscle-specific antibody, distinguishes between cellular leiomyoma and endometrial stromal sarcoma. *Am J Surg Pathol* 25: 253-258.

2489. Russell P (1979). The pathological assessment of ovarian neoplasms. I: Introduction to the common 'epithelial' tumours and analysis of benign 'epithelial' tumours. *Pathology* 11: 5-26.

2490. Russell P (1979). The pathological assessment of ovarian neoplasms. II: The proliferating 'epithelial' tumours. *Pathology* 11: 251-282.

2491. Russell P, Merkur H (1979). Proliferating ovarian "epithelial" tumours: a clinico-pathological analysis of 144 cases. *Aust N Z J Obstet Gynaecol* 19: 45-51.

2492. Russell P, Wills EJ, Watson G, Lee J, Geraghty T (1995). Monomorphic (basal cell) salivary adenoma of ovary: report of a case. *Ultrastruct Pathol* 19: 431-438.

2493. Russell PA, Pharoah PD, De Foy K, Ramus SJ, Symmonds I, Wilson A, Scott I, Ponder BA, Gayther SA (2000). Frequent loss of BRCA1 mRNA and protein expression in sporadic ovarian cancers. *Int J Cancer* 87: 317-321.

2494. Russo L, Woolmough E, Heatley MK (2000). Structural and cell surface antigen expression in the rete ovarii and epoophoron differs from that in the Fallopian tube and in endometriosis. *Histopathology* 37: 64-69.

2495. Rutgers JL, Scully RE (1988). Cysts (cystadenomas) and tumors of the rete ovarii. *Int J Gynecol Pathol* 7: 330-342.

2496. Rutgers JL, Scully RE (1988). Ovarian mixed-epithelial papillary cystadenomas of borderline malignancy of mullerian type. A clinicopathologic analysis. *Cancer* 61: 546-554.

2497. Rutgers JL, Scully RE (1988). Ovarian mullerian mucinous papillary cystadenomas of borderline malignancy. A clinicopathologic analysis. *Cancer* 61: 340-348.

2498. Rutgers JL, Scully RE (1991). The androgen insensitivity syndrome (testicular feminization): a clinicopathologic study of 43 cases. *Int J Gynecol Pathol* 10: 126-144.

2499. Rutledge F (1967). Cancer of the vagina. *Am J Obstet Gynecol* 97: 635-655.
2500. Rutqvist LE, Wallgren A (1983). Influence of age on outcome in breast carcinoma. *Acta Radiol Oncol* 22: 289-294.
2501. Rywlin AM, Simmons RJ, Robinson MJ (1969). Leiomyoma of vagina recurrent in pregnancy: a case with apparent hormone dependency. *South Med J* 62: 1449-1451.
2502. Sabini G, Chumas JC, Mann WJ (1992). Steroid hormone receptors in endometrial stromal sarcomas. A biochemical and immunohistochemical study. *Am J Clin Pathol* 97: 381-386.
2503. Safe SH (1997). Xenoestrogens and breast cancer. *N Engl J Med* 337: 1303-1304.
2504. Saffos RO, Rhatigan RM, Scully RE (1980). Metaplastic papillary tumor of the fallopian tube--a distinctive lesion of pregnancy. *Am J Clin Pathol* 74: 232-236.
2505. Sagebiel R.W. (1969). Ultrastructural observations on epidermal cells in Paget's disease of the breast. *Am J Pathol* 1: 49-64.
2506. Sahin A, Benda JA (1988). Primary ovarian Wilms' tumor. *Cancer* 61: 1460-1463.
2507. Sahin AA, Silva EG, Ordonez NG (1989). Alveolar soft part sarcoma of the uterine cervix. *Mod Pathol* 2: 676-680.
2508. Saigo PE, Rosen PP (1981). Mammary carcinoma with "choriocarcinomatous" features. *Am J Surg Pathol* 5: 773-778.
2509. Sainsbury JR, Farndon JR, Needham GK, Malcolm AJ, Harris AL (1987). Epidermal-growth-factor receptor status as predictor of early recurrence of and death from breast cancer. *Lancet* 1: 1398-1402.
2510. Saint Aubain SN, Larsimont D, Cluydts N, Heymans O, Verhest A (1997). Pseudoangiomatous hyperplasia of mammary stroma in an HIV patient. *Gen Diagn Pathol* 143: 251-254.
2511. Sainz dlC, Eichhorn JH, Rice LW, Fuller AF Jr., Nikrui N, Goff BA (1996). Histologic transformation of benign endometriosis to early epithelial ovarian cancer. *Gynecol Oncol* 60: 238-244.
2512. Saitoh A, Tsutsumi Y, Osamura RY, Watanabe K (1989). Sclerosing stromal tumor of the ovary. Immunohistochemical and electron-microscopic demonstration of smooth-muscle differentiation. *Arch Pathol Lab Med* 113: 372-376.
2513. Sakamoto A, Sasaki H, Furusato M, Suzuki M, Hirai Y, Tsugane S, Fukushima M, Terashima Y (1994). Observer disagreement in histological classification of ovarian tumors in Japan. *Gynecol Oncol* 54: 54-58.
2514. Sakuragi N, Satoh C, Takeda N, Hareyama H, Takeda M, Yamamoto R, Fujimoto T, Oikawa M, Fujino T, Fujimoto S (1999). Incidence and distribution pattern of pelvic and paraaortic lymph node metastasis in patients with Stages IB, IIA, and IIB cervical carcinoma treated with radical hysterectomy. *Cancer* 85: 1547-1554.
2515. Salazar H, Kanbour A, Tobon H, Gonzalez-Angulo A (1974). Endoderm cell derivatives in embryonal carcinoma of the ovary: an electron microscopic study of two cases. *Am J Pathol* 74: 108 A.
2516. Salovaara R, Loukola A, Kristo P, Kaariainen H, Ahtola H, Eskelinen M, Harkonen N, Julkunen R, Kangas E, Ojala S, Tulikoura J, Valkamo E, Jarvinen H, Mecklin JP, Aaltonen LA, de la CA (2000). Population-based molecular detection of hereditary nonpolyposis colorectal cancer. *J Clin Oncol* 18: 2193-2200.
2517. Saltzstein SL (1974). Clinically occult inflammatory carcinoma of the breast. *Cancer* 34: 382-388.
2518. Salvesen HB, MacDonald N, Ryan A, Iversen OE, Jacobs IJ, Akslen LA, Das S (2000). Methylation of hMLH1 in a population-based series of endometrial carcinomas. *Clin Cancer Res* 6: 3607-3613.
2519. Samanth KK, Black WC, III (1970). Benign ovarian stromal tumors associated with free peritoneal fluid. *Am J Obstet Gynecol* 107: 538-545.
2520. Samuels TH, Miller NA, Manchul LA, DeFreitas G, Panzarella T (1996). Squamous cell carcinoma of the breast. *Can Assoc Radiol J* 47: 177-182.
2521. Sanchez AG, Villanueva AG, Redondo C (1986). Lobular carcinoma of the breast in a patient with Klinefelter's syndrome. A case with bilateral, synchronous, histologically different breast tumors. *Cancer* 57: 1181-1183.
2522. Sander CM (1993). Angiomatous malformation of placental chorionic stem vessels and pseudo-partial molar placentas: report of five cases. *Pediatr Pathol* 13: 621-633.
2523. Sangwan K, Khosla AH, Hazra PC (1996). Leiomyoma of the vagina. *Aust N Z J Obstet Gynaecol* 36: 494-495.
2524. Sanjeevi CB, Hjelmstrom P, Hallmans G, Wiklund F, Lenner P, Angstrom T, Dillner J, Lernmark A (1996). Different HLA-DR-DQ haplotypes are associated with cervical intraepithelial neoplasia among human papillomavirus type-16 seropositive and seronegative Swedish women. *Int J Cancer* 68: 409-414.
2525. Sankaranarayanan R, Black RJ, Parkin DM (1998). *Cancer Survival in Developing Countries.* IARC: Lyon.
2526. Sankila R, Aaltonen LA, Jarvinen HJ, Mecklin JP (1996). Better survival rates in patients with MLH1-associated hereditary colorectal cancer. *Gastroenterology* 110: 682-687.
2527. Sano T, Oyama T, Kashiwabara K, Fukuda T, Nakajima T (1998). Expression status of p16 protein is associated with human papillomavirus oncogenic potential in cervical and genital lesions. *Am J Pathol* 153: 1741-1748.
2528. Santesson L, Kottmeier HL (1968). General classification of ovarian tumours. In: Ovarian Cancer, Gentil F, Junquiera AC, eds., Springer-Verlag: New York , pp. 1-8.
2529. Santeusanio G, Schiaroli S, Anemona L, Sesti F, Valli E, Piccione E, Spagnoli LG (1991). Carcinoma of the vulva with sarcomatoid features: a case report with immunohistochemical study. *Gynecol Oncol* 40: 160-163.
2530. Santini D, Gelli MC, Mazzoleni G, Ricci M, Severi B, Pasquinelli G, Pelusi G, Martinelli G (1989). Brenner tumor of the ovary: a correlative histologic, histochemical, immunohistochemical, and ultrastructural investigation. *Hum Pathol* 20: 787-795.
2531. Santos MJ, Gonzalez SS, Carretero AL (2000). Breast metastases from embryonal rhabdomyosarcoma: apropos 2 cases and a review of the literature. *Rev Clin Esp* 200: 21-25.
2532. Sanz-Ortega J, Chuaqui R, Zhuang Z, Sobel ME, Sanz-Esponera J, Liotta LA, Emmert-Buck MR, Merino MJ (1995). Loss of heterozygosity on chromosome 11q13 in microdissected human male breast carcinomas. *J Natl Cancer Inst* 87: 1408-1410.
2533. Sapino A, Bussolati G (2002). Is detection of endocrine cells in breast adenocarcinoma of diagnostic and clinical significance? *Histopathology* 40: 211-214.
2534. Sapino A, Frigerio A, Peterse JL, Arisio R, Coluccia C, Bussolati G (2000). Mammographically detected in situ lobular carcinomas of the breast. *Virchows Arch* 436: 421-430.
2535. Sapino A, Righi L, Cassoni P, Papotti M, Gugliotta P, Bussolati G (2001). Expression of apocrine differentiation markers in neuroendocrine breast carcinomas of aged women. *Mod Pathol* 14: 768-776.
2536. Sapino A, Righi L, Cassoni P, Papotti M, Pietribiasi F, Bussolati G (2000). Expression of the neuroendocrine phenotype in carcinomas of the breast. *Semin Diagn Pathol* 17: 127-137.
2536 a. Sartwell PE, Arthes FG, Tonascia JA (1978). Benign and malignant breast tumours: epidemiological similarities. *Int J Epidemiol* 7: 217-221.
2537. Sasano H, Mason JI, Sasaki E, Yajima A, Kimura N, Namiki T, Sasano N, Nagura H (1990). Immunohistochemical study of 3 beta-hydroxysteroid dehydrogenase in sex cord-stromal tumors of the ovary. *Int J Gynecol Pathol* 9: 352-362.
2538. Sasano H, Sato S, Yajima A, Akama J, Nagura H (1997). Adrenal rest tumor of the broad ligament: case report with immunohistochemical study of steroidogenic enzymes. *Pathol Int* 47: 493-496.
2539. Sasco AJ, Lowenfels AB, Pasker-de Jong P (1993). Epidemiology of male breast cancer. A meta-analysis of published case-control studies and discussion of selected aetiological factors. *Int J Cancer* 53: 538-549.
2540. Sashiyama H, Abe Y, Miyazawa Y, Nagashima T, Hasegawa M, Okuyama K, Kuwahara T, Takagi T (1999). Primary Non-Hodgkin's Lymphoma of the Male Breast: A Case Report. *Breast Cancer* 6: 55-58.
2541. Sastre-Garau X, Jouve M, Asselain B, Vincent-Salomon A, Beuzeboc P, Dorval T, Durand JC, Fourquet A, Pouillart P (1996). Infiltrating lobular carcinoma of the breast. Clinicopathologic analysis of 975 cases with reference to data on conservative therapy and metastatic patterns. *Cancer* 77: 113-120.
2542. Satake T, Matsuyama M (1991). Endocrine cells in a normal breast and non-cancerous breast lesion. *Acta Pathol Jpn* 41: 874-878.
2543. Sato N, Tsunoda H, Nishida M, Morishita Y, Takimoto Y, Kubo T, Noguchi M (2000). Loss of heterozygosity on 10q23.3 and mutation of the tumor suppressor gene PTEN in benign endometrial cyst of the ovary: possible sequence progression from benign endometrial cyst to endometrioid carcinoma and clear cell carcinoma of the ovary. *Cancer Res* 60: 7052-7056.
2544. Sau P, Solis J, Lupton GP, James WD (1989). Pigmented breast carcinoma. A clinical and histopathologic simulator of malignant melanoma. *Arch Dermatol* 125: 536-539.
2545. Savey L, Lasser P, Castaigne D, Michel G, Bognel C, Colau JC (1996). [Krukenberg tumors. Analysis of a series of 28 cases]. *J Chir (Paris)* 133: 427-431.
2546. Savitsky K, Bar-Shira A, Gilad S, Rotman G, Ziv Y, Vanagaite L, Tagle DA, Smith S, Uziel T, Sfez S, Ashkenazi M, Pecker I, frydman M, Harnik R, Patanjali SR, Simmons A, Clines GA, Sartiel A, Gatti RA, Chessa L, Sanal O, Lavin MF, Jaspers NGJ, Malcolm A, Taylor R, Arlett CF, Miki T, Weissman SM, Lovett M, Collins FS, Shiloh H. (1995). A single ataxia telangiectasia gene with a product similar to PI-3 kinase. *Science* 268: 1749-1753.
2547. Savitsky K, Platzer M, Uziel T, Gilad S, Sartiel A, Rosenthal A, Elroy-Stein O, Shiloh Y, Rotman G (1997). Ataxia-telangiectasia: structural diversity of untranslated sequences suggests complex post-transcriptional regulation of ATM gene expression. *Nucleic Acids Res* 25: 1678-1684.
2548. Scarff RW, Torloni H (1968). *International Histological Classification of Tumours,* n°2. Histological Typing of Breast Tumours. World Health Organization: Geneva.
2549. Scatarige JC, Hsiu JG, de la TR, Cramer MS, Siddiky MA, Jaffe AH (1987). Acoustic shadowing in benign granular cell tumor (myoblastoma) of the breast. *J Ultrasound Med* 6: 545-547.
2550. Schammel DP, Silver SA, Tavassoli FA (1999). Combined endometrial stromal/smooth muscle neoplasms of the uterus: clinicopathologic study of 38 cases. *Mod Pathol* 12: 124A.
2551. Schammel DP, Tavassoli FA (1998). Uterine angiosarcomas: a morphologic and immunohistochemical study of four cases. *Am J Surg Pathol* 22: 246-250.
2552. Scheidbach H, Dworak O, Schmucker B, Hohenberger W (2000). Lobular carcinoma of the breast in an 85-year-old man. *Eur J Surg Oncol* 26: 319-321.
2553. Scheistroen M, Trope C, Kaern J, Pettersen EO, Alfsen GC, Nesland JM (1997). DNA ploidy and expression of p53 and C-erbB-2 in extramammary Paget's disease of the vulva. *Gynecol Oncol* 64: 88-92.
2554. Scheithauer B, Woodruff JM (1999). *Tumours of the Peripheral Nervous System.* AFIP: Washington, DC.
2555. Schell SR, Montague ED, Spanos WJ Jr., Tapley ND, Fletcher GH, Oswald MJ (1982). Bilateral breast cancer in patients with initial stage I and II disease. *Cancer* 50: 1191-1194.
2556. Schernhammer ES, Laden F, Speizer FE, Willett WC, Hunter DJ, Kawachi I, Colditz GA (2001). Rotating night shifts and risk of breast cancer in women participating in the nurses' health study. *J Natl Cancer Inst* 93: 1563-1568.
2556a. Schildkraut JM, Risch N, Thompson WD (1989). Evaluating genetic association among ovarian, breast, and endometrial cancer: evidence for a breast/ovarian cancer relationship. *Am J Hum Genet* 45: 521-529.
2557. Schildkraut JM, Thompson WD (1988). Familial ovarian cancer: a population-based case-control study. *Am J Epidemiol* 128: 456-466.
2558. Schlesinger C, Kamoi S, Ascher SM, Kendell M, Lage JM, Silverberg SG (1998). Endometrial polyps: a comparison study of patients receiving tamoxifen with two control groups. *Int J Gynecol Pathol* 17: 302-311.

2559. Schlesinger C, Silverberg SG (1999). Endocervical adenocarcinoma in situ of tubal type and its relation to atypical tubal metaplasia. *Int J Gynecol Pathol* 18: 1-4.
2560. Schmidt-Kittler O, Ragg T, Daskalakis A, Granzow M, Ahr A, Blankenstein TJ, Kaufmann M, Diebold J, Arnholdt H, Muller P, Bischoff J, Harich D, Schlimok G, Riethmuller G, Eils R, Klein CA (2003). From latent disseminated cells to overt metastasis: genetic analysis of systemic breast cancer progression. *Proc Natl Acad Sci USA* 100: 7737-7742.
2561. Schmitt FC, Ribeiro CA, Alvarenga S, Lopes JM (2000). Primary acinic cell-like carcinoma of the breast--a variant with good prognosis? *Histopathology* 36: 286-289.
2562. Schmitz MJ, Hendricks DT, Farley J, Taylor RR, Geradts J, Rose GS, Birrer MJ (2000). p27 and cyclin D1 abnormalities in uterine papillary serous carcinoma. *Gynecol Oncol* 77: 439-445.
2563. Schmutte C, Marinescu RC, Copeland NG, Jenkins NA, Overhauser J, Fishel R (1998). Refined chromosomal localization of the mismatch repair and hereditary nonpolyposis colorectal cancer genes hMSH2 and hMSH6. *Cancer Res* 58: 5023-5026.
2564. Schnarkowski P, Kessler M, Arnholdt H, Helmberger T (1997). Angiosarcoma of the breast: mammographic, sonographic, and pathological findings. *Eur J Radiol* 24: 54-56.
2565. Schneider A, de Villiers EM, Schneider V (1987). Multifocal squamous neoplasia of the female genital tract: significance of human papillomavirus infection of the vagina after hysterectomy. *Obstet Gynecol* 70: 294-298.
2566. Schneider C, Wight E, Perucchini D, Haller U, Fink D (2000). Primary carcinoma of the fallopian tube. A report of 19 cases with literature review. *Eur J Gynaecol Oncol* 21: 578-582.
2567. Schneider JA (1989). Invasive papillary breast carcinoma: mammographic and sonographic appearance. *Radiology* 171: 377-379.
2568. Schneider V, Zimberg ST, Kay S (1981). The pigmented portio: benign lentigo of the uterine cervix. *Diagn Gynecol Obstet* 3: 269-272.
2569. Schnitt SJ (1997). Morphologic risk factors for local recurrence in patients with invasive breast cancer treated with conservative surgery and radiation therapy. *Breast J.* 3: 261-266.
2570. Schnitt SJ, Connolly JL, Recht A, Silver B, Harris JR (1989). Influence of infiltrating lobular histology on local tumor control in breast cancer patients treated with conservative surgery and radiotherapy. *Cancer* 64: 448-454.
2571. Schnitt SJ, Connolly JL, Tavassoli FA, Fechner RE, Kempson RL, Gelman R, Page DL (1992). Interobserver reproducibility in the diagnosis of ductal proliferative breast lesions using standardized criteria. *Am J Surg Pathol* 16: 1133-1143.
2572. Schnuch A (1993). [Post hoc or propter hoc? On the heuristics of side-effects in the example of gynecomastia]. *Dtsch Med Wochenschr* 118: 796-803.
2573. Schorge JO, Lee KR, Sheets EE (2000). Prospective management of stage IA(1) cervical adenocarcinoma by conization alone to preserve fertility: a preliminary report. *Gynecol Oncol* 78: 217-220.
2574. Schorge JO, Miller YB, Qi LJ, Muto MG, Welch WR, Berkowitz RS, Mok SC (2000). Genetic alterations of the WT1 gene in papillary serous carcinoma of the peritoneum. *Gynecol Oncol* 76: 369-372.
2575. Schorge JO, Muto MG, Lee SJ, Huang LW, Welch WR, Bell DA, Keung EZ, Berkowitz RS, Mok SC (2000). BRCA1-related papillary serous carcinoma of the peritoneum has a unique molecular pathogenesis. *Cancer Res* 60: 1361-1364.
2576. Schorge JO, Muto MG, Welch WR, Bandera CA, Rubin SC, Bell DA, Berkowitz RS, Mok SC (1998). Molecular evidence for multifocal papillary serous carcinoma of the peritoneum in patients with germline BRCA1 mutations. *J Natl Cancer Inst* 90: 841-845.
2577. Schottenfeld D, Lilienfeld AM, Diamond H (1963). Some observations on the epidemiology of breast cancer among males. *Am J Publ Hlth* 53: 890-897.
2578. Schrager CA, Schneider D, Gruener AC, Tsou HC, Peacocke M (1998). Clinical and pathological features of breast disease in Cowden's syndrome: an underrecognized syndrome with an increased risk of breast cancer. *Hum Pathol* 29: 47-53.
2579. Schuh ME, Nemoto T, Penetrante RB, Rosner D, Dao TL (1986). Intraductal carcinoma. Analysis of presentation, pathologic findings, and outcome of disease. *Arch Surg* 121: 1303-1307.
2580. Schultz DM (1957). A malignant, melonotic neoplasm of the uterus, resembling the "retinal anlage" tumours. *Arch Pathol* 28: 524-532.
2581. Schurch W, Potvin C, Seemayer TA (1985). Malignant myoepithelioma (myoepithelial carcinoma) of the breast: an ultrastructural and immunocytochemical study. *Ultrastruct Pathol* 8: 1-11.
2582. Schuuring E, Verhoeven E, van Tinteren H, Peterse JL, Nunnink B, Thunnissen FB, Devilee P, Cornelisse CJ, Van de Vijver MJ, Mooi WJ, Michalides RJAM. (1992). Amplification of genes within the chromosome 11q13 region is indicative of poor prognosis in patients with operable breast cancer. *Cancer Res* 52: 5229-5234.
2583. Schwartz GF, Feig SA, Rosenberg AL, Patchefsky AS, Schwartz AB (1984). Staging and treatment of clinically occult breast cancer. *Cancer* 53: 1379-1384.
2584. Schwartz GF, Patchefsky AS, Finklestein SD, Sohn SH, Prestipino A, Feig SA, Singer JS (1989). Nonpalpable in situ ductal carcinoma of the breast. Predictors of multicentricity and microinvasion and implications for treatment. *Arch Surg* 124: 29-32.
2585. Schwartz IS, Strauchen JA (1990). Lymphocytic mastopathy. An autoimmune disease of the breast? *Am J Clin Pathol* 93: 725-730.
2586. Schwartz PE (2000). Surgery of germ cell tumours of the ovary. *Forum (Genova)* 10: 355-365.
2587. Schwartz PE, Chambers SK, Chambers JT, Kohorn E, McIntosh S (1992). Ovarian germ cell malignancies: the Yale University experience. *Gynecol Oncol* 45: 26-31.
2588. Schwartz PE, Smith JP (1976). Treatment of ovarian stromal tumors. *Am J Obstet Gynecol* 125: 402-411.
2589. Schweizer P, Moisio AL, Kuismanen SA, Truninger K, Vierumaki R, Salovaara R, Arola J, Butzow R, Jiricny J, Peltomaki P, Nystrom-Lahti M (2001). Lack of MSH2 and MSH6 characterizes endometrial but not colon carcinomas in hereditary nonpolyposis colorectal cancer. *Cancer Res* 61: 2813-2815.
2590. Scopsi L, Andreola S, Pilotti S, Bufalino R, Baldini MT, Testori A, Rilke F (1994). Mucinous carcinoma of the breast. A clinicopathologic, histochemical, and immunocytochemical study with special reference to neuroendocrine differentiation. *Am J Surg Pathol* 18: 702-711.
2591. Scopsi L, Andreola S, Saccozzi R, Pilotti S, Boracchi P, Rosa P, Conti AR, Manzari A, Huttner WB, Rilke F (1991). Argyrophilic carcinoma of the male breast. A neuroendocrine tumor containing predominantly chromogranin B (secretogranin I). *Am J Surg Pathol* 15: 1063-1071.
2592. Scott SP, Bendix R, Chen P, Clark R, Dork T, Lavin MF (2002). Missense mutations but not allelic variants alter the function of ATM by dominant interference in patients with breast cancer. *Proc Natl Acad Sci USA* 99: 925-930.
2593. Scully R, Anderson SF, Chao DM, Wei W, Ye L, Young RA, Livingston DM, Parvin JD (1997). BRCA1 is a component of the RNA polymerase II holoenzyme. *Proc Natl Acad Sci USA* 94: 5605-5610.
2594. Scully R, Chen J, Ochs RL, Keegan K, Hoekstra M, Feunteun J, Livingston DM (1997). Dynamic changes of BRCA1 subnuclear location and phosphorylation state are initiated by DNA damage. *Cell* 90: 425-435.
2595. Scully R, Chen J, Plug A, Xiao Y, Weaver D, Feunteun J, Ashley T, Livingston DM (1997). Association of BRCA1 with Rad51 in mitotic and meiotic cells. *Cell* 88: 265-275.
2596. Scully R, Ganesan S, Brown M, De Caprio JA, Cannistra SA, Feunteun J, Schnitt S, Livingston DM (1996). Location of BRCA1 in human breast and ovarian cancer cells. *Science* 272: 123-126.
2597. Scully R, Ganesan S, Vlasakova K, Chen J, Socolovsky M, Livingston DM (1999). Genetic analysis of BRCA1 function in a defined tumor cell line. *Mol Cell* 4: 1093-1099.
2598. Scully RE (1970). Gonadoblastoma. A review of 74 cases. *Cancer* 25: 1340-1356.
2599. Scully RE (1970). Sex cord tumor with annular tubules a distinctive ovarian tumor of the Peutz-Jeghers syndrome. *Cancer* 25: 1107-1121.
2600. Scully RE, Bell DA, Abu-Jawdeh GM (1995). Update on early ovarian cancer and cancer developing in benign ovarian tumors. In: *Ovarian Cancer 3,* P Mason, F Sharp, T Blackett, J Berek (eds.), Chapman and Hall: London, pp. 139-144.
2601. Scully RE, Bonfiglio TA, Kurman RJ, Silverberg SG, Wilkinson EJ (1994). *World Health Organization: Histological Typing of Female Tract Tumours.* 2nd ed. Springer-Verlag: Berlin.
2602. Scully RE, Bonfiglio TA, Kurman RJ, Silverberg SG, Wilkinson EJ (1994). Uterine corpus. In: *World Health Organization: Histological Typing of Female Genital Tract Tumors,* Springer-Verlag: New York , pp. 13-31.
2603. Scully RE, Galdabini JJ, McNeely BU (1976). Case records of the Massachusetts General Hospital. Weekly clinicopathological exercises. Case 14-1976. *N Engl J Med* 294: 772-777.
2604. Scully RE, Sobin LH (1999). World Health Organization: *Histological Typing of Ovarian Tumours.* 2nd ed. Spinger-Verlag: Berlin.
2605. Scully RE, Young RH, Clement PB (1998). *Atlas of Tumor Pathology Tumors of the Ovary, Maldeveloped Gonads, Fallopian Tube, and Broad Ligament.* 3rd ed. AFIP: Washington,D.C.
2606. Scurry J, Beshay V, Cohen C, Allen D (1998). Ki67 expression in lichen sclerosus of vulva in patients with and without associated squamous cell carcinoma. *Histopathology* 32: 399-404.
2607. Scurry J, Brand A, Planner R, Dowling J, Rode J (1996). Vulvar Merkel cell tumor with glandular and squamous differentiation. *Gynecol Oncol* 62: 292-297.
2608. Scurry J, Craighead P, Duggan M (2000). Histologic study of patterns of cervical involvement in FIGO stage II endometrial carcinoma. *Int J Gynecol Cancer* 10: 497-502.
2609. Scurry J, Planner R, Grant P (1991). Unusual variants of vaginal adenosis: a challenge for diagnosis and treatment. Gynecol Oncol 41: 172-177.
2610. Scurry JP, Brown RW, Jobling T (1996). Combined ovarian serous papillary and hepatoid carcinoma. *Gynecol Oncol* 63: 138-142.
2611. Sebek BA (1984). Cavernous hemangioma of the female breast. *Cleve Clin Q* 51: 471-474.
2612. Seckl MJ, Mulholland PJ, Bishop AE, Teale JD, Hales CN, Glaser M, Watkins S, Seckl JR (1999). Hypoglycemia due to an insulin-secreting small-cell carcinoma of the cervix. *N Engl J Med* 341: 733-736.
2613. Secreto G, Zumoff B (1994). Abnormal production of androgens in women with breast cancer. *Anticancer Res* 14: 2113-2117.
2614. Sedlis A (1961). Primary carcinoma of the Fallopian tube. *Obstet Gynecol Surv* 16: 209-226.
2615. Segal GH, Hart WR (1992). Ovarian serous tumors of low malignant potential (serous borderline tumors). The relationship of exophytic surface tumor to peritoneal "implants". *Am J Surg Pathol* 16: 577-583.
2616. Segawa T, Sasagawa T, Yamazaki H, Sakaike J, Ishikawa H, Inoue M (1999). Fragile histidine triad transcription abnormalities and human papillomavirus E6-E7 mRNA expression in the development of cervical carcinoma. *Cancer* 85: 2001-2010.
2617. Seidman JD (1994). Mucinous lesions of the fallopian tube. A report of seven cases. *Am J Surg Pathol* 18: 1205-1212.
2618. Seidman JD (1996). Prognostic importance of hyperplasia and atypia in endometriosis. *Int J Gynecol Pathol* 15: 1-9.
2619. Seidman JD (1996). Unclassified ovarian gonadal stromal tumors. A clinicopathologic study of 32 cases. *Am J Surg Pathol* 20: 699-706.
2620. Seidman JD, Abbondanzo SL, Bratthauer GL (1995). Lipid cell (steroid cell) tumor of the ovary: immunophenotype with analysis of potential pitfall due to endogenous biotin-like activity. *Int J Gynecol Pathol* 14: 331-338.
2621. Seidman JD, Ashton M, Lefkowitz M (1996). Atypical apocrine adenosis of the breast: a clinicopathologic study of 37 patients with 8.7-year follow-up. *Cancer* 77: 2529-2537.

2622. Seidman JD, Borkowski A, Aisner SC, Sun CC (1993). Rapid growth of pseudoangiomatous hyperplasia of mammary stroma in axillary gynecomastia in an immunosuppressed patient. *Arch Pathol Lab Med* 117: 736-738.
2623. Seidman JD, Elsayed AM, Sobin LH, Tavassoli FA (1993). Association of mucinous tumors of the ovary and appendix. A clinicopathologic study of 25 cases. *Am J Surg Pathol* 17: 22-34.
2624. Selim AG, Wells CA (1999). Immunohistochemical localisation of androgen receptor in apocrine metaplasia and apocrine adenosis of the breast: relation to oestrogen and progesterone receptors. *J Clin Pathol* 52: 838-841.
2625. Seltzer VL, Levine A, Spiegel G, Rosenfeld D, Coffey EL (1990). Adenofibroma of the uterus: multiple recurrences following wide local excision. *Gynecol Oncol* 37: 427-431.
2626. Seltzer VL, Molho L, Fougner A, Hong P, Kereszti B, Gero M, Spitzer M (1988). Parovarian cystadenocarcinoma of low-malignant potential. *Gynecol Oncol* 30: 216-221.
2627. Semczuk A, Baranowski W, Berbec H, Marzec B, Skomra D, Miturski R (1999). Analysis of p53 and K-ras genes and their proteins in a sarcoma botryoides of the uterine cervix. *Eur J Gynaecol Oncol* 20: 311-314.
2628. Sengupta BS (1981). Vulval cancer following or co-existing with chronic granulomatous diseases of vulva. An analysis of its natural history, clinical manifestation and treatment. *Trop Doct* 11: 110-114.
2629. Senzaki H, Kiyozuka Y, Mizuoka H, Yamamoto D, Ueda S, Izumi H, Tsubura A (1999). An autopsy case of hepatoid carcinoma of the ovary with PIVKA-II production: immunohistochemical study and literature review. *Pathol Int* 49: 164-169.
2630. Seong C, Kirby RW (1987). Leydig-cell tumour of the ovary en a multiple endocrine neoplasia syndrome. *J Obstet Gynaecol* 7: 295-296.
2631. Serova OM, Mazoyer S, Puget N, Dubois V, Tonin P, Shugart YY, Goldgar D, Narod SA, Lynch HT, Lenoir GM (1997). Mutations in BRCA1 and BRCA2 in breast cancer families: are there more breast cancer-susceptibility genes? *Am J Hum Genet* 60: 486-495.
2632. Shabb NS, Tawil A, Mufarrij A, Obeid S, Halabi J (1997). Mammary carcinoma with osteoclastlike giant cells cytologically mimicking benign breast disease. A case report. *Acta Cytol* 41: 1284-1288.
2633. Shanks JH, Harris M, Banerjee SS, Eyden BP, Joglekar VM, Nicol A, Hasleton PS, Nicholson AG (2000). Mesotheliomas with deciduoid morphology: a morphologic spectrum and a variant not confined to young females. *Am J Surg Pathol* 24: 285-294.
2634. Sharma A, Pratap M, Sawhney VM, Khan IU, Bhambhani S, Mitra AB (1999). Frequent amplification of C-erbB2 (HER-2/Neu) oncogene in cervical carcinoma as detected by non-fluorescence in situ hybridization technique on paraffin sections. *Oncology* 56: 83-87.
2635. Shashi V, Golden WL, Kap-Herr C, Andersen WA, Gaffey MJ (1994). Interphase fluorescence in situ hybridization for trisomy 12 on archival ovarian sex cord-stromal tumors. *Gynecol Oncol* 55: 349-354.
2636. Shatz P, Bergeron C, Wilkinson EJ, Arseneau J, Ferenczy A (1989). Vulvar intraepithelial neoplasia and skin appendage involvement. *Obstet Gynecol* 74: 769-774.
2637. Shaw JA, Dabbs DJ, Geisinger KR (1992). Sclerosing stromal tumor of the ovary: an ultrastructural and immunohistochemical analysis with histogenetic considerations. *Ultrastruct Pathol* 16: 363-377.
2638. Sheikh MS, Rochefort H, Garcia M (1995). Overexpression of p21WAF1/CIP1 induces growth arrest, giant cell formation and apoptosis in human breast carcinoma cell lines. *Oncogene* 11: 1899-1905.
2639. Shen JT, d'Ablaing G, Morrow CP (1982). Alveolar soft part sarcoma of the vulva: report of first case and review of literature. *Gynecol Oncol* 13: 120-128.
2640. Shen T, Zhuang Z, Gersell DJ, Tavassoli FA (2000). Allelic Deletion of VHL Gene Detected in Papillary Tumors of the Broad Ligament, Epididymis, and Retroperitoneum in von Hippel-Lindau Disease Patients. *Int J Surg Pathol* 8: 207-212.
2641. Shenson DL, Gallion HH, Powell DE, Pieretti M (1995). Loss of heterozygosity and genomic instability in synchronous endometrioid tumors of the ovary and endometrium. *Cancer* 76: 650-657.
2642. Shepherd JH (1989). Revised FIGO staging for gynaecological cancer. *Br J Obstet Gynaecol* 96: 889-892.
2643. Shepherd JJ, Wright DH (1967). Burkitt's tumour presenting as bilateral swelling of the breast in women of child-bearing age. *Br J Surg* 54: 776-780.
2644. Sheppard DG, Libshitz HI (2001). Post-radiation sarcomas: a review of the clinical and imaging features in 63 cases. *Clin Radiol* 56: 22-29.
2645. Sherman JE, Smith JW (1981). Neurofibromas of the breast and nipple-areolar area. *Ann Plast Surg* 7: 302-307.
2646. Sherman ME, Bitterman P, Rosenshein NB, Delgado G, Kurman RJ (1992). Uterine serous carcinoma. A morphologically diverse neoplasm with unifying clinicopathologic features. *Am J Surg Pathol* 16: 600-610.
2647. Sherman ME, Bur ME, Kurman RJ (1995). p53 in endometrial cancer and its putative precursors: evidence for diverse pathways of tumorigenesis. *Hum Pathol* 26: 1268-1274.
2648. Sherman ME, Sturgeon S, Brinton LA, Potischman N, Kurman RJ, Berman ML, Mortel R, Twiggs LB, Barrett RJ, Wilbanks GD (1997). Risk factors and hormone levels in patients with serous and endometrioid uterine carcinomas. *Mod Pathol* 10: 963-968.
2649. Sheth NA, Saruiya JN, Ranadive KJ, Sheth AR (1974). Ectopic production of human chorionic gonadotrophin by human breast tumours. *Br J Cancer* 30: 566-570.
2650. Sheth S, Hamper UM, Kurman RJ (1993). Thickened endometrium in the post-menopausal woman: sonographic-pathologic correlation. *Radiology* 187: 135-139.
2651. Sheu BC, Lin HH, Chen CK, Chao KH, Shun CT, Huang SC (1995). Synchronous primary carcinomas of the endometrium and ovary. *Int J Gynaecol Obstet* 51: 141-146.
2652. Shevchuk MM, Fenoglio CM, Lattes R, Frick HC, Richart RM (1978). Malignant mixed tumor of the vagina probably arising in mesonephric rests. *Cancer* 42: 214-223.
2653. Sheyn I, Mira JL, Bejarano PA, Husseinzadeh N (2000). Metastatic female adnexal tumor of probable Wolffian origin: a case report and review of the literature. *Arch Pathol Lab Med* 124: 431-434.
2654. Shidara Y, Karube A, Watanabe M, Satou E, Uesaka Y, Matsuura T, Tanaka T (2000). A case report: verrucous carcinoma of the endometrium--the difficulty of diagnosis, and a review of the literature. *J Obstet Gynaecol Res* 26: 189-192.
2655. Shigematsu T, Kamura T, Arima T, Wake N, Nakano H (2000). DNA polymorphism analysis of a pure non-gestational choriocarcinoma of the ovary: case report. *Eur J Gynaecol Oncol* 21: 153-154.
2656. Shigeta H, Taga M, Kurogi K, Kitamura H, Motoyama T, Gorai I (1999). Ovarian strumal carcinoid with severe constipation: immunohistochemical and mRNA analyses of peptide YY. *Hum Pathol* 30: 242-246.
2657. Shih HA, Couch FJ, Nathanson KL, Blackwood MA, Rebbeck TR, Armstrong KA, Calzone K, Stopfer J, Seal S, Stratton MR, Weber BL (2002). BRCA1 and BRCA2 mutation frequency in women evaluated in a breast cancer risk evaluation clinic. *J Clin Oncol* 20: 994-999.
2658. Shih IM, Kurman RJ (1998). Epithelioid trophoblastic tumor: a neoplasm distinct from choriocarcinoma and placental site trophoblastic tumor simulating carcinoma. *Am J Surg Pathol* 22: 1393-1403.
2659. Shih IM, Kurman RJ (2001). The pathology of intermediate trophoblastic tumors and tumor-like lesions. *Int J Gynecol Pathol* 20: 31-47.
2660. Shiloh Y, Kastan MB (2001). ATM: genome stability, neuronal development, and cancer cross paths. *Adv Cancer Res* 83: 209-254.
2661. Shin SJ, DeLellis RA, Rosen PP (2001). Small cell carcinoma of the breast--additional immunohistochemical studies. *Am J Surg Pathol* 25: 831-832.
2662. Shin SJ, DeLellis RA, Ying L, Rosen PP (2000). Small cell carcinoma of the breast: a clinicopathologic and immunohistochemical study of nine patients. *Am J Surg Pathol* 24: 1231-1238.
2663. Shin SJ, Kanomata N, Rosen PP (2000). Mammary carcinoma with prominent cytoplasmic lipofuscin granules mimicking melanocytic differentiation. *Histopathology* 37: 456-459.
2664. Shivas AA, Douglas JG (1972). The prognostic significance of elastosis in breast carcinoma. *J R Coll Surg Edinb* 17: 315-320.
2665. Shokeir MO, Noel SM, Clement PB (1996). Malignant mullerian mixed tumor of the uterus with a prominent alpha-fetoprotein-producing component of yolk sac tumor. *Mod Pathol* 9: 647-651.
2666. Shoker BS, Jarvis C, Clarke RB, Anderson E, Munro C, Davies MP, Sibson DR, Sloane JP (2000). Abnormal regulation of the oestrogen receptor in benign breast lesions. *J Clin Pathol* 53: 778-783.
2667. Shoker BS, Jarvis C, Sibson DR, Walker C, Sloane JP (1999). Oestrogen receptor expression in the normal and precancerous breast. *J Pathol* 188: 237-244.
2668. Shousha S, Backhous CM, Alaghband-Zadeh J, Burn I (1986). Alveolar variant of invasive lobular carcinoma of the breast. A tumor rich in estrogen receptors. *Am J Clin Pathol* 85: 1-5.
2669. Shousha S, Coady AT, Stamp T, James KR, Alaghband-Zadeh J (1989). Oestrogen receptors in mucinous carcinoma of the breast: an immunohistological study using paraffin wax sections. *J Clin Pathol* 42: 902-905.
2670. Shousha S, Schoenfeld A, Moss J, Shore I, Sinnett HD (1994). Light and electron microscopic study of an invasive cribriform carcinoma with extensive microcalcification developing in a breast with silicone augmentation. *Ultrastruct Pathol* 18: 519-523.
2671. Sieinski W (1989). Lipomatous neometaplasia of the uterus. Report of 11 cases with discussion of histogenesis and pathogenesis. *Int J Gynecol Pathol* 8: 357-363.
2672. Sigurdsson K, Hrafnkelsson J, Geirsson G, Gudmundsson J, Salvarsdottir A (1991). Screening as a prognostic factor in cervical cancer: analysis of survival and prognostic factors based on Icelandic population data, 1964-1988. *Gynecol Oncol* 43: 64-70.
2673. Sijmons RH, Kiemeney LA, Witjes JA, Vasen HF (1998). Urinary tract cancer and hereditary nonpolyposis colorectal cancer: risks and screening options. *J Urol* 160: 466-470.
2674. Sillman FH, Fruchter RG, Chen YS, Camilien L, Sedlis A, McTigue E (1997). Vaginal intraepithelial neoplasia: risk factors for persistence, recurrence, and invasion and its management. *Am J Obstet Gynecol* 176: 93-99.
2675. Silva EG, Jenkins R (1990). Serous carcinoma in endometrial polyps. *Mod Pathol* 3: 120-128.
2676. Silva EG, Robey-Cafferty SS, Smith TL, Gershenson DM (1990). Ovarian carcinomas with transitional cell carcinoma pattern. *Am J Clin Pathol* 93: 457-465.
2677. Silva EG, Tornos C, Bailey MA, Morris M (1991). Undifferentiated carcinoma of the ovary. *Arch Pathol Lab Med* 115: 377-381.
2678. Silver SA, Cheung AN, Tavassoli FA (1999). Oncocytic metaplasia and carcinoma of the endometrium: an immunohistochemical and ultrastructural study. *Int J Gynecol Pathol* 18: 12-19.
2679. Silver SA, Devouassoux-Shisheboran M, Mezzetti TP, Tavassoli FA (2001). Mesonephric adenocarcinomas of the uterine cervix: a study of 11 cases with immunohistochemical findings. *Am J Surg Pathol* 25: 379-387.
2680. Silver SA, Tavassoli FA (1998). Mammary ductal carcinoma in situ with microinvasion. *Cancer* 82: 2382-2390.
2681. Silver SA, Tavassoli FA (1998). Primary osteogenic sarcoma of the breast: a clinicopathologic analysis of 50 cases. *Am J Surg Pathol* 22: 925-933.
2682. Silver SA, Tavassoli FA (2000). Glomus tumor arising in a mature teratoma of the ovary: report of a case simulating a metastasis from cervical squamous carcinoma. *Arch Pathol Lab Med* 124: 1373-1375.
2683. Silver SA, Tavassoli FA (2000). Pleomorphic carcinoma of the breast: clinicopathological analysis of 26 cases of an unusual high-grade phenotype of ductal carcinoma. *Histopathology* 36: 505-514.
2684. Silver SA, Wiley JM, Perlman EJ (1994). DNA ploidy analysis of pediatric germ cell tumors. *Mod Pathol* 7: 951-956.
2685. Silverberg SG (1971). Brenner tumor of the ovary. A clinicopathologic study of 60 tumors in 54 women. *Cancer* 28: 588-596.

2686. Silverberg SG (1999). Protocol for the examination of specimens from patients with carcinomas of the endometrium: a basis for checklists. Cancer Committee, College of American Pathologists. *Arch Pathol Lab Med* 123: 28-32.
2687. Silverberg SG (2000). Histopathologic grading of ovarian carcinoma: a review and proposal. *Int J Gynecol Pathol* 19: 7-15.
2688. Silverberg SG (2000). Problems in the differential diagnosis of endometrial hyperplasia and carcinoma. *Mod Pathol* 13: 309-327.
2689. Silverberg SG, Chitale AR (1973). Assessment of significance of proportions of intraductal and infiltrating tumor growth in ductal carcinoma of the breast. *Cancer* 32: 830-837.
2690. Silverberg SG, Kay S, Koss LG (1971). Postmastectomy lymphangiosarcoma: ultrastructural observations. *Cancer* 27: 100-108.
2691. Silverberg SG, Kurman RJ (1992). *Atlas of Tumour Pathology. Tumours of the uterine corpus and gestational trophoblastic disease,* AFIP: Washington DC.
2692. Silverberg SG, Major FJ, Blessing JA, Fetter B, Askin FB, Liao SY, Miller A (1990). Carcinosarcoma (malignant mixed mesodermal tumor) of the uterus. A Gynecologic Oncology Group pathologic study of 203 cases. *Int J Gynecol Pathol* 9: 1-19.
2693. Silverberg SG, Willson MA, Board JA (1971). Hemangiopericytoma of the uterus: an ultrastructural study. *Am J Obstet Gynecol* 110: 397-404.
2694. Silverman EM, Oberman HA (1974). Metastatic neoplasms in the breast. *Surg Gynecol Obstet* 138: 26-28.
2695. Silverstein MJ, Gierson ED, Colburn WJ, Rosser RJ, Waisman JR, Gamagami P (1991). Axillary lymphadenectomy for intraductal carcinoma of the breast. *Surg Gynecol Obstet* 172: 211-214.
2696. Silverstein MJ, Lewinsky BS, Waisman JR, Gierson ED, Colburn WJ, Senofsky GM, Gamagami P (1994). Infiltrating lobular carcinoma. Is it different from infiltrating duct carcinoma? *Cancer* 73: 1673-1677.
2697. Simkin PH, Ramirez LA, Zweizig SL, Afonso SA, Fraire AE, Khan A, Dunn AD, Dunn JT, Braverman LE (1999). Monomorphic teratoma of the ovary: a rare cause of triiodothyronine toxicosis. *Thyroid* 9: 949-954.
2698. Simpson JF, Page DL, Dupont WD (1990). Apocrine adenosis - a mimmic of mammary carcinoma. *Surgical Pathology* 3: 289-299.
2699. Simpson JF, Page DL, Dupont WD (1990). Apocrine adenosis - an occasional mimicker of breast carcinoma. *Mod Pathol* 3.
2700. Simpson JF, Quan DE, O'Malley F, Odom-Maryon T, Clarke PE (1997). Amplification of CCND1 and expression of its protein product, cyclin D1, in ductal carcinoma in situ of the breast. *Am J Pathol* 151: 161-168.
2701. Simpson JL, Michael H, Roth LM (1998). Unclassified sex cord-stromal tumors of the ovary: a report of eight cases. *Arch Pathol Lab Med* 122: 52-55.
2702. Simpson RH, Cope N, Skalova A, Michal M (1998). Malignant adenomyoepithelioma of the breast with mixed osteogenic, spindle cell, and carcinomatous differentiation. *Am J Surg Pathol* 22: 631-636.
2703. Simpson T, Thirlby RC, Dail DH (1992). Surgical treatment of ductal carcinoma in situ of the breast. 10- to 20-year follow-up. *Arch Surg* 127: 468-472.
2704. Simsek T, Trak B, Tunc M, Karaveli S, Uner M, Sonmez C (1998). Primary pure choriocarcinoma of the ovary in reproductive ages: a case report. *Eur J Gynaecol Oncol* 19: 284-286.
2705. Singer A, Monaghan J (2000). *Lower Genital Tract Precancer. Colposcopy, Pathology and Treatment.* 2nd ed. Blackwell Science Ltd: Oxford.
2706. Singer G, Kurman RJ, Chang HW, Cho SK, Shih I (2002). Diverse tumorigenic pathways in ovarian serous carcinoma. *Am J Pathol* 160: 1223-1228.
2707. Singer G, Oldt R, III, Cohen Y, Wang BG, Sidransky D, Kurman RJ, Shih I (2003). Mutations in BRAF and KRAS characterize the development of low-grade ovarian serous carcinoma. *J Natl Cancer Inst* 95: 484-486.
2708. Singh TT, Hopkins MP, Price J, Schuen R (1992). Myxoid liposarcoma of the broad ligament. Int J Gynecol Cancer 2: 220-223.
2709. Singhal S, Sharma S, De S, Kumar L, Chander S, Rath GK, Gupta SD (1990). Adult embryonal rhabdomyosarcoma of the vagina complicating pregnancy: a case report and review of the literature. Asia Oceania J Obstet Gynaecol 16: 301-306.
2710. Sinkre P, Albores-Saavedra J, Miller DS, Copeland LJ, Hameed A (2000). Endometrial endometrioid carcinomas associated with Ewing sarcoma/peripheral primitive neuroectodermal tumor. *Int J Gynecol Pathol* 19: 127-132.
2711. Sinkre P, Miller DS, Milchgrub S, Hameed A (2000). Adenomyofibroma of the endometrium with skeletal muscle differentiation. *Int J Gynecol Pathol* 19: 280-283.
2712. Sinniah R, O'Brien FV (1973). Pigmented progonoma in a dermoid cyst of the ovary. *J Pathol* 109: 357-359.
2713. Siriaunkgul S, Robbins KM, McGowan L, Silverberg SG (1995). Ovarian mucinous tumors of low malignant potential: a clinicopathologic study of 54 tumors of intestinal and mullerian type. *Int J Gynecol Pathol* 14: 198-208.
2714. Sirota RL, Dickersin GR, Scully RE (1981). Mixed tumors of the vagina. A clinicopathological analysis of eight cases. *Am J Surg Pathol* 5: 413-422.
2715. Sit AS, Price FV, Kelley JL, Comerci JT, Kunschner AJ, Kanbour-Shakir A, Edwards RP (2000). Chemotherapy for malignant mixed Mullerian tumors of the ovary. *Gynecol Oncol* 79: 196-200.
2716. Sjostedt S, Whalen T (1961). Prognosis of granulosa cell tumours. Acta Obstet Gynecol Scand 40(suppl 6): 3-26.
2717. Skelton H, Smith KJ (2001). Spindle cell epithelioma of the vagina shows immunohistochemical staining supporting its origin from a primitive/progenitor cell population. *Arch Pathol Lab Med* 125: 547-550.
2718. Skinnider BF, Clement PB, MacPherson N, Gascoyne RD, Viswanatha DS (1999). Primary non-Hodgkin's lymphoma and malakoplakia of the vagina: a case report. *Hum Pathol* 30: 871-874.
2719. Slamon DJ, Clark GM, Wong SG, Levin WJ, Ullrich A, McGuire WL (1987). Human breast cancer: correlation of relapse and survival with amplification of the HER-2/neu oncogene. *Science* 235: 177-182.
2720. Slanetz PJ, Whitman GJ, Halpern EF, Hall DA, McCarthy KA, Simeone JF (1997). Imaging of fallopian tube tumors. *AJR Am J Roentgenol* 169: 1321-1324.
2720a. Slattery ML, Kerber RA (1993). A comprehensive evaluation of family history and breast cancer risk. The Utah Population Database. *JAMA* 270: 1563-1568.
2721. Sloan D (1988). Diagnosis of a tumor with an unusual presentation in the pelvis. *Am J Obstet Gynecol* 159: 826-827.
2722. Sloane JP (2001). *Biopsy Pathology of the Breast.* 2nd ed. Arnold: London.
2723. Sloane JP, Amendoeira I, Apostolikas N, Bellocq JP, Bianchi S, Boecker W, Bussolati G, Coleman D, Connolly CE, Dervan P, Eusebi V, De Miguel C, Drijkoningen M, Elston CW, Faverley D, Gad A, Jacquemier J, Lacerda M, Martinez-Penuela J, Munt C, Peterse JL, Rank F, Sylvan M, Tsakraklides V, Zafrani B (1998). Consistency achieved by 23 European pathologists in categorizing ductal carcinoma in situ of the breast using five classifications. European Commission Working Group on Breast Screening Pathology. *Hum Pathol* 29: 1056-1062.
2724. Sloane JP, Amendoeira I, Apostolikas N, Bellocq JP, Bianchi S, Boecker W, Bussolati G, Coleman D, Connolly CE, Eusebi V, De Miguel C, Dervan P, Drijkoningen R, Elston CW, Faverly D, Gad A, Jacquemier J, Lacerda M, Martinez-Penuela J, Munt C, Peterse JL, Rank F, Sylvan M, Tsakraklides V, Zafrani B (1999). Consistency achieved by 23 European pathologists from 12 countries in diagnosing breast disease and reporting prognostic features of carcinomas. European Commission Working Group on Breast Screening Pathology. *Virchows Arch* 434: 3-10.
2725. Sloane JP, Mayers MM (1993). Carcinoma and atypical hyperplasia in radial scars and complex sclerosing lesions: importance of lesion size and patient age. *Histopathology* 23: 225-231.
2726. Sloboda J, Zaviacic M, Jakubovsky J, Hammar E, Johnsen J (1998). Metastasizing adenocarcinoma of the female prostate (Skene's paraurethral glands). Histological and immunohistochemical prostate markers studies and first ultrastructural observation. *Pathol Res Pract* 194: 129-136.
2727. Slomovitz BM, Caputo TA, Gretz HF, III, Economos K, Tortoriello DV, Schlosshauer PW, Baergen RN, Isacson C, Soslow RA (2002). A comparative analysis of 57 serous borderline tumors with and without a noninvasive micropapillary component. *Am J Surg Pathol* 26: 592-600.
2728. Smit VT, Cornelisse CJ, De Jong D, Dijkshoorn NJ, Peters AA, Fleuren GJ (1988). Analysis of tumor heterogeneity in a patient with synchronously occurring female genital tract malignancies by DNA flow cytometry, DNA fingerprinting, and immunohistochemistry. *Cancer* 62: 1146-1152.
2729. Smith-Warner SA, Spiegelman D, Yaun SS, van den Brandt PA, Folsom AR, Goldbohm RA, Graham S, Holmberg L, Howe GR, Marshall JR, Miller AB, Potter JD, Speizer FE, Willett WC, Wolk A, Hunter DJ (1998). Alcohol and breast cancer in women: a pooled analysis of cohort studies. *JAMA* 279: 535-540.
2730. Smith BH, Taylor HB (1969). The occurrence of bone and cartilage in mammary tumors. *Am J Clin Pathol* 51: 610-618.
2731. Smith DR, Ji CY, Goh HS (1996). Prognostic significance of p53 overexpression and mutation in colorectal adenocarcinomas. *Br J Cancer* 74: 216-223.
2732. Smith HO, Qualls CR, Romero AR, Webb JC, Dorin MH, Padilla LA, Key CR (2002). Is there a difference in survival for IA1 and IA2 adenocarcinoma of the uterine cervix? *Gynec Oncol* 85: 229-241.
2733. Smith J, Munoz N, Herrero R, Eluf-Neto J, Ngelangel C, Franceschi S, Bosch FX, Walboomers JM, Peeling RW (2002). Evidence for Chlamydia trachomatis as a human papillomavirus cofactor in the etiology of invasive cervical cancer in Brazil and the Philippines. *J Infect Dis* 185: 324-331.
2734. Smith JS, Herrero R, Bosetti C, Munoz N, Bosch FX, Eluf-Neto J, Castellsague X, Meijer CJ, van den Brule AJ, Franceschi S, Ashley R (2002). Herpes simplex virus-2 as a human papillomavirus cofactor in the etiology of invasive cervical cancer. *J Natl Cancer Inst* 94: 1604-1613.
2735. Smith TM, Lee MK, Szabo CI, Jerome N, McEuen M, Taylor M, Hood L, King MC (1996). Complete genomic sequence and analysis of 117 kb of human DNA containing the gene BRCA1. *Genome Res* 6: 1029-1049.
2736. Smith YR, Quint EH, Hinton EL (1998). Recurrent benign mullerian papilloma of the cervix. *J Pediatr Adolesc Gynecol* 11: 29-31.
2737. Snyder RR, Norris HJ, Tavassoli F (1988). Endometrioid proliferative and low malignant potential tumors of the ovary. A clinicopathologic study of 46 cases. *Am J Surg Pathol* 12: 661-671.
2738. Soares J, Tomasic G, Bucciarelli E, Eusebi V (1994). Intralobular growth of myoepithelial cell carcinoma of the breast. *Virchows Arch* 425: 205-210.
2739. Sobin LH, Wittekind CH (1997). *Breast Tumours in TNM.* 5th ed. Wiley-Liss: New York.
2740. Sodha N, Houlston RS, Bullock SL, Yuille MA, Chu C, Turner G, Eeles RA (2002). Increasing evidence that germline mutations in CHEK2 do not cause Li-Fraumeni syndrome. *Hum Mutat* 20: 460-462.
2741. Sodha N, Houlston RS, Williams R, Yuille MA, Mangion J, Eeles RA (2002). A robust method for detecting CHK2/RAD53 mutations in genomic DNA. *Hum Mutat* 19: 173-177.
2742. Sodha N, Williams R, Mangion J, Bullock SL, Yuille MR, Eeles RA (2000). Screening hCHK2 for mutations. *Science* 289: 359.
2743. Soga J, Osaka M, Yakuwa Y (2000). Carcinoids of the ovary: an analysis of 329 reported cases. *J Exp Clin Cancer Res* 19: 271-280.
2744. Solin LJ, Fowble BL, Yeh IT, Kowalyshyn MJ, Schultz DJ, Weiss MC, Goodman RL (1992). Microinvasive ductal carcinoma of the breast treated with breast-conserving surgery and definitive irradiation. *Int J Radiat Oncol Biol Phys* 23: 961-968.
2745. Somasundaram K, Zhang H, Zeng YX, Houvras Y, Peng Y, Zhang H, Wu GS, Licht JD, Weber BL, El Deiry WS (1997). Arrest of the cell cycle by the tumour-suppressor BRCA1 requires the CDK-inhibitor p21WAF1/CiP1. *Nature* 389: 187-190.

2746. Somerville JE, Clarke LA, Biggart JD (1992). c-erbB-2 overexpression and histological type of in situ and invasive breast carcinoma. *J Clin Pathol* 45: 16-20.

2747. Sonnendecker HE, Cooper K, Kalian KN (1994). Primary fallopian tube adenocarcinoma in situ associated with adjuvant tamoxifen therapy for breast carcinoma. *Gynecol Oncol* 52: 402-407.

2748. Sonoda Y, Saigo PE, Federici MG, Boyd J (2000). Carcinosarcoma of the ovary in a patient with a germline BRCA2 mutation: evidence for monoclonal origin. *Gynecol Oncol* 76: 226-229.

2749. Sood AK, Sorosky JI, Gelder MS, Buller RE, Anderson B, Wilkinson EJ, Benda JA, Morgan LS (1998). Primary ovarian sarcoma: analysis of prognostic variables and the role of surgical cytoreduction. *Cancer* 82: 1731-1737.

2750. Soomro S, Shousha S, Taylor P, Shepard HM, Feldmann M (1991). c-erbB-2 expression in different histological types of invasive breast carcinoma. *J Clin Pathol* 44: 211-214.

2751. Sorbe B, Risberg B, Thornthwaite J (1994). Nuclear morphometry and DNA flow cytometry as prognostic methods for endometrial carcinoma. *Int J Gynecol Cancer* 4: 94-100.

2752. Sordillo PP, Chapman R, Hajdu SI, Magill GB, Golbey RB (1981). Lymphangiosarcoma. *Cancer* 48: 1674-1679.

2753. Soreide JA, Anda O, Eriksen L, Holter J, Kjellevold KH (1988). Pleomorphic adenoma of the human breast with local recurrence. *Cancer* 61: 997-1001.

2754. Sorensen FB, Paulsen SM (1987). Glycogen-rich clear cell carcinoma of the breast: a solid variant with mucus. A light microscopic, immunohistochemical and ultrastructural study of a case. *Histopathology* 11: 857-869.

2755. Sorensen HT, Friis S, Olsen JH, Thulstrup AM, Mellemkjaer L, Linet M, Trichopoulos D, Vilstrup H, Olsen J (1998). Risk of breast cancer in men with liver cirrhosis. *Am J Gastroenterol* 93: 231-233.

2756. Sorlie T, Perou CM, Tibshirani R, Aas T, Geisler S, Johnsen H, Hastie T, Eisen MB, van de Rijn M, Jeffrey SS, Thorsen T, Quist H, Matese JC, Brown PO, Botstein D, Eystein LP, Borresen-Dale AL (2001). Gene expression patterns of breast carcinomas distinguish tumor subclasses with clinical implications. *Proc Natl Acad Sci USA* 98: 10869-10874.

2757. Sorlie T, Tibshirani R, Parker J, Hastie T, Marron JS, Nobel A, Deng S, Johnsen H, Pesich R, Geisler S, Demeter J, Perou CM, Lonning PE, Brown PO, Borresen-Dale AL, Botstein D (2003). Repeated observation of breast tumor subtypes in independent gene expression data sets. Proc Natl Acad Sci USA 100: 8418-8423.

2758. Soslow RA, Rouse RV, Hendrickson MR, Silva EG, Longacre TA (1996). Transitional cell neoplasms of the ovary and urinary bladder: a comparative immunohistochemical analysis. *Int J Gynecol Pathol* 15: 257-265.

2759. Soussi T (1996). The p53 tumour suppressor gene: a model for molecular epidemiology of human cancer. *Mol Med Today* 2: 32-37.

2760. Soussi T, Beroud C (2001). Assessing TP53 status in human tumours to evaluate clinical outcome. *Nat Rev Cancer* 1: 233-240.

2761. Soussi T, Dehouche K, Beroud C (2000). p53 website and analysis of p53 gene mutations in human cancer: forging a link between epidemiology and carcinogenesis. *Hum Mutat* 15: 105-113.

2762. Spagnolo DV, Shilkin KB (1983). Breast neoplasms containing bone and cartilage. *Virchows Arch A Pathol Anat Histopathol* 400: 287-295.

2763. Spatz A, Bouron D, Pautier P, Castaigne D, Duvillard P (1998). Primary yolk sac tumor of the endometrium: a case report and review of the literature. *Gynecol Oncol* 70: 285-288.

2764. Spiegel GW (1995). Endometrial carcinoma in situ in postmenopausal women. *Am J Surg Pathol* 19: 417-432.

2765. Spitz DJ, Reddy VB, Gattuso P (1999). Fine-needle aspiration of pseudoangiomatous stromal hyperplasia of the breast. Diagn Cytopathol 20: 323-324.

2766. Spitzer M (1999). Lower genital tract intraepithelial neoplasia in HIV-infected women: guidelines for evaluation and management. *Obstet Gynecol Surv* 54: 131-137.

2767. Sreenan JJ, Hart WR (1995). Carcinosarcomas of the female genital tract. A pathologic study of 29 metastatic tumors: further evidence for the dominant role of the epithelial component and the conversion theory of histogenesis. *Am J Surg Pathol* 19: 666-674.

2768. Srigley JR, Colgan TJ (1988). Multifocal and diffuse adenomatoid tumor involving uterus and fallopian tube. *Ultrastruct Pathol* 12: 351-355.

2769. Srivatsa PJ, Keeney GL, Podratz KC (1994). Disseminated cervical adenoma malignum and bilateral ovarian sex cord tumors with annular tubules associated with Peutz-Jeghers syndrome. *Gynecol Oncol* 53: 256-264.

2770. Ssali JC, Gakwaya A, Katongole-Mbidde F (1995). Risk factors for breast cancer in Ugandan women: a case-control study. *East Central Afr J Surg* 1: 9-13.

2771. Staebler A, Heselmeyer-Haddad K, Bell K, Riopel M, Perlman E, Ried T, Kurman RJ (2002). Micropapillary serous carcinoma of the ovary has distinct patterns of chromosomal imbalances by comparative genomic hybridization compared with atypical proliferative serous tumors and serous carcinomas. *Hum Pathol* 33: 47-59.

2772. Staebler A, Lax SF, Ellenson LH (2000). Altered expression of hMLH1 and hMSH2 protein in endometrial carcinomas with microsatellite instability. *Hum Pathol* 31: 354-358.

2773. Stalsberg H, Blom PE, Bostad LH, Westgaard G (1983). *An International Survey of Distributions of Histologic Types of Tumours of the Testis and Ovary (Ovarian tumours and endometriosis in Norway General Hospital material)*. UICC: Geneva.

2774. Stambolic V, Suzuki A, de la Pompa JL, Brothers GM, Mirtsos C, Sasaki T, Ruland J, Penninger JM, Siderovski DP, Mak TW (1998). Negative regulation of PKB/Akt-dependent cell survival by the tumor suppressor PTEN. *Cell* 95: 29-39.

2775. Stankovic T, Kidd AM, Sutcliffe A, McGuire GM, Robinson P, Weber P, Bedenham T, Bradwell AR, Easton DF, Lennox GG, Haites N, Byrd PJ, Taylor AM (1998). ATM mutations and phenotypes in ataxia-telangiectasia families in the British Isles: expression of mutant ATM and the risk of leukemia, lymphoma, and breast cancer. *Am J Hum Genet* 62: 334-345.

2775a. Stapleton JJ, Holser MH, Linder LE (1981). Paramesonephric papillary serous cystadenocarcinoma. A case report with scanning electron microscopy. *Acta Cytol* 25: 310-316.

2776. Starink TM, van der Veen JP, Arwert F, de Waal LP, de Lange GG, Gille JJ, Eriksson AW (1986). The Cowden syndrome: a clinical and genetic study in 21 patients. *Clin Genet* 29: 222-233.

2777. Steck PA, Pershouse MA, Jasser SA, Yung WK, Lin H, Ligon AH, Langford LA, Baumgard ML, Hattier T, Davis T, Frye C, Hu R, Swedlund B, Teng DH, Tavtigian SV (1997). Identification of a candidate tumour suppressor gene, MMAC1, at chromosome 10q23.3 that is mutated in multiple advanced cancers. *Nat Genet* 15: 356-362.

2778. Steeper TA, Piscioli F, Rosai J (1983). Squamous cell carcinoma with sarcoma-like stroma of the female genital tract. Clinicopathologic study of four cases. *Cancer* 52: 890-898.

2779. Steeper TA, Rosai J (1983). Aggressive angiomyxoma of the female pelvis and perineum. Report of nine cases of a distinctive type of gynecologic soft-tissue neoplasm. *Am J Surg Pathol* 7: 463-475.

2780. Steeper TA, Wick MR (1986). Minimal deviation adenocarcinoma of the uterine cervix ("adenoma malignum"). An immunohistochemical comparison with microglandular endocervical hyperplasia and conventional endocervical adenocarcinoma. *Cancer* 58: 1131-1138.

2781. Stefani M, Speranza N (1970). [A case of cylindroma of the vagina]. *Riv Anat Patol Oncol* 36: 77-105.

2782. Stehman FB, Bundy BN, Disaia PJ, Keys HM, Larson JE, Fowler WC (1991). Carcinoma of the cervix treated with radiation therapy. I. A multi-variate analysis of prognostic variables in the Gynecologic Oncology Group. *Cancer* 67: 2776-2785.

2783. Stehman FB, Bundy BN, Dvoretsky PM, Creasman WT (1992). Early stage I carcinoma of the vulva treated with ipsilateral superficial inguinal lymphadenectomy and modified radical hemivulvectomy: a prospective study of the Gynecologic Oncology Group. *Obstet Gynecol* 79: 490-497.

2784. Steingaszner LC, Enzinger FM, Taylor HB (1965). Hemangiosarcoma of the breast. *Cancer* 18: 352-361.

2785. Stenkvist B, Bengtsson E, Dahlqvist B, Eklund G, Eriksson O, Jarkrans T, Nordin B (1982). Predicting breast cancer recurrence. *Cancer* 50: 2884-2893.

2786. Stenwig JT, Hazekamp JT, Beecham JB (1979). Granulosa cell tumors of the ovary. A clinicopathological study of 118 cases with long-term follow-up. *Gynecol Oncol* 7: 136-152.

2787. Stephenson TJ, Mills PM (1986). Adenomatoid tumours: an immunohistochemical and ultrastructural appraisal of their histogenesis. *J Pathol* 148: 327-335.

2788. Sternberg WH, Barclay DL (1966). Luteoma of pregnancy. *Am J Obstet Gynecol* 95: 165-184.

2789. Sternberg WH, Roth LM (1973). Ovarian stromal tumors containing Leydig cells. I. Stromal-Leydig cell tumor and non-neoplastic transformation of ovarian stroma to Leydig cells. *Cancer* 32: 940-951.

2790. Stettner AR, Hartenbach EM, Schink JC, Huddart R, Becker J, Pauli R, Long R, Laxova R (1999). Familial ovarian germ cell cancer: report and review. *Am J Med Genet* 84: 43-46.

2791. Stevens RG (1987). Electric power use and breast cancer: a hypothesis. *Am J Epidemiol* 125: 556-561.

2792. Stewart CJ, Nandini CL, Richmond JA (2000). Value of A103 (melan-A) immunostaining in the differential diagnosis of ovarian sex cord stromal tumours. *J Clin Pathol* 53: 206-211.

2793. Stewart FW, Treves N (1949). Lymphangiosarcoma in postmastectomy lymphedema. A report of six cases of elephantiasis chirurgica. *Cancer* 1: 64-81.

2794. Stock RJ, Zaino R, Bundy BN, Askin FB, Woodward J, Fetter B, Paulson JA, Disaia PJ, Stehman FB (1994). Evaluation and comparison of histopathologic grading systems of epithelial carcinoma of the uterine cervix: Gynecologic Oncology Group studies. *Int J Gynecol Pathol* 13: 99-108.

2795. Stocks LH, Patterson FM (1976). Inflammatory carcinoma of the breast. *Surg Gynecol Obstet* 143: 885-889.

2796. Stomper PC, Connolly JL (1992). Ductal carcinoma in situ of the breast: correlation between mammographic calcification and tumor subtype. *AJR Am J Roentgenol* 159: 483-485.

2797. Stone GC, Bell DA, Fuller A, Dickersin GR, Scully RE (1986). Malignant schwannoma of the ovary. Report of a case. *Cancer* 58: 1575-1582.

2798. Storm HH, Jensen OM (1986). Risk of contralateral breast cancer in Denmark 1943-80. *Br J Cancer* 54: 483-492.

2799. Storm HH, Olsen J (1999). Risk of breast cancer in offspring of male breast-cancer patients. *Lancet* 353: 209.

2800. Stratton JF, Gayther SA, Russell P, Dearden J, Gore M, Blake P, Easton D, Ponder BA (1997). Contribution of BRCA1 mutations to ovarian cancer. *N Engl J Med* 336: 1125-1130.

2801. Stratton JF, Pharoah P, Smith SK, Easton D, Ponder BA (1998). A systematic review and meta-analysis of family history and risk of ovarian cancer. *Br J Obstet Gynaecol* 105: 493-499.

2802. Stratton JF, Thompson D, Bobrow L, Dalal N, Gore M, Bishop DT, Scott I, Evans G, Daly P, Easton DF, Ponder BA (1999). The genetic epidemiology of early-onset epithelial ovarian cancer: a population-based study. *Am J Hum Genet* 65: 1725-1732.

2803. Straughn JM Jr., Richter HE, Conner MG, Meleth S, Barnes MN (2001). Predictors of outcome in small cell carcinoma of the cervix--a case series. *Gynecol Oncol* 83: 216-220.

2804. Sturgeon SR, Brinton LA, Devesa SS, Kurman RJ (1992). In situ and invasive vulvar cancer incidence trends (1973 to 1987). *Am J Obstet Gynecol* 166: 1482-1485.

2805. Sturgeon SR, Sherman ME, Kurman RJ, Berman ML, Mortel R, Twiggs LB, Barrett RJ, Wilbanks GD, Brinton LA (1998). Analysis of histopathological features of endometrioid uterine carcinomas and epidemiologic risk factors. Cancer Epidemiol Biomarkers Prev 7: 231-235.

2806. Stutz JA, Evans AJ, Pinder S, Ellis IO, Yeoman LJ, Wilson AR, Sibbering DM (1994). The radiological appearances of invasive cribriform carcinoma of the breast. Nottingham Breast Team. *Clin Radiol* 49: 693-695.

2807. Su TH, Wang JC, Tseng HH, Chang CP, Chang TA, Wei HJ, Chang JG (1998). Analysis of FHIT transcripts in cervical and endometrial cancers. *Int J Cancer* 76: 216-222.

2808. Su Y, Swift M (2000). Mortality rates among carriers of ataxia-telangiectasia mutant alleles. *Ann Intern Med* 133: 770-778.

2809. Su Y, Swift M (2001). Outcomes of adjuvant radiation therapy for breast cancer in women with ataxia-telangiectasia mutations. *JAMA* 286: 2233-2234.

2810. Su YN, Cheng WF, Chen CA, Lin TY, Hsieh FJ, Cheng SP, Hsieh CY (1999). Pregnancy with primary tubal placental site trophoblastic tumor--A case report and literature review. *Gynecol Oncol* 73: 322-325.

2811. Suarez A, Palacios J, Burgos E, Gamallo C (1993). Signet-ring stromal tumor of the ovary: a histochemical, immunohistochemical and ultrastructural study. *Virchows Arch A Pathol Anat Histopathol* 422: 333-336.

2812. Suarez VD, Gimenez PA, Rio SM (1990). Vaginal rhabdomyoma and adenosis. *Histopathology* 16: 393-394.

2813. Sugiyama T, Ohta S, Nishida T, Okura N, Tanabe K, Yakushiji M (1998). Two cases of endometrial adenocarcinoma arising from atypical polypoid adenomyoma. *Gynecol Oncol* 71: 141-144.

2814. Sullivan JJ, Magee HR, Donald KJ (1977). Secretory (juvenile) carcinoma of the breast. *Pathology* 9: 341-346.

2815. Sumpio BE, Jennings TA, Merino MJ, Sullivan PD (1987). Adenoid cystic carcinoma of the breast. Data from the Connecticut Tumor Registry and a review of the literature. *Ann Surg* 205: 295-301.

2816. Suster S, Moran CA, Hurt MA (1991). Syringomatous squamous tumors of the breast. *Cancer* 67: 2350-2355.

2817. Suzuki A, de la Pompa JL, Stambolic V, Elia AJ, Sasaki T, del Barco Barrantes I, Ho A, Wakeham A, Itie A, Khoo W, Fukumoto M, Mak TW (1998). High cancer susceptibility and embryonic lethality associated with mutation of the PTEN tumor suppressor gene in mice. *Curr Biol* 8: 1169-1178.

2818. Swanson GP, Dobin SM, Arber JM, Arber DA, Capen CV, Diaz JA (1997). Chromosome 11 abnormalities in Bowen disease of the vulva. *Cancer Genet Cytogenet* 93: 109-114.

2819. Swift M, Morrell D, Massey RB, Chase CL (1991). Incidence of cancer in 161 families affected by ataxia-telangiectasia. *N Engl J Med* 325: 1831-1836.

2820. Swift M, Reitnauer PJ, Morrell D, Chase CL (1987). Breast and other cancers in families with ataxia-telangiectasia. *N Engl J Med* 316: 1289-1294.

2821. Switzer JM, Weckstein ML, Campbell LF, Curtis KL, Powaser JT (1984). Ovarian hydatidiform mole. *J Ultrasound Med* 3: 471-473.

2822. Sworn MJ, Hammond GT, Buchanan R (1979). Mixed mesenchymal sarcoma of the broad ligament: case report. *Br J Obstet Gynaecol* 86: 403-406.

2823. Symonds RP, Habeshaw T, Paul J, Kerr DJ, Darling A, Burnett RA, Sotsiou F, Linardopoulos S, Spandidos DA (1992). No correlation between ras, c-myc and c-jun proto-oncogene expression and prognosis in advanced carcinoma of cervix. *Eur J Cancer* 28A: 1615-1617.

2824. Szabo CI, King MC (1997). Population genetics of BRCA1 and BRCA2. *Am J Hum Genet* 60: 1013-1020.

2825. Szabo CI, Wagner LA, Francisco LV, Roach JC, Argonza R, King MC, Ostrander EA (1996). Human, canine and murine BRCA1 genes: sequence comparison among species. *Hum Mol Genet* 5: 1289-1298.

2826. Szarewski A, Cuzick J (1998). Smoking and cervical neoplasia: a review of the evidence. *J Epidem Biostat* 3: 229-256.

2827. Szukala SA, Marks JR, Burchette JL, Elbendary AA, Krigman HR (1999). Co-expression of p53 by epithelial and stromal elements in carcinosarcoma of the female genital tract: an immunohistochemical study of 19 cases. *Int J Gynecol Cancer* 9: 131-136.

2828. Szulman AE, Surti U (1978). The syndromes of hydatidiform mole. I. Cytogenetic and morphologic correlations. *Am J Obstet Gynecol* 131: 665-671.

2829. Szulman AE, Surti U (1978). The syndromes of hydatidiform mole. II. Morphologic evolution of the complete and partial mole. *Am J Obstet Gynecol* 132: 20-27.

2830. Szych C, Staebler A, Connolly DC, Wu R, Cho KR, Ronnett BM (1999). Molecular genetic evidence supporting the clonality and appendiceal origin of Pseudomyxoma peritonei in women. *Am J Pathol* 154: 1849-1855.

2831. Szyfelbein WM, Young RH, Scully RE (1994). Cystic struma ovarii: a frequently unrecognized tumor. A report of 20 cases. *Am J Surg Pathol* 18: 785-788.

2832. Szyfelbein WM, Young RH, Scully RE (1995). Struma ovarii simulating ovarian tumors of other types. A report of 30 cases. *Am J Surg Pathol* 19: 21-29.

2833. Tagaya N, Kodaira H, Kogure H, Shimizu K (1999). A case of phyllodes tumor with bloody nipple discharge in juvenile patient. *Breast Cancer* 6: 207-210.

2834. Tai LH, Tavassoli FA (2002). Endometrial polyps with atypical (bizarre) stromal cells. *Am J Surg Pathol* 26: 505-509.

2835. Takahashi M, Kigawa J, Ishihara K, Shimada M, Kamei T, Terakawa N (2002). Hydrotubation for diagnosing carcinoma in situ of the fallopian tube. A case report. *Acta Cytol* 46: 735-737.

2836. Takahashi O, Shibata S, Hatazawa J, Takisawa J, Sato H, Ota H, Tanaka T (1998). Mature cystic teratoma of the uterine corpus. *Acta Obstet Gynecol Scand* 77: 936-938.

2837. Takahashi T, Moriki T, Hiroi M, Nakayama H (1998). Invasive lobular carcinoma of the breast with osteoclastlike giant cells. A case report. *Acta Cytol* 42: 734-741.

2838. Takemori M, Nishimura R, Yasuda D, Sugimura K (1997). Carcinosarcoma of the uterus: magnetic resonance imaging. *Gynecol Obstet Invest* 43: 139-141.

2839. Takeshima N, Tabata T, Nishida H, Furuta N, Tsuzuku M, Hirai Y, Hasumi K (2001). Peripheral primitive neuroectodermal tumor of the vulva: report of a case with imprint cytology. *Acta Cytol* 45: 1049-1052.

2840. Takeuchi K, Murata K, Funaki K, Fujita I, Hayakawa Y, Kitazawa S (2000). Liposarcoma of the uterine cervix: case report. *Eur J Gynaecol Oncol* 21: 290-291.

2841. Takeuchi S (1982). Nature of invasive mole and its rational management. *Semin Oncol* 9: 181-186.

2842. Takeuchi S, Ishihara N, Ohbayashi C, Itoh H, Maruo T (1999). Stromal Leydig cell tumor of the ovary. Case report and literature review. *Int J Gynecol Pathol* 18: 178-182.

2843. Talamonti MS (1996). Management of ductal carcinoma in situ. *Semin Surg Oncol* 12: 300-313.

2844. Talerman A (1972). A distinctive gonadal neoplasm related to gonadoblastoma. *Cancer* 30: 1219-1224.

2845. Talerman A (1972). A mixed germ cell-sex cord stroma tumor of the ovary in a normal female infant. *Obstet Gynecol* 40: 473-478.

2846. Talerman A (1974). Gonadoblastoma associated with embryonal carcinoma. *Obstet Gynecol* 43: 138-142.

2847. Talerman A (1980). The pathology of gonadal neoplasms composed of germ cells and sex cord stroma derivatives. *Pathol Res Pract* 170: 24-38.

2848. Talerman A (1994). Germ cell tumours of the ovary. In: *Blaustein's Pathology of the Female Genital Tract, RJ Kurman (ed.), 4th* ed. Springer-Verlag: New York, pp. 849-914.

2849. Talerman A (2002). Mixed germ cell-sex cord stromal tumours. In: Haines and Taylor, Gynaecological and Obstetrical Pathology, 5th ed. Churchill Livingstone: Edingburgh.

2850. Talerman A (2002). Mixed germ cell tumors of the ovary. In: *Blaustein's Pathology of the Female Genital Tract, RJ Kurman, A Blaustein (eds.), 5th ed.* Springer Verlag: New York.

2851. Talerman A, Auerbach WM, van Meurs AJ (1981). Primary chondrosarcoma of the ovary. *Histopathology* 5: 319-324.

2852. Talerman A, van der Harten JJ (1977). Mixed germ cell-sex cord stroma tumor of the ovary associated with isosexual precocious puberty in a normal girl. *Cancer* 40: 889-894.

2853. Tallini G, Price FV, Carcangiu ML (1993). Epithelioid angiosarcoma arising in uterine leiomyomas. *Am J Clin Pathol* 100: 514-518.

2854. Tallini G, Vanni R, Manfioletti G, Kazmierczak B, Faa G, Pauwels P, Bullerdiek J, Giancotti V, Van den Berghe H, Dal Cin P (2000). HMGI-C and HMGI(Y) immunoreactivity correlates with cytogenetic abnormalities in lipomas, pulmonary chondroid hamartomas, endometrial polyps, and uterine leiomyomas and is compatible with rearrangement of the HMGI-C and HMGI(Y) genes. *Lab Invest* 80: 359-369.

2855. Talwar S, Prasad N, Gandhi S, Prasad P (1999). Haemangiopericytoma of the adult male breast. *Int J Clin Pract* 53: 485-486.

2856. Tambouret R, Bell DA, Young RH (2000). Microcystic endocervical adenocarcinomas: a report of eight cases. *Am J Surg Pathol* 24: 369-374.

2857. Tamimi HK, Bolen JW (1984). Enchondromatosis (Ollier's disease) and ovarian juvenile granulosa cell tumor. *Cancer* 53: 1605-1608.

2858. Tamura S, Enjoji M (1988). Elastosis in neoplastic and non-neoplastic tissues from patients with mammary carcinoma. *Acta Pathol Jpn* 38: 1537-1546.

2859. Tanaka Y, Sasaki Y, Nishihira H, Izawa T, Nishi T (1992). Ovarian juvenile granulosa cell tumor associated with Maffucci's syndrome. *Am J Clin Pathol* 97: 523-527.

2860. Tang CK, Toker C, Ances IG (1979). Stromomyoma of the uterus. *Cancer* 43: 308-316.

2861. Tariel D, Body G, Fetissof F, Menard F, Lansac J (1986). [Postoperative vaginal pseudosarcoma. Apropos of a case]. *J Gynecol Obstet Biol Reprod (Paris)* 15: 769-771.

2862. Taruscio D, Carcangiu ML, Ward DC (1993). Detection of trisomy 12 on ovarian sex cord stromal tumors by fluorescence in situ hybridization. *Diagn Mol Pathol* 2: 94-98.

2863. Tashiro H, Isacson C, Levine R, Kurman RJ, Cho KR, Hedrick L (1997). p53 gene mutations are common in uterine serous carcinoma and occur early in their pathogenesis. *Am J Pathol* 150: 177-185.

2864. Tasseron EW, van der Esch EP, Hart AA, Brutel de la Riviere G, Aartsen EJ (1992). A clinicopathological study of 30 melanomas of the vulva. *Gynecol Oncol* 46: 170-175.

2865. Tateno H, Sasano N (1983). An International Survey of Distribution of Histologic Types Tumours of the Testis and Ovary (Ovarian Tumours in Sendai Japan. General Hospital Material). UICC Technical Report Series: Genova.

2866. Tavassoli FA (1986). Melanotic paraganglioma of the uterus. *Cancer* 58: 942-948.

2867. Tavassoli FA (1988). Serous tumor of low malignant potential with early stromal invasion (serous LMP with microinvasion). *Mod Pathol* 1: 407-414.

2868. Tavassoli FA (1991). Myoepithelial lesions of the breast. Myoepitheliosis, adenomyoepithelioma, and myoepithelial carcinoma. *Am J Surg Pathol* 15: 554-568.

2869. Tavassoli FA (1992). Carcinoma with osteoclastic giant cells. In: *Pathology of the Breast,* Appleton and Lange: Norwalk, Connecticut.

2870. Tavassoli FA (1992). Glycogen-rich (clear-cell) carcinoma. In: *Pathology of the Breast,* Appleton and Lange: Norwalk, Connecticut .

2871. Tavassoli FA (1992). Mesenchymal lesions. In: *Pathology of the Breast,* Tavassoli FA, ed., First edition ed. Appleton and Lange: Norwalk , pp. 557-558.

2872. Tavassoli FA (1992). Metastatic carcinoma. In: *Pathology of the Breast,* Appleton and Lange: Norwalk, Connecticut.

2873. Tavassoli FA (1992). Papillary lesions. In: *Pathology of the Breast,* Appleton and Lange: Stamford , pp. 193-228.

2874. Tavassoli FA (1992). Pathology of the Breast. Appleton and Lange: Stanford.

2875. Tavassoli FA (1999). Myoepithelial lesions. In: *Pathology of the Breast,* 2nd ed. Appleton and Lange: Hartford, pp. 763-791.

2876. Tavassoli FA (1999). *Pathology of the Breast.* 2nd ed. Appleton-Lange: Stamford.

2877. Tavassoli FA, Andrade R, Merino M (1990). Retiform wolffian adenoma. In: *Progress in Surgical Pathology,* CM Fenoglio-Preiser, M Wolfe, F Rilke (eds.), Field & Wood Medica Publishers inc: New York, pp. 121-136.

2878. Tavassoli FA, Andradre R, Merino M (1990). Retiform wolffian adenoma. *Progress in Surgical Pathology*. Field & Wood Medical Publishers: New York.

2879. Tavassoli FA, Norris HJ (1979). Smooth muscle tumors of the vagina. *Obstet Gynecol* 53: 689-693.

2880. Tavassoli FA, Norris HJ (1979). Smooth muscle tumors of the vulva. *Obstet Gynecol* 53: 213-217.

2881. Tavassoli FA, Norris HJ (1980). Secretory carcinoma of the breast. *Cancer* 45: 2404-2413.

2882. Tavassoli FA, Norris HJ (1980). Sertoli tumors of the ovary. A clinicopathologic study of 28 cases with ultrastructural observations. *Cancer* 46: 2281-2297.

2883. Tavassoli FA, Norris HJ (1981). Mesenchymal tumours of the uterus. VII. A clinicopathological study of 60 endometrial stromal nodules. *Histopathology* 5: 1-10.

2884. Tavassoli FA, Norris HJ (1983). Microglandular adenosis of the breast. A clinicopathologic study of 11 cases with ultrastructural observations. *Am J Surg Pathol* 7: 731-737.

2885. Tavassoli FA, Norris HJ (1986). Mammary adenoid cystic carcinoma with sebaceous differentiation. A morphologic study of the cell types. *Arch Pathol Lab Med* 110: 1045-1053.

2886. Tavassoli FA, Norris HJ (1990). A comparison of the results of long-term follow-up for atypical intraductal hyperplasia and intraductal hyperplasia of the breast. *Cancer* 65: 518-529.

2887. Tavassoli FA, Norris HJ (1994). Intraductal apocrine carcinoma: a clinicopathologic study of 37 cases. *Mod Pathol* 7: 813-818.

2888. Tavassoli FA, Purcell CA, Bratthauer GL, Man Y (1996). Androgen receptor expression along with loss of bcl-2, ER and PR expression in benign and malignant apocrine lesions of the breast: implications for therapy. *Breast Jour* 2: 261-269.

2889. Tavassoli FA, Weiss S (1981). Hemangiopericytoma of the breast. *Am J Surg Pathol* 5: 745-752.

2890. Tavassoli FA, Yeh IT (1988). Surgical pathology of the ovary: a review of selected tumors. *Mod Pathol* 1: 140-167.

2891. Tavtigian SV, Simard J, Rommens J, Couch F, Shattuck-Eidens D, Neuhausen S, Merajver S, Thorlacius S, Offit K, Stoppa-Lyonnet D, Belanger C, Bell R, Berry S, Bogden R, Chen Q, Davis T, Dumont M, Frye C, Hattier T, Jammulapati S, Janecki T, Jiang P, Kehrer R, Leblanc JF, Mitchell JT, McArthur Morrisson J, Nguyen K, Peng Y, Samson C, Shroeder M, Snyder SC, Steele L, Stringfellow M, Stroup C, Swedlund B, Swensen J, Teng D, Thomas A, Tran T, Tran T, Tranchant M, Weaver Feldhaus J, Wong AKC, Shizuya H, Eyfjord JE, Cannon Albright L, Labrie F, Skolnick MH, Weber B, Kamb A, Goldgar DE (1996). The complete BRCA2 gene and mutations in chromosome 13q-linked kindreds. *Nat Genet* 12: 333-337.

2892. Taxy JB, Trujillo YP (1994). Breast cancer metastatic to the uterus. Clinical manifestations of a rare event. *Arch Pathol Lab Med* 118: 819-821.

2893. Taylor CE, Tuttle HK (1944). Melanocarcinoma of the cervix uteri and vaginal vault. *Arch Pathol* 38: 60-61.

2894. Taylor HB, Robertson A.G. (1965). Adenomas of the nipple. *Cancer* 18: 995-1002.

2894a. Taylor HCJ (1929). Malignant and semimalignant tumors of the ovary. *Surg Gynecol Obstet* 48: 204-230.

2895. Taylor RN, Lacey CG, Shuman MA (1985). Adenocarcinoma of Skene's duct associated with a systemic coagulopathy. *Gynecol Oncol* 22: 250-256.

2896. Teilum G (1965). Endodermal sinus of the ovary and testis: comparative morphogenesis of the so-called mesonephroma ovarii (Schiller) and extraembryonic (yolk sac allantoic) structures of the rat's placenta. *Cancer* 12: 1091-1105.

2897. Teixeira MR, Kristensen GB, Abeler VM, Heim S (1999). Karyotypic findings in tumors of the vulva and vagina. *Cancer Genet Cytogenet* 111: 87-91.

2898. Tempany CM, Zou KH, Silverman SG, Brown DL, Kurtz AB, McNeil BJ (2000). Staging of advanced ovarian cancer: comparison of imaging modalities--report from the Radiological Diagnostic Oncology Group. *Radiology* 215: 761-767.

2899. Terada S, Suzuki N, Uchide K, Shozu M, Akasofu K (1993). Parovarian fibroma with heterotopic bone formation of probable wolffian origin. *Gynecol Oncol* 50: 115-118.

2900. Terzakis JA, Opher E, Melamed J, Santagada E, Sloan D (1990). Pigmented melanocytic schwannoma of the uterine cervix. *Ultrastruct Pathol* 14: 357-366.

2901. Tetu B, Bonenfant JL (1991). Ovarian myxoma. A study of two cases with long-term follow-up. *Am J Clin Pathol* 95: 340-346.

2902. Tetu B, Silva EG, Gershenson DM (1987). Squamous cell carcinoma of the ovary. *Arch Pathol Lab Med* 111: 864-866.

2903. Tewari K, Cappuccini F, Disaia PJ, Berman ML, Manetta A, Kohler MF (2000). Malignant germ cell tumors of the ovary. *Obstet Gynecol* 95: 128-133.

2904. Thakur S, Zhang HB, Peng Y, Le H, Carroll B, Ward T, Yao J, Farid LM, Couch FJ, Wilson RB, Weber BL (1997). Localization of BRCA1 and a splice variant identifies the nuclear localization signal. *Mol Cell Biol* 17: 444-452.

2905. The European Commission (1996). *European Guidelines for Quality Assurance in Mammography Screening*. 2nd ed. The European Commission: Luxembourg.

2906. Thomas DB, Jimenez LM, McTiernan A, Rosenblatt K, Stalsberg H, Stemhagen A, Thompson WD, Curnen MG, Satariano W, Austin DF, et al. (1992). Breast cancer in men: risk factors with hormonal implications. *Am J Epidemiol* 135: 734-748.

2907. Thomas EJ, Campbell IG (2000). Molecular genetic defects in endometriosis. *Gynecol Obstet Invest* 50 Suppl 1: 44-50.

2908. Thomas GM (2000). Concurrent chemotherapy and radiation for locally advanced cervical cancer: the new standard of care. *Semin Radiat Oncol* 10: 44-50.

2909. Thomas HV, Key TJ, Allen DS, Moore JW, Dowsett M, Fentiman IS, Wang DY (1997). A prospective study of endogenous serum hormone concentrations and breast cancer risk in premenopausal women on the island of Guernsey. *Br J Cancer* 75: 1075-1079.

2910. Thomas JP, Timbal Y, Wannin G, Dumurgier C (1973). [Schwannoglioma of the broad ligament]. *J Urol Nephrol (Paris)* 79: 933-935.

2911. Thomas M, Pim D, Banks L (1999). The role of the E6-p53 interaction in the molecular pathogenesis of HPV. *Oncogene* 18: 7690-7700.

2912. Thomas NA, Choong DY, Jokubaitis VJ, Neville PJ, Campbell IG (2001). Mutation of the ST7 tumor suppressor gene on 7q31.1 is rare in breast, ovarian and colorectal cancers. *Nat Genet* 29: 379-380.

2912a. Thomason RW, Rush W, Dave H (1995). Transitional cell carcinoma arising within a paratubal cyst: report of a case. *Int J Gynecol Pathol* 14: 270-273.

2913. Thompson D, Easton D (2001). Variation in cancer risks, by mutation position, in BRCA2 mutation carriers. *Am J Hum Genet* 68: 410-419.

2914. Thompson D, Easton D (2002). Variation in BRCA1 cancer risks by mutation position. Cancer Epidemiol Biomarkers Prev 11: 329-336.

2915. Thompson D, Easton DF (2002). Cancer incidence in BRCA1 mutation carriers. *J Natl Cancer Inst* 94: 1358-1365.

2916. Thompson M, Husemeyer R (1981). Carcinofibroma--a variant of the mixed Mullerian tumour. Case report. *Br J Obstet Gynaecol* 88: 1151-1155.

2917. Thompson ME, Jensen RA, Obermiller PS, Page DL, Holt JT (1995). Decreased expression of BRCA1 accelerates growth and is often present during sporadic breast cancer progression. *Nat Genet* 9: 444-450.

2918. Thompson WD, Schildkraut JM (1991). Family history of gynaecological cancers: relationships to the incidence of breast cancer prior to age 55. *Int J Epidemiol* 20: 595-602.

2919. Thor AD, Young RH, Clement PB (1991). Pathology of the fallopian tube, broad ligament, peritoneum, and pelvic soft tissues. *Hum Pathol* 22: 856-867.

2920. Thorlacius S, Sigurdsson S, Bjarnadottir H, Olafsdottir G, Jonasson JG, Tryggvadottir L, Tulinius H, Eyfjord JE (1997). Study of a single BRCA2 mutation with high carrier frequency in a small population. *Am J Hum Genet* 60: 1079-1084.

2921. Thorlacius S, Struewing JP, Hartge P, Olafsdottir GH, Sigvaldason H, Tryggvadottir L, Wacholder S, Tulinius H, Eyfjord JE (1998). Population-based study of risk of breast cancer in carriers of BRCA2 mutation. *Lancet* 352: 1337-1339.

2922. Thurlbeck WM, Scully RE (1960). Solid teratoma of the ovary. A clinicopathological analysis of 9 cases. *Cancer* 13: 804-811.

2923. Tietze L, Gunther K, Horbe A, Pawlik C, Klosterhalfen B, Handt S, Merkelbach-Bruse S (2000). Benign metastasizing leiomyoma: a cytogenetically balanced but clonal disease. *Hum Pathol* 31: 126-128.

2924. Tiltman AJ (1980). Adenomatoid tumours of the uterus. *Histopathology* 4: 437-443.

2925. Tiltman AJ (1998). Leiomyomas of the uterine cervix: a study of frequency. *Int J Gynecol Pathol* 17: 231-234.

2926. Tiltman AJ, Allard U (2001). Female adnexal tumours of probable Wolffian origin: an immunohistochemical study comparing tumours, mesonephric remnants and paramesonephric derivatives. *Histopathology* 38: 237-242.

2927. Tirkkonen M, Kainu T, Loman N, Johannsson OT, Olsson H, Barkardottir RB, Kallioniemi OP, Borg A (1999). Somatic genetic alterations in BRCA2-associated and sporadic male breast cancer. *Genes Chromosomes Cancer* 24: 56-61.

2928. Tjarks M, Van Voorhis BJ (2000). Treatment of endometrial polyps. *Obstet Gynecol* 96: 886-889.

2929. Tobon H, Murphy AI (1977). Benign blue nevus of the vagina. *Cancer* 40: 3174-3176.

2930. Todorov S (1980). Polyposis of the uterine cervix. *Jugosl Ginekol Opstet* 19: 183-186.

2931. Tohya T, Katabuchi H, Fukuma K, Fujisaki S, Okamura H (1991). Angiosarcoma of the vagina. A light and electronmicroscopy study. *Acta Obstet Gynecol Scand* 70: 169-172.

2932. Toikkanen S (1981). Primary squamous cell carcinoma of the breast. *Cancer* 48: 1629-1632.

2933. Toikkanen S, Eerola E, Ekfors TO (1988). Pure and mixed mucinous breast carcinomas: DNA stemline and prognosis. *J Clin Pathol* 41: 300-303.

2934. Toikkanen S, Kujari H (1989). Pure and mixed mucinous carcinomas of the breast: a clinicopathologic analysis of 61 cases with long-term follow-up. *Hum Pathol* 20: 758-764.

2935. Toikkanen S, Pylkkanen L, Joensuu H (1997). Invasive lobular carcinoma of the breast has better short- and long-term survival than invasive ductal carcinoma. *Br J Cancer* 76: 1234-1240.

2936. Toki T, Kurman RJ, Park JS, Kessis T, Daniel RW, Shah KV (1991). Probable non-papillomavirus etiology of squamous cell carcinoma of the vulva in older women: a clinicopathologic study using in situ hybridization and polymerase chain reaction. *Int J Gynecol Pathol* 10: 107-125.

2937. Toki T, Zhai Y-L, Park JS, Fujii S (1999). Infrequent occurence of high-risk human papillomavirus and of p53 mutation in minimal deviation adenocarcinoma of the cervix. *Int J Gynecol Pathol* 18: 215-219.

2938. Tokunaga M, Land CE, Yamamoto T, Asano M, Tokuoka S, Ezaki H, Nishimori I (1987). Incidence of female breast cancer among atomic bomb survivors, Hiroshima and Nagasaki, 1950-1980. *Radiat Res* 112: 243-272.

2938a. Tommasino M (2001). Early genes of human papillomaviruses. In: *Encyclopedic Reference of Cancer*. Springer-Verlag: Heidelberg, p. 270.

2939. Tonin P, Moslehi R, Green R, Rosen B, Cole D, Boyd N, Cutler C, Margolese R, Carter R, McGillivray B, Ives E, Labrie F, Gilchrist D, Morgan K, Simard J, Narod SA. (1995). Linkage analysis of 26 Canadian breast and breast-ovarian cancer families. *Hum Genet* 95: 545-550.

2940. Topalovski M, Crisan D, Mattson JC (1999). Lymphoma of the breast. A clinicopathologic study of primary and secondary cases. *Arch Pathol Lab Med* 123: 1208-1218.

2941. Tornos C, Silva EG, Khorana SM, Burke TW (1994). High-stage endometrioid carcinoma of the ovary. Prognostic significance of pure versus mixed histologic types. *Am J Surg Pathol* 18: 687-693.

2942. Tornos C, Silva EG, Ordonez NG, Gershenson DM, Young RH, Scully RE (1995). Endometrioid carcinoma of the ovary with a prominent spindle-cell component, a source of diagnostic confusion. A report of 14 cases. *Am J Surg Pathol* 19: 1343-1353.
2943. Tot T (2000). The cytokeratin profile of medullary carcinoma of the breast. *Histopathology* 37: 175-181.
2944. Towfighi J, Simmonds MA, Davidson EA (1983). Mucin and fat emboli in mucinous carcinomas. Cause of hemorrhagic cerebral infarcts. *Arch Pathol Lab Med* 107: 646-649.
2945. Traiman P, Bacchi CE, De Luca LA, Uemura G, Nahas NJ, Nahas EA, Pontes A (1999). Vulvar carcinoma in young patients and its relationship with genital warts. *Eur J Gynaecol Oncol* 20: 191-194.
2946. Treffers PE, Hanselaar AG, Helmerhorst TJ, Koster ME, van Leeuwen FE (2001). [Consequences of diethylstilbestrol during pregnancy; 50 years later still a significant problem]. *Ned Tijdschr Geneeskd* 145: 675-680.
2947. Treilleux T, Mignotte H, Clement-Chassagne C, Guastalla P, Bailly C (1999). Tamoxifen and malignant epithelial-nonepithelial tumours of the endometrium: report of six cases and review of the literature. *Eur J Surg Oncol* 25: 477-482.
2948. Tremblay G, Pearse AGE (2001). Histochemistry of oxidative enzyme systems in human thyroid with special reference to Askanazy cells. *J Pathol Bacteriol* 80: 353-358.
2949. Trimble EL (1996). Melanomas of the vulva and vagina. *Oncology (Huntingt)* 10: 1017-1023.
2950. Trimble EL, Lewis JL Jr., Williams LL, Curtin JP, Chapman D, Woodruff JM, Rubin SC, Hoskins WJ (1992). Management of vulvar melanoma. *Gynecol Oncol* 45: 254-258.
2951. Trivedi P, Dave K, Shah M, Karelia N, Patel D, Wadhwa M (1998). Hepatoid carcinoma of the ovary--a case report. *Eur J Gynaecol Oncol* 19: 167-169.
2952. Trojani M, De Mascarel I, Coquet M, Coindre JM, De Mascarel A (1989). [Osteoclastic type giant cell carcinoma of the breast]. *Ann Pathol* 9: 189-194.
2953. Trojani M, Guiu M, Trouette H, De Mascarel I, Cocquet M (1992). Malignant adenomyoepithelioma of the breast. An immunohistochemical, cytophotometric, and ultrastructural study of a case with lung metastases. *Am J Clin Pathol* 98: 598-602.
2954. Troncone G, Martinez JC, Palombini L, De Rosa G, Mugica C, Rodriguez JA, Zeppa P, Di Vizio D, Lucariello A, Piris MA (1998). Immunohistochemical expression of mdm2 and p21WAF1 in invasive cervical cancer: correlation with p53 protein and high risk HPV infection. *J Clin Pathol* 51: 754-760.
2955. Tsang WY, Chan JK (1996). Endocrine ductal carcinoma in situ (E-DCIS) of the breast: a form of low-grade DCIS with distinctive clinicopathologic and biologic characteristics. *Am J Surg Pathol* 20: 921-943.
2956. Tsang WYW, Chan JKC (1996). Endocrine ductal carcinoma in situ (E-DCIS) of the breast: a form of low-grade DCIS with distinctive clinicopathologic and biologic characteristics. *Am J Surg Pathol* 20: 921-943.
2957. Tseng CJ, Pao CC, Tseng LH, Chang CT, Lai CH, Soong YK, Hsueh S, Jyu-Jen H (1997). Lymphoepithelioma-like carcinoma of the uterine cervix: association with Epstein-Barr virus and human papillomavirus. *Cancer* 80: 91-97.
2958. Tsongalis GJ, Ried A Jr. (2001). HER2: the neu prognostic marker for breast cancer. *Crit Rev Clin Lab Sci* 38: 167-182.
2959. Tsou HC, Teng DH, Ping XL, Brancolini V, Davis T, Hu R, Xie XX, Gruener AC, Schrager CA, Christiano AM, Eng C, Steck P, Ott J, Tavtigian SV, Peacocke M (1997). The role of MMAC1 mutations in early-onset breast cancer: causative in association with Cowden syndrome and excluded in BRCA1-negative cases. *Am J Hum Genet* 61: 1036-1043.
2960. Tsuda H, Callen DF, Fukutomi T, Nakamura Y, Hirohashi S (1994). Allele loss on chromosome 16q24.2-qter occurs frequently in breast cancers respectively of differences in phenotype and extent of spread. *Cancer Res* 54: 513-517.
2961. Tsuda H, Takarabe T, Susumu N, Inazawa J, Okada S, Hirohashi S (1997). Detection of numerical and structural alterations and fusion of chromosomes 16 and 1 in low-grade papillary breast carcinoma by fluorescence in situ hybridization. *Am J Pathol* 151: 1027-1034.
2962. Tsuda HH (2001). Prognostic and predictive value of c-erbB-2 (HER-2/neu) gene amplification in human breast cancer. *Breast Cancer* 8: 38-44.
2963. Tsuji T, Kawauchi S, Utsunomiya T, Nagata Y, Tsuneyoshi M (1997). Fibrosarcoma versus cellular fibroma of the ovary: a comparative study of their proliferative activity and chromosome aberrations using MIB-1 immunostaining, DNA flow cytometry, and fluorescence in situ hybridization. *Am J Surg Pathol* 21: 52-59.
2964. Tsukamoto N, Nakamura M, Ishikawa H (1976). Case report: sclerosing stromal tumor of the ovary. *Gynecol Oncol* 4: 335-339.
2965. Tsuura Y, Hiraki H, Watanabe K, Igarashi S, Shimamura K, Fukuda T, Suzuki T, Seito T (1994). Preferential localization of c-kit product in tissue mast cells, basal cells of skin, epithelial cells of breast, small cell lung carcinoma and seminoma/dysgerminoma in human: immunohistochemical study on formalin-fixed, paraffin-embedded tissues. *Virchows Arch* 424: 135-141.
2966. Tuncer ZS, Vegh GL, Fulop V, Genest DR, Mok SC, Berkowitz RS (2000). Expression of epidermal growth factor receptor-related family products in gestational trophoblastic diseases and normal placenta and its relationship with development of postmolar tumor. *Gynecol Oncol* 77: 389-393.
2967. Twiggs LB, Okagaki T, Phillips GL, Stroemer JR, Adcock LL (1981). Trophoblastic pseudotumor-evidence of malignant disease potential. *Gynecol Oncol* 12: 238-248.
2968. Tyagi SP, Saxena K, Rizvi R, Langley FA (1979). Foetal remnants in the uterus and their relation to other uterine heterotopia. *Histopathology* 3: 339-345.
2969. Uchiyama M, Iwasaka T, Matsuo N, Hachisuga T, Mori M, Sugimori H (1997). Correlation between human papillomavirus positivity and p53 gene overexpression in adenocarcinoma of the uterine cervix. *Gynecol Oncol* 65: 23-29.
2970. Ueda G, Fujita M, Ogawa H, Sawada M, Inoue M, Tanizawa O (1993). Adenocarcinoma in a benign cystic teratoma of the ovary: report of a case with a long survival period. *Gynecol Oncol* 48: 259-263.
2971. Ueda H, Togashi K, Konishi I, Kataoka ML, Koyama T, Fujiwara T, Kobayashi H, Fujii S, Konishi J (1999). Unusual appearances of uterine leiomyomas: MR imaging findings and their histopathologic backgrounds. Radiographics 19 Spec No: S131-S145.
2972. Uehara T, Izumo T, Kishi K, Takayama S, Kasuga T (1991). Stromal melanocytic foci ("blue nevus") in step sections of the uterine cervix. *Acta Pathol Jpn* 41: 751-756.
2973. Uehara T, Takayama S, Takemura T, Kasuga T (1991). Foci of stromal melanocytes (so-called blue naevus) of the uterine cervix in Japanese women. *Virchows Arch A Pathol Anat Histopathol* 418: 327-331.
2974. Uehira K, Hashimoto H, Tsuneyoshi M, Enjoji M (1993). Transitional cell carcinoma pattern in primary carcinoma of the fallopian tube. *Cancer* 72: 2447-2456.
2975. Ueki M, Sano T, Okamura S, Iito Y, Kitsuki K, Sugimoto O (1982). [Clinical diagnosis of well differentiated cervical adenocarcinoma with plentiful mucous secretion]. *Nippon Sanka Fujinka Gakkai Zasshi* 34: 1846-1852.
2976. UICC (2002). *TNM classification of malignant tumors.* Sixth ed. John Wiley & Sons: New York.
2977. Ulbright TM, Alexander RW, Kraus FT (1981). Intramural papilloma of the vagina: evidence of Mullerian histogenesis. *Cancer* 48: 2260-2266.
2978. Ulbright TM, Roth LM (1985). Metastatic and independent cancers of the endometrium and ovary: a clinicopathologic study of 34 cases. *Hum Pathol* 16: 28-34.
2979. Ulbright TM, Roth LM, Brodhecker CA (1986). Yolk sac differentiation in germ cell tumors. A morphologic study of 50 cases with emphasis on hepatic, enteric, and parietal yolk sac features. *Am J Surg Pathol* 10: 151-164.
2980. Ulbright TM, Roth LM, Stehman FB (1984). Secondary ovarian neoplasia. A clinicopathologic study of 35 cases. *Cancer* 53: 1164-1174.
2981. Underwood PB Jr., Smith RT (1971). Carcinoma of the vagina. *JAMA* 217: 46-52.
2982. Unkila-Kallio L, Tiitinen A, Wahlstrom T, Lehtovirta P, Leminen A (2000). Reproductive features in women developing ovarian granulosa cell tumour at a fertile age. *Hum Reprod* 15: 589-593.
2983. Uziel T, Savitsky K, Platzer M, Ziv Y, Helbitz T, Nehls M, Boehm T, Rosenthal A, Shiloh Y, Rotman G (1996). Genomic Organization of the ATM gene. *Genomics* 33: 317-320.
2984. Vahteristo P, Bartkova J, Eerola H, Syrjakoski K, Ojala S, Kilpivaara O, Tamminen A, Kononen J, Aittomaki K, Heikkila P, Holli K, Blomqvist C, Bartek J, Kallioniemi OP, Nevanlinna H (2002). A CHEK2 genetic variant contributing to a substantial fraction of familial breast cancer. *Am J Hum Genet* 71: 432-438.
2985. Vaizey C, Burke M, Lange M (1999). Carcinoma of the male breast - a review of 91 patients from the Johannesburg Hospital breast clinics. *S Afr J Surg* 37: 6-8.
2986. van't Veer LJ, Dai H, Van de Vijver MJ, He YD, Hart AA, Mao HL, van der Kooy K, Marton MJ, Witteveen AT, Schreiber GJ, Kerkhoven RM, Roberts C, Linsley PS, Bernards R, Friend SH (2002). Gene expression profiling predicts clinical outcome of breast cancer. *Nature* 415: 530-536.
2987. van Belzen MJ, Hiel JA, Weemaes CM, Gabreels FJ, van Engelen BG, Smeets DF, van den Heuvel LP (1998). A double missense mutation in the ATM gene of a Dutch family with ataxia telangiectasia. *Hum Genet* 102: 187-191.
2988. Van Bogaert LJ, Maldague P (1977). Histologic variants of lipid-secreting carcinoma of the breast. *Virchows Arch A Pathol Anat* 375: 345-353.
2989. Van de Vijver MJ (1999). The pathology of familial breast cancer: The pre-BRCA1/BRCA2 era: historical perspectives. *Breast Cancer Res* 1: 27-30.
2990. Van de Vijver MJ, He YD, van't Veer LJ, Dai H, Hart AA, Voskuil DW, Schreiber GJ, Peterse JL, Roberts C, Marton MJ, Parrish M, Atsma D, Witteveen A, Glas A, Delahaye L, van der Velde T, Bartelink H, Rodenhuis S, Rutgers ET, Friend SH, Bernards R (2002). A gene-expression signature as a predictor of survival in breast cancer. *N Engl J Med* 347: 1999-2009.
2991. van der Putte SC (1994). Mammary-like glands of the vulva and their disorders. *Int J Gynecol Pathol* 13: 150-160.
2992. van der Putte SC, van Gorp LH (1994). Adenocarcinoma of the mammary-like glands of the vulva: a concept unifying sweat gland carcinoma of the vulva, carcinoma of supernumerary mammary glands and extramammary Paget's disease. *J Cutan Pathol* 21: 157-163.
2993. van Diest PJ, Baak JPA (1991). The morphometric prognostic index is the strongest prognosticator in premenopausal lymph node-negative and lymph node-positive breast cancer patients. *Hum Pathol* 22: 326-330.
2994. Van Dorpe J, De Pauw A, Moerman P (1998). Adenoid cystic carcinoma arising in an adenomyoepithelioma of the breast. *Virchows Arch* 432: 119-122.
2995. Van Hoeven KH, Drudis T, Cranor ML, Erlandson RA, Rosen PP (1993). Low-grade adenosquamous carcinoma of the breast. A clinicopathologic study of 32 cases with ultrastructural analysis. *Am J Surg Pathol* 17: 248-258.
2996. van Ingen G, Schoemaker J, Baak JP (1991). A testosterone-producing tumour in the mesovarium. *Pathol Res Pract* 187: 362-370.
2997. Vanderstichele S, Elhage A, Verbert-Scherrer A, Robert Y, Querleu D, Crepin G (1996). [Granulosa cell tumors: a case located in the broad ligament of the uterus with normal ovaries]. *J Gynecol Obstet Biol Reprod (Paris)* 25: 47-52.
2998. Vang R, Kempson RL (2002). Perivascular epithelioid cell tumor ('PEComa') of the uterus: a subset of HMB-45-positive epithelioid mesenchymal neoplasms with an uncertain relationship to pure smooth muscle tumors. *Am J Surg Pathol* 26: 1-13.
2999. Vang R, Medeiros LJ, Fuller GN, Sarris AH, Deavers M (2001). Non-Hodgkin's lymphoma involving the gynecologic tract: a review of 88 cases. *Adv Anat Pathol* 8: 200-217.
3000. Vang R, Medeiros LJ, Ha CS, Deavers M (2000). Non-Hodgkin's lymphomas involving the uterus: a clinicopathologic analysis of 26 cases. *Mod Pathol* 13: 19-28.

3001. Vang R, Medeiros LJ, Silva EG, Gershenson DM, Deavers M (2000). Non-Hodgkin's lymphoma involving the vagina: a clinicopathologic analysis of 14 patients. *Am J Surg Pathol* 24: 719-725.

3002. Vang R, Taubenberger JK, Mannion CM, Bijwaard K, Malpica A, Ordonez NG, Tavassoli FA, Silver SA (2000). Primary vulvar and vaginal extraosseous Ewing's sarcoma/peripheral neuroectodermal tumor: diagnostic confirmation with CD99 immunostaining and reverse transcriptase-polymerase chain reaction. *Int J Gynecol Pathol* 19: 103-109.

3003. Vang R, Whitaker BP, Farhood AI, Silva EG, Ro JY, Deavers MT (2001). Immunohistochemical analysis of clear cell carcinoma of the gynecologic tract. *Int J Gynecol Pathol* 20: 252-259.

3004. Vanni R, Faa G, Dettori T, Melis GB, Dumanski JP, O'Brien KP (2000). A case of dermatofibrosarcoma protuberans of the vulva with a COL1A1/PDGFB fusion identical to a case of giant cell fibroblastoma. *Virchows Arch* 437: 95-100.

3005. Vardi JR, Tovell HM (1980). Leiomyosarcoma of the uterus: clinicopathologic study. *Obstet Gynecol* 56: 428-434.

3006. Varga Z, Kolb SA, Flury R, Burkhard R, Caduff R (2000). Sebaceous carcinoma of the breast. *Pathol Int* 50: 63-66.

3007. Vasen HF (2000). Clinical diagnosis and management of hereditary colorectal cancer syndromes. *J Clin Oncol* 18: 81S-92S.

3008. Vasen HF, Mecklin JP, Khan PM, Lynch HT (1991). The International Collaborative Group on Hereditary Non-Polyposis Colorectal Cancer (ICG-HNPCC). *Dis Colon Rectum* 34: 424-425.

3009. Vasen HF, Stormorken A, Menko FH, Nagengast FM, Kleibeuker JH, Griffioen G, Taal BG, Moller P, Wijnen JT (2001). MSH2 mutation carriers are at higher risk of cancer than MLH1 mutation carriers: a study of hereditary nonpolyposis colorectal cancer families. *J Clin Oncol* 19: 4074-4080.

3010. Vasen HF, Watson P, Mecklin JP, Lynch HT (1999). New clinical criteria for hereditary nonpolyposis colorectal cancer (HNPCC, Lynch syndrome) proposed by the International Collaborative group on HNPCC. *Gastroenterology* 116: 1453-1456.

3011. Vasen HF, Wijnen JT, Menko FH, Kleibeuker JH, Taal BG, Griffioen G, Nagengast FM, Meijers-Heijboer EH, Bertario L, Varesco L, Bisgaard ML, Mohr J, Fodde R, Khan PM (1996). Cancer risk in families with hereditary nonpolyposis colorectal cancer diagnosed by mutation analysis. *Gastroenterology* 110: 1020-1027.

3012. Vaughn JP, Cirisano FD, Huper G, Berchuck A, Futreal PA, Marks JR, Iglehart JD (1996). Cell cycle control of BRCA2. *Cancer Res* 56: 4590-4594.

3013. Vega de la G. (1976). Signet ring cell carcinoma of the uterine cervix. *Patologia* 14: 193-196.

3014. Vegh GL, Fulop V, Liu Y, Ng SW, Tuncer ZS, Genest DR, Paldi-Haris P, Foldi J, Mok SC, Berkowitz RS (1999). Differential gene expression pattern between normal human trophoblast and choriocarcinoma cell lines: downregulation of heat shock protein-27 in choriocarcinoma in vitro and in vivo. *Gynecol Oncol* 75: 391-396.

3015. Velasco-Oses A, Alonso-Alvaro A, Blanco-Pozo A, Nogales FF Jr. (1988). Ollier's disease associated with ovarian juvenile granulosa cell tumor. *Cancer* 62: 222-225.

3016. Veliath AJ, Hannah P, Ratnakar C, Jayanthi K, Aurora AL (1978). Primary liposarcoma of the cervix: a case report. *Int J Gynaecol Obstet* 16: 75-79.

3017. Venable JG, Schwartz AM, Silverberg SG (1990). Infiltrating cribriform carcinoma of the breast: a distinctive clinicopathologic entity. *Hum Pathol* 21: 333-338.

3018. Venkitaraman AR (2002). Cancer susceptibility and the functions of BRCA1 and BRCA2. *Cell* 108: 171-182.

3019. Venkitaraman AR (2003). A growing network of cancer-susceptibility genes. *N Engl J Med* 348: 1917-1919.

3020. Vergier B, Trojani M, De Mascarel I, Coindre JM, Le Treut A (1991). Metastases to the breast: differential diagnosis from primary breast carcinoma. *J Surg Oncol* 48: 112-116.

3021. Verhest A, Nedoszytko B, Noel JC, Dangou JM, Simon P, Limon J (1992). Translocation (6;16) in a case of granulosa cell tumor of the ovary. *Cancer Genet Cytogenet* 60: 41-44.

3022. Verhoog LC, Brekelmans CT, Seynaeve C, van den Bosch LM, Dahmen G, van Geel AN, Tilanus-Linthorst MM, Bartels CC, Wagner A, van den Ouweland A, Devilee P, Meijers-Heijboer EJ, Klijn JG (1998). Survival and tumour characteristics of breast-cancer patients with germline mutations of BRCA1. *Lancet* 351: 316-321.

3023. Verhoog LC, van den Ouweland AM, Berns E, Veghel-Plandsoen MM, van Staveren IL, Wagner A, Bartels CC, Tilanus-Linthorst MM, Devilee P, Seynaeve C, Halley DJ, Niermeijer MF, Klijn JG, Meijers-Heijboer H (2001). Large regional differences in the frequency of distinct BRCA1/BRCA2 mutations in 517 Dutch breast and/or ovarian cancer families. *Eur J Cancer* 37: 2082-2090.

3024. Veridiano NP, Gal D, Delke I, Rosen Y, Tancer ML (1980). Gestational choriocarcinoma of the ovary. *Gynecol Oncol* 10: 235-240.

3025. Viacava P, Naccarato AG, Nardini V, Bevilacqua G (1995). Breast carcinoma with osteoclast-like giant cells: immunohistochemical and ultrastructural study of a case and review of the literature. *Tumori* 81: 135-141.

3026. Vicandi B., Jimenez-Hefferman J.A., Lopez-Ferrer P., Ortega L., Viguer J.M. (1998). Nodular pseudoangiomatous stromal hyperplasia of the breast. Cytologic features. *Acta Cytol* 42: 335-341.

3027. Vivian JB, Tan EG, Frayne JR, Waters ED (1993). Bilateral liposarcoma of the breast. *Aust N Z J Surg* 63: 658-659.

3028. Vizcaino AP, Moreno V, Bosch FX, Munoz N, Barros-Dios XM, Parkin DM (1998). International trends in the incidence of cervical cancer: I. Adenocarcinoma and adenosquamous cell carcinomas. *Int J Cancer* 75: 536-545.

3029. Vizcaino I, Torregrossa AHV, Morote V, Crenades A, Torres V, Olmos S, Molins C (2001). Metastasis to the breast from extramammary malignancies: a report of four cases and a review of literature. *Eur Radiol* 11: 802-806.

3030. Vleminckx K, Vakaet L Jr., Mareel M, Fiers W, van Roy F (1991). Genetic manipulation of E-cadherin expression by epithelial tumor cells reveals an invasion suppressor role. *Cell* 66: 107-119.

3031. Voet RL, Lifshitz S (1982). Primary clear cell adenocarcinoma of the fallopian tube: light microscopic and ultrastructural findings. *Int J Gynecol Pathol* 1: 292-298.

3032. Vortmeyer AO, Devouassoux-Shisheboran M, Li G, Mohr V, Tavassoli F, Zhuang Z (1999). Microdissection-based analysis of mature ovarian teratoma. *Am J Pathol* 154: 987-991.

3033. Vos A, Oosterhuis JW, de Jong B, Castedo SM, Hollema H, Buist J, Aalders JG (1990). Karyotyping and DNA flow cytometry of metastatic ovarian yolk sac tumor. *Cancer Genet Cytogenet* 44: 223-228.

3034. Vos CB, Cleton-Jansen AM, Berx G, de Leeuw WJ, ter Haar NT, van Roy F, Cornelisse CJ, Peterse JL, Van de Vijver MJ (1997). E-cadherin inactivation in lobular carcinoma in situ of the breast: an early event in tumorigenesis. *Br J Cancer* 76: 1131-1133.

3035. Vos CB, ter Haar NT, Peterse JL, Cornelisse CJ, Van de Vijver MJ (1999). Cyclin D1 gene amplification and overexpression are present in ductal carcinoma in situ of the breast. *J Pathol* 187: 279-284.

3036. Vos CB, ter Haar NT, Rosenberg C, Peterse JL, Cleton-Jansen AM, Cornelisse CJ, Van de Vijver MJ (1999). Genetic alterations on chromosome 16 and 17 are important features of ductal carcinoma in situ of the breast and are associated with histologic type. *Br J Cancer* 81: 1410-1418.

3037. Vuitch MF, Rosen PP, Erlandson RA (1986). Pseudoangiomatous hyperplasia of mammary stroma. *Hum Pathol* 17: 185-191.

3038. Wadhwa J, Dawar R, Kumar L (1999). Ovarian carcinoma metastatic to the breast. *Clin Oncol (R Coll Radiol)* 11: 419-421.

3039. Wagner A, Hendriks Y, Meijers-Heijboer EJ, de Leeuw WJ, Morreau H, Hofstra R, Tops C, Bik E, Brocker-Vriends AH, van der Meer C, Lindhout D, Vasen HF, Breuning MH, Cornelisse CJ, van Krimpen C, Niermeijer MF, Zwinderman AH, Wijnen J, Fodde R (2001). Atypical HNPCC owing to MSH6 germline mutations: analysis of a large Dutch pedigree. *J Med Genet* 38: 318-322.

3040. Wagner I, Bettendorf U (1980). Extraovarian Brenner tumor. Case report and review. *Arch Gynecol* 229: 191-196.

3041. Waha A, Sturne C, Kessler A, Koch A, Kreyer E, Fimmers R, Wiestler OD, von Deimling A, Krebs D, Schmutzler RK (1998). Expression of the ATM gene is significantly reduced in sporadic breast carcinomas. *Int J Cancer* 78: 306-309.

3042. Wahner-Roedler DL, Sebo TJ, Gisvold JJ (2001). Hamartomas of the breast: clinical, radiologic, and pathologic manifestations. *Breast J* 7: 101-105.

3043. Waite KA, Eng C (2002). Protean PTEN: form and function. *Am J Hum Genet* 70: 829-844.

3044. Walboomers JM, Jacobs MV, Manos MM, Bosch FX, Kummer JA, Shah KV, Snijders PJ, Peto J, Meijer CJ, Munoz N (1999). Human papillomavirus is a necessary cause of invasive cervical cancer worldwide. *J Pathol* 189: 12-19.

3045. Waldman FM, Devries S, Chew KL, Moore DH, Kerlikowske K, Ljung BM (2000). Chromosomal alterations in ductal carcinomas in situ and their in situ recurrences. *J Natl Cancer Inst* 92: 313-320.

3046. Waldman FM, Hwang ES, Etzell J, Eng C, Devries S, Bennington J, Thor A (2001). Genomic alterations in tubular breast carcinomas. *Hum Pathol* 32: 222-226.

3047. Walford N, ten Velden J (1989). Histiocytoid breast carcinoma: an apocrine variant of lobular carcinoma. *Histopathology* 14: 515-522.

3048. Walker RA, Jones JL, Chappell S, Walsh T, Shaw JA (1997). Molecular pathology of breast cancer and its application to clinical management. *Cancer Metastasis Rev* 16: 5-27.

3049. Walsh MM, Bleiweiss IJ (2001). Invasive micropapillary carcinoma of the breast: eighty cases of an underrecognized entity. *Hum Pathol* 32: 583-589.

3050. Walt H, Hornung R, Fink D, Dobler-Girdziunaite D, Stallmach T, Spycher MA, Maly F, Haller U, Burki N (2001). Hypercalcemic-type of small cell carcinoma of the ovary: characterization of a new tumor line. *Anticancer Res* 21: 3253-3259.

3051. Walter A (1982). Benign teratoma of the Fallopian tube. *Aust N Z J Obstet Gynaecol* 22: 245-247.

3052. Wang H, Douglas W, Lia M, Edelmann W, Kucherlapati R, Podsypanina K, Parsons R, Ellenson LH (2002). DNA mismatch repair deficiency accelerates endometrial tumorigenesis in Pten heterozygous mice. *Am J Pathol* 160: 1481-1486.

3053. Wang WW, Spurdle AB, Kolachana P, Bove B, Modan B, Ebbers SM, Suthers G, Tucker MA, Kaufman DJ, Doody MM, Tarone RE, Daly M, Levavi H, Pierce H, Chetrit A, Yechezkel GH, Chenevix-Trench G, Offit K, Godwin AK, Struewing JP (2001). A single nucleotide polymorphism in the 5' untranslated region of RAD51 and risk of cancer among BRCA1/2 mutation carriers. *Cancer Epidemiol Biomarkers Prev* 10: 955-960.

3054. Wang Y, Cortez D, Yazdi P, Neff N, Elledge SJ, Qin J (2000). BASC, a super complex of BRCA1-associated proteins involved in the recognition and repair of aberrant DNA structures. *Genes Dev* 14: 927-939.

3055. Ward BA, McKhann CF, Ravikumar TS (1992). Ten-year follow-up of breast carcinoma in situ in Connecticut. *Arch Surg* 127: 1392-1395.

3056. Ward BE, Cooper PH, Subramony C (1989). Syringomatous tumor of the nipple. *Am J Clin Pathol* 92: 692-696.

3057. Ward BE, Saleh AM, Williams JV, Zitz JC, Crum CP (1992). Papillary immature metaplasia of the cervix: a distinct subset of exophytic cervical condyloma associated with HPV-6/11 nucleic acids. *Mod Pathol* 5: 391-395.

3058. Ward RM, Evans HL (1986). Cystosarcoma phyllodes. A clinicopathologic study of 26 cases. Cancer 58: 2282-2289.

3059. Wargotz ES, Deos PH, Norris HJ (1989). Metaplastic carcinomas of the breast. II. Spindle cell carcinoma. *Hum Pathol* 20: 732-740.

3060. Wargotz ES, Norris HJ (1989). Metaplastic carcinomas of the breast. I. Matrix-producing carcinoma. *Hum Pathol* 20: 628-635.

3061. Wargotz ES, Norris HJ (1990). Metaplastic carcinomas of the breast. IV. Squamous cell carcinoma of ductal origin. *Cancer* 65: 272-276.
3062. Wargotz ES, Norris HJ (1990). Metaplastic carcinomas of the breast: V. Metaplastic carcinoma with osteoclastic giant cells. *Hum Pathol* 21: 1142-1150.
3063. Wargotz ES, Norris HJ, Austin RM, Enzinger FM (1987). Fibromatosis of the breast. A clinical and pathological study of 28 cases. *Am J Surg Pathol* 11: 38-45.
3064. Wargotz ES, Silverberg SG (1988). Medullary carcinoma of the breast: a clinicopathologic study with appraisal of current diagnostic criteria. Hum Pathol 19: 1340-1346.
3065. Warner E, Foulkes W, Goodwin P, Meschino W, Blondal J, Paterson C, Ozcelik H, Goss P, Allingham-Hawkins D, Hamel N, Di Prospero L, Contiga V, Serruya C, Klein M, Moslehi R, Honeyford J, Liede A, Glendon G, Brunet JS, Narod S (1999). Prevalence and penetrance of BRCA1 and BRCA2 gene mutations in unselected Ashkenazi Jewish women with breast cancer. *J Natl Cancer Inst* 91: 1241-1247.
3066. Warner NE (1969). Lobular carcinoma of the breast. *Cancer* 23: 840-846.
3067. Watanabe Y, Nakajima H, Nozaki K, Ueda H, Obata K, Hoshiai H, Noda K (2001). Clinicopathologic and immunohistochemical features and microsatellite status of endometrial cancer of the uterine isthmus. *Int J Gynecol Pathol* 20: 368-373.
3068. Waterhouse J, Muir CS, Correa P, Powell J (1976). Cancer Incidence in Five Continents (IARC Scientific Publications n°15). IARC: Lyon.
3069. Watkin W, Silva EG, Gershenson DM (1992). Mucinous carcinoma of the ovary. Pathologic prognostic factors. *Cancer* 69: 208-212.
3070. Watson P, Lin KM, Rodriguez-Bigas MA, Smyrk T, Lemon S, Shashidharan M, Franklin B, Karr B, Thorson A, Lynch HT (1998). Colorectal carcinoma survival among hereditary nonpolyposis colorectal carcinoma family members. *Cancer* 83: 259-266.
3071. Watson P, Vasen HF, Mecklin JP, Jarvinen H, Lynch HT (1994). The risk of endometrial cancer in hereditary nonpolyposis colorectal cancer. *Am J Med* 96: 516-520.
3072. Watt AC, Haggar AM, Krasicky GA (1984). Extraosseous osteogenic sarcoma of the breast: mammographic and pathologic findings. *Radiology* 150: 34.
3073. Waxman M (1979). Pure and mixed Brenner tumors of the ovary: clinicopathologic and histogenetic observations. *Cancer* 43: 1830-1839.
3074. Waxman M, Vuletin JC, Urcuyo R, Belling CG (1979). Ovarian low-grade stromal sarcoma with thecomatous features: a critical reappraisal of the so-called "malignant thecoma". *Cancer* 44: 2206-2217.
3075. Way S (1948). Primary carcinoma of the vagina. *J Obstet Br Emp* 55: 739.
3076. Webb JC, Key CR, Qualls CR, Smith HO (2001). Population-based study of microinvasive adenocarcinoma of the uterine cervix. *Obstet Gynecol* 97: 701-706.
3077. Webb LA, Young JR (1996). Case report: haemangioma of the breast--appearances on mammography and ultrasound. *Clin Radiol* 51: 523-524.
3078. Webb MJ, Symmonds RE, Weiland LH (1974). Malignant fibrous histiocytoma of the vagina. *Am J Obstet Gynecol* 119: 190-192.
3079. Weber AM, Hewett WF, Gajewski WH, Curry SL (1993). Malignant mixed mullerian tumors of the fallopian tube. *Gynecol Oncol* 50: 239-243.
3080. Wei LH, Huang CY, Cheng SP, Chen CA, Hsieh CY (2001). Carcinosarcoma of ovary associated with previous radiotherapy. *Int J Gynecol Cancer* 11: 81-84.
3081. Weidner N (1990). Benign breast lesions that mimic malignant tumors: analysis of five distinct lesions. *Semin Diagn Pathol* 7: 90-101.
3082. Weidner N, Semple JP (1992). Pleomorphic variant of invasive lobular carcinoma of the breast. *Hum Pathol* 23: 1167-1171.
3083. Weigand RA, Isenberg WM, Russo J, Brennan MJ, Rich MA (1982). Blood vessel invasion and axillary lymph node involvement as prognostic indicators for human breast cancer. *Cancer* 50: 962-969.
3084. Weinberg E, Hoisington S, Eastman AY, Rice DK, Malfetano J, Ross JS (1993). Uterine cervical lymphoepithelial-like carcinoma. Absence of Epstein-Barr virus genomes. *Am J Clin Pathol* 99: 195-199.
3085. Weir MM, Bell DA, Young RH (1997). Transitional cell metaplasia of the uterine cervix and vagina: an underrecognized lesion that may be confused with high-grade dysplasia. A report of 59 cases. *Am J Surg Pathol* 21: 510-517.
3086. Weiss SW (1994). *Histological Typing of Soft Tissue Tumours.* 2nd ed. Springer: Berlin Heidelberg, New York.
3087. Weiss SW, Tavassoli FA (1988). Multicystic mesothelioma. An analysis of pathologic findings and biologic behavior in 37 cases. *Am J Surg Pathol* 12: 737-746.
3088. Weissberg JB, Huang DD, Swift M (1998). Radiosensitivity of normal tissues in ataxia-telangiectasia heterozygotes. *Int J Radiat Oncol Biol Phys* 42: 1133-1136.
3089. Weitmann HD, Knocke TH, Kucera H, Potter R (2001). Radiation therapy in the treatment of endometrial stromal sarcoma. *Int J Radiat Oncol Biol Phys* 49: 739-748.
3090. Weitzner S, Nascimento AG, Scanlon LJ (1979). Intramammary granular cell myoblastoma. *Am Surg* 45: 34-37.
3091. Wellings SR, Jensen HM, Marcum RG (1975). An atlas of subgross pathology of the human breast with special reference to possible precancerous lesions. *J Natl Cancer Inst* 55: 231-273.
3092. Wells CA, Ferguson DJ (1988). Ultrastructural and immunocytochemical study of a case of invasive cribriform breast carcinoma. *J Clin Pathol* 41: 17-20.
3093. Wells CA, McGregor IL, Makunura CN, Yeomans P, Davies JD (1995). Apocrine adenosis: a precursor of aggressive breast cancer? *J Clin Pathol* 48: 737-742.
3094. Wells CA, Nicoll S, Ferguson DJ (1986). Adenoid cystic carcinoma of the breast: a case with axillary lymph node metastasis. *Histopathology* 10: 415-424.
3095. Wen WH, Reles A, Runnebaum IB, Sullivan-Halley J, Bernstein L, Jones LA, Felix JC, Kreienberg R, el Naggar A, Press MF (1999). p53 mutations and expression in ovarian cancers: correlation with overall survival. *Int J Gynecol Pathol* 18: 29-41.
3096. Weng L, Brown J, Eng C (2001). PTEN induces apoptosis and cell cycle arrest through phosphoinositol-3-kinase/Akt-dependent and -independent pathways. *Hum Mol Genet* 10: 237-242.
3097. Weng LP, Brown JL, Baker KM, Ostrowski MC, Eng C (2002). PTEN blocks insulin-mediated ETS-2 phosphorylation through MAP kinase, independently of the phosphoinositide 3-kinase pathway. *Hum Mol Genet* 11: 1687-1696.
3098. Weng LP, Smith WM, Brown JL, Eng C (2001). PTEN inhibits insulin-stimulated MEK/MAPK activation and cell growth by blocking IRS-1 phosphorylation and IRS-1/Grb-2/Sos complex formation in a breast cancer model. *Hum Mol Genet* 10: 605-616.
3099. Werling RW, Hwang H, Yaziji H, Gown AM (2003). Immunohistochemical distinction of invasive from noninvasive breast lesions: a comparative study of p63 versus calponin and smooth muscle myosin heavy chain. *Am J Surg Pathol* 27: 82-90.
3100. Werner M, Mattis A, Aubele M, Cummings M, Zitzelsberger H, Hutzler P, Hofler H (1999). 20q13.2 amplification in intraductal hyperplasia adjacent to in situ and invasive ductal carcinoma of the breast. *Virchows Arch* 435: 469-472.
3101. Werness BA, Dicioccio RA (2002). Transitional cell ovarian carcinoma in a BRCA1 mutation carrier. *Obstet Gynecol* 100: 385.
3102. Werness BA, Ramus SJ, Whittemore AS, Garlinghouse-Jones K, Oakley-Girvan I, Dicioccio RA, Tsukada Y, Ponder BA, Piver MS (2000). Histopathology of familial ovarian tumors in women from families with and without germline BRCA1 mutations. *Hum Pathol* 31: 1420-1424.
3103. Werness BA, Ramus SJ, Whittemore AS, Garlinghouse-Jones K, Oakley-Girvan I, Dicioccio RA, Tsukada Y, Ponder BA, Piver MS (2000). Primary ovarian dysgerminoma in a patient with a germline BRCA1 mutation. *Int J Gynecol Pathol* 19: 390-394.
3104. West M, Blanchette C, Dressman H, Huang E, Ishida S, Spang R, Zuzan H, Olson JA Jr., Marks JR, Nevins JR (2001). Predicting the clinical status of human breast cancer by using gene expression profiles. *Proc Natl Acad Sci USA* 98: 11462-11467.
3104a. Westenend PJ, Liem SJ (2001). Adenosis tumor of the breast containing ductal carcinoma in situ, a pitfall in core needle biopsy. *Breast J* 7: 200-201.
3105. Wheeler DT, Bell KA, Kurman RJ, Sherman ME (2000). Minimal uterine serous carcinoma: diagnosis and clinicopathologic correlation. *Am J Surg Pathol* 24: 797-806.
3106. Wheeler JE, Enterline HT (1976). Lobular carcinoma of the breast in situ and infiltrating. *Pathol Annu* 11: 161-188.
3107. Wheeler JE, Enterline HT, Roseman JM, Tomasulo JP, McIlvaine CH, Fitts WT Jr., Kirshenbaum J (1974). Lobular carcinoma in situ of the breast. Long-term followup. *Cancer* 34: 554-563.
3108. Wheelock JB, Goplerud DR, Dunn LJ, Oates JF, III (1984). Primary carcinoma of the Bartholin gland: a report of ten cases. *Obstet Gynecol* 63: 820-824.
3109. Wheelock JB, Krebs HB, Schneider V, Goplerud DR (1985). Uterine sarcoma: analysis of prognostic variables in 71 cases. *Am J Obstet Gynecol* 151: 1016-1022.
3110. Whiteman DC, Murphy MF, Verkasalo PK, Page WF, Floderus B, Skytthe A, Holm NV (2000). Breast cancer risk in male twins: joint analyses of four twin cohorts in Denmark, Finland, Sweden and the United States. *Br J Cancer* 83: 1231-1233.
3111. WHO Technical Report Series (1983). *WHO Scientific Group*: Gestional trophoblastic diseases. WHO:
3112. Wick MR, Goellner JR, Wolfe JT, III, Su WP (1985). Vulvar sweat gland carcinomas. *Arch Pathol Lab Med* 109: 43-47.
3113. Wick MR, Lillemoe TJ, Copland GT, Swanson PE, Manivel JC, Kiang DT (1989). Gross cystic disease fluid protein-15 as a marker for breast cancer: immunohistochemical analysis of 690 human neoplasms and comparison with alpha-lactalbumin. *Hum Pathol* 20: 281-287.
3114. Wijnen J, de Leeuw W, Vasen H, van der Klift H, Moller P, Stormorken A, Meijers-Heijboer H, Lindhout D, Menko F, Vossen S, Moslein G, Tops C, Brocker-Vriends A, Wu Y, Hofstra R, Sijmons R, Cornelisse C, Morreau H, Fodde R (1999). Familial endometrial cancer in female carriers of MSH6 germline mutations. *Nat Genet* 23: 142-144.
3115. Wijnen J, Khan PM, Vasen H, Menko F, van der Klift H, van den Broek M, Leeuwen-Cornelisse I, Nagengast F, Meijers-Heijboer EJ, Lindhout D, Griffioen G, Cats A, Kleibeuker J, Varesco L, Bertario L, Bisgaard ML, Mohr J, Kolodner R, Fodde R (1996). Majority of hMLH1 mutations responsible for hereditary nonpolyposis colorectal cancer cluster at the exonic region 15-16. *Am J Hum Genet* 58: 300-307.
3116. Wijnen J, van der Klift H, Vasen H, Khan PM, Menko F, Tops C, Meijers HH, Lindhout D, Moller P, Fodde R (1998). MSH2 genomic deletions are a frequent cause of HNPCC. *Nat Genet* 20: 326-328.
3117. Wijnen JT, Vasen HF, Khan PM, Zwinderman AH, van der Klift H, Mulder A, Tops C, Moller P, Fodde R (1998). Clinical findings with implications for genetic testing in families with clustering of colorectal cancer. *N Engl J Med* 339: 511-518.
3118. Wijnmaalen A, van Ooijen B, van Geel BN, Henzen-Logmans SC, Treurniet-Donker AD (1993). Angiosarcoma of the breast following lumpectomy, axillary lymph node dissection, and radiotherapy for primary breast cancer: three case reports and a review of the literature. *Int J Radiat Oncol Biol Phys* 26: 135-139.
3119. Wilkinson EJ (2000). Protocol for the examination of specimens from patients with carcinomas and malignant melanomas of the vulva: a basis for checklists. Cancer Committee of the American College of Pathologists. *Arch Pathol Lab Med* 124: 51-56.
3120. Wilkinson EJ (2002). *Premalignant and Malignant Tumours of the vulva. In: Blaustein's Pathology of the Female Genital Tract.* 5th ed. Springer-Verlag: New York.
3121. Wilkinson EJ, Brown H (2002). Vulvar Paget disease of urothelial origin: a report of three cases and proposed classification of vulvar Paget disease. *Hum Pathol* 33: 549-554.
3122. Wilkinson EJ, Croker BP, Friedrich EG Jr., Franzini DA (1988). Two distinct pathologic types of giant cell tumor of the vulva. A report of two cases. *J Reprod Med* 33: 519-522.
3123. Wilkinson EJ, Friedrich EG Jr., Fu YS (1981). Multicentric nature of vulvar carcinoma in situ. *Obstet Gynecol* 58: 69-74.
3124. Wilkinson EJ, Stone IK (1994). *Atlas of Vulvar Disease.* Williams and WIlkins: Baltimore, Maryland.

3125. Willemsen W, Kruitwagen R, Bastiaans B, Hanselaar T, Rolland R (1993). Ovarian stimulation and granulosa-cell tumour. *Lancet* 341: 986-988.

3126. Willen R, Bekassy A, Carlen B, Bozoky B, Cajander S (1999). Cloacogenic adenocarcinoma of the vulva. *Gynecol Oncol* 74: 298-301.

3127. Willett GD, Kurman RJ, Reid R, Greenberg M, Jenson AB, Lorincz AT (1989). Correlation of the histologic appearance of intraepithelial neoplasia of the cervix with human papillomavirus types. Emphasis on low grade lesions including so-called flat condyloma. *Int J Gynecol Pathol* 8: 18-25.

3128. Williamson JD, Colome MI, Sahin A, Ayala AG, Medeiros LJ (2000). Pagetoid Bowen disease: a report of 2 cases that express cytokeratin 7. *Arch Pathol Lab Med* 124: 427-430.

3129. Willsher PC, Leach IH, Ellis IO, Bell JA, Elston CW, Bourke JB, Blamey RW, Robertson JF (1997). Male breast cancer: pathological and immunohistochemical features. *Anticancer Res* 17: 2335-2338.

3130. Wilson CA, Ramos L, Villasenor MR, Anders KH, Press MF, Clarke K, Karlan B, Chen JJ, Scully R, Livingston D, Zuch RH, Kanter MH, Cohen S, Calzone FJ, Slamon DJ (1999). Localization of human BRCA1 and its loss in high-grade, non-inherited breast carcinomas. *Nat Genet* 21: 236-240.

3131. Wilson RB, Hunter JSJ, Dockerty MB (1961). Chorioadenoma destruens. *Am J Obstet Gynecol* 81: 546-559.

3132. Wilson TM, Ewel A, Duguid JR, Eble JN, Lescoe MK, Fishel R, Kelley MR (1995). Differential cellular expression of the human MSH2 repair enzyme in small and large intestine. *Cancer Res* 55: 5146-5150.

3133. Winchester DJ, Chang HR, Graves TA, Menck HR, Bland KI, Winchester DP (1998). A comparative analysis of lobular and ductal carcinoma of the breast: presentation, treatment, and outcomes. *J Am Coll Surg* 186: 416-422.

3134. Wingren S, van den Heuvel A, Gentile M, Olsen K, Hatschek T, Soderkvist P (1997). Frequent allelic losses on chromosome 13q in human male breast carcinomas. *Eur J Cancer* 33: 2393-2396.

3135. Winkler B, Alvarez S, Richart RM, Crum CP (1984). Pitfalls in the diagnosis of endometrial neoplasia. *Obstet Gynecol* 64: 185-194.

3136. Wiseman C, Liao KT (1972). Primary lymphoma of the breast. *Cancer* 29: 1705-1712.

3137. Wohlfahrt J, Melbye M (2001). Age at any birth is associated with breast cancer risk. *Epidemiology* 12: 68-73.

3138. Wolber RA, Talerman A, Wilkinson EJ, Clement PB (1991). Vulvar granular cell tumors with pseudocarcinomatous hyperplasia: a comparative analysis with well-differentiated squamous carcinoma. *Int J Gynecol Pathol* 10: 59-66.

3139. Wolfson AH, Wolfson DJ, Sittler SY, Breton L, Markoe AM, Schwade JG, Houdek PV, Averette HE, Sevin BU, Penalver M, Duncan RC, Ganjei P. (1994). A multivariate analysis of clinicopathologic factors for predicting outcome in uterine sarcomas. *Gynecol Oncol* 52: 56-62.

3140. Wong JH, Kopald KH, Morton DL (1990). The impact of microinvasion on axillary node metastases and survival in patients with intraductal breast cancer. *Arch Surg* 125: 1298-1301.

3141. Wong SY, Kernohan NM, Walker F (1990). Breast cancers with extremely high oestrogen receptor protein status. *Histopathology* 16: 125-132.

3142. Woodard BH, Brinkhous AD, McCarty KS, Sr., McCarty KS Jr. (1980). Adenosquamous differentiation in mammary carcinoma: an ultrastructural and steroid receptor study. *Arch Pathol Lab Med* 104: 130-133.

3143. Woodman CB, Collins S, Winter H, Bailey A, Ellis J, Prior P, Yates M, Rollason TP, Young LS (2001). Natural history of cervical human papillomavirus infection in young women: a longitudinal cohort study. *Lancet* 357: 1831-1836.

3144. Woodruff JD, Dietrich D, Genadry R, Parmley TH (1981). Proliferative and malignant Brenner tumors. Review of 47 cases. *Am J Obstet Gynecol* 141: 118-125.

3145. Woodruff JD, Julian CG (1969). Multiple malignancy in the upper genital canal. *Am J Obstet Gynecol* 103: 810-822.

3146. Woodruff JD, Rauh JT, Markley RL (1966). Ovarian struma. *Obstet Gynecol* 27: 194-201.

3147. Woods DB, Vousden KH (2001). Regulation of p53 function. *Exp Cell Res* 264: 56-66.

3148. Woods ER, Helvie MA, Ikeda DM, Mandell SH, Chapel KL, Adler DD (1992). Solitary breast papilloma: comparison of mammographic, galactographic, and pathologic findings. *AJR Am J Roentgenol* 159: 487-491.

3149. Woodward AH, Ivins JC, Soule EH (1972). Lymphangiosarcoma arising in chronic lymphedematous extremities. *Cancer* 30: 562-572.

3150. Woolas R, Smith J, Paterson JM, Sharp F (1997). Fallopian tube carcinoma: an under-recognized primary neoplasm. *Int J Gynecol Cancer* 7: 284-288.

3151. Woolcott RJ, Henry RJ, Houghton CR (1988). Malignant melanoma of the vulva. Australian experience. *J Reprod Med* 33: 699-702.

3152. Wooster R, Mangion J, Eeles R, Smith S, Dowsett M, Averill D, Barrett-Lee P, Easton DF, Ponder BA, Stratton MR (1992). A germline mutation in the androgen receptor gene in two brothers with breast cancer and Reifenstein syndrome. *Nat Genet* 2: 132-134.

3153. World Cancer Research Fund.American Institute for Cancer Research (1997). *Food, Nutrition and the Prevention of Cancer: a Global Perspective*. American Institute for Cancer Research: Washington DC.

3154. *World Health Organization (1981). International Histological Classification of Tumours: Histologic Types of Breast Tumours.* Geneva.

3155. World Health Organization (2000). World Health Organisation 1997-1999 World Health Statistics Annual. http://www who int/whosis.

3156. Worsham MJ, Van Dyke DL, Grenman SE, Grenman R, Hopkins MP, Roberts JA, Gasser KM, Schwartz DR, Carey TE (1991). Consistent chromosome abnormalities in squamous cell carcinoma of the vulva. *Genes Chromosomes Cancer* 3: 420-432.

3157. Wotherspoon AC, Finn TM, Isaacson PG (1995). Trisomy 3 in low-grade B-cell lymphomas of mucosa-associated lymphoid tissue. *Blood* 85: 2000-2004.

3158. Wrba F, Ellinger A, Reiner G, Spona J, Holzner JH (1988). Ultrastructural and immunohistochemical characteristics of lipid-rich carcinoma of the breast. *Virchows Arch A Pathol Anat Histopathol* 413: 381-385.

3159. Wright CV, Shier MR (2000). Colposcopy of Adenocarcinoma in situ and Adenocarcinoma of the Cervix. Differentiation from Other Cervical Lesions. Biomedical Communications: Houston.

3160. Wu Y, Berends MJ, Mensink RG, Kempinga C, Sijmons RH, Der Zee AG, Hollema H, Kleibeuker JH, Buys CH, Hofstra RM (1999). Association of hereditary nonpolyposis colorectal cancer-related tumors displaying low microsatellite instability with MSH6 germline mutations. *Am J Hum Genet* 65: 1291-1298.

3161. Wu Y, Berends MJ, Post JG, Mensink RG, Verlind E, Van Der Sluis T, Kempinga C, Sijmons RH, van der Zee AG, Hollema H, Kleibeuker JH, Buys CH, Hofstra RM (2001). Germline mutations of EXO1 gene in patients with hereditary nonpolyposis colorectal cancer (HNPCC) and atypical HNPCC forms. *Gastroenterology* 120: 1580-1587.

3162. Wu Y, Berends MJ, Sijmons RH, Mensink RG, Verlind E, Kooi KA, Van Der Sluis T, Kempinga C, dDer Zee AG, Hollema H, Buys CH, Kleibeuker JH, Hofstra RM (2001). A role for MLH3 in hereditary nonpolyposis colorectal cancer. *Nat Genet* 29: 137-138.

3163. Wurdinger S, Schutz K, Fuchs D, Kaiser WA (2001). Two cases of metastases to the breast on MR mammography. *Eur Radiol* 11: 802-806.

3164. Wyatt SW, Lancaster M, Bottorff D, Ross F (2001). History of tobacco use among Kentucky women diagnosed with invasive cervical cancer: 1997-1998. *J Ky Med Assoc* 99: 537-539.

3165. Wysocka B, Serkies K, Debniak J, Jassem J, Limon J (1999). Sertoli cell tumor in androgen insensitivity syndrome--a case report. *Gynecol Oncol* 75: 480-483.

3166. Xu B, Kim S, Kastan MB (2001). Involvement of Brca1 in S-phase and G(2)-phase checkpoints after ionizing irradiation. *Mol Cell Biol* 21: 3445-3450.

3167. Xu X, Wagner KU, Larson D, Weaver Z, Li C, Ried T, Hennighausen L, Wynshaw-Boris A, Deng CX (1999). Conditional mutation of Brca1 in mammary epithelial cells results in blunted ductal morphogenesis and tumour formation. *Nat Genet* 22: 37-43.

3168. Yaghsezian H, Palazzo JP, Finkel GC, Carlson JA Jr., Talerman A (1992). Primary vaginal adenocarcinoma of the intestinal type associated with adenosis. *Gynecol Oncol* 45: 62-65.

3169. Yakirevich E, Izhak OB, Rennert G, Kovacs ZG, Resnick MB (1999). Cytotoxic phenotype of tumor infiltrating lymphocytes in medullary carcinoma of the breast. *Mod Pathol* 12: 1050-1056.

3170. Yakirevich E, Maroun L, Cohen O, Izhak OB, Rennert G, Resnick MB (2000). Apoptosis, proliferation, and Fas (APO-1, CD95)/Fas ligand expression in medullary carcinoma of the breast. *J Pathol* 192: 166-173.

3171. Yamamoto Y, Akagi A, Izumi K, Kishi Y (1995). Carcinosarcoma of the uterine body of mesonephric origin. *Pathol Int* 45: 303-309.

3172. Yamashita K, Wake N, Araki T, Ichinoe K, Makoto K (1979). Human lymphocyte antigen expression in hydatidiform mole: androgenesis following fertilization by a haploid sperm. *Am J Obstet Gynecol* 135: 597-600.

3173. Yamauchi H, Stearns V, Hayes DF (2001). When is a tumor marker ready for prime time? A case study of c-erbB-2 as a predictive factor in breast cancer. *J Clin Oncol* 19: 2334-2356.

3174. Yanai-Inbar I, Scully RE (1987). Relation of ovarian dermoid cysts and immature teratomas: an analysis of 350 cases of immature teratoma and 10 cases of dermoid cyst with microscopic foci of immature tissue. *Int J Gynecol Pathol* 6: 203-212.

3175. Yang B, Hart WR (2000). Vulvar intraepithelial neoplasia of the simplex (differentiated) type: a clinicopathologic study including analysis of HPV and p53 expression. *Am J Surg Pathol* 24: 429-441.

3176. Yang WT, Suen M, Metreweli C (1997). Sonographic features of benign papillary neoplasms of the breast: review of 22 patients. *J Ultrasound Med* 16: 161-168.

3177. Yannacou N, Gerolymatos A, Parissi-Mathiou P, Chranioti S, Perdikis T (2000). Carcinosarcoma of the uterine cervix composed of an adenoid cystic carcinoma and an homologous stromal sarcoma. A case report. *Eur J Gynaecol Oncol* 21: 292-294.

3178. Yarden RI, Pardo-Reoyo S, Sgagias M, Cowan KH, Brody LC (2002). BRCA1 regulates the G2/M checkpoint by activating Chk1 kinase upon DNA damage. *Nat Genet* 30: 285-289.

3179. Yazigi R, Sandstad J, Munoz AK (1988). Breast cancer metastasizing to the uterine cervix. *Cancer* 61: 2558-2560.

3180. Yaziji H, Gown AM (2001). Immunohistochemical analysis of gynecologic tumors. *Int J Gynecol Pathol* 20: 64-78.

3181. Yaziji H, Gown AM, Sneige N (2000). Detection of stromal invasion in breast cancer: the myoepithelial markers. *Adv Anat Pathol* 7: 100-109.

3182. Yilmaz AG, Chandler P, Hahm GK, O'Toole RV, Niemann TH (1999). Melanosis of the uterine cervix: a report of two cases and discussion of pigmented cervical lesions. *Int J Gynecol Pathol* 18: 73-76.

3183. Yip CH, Wong KT, Samuel D (1997). Bilateral plasma cell granuloma (inflammatory pseudotumour) of the breast. *Aust N Z J Surg* 67: 300-302.

3184. Yokoyama Y, Sato S, Futagami M, Saito Y (2000). Solitary metastasis to the uterine cervix from the early gastric cancer: a case report. *Eur J Gynaecol Oncol* 21: 469-471.

3185. Yoonessi M (1979). Carcinoma of the fallopian tube. *Obstet Gynecol Surv* 34: 257-270.

3186. Yoonessi M, Abell MR (1979). Brenner tumors of the ovary. *Obstet Gynecol* 54: 90-96.

3187. Yoshino K, Enomoto T, Nakamura T, Nakashima R, Wada H, Saitoh J, Noda K, Murata Y (1998). Aberrant FHIT transcripts in squamous cell carcinoma of the uterine cervix. *Int J Cancer* 76: 176-181.

3188. Yoshino K, Enomoto T, Nakamura T, Sun H, Ozaki K, Nakashima R, Wada H, Saitoh J, Watanabe Y, Noda K, Murata Y (2000). FHIT alterations in cancerous and non-cancerous cervical epithelium. *Int J Cancer* 85: 6-13.

3189. Yoshioka T, Tanaka T (2000). Mature solid teratoma of the fallopian tube: case report. *Eur J Obstet Gynecol Reprod Biol* 89: 205-206.
3190. Yoshiura K, Kanai Y, Ochiai A, Shimoyama Y, Sugimura T, Hirohashi S (1995). Silencing of the E-cadherin invasion-suppressor gene by CpG methylation in human carcinomas. *Proc Natl Acad Sci USA* 92: 7416-7419.
3191. Young JLJr, Percy CL, Asire AJ (1981). *Surveillance, Epidemiology and End results: Incidence and mortality data: 1973-1977.* NCI Monogr.
3192. Young RH, Clement PB (1988). Adenomyoepithelioma of the breast. A report of three cases and review of the literature. *Am J Clin Pathol* 89: 308-314.
3193. Young RH, Clement PB (2000). Endocervicosis involving the uterine cervix: a report of four cases of a benign process that may be confused with deeply invasive endocervical adenocarcinoma. *Int J Gynecol Pathol* 19: 322-328.
3194. Young RH, Clement PB, Scully RE (1988). Calcified thecomas in young women. A report of four cases. *Int J Gynecol Pathol* 7: 343-350.
3195. Young RH, Dickersin GR, Scully RE (1984). Juvenile granulosa cell tumor of the ovary. A clinicopathological analysis of 125 cases. *Am J Surg Pathol* 8: 575-596.
3196. Young RH, Dudley AG, Scully RE (1984). Granulosa cell, Sertoli-Leydig cell, and unclassified sex cord-stromal tumors associated with pregnancy: a clinicopathological analysis of thirty-six cases. *Gynecol Oncol* 18: 181-205.
3197. Young RH, Gersell DJ, Clement PB, Scully RE (1992). Hepatocellular carcinoma metastatic to the ovary: a report of three cases discovered during life with discussion of the differential diagnosis of hepatoid tumors of the ovary. *Hum Pathol* 23: 574-580.
3198. Young RH, Gersell DJ, Roth LM, Scully RE (1993). Ovarian metastases from cervical carcinomas other than pure adenocarcinomas. A report of 12 cases. *Cancer* 71: 407-418.
3199. Young RH, Gilks CB, Scully RE (1991). Mucinous tumors of the appendix associated with mucinous tumors of the ovary and pseudomyxoma peritonei. A clinicopathological analysis of 22 cases supporting an origin in the appendix. *Am J Surg Pathol* 15: 415-429.
3200. Young RH, Hart WR (1989). Metastases from carcinomas of the pancreas simulating primary mucinous tumors of the ovary. A report of seven cases. *Am J Surg Pathol* 13: 748-756.
3201. Young RH, Kleinman GM, Scully RE (1981). Glioma of the uterus. Report of a case with comments on histogenesis. Am *J Surg Pathol* 5: 695-699.
3202. Young RH, Kurman RJ, Scully RE (1988). Proliferations and tumors of intermediate trophoblast of the placental site. *Semin Diagn Pathol* 5: 223-237.
3203. Young RH, Kurman RJ, Scully RE (1990). Placental site nodules and plaques. A clinicopathologic analysis of 20 cases. *Am J Surg Pathol* 14: 1001-1009.
3204. Young RH, Oliva E, Scully RE (1994). Small cell carcinoma of the ovary, hypercalcemic type. A clinicopathological analysis of 150 cases. *Am J Surg Pathol* 18: 1102-1116.
3205. Young RH, Prat J, Scully RE (1980). Epidermoid cyst of the ovary. A report of three cases with comments on histogenesis. *Am J Clin Pathol* 73: 272-276.
3206. Young RH, Prat J, Scully RE (1982). Ovarian endometrioid carcinomas resembling sex cord-stromal tumors. A clinicopathological analysis of 13 cases. *Am J Surg Pathol* 6: 513-522.
3207. Young RH, Prat J, Scully RE (1982). Ovarian Sertoli-Leydig cell tumors with heterologous elements. I. Gastrointestinal epithelium and carcinoid: a clinicopathologic analysis of thirty-six cases. *Cancer* 50: 2448-2456.
3208. Young RH, Prat J, Scully RE (1984). Endometrioid stromal sarcomas of the ovary. A clinicopathologic analysis of 23 cases. *Cancer* 53: 1143-1155.
3209. Young RH, Scully RE (1983). Ovarian Sertoli-Leydig cell tumors with a retiform pattern: a problem in histopathologic diagnosis. A report of 25 cases. *Am J Surg Pathol* 7: 755-771.
3210. Young RH, Scully RE (1983). Ovarian sex cord-stromal tumors with bizarre nuclei: a clinicopathologic analysis of 17 cases. *Int J Gynecol Pathol* 1: 325-335.
3211. Young RH, Scully RE (1983). Ovarian stromal tumors with minor sex cord elements: a report of seven cases. *Int J Gynecol Pathol* 2: 227-234.
3212. Young RH, Scully RE (1983). Ovarian tumors of probable wolffian origin. A report of 11 cases. Am J Surg Pathol 7: 125-135.
3213. Young RH, Scully RE (1984). Endodermal sinus tumor of the vagina: a report of nine cases and review of the literature. Gynecol Oncol 18: 380-392.
3214. Young RH, Scully RE (1984). Fibromatosis and massive edema of the ovary, possibly related entities: a report of 14 cases of fibromatosis and 11 cases of massive edema. *Int J Gynecol Pathol* 3: 153-178.
3215. Young RH, Scully RE (1984). Ovarian Sertoli cell tumors: a report of 10 cases. *Int J Gynecol Pathol* 2: 349-363.
3216. Young RH, Scully RE (1984). Well-differentiated ovarian Sertoli-Leydig cell tumors: a clinicopathological analysis of 23 cases. *Int J Gynecol Pathol* 3: 277-290.
3217. Young RH, Scully RE (1985). Ovarian Sertoli-Leydig cell tumors. A clinicopathological analysis of 207 cases. *Am J Surg Pathol* 9: 543-569.
3218. Young RH, Scully RE (1987). Ovarian steroid cell tumors associated with Cushing's syndrome: a report of three cases. *Int J Gynecol Pathol* 6: 40-48.
3219. Young RH, Scully RE (1988). Mucinous ovarian tumors associated with mucinous adenocarcinomas of the cervix. A clinicopathological analysis of 16 cases. *Int J Gynecol Pathol* 7: 99-111.
3220. Young RH, Scully RE (1988). Urothelial and ovarian carcinomas of identical cell types: problems in interpretation. A report of three cases and review of the literature. *Int J Gynecol Pathol* 7: 197-211.
3221. Young RH, Scully RE (1990). Ovarian metastases from carcinoma of the gallbladder and extrahepatic bile ducts simulating primary tumors of the ovary. A report of six cases. *Int J Gynecol Pathol* 9: 60-72.
3222. Young RH, Scully RE (1990). Sarcomas metastatic to the ovary: a report of 21 cases. *Int J Gynecol Pathol* 9: 231-252.
3223. Young RH, Scully RE (1991). Malignant melanoma metastatic to the ovary. A clinicopathologic analysis of 20 cases. *Am J Surg Pathol* 15: 849-860.
3224. Young RH, Scully RE (1992). Uterine carcinomas simulating microglandular hyperplasia. A report of six cases. *Am J Surg Pathol* 16: 1092-1097.
3225. Young RH, Scully RE (1993). Minimal-deviation endometrioid adenocarcinoma of the uterine cervix. A report of five cases of a distinctive neoplasm that may be misinterpreted as benign. *Am J Surg Pathol* 17: 660-665.
3226. Young RH, Scully RE (1994). Metastatic tumours of the ovary. In: *Blaustein's Pathology of the Female Genital Tract*, Kurman RJ, ed., 4th ed. Springer-Verlag: New York , pp. 939-974.
3227. Young RH, Scully RE, McCluskey RT (1985). A distinctive glomerular lesion complicating placental site trophoblastic tumor: report of two cases. *Hum Pathol* 16: 35-42.
3228. Young RH, Treger T, Scully RE (1986). Atypical polypoid adenomyoma of the uterus. A report of 27 cases. *Am J Clin Pathol* 86: 139-145.
3229. Young TW, Thrasher TV (1982). Nonchromaffin paraganglioma of the uterus. A case report. *Arch Pathol Lab Med* 106: 608-609.
3230. Youngs LA, Taylor HB (1967). Adenomatoid tumors of the uterus and fallopian tube. *Am J Clin Pathol* 48: 537-545.
3231. Youngson BJ, Cranor M, Rosen PP (1994). Epithelial displacement in surgical breast specimens following needling procedures. *Am J Surg Pathol* 18: 896-903.
3232. Yu GH, Fishman SJ, Brooks JS (1993). Cellular angiolipoma of the breast. *Mod Pathol* 6: 497-499.
3233. Yuan CC, Wang PH, Lai CR, Yen MS, Chen CY, Juang CM (1998). Prognosis-predicting system based on factors related to survival of cervical carcinoma. *Int J Gynaecol Obstet* 63: 163-167.
3234. Zabernigg A, Muller-Holzner E, Gasc JM, Gattringer C (1997). An unusual case of a renin-producing tumour of the fallopian tube. *Eur J Cancer* 33: 1709.
3235. Zafrani B, Aubriot MH, Mouret E, de Cremoux P, De Rycke Y, Nicolas A, Boudou E, Vincent-Salomon A, Magdelenat H, Sastre-Garau X (2000). High sensitivity and specificity of immunohistochemistry for the detection of hormone receptors in breast carcinoma: comparison with biochemical determination in a prospective study of 793 cases. *Histopathology* 37: 536-545.
3236. Zahradka M, Zahradka W, Mach S (1989). [Stromal sarcoma of the vagina]. *Zentralbl Gynakol* 111: 1450-1454.
3237. Zaidi SN, Conner MG (2001). Primary vulvar adenocarcinoma of cloacogenic origin. *South Med J* 94: 744-746.
3238. Zaino RJ, Kurman RJ, Diana KL, Morrow CP (1995). The utility of the revised International Federation of Gynecology and Obstetrics histologic grading of endometrial adenocarcinoma using a defined nuclear grading system. A Gynecologic Oncology Group study. *Cancer* 75: 81-86.
3239. Zaino RJ, Unger ER, Whitney C (1984). Synchronous carcinomas of the uterine corpus and ovary. *Gynecol Oncol* 19: 329-335.
3240. Zaki I, Dalziel KL, Solomonsz FA, Stevens A (1996). The under-reporting of skin disease in association with squamous cell carcinoma of the vulva. *Clin Exp Dermatol* 21: 334-337.
3241. Zaloudek C, Hayashi GM, Ryan IP, Powell CB, Miller TR (1997). Microglandular adenocarcinoma of the endometrium: a form of mucinous adenocarcinoma that may be confused with microglandular hyperplasia of the cervix. *Int J Gynecol Pathol* 16: 52-59.
3242. Zaloudek C, Norris HJ (1982). Granulosa tumors of the ovary in children: a clinical and pathologic study of 32 cases. *Am J Surg Pathol* 6: 503-512.
3243. Zaloudek C, Norris HJ (1984). Sertoli-Leydig tumors of the ovary. A clinicopathologic study of 64 intermediate and poorly differentiated neoplasms. *Am J Surg Pathol* 8: 405-418.
3244. Zaloudek C, Oertel YC, Orenstein JM (1984). Adenoid cystic carcinoma of the breast. *Am J Clin Pathol* 81: 297-307.
3245. Zaloudek CJ, Norris HJ (1981). Adenofibroma and adenosarcoma of the uterus: a clinicopathologic study of 35 cases. *Cancer* 48: 354-366.
3246. Zaloudek CJ, Tavassoli FA, Norris HJ (1981). Dysgerminoma with syncytiotrophoblastic giant cells. A histologically and clinically distinctive subtype of dysgerminoma. *Am J Surg Pathol* 5: 361-367.
3247. Zamecnik M, Michal M (1998). Endometrial stromal nodule with retiform sex-cord-like differentiation. *Pathol Res Pract* 194: 449-453.
3248. Zamecnik M, Michal M, Curik R (2000). Adenoid cystic carcinoma of the ovary. *Arch Pathol Lab Med* 124: 1529-1531.
3249. Zanella M, Falconieri G, Lamovec J, Bittesini L (1998). Pseudoangiomatous hyperplasia of the mammary stroma: true entity or phenotype? *Pathol Res Pract* 194: 535-540.
3250. Zanetta G, Rota SM, Lissoni A, Chiari S, Bratina G, Mangioni C (1999). Conservative treatment followed by chemotherapy with doxorubicin and ifosfamide for cervical sarcoma botryoides in young females. *Br J Cancer* 80: 403-406.
3251. Zanetta GM, Webb MJ, Li H, Keeney GL (2000). Hyperestrogenism: a relevant risk factor for the development of cancer from endometriosis. *Gynecol Oncol* 79: 18-22.
3252. Zhang J, Young RH, Arseneau J, Scully RE (1982). Ovarian stromal tumors containing lutein or Leydig cells (luteinized thecomas and stromal Leydig cell tumors)--a clinicopathological analysis of fifty cases. *Int J Gynecol Pathol* 1: 270-285.
3253. Zhao S, Kato N, Endoh Y, Jin Z, Ajioka Y, Motoyama T (2000). Ovarian gonadoblastoma with mixed germ cell tumor in a woman with 46, XX karyotype and successful pregnancies. *Pathol Int* 50: 332-335.
3254. Zhao X, Wei YQ, Kariya Y, Teshigawara K, Uchida A (1995). Accumulation of gamma/delta T cells in human dysgerminoma and seminoma: roles in autologous tumor killing and granuloma formation. *Immunol Invest* 24: 607-618.
3255. Zheng L, Pan H, Li S, Flesken-Nikitin A, Chen PL, Boyer TG, Lee WH (2000). Sequence-specific transcriptional corepressor function for BRCA1 through a novel zinc finger protein, ZBRK1. *Mol Cell* 6: 757-768.

3256. Zheng W, Khurana R, Farahmand S, Wang Y, Zhang ZF, Felix JC (1998). p53 immunostaining as a significant adjunct diagnostic method for uterine surface carcinoma: precursor of uterine papillary serous carcinoma. *Am J Surg Pathol* 22: 1463-1473.

3257. Zheng W, Wolf S, Kramer EE, Cox KA, Hoda SA (1996). Borderline papillary serous tumour of the fallopian tube. *Am J Surg Pathol* 20: 30-35.

3258. Zhong Q, Chen CF, Li S, Chen Y, Wang CC, Xiao J, Chen PL, Sharp ZD, Lee WH (1999). Association of BRCA1 with the hRad50-hMre11-p95 complex and the DNA damage response. *Science* 285: 747-750.

3259. Zhou H, Kuang J, Zhong L, Kuo WL, Gray JW, Sahin A, Brinkley BR, Sen S (1998). Tumour amplified kinase STK15/BTAK induces centrosome amplification, aneuploidy and transformation. *Nat Genet* 20: 189-193.

3260. Zhou X, Hampel H, Thiele H, Gorlin RJ, Hennekam RC, Parisi M, Winter RM, Eng C (2001). Association of germline mutation in the PTEN tumour suppressor gene and Proteus and Proteus-like syndromes. *Lancet* 358: 210-211.

3261. Zhou XP, Kuismanen S, Nystrom-Lahti M, Peltomaki P, Eng C (2002). Distinct PTEN mutational spectra in hereditary non-polyposis colon cancer syndrome-related endometrial carcinomas compared to sporadic microsatellite unstable tumors. *Hum Mol Genet* 11: 445-450.

3262. Zhou XP, Woodford-Richens K, Lehtonen R, Kurose K, Aldred M, Hampel H, Launonen V, Virta S, Pilarski R, Salovaara R, Bodmer WF, Conrad BA, Dunlop M, Hodgson SV, Iwama T, Jarvinen H, Kellokumpu I, Kim JC, Leggett B, Markie D, Mecklin JP, Neale K, Phillips R, Piris J, Rozen P, Houlston RS, Aaltonen LA, Tomlinson IP, Eng C (2001). Germline mutations in BMPR1A/ALK3 cause a subset of cases of juvenile polyposis syndrome and of Cowden and Bannayan-Riley-Ruvalcaba syndromes. *Am J Hum Genet* 69: 704-711.

3263. Zhu WY, Leonardi C, Penneys NS (1992). Detection of human papillomavirus DNA in seborrheic keratosis by polymerase chain reaction. *J Dermatol Sci* 4: 166-171.

3264. Zhu XL, Hartwick W, Rohan T, Kandel R (1998). Cyclin D1 gene amplification and protein expression in benign breast disease and breast carcinoma. *Mod Pathol* 11: 1082-1088.

3265. Zhuang Z, Merino MJ, Chuaqui R, Liotta LA, Emmert-Buck MR (1995). Identical allelic loss on chromosome 11q13 in microdissected in situ and invasive human breast cancer. *Cancer Res* 55: 467-471.

3266. Ziegler RG, Hoover RN, Pike MC, Hildesheim A, Nomura AM, West DW, Wu-Williams AH, Kolonel LN, Horn-Ross PL, Rosenthal JF, Hyer MB. (1993). Migration patterns and breast cancer risk in Asian-American women. *J Natl Cancer Inst* 85: 1819-1827.

3267. Zollo JD, Zeitouni NC (2000). The Roswell Park Cancer Institute experience with extramammary Paget's disease. *Br J Dermatol* 142: 59-65.

3268. Zotalis G, Nayar R, Hicks DG (1998). Leiomyomatosis peritonealis disseminata, endometriosis, and multicystic mesothelioma: an unusual association. *Int J Gynecol Pathol* 17: 178-182.

3269. Zou A, Marschke KB, Arnold KE, Berger EM, Fitzgerald P, Mais DE, Allegretto EA (1999). Estrogen receptor beta activates the human retinoic acid receptor alpha-1 promoter in response to tamoxifen and other estrogen receptor antagonists, but not in response to estrogen. *Mol Endocrinol* 13: 418-430.

3270. Zuntova A, Motlik K, Horejsi J, Eckschlager T (1992). Mixed germ cell-sex cord stromal tumor with heterologous structures. *Int J Gynecol Pathol* 11: 227-233.

3271. Zweemer RP, van Diest PJ, Verheijen RH, Ryan A, Gille JJ, Sijmons RH, Jacobs IJ, Menko FH, Kenemans P (2000). Molecular evidence linking primary cancer of the fallopian tube to BRCA1 germline mutations. *Gynecol Oncol* 76: 45-50.

3272. Zweemer RP, Verheijen RH, Gille JJ, van Diest PJ, Pals G, Menko FH (1998). Clinical and genetic evaluation of thirty ovarian cancer families. *Am J Obstet Gynecol* 178: 85-90.

3273. Zwijsen RM, Wientjens E, Klompmaker R, van der Sman J, Bernards R, Michalides RJ (1997). CDK-independent activation of estrogen receptor by cyclin D1. *Cell* 88: 405-415.

Subject index

MPNST, *see* Malignant peripheral nerve sheath tumour

MRE11, 341

MSH2, 53, 118, 132, 337, 342, 358-361

MSH6, 53, 337, 342, 358-361

MSI, 53, 359-361

MSI-H, 360, 361

Mucin producing carcinoma, 30

Mucinous adenocarcinoma, 124, 206, 212, 221, 224, 272, 273, 297, 300

Mucinous borderline tumour, 124-126, 128, 145, 193

Mucinous borderline tumour, intestinal type, 125

Mucinous carcinoid, 171, 173, 195

Mucinous carcinoma, 30, 31, 34, 35, 57, 80, 124-126, 128, 195, 206, 226, 339

Mucinous cystadenocarcinofibroma, 124

Mucinous cystadenocarcinoma, 30-32, 145

Mucinous cystadenoma, 124-127, 129, 143, 156, 175, 209, 212

Mucinous cystic tumours with mural nodules, 127

Mucinous tumour of borderline malignancy, endocervical-like, 126

Mucinous tumour of borderline malignancy, intestinal type, 125

Mucinous tumour of low malignant potential, endocervical-like, 126

Mucinous tumour of low malignant potential, intestinal type, 125

Mucocoele-like lesion, 31

Mucoepidermoid carcinoma, 39, 277

Mucoid carcinoma, 30, 42

Mucosal/acral lentiginous melanoma, 331

Muir-Torre syndrome, 132

MUL, 51

Müllerian papilloma, 276, 300

Multicystic mesothelioma, 197, 198

Multilocular peritoneal inclusion cyst, 198

Multinodular goitre, 356

Multinucleated giant cells, 92, 99, 207

Multiple facial trichilemmomas, 356

Multiple hamartoma syndrome, 355

MutL homologue 1, 359

MutL homologue 3, 359

MutS homologue 2, 359

MutS homologue 6, 359

Myc, 250, 266

Myoepithelial carcinoma, 40, 86, 88, 92

Myoepitheliosis, 86

Myofibroblastoma, 91

Myoglobin, 246, 302

Myoid hamartoma, 103

Myxoid leiomyoma, 236, 241

Myxoid leiomyosarcoma, 238

Myxoma, 182, 187, 244

N

NCOA3 (AIB1), 51, 343, 350

Neuroblastoma, 51, 174, 334

Neuroendocrine carcinoma, 30, 43, 184, 279, 333

Neuroendocrine tumours, 32, 144, 277, 279

Neurofibroma, 94, 329, 330

Neuron-specific enolase, 200, 255

Nevoid basal cell carcinoma syndrome, 151

NFKB / NF-kappaB, 352, 362

Nipple adenoma, 81, 104

Nipple discharge, 68, 74, 76, 77, 85, 92, 97, 101, 112

Nipple duct adenoma, 104

Nodular adenosis with apocrine metaplasia, 85

Nodular hidradenoma, 324, 325

Nodular melanoma, 331

Nodular theca-lutein hyperplasia of pregnancy, 188

Non-encapsulated sclerosing lesion, 83

Non-gestational choriocarcinoma, 163, 167, 168

Non-keratinizing, squamous cell carcinoma, 266, 267, 316, 317

Non-medullary thyroid cancer, 355

Nuclear grooves, 86, 147

O

O6-Methylguanine DNA ethyltransferase (O6MGMT) 353

Ollier disease, 149

Oncocytic carcinoma, 43

Ordinary intraductal hyperplasia, 65

Osteosarcoma, 40, 97, 98, 101, 175, 188, 244, 246, 282

Ovarian tumour of probable wolffian origin, 186

Ovarian wolffian tumour, 182, 186

P

p14ARF, 353

p16/CDKN2a/p16INK4, 270, 353

p21, 250, 341, 348

p27, 58

p63, 86

p73, 362

Paget disease, 23, 35, 41, 63, 68, 105, 112, 174, 319, 321, 322, 324, 332, 352

Paget disease of the nipple, 35, 41, 105

Pagetoid spread, 332, 333

Paneth cell, 45, 125-127, 272, 276

Papillary adenoma, 104

Papillary carcinoma, non-invasive, 78

Papillary ductal carcinoma in situ, 79

Papillary hidradenoma, 321, 323

Papillary intraductal carcinoma, 32, 34, 79

Papillary squamous cell carcinoma, 267

Papilloma, 76-79, 119, 209, 296

Papillomatosis, 76, 104, 271, 296

Papillomatosis of the nipple, 104

Paraganglioma, 182, 187, 255, 283

Parasitic leiomyoma, 239

Parathyroid hormone-related protein, 138

Partial hydatidiform mole, 254

PAT1, 51

PDGFRL, 52

Peau d'orange, 48

PEComa, 243

Peptide YY, 172

Periductal stromal sarcoma, 100, 102

Peripheral papilloma, 76-78, 83

Peripheral primitive neuroectodermal tumour, 244, 255, 309, 334

Peritoneal mesothelioma, 185,197, 199

Peritoneal mucinous carcinomatosis, 128

Peritoneal tumours, 197

Perivascular epithelioid cell tumour, 243

Peutz-Jeghers syndrome, 156-158, 208, 273

Phaeochromocytoma, 187

Phosphoinositol-3-kinase, 357

Phyllodes tumour, 96, 97, 99-101, 103, 247, 352

Pigmented progonoma, 175

PIVKA-II (protein induced by vitamin K absence), 184

Placental alkaline phosphatase, 196